SCIENCE

NEW SERIES. VOLUME LXVII

JANUARY-JUNE, 1928

NEW YORK
THE SCIENCE PRESS
1928

THE SCIENCE PRESS PRINTING COMPANY
LANCASTER, PA.

CONTENTS AND INDEX

NEW SERIES. VOL. LXVII—JANUARY TO JUNE, 1928

THE NAMES OF CONTRIBUTORS ARE PRINTED IN SMALL CAPITALS

ABBOT, C. G., Variation in Solar Radiation, 634
Absolute Zero of Temperature, R. D. KLEEMAN, 69, 420
Academies of Science, State, 195
Academy of Science, Ind., H. F. DIETZ, 140, 636; Ohio, W. H. ALEXANDER, 538; Ky., A. M. PETER, 614; N. D., 614; N. C., H. R. TOTTEN, 635; Kans., G. E. JOHNSON, 636; Sciences, Natl., 425, 459, W. W. CAMPBELL, 482; Belgium, Award of Prizes, 622
Acoustics of Auditoriums, F. R. WATSON, 335
Acquired Character, in Flax, B. B. ROBINSON, 242
ADAMS, F. D., Rainfall and Run-off, 500
ADAMS, L. A., Banana Stowaways, 218
ADAMS, W. S., Twenty Years of Physical Astron., 637
Agassiz, Louis, H. F. OSBORN, 523
Agricultural Experiment Station, C. G. WILLIAMS, 519
Agriculture, U. S. Dept. of, 1929 Budget, 186; Week on, at Inst. of Chemistry, C. D. HURD, 549
Agronomic Jabberwocky, J. H. KEMPTON, 629
ALEXANDER, W. H., Ohio Academy of Science, 538
ALLARD, H. A., Musical Technique of the Katydid, 613
ALLEN, E., Chromosomes of Moina Macrocopa, 18
ALLISON, V. C., Deposits in Jacobs Cavern, 70
American Association for the Advancement of Science, A—113; B—114; C—115; D—116; E—116; F—118, 141; G—21, 120; F and G—124; H—1, 125; I—24, 126; K—126; L—126; M—5, 127; N—47, 128, 385; O—128; Q—129; Organizations not related to any section, 130; Officers, 11, 97; Nashville Meeting, General Reports, 77, Prize, 81, News Service, 83, Council Roll, 85, Legislative and Executive Proceedings, 88, Roll Executive Committee, 88, Annual Conference Section and Society Secretaries, 91, Report of the Treasurer, 91, Resolutions, 91, Financial Report, 93, Report of Committee on Place of Science in Education, 95, Grants for Research, 96, Special Notes, 99, 131, Response to Address of Welcome, A. A. NOYES, 109, Reports of Sessions of Sections and Societies, 113; Future Annual Meetings, 98; The Newly Elected President, B. E. LIVINGSTON, 111; Science and the Newspapers, W. E. RITTER, 279; Science Week in New York, H. F. OSBORN, 411; New York Meeting, B. E. LIVINGSTON, 432; and Affiliated Societies, G. T. HARGITT, 481; Spring Meeting of the Executive Committee, B. E. LIVINGSTON, 516
Americanists, International Council of, F. BOAS, 503
Amphibian Record from Kansas, C. E. BURT, 630
ANDREWS, E. A., Tree Frogs and Pitcher Plants, 269
Ångström in English, E. F. B. FRIES, 652
Anthropology and Medicine, A. HRDLIČKA, 385
Antiquity of Man in Oklahoma, O. P. HAY, 442
Apparatus, W. SOUDER, 298
Apportionment of Representatives, E. V. HUNTINGTON, 509; W. F. WILLCOX, 581
Archimedes and Trigonometry, G. A. MILLER, 555
Arctic, Exploration of, by Airship, I. TOLMACHOFF, 363
Arnold Arboretum, 209
ARNOLD, C. A., Devonian Plants, 276
Artifacts, Pseudo-, N. C. NELSON, 316
Ascaris, Physiology of, J. F. MUELLER, 590
ASHLEY, G. H., Geology and the World at Large, 21
Aspirator, A Constant Rate, C. F. HOTTES and A. L. HAFENRICHTER, 320
Astronomical Soc. of the Pacific, Lectures, 504
Astronomy, Physical, Twenty Years of, W. S. ADAMS, 637
Atmospheric Phenomenon, B. W. BARTLETT, 195
Atom Building, R. A. MILLIKAN and G. H. CAMERON, 401
Atoms, Orientation of, T. H. JOHNSON, 37
Aurora of March 28, 1928, H. T. STETSON, 394
Australasian Assoc., Address of the President, 138

BAKER, W. C., The Adhesion of Mercury to Glass, 74
BALDWIN, H. I., Journal of Swedish Forestry Soc., 152
Banana Stowaways, L. A. ADAMS, 218; G. WAGNER, 422; E. R. WARREN, 422
BANTA, A. M. and T. R. WOOD, The Cladocera Male, 18
BARGER, G., International Relations in Science, 405
Barnes, Charles Reid, Award of Life Membership in the Amer. Soc. of Plant Physiologists, 264
BARNEY, I., Romance of the Sun, M. Proctor, 444
Barnum, William, I. M. GREY, 548
Barro Colorado Island Station, V. KELLOGG, 389
BARTLETT, B. W., Atmospheric Phenomenon, 195
BARUS, C., Cathode and Anode Points, 248; The Little Circle of Reference, 530
BASS, C. C., Parasitology and the South, 454
Bather, F. A., Dr., 17
BATSON, O. V., The Anatomy of the Corium, 198
Battelle Memorial Institute, 62
Bayliss, William M., Proposed Memorial to, 414
BEAN, R. B., Stature throughout the World, 1
BEARCE, H. W., The Liter and Cubic Decimeter, 511
BEAUMONT, A. B., and G. J. LARSINOS, Growing Small-seeded Plants under Sterile Conditions, 350
Bees, Foulbrood of, A. G. LOCHHEAD, 159
BEHREND, B. A., Scientific Research, 272
Belgium Acad. of Sciences, Award of Prizes, 622
"Believe," a Word to Replace, E. C. L. MILLER, 319
BENEDICT, H. C., Teeth in Ultra-Violet Rays, 442
BERKEY, C. P., Geological Society of America, 140
BERMAN, L., Psycho-Endocrinology, 195
BERRY, E. W., Paläobotanik, M. Hirmer, 319
Berthelot, Marcelin, A. SEIDELL, 180, 497
Biological, Station, Alexandrovsk, R. B. HARVEY, 158; Survey, Bureau of, Budget, 288; Sciences, 290
Biologists, Lake Erie, Conference of, E. HIGGINS, 309
Biology, The Importance of, W. W. LEPESCHKIN, 59; Colorimetric Methods in, F. B. SUMNER, 271; Federation of Amer. Societies of, E. D. BROWN, 496
BISSELL, M. H., Climate, C. E. P. Brooks, 298
BLACK, D., Hominid Remains of Quaternary Age, 135
BLACKWELDER, E., A Plate that Penetrates Haze, 275
BLISS, S., The Amide Nitrogen of Blood, 515
Blood, The Amide Nitrogen of, S. BLISS, 515; Serum, Modification of the Viscosity of, L. DU NOÜY, 563
BOAS, F., International Congress of Americanists, 503
BODMAN, G. B., Soil Color Analysis, 446
Boiling-Point and Latent Heat, J. B. NATHANSON, 583
BOLAND, J. C., Immobilization of Paramecium, 654
Boron and Tomato Plant, E. S. JOHNSON and W. H. DORE, 324
Bosmans, Henri, F. CAJORI, 362
Botanists, Taxonomic, A. S. HITCHCOCK, 431
BOUYOUCOS, C. J., Soil Moisture, 167; Soils Analysis, 587
BRADLEY, W. H., Zeolite in Green River Formation, 73
BRANSON, E. B., and M. G. MEHL, Triassic Fossils, 325
BRASCH, F. E., Commemoration of Newton, 255
BREDER, C. M., JR., Fresh-Water Jelly-Fish, 241
British Association, Glasgow Meeting, 599

BRODY, S., Growth Curves, 43
BROWN, E. D., The Federation of American Societies of Experimental Biology, 496
BROWNE, C. A., Eye Soreness, 510
Bulletins, The User of, L. O. HOWARD, 40
Burette Cleaner, F. H. FISH, 654
Burgess, Edward Sandford, T. E. HAMILTON, 388; W. K. FISHER, 501
BURT, C. E., Amphibian Record from Kansas, 620

CAJORI, F., Henri Bosmans, 362
California, Univ. of, The Giannini Foundation, 289
CAMPBELL, A. S., A Plankton Bucket, 322
CAMPBELL, W. W., National Academy of Sciences, 482
Cancer, Research, 185; and Ovarian Secretion, W. S. MURRAY, 396
Canker, Coryneum, of Cypress, W. W. WAGENER, 584
Carbohydrate from Seaweed, L. H. CRETCHER and W. L. NELSON, 537
CARLSON, A. J., The Physiologic Life, 355
Carnegie Institution, Appointments, 483
CAROTHERS, E. E., The Collodion Method, 400
CARTY, J. J., Ideals of the Engineer, 307
Carty, J. J., Presentation of Medals, 132
Cathode and Anode Points, C. BARUS, 248
CATTELL, J. MCK., The Scientific Men of Harvard and of Columbia, 136; Early Psychological Laboratories, 543; Corrections to the Biographical Directory of American Men of Science, 585
Cells, in Heart-wood of Trees, J. H. FAULL, 296; Living, Centuries Old, D. T. MACDOUGAL and J. G. BROWN, 447
Cereals, Embryoless Seeds in, M. E. LYON, 652
Chart, Prehistory, E. A. HOOTON, 297
Charts in the Natural Sciences, Use of, A. C. NOÉ, 571
Chemical Soc., Amer., Officers, 10; St. Louis Meeting, 235, 364
Chemistry, The Institute of, 100; Bureau of, Budget, 288; and the Berthelot Centenary, A. SEIDELL, 497
Children who Run on All Fours, A. HRDLIČKA, 273
Chloroplast Pigments, Measuring, H. B. SPRAGUE, 167
Chromosomes, of Moina Macrocopa, E. ALLEN, 18; of the Killifish, A. C. FRASER and M. GORDON, 470
CLAASSEN, P. W., Wild Life Preserve, 651
Cladocera Male, A. M. BANTA and T. R. WOOD, 18
CLARK, H. L., Zoology, W. J. Dakin, 105
Cleavage, Determining the Rate of, E. A. WOLF, 611
Coal, Bituminous, Conference on, 524
Coast and Geodetic Survey, 32; G. O. SMITH, 67; B. WILLIS and E. B. MATHEWS, 100
Colds, Fund for Study of, 62
COLE, E. C., Narcotizing Earthworms, 492
COLE, R., The Medical Sciences, 47
Collisions of the Second Kind, J. R. NIELSEN, 651
Collodion Method, E. E. CAROTHERS, 400
Colloid Symposium, Sixth National, 524
Colophonium Wax, R. R. DURANT, 490
Colorimetry, Bibliography of, I. G. PRIEST, 39
Columbia Univ., Salaries at, 415; Reorganization of Department of Zoology, 576
COLWELL, R. C., Sharp Rattling in Steam Pipes, 397
Commonwealth Fund, Appropriations, 339
CONDON, E. U., Statistics of Vocabulary, 300
Conjugation in Paramecium, D. H. WENRICH and C. C. WANG, 270
COOK, H. J., Man's Antiquity in Oklahoma, 371
COOLEY, R. A. and G. M. KOHLS, Egg Laying of Ixodiphagus in Larval Ticks, 656
Coolidge, W. D., Presentation of Edison Medal, 132
Cooperation, Intellectual, and Biology, J. E. DE VOS VAN STEENWIJK, 633
CORI, C. F., Ernest J. Lesser, 523
Corium, The Anatomy of, O. V. BATSON, 198
Correlations, A Method for, C. D. MURRAY, 588
COULTER, J. M., Flora of Canal Zone, P. C. Standley, 423
COURTNEY, W. D., Dehydrating Apparatus, 653
COWLES, R. B., Varanus Niloticus, 317
Cows, Dairy, W. L. GAINES, 353
CRAMPTON, H. E., Differentiation of Species, 615
CRETCHER, L. H., and W. L. NELSON, Seaweed, 537
Cruise of the Non-magnetic Yacht, J. A. FLEMING, 478
Crustal Movements of the Earth, J. L. GILLSON, 608
CURTIS, W. C., Old Problems and a New Technique, 141
Cuticula of Nematodes, The, T. B. MAGATH, 194

Dairy Congress, International, 645
DAKIN, W. J., "General Zoology," 465
Dakin, W. J., Zoology, H. L. CLARK, 105
Daly Medal, Presentation to Alois Musil, 289
"Data," R. H. SMITH, 70; C. LADD-FRANKLIN, 444; F. L. WELLS, 491; Datum, F. E., 631
DAVIS, H., "Visible Radiation from Nerve Fiber," 69
DAVIS, W., Annual Meeting of Science Service, 482
DAVIS, W. H. and F. A. MACLAUGHLIN, Determining the Color of Objects in Microscopic Mounts, 71
Deafness in Pre-Columbian Peru, R. L. MOODIE, 464
Decimeter, Cubic, and the Liter, H. W. BEARCE, 511
Decorah Formation, Divisions of the, G. M. KAY, 16
Dehydrating Apparatus, W. D. COURTNEY, 653
Devonian Plants, C. A. ARNOLD, 276
DIETZ, H. F., Indiana Acad. of Science, 140, 636
Discussion and Correspondence, 15, 37, 67, 104, 135, 158, 192, 215, 241, 269, 295, 315, 345, 370, 394, 420, 442, 464, 488, 509, 530, 555, 581, 605, 628, 651
DUNLAP, K., Habit Formation, 360
DURANT, R. R., Colophonium Wax, 490
Dynamo, The Earliest, H. W. WILEY, 532

Earthworms, Narcotizing, E. C. COLE, 492
EATON, P. and C. S. STIRRETT, Reproduction in Rats, 555
EATON, T. H., Research and Training, 619
EBELING, A. H., Gewebezellen, A. Fischer, 374
EGGERS, H. E., Origin of Tumors, 193
Einthoven, Willem, H. B. WILLIAMS, 456
Elasmobranchs, E. M. KAPP, 513
Elect. Discharge, Chemical Action in, S. C. LIND, 565
Electrochemical Soc., Amer., 310
Ella Sachs Plotz Foundation, 152
Embryos, Chick, Mounting, J. W. MAVOR, 445
Engineer, Ideals of the, J. J. CARTY, 307
Engineering; The Functions of Section M, C. R. RICHARDS, 5; Congress, World, 235, 646
Ethnological Research, 525
Ethnology, Amer. Bureau of, 458
Ethylene as a Ripener of Fruits, R. B. HARVEY, 421
EVE, A. S., Applied Geophysics, 192
Eye Soreness, C. A. BROWNE, 510

Faraday Memorial Fund, 234
FAULL, J. H., Cells in Heart-wood of Trees, 296
FENNER, C. N., The Beginning of Winter, 243
Field Museum Paleontological Expeditions to South America, E. S. RIGGS, 585
FISH, F. H., A Burette Cleaner, 654
FISHER, W. K., Edward Sandford Burgess, 501
FISKE, C. H., and Y. SUBBAROW, Phosphocreatine, 169
Fixative and Stain for Flagella, L. E. NOLAND, 535
FLEMING, J. A., Cruise of the Non-magnetic Yacht, 478
Floods in Mississippi Basin, A. J. HENRY, 15
Folk Songs, Collecting, M. METFESSEL, 28
FORBES, W. T. M., Lepidoptera of New York, 347; What is a Name?, 373
Forest Research, Enlarged Program of, 648
Forestry, Soc. Swedish, Journal of, H. I. BALDWIN, 152; Yale School of, 415; Advances in United States, 437
Fossil Tracks on the North Rim of the Grand Canyon, C. W. GILMORE and G. E. STURDEVANT, 216
Fossils, Triassic, E. B. BRANSON and M. G. MEHL, 325
Franck, J., Symposium in Honor of, 63

Franklin Institute, Award of Medals, 525
FRASER, A. C., and M. GORDON, Crossing-over between Chromosomes of the Killifish, 470
FRIEDEMANN, T. E., Starvation Ketosis of Primates, 221
FRIES, E. F. B., Ångström in English, 652
Fungi, Sexual Stage of, F. L. STEVENS, 514
Fungicidal Factor of Sulphur, H. C. YOUNG and R. WILLIAMS, 19

GAGER, C. S., Wellesley College and Bot. Education, 171
GAINES, W. L., Dairy Cows, 353
Galilei or Galileo?, A. KAMPMEIER, 422
GARDNER, I. C., Optical Instruments and Products, 600
Garman, Samuel, D. S. JORDAN and T. BARBOUR, 232
GARVER, M. M., Philosophy or Irony, 297
Gas Reactions, Molecular Diameters in, R. C. TOLMAN, D. M. YOST and R. G. DICKINSON, 241
GELFAN, S., A Bioelectric Potential, 589
General Education Board, 390
Genesis and Evolution, 162
Geodetic and Geophysical Union, C. LALLEMAND, 196
Geologic Age by Lead Uranium Ratios, A. C. LANE, 631
Geological Soc. of Amer., C. P. BERKEY, 140
Geology, and the World, G. H. ASHLEY, 21; of Sonora, G. J. MITCHELL, 373
Geophysical Union, Amer., 390
Geophysics, Applied, A. S. EVE, 192
Georgia Experiment Station, T. H. MCHATTON, 264
Gestation in the Monkey, C. G. HARTMAN, 15
Gibbs, Willard, Works, 389; Medal, Award of, 550
GILBERT, A. H., Potato Tuber Necrosis, 464
Gilbert, Charles Henry, D. S. JORDAN, 644
GILLSON, J. L., Crustal Movements of the Earth, 608
GILMORE, C. W. and G. E. STURDEVANT, Fossil Tracks on the North Rim of the Grand Canyon, 216
Gladiolus, Rot of, L. MCCULLOCH and C. THOM, 216
Glands, Parathyroid, as Influenced by Selective Solar Radiation, G. M. HIGGINS and C. SHEARD, 536
Glass Tubing, Cutting, H. E. SEEMANN, 107; I. P. TOLMACHOFF, 299; J. L. ST. JOHN, 561
GOODPASTURE, E. W., Pathology of Virus Disease, 591
GOODSPEED, T. H., and A. R. OLSON, Progenies from X-rayed Sex Cells of Tobacco, 46
Gravitation, Newtonian Constant of, T. E. STERN, 377
GREENE, C. W., Comparative Physiol., C. G. Rogers, 399
Greenland, Oxford Expedition to, 502
GREY, I. M., William Barnum, 548
von Groth, Paul Heinrich, E. H. KRAUS, 150
Grouse, Ruffed, B. R. HEADSTROM, 373
Growth, Curves, S. BRODY, 43; Food, W. C. ROSE, 488
Guggenheim Foundation, Award of Fellowships by, 340

Habit Formation, K. DUNLAP, 360
HALL, W. T., Oxidation-Reduction Reactions, 315
HAMILTON, T. E., Edward Sandford Burgess, 388
HAMMETT, F. S., Plant Solution-Culture Work, 106
HANSON, F. B., X-Rays and Return Gene Mutations, 562
HARGITT, G. T., Secretaries' Conference of the Amer. Assoc. and Affiliated Societies, 481
Harkins, W. D., Award of Willard Gibbs Medal to, 550
HARSHBERGER, J. W., Colorado Plants, F. Ramaley, 467
HARTMAN, C. G., Gestation in the Monkey, 15
Hartwell, B. L. and the R. I. Agric. Exper. Station, 437
Harvard, Observatory, South African Station of, H. SHAPLEY, 297; Univ., Milton Research Awards, 364; Appointments and Promotions, 623
HARVEY, R. B., Alexandrovsk Biological Station, 158; Ethylene as a Ripener of Fruits, 421
Hatch, One Hundred per cent., R. C. JACKSON, 444
HAWKINS, A. C., Crystallographic Tables, V. Goldschmidt and S. G. Gordon, 653
HAY, O. P., Antiquity of Man in Oklahoma, 442; Preparation of Specimens by Filtration of Paraffin, 557
HEADSTROM, B. R., Mallard Ducks, 318; Ruffed Grouse, 373; An Ancient Walrus Skull, 608
Health Commissioner of Chicago, 153
HENRY, A. J., Floods in Miss., 15; Weather Reports, 512
HESS, A. F., Rickets, 333
HEWATT, W. G., The Eastland Horned "Toad," 348
HIGGINS, E., Conference of Lake Erie Biologists, 309
HIGGINS, G. M. and C. SHEARD, The Parathyroid Glands as Influenced by Selective Solar Radiation, 536
HILL, S. E., Diffusion of Oxygen through Rubber, 374
History, A Layman's View of, H. C. TAYLOR, 227
HITCHCOCK, A. S., Taxonomic Botanists, 431
HOLLAND, W. J., "Exit the Tentamen," 161
HOLM, G. E., Vitamins and the Oxidation of Fats, 424
HOLMES, H. N., Place of Research in the College, 539
Hominid Remains of Quaternary Age, D. BLACK, 135
HOOTON, E. A., A Prehistory Chart, 297
HOPKINS, B. S., Research, An Educational Asset, 427
HOTELLING, H., Statistics and Their Metrization, 149
HOTTES, C. F. and A. L. HAFENRICHTER, A Constant Rate Aspirator, 320
HOWARD, L. O., The User of Bulletins, 40; Malaria, 136; Biology of Insects, G. H. Carpenter, 467
Howard, L. O., Dinner in Honor of, 211
HRDLIČKA, A., Children Who Run on All Fours, 273; Anthropology and Medicine, 385
Humidity, Taciturnity, E. A. VUILLEUMIER, 608
HUNGATE, J. W., Northwest Scientific Assoc., 32
HUNT, C. H., Vitamin B, 556
HUNTINGTON, E. V., The Reapportionment Bill, 509
Huntington, George Sumner, C. F. W. MCCLURE, 301
HURD, C. D., Agriculture at the Inst. of Chemistry, 549
Hydrogen, Atomic, and Indust. Research, I. LANGMUIR, 201

Ichnology of Texas, R. L. MOODIE, 215
Illustrations, Reproducing, E. P. JONES, 535
Indiana Acad. of Science, H. F. DIETZ, 140, 636
Inertia Dyadic, I. F. MORRISON, 630
Infantile Paralysis, Research on, Committee for, 574
Institute of Chemistry, Agriculture at, C. D. HURD, 549
Interference, A. G. SIMSON, 16
International, Population Union, R. PEARL, 435; Conferences in 1928, 436
Ionic Migration Method, J. KENDALL, 163
Italy, National Research Council of, 233
Ixodiphagus Caucurtei, F. LARROUSSE, A. G. KING and S. B. WOLBACH, 351; in Larval Ticks, Egg Laying of, R. A. COOLEY, and G. M. KOHLS, 656

JACKSON, R. C., One Hundred per cent. Hatch, 444
Jacobs Cavern, Deposits in, V. C. ALLISON, 70
JAMES, L. H. and D. J. PRICE, Heating Hay, 322
Jelly-Fish, Fresh-Water, C. M. BREDER, JR., 241
JOFFE, J. S., Soil Science Publication in Russia, 105
JOHNSON, G. E., Kansas Academy of Science, 636
JOHNSON, P. L., Transferring Protozoa, 299
JOHNSON, T. H., Orientation of Atoms, 37
JOHNSTON, E. S. and W. H. DORE, Boron and the Growth of the Tomato Plant, 324
JONES, E. P., Reproducing Illustrations, 535
JONES, W. B., Eugene Allen Smith, 7
JORDAN, D. S., Charles Henry Gilbert, 644; and T. BARBOUR, Samuel Garman, 232
JORDAN, H. E., Physiology and Pathology of the Bone, R. Leriche and A. Policard, 70

KAMM, O., Pituitary Extracts, 199
KAMPMEIER, A., Galilei or Galileo, 422
Kansas Academy of Science, G. E. JOHNSON, 636
KAPP, E. M., Elasmobranchs, 513
KARPINSKI, L. C., Mathematics of the Greeks, 241
KARSNER, H. T., Wings for the Spirit, 251
Katydid, Musical Technique of, H. A. ALLARD, 613
KAY, G. M., The Decorah Formation, 16
KELLOGG, V., The Fourth Pacific Science Congress, 340; Barro Colorado Island Station, 389
KEMPTON, J. H., Agronomic Jabberwocky, 629

KENDALL, E. C., Biological Oxidations, 379
KENDALL, J., The Ionic Migration Method, 163
KENNEDY, F., Neurology and the Teaching of Med., 178
Kentucky Acad. of Science, A. M. PETER, 614
KLEEMAN, R. D., Absolute Zero of Temperature, 69; Condensed Substances near Absolute Zero, 420; The Constant of Mass Action, 295; Cosmic Radiation, 512
KOFOID, C. A., Freshwater Algae, G. S. West, 373
KOPELOFF, N., The Pronunciation of "Research," 319
KORFF, S. A., Hardness and Melting-points, 370
KOTILA, J. E., Rhizoctonia Cells, 490
KRAUS, E. H., Paul Heinrich von Groth, 150

LADD-FRANKLIN, C., Radiation from Nerve, 162; More Data, 444
LALLEMAND, C., Geodetic and Geophysical Union, 196
LANE, A. C., Geologic Age by Lead Uranium Ratios, 631
LANGMUIR, I., Atomic Hydrogen and Indust. Research, 201
Laplace Memorial, G. W. LITTLEHALES, 422
LARGE, T., Regional Scientific Societies, 272
LARROUSSE, F., A. G. KING and S. B. WOLBACH, Ixodiphagus Caucurtei, 351
Lasker Foundation for Medical Research, 549
LEECH, P. N., The Pronunciation of "Research," 466
LEPESCHKIN, W. W., The Importance of Biology, 59
Lepidoptera of New York, W. T. M. FORBES, 347
Lesser, Ernest J., C. F. CORI, 523
Life Sciences, New Building at Univ. of Calif., 63
Light, Reflection of, from Leaves, C. A. SHULL, 107
LILLIE, F. R., National Research Fellowships, 290
LILLIE, R. S., Physiological Rhythms and the Rhythmical Reactions in Inorganic Systems, 593
LIND, S. C., Chemical Action in Electrical Discharge, 565
LITTLEHALES, G. W., A Memorial to Laplace, 422
LIVINGSTON, B. E., Amer. Assoc., Newly Elected President, 111; N. Y. Meeting, 432; Spring Meeting of Executive Committee, 516
LOCHHEAD, A. G., European Foulbrood of Bees, 159
LOEB, L., Ovarian Secretion and Tumor Incidence, 104, 605
LOEB, L. B., Multiple Charged Radioactive Ions, 468
London Zoological Soc., Centenary of, 599
LYON, M. E., Embryoless Seeds in Cereals, 652

MCADIE, A., Manual of Meteorology, N. Shaw, 632
MCCAY, C. M., F. C. BING and W. E. DILLEY, The Nutrition of Trout, 249
MCCLURE, C. F. W., George Sumner Huntington, 301
MCCREA, A., Ultra-Violet Light and Digitalis, 277
MCCULLOCH, L. and C. THOM, Corm Rot of Gladiolus, 216
MACCURDY, G. G., School of Prehistoric Research, 219
MACDOUGAL, D. T. and J. G. BROWN, Cells, 447
MACDOUGALL, M. S., Chilodon and Ultra-Violet Light, 425
MCHATTON, T. H., Georgia State Coll. Exper. Sta., 264
MCKINNEY, H. H., Centrifuging Filterable Viruses, 271
MCLAUGHLIN, A. R., A Modified Erlanger Sphygmomanometer, 72; A Universal Muscle Lever, 349
MAGATH, T. B., The Cuticula of Nematodes, 194; Host of the Broad Tapeworm, 652
MAGISTAD, O. C., Musical Salt Solutions, 217
MAGRUDER, W. T., Pronunciation of "Research," 466
Malaria, L. O. HOWARD, 136; A. M. STIMSON, 449
Mallard Ducks, B. R. HEADSTROM, 318
MALUMPHY, T. L., Infiltrating Pig Embryos, 197
Man, Antiquity of, L. SPIER, 160; H. J. COOK, 371
Mass Action, The Constant of, R. D. KLEEMAN, 295
Mathematical, Operations, G. A. MILLER, 104; Symbols, Standard, 549
Mathematics—Too Little and Too Much, E. B. WILSON, 52; of the Greeks, L. C. KARPINSKI, 241
MAURY, C. J., Trinitasia—A New Molluscan Genus, 318; The Brasso Fossiliferous Miocene of Trinidad, 348
MAVOR, J. W., Mounting Chick Embryos, 445
Medal, Nichols, Presentation to H. S. Taylor; John Fritz, to J. J. Carty; Edison, to W. D. Coolidge, 132
Medical, Lectures, 10; Sciences, R. COLE, 47; School and Hospital, Post-Graduate, Reorganization, 363; Assoc., Amer., Grants for Research, 416
Medicine, Tropical, 10; New Laboratories for the Faculty of, at Paris, 31; Teaching of, and Neurology, F. KENNEDY, 178; Yale School of, New Building, 186; and Anthropology, A. HRDLIČKA, 385
Mercury, The Adhesion of, to Glass, W. C. BAKER, 74
MERRILL, G. P., The Siberian Meteorite, 489
Meteor, Daylight, A. B. REAGAN, 16
Meteorite, R. W. STONE, 40; Siberian, G. P. MERRILL, 489
METFESSEL, M., Collecting Folk Songs, 28
Microscopic Mounts, Determining the Color of Objects in, W. H. DAVIS and F. A. MACLAUGHLIN, 71
MILES, W. R., Alcohol and Longevity, R. Pearl, 557
MILLER, E. C. L., A Word to Replace "Believe," 319
MILLER, G. A., Mathematical Operations, 104; Archimedes and Trigonometry, 555
MILLIKAN, R. A. and G. H. CAMERON, Atom Building, 401
Minnesota, Univ. of, Building for Plant Industry, 504
MITCHELL, G. J., The Geology of Sonora, 373
Molecular Diameters in Gas Reactions, R. C. TOLMAN, D. M. YOST and R. G. DICKINSON, 241
Molluscan Genus, New,—Trinitasia, C. J. MAURY, 317
Molluscs, Temp. for Spawning, T. C. NELSON, 220
MOODIE, R. L., The Ichnology of Texas, 215; The Cephalaspidae, E. A. S. Stensiö, 348; Deafness in Pre-Columbian Peru, 464
MORRISON, I. F., Inertia Dyadic, 630
MUELLER, J. F., Physiology of *Ascaris*, 590
MUGRAGE, E. R., James Campbell Todd, 208
MUNRO, W. B., Physics and Politics, 223
MURRAY, C. D., Method of Picking up Correlations, 588
MURRAY, W. S., Ovarian Secretion and Cancer, 396
Muscle Lever, Universal, A. R. MCLAUGHLIN, 349
Museum, Amer., of Natural History, 503
Museums, Amer. Assoc. of, 459
Musil, Alois, Presentation of Daly Medal to, 289
Mutant Meadow Mouse, R. D. and A. SVIHLA, 531
Mutations, The Production of, A. WEINSTEIN, 376; Gene, The Effect of X-Rays on, F. B. HANSON, 562

Name, What is a?, W. T. M. FORBES, 373
NATHANSON, J. B., Boiling-Point and Latent Heat, 583
National, Research, Fellows, 132; Council of Italy, 233; Acad. of Sci., 425, 459, W. W. CAMPBELL, 482
NELSON, N. C., Pseudo-Artifacts, 316
NELSON, T. C., Critical Temperatures for Spawning, 220
Nerve Impulse, Conduction of the, L. E. TRAVIS, 41
NEWCOMER, E. J., The Western Oil-Spray Project, 560
NEWTON, A. J., The Royal Photographic Soc., 608
Newton, Bi-centenary of, F. E. BRASCH, 255
NICHOLS, J. T., Re Speciation, 346
Nichols Medal, Presentation to H. S. Taylor, 132
NIELSEN, J. R., Collisions of the Second Kind, 651
NOÉ, A. C., Use of Charts in the Natural Sciences, 571
NOLAND, L. E., Fixative and Stain for Flagella, 535
North Carolina Acad. of Science, H. R. TOTTEN, 635
North Dakota Acad. of Science, 614
Northwest Sci. Assoc., J. W. HUNGATE, 32
DU NOÜY, L., Modification of the Viscosity Serum, 563; The Ring Method in Changing Surface Tension, 607
NOYES, A. A., Response to Address of Welcome at Nashville Meeting of the Amer. Assoc., 109
"Nutrilites," R. J. WILLIAMS, 607
Nutrition of Trout, Factor H in the, C. M. MCCAY, F. C. BING and W. E. DILLEY, 249
Nutritional Anemia and Beef Liver, J. WADDELL, C. A. ELVEHJEM, H. STEENBOCK and E. B. HART, 139

Observatory, Harvard, South African Station of, 61
Oceanographic, Bingham, Collection at Yale Univ., 622

OGDEN, J. G., Frank W. Very, 262
Ohio Acad. of Science, W. H. ALEXANDER, 538
Oil-Spray Project, Western, E. J. NEWCOMER, 560
Oklahoma Geological Survey Field Parties, 623
Optical, Glass, casting of a Large Disk of, 263; Instruments and Products, Exhibit, I. C. GARDNER, 600
ORTON, J. H., Transplantation of the Oyster, 582
OSBORN, H. F., Antiquity of Man, J. R. Moir, 273; Science Week in New York, 411; Louis Agassiz, 523; The Plateau Habitat of the Pro-Dawn Man, 570
Osmosis, What is It?, O. K. STARK, 556
OSTERUD, H. L. and K. F. BASCOM, Sarcocystis, 531
Oxford Expedition to Greenland, 502
Oxidation-Reduction Reactions, W. T. HALL, 315
Oxidations, Biological, E. C. KENDALL, 379
Oxygen, Diffusion of, through Rubber, S. E. HILL, 374
Oyster, Transplantation of, J. H. ORTON, 582

Pacific Science Congress, The Fourth, V. KELLOGG, 340
Paleontology, W. B. SCOTT, 327
Pan-American Geodetic Institute, 185
Pan-Pacific Congress, 153
Paraffin, in Preparation of Biological Specimens, O. P. HAY, 557
Paramecium, Immobilization of, J. C. BOLAND, 654
Parasitology, C. C. BASS, 454
PARKER, F. W., Water Soluble Phosphorus in Soils, 402
Patagonia, Princeton Expeditions to, 575
Pathology of Virus Diseases, E. W. GOODPASTURE, 591
Peabody, Francis W., 33
PEARL, R., International Population Union, 435
Pentathionic Acid, H. C. YOUNG and R. WILLIAMS, 19
Periodic Hardness and Melting-points, S. A. KORFF, 370
PETER, A. M., Kentucky Acad. of Science, 614
Philosophical Soc., Amer., Annual Meeting, 403
Philosophy or Irony, M. M. GARVER, 297
Phosphocreatine, C. H. FISKE and Y. SUBBAROW, 169
Phosphorus, Water Soluble, in Soils, F. W. PARKER, 402
Photography, International Congress of, 458
Physical Sciences, New Buildings at Univ. of Chicago, 99
Physicians and Surgeons, Coll. of, Gifts to, 210
Physics and Politics, W. B. MUNRO, 223
Physiologic Life, The, A. J. CARLSON, 355
PIETSCHMANN, V., X-Ray in Biolog. Investigations, 610
Pig Embryos, Infiltrating, T. L. MALUMPHY, 197
Pituitary Extracts, O. KAMM, 199
Plankton Bucket, A. S. CAMPBELL, 322
Plant Solution-Culture Work, F. S. HAMMETT, 106
Plants, Malnutrition in, F. J. SIEVERS, 286; Small-seeded, Growing under Sterile Conditions, A. B. BEAUMONT and G. J. LARSINOS, 350
Plate that Penetrates Haze, E. BLACKWELDER, 275
POKROWSKI, G. I., Sun's Activity and Biol. Factors, 397
Population, U. S., 339; Union, Internat., R. PEARL, 435
Potato Tuber Necrosis, A. H. GILBERT, 464
Potential, Bioelectric, S. GELFAN, 589
PRATT, H. S., Harris Hawthorne Wilder, 479
Precambrian Life, D. WHITE, 620
Prehistoric Research, School of, G. G. MACCURDY, 219
PRIEST, I. G., Bibliography of Colorimetry, 39
Primates, Starvation Ketosis of, T. E. FRIEDEMANN, 221
Pro-Dawn Man, Plateau Habitat of, H. F. OSBORN, 570
Propagation of the Apple by Seed, C. F. SWINGLE, 296
Protozoa, Transferring, P. L. JOHNSON, 299
Psycho-Endocrinology, L. BERMAN, 195
Psychological Laboratories, Early, J. McK. CATTELL, 543
Psychology, Congress of, 33
Publication, What Constitutes It?, C. W. STILES, 471
Pure Science, Research Fund at Princeton Univ., 99
Purposive Action, M. F. WASHBURN, 24

Quails, Potato Bugs and Other Things, N. L. WILLET, 532
Quotations, 17, 162, 195, 243, 466

Radiation, Cosmic, R. D. KLEEMAN, 512
Radioactive Ions, Multiple Charged, L. B. LOEB, 468
Rainfall and Run-off, F. D. ADAMS, 500
Rats, Reproduction in, P. EATON and C. S. STIRRETT, 555
REAGAN, A. B., A Daylight Meteor, 16
Reference, The Little Circle of, C. BARUS, 530
Regulator, Water, Modified, T. SKOGSBERG, 275
Reports, 138, 196, 219, 560, 585, 608, 633
Research, Scientific, B. A. BEHREND, 272; National Fellowships, F. R. LILLIE, 290; The Pronunciation of, N. KOPELOFF, 319, E. E. SLOSSON, 465, P. N. LEECH, 466; W. T. MAGRUDER, 466; an Educational Asset, B. S. HOPKINS, 427; A "Data" of, F. L. WELLS, 491; in the College, Place of, H. N. HOLMES, 539; More, J. S. STEVENS, W. H. KUN and E. H. MCCLELLAND, 584; and the Training of the Researcher, T. H. EATON, 619; Plus News, E. E. SLOSSON and W. DAVIS, 628
Retina of Mammals, Changes in, G. L. WALLS, 655
Rhizoctonia, J. E. KOTILA, 490
Rhythms, Physiological, and the Rhythmical Reaction in Inorganic Systems, R. S. LILLIE, 593
RICE, B. B., The Vacuome of Plant Cells, 561
RICHARDS, C. R., Functions of Sect. M—Engineering, 5
Rickets, A. F. HESS, 333
RIGGS, E. S., Field Museum Expeditions, 585
RITTER, W. E., Science and the Newspapers, 279
ROBINSON, B. B., Acquired Character in Flax, 242
Rockefeller Foundation, 458
ROMBERG, A. and L. W. BLAU, Weight and Humidity, 347
Rose, Joseph Nelson, W. TRELEASE, 598
ROSE, W. C., Food and Growth, 488
Royal, Photographic Society, A. J. NEWTON, 608; Society of Edinburgh, 310

ST. JOHN, J. L., Cutting Glass Tubing, 561
Salt Solutions, O. C. MAGISTAD, 217
Santa Catalina Natural Area, Dedication of, 575
Sarcocystis, H. L. OSTERUD and K. F. BASCOM, 531
SCHUCHERT, C., Brachiopod and Genera, J. A. Thomson, 491
Science, and the Newspapers, W. E. RITTER, 279; and Secretaries, B. WILLIS, 345; International Relations in, G. BARGER, 405; Week in New York, H. F. OSBORN, 411; Popular, 466; Service, Meeting, W. DAVIS, 482
Sciences, Nat. Acad. of, 425, 459, W. W. CAMPBELL, 482
Scientific, Events, 10, 31, 61, 99, 132, 152, 185, 209, 233, 263, 288, 309, 339, 363, 389, 414, 435, 458, 481, 502, 524, 548, 574, 599, 622, 645; Notes and News, 12, 34, 63, 101, 133, 154, 187, 211, 236, 265, 290, 311, 341, 365, 391, 416, 437, 460, 483, 505, 526, 550, 577, 601, 624, 647; Books, 41, 70, 105, 218, 244, 273, 298, 319, 348, 373, 398, 423, 444, 467, 491, 533, 577, 632, 653; Apparatus and Laboratory Methods, 71, 106, 167, 197, 275, 299, 320, 349, 374, 400, 445, 492, 512, 535, 561, 587, 600, 653; Men of Harvard and of Columbia, J. McK. CATTELL, 136; Societies, Regional, T. LARGE, 272; Obscurity, E. E. SLOSSON, 398
SCOTT, W. B., Paleontology, 327
Secretaries' Conf. of Amer. Assoc., G. T. HARGITT, 481
SEEMANN, H. E., Cutting Glass Tubing, 107
SEIDELL, A., Marcelin Berthelot, 180; Centenary, 497
SEIFRIZ, W., Biochemical Methods, C. A. Morrow, 533
SHAPLEY, H., African Station of Harvard Obs., 297
SHAW, F. W., Undulant Fever in America, 217
SHEARD, C. and G. M. HIGGINS, Solar Radiations, 493
SHULL, C. A., Reflection of Light from Leaves, 107
SIEVERS, F. J., Malnutrition in Plants, 286
Sigma, Pi Sigma, 538; Xi, New Chapters, 311
SIMSON, A. G., Interference, 16
SKOGSBERG, T., Modified Water Regulator, 275
Skull, Clear Creek, Identity of, H. S. THATCHER, 38
Sleeping Sickness in Africa, Expedition to Combat, 263
SLOSSON, E. E., Scientific Obscurity, 398; The Pronunciation of "Research," 465; and W. DAVIS, Research Plus News, 628
Smith, Eugene Allen, W. B. JONES, 7

SMITH, G. O., The U. S. Coast and Geodetic Survey, 67
SMITH, R. H., The Mispronunciation of "Data," 70
SMITH, S. L., Vitamin B, 494
Societies and Acad., 140, 403, 425, 496, 538, 614, 635
Soil, Science Publication in Russia, J. S. JOFFE, 105; Moisture, G. J. BOUYOUCOS, 167; Color Analysis, G. B. BODMAN, 446
Soils, Making an Analysis of, G. J. BOUYOUCOS, 587
Solar Radiations and Growth, C. SHEARD and G. M. HIGGINS, 493; Variation in, C. G. ABBOT, 634
SOUDER, W., Apparatus, 298
Sound, The Velocity of, P. I. WOLD and G. R. STIBITZ, 218; Secondary, and Hearing, E. G. WEVER, 612
Special Articles, 18, 41, 73, 107, 139, 169, 198, 220, 248, 276, 300, 322, 351, 376, 401, 424, 447, 468, 493, 514, 536, 562, 589, 612, 634, 655
Speciation, Re, J. T. NICHOLS, 346
Species, Differentiation of, H. E. CRAMPTON, 615
Sphygmomanometer, A. R. MCLAUGHLIN, 72
SPIER, L., Antiquity of Man in Oklahoma, 160
SPRAGUE, H. B., Measuring Chloroplast Pigments, 167
STARK, O. K., What is Osmosis?, 556
Starling, Ernest H., Proposed Memorial to, 414
Statistics, Spaces of, and Their Metrization, H. HOTELLING, 149; of Vocabulary, E. U. CONDON, 300
Stature throughout the World, R. B. BEAN, 1
Steam Pipes, Sharp Rattling in, R. C. COLWELL, 397
STEENWIJK, J. E. DE VOS VAN, Intellectual Cooperation and Biology, 633
STERN, T. E., Newtonian Constant of Gravitation, 377
STETSON, H. T., Stars and Atoms, A. S. EDDINGTON, 41; Nathaniel Bowditch, A. Stanford, 218; The Aurora of March 28, 1928, 394
STEVENS, F. L., The Sexual Stage of Fungi, 514
STEVENS, J. S., W. H. KUN and E. H. MCCLELLAND, More Research, 584
Stevens, Walter Le Conte, B. A. WOOTEN, 413
STILES, C. W., Zoological Nomenclature, 17; What Constitutes Publication?, 471
STIMSON, A. M., Malaria, 449
STONE, R. W., No Meteorite, 40
STORER, T. I., Pacific States, Birds, R. Hoffmann, 398
SUMNER, F. B., Colorimetric Methods in Biology, 271
Sun's Activity and Biolog. Factors, G. I. POKROWSKI, 397
SVIHLA, R. D., and A. SVIHLA, Mutant Mouse, 531
SWINGLE, C. F., Propagation of the Apple by Seed, 296

Tapeworm, Broad, Host of, T. B. MAGATH, 652
TAYLOR, H. O., A Layman's View of History, 227
Taylor, H. S., Presentation of Nichols Medal to, 132
Technique, New and Old Problems, W. C. CURTIS, 141
Teeth, in Ultra-Violet Rays, H. C. BENEDICT, 442
Tension, Surface, Ring Method in, L. DU NOÜY, 607
"Tentamen," Exit, W. J. HOLLAND, 161
THATCHER, H. S., Identity of Clear Creek Skull, 38
"Toad," the Eastland Horned, W. G. HEWATT, 348
Todd, James Campbell, E. R. MUGRAGE, 208
TOLMACHOFF, I. P., Cutting Glass Tubing, 299; Exploration of the Arctic Regions by Airship, 363
TOLMAN, R. C., D. M. YOST and R. G. DICKINSON, Molecular Diameters in Gas Reactions, 241
Tooth Gone Wrong, One, 243
TOTTEN, H. R., N. C. Academy of Science, 635
TRAVIS, L. E., Conduction of the Nerve Impulse, 41
TREASHER, R. C., "Washboard" Effect in Roads, 395
Tree Frogs and Pitcher Plants, E. A. ANDREWS, 269
TRELEASE, W., Joseph Nelson Rose, 598
Trinidad, Fossiliferous Miocene of, C. J. MAURY, 348
Tumors, Origin of, H. E. EGGERS, 193; and Ovarian Secretion, L. LOEB, 104, 605

Ultra-Violet Light, and Digitalis Purpurea, A. MCCREA, 277; in Chilodon uncinatus, M. S. MACDOUGALL, 425
Undulant Fever in America, F. W. SHAW, 217
University and Educational Notes, 14, 37, 67, 103, 135, 158, 191, 215, 240, 269, 295, 314, 344, 369, 394, 420, 441, 463, 487, 508, 530, 554, 580, 605, 627, 650

Vacuome of Plant Cells, B. B. RICE, 561
Vaporization of Water, Latent Heat of, and Boiling Point, J. B. NATHANSON, 583
Varanus Niloticus, R. B. COWLES, 317
Very, Frank W., J. G. OGDEN, 262
Viruses, Filterable, Centrifuging, H. H. MCKINNEY, 271
Visible Radiation from an Excited Nerve Fiber, H. DAVIS, 69; C. LADD-FRANKLIN, 162
Vitamin B, S. L. SMITH, 494; C. H. HUNT, 556
Vitamins and the Oxidation of Fats, G. E. HOLM, 424
VUILLEUMIER, E. A., Humidity and Taciturnity, 608

WADDELL, J., C. A. ELVEHJEM, H. STEENBOCK and E. B. HART, Nutritional Anemia, 139
WAGENER, W. W., Coryneum Canker of Cypress, 584
WAGNER, G., Banana Stowaways, 422
WALLS, G. L., Changes in the Retina of Mammals, 655
Walrus Skull, Ancient, B. R. HEADSTROM, 608
WARREN, E. R., Banana Stowaways, 422
"Washboard" Effect in Dirt Roads, R. C. TREASHER, 395; E. WILSON, 396
WASHBURN, M. F., Purposive Action, 24
WATSON, F. R., Acoustics of Auditoriums, 335
Weather Reports, 210; A. J. HENRY, 512
Weight and Humidity, A. ROMBERG and L. W. BLAU, 347
WEINSTEIN, A., The Production of Mutations, 376
Wellesley College and Bot. Education, C. S. GAGER, 171
WELLS, F. L., A "Data" of Research, 491
WENRICH, D. H. and C. C. WANG, Conjugation in Paramecium, 270
WEVER, E. G., Secondary Sound and Hearing, 612
WHITE, D., Precambrian Life, 620
Wild-Life, Refuge, 645; Preserve, P. W. CLAASSEN, 651
Wilder, Harris Hawthorne, H. S. PRATT, 479
WILEY, H. W., The Earliest Dynamo, 532
WILLCOX, W. F., Apportionment of Representatives, 581
WILLET, N. L., Quails and Other Things, 532
WILLIAMS, C. G., Agricultural Experiment Station, 519
WILLIAMS, H. B., Willem Einthoven, 456
WILLIAMS, R. J., "Nutrilites," 607
WILLIS, B., Science and Secretaries, 345; and E. B. MATHEWS, U. S. Coast and Geodetic Survey, 100
WILSON, E., "Washboard" Effect in Dirt Roads, 396
WILSON, EDWIN B., Too Little Mathematics and Too Much, 52; Abilities of Man, C. Spearman, 244
WILSON, J. F., Medullated Wool Fiber, 512
Wings for the Spirit, H. T. KARSNER, 251
Winter, The Beginning of, C. N. FENNER, 243
WOLD, P. I. and G. R. STIBITZ, Velocity of Sound, 218
WOLF, E. A., Determining the Rate of Cleavage, 611
Wool Fiber, Medullated, J. F. WILSON, 512
WOOTEN, B. A., Walter LeConte Stevens, 413

X-ray in Biological Investigations, V. PIETSCHMANN, 610
X-rayed Sex Cells, T. H. GOODSPEED and A. R. OLSON, 46

Yale Foundation for Study of Children's Diseases, 646
YOUNG, H. C. and R. WILLIAMS, Pentathionic Acid, 19

Zeolite in Green River Formation, W. H. BRADLEY, 73
Zoological, Nomenclature, C. W. STILES, 17; Society, London, Centenary of, 599
"Zoology, General," W. J. DAKIN, 465

SCIENCE

VOL. LXVII JANUARY 6, 1928 NO. 1723

CONTENTS

The American Association for the Advancement of Science:

Stature throughout the World: PROFESSOR R. BENNETT BEAN ... 1

The Functions of Section M—Engineering: PROFESSOR CHARLES RUSS RICHARDS ... 5

Eugene Allen Smith: DR. WALTER B. JONES ... 7

Scientific Events:

The London School of Hygiene and Tropical Medicine; Free Public Lectures on Medical Subjects; Officers of the American Chemical Society; Officers of the American Association for the Advancement of Science ... 10

Scientific Notes and News ... 12

University and Educational Notes ... 14

Discussion and Correspondence:

The Period of Gestation in the Monkey: DR. CARL G. HARTMAN. *The Floods of 1927 in the Mississippi River Basin:* A. J. HENRY. *Divisions of the Decorah Formation:* G. MARSHALL KAY. *A Daylight Meteor:* DR. ALBERT B. REAGAN. *Interference?* A. GAEL SIMSON ... 15

Quotations:

Dr. F. A. Bather ... 17

Amendments to the International Rules of Zoological Nomenclature: DR. C. W. STILES ... 17

Special Articles:

The Chromosomes of Moina Macrocopa: DR. EZRA ALLEN. *Genetic Evidence that the Cladocera Male is Diploid:* DR. ARTHUR M. BANTA and THELMA R. WOOD. *Pentathionic Acid, the Fungicidal Factor of Sulphur:* DR. H. C. YOUNG and ROBERT WILLIAMS ... 18

Science News ... x

SCIENCE: A Weekly Journal devoted to the Advancement of Science, edited by J. McKeen Cattell and published every Friday by

THE SCIENCE PRESS

New York City: Grand Central Terminal.

Lancaster, Pa. Garrison, N. Y.

Annual Subscription, $6.00. Single Copies, 15 Cts.

SCIENCE is the official organ of the American Association for the Advancement of Science. Information regarding membership in the Association may be secured from the office of the permanent secretary, in the Smithsonian Institution Building, Washington, D. C.

Entered as second-class matter July 18, 1923, at the Post Office at Lancaster, Pa., under the Act of March 8, 1879.

STATURE THROUGHOUT THE WORLD[1]

A GENERAL survey of stature has been started in connection with a study of old Americans in Virginia and this report is a condensed summary of the preliminary work. Only males are considered.

Stature is a complex dependent upon the growth of various parts of the body, chiefly bone and cartilage. This growth is partly regulated by the endocrines of the hypophysis and thyroid, and it is influenced by a great number of factors, such as food, water, habit and habitat. It is impossible to measure each factor that enters into the life history of each individual, therefore mass statistics are used, and only general results and conclusions may be given.

The records have been obtained from various sources, and many of them are of men below the age of 25 years who therefore had not finished their growth. In general there is no distinction as to age; all ages are included, from near adult to the old, although the majority are between the ages of 20 and 30 years. The technique of measuring is not always the same in gathering the records, therefore they may not all be fairly comparable. The method of grouping them by the median of group means or averages should prevent any gross errors as the result of technique or the selection of individuals.

Group medians are used throughout because this affords the fairest average stature. There are 326 groups from Europe and the median of the group averages is 169.4 centimeters. The extremes are one group of "Indigent French" with a stature of 156.0 centimeters, and one group of "Scotch Farmers" with a stature of 181.2 centimeters. There are two distinct modes, one at 166.0 centimeters and the other at 170.0 centimeters. This is clearly indicated by the median for southern Europe at 165.5 centimeters, and that for northern Europe at 170.6 centimeters, with middle Europe at 166.6 centimeters.

The median of 135 groups in Asia is 161.1 centimeters, with extremes of one group of Negritos from southern India at 148.0 centimeters, and one group of Ainos with a stature of 172.0 centimeters. Persians and Turks are not included in Asia but are put

[1] Address of the vice-president and chairman of Section H—Anthropology, American Association for the Advancement of Science, Nashville, December, 1927.

with Europe. There are three groups of these at 165.0, 173.0 and 175.0 centimeters. The Asiatics, except for the Negritos, are more homogeneous than the Europeans, if we leave out the Persians and Turks, although the Ainos should also be excluded because they are modified Europeans. Under such circumstances the extremes for Asia would be one group of Malays with a stature of 154.0 centimeters, and one group of Tibetans with a stature of 162.5 centimeters. The stature increases from Asia to Europe through the Persians with a stature of 166.0 centimeters and the Turks with a stature of 168.0 to 175.0 centimeters.

The median of 245 groups in Africa is 170.0 centimeters, with extremes of one group of Negrillos with a stature of 130.0 centimeters, and one group of Somalis with a stature of 180.3 centimeters. The spread of the curve is greater for Africa than for Europe, and it is skew for tall stature, trailing in the low. This would show that there are more negroid stocks in Africa than true Negroes and Negrillos, who are not so tall as the negroid stocks.

The median of 126 groups of North American Indians is 165.0 centimeters, and extremes of one group of "Partial Albino" Central American Indians with a stature of 145.7 centimeters, and one group of the Winnipeg Indians with a stature of 180.0 centimeters. The curve is irregular with three distinct nodes at 156.3, 163.8 and 173.8 centimeters.

The median of 38 groups of South American Indians is 160.0 centimeters with extremes of one group of Aymaras with a stature of 148.0 centimeters and one group of Patagonians with a stature of 185.0 centimeters.

The median stature of 152 groups from the Pacific Islands is 159.0 centimeters, with extremes of one group of Negritos with a stature of 139.7 centimeters and one group of Australians with a stature of 185.0 centimeters. The curve has a mode at 160.0 centimeters and a submode at 170.0 centimeters.

The tall statures of the Patagonians, Australians and Somalis may have been the result of the selection of extremely tall persons to be measured. This seems to have been the case with the Patagonians, especially, because several groups had statures from 171 to 175 centimeters.

Europe

Stature in Europe has its summit in Scandinavia of 172.5 centimeters, with Great Britain a close second at 171.0 centimeters, and Denmark, Germany and Turkey following with about 170.0 centimeters. Some may object to putting Turkey and Persia in Europe, but their similarity in many physical characters and their similarity of stock and origin have led me to do this. Low stature has its extreme at 155.0 and 157.5 centimeters among the Lapps and northern Russians, who might well be put with Asia. The Italians and Jews come next with a stature of 164.0 centimeters followed by the Russians and French at about 165.0 centimeters. Central Europe, which includes Belgium, Switzerland, and the Balkans, has a stature of 167.0 centimeters, and Greece has about the same.

It may be said that in general stature in Europe is low in the north as among the Lapps and northern Russians, and low in the south as among the Italians and Jews, and it is higher in between. The Scotch have the highest individual statures, it is high in England, and higher in the United States, especially among the Old Americans of British origin. There is evidence of two areas of high stature in Europe, the one in Scandinavia, North Germany and the British Isles, the other about the interior littoral of the Atlantic and Mediterranean. The former are called the Nordic or Teutonic Peoples, and the latter are called the Littoral, Adriatic and Dinaric Peoples. There is also evidence of two areas of small stature the one toward the Arctic zone and the other toward the Tropics. The restless activity by the cold, moist, cloudy Baltic region, or the steppe and mountain, had some influence in molding the tall stature, whereas the extreme cold of the far north and the heat of the Mediterranean with civilization had some influence in making the stature small. Through these influences selection acted, and heredity carried on the result.

There are pockets of high and low stature in Europe and in the other continents, as demonstrated by Wissler for the American Indian. These "patches" may be the centers of radiation for the culture, or centers of compression by the tribes from without. Ripley presents evidences of the crazy quilt effect of stature distribution in Europe, and discusses at some length the effects of race and environment. He gives the results of "misery spots," "artificial selection," "natural emigrants," "occupation or professions," and the "habits of life or of the nature of employment." These all have their influence in a minor way. Visualizing the whole continent brings out major influences. It is only by getting out of the woods that the forest may be seen.

Asia

The summit of stature is found in China, 162.0 centimeters, India 164.0 centimeters and Tibet, 162.5 centimeters: and the lowest stature is found among the Negritos, 148.0 centimeters, and in the Malay peninsula, 154.0 centimeters. The Mongolians and Siberians in the north have about the same stature as the Indo-Chinese and southern Indians in the south, 159.0 centimeters. Tall statures are found about the high plateaus of western Asia and this is less in the north and south as well as in Japan, and in the latter the stature is also about 159.0 centimeters. The stature changes from 164.0 in northern India to 157.5 in southern India and 148.0 among the Negritos of southern India and the Malay peninsula. The Malays are closer to the Negritos in stature than any other people and the Indo-Chinese are closer to the Malays. These relations become more distinct when the peoples of the Pacific Islands are studied.

PACIFIC ISLANDS

The summit of stature in the Pacific Islands is reached in certain groups of Polynesians where it is 172.0 centimeters, and the extreme of low stature among the Negritos where it is as low as 139.7 centimeters. A few small groups of individuals among the Australians have a stature of 185.0 centimeters. The stature of all the groups of Malays is 159.0 centimeters and that of the Senoi or Sakai is 152.5, whereas the stature of the Negritos nearby is 148.0 centimeters. The Senoi or Sakai are so manifestly crosses between the Malays and Negritos that their stature is easily explicable. There are two distinct types among the Polynesians, the European and the Malay, and there are two distinct groups of stature, the one at 161.0 centimeters and the other at 172.0 centimeters, with no intervening groups between 165.0 and 170.0 centimeters. The stature of the Melanesians is 161.5 centimeters and the stature of the Australians is 167.0 centimeters. The latter shows the European influence through the "Hairy Men." Groups of hairy men are found in a broad zone from Russia to Australia, with remnants in Japan and the Philippines.

There is tall stature in Asia about the great plateaus bordering on Persia and Turkey, and small stature toward the Arctic and Tropic zones, with smaller statures in the Pacific Islands among the Negritos and Malays. The Malays are mixtures of the Asiatic, Negrito and European. There is tall stature among the Polynesians and Australians, with less tall stature among the Melanesians. The Polynesians are mixtures of the Europeans, Malays and Melanesians with more European than other stocks, and the Australians are mixtures of the Melanesians, Malays and Europeans with more of the Negroid than other stocks. In Australia there is apparently a tall negro element different from the Negrito. This, however, may be more apparent than real.

AFRICA

The summit of stature in Africa is found among the Bantus of eastern Africa, along the upper Nile region and among the great lakes, as well as in North Africa, where the group average of 185 centimeters is not uncommon and in one group of Somalis the stature is 185.3 centimeters. Low stature has its extreme among the Negrillos and Bushmen, with a low of 130.0 centimeters for the former and of 142.5 centimeters for the latter. The median for 102 groups of North Africa and 48 groups of East Africa is 171.0 centimeters which is the same as that of the Bantus. The median for 21 groups of Negrillos is 147.5 centimeters. Between the extremes of high and low stature are the Bushmen, 156.0, True Negroes 161.0, Berbers 164.0, and Bantus mixed with True Negroes 166.5 centimeters. If one approach the Negrillos from any side there is a gradual transition from a high to a low stature and other changes accompany this, from the True Negro on the west, the Bantu on the east, the Hottentot and Bushman on the south, and the Europeanized Hamitic and Semitic Negroid on the north.

Tall stocks have been coming into Africa from Asia and Europe throughout historic time and probably before, and these stocks have mixed with the Negroes to produce the tall peoples of Africa. The tropic conditions in central Africa have dwarfed the True Negro into the Negrillo, and the True Negro has also become dwarfed.

NORTH AMERICA

North America is divided into five parts, Eskimo, Canada, United States, Mexico and Central America. There is a gradual increase in stature from the Eskimos through Canada to the United States, and a sudden decrease through Mexico to Central America. The summit of stature is reached among the Winnipeg Indians of Canada, 180.2 centimeters, and the Dakotas, 178.0 centimeters, and Apaches, 176.2 centimeters, in the United States. Low stature has its extreme among the San Blas Indians of South America. Starr gives the stature of 2,276 Mexican and Central American Indians as 157.5 centimeters. The low stature towards the arctic and tropic zones in North America indicates as elsewhere that those zones do not favor tall stature.

SOUTH AMERICA

Stature in South America has its summit in Patagonia, where several groups attain the stature of 185.0 centimeters. Other groups of Patagonians average between 171.0 and 175.0 centimeters. Probably tall members of the tribe were measured in the groups with statures of 185.0 centimeters. Low stature has its extreme among the Aymaras, Quechuas and Machigangas of the interior tropic zone and among the Fuegians at the southern extremity of South America towards the arctic zone. We have something similar to this condition in Africa in the low stature of the Negrillo in the jungles, high stature in the southeast, and low stature in the south among isolated groups of Bushmen and Hottentots. Steppes, pampas and fertile regions in temperate zones produce high statures. Jungle and infertile cold regions produce low statures. This is but an expression of the fittest for each region, who survive.

Old American Whites of Virginia

For the past few years I have been making a study of the Old Americans in Virginia, and in this study have measured several thousand men, women and children from Tidewater, Piedmont and Mountain sections of the state. There is a difference in the stature of the Tidewater section on the one hand and the Piedmont and Mountain sections on the other. The stature from all three sections is 173.7 centimeters. The tallest group is that of the leading farmers of Albemarle County in the Piedmont section of the state where the stature is 176.2 centimeters with extremes of 165.1 and 190.4 centimeters, and the smallest group is from Tidewater where the stature is 170.7 centimeters with extremes of 160.6 and 181.6 centimeters.

The tall stature in the Piedmont and Mountain sections of the state may be the result of the stock from which they were derived. The Scotch, or Scotch-Irish as they are called, have been traced through Pennsylvania, Virginia, North Carolina, Tennessee, Kentucky, Missouri and to the Pacific Coast. They were pioneers in the colonial period and acted as a buffer between the Indians and the colonists on the Atlantic seaboard. Later they aided largely in the settlement of the west. They have been the tallest men of the United States. During the Revolution Virginia furnished some of the tallest men of the army in Morgan's Rangers, and such pioneers as Washington, Jefferson and Marshall, who were over six feet tall; during the War between the States the tallest soldiers were from Kentucky, the sons of Virginia, and during the World War the tallest soldiers came from Missouri. California is celebrated for its tall men.

The tall stature of Piedmont and Mountain may be the result of other factors than the stock of people, but this is one factor. The small stature of Tidewater may be partly the result of malaria and dysentery in the earlier colonial period, leaving a sturdier and stockier kind, and the moving out of the tall active, restless pioneer into the open spaces of the west where they joined the Scotch in maintaining the tall stature. A long experience among the mountaineers showed me their tall stature, and the recent measurements confirmed it. The examination and measurement of several hundred mountain children showed their superior physique. They had no malnutrition and they proved to be the best developed of all Virginia children so far measured.

The University of Virginia Free Dispensary provided the examination of some poor whites from Charlottesville and the surrounding district. The stature is 172.9 centimeters with extremes of 157.6 and 187.1. This is a heterogeneous group, although the extremes are not so great as in the morgue subjects measured at autopsy in the Charity Hospital, New Orleans, where the stature was 171.1 centimeters and the extremes 157.0 and 190.0 centimeters. Is the submerged tenth made up of extremes? The low stature of this group may be the result of disease or malnutrition, but the stature is not so low as that of the business men of Charlottesville, which is 171.0 centimeters, with extremes of 160.6 and 180.0 centimeters. This is a group comparable in social position with the Albemarle farmers, living in the same community, and with equal if not better opportunity for proper nourishment. It has been recognized that clerks are smaller than laborers and merchants than farmers. This is a difference of type and not the result of nourishment. The tall, active, restless pioneer develops the country, then the small, quiet, sedentary citizen builds towns and conducts its business. The pioneer may develop business, but usually lives in the country and the small man is left in the city. This is the selection by the fittest for what is for their best good.

A comparison of soldiers and students shows a difference in stature in favor of the students of about 3 centimeters. The students have a stature of 174.2 centimeters with extremes of 160.2 and 189.7 centimeters, and the soldiers have a stature of 171.0 centimeters with extremes of 152.0 and 191.0 centimeters. The students were University of Virginia men over 20 years of age, and the soldiers were engineers of the Truck Camp near-by also over 20 years of age. The students were more of the hypermorph type which is taller, whereas the soldiers were more of the mesomorph type which is not so tall.

Summary

Tropic jungle life has an influence that decreases stature, and so has Arctic cold and waste. In each there is difficulty in procuring proper food, and discomfort in the extreme.

The active life of the temperate zone with its comforts and abundant food supply produces the tallest statures.

The greatest extremes of small stature are found among the Negrillos of Central Africa and the Aymaras of Central South America, in the jungles of excessive heat and poor food supply. Next to these come the Eskimos, Lapps and Siberians, with ice and excessive cold and poor food supply. On the other hand, the littoral and southern Baltic regions in Europe, the western part of Asia, eastern Africa, and the plains and pampas of the Americas with their active life, abundant food supply and temperate climate produce the tallest statures.

Certain stocks may move into areas for which they are not fitted and remain for a time, and such conditions exist throughout the world to-day where recent movements of peoples have taken place, but ultimately there is a survival of the stock best fitted for the environment, and the unfitted stocks disappear by amalgamation, eradication or dispersal.

Sea areas and probably sea food have an influence in reducing stature. The present Mediterranean peoples and the primordial British have small statures and so does Japan, yet they came from taller continental stocks. The Central Americans and Fuegians are smaller than the continental peoples near-by. The Malays and southern Asiatics are smaller than the peoples of the interior of the continent. Other instances might be cited.

There is some evidence that the seaboard statures of the United States are less than those of the interior, but other factors enter here.

Looked at in its broadest sense, environment molds the individual, selection retains the fittest under different environments, and heredity carries on the results.

R. BENNETT BEAN

THE FUNCTIONS OF SECTION M—ENGINEERING[1]

FROM time to time during the ages of his development man has accidentally discovered or invented various devices and processes that have enabled him to raise himself above the level of the rest of the animal kingdom, to better cope with the forces of nature and to adapt himself to his environment. With slowly accumulated experience he improved and developed these devices and processes until they came into general use among his fellows. Each forward step in man's ascent has been thus marked by some epoch-making discovery that expanded his power and improved his status. Doubtless from the beginning some men more than their fellows were endowed with powers of observation, deduction and ingenuity, and it is to them that the real progress of the race has been due. To such men various types of construction work were intrusted, and their experience and knowledge were passed on from generation to generation by a kind of apprenticeship and by word of mouth. Master craftsmen were thus developed who possessed some knowledge of materials and the design and construction of structures. It was from such ancestors that the modern engineer sprang.

Naturally with advancing knowledge of science, the work of the engineer—as the master craftsman came to be called—was profoundly affected. The uncertainties of his work were reduced and gradually analytical methods with reliable scientific data replaced the method of trial and error, although, alas! the latter is still employed in an altogether unjustifiable degree by engineers and by many industries. Frequently in the solution of an industrial problem it is necessary to guess because of the indeterminate nature of the problem. If one continues to guess as the problem recurs, it indicates a low order of intelligence and foresight among those who are responsible for the answer.

As a class engineers are now more concerned with the adaptation of existing knowledge to their needs than with the extension of knowledge. Occasionally their needs are such that they are, perforce, led to explore somewhat the boundaries between the known and the unknown, but they are generally content if this process develops empirical relations that satisfy for the moment their peculiar requirements or if some difficulty in design or operation is temporarily met. While for a time empirical methods may be sufficient, sooner or later every engineer and every industry will recognize the necessity for precise knowledge of processes and materials and for exact methods of analysis that can only be supplied through the aid of the fundamental sciences. No industry can feel secure until it is fully aware of the scientific basis of its various activities. Accretions to knowledge result from scientific research and developments in industry follow the adaptation of such knowledge through industrial research. Upon the combined result of scientific and industrial research depends the progress of civilization and the improvement of man's status.

Until recently men responsible for the design and construction of structures and for the control of industry were trained as apprentices and their effectiveness depended upon their natural adaptability for such work and their practical experience. The devel-

[1] Address of the vice-president and chairman of the Section of Engineering, American Association for the Advancement of Science, Nashville, December, 1927.

opment of scientific and technical education has, however, greatly modified the training of such men and it has increased their efficiency. The advancement of science has been so rapid during recent years that now even the best product of a technical school is only moderately well equipped to avail himself of the latest achievements of physicists, chemists and other specialists in the fundamental sciences. More and more the engineer must work in close cooperation with those concerned with these sciences, and, for certain classes of work, his own training will need to be greatly modified and expanded.

The dawning of a professional consciousness among American engineers dates from the organization of the American Society of Civil Engineers in 1852. This society was designed as a medium for enlarging the acquaintanceship among engineers and for the interchange of professional knowledge and experience. In 1852 there were few men other than civil engineers and military engineers who were engaged in activities of an engineering nature. There were millwrights, the antecedents of the mechanical engineer, who were versed in the installation and utilization of machinery, but a class consciousness among such men that would raise them above the level of the artisan had not yet developed. The rapid expansion of knowledge of the physical sciences and of industry that began in the latter half of the nineteenth century, increased the need for men competent to meet the expanding problems of industry and so specialized the work of the engineer that various divisions of the profession soon came to be recognized. It was inevitable that such specialization would develop a need for the organization of additional societies designed to promote the interests of these newer divisions of engineering and of the men concerned with them. Thus, the American Institute of Mining Engineers, whose name was recently changed to the American Institute of Mining and Metallurgical Engineers, was organized in 1871, the American Society of Mechanical Engineers in 1880, and the American Institute of Electrical Engineers in 1884. While these four organizations, which have come to be called the "founder societies," have taken leadership among engineering organizations, it is interesting to note that one society, the Western Society of Engineers, was organized in 1860, soon after the founding of the American Society of Civil Engineers. With the continued and rapidly increasing knowledge of science and its applications to the engineering industries, there has been during the present century a tremendous expansion in the number of specialized national engineering organizations, such as the American Society of Refrigerating Engineers, the American Society of Heating and Ventilating Engineers and the Institute of Radio Engineers and of local clubs and societies until there are now, I am told, over six hundred engineering societies of all kinds in the United States.

In 1874, Articles of Incorporation of the American Association for the Advancement of Science were granted by the commonwealth of Massachusetts. The purpose of the association, as defined by the constitution adopted on December 29, 1919, is "to promote intercourse among those who are cultivating science in different parts of America, to cooperate with other scientific societies and institutions, to give a stronger and more general impulse and more systematic direction to scientific research and to procure for the labors of scientific men increased facilities and a wider usefulness." In 1881 the association organized Section D, to promote interest in mechanical science; in 1885 the name of this section was changed to Mechanical Science and Engineering; in 1912 the section name was again changed to Section D (Engineering), and in 1919, when the new constitution was adopted, the old section became known as Section M (Engineering).

The functions of Section M have never been clearly defined. Presumably it was organized to promote the knowledge of engineering and to advance the interests of engineers, thus placing engineering in a class with those sections of the association that represent the fundamental sciences. Engineering, however, can not be classed as a fundamental science, although it is concerned with the application of such sciences to the constructive and industrial arts. It has often been characterized as an applied science, although the term would seem to be a misnomer, for there is no other science than pure science.

The manner in which the section can promote effectively the interests of engineers is by no means clear. When one considers the infinite variety of engineering associations that already exist it seems unlikely that Section M will function effectively if it is simply one of over six hundred engineering societies, each having very much the same aims. The mechanical engineer will pledge his allegiance to one or more national and local associations that are devoted to the particular interests, and especially to the technique, of his own profession; and so with the adherents of each of the other divisions of engineering. No profit will accrue from the continued multiplication of engineering associations; in fact, engineers generally recognize that the profession has already gone too far in the organization of national professional societies and that it would be a very great advantage to them if the number of such organizations could be greatly reduced. Apparently Section M has generally been considered as simply a non-specialized technical society with functions similar to those of any other engineering society. So long as this conception of the purposes of the section exists it is inconceivable that it will occupy a position of any importance in the minds of engineers. Unless, therefore, its characteristics can be so modified that it occupies a place among its sister organizations that is unique, it has no justification for continued existence.

As has already been explained, the engineer is concerned with the adaptation of existing knowledge to the needs of the constructive arts; while the fundamental scientist is concerned with the advancement of learning through scientific research, and is rarely interested in the practical application of the results of his work. Because of the nature of their professional duties very few engineers find the time or the opportunity to keep abreast of the advances in abstract knowledge after the completion of their formal training, and, as a consequence, they are unacquainted with, if not positively indifferent to, the newer developments in science that might revolutionize their own work if these developments could be quickly assimilated and adapted to use.

There is, then, an opportunity for Section M to occupy a place of peculiar usefulness as the common meeting ground of the creators of scientific knowledge and of those who adapt such knowledge to the use and benefit of mankind. I would, therefore, suggest that a serious effort be made to so modify the aims of the section that it will effectively promote the association of scientists and engineers, and enable the latter to voice his scientific needs and his achievements in adapting science to industry, and the former to attempt to forecast the possible practical applications of some new theory that has been recently developed or of a discovery which, if it can be made useful, will be revolutionary in its character. I recognize the difficulties that are inherent to this plan but I hope that they may be overcome. Under such an arrangement it would seem to me that the programs for the section meetings might very properly include papers presented by representatives of the different divisions of engineering that will present the latest applications of scientific knowledge in each of these divisions, and by the exponents of the fundamental sciences that will present and interpret the possible applications of the latest discoveries in the several sciences. The advantages of such programs would seem to be obvious for, as has already been explained, the older societies are generally more concerned with the technique of engineering than with its theoretical or fundamental scientific basis.

In addition to programs for the meetings of Section M, such as I have just described, it would seem desirable that the American Association for the Advancement of Science foster the publication of a journal that will endeavor to present in a popular form the latest scientific data and discoveries with suggestions of their possible applications, so that engineers and those who are responsible for the management of our industries may more quickly than formerly have access to and utilize such information.

If, therefore, Section M can in some manner establish a bond of interest and sympathy between engineers and scientists so that the former will become more scientific and the latter more practical, the future of the section will become secure.

CHARLES RUSS RICHARDS
LEHIGH UNIVERSITY

EUGENE ALLEN SMITH

EUGENE ALLEN SMITH became State geologist of Alabama on April 18, 1873, and served continuously in that capacity until his death on September 7, of this year, or more than fifty-four years' service. Michael Tuomey was the first State geologist, appointed to the place when the State Legislature of 1847–48 created the department, with final approval on January 4, 1848. However, from the results accomplished by the Smith survey, it would seem that Eugene Allen Smith was also the Geological Survey of Alabama. He did not write all its reports, but he certainly dominated the entire program and policy of the survey. He published some very long and detailed accounts of Alabama's natural resources, to which almost all of his writings were confined, but most of his contributions were in the form of short and concise accounts, rather than exhaustive monographs. Furthermore, his writings cover a wide variety of subjects from the oldest rocks in the crystalline area to the recent sands at the seashore; from the metals to clays and sulphur; from agriculture to gold mining. In addition to his writings which found their way into print, he must have issued thousands of volumes in the form of letters and reports. No matter how unimportant the sample or the inquiry, it was his habit of sending back a courteous and complete reply. The office is filled with a tremendous mass of correspondence, including many volumes of copies made by presses in the days before carbon paper and the typewriter.

Eugene Allen Smith was born at Washington, Autauga County, Alabama, October 27, 1841, the son of Samuel Parrish and Adelaide Julia (Allen) Smith. On his mother's side his ancestry is traceable back to Governor William Bradford through Allyns, Phelps, Bishop, Fitch, Walcott and others. He attended the private school at Prattville and entered the public schools of Philadelphia at the age of 11. His work in the Philadelphia schools was a great inspiration to him, and in his own words: "I read three or four pages of Latin each day just because my instructor liked for me to do so." It was also in Philadelphia that he composed and edited "The Half-Yankee Boy," several copies of which have been preserved. This interesting newspaper consisted of a double sheet or four pages, filled with excerpts from various sources, and on a wide variety of subjects. These were carefully lettered in ink and comprise one of the many clever and original ideas which filled his life. It was during this period between the Prattville schools and college that he developed a passion for carving. He used a penknife with amazing dexterity, as is attested to by the numerous articles left in his personal effects. Perhaps his most beautiful work was done on peach seeds, while some very nice things were done in wood. His designs were original and artistic, and the craftsmanship inspired.

At the age of nineteen he entered the junior class at the University of Alabama, where he received the A.B. degree in 1862. In April of that year all of the members of his class were sent to various parts of the state as instructors for drilling recruits. He was sent to Greenville and enlisted in Company K, the company which he was drilling, as a private. He was later elected a second lieutenant in this company, and was later detailed by President Davis as state captain and instructor in tactics at the University of Alabama. He served in this capacity from December, 1862, until April, 1865. Somehow the war and its heavy blow to the South had not entirely upset his life and plans, and he managed to go to Germany in October, 1865, to continue his studies. He spent a few months at the University of Berlin, a similar period at Göttingen and then went to Heidelberg. From the latter university he received the degrees of master of arts and doctor of philosophy *summa cum laude,* in 1868. While in Europe he spent his summers in travel, and, as would be expected, allowed the art galleries to consume a good bit of that time. Usually on these jaunts he was accompanied by some of his fellow students, "not because of their interest, but because they were on allowances also!"

Upon his return to America in December, 1868, he went to the University of Mississippi as assistant professor of chemistry, and was associated with the geological survey of the state, which was under the charge of Eugene Woldemar Hilgard. There can be no doubt but that Hilgard instilled in him much of his interest in geology. His first work was embodied in his report on the Mississippi bottoms. He remained at the University of Mississippi until May, 1871, when he was elected professor of chemistry and mineralogy in the University of Alabama. He was instructed by the trustees of the university to spend such time as was not required by his duties as a professor in the university to the study of the natural resources of the state, which he did at his own expense. It might be said in passing that the University of Alabama has always taken the lead in this important work.

In 1873 the Legislature passed an act "To revive and complete the Geological and Agricultural Survey of Alabama," and made a special appropriation of $2,200 for the purchase of an ambulance, team and other equipment. In addition to this, the sum of $800 was appropriated for chemical apparatus for the analysis of soil and ores, and $500 annually for a period of ten years for the expenses of the survey. Eugene A. Smith was appointed state geologist, to receive no compensation since his salary as a professor in the university was regarded as being sufficient remuneration for the added duties. During this decade he was assisted by Henry McCalley, of Huntsville, who gave his services to the work of the survey gratuitously. Much of the state was visited, and the results incorporated in the rather detailed reports of progress, and many shorter contributions which were published in various scientific journals.

He devoted the first part of this period to the metamorphic region, studying the formations at that time thought to be Pre-Cambrian. Later, he gave considerable attention to the coal and iron regions of the present Birmingham district, calling attention for the first time to the vast areas underlain by coal. The brown ores of Bibb, Shelby, Talladega and Calhoun Counties received all the consideration given iron ores since red ores were regarded as too low grade to be used as a source of iron. During the latter part of this decade, he was appointed special agent in the division devoted to cotton culture, for the 1880 census. This work carried him into the Coastal Plain country for his first intimate glimpse of the wonderful sections along the Alabama and Tombigbee Rivers. In addition to his reports for the census, he published his very fine and comprehensive "Report for 1881–82, embracing an account of the agricultural features of the State." All this had been accomplished on an appropriation of $500 annually!

In 1883 the wonderful work of the survey prompted the legislature to increase the annual appropriation to $5,000. This made it possible to do more efficient work, and to accomplish even greater results. McCalley was given general charge of the Warrior Coal Field, while Smith delved into the problems of the younger formations of the state, a work which perhaps gave him his greatest accomplishment and certainly his greatest enjoyment. Many field seasons were spent in the Coastal Plain region, and several reports record the results.

In 1891 the annual appropriation of the survey was increased to $7,500 and the work continued to enlarge and expand, and grow in importance. Reports appeared more frequently and on a greater variety of subjects. Smith had a large and important share in all this work, besides being charged with all administrative duties. With the natural enlargement of the work, the legislature in 1919 increased the annual appropriation to $12,600, where it remained until his death. His fast increasing duties as state geologist made it necessary for him to give up his work in the university in 1913, and he was made professor emeritus, and subsequently devoted all his energies to the work of the survey. For the first time in 1906 the state gave financial support to the state geologist, and $1,500 was designated as his salary. This was increased, over his protest, to $4,000 in 1919. His plea was that if there was anything available, he wanted it for the survey and not for himself. As the result of his final request of the legislature, the annual appropriation was increased to $50,000, and his survey was assured of adequate support for the first time in its history. The final passage of this bill was recorded during the first day of his fatal illness, but he had full knowledge of its successful voyage through the law-making channels.

His quarters at the University had evolved from a small laboratory in the basement of Wood's Hall, and later the lower floor of Garland Hall, to the handsome building which bears his name. This structure was completed in 1910, and houses the survey and the museum, with the departments of geology and biology occupying parts of the wings. He made the building and its surroundings the beauty spot of the campus, using his full knowledge of flowers and shrubbery to the very best advantage. Thus in the midst of an environment his very own, he was stricken on August 29 while at the breakfast table with an internal malady and had to be taken to the hospital for an immediate operation. The operation was successful, but his vitality was too low to allow him to recover from the shock. He succumbed at 4:30 P. M., on September 7, and was buried the following afternoon.

He was a life member of the American Association for the Advancement of Science, and was vice-president and chairman of Section E (Geology) in 1904 and elected again in 1926, which he declined because of his age. He was appointed honorary commissioner at the Paris Exposition in 1878; was a member of the council of the Geological Society of America from 1892–95, vice-president in 1906 and president in 1913; was honorary life-member of the American Institute of Mining and Metallurgical Engineers and received numerous other honors during his long and colorful career. Perhaps one of the greatest honors and distinctions came from the law makers of his own state, when he was named specifically in the statutes as state geologist. His resignation could only have been received by the State Legislature.

He always took an active interest in all of the affairs of the university, appearing at all its functions, especially the athletic contests. He would never go into enemy territory to a football game, saying "there is trouble enough at home without going away to hunt for it!" He enjoyed most the baseball games in which there was an abundance of base hits. The university loses one of its most loyal friends.

His bibliography carries more than 120 entries, which comprise about 5,000 pages, with hundreds of maps and illustrations. His contributions have been as valuable as voluminous, and his further achievement in directing the complicated affairs of the survey in such a way as to keep it intact for more than half a century and amply providing for its future constitutes an accomplishment which stands on its own merits.

The phenomenal development of the mineral industries of Alabama, which accompanied the progress of the work of the survey, must have given him a great deal of pleasure and satisfaction, but he never gave voice to any such emotion. The annual production of coal had gone from almost nothing to over 20,000,000 tons. Industrial plants emerged from the hillsides like mushrooms, and great mines and quarries were everywhere. He was directly responsible for the location of the cement plant at Spocari, near Demopolis, and he and Watt T. Brown brought about the establishment of the Ragland plant. These proved that cement could be successfully made in Alabama, and the growth of this industry has been remarkable. Surely his reward was in watching this progress in the development of the state he loved and for which he had devoted his life, without ever a thought of himself. He died, poor in this world's goods, but rich in its honor. His achievements had won for him the love and respect of all who knew him. His simple and beautiful life, his modesty and genial nature endeared him to his associates as "The Little Doctor." He had outlived all his contemporaries, passing from this life with the full knowledge that he had done everything he could for his work and for the state.

WALTER B. JONES,
State Geologist

ALABAMA

SCIENTIFIC EVENTS

THE LONDON SCHOOL OF HYGIENE AND TROPICAL MEDICINE

A NEW department has been added to the London School of Hygiene and Tropical Medicine for an advanced course in bacteriology and immunology. A house has been secured for the purpose in Gordon Square, over the school in Endsleigh Gardens, and students will be prepared for the new diploma in bacteriology of London University. It will be opened next month, and the course of study will include the bacteriology of public health and of industry.

Another new department is to be opened in connection with the school, at the National Institute for Medical Research, at Hampstead, for special instruction in epidemiology and vital statistics. Other important developments are contemplated in the activities of the institution, but these can not be carried out until the completion of the new school, towards which the trustees of the Rockefeller Foundation gave $2,000,000. Good progress is being made with the building, which is being erected in Bloomsbury, near the British Museum, and, although it is not expected to be finished until 1929, it is hoped that a part will be ready for occupation by October of this year. In the new building the school will be one of the most important institutions in the world for research into various problems relating to health, both in temperate and tropical climates. The training of students in general public health work will be an outstanding feature of its activities, and, with a department which will act as a coordinating center for research in different countries, the school is expected to have a world-wide influence in the promotion of public health services.

Steps are also being taken to provide more efficient clinical teaching in tropical diseases, and an important proposal associated with the future work of the school relates to the erection of a hospital for tropical diseases. Such an institution is regarded as an urgent necessity, and it is hoped to raise sufficient funds to provide a suitable building in close proximity to the new school.

FREE PUBLIC LECTURES ON MEDICAL SUBJECTS

THE faculty of medicine of Harvard University offers a course of free public lectures on medical subjects, to be given at the medical school on Sunday afternoons, beginning January 8 and ending March 25, 1928. The lectures will begin at four o'clock.

January 8.—*Maintaining physical efficiency by work and play:* NORMAN W. FRADD, instructor in physical education.

January 15.—*Gas poisoning, electric shock and drowning:* DR. CECIL K. DRINKER, professor of physiology and assistant dean of the School of Public Health.

January 22.—*The laws of the heart:* DR. ALFRED C. REDFIELD, assistant professor of physiology.

January 29.—*The importance of diet in the treatment of anemia:* DR. GEORGE R. MINOT, clinical professor of medicine.

February 5.—*Aptitude measurements in vocational guidance:* JOHNSON O'CONNOR, in charge of the human engineering department, General Electric Company, West Lynn.

February 12.—*The child meets the family:* DR. HALLOWELL DAVIS, assistant professor of physiology.

February 19.—*Infantile paralysis:* DR. WILLIAM L. AYCOCK, associate in preventive medicine and hygiene.

February 26.—*Restoration of function in the mouth and teeth as a health measure:* DR. FRED A. BECKFORD, professor of prosthetic dentistry.

March 4.—*Brain disorders from the surgical standpoint:* DR. GILBERT HORRAX, instructor in surgery.

March 11.—*Cancer:* DR. DANIEL F. JONES, associate in surgery.

March 18.—*Public health aspects of canned food:* HENRY M. LOOMIS, secretary of the National Canners' Association, Washington, D. C.

March 25.—*Health conditions in Equatorial Africa contrasted with those in countries where sanitation prevails:* DR. RICHARD P. STRONG, professor of tropical medicine.

At Stanford University Medical School the forty-sixth courses of popular medical lectures will be given at Lane Hall on alternate Friday evenings as follows:

January 13.—*Psycho-analysis:* DR. JAMES L. WHITNEY.

January 27.—*Infantile paralysis:* DR. RUSSELL VAN ARSDALE LEE.

February 10.—*Cults, quacks and cures:* DR. EDGAR L. GILCREEST.

February 24.—*Chinese medicine:* DR. EMMET RIXFORD.

March 9.—*Protection against tuberculosis:* DR. FREDERICK EBERSON.

March 23.—*Prevention of heart disease:* DR. WILLIAM DOCK.

OFFICERS OF THE AMERICAN CHEMICAL SOCIETY

IN addition to the election of Dr. Samuel Wilson Parr, professor of industrial chemistry at the University of Illinois, president of the American Chemical Society, W. D. Bigelow, director of the research laboratories of the National Canners' Association, was reelected a director of the society from the fourth district and E. C. Franklin, professor of chemistry in

Stanford University, was again chosen a director from the sixth district.

The following were elected councillors-at-large: Edward Mallinckrodt, Jr., vice-president of the Mallinckrodt Chemical Works, St. Louis; Professor Harry N. Holmes, head of the department of chemistry in Oberlin College; Treat B. Johnson, professor of organic chemistry at Yale University.

Balloting for the fourth councillor resulted in a tie between William J. Hale, director of organic chemical research, Dow Chemical Company, Midland, Mich., and Joel H. Hildebrand, professor of chemistry in the University of California. The tie will be broken by vote of the society's council at the meeting in St. Louis early in April.

The election of officers of the professional divisions of the society was also announced.

DIVISION OF INDUSTRIAL AND ENGINEERING CHEMISTRY—R. J. McKay, New York, *chairman;* R. E. Wilson, Whiting, Ind., *vice-chairman;* E. M. Billings, Rochester, N. Y., *secretary-treasurer.*

PAINT AND VARNISH DIVISION—W. T. Pearce, Fargo, N. D., *chairman;* P. E. Marling, Dayton, Ohio, *vice-chairman;* E. W. Boughton, New York, *secretary-treasurer.*

DIVISION OF AGRICULTURAL AND FOOD CHEMISTRY—F. C. Blanck, Washington, *chairman;* R. C. Roark, Washington, *vice-chairman;* C. S. Brinton, Philadelphia, *secretary.*

DIVISION OF BIOLOGICAL CHEMISTRY—P. E. Howe, Washington, *chairman;* M. X. Sullivan, Washington, *secretary.*

DIVISION OF CELLULOSE CHEMISTRY—L. E. Wise, Syracuse, N. Y., *chairman;* J. L. Parsons, Erie, Pa., *vice-chairman.*

DIVISION OF CHEMICAL EDUCATION—B. S. Hopkins, Urbana, Ill., *chairman;* H. R. Smith, Chicago, *vice-chairman;* R. A. Baker, Syracuse, N. Y., *secretary;* J. L. Wood, St. Louis, *assistant secretary;* E. M. Billings, Rochester, N. Y., *treasurer.*

FERTILIZER DIVISION—E. W. Magruder, Norfolk, Va., *chairman;* W. H. Ross, Washington, *vice-chairman;* H. C. Moore, Chicago, *secretary.*

DIVISION OF HISTORY OF CHEMISTRY—L. C. Newell, Boston, *chairman;* T. L. Davis, Cambridge, Mass., *secretary.*

DYE DIVISION—M. L. Crossley, Bound Brook, N. J., *chairman;* E. B. Bolton, Wilmington, Del., *vice-chairman;* H. T. Herrick, Washington, *secretary.*

ORGANIC DIVISION—W. L. Evans, Columbus, Ohio, *chairman;* F. C. Whitmore, Evanston, Ill., *secretary.*

DIVISION OF GAS AND FUEL CHEMISTRY—A. C. Fieldner, Pittsburgh, *chairman;* S. P. Burke, New York, *vice-chairman;* O. O. Malleis, Pittsburgh, *secretary-treasurer.*

DIVISION OF MEDICINAL CHEMISTRY—A. W. Dox, Detroit, *chairman;* F. Fenger, Chicago, *vice-chairman;* A. E. Osterberg, Rochester, Minn., *secretary.*

PETROLEUM DIVISION—J. B. Hill, Philadelphia, *chairman;* F. W. Padgett, University of Oklahoma, *vice-chairman;* C. L. Johnson, Kansas City, *secretary-treasurer.*

SUGAR DIVISION—F. J. Bates, Washington, *chairman;* F. W. Zerban, New York, *secretary-treasurer.*

DIVISION OF WATER, SEWAGE AND SANITATION CHEMISTRY—S. E. Coburn, Boston, *chairman;* W. D. Collins, Washington, *secretary.*

RUBBER DIVISION—H. L. Fisher, New York, *chairman;* A. H. Smith, Akron, Ohio, *vice-chairman;* H. E. Simmons, Akron, Ohio, *secretary-treasurer.*

DIVISION OF COLLOID CHEMISTRY—H. B. Weiser, Houston, Texas, *chairman;* F. E. Bartell, University of Michigan, *secretary.*

OFFICERS OF THE AMERICAN ASSOCIATION FOR THE ADVANCEMENT OF SCIENCE

A FULL account of the Nashville meeting of the American Association for the Advancement of Science by the permanent secretary will be printed in the issues of SCIENCE for January 27 and February 3. Officers were elected as follows:

President

Henry Fairfield Osborn, president of the American Museum of Natural History.

Vice-presidents and Chairmen of the Sections

A—Mathematics: R. C. Archibald, Brown University.
B—Physics: P. W. Bridgman, Harvard University.
C—Chemistry: C. E. K. Mees, Eastman Kodak Company.
D—Astronomy: J. S. Plaskett, Dominion Astrophysical Observatory, Victoria, B. C.
E—Geology and Geography: Frank Leverett, University of Michigan.
F—Zoological Sciences: M. F. Guyer, University of Wisconsin.
G.—Botanical Sciences: C. E. Allen, University of Wisconsin.
H—Anthropology: Fay-Cooper Cole, University of Chicago.
I—Psychology: H. C. Warren, Princeton University.
M—Engineering: R. L. Sackett, Pennsylvania State College.
N—Medical Sciences: A. J. Goldforb, College of the City of New York.
O—Agriculture: C. A. Mooers, University of Tennessee.
Q—Education: Truman L. Kelley, Leland Stanford University.

Secretaries of Sections

Sect. A (Math.): C. N. Moore, University of Cincinnati.
Sect. N (Med.): H. Austin, University of Pennsylvania.
Sect. H (Anthrop.): C. H. Danforth, Stanford University.

Members of the Council

A. H. Compton, University of Chicago.
Austin H. Clark, Smithsonian Institution.

Members of the Executive Committee

John Johnston, U. S. Steel Corporation.
David R. Curtiss, Northwestern University.

Committee on Grants

Kail Kellerman, Bureau of Plant Industry.
W. S. Adams, Mount Wilson Observatory.

Board of Trustees of Science Service

J. McKeen Cattell.

Finance Committee

A. L. Day (reelected).

SCIENTIFIC NOTES AND NEWS

DR. H. J. MULLER, professor of zoology at the University of Texas, has been awarded the $1,000 prize of the American Association for the Advancement of Science for his paper on "The Effects of X-radiation on Genes and Chromosomes," read at the Nashville meeting.

AT the meeting of the Geological Society of America held in Cleveland from December 29 to 31 the Penrose gold medal of the society was conferred upon Professor Emeritus T. C. Chamberlin, of the University of Chicago, in recognition of his distinguished contributions to geology.

SIR ERNEST RUTHERFORD, Cavendish professor of experimental physics and director of the Cavendish Laboratory at the University of Cambridge, has been elected a foreign associate member of the French Academy of Sciences. He was already a corresponding member of the academy.

THE council of the British Physical Society has awarded the Duddell medal for 1927 to Dr. F. E. Smith, F.R.S., director of scientific research at the Admiralty. This medal is given annually for work in connection with the development of scientific instruments or of materials used in their manufacture.

C. TATE REGAN, director of the British Museum (Natural History), and Dr. F. A. Bather, keeper of the department of geology in the museum, have been elected as honorary members of the Yorkshire Philosophical Society.

PROFESSOR P. KOEBE, of Leipzig, has been elected a member of the Saxon Academy of Sciences.

THE King of Belgium will confer upon M. Braillard, the president of the technical commission of the Union International de Radiophonie, the decoration of Chevalier of the Order of Leopold in recognition of his services to the cause of radio broadcasting.

PROFESSOR EDWIN G. BORING, director of the psychological laboratory at Harvard University, has been elected president of the American Psychological Association.

DR. MARSHALL H. SAVILLE, professor of American archeology at Columbia University, was elected president of the American Anthropological Association at the annual meeting held at Andover, Mass.

MISS ALICE C. EVENS, of the U. S. Hygienic Laboratory, Washington, was elected president of the Society of American Bacteriologists at the recent annual meeting in Rochester. Miss Evens is at present confined to a hospital with Malta fever, acquired during experimentation on the disease.

DR. C. MACFIE CAMPBELL, professor of psychiatry in the Harvard Medical School, has been reelected president of the Massachusetts Society for Mental Hygiene.

AT the annual meeting of the Royal Academy of Medicine in Ireland, Sir William Taylor was elected president, and Louis L. Cassidy, the secretary for foreign correspondence.

AT its annual meeting in Chicago in November, the American Society of Animal Production elected E. W. Sheets, chief of the division of animal husbandry of the U. S. Bureau of Animal Industry, *president*. H. T. Gramlich, head of the department of animal husbandry, University of Nebraska, was made *vice-president,* and James R. Wiley, professor of animal husbandry, Purdue University, *secretary-treasurer*.

PRESIDENT COOLIDGE has approved senate joint resolution no. 48 and senate joint resolution no. 49, providing for the filling of two vacancies on the board of regents of the Smithsonian Institution by the appointment of the Hon. Charles Evans Hughes and Dr. John C. Merriam.

DR. WILLIAM J. HALE, director of organic research of the Dow Chemical Company and past-chairman of the division of chemistry and chemical technology of the National Research Council, has been appointed chairman of a committee of the division to foster cooperative researches between industries and academic institutions. This cooperative plan was instituted by Dr. Hale while he was chairman of the division.

THE newly-organized economic committee of the League of Nations has appointed a subcommittee to prepare a program of inquiry into the economic employment of the riches of the sea. This committee will consist of Sir Sydney Chapman (Great Britain), M. Serruys (France), M. Jahn (Norway) and Mr. Ito (Japan). The main object of this inquiry is to decide whether and under what conditions, and in what waters, the production of marine fauna might be organized.

IN honor of Dr. Marston Taylor Bogert, professor of chemistry at Columbia University and first Carnegie professor in international relations, the Czechoslovak Prague Rotary Club recently gave a dinner at which Professor Bogert delivered an address on "Chemistry and War."

PROFESSOR GORDON H. TRUE, of the animal husbandry division at the University of California, was the guest of honor at the annual dinner of the American Society of Animal Production at the Saddle and Sirloin Club, Chicago.

A DINNER was recently given in New Orleans in honor of Dr. Isaac M. Cline, meteorologist in charge of the New Orleans headquarters of the U. S. Weather Bureau, at which R. C. Watkins, vice-president and general manager of the Southern Pacific Lines, presented to Dr. Cline, on behalf of his company, a bronze tablet eulogizing his services in connection with the recent Mississippi Valley flood.

DR. WALTER M. BRICKNER is relinquishing the editorship of the *American Journal of Surgery* with the December issue. Dr. Brickner has conducted this journal since its establishment twenty-three years ago.

THE following joined the scientific staff of *Biological Abstracts* during 1927: Dr. Ezra Allen, Mr. Frank Haimbach, Dr. Nellie M. Payne, Dr. Oran Raber, Dr. George Hume Smith. The other members of the central editorial staff are: Dr. Mary Jones Fisher, Dr. Frederick V. Rand and Dr. J. R. Schramm.

DR. LUDLOW GRISCOM, who recently resigned as assistant curator of ornithology in the American Museum of Natural History, has been appointed research curator of zoology in the museum of comparative zoology at Harvard University, and not assistant director as has been incorrectly reported.

DR. JOHN RYAN DEVEREUX, of Chevy Chase, Md., has been appointed medical director for the Catholic Near East Welfare Association, and will leave for Europe within a few days to make a survey of sanitary and public health conditions in the Balkans for the association.

DR. THOMAS STOCKHAM BAKER, president of the Carnegie Institute of Technology, in Pittsburgh, expects to spend six weeks in Europe during February, March and April, to organize plans for the Second International Conference on Bituminous Coal at Pittsburgh.

G. PROCTOR COOPER sailed from New York on December 3 for Central America where he will make a study of forest conditions and collect specimens of woods and plants for the Yale School of Forestry, the New York Botanical Garden and the Field Museum of Natural History. The trip is made possible through the cooperation of the three institutions and of the United Fruit Company.

DR. WILLIAM TRELEASE, retired professor of botany at the University of Illinois, has returned from a half-year's stay in the European herbaria, where he has been accumulating data for a monograph on the American *Piperaceae* or true peppers.

DR. KURT KOFFKA, formerly professor of psychology at the University of Giessen and now holder of the William Allan Neilson chair of research at Smith College expected to arrive in the United States on January 3 and will begin his work after the Christmas holidays. Dr. Alexander Mintz, Russian psychologist, who is to be research associate to Dr. Koffka, has already arrived, together with Richard E. Hill, another research assistant.

DR. JOHN W. EVANS, F.R.S., left England on November 18 for Egypt and Palestine to undertake geological work for the Egyptian government and for the Zionist Board.

DR. JASPER C. BARNES, dean and head of the department of psychology and education of Maryville College, will give courses in psychology in the University of Wyoming during the next summer quarter.

THE fourth Ludvig Hektoen lecture of the Billings foundation of the Institute of Medicine of Chicago will be given by Dr. Francis Peyton Rous, of the Rockefeller Institute, January 27, at the City Club, on "The Genesis of Gallstones." The fourth Lewis Linn McArthur Lecture of the Billings Foundation will be given February 24, by Dr. Frank C. Mann, of the Mayo Clinic, Rochester, Minn., on "Experimental Peptic Ulcer."

DR. FRANKLIN C. MCLEAN, professor of medicine in the University of Chicago, addressed the Milwaukee Academy of Medicine on November 22, on "Some Problems in Edema."

PROFESSOR EINAR HILLE, of the department of mathematics of Princeton University, lectured on December 9 and 15 at the Bartol Research Foundation, on "Boundary Problems in Differential Equations with Special Reference to their Application to Schrödinger's Wave Equation." Professor Arnold Dresden, of the mathematical department of Swarthmore College, will give a lecture on January 10 at the foundation on "Special Devices used in the Solution of Problems by the Matrix Mechanics."

TRIBUTE was paid to the memory of a former U. S. Forest Service official, Major Frank A. Fenn, by the

United States Geographic Board at its November meeting, by naming for him a mountain in the Bitterroot Range in northern Idaho. Fenn Mountain lies within the Selway National Forest, near Kooskia, Idaho, where Major Fenn spent the last years of his life.

Dartmouth's new dormitory, being constructed on Tuck Drive at Hanover, will be known as "Gile Hall" in memory of the late Dr. John M. Gile, who was for many years dean of the Dartmouth Medical School and a trustee of the college.

Nature notes that on December 23 occurred the centenary of the death of Robert Woodhouse, the Cambridge mathematician, who was successively Lucasian and Plumian professor and was also the first director of the Cambridge Observatory.

Dr. Walter Le Conte Stevens, emeritus professor of physics at Washington and Lee University, died on December 29, aged seventy-nine years.

Dr. Ruliff Stephen Holway, emeritus professor of physical geography at the University of California, died on December 2.

Dr. Harry N. Gardiner, professor emeritus of philosophy at Smith College, was struck by an automobile on December 29 and died a few hours later. Dr. Gardiner was seventy-two years of age.

Dr. J. A. Kiernan, chief of the tuberculosis eradication division of the U. S. Bureau of Animal Industry, died on December 13, aged fifty-four years.

Dr. Albert Robin, professor of pathology and hygiene at Temple University, died on December 23 in the fifty-fourth year of his age.

According to *Nature*, Professor Archibald Liversidge, emeritus professor of chemistry in the University of Sydney, who died on September 26, leaving an estate of the value of £46,000, bequeathed to the University of Sydney two sums of money, £2,000 and £500, towards a scholarship and for the advancemenet of science in Sydney, respectively. Other bequests include £1,000 and £500 to Christ's College, Cambridge, towards a scholarship and a research lectureship in chemistry, respectively; £1,000 to the Royal School of Mines, towards a scholarship; £500 each to the Royal Society of New South Wales and to the Australasian Association, and also to the Chemical Society of London, towards research lectureships in chemistry, as well as a further £100 and his unpublished papers on scientific and chemical matters.

Among the public bequests willed by the late Mrs. Marrvat, of Dundee, is £200,000 for the foundation of traveling scholarships in engineering, electricity, aeronautics and music, to be open to natives of Scotland only, and to be known as "Sir James Caird's traveling scholarships."

UNIVERSITY AND EDUCATIONAL NOTES

Yale University's two-year drive for a \$20,000,000 addition to its endowment fund ended on December 31 with the goal exceeded by \$810,000.

Following the assumption of the duties of his office by the new dean of the Medical School of the University of California, Dr. Langley Porter, it was determined by the board of regents that all departments of the medical school be brought together on Parnassus Heights, San Francisco. This means that those medical school activities now conducted within a few departments on the Berkeley campus, such as pharmacology, biochemistry, bacteriology, etc., will be transferred to San Francisco as rapidly as space to accommodate them on Parnassus Heights becomes available.

Professor F. J. Sievers, head of the department of soils at the State College of Washington and chief of the division of soils at the Washington Agricultural Experiment Station, has been elected director of the Massachusetts Agricultural Experiment Station, at Amherst, with duties beginning February 1.

G. C. Shaad, professor of electrical engineering at the University of Kansas, has been appointed dean of the school of engineering and architecture.

B. M. Gonzales, head of the department of animal husbandry in the Philippine College of Agriculture, has been appointed acting dean of the college.

C. E. Lampman, of the University of Wisconsin, has been appointed head of the poultry department at the University of Idaho.

Dr. Otto Rahn, formerly head of the dairy physics department in the agricultural experiment station at Kiel, Germany, has been appointed professor of bacteriology in the Cornell Agricultural College.

Dr. Peter Kronfeld, of Vienna, until recently an assistant in the eye clinic of Professor Josef Muller, has been appointed assistant professor of ophthalmology at the University of Chicago. The appointment of Dr. Kronfeld is the first research appointment made under the Kuppenheimer Foundation, for which Mr. Louis Kuppenheimer recently gave the University of Chicago \$250,000.

The following appointments have been made at the University of California: G. B. Harris, assistant in anthropology; T. W. Koch, assistant in geology, and Beryl Kautz, assistant in paleontology.

DR. A. K. MACBETH, reader in chemistry in the department of science at the University of Oxford, has been appointed professor of chemistry in the University of Adelaide, South Australia.

DISCUSSION AND CORRESPONDENCE

THE PERIOD OF GESTATION IN THE MONKEY, MACACUS RHESUS

So far as we know, there is no exact record on the length of the period of gestation in any primate other than man; hence the following report of mating and parturition in *Macacus rhesus* will prove of interest.

For over a year the female in question had been found to menstruate regularly in cycles of 26 days. The successful mating took place from the ninth to the twelfth day after the beginning of the last menstrual period and just before the leucocyte count of the vaginal content had reached zero. This is also about the time at which Corner (1923) and Allen (1927) had found ova in the Fallopian tube of the same species of monkey. For theoretical reasons, therefore, it is almost certain that conception took place within the three-day period when the female was left with the male. A male rhesus was born almost exactly six lunar months after conception.

From the fourteenth to the thirty-seventh day after conception the vaginal content of the prospective mother showed slight admixture of red blood cells. This phenomenon is regarded as the "placental sign," discovered by Long and Evans (1920) in the rat and interpreted as slight leakage from the developing placenta. In the rat the sign is infallible. The finding of a slight bleeding under similar conditions in the monkey arouses the hope that an easily ascertainable sign may be found in the first six weeks of human gestation. After the disappearance of the erythrocytes there followed a period of massive vaginal leucocytosis.

Details concerning the phenomena outlined above will be discussed in a fuller account to appear elsewhere.

CARL G. HARTMAN
CARNEGIE INSTITUTION OF WASHINGTON,
BALTIMORE, MARYLAND

THE FLOODS OF 1927 IN THE MISSISSIPPI BASIN

THE flood of 1927 whether measured by the volume of water carried, the area overflowed or the economic loss produced was the greatest of recorded history in the Mississippi Basin.

A full account is given by H. C. Frankenfield and others in a *Monthly Weather Review Supplement.* The setting for the flood was produced by heavy rains that fell as far back as the second week of August, 1926, over Kansas and Oklahoma and thence eastward to and including the greater part of the Ohio Valley. These rains so thoroughly saturated the soil throughout the middle drainage of the Mississippi that further heavy rains coming in September and October, 1926, caused general and in some cases destructive floods in the drainage above Cairo, Ill. The distribution of the rainfall from August to December, 1926, was such as to keep the main river and its tributaries at relatively high stages in a season when stages are normally low. Superposed on these conditions a record-breaking flood occurred in the Cumberland River late in December, 1926, continuing until early January, 1927, and thus the foundation was laid for a serious spring flood in the Mississippi, conditioned only upon the amount and distribution in time and space of the rains of January to April, both inclusive. It so happened that heavy rains fell in March and April and in such sequence as to produce a catastrophic flood in the lower Mississippi Valley. The rains of the third and fourth week of January, 1927, started a flood wave in the Ohio which continued down-river to New Orleans, reaching that place in 38 days. This was the second of a series of flood waves that passed down the river during the interval January–June, 1927, due to heavy rains in the middle drainage area. After the middle of March heavy rains fell between the mouth of the Des Moines and the mouth of the Ohio and during the last week of the month heavy rains also fell over the Missouri Valley south of Omaha, especially over the Kansas and Osage basins. These and other rains resulted in a crest stage at Cairo, Ill., of 52.8 feet on March 25 and that stage was followed by the maximum crest of 56.4 feet on April 20, and by lesser crests of 44.0 feet on May 19 and 49.7 feet on June 8. The characteristic feature of the 1927 flood was a series of flood waves as indicated by the data just given for Cairo, Ill. Higher stages than those recorded would have been experienced had the levees held.

The report contains an estimated stage that would have been recorded had the levees held all along the line. It also submits and discusses the maximum possible stage on the main river under the most favorable conditions. Space does not permit touching in detail upon these phases of the subject.

The progress of the several flood waves was accurately forecast by the Weather Bureau, at least a week, and, in some cases two weeks, in advance; the unique service, however, was furnished when the necessity arose of forecasting the depth of the wave of crevasse water that passed overland through the Atchafalaya Basin to the Gulf of Mexico. In the absence of a contour map for Louisiana, one had to be constructed, over-night, so to speak, by the New

Orleans Weather Bureau Office. By the aid of this map the Bureau was able to give timely warning of the flooding of parts of the Atchafalaya Basin and towns therein that never before in the 200 years since settlement of the region had been reached by flood waters.

A. J. Henry

DIVISIONS OF THE DECORAH FORMATION

In studying the stratigraphy and paleontology of the Ordovician Decorah formation in northeastern Iowa, it has been found advisable to divide the formation into three members, here named and defined. The lowest of the three, the Spechts Ferry member, has as its type locality the ravine southwest of the C. M. and St. P. railroad station of Spechts Ferry, Dubuque County, Iowa, at which place the eight and one half feet of shales and interbedded limestones form a lithologic unit lying above the "Platteville" limestone; the "Platteville" of Iowa does not include the uppermost beds of the typical Platteville of southwestern Wisconsin. The Spechts Ferry member includes the "glass rock" and overlying shales at the top of the typical Platteville. The member is of latest Black River (Watertown) age.

The middle member of the Decorah formation, here named the Guttenberg, consists of about fifteen and one half feet of brownish, fine-textured limestone at its type section in the bluff of the Mississippi River just northwest of the town of Guttenberg, Clayton County, Iowa; northward from this locality this limestone grades into shale. In northwestern Illinois the Guttenberg is the "oil rock" member at the base of the Galena formation.

In the N. W. ¼ of sec. 35, T. 96 N., R. 4 W., the Guttenberg limestone is overlain by sixteen feet of calcareous shale and argillaceous limestone that constitute the type section of the top member of the Decorah, here named the Ion member. The type locality is about a mile southwest of the hamlet of Ion, Allamakee County, Iowa. The Ion beds become more argillaceous to the northward, more calcareous to the southeastward.

The limestones of the two upper members of the Decorah have been irregularly dolomitized in the southeast part of their Iowa outcrop. The Guttenberg and Ion members are of basal Trenton (Rockland) age.

The Decorah formation thus consists of three members, in descending order, the Ion, Guttenberg and Spechts Ferry members, the type localities of which have been designated.

G. Marshall Kay

Columbia University

A DAYLIGHT METEOR

I read with interest the two notes that appeared in Science, entitled "A Daylight Meteor," the one of William L. Bryant which appeared in the issue of July 22, 1927, and that of Frederick H. Getman of October 14, 1927. These recall a daylight meteor which I saw in May, 1890.

I was working in a gravel pit at Maxwell, near Des Moines, Iowa, when my attention was drawn to a streak of bright red which dashed from 15 degrees west of the zenith toward the northeast, like a streak of lightning out of a clear sky, for there was not a cloud in sight. I called other workers' attention to it, all concluding that it alighted six or eight miles about north of us—when the papers the next day gave an account of its falling 400 miles distant, in northern Minnesota. The papers also stated that it exploded just before reaching the ground, and that the concussion caused by same broke out all the window lights in several small settlements in the vicinity of where it fell.

This meteor left a trail of smoke (and dust?) behind it which drifted about in the sky all the rest of the afternoon, not having settled at dark that night. This streak of smoke first appeared in a straight line along the line the meteor had fallen, then became wavy, showing different currents of air acting upon it.

Albert B. Reagan

Indian Field Service, Arizona

INTERFERENCE?

While on a large forest fire on the Columbia National Forest in Washington, August, 1927, an unusual optical phenomenon was observed shortly after noon one day. The sky was clear save for the smoke column from the fire. This column was very compact, so much so that the upper protuberances had the appearance of burnished metal and the disc of the sun was not discernible through the smoke. The angle of the sun with respect to the observer was slightly below the top of the smoke column. On the N or NNW side of the top of the column there was a broad band of black. This band did not quite touch the smoke column, there was a narrow ribbon of blue sky visible in between, but it extended outward for several hundred feet, assuming that it was a mile or mile and a quarter distant. The band did not appear to be a shadow, there could have been nothing behind it but blue sky yet it seemed as opaque as a strip of black cloth hung in the sky. It is unfortunate that a camera was not available as it probably would have photographed with good definition.

Perhaps someone can explain the optics of this odd phenomenon.

A. GAEL SIMSON

QUOTATIONS

DR. F. A. BATHER

IN February next, after forty years' service in the British Museum (Natural History), Dr. F. A. Bather retires from the post of keeper of the department of geology. His vigorous and cheery personality will be missed by geologists visiting the museum no less than by his colleagues. Educated at Winchester and Oxford, he joined the staff of the British Museum in 1887 as assistant in the department of geology and was placed in charge of the echinoderma. After becoming assistant keeper, and later deputy keeper, he succeeded Sir Arthur Smith Woodward as keeper of the department in 1924. Dr. Bather was elected F.R.S. in 1909; was awarded the Lyell medal by the Geological Society in 1911; has been president of section C of the British Association and of the Museums Association; he is now president of the Geological Society. Dr. Bather's original work on the paleontology of the echinoderms has gained him a world-wide reputation, and amongst the distinguished paleontologists of to-day he stands in the front rank. His memoirs and papers are too well known to need mention here; not only are they models of scientific method, but also they possess a literary charm seldom found in the writings of scientific authors.

In his presidential addresses to section C of the British Association at Cardiff (1920), and to the Geological Society last February, Dr. Bather dealt in a masterly manner with the principles of paleontology, and his listeners felt that those addresses were worthy of Huxley. Dr. Bather does more than look on fossils from the point of view of a morphologist and evolutionist; as is so well shown in his "Caradocian Cystidea of Girvan," he regards them as animals which once lived, and endeavors to correlate form with function, morphology with physiology. For several years Dr. Bather contributed the section on Echinoderma to the *Zoological Record;* although these are masterpieces of bibliography and analysis, one can not avoid a feeling of regret that so much of his time was taken away from original research. In another direction, by the active interest which he has taken in the work of the Museums Association, Dr. Bather has rendered good service to his country; he has contributed many papers to the association's journal dealing with the preparation and exhibition of specimens and other matters of importance to the curators of provincial museums. After his release from the cares and responsibilities of office, all who know Dr. Bather, whether personally or only from his writings, will fervently hope that leisure and health will enable him to continue for many years his splendid work in paleontology.—*Nature.*

AMENDMENTS TO THE INTERNATIONAL RULES OF ZOOLOGICAL NOMENCLATURE

UPON unanimous recommendation by the International Commission on Zoological Nomenclature, the International Zoological Congress, which met at Budapest, Hungary, September 4–9, 1927, adopted a very important amendment to Article 25 (Law of Priority) which makes this Article, as amended, read as follows (*italicized type represents the amendment; Roman type represents the old wording*):

Article 25.—The valid name of a genus or species can be only that name under which it was first designated on the condition:

(a) That (*prior to January 1, 1931*) this name was published and accompanied by an indication, or a definition, or a description; and

(b) That the author has applied the principles of binary nomenclature.

(c) *But no generic name nor specific name, published after December 31, 1930, shall have any status of availability (hence also of validity) under the Rules, unless and until it is published either*

(1) *with a summary of characters (seu diagnosis; seu definition; seu condensed description) which differentiate or distinguish the genus or the species from other genera or species;*

(2) *or with a definite bibliographic reference to such summary of characters (seu diagnosis; seu definition; seu condensed description). And further*

(3) *in the case of a generic name, with the definite unambiguous designation of the type species (seu genotype; seu autogenotype; seu orthotype).*

The purpose of this amendment is to inhibit two of the most important factors which heretofore have produced confusion in scientific names. The date, January 1, 1931, was selected (instead of making the amendment immediately effective) in order to give authors ample opportunity to accommodate themselves to the new rule.

The commission unanimously adopted the following resolution:

(a) It is requested that an author who publishes a name as new shall definitely state that it is new, that this be stated in only one (*i.e.,* in the first) publication, and that the date of publication be not added to the name in its first publication.

(b) It is requested that an author who *quotes* a generic name, or a specific name, or a subspecific name, shall add at least once the author and year of publication of the quoted name or a full bibliographic reference.

The foregoing resolution was adopted in order to inhibit the confusion which has frequently resulted from the fact that authors have occasionally published a given name as "new" in two to five or more different articles of different dates—up to five years in exceptional cases.

The three propositions submitted by Dr. Franz Poche, of Vienna, failed to receive the necessary number of votes in commission to permit of their being recommended to the Congress. Out of a possible 18 votes for each proposition, Poche's proposition I received 9 votes, II received 6 votes, and III received 7 votes.

Zoological, medical and veterinary journals throughout the world are requested to give to the foregoing the widest possible publicity in order to avoid confusion and misunderstanding.

C. W. Stiles,
Secretary to Commission

SPECIAL ARTICLES

A NOTE ON THE CHROMOSOMES OF MOINA MACROCOPA

Banta and Brown[1] have shown that this cladoceran as well as certain others may be induced to increase the number of males by crowding parthenogenetic mothers. In order to study chromosomal evidence, several hundred parthenogenetic and sexual females have been sectioned. The most favorable time for observing the chromosomes is just before and after the eggs are laid.

The nucleus of the young egg is characterized by a number of deeply-staining granules, which increase in number and size until they fill the nucleus excepting a thin space beneath the membrane. This substance is not chromatin, as it does not react to chromatin stains after fixation in Gilson's fluid. Shortly before the eggs are laid, the mass breaks up into very fine granules, forming a homogeneous material which extends to the nuclear membrane. It gradually loses its staining properties until it appears relatively faint. At this stage there appears near one side a small, faintly-outlined spindle with a few irregularly shaped bits of chromatin within it. At about this time the nuclear membrane begins to dissolve, and the granular substance mingles with the yolk. In it very small, apparently ellipsoid chromosomes appear, and at a little later stage a well-defined spindle appears at the periphery of the egg, lying usually at right angles to the egg membrane.

1 Banta, A. M. and Brown, L. A. 1923. Some data on control of sex in Cladocera. Eugenics, Genetics and the Family, Vol. 1.

After the egg is laid, the first division occurs: in the parthenogenetic egg without reduction in the number of chromosomes. In the sexual egg, the first maturation division results in the haploid number, which is 11. The diploid number is 22 in both types of egg. In the eggs of crowded mothers which should produce a high percentage of males, no evidence has yet been obtained indicating that the male number of chromosomes is haploid. Several such crowded mothers have been studied.

The chromosomes have not been seen in the form of rods. They are too small to determine whether tetrads are formed in the maturation divisions. It does not seem that their nearly spherical shape can be accounted for by faulty technique, as the tissues in general are in excellent condition.

With the exception of Schräder's work,[2] the number of chromosomes reported for Cladocera is not more than 8 or 8–10. Schräder reports 24. The chromosomes in *Moina macrocopa* have been previously studied, so far as the author can learn, only by Weismann and Ischikawa,[3] who report 4 in the females of *Moina paradoxa* (now *M. macrocopa*) and *M. rectirostris.*

The sperm cells in *Moina macrocopa* are extremely small in all stages, and thus far have yielded no satisfactory pictures of chromosomes.

Ezra Allen

Carnegie Institution for Experimental Evolution

GENETIC EVIDENCE THAT THE CLADOCERA MALE IS DIPLOID

Cladocera males have long been supposed to be diploid in chromosome make-up. Because of the difficulty of Cladocera material for cytological study, not much evidence on this point has been produced. Chambers (1913, Biol. Bull; 25, p. 134) reported the male Simocephalus vetulus as having "considerably more than eight" chromosomes, which number he found in spermatogenesis. Miss Taylor (1914, Zool. Anz.; 45, p. 21) gave 8 or 10 as the diploid number in male *Daphnia pulex* and 4 or 5 as the reduced number in spermatogenesis. In view of the much larger chromosome numbers, 24 in females, found in material of a *Daphnia pulex* type studied by Schrader (1925, Zeit. ind. Abs.-u. Vererbungslehre; 40, p. 1) and by Dr. Ezra Allen in Moina macrocopa (about 20 in females) compared with the reports of these earlier workers, verification of the supposed diploid condition of the Cladocera male seemed desirable.

We are now in a position to report genetical evi-

2 Schräder, F. 1925. The cytology of pseudosexual eggs in a species of Daphnia. Zeit. f. induktive Abstammungs- und Vererbungslehre, Bd. XL, Heft 1/2.

3 Weismann, A., and Ischikawa, C. 1891. Ueber die Paracopulation in Daphnidenei. *Zoöl. Jahrb. Bd. 4.*

dence on this point. Individual males of *Daphnia longispina* from three different lines which were known to be heterozygous for one or more mutant characters were mated with (usually) 8 to 16 sexual egg bearing females of a stock known not to carry these (dominant) mutant characters. These sexual eggs hatch poorly but from four such crosses (all of these crosses from which we have reared more than a single individual) we have had offspring of two classes—those with, and those without the mutant character. In two of these crosses, two dominant mutant characters were involved and segregation in the male occurred for both characters.

Since it is obvious that chromatic reduction and segregation are not to be expected in a haploid male, the demonstration of segregation in these males constitutes genetic evidence that they are diploid.

ARTHUR M. BANTA,
THELMA R. WOOD

CARNEGIE INSTITUTION
OF WASHINGTON,
COLD SPRING HARBOR, L. I.

PENTATHIONIC ACID, THE FUNGICIDAL FACTOR OF SULPHUR

IN a previous paper (Young, '22)[1] it is pointed out that pentathionic acid is the fungicidal factor accompanying sulphur. It is further stated that this acid is a product of oxidized sulphur resulting only when oxygen and water are present. These earlier tests proved also that particulate sulphur is more readily oxidized and consequently more fungicidal than ordinary sulphur. This work was confirmed in the main by Tisdale ('25),[2] and its practical application by Lee and Martin ('27).[3] The conclusions have been questioned by some English workers ('25).[4]

During the present summer, the writers continued this investigation with the aim in view of ascertaining the definite chemical relationship of the toxic factor of sulphur to sulphur itself and to determine the effect of certain factors influencing this relationship. We assumed at the outset that the conclusion reached by Freundlich and Scholz ('22)[5] that pentathionic acid is a peptizing agent for sulphur made by the reaction of H_2S and SO_2 and confirmed by Kruyt ('27),[6] the latter giving a simple diagram of the structure of the sulphur particle peptized by the pentathionic acid $(S)S_5O_6=\begin{matrix}H+\\H+\end{matrix}$, is correct. In all previous work it was generally supposed that pentathionic acid is peculiar to colloidal forms of sulphur. However, if a test for pentathionic acid (the ammoniacal silver nitrate test given in Mellar's Modern Inorganic Chemistry) is applied to sulphur the characteristic brown color develops and slowly changes to black. Hydrogen sulfide, or the sulfide ion, is the only sulphur compound that might give the same test. When flowers or flour of sulphur is treated with lead acetate, copper sulfate, or silver nitrate, no precipitate of the respective sulfides appears. Sulphur treated with ammoniacal copper sulfate gives no precipitate even on standing; likewise, no sulfide ion is obtained when sulphur is treated with ammonium hydroxide for several hours. Moreover, known solutions of sulfite, sulfate or thiosulfate ions do not respond to the above test for pentathionic acid. It can only be concluded that ordinary forms of sulphur have associated with them pentathionic acid. Our tests showed further that the acid is adsorbed quite completely by the sulphur particle, so much so that none can be washed off, as can be done in the case of hydrophilic colloidal sulphur using a simple ultra filter. The ordinary particle of sulphur flour is hydrophobic, partly because the pentathionic acid is too small in amount to effect hydration to an observable extent. However, when pentathionic acid is added to amorphous sulphur, it, along with other factors, causes complete hydration.

Strong ammonia destroys pentathionic acid if treated for some time, breaking it down to thiosulfate. Freundlich and Scholz used this treatment in determining the acid quantitatively by titrating the thiosulfate with iodine. They give the following reactions:

$$2NH_4OH + H_2S_5O_6 \rightarrow (NH_4)_2S_3O_6 + S_2 + H_2O$$

$$2(NH_4)_2S_3O_6 + 6NH_4OH \rightarrow (NH_4)_2S_2O_3 + 4(NH_4)_2SO_3 + 3H_2O + 4S$$

$$2(NH_4)_2S_3O_6 + 6NH_4OH \rightarrow 5(NH_4)_2S_2O_3 + 3H_2O$$

On the other hand, strong ammonia does not completely destroy the $S_5O_6=$ ion on the sulphur particle. In this case, we are not dealing with free pentathionic acid but with strongly adsorbed $S_5O_6=$ which is not free. Consequently, when the pentathionic acid test is used on ammonia-treated sulphur, the nega-

[1] Young, H. C. The toxic property of sulphur. Ann. Mo. Bot. Gard. 9: 403–435, 1922.

[2] Tisdale, L. E. Colloidal sulphur: preparation and toxicity. Ann. Mo. Bot. Gard. 12: 381–418, 1925.

[3] Lee, H. Atherton, and J. P. Martin. The development of more effective dust fungicides by adding oxidizing agents to sulphur. SCIENCE 66: 178, 1927.

[4] Discussion on "The fungicidal action of sulphur." Ann. of Apl. Biol. 13: 308–318, 1925.

[5] Freundlich, H., and P. Scholz. Ueber hydrophobe und hydrophile Sole des Schwefels. Koll. Beih. 16: 234–266, 1922.

[6] Kruyt, H. R. "Colloids" translated by H. S. Van Klooster. John Wiley & Son (Inc.) Page 238, 1927.

tive $S_5O_6=$ ion and the negative sulphur particle attract the positive $Ag(NH_3)_2+$ ion which reacts with the $S_5O_6=$ to form the characteristic compound which is in the end Ag_2S. A parallel case of the difference of reactions from normal under conditions of powerful adsorption is that a quantity of HCl sufficient to invert sugar will not do so when in a system adsorbed by charcoal.

Since pentathionic acid is present on most forms of sulphur and such forms of sulphur show a degree of toxicity, it is reasonable to assume that the acid is, or contains, the toxic factor. A complete proof of this was obtained by freeing sulphur of this acid and testing it for toxicity. At the outset it was found that when pure pentathionic acid was treated with strong ammonia, then brought back to pH6, or even more acid with HCl, the spores of *S. cinerea* and *V. inequalis* germinated as freely as in the checks. When sulphur was treated with strong ammonia and brought back to pH6, immediate germination tests were positive, but the suspension soon became toxic. Sulphur in the presence of oxygen and moisture is a continual source of pentathionic acid until equilibrium is reached. When the reaction was kept between pH7–7.5, the suspension was only slightly toxic. The oxidation of sulphur probably proceeds as follows:

$$S + O_2 \rightarrow SO_2$$
$$SO_2 + H_2O \rightleftarrows H_2SO_3$$
$$H_2SO_3 + S \rightleftarrows H_2S_2O_3$$
$$5H_2S_2O_3 \rightarrow 2H_2S_5O_6 + 3H_2O$$

In view of these reactions, which indicate the formation of pentathionic acid at the expense of sulphur, oxygen, and water, and those showing the alternate breakdown of this acid by ammonia into ammonium thiosulphate and sulphur, the difficulty Freundlich and Scholz experienced when trying to estimate pentathionic acid in the presence of sulphur can be explained. The reactions also account for the fact that although a solution of pentathionic acid with an added excess of ammonia fails to give a positive test for $S_5O_6=$, the free sulphur thrown down as indicated in the step reactions develops sufficient $S_5O_6=$ to give a positive test on standing. This entire procedure can account for the way ammonia gradually dissolves sulphur.

Sulphur prepared from H_2S and SO_2 is affected by strong ammonia in the same way except that the $S_5O_6=$ ion is much more abundant, reacting more quickly to the pentathionic acid test and recurring more quickly after the sulphur has been treated with ammonia.

Pure pentathionic acid is not so completely destroyed with bases such as $Ca(OH)_2$, KOH, or NaOH. These react directly, each forming the respective pentathionate which gives a positive test. They were non-toxic to the organism used but regained their toxicity when brought to pH6, or below, with HCl. All the germination tests were made in hanging-drop cultures in Van Tieghen cells, and results are given in the table.

GERMINATION TESTS WITH VARIOUS TYPES OF SULPHUR

Treatment	Germination S. Cinerea	Germination V. inequalis
	%	%
1. Pentathionic acid, .062%	0	0
2. " " .03 %	2	trace
3. " " .0075	4	5
4. Pentathionic acid .03% + strong ammonia, then acidified to pH6 with HCl	80	......
5. Pentathionic acid .03% + CaOH then brought back to neutral pH7 with HCl	72	......
6. Pentathionic acid .03% + CaOH then brought back to pH5 with HCl	trace	......
7. Check-distilled water to pH7 with slight $Ca(OH)_2$	80	70
8. Ground flour of sulphur treated with strong ammonia then thoroughly washed with O_2 free water	27	......
9. Ground flour of sulphur washed with O_2 free water	1.6	......
10. Ground flour of sulphur treated with $Ca(OH)_2$ then brought to 6.4 with HCl	5	......
11. Ground flour of sulphur treated with gelatin to aid wetting	trace	......

It is quite evident from the above results that pentathionic acid is the toxic factor of sulphur and that this compound is quite sensitive to basic materials. They further show that the natural oxidation and dissolving of sulphur gives a continuous yield of pentathionic acid. Particulate sulphur oxidizes more readily as would be expected in such systems, and consequently is more toxic. The results explain why failures occur with so many commercial dusts and sprays which have been made up more from the standpoint of spreading and sticking than maintaining toxicity. Basic compounds aid in spreading and sticking but inhibit toxicity.

H. C. YOUNG
ROBERT WILLIAMS

SCIENCE

VOL. LXVII JANUARY 13, 1928 No. 1724

CONTENTS

American Association for the Advancement of Science:
Geology and the World at Large: PROFESSOR GEORGE H. ASHLEY ... 21
Purposive Action: PROFESSOR MARGARET FLOY WASHBURN ... 24
The Collecting of Folk Songs by Phonophotography: DR. MILTON METFESSEL ... 28
Scientific Events:
New Laboratories for the Faculty of Medicine at Paris; Proposed Transfer of the Geodetic Work of the U. S. Coast and Geodetic Survey; Annual Meeting of the Northwest Scientific Association; Resolutions on the Death of Dr. Francis W. Peabody; The Ninth International Congress of Psychology ... 31
Scientific Notes and News ... 34
University and Educational Notes ... 37
Discussion and Correspondence:
On the Mechanism of Orientation of Atoms in Magnetic and Electric Fields: THOMAS H. JOHNSON. *The Identity of the Clear Creek Skull:* HARVEY S. THATCHER. *Bibliography of Colorimetry:* DR. IRWIN G. PRIEST. *No Meteorite:* R. W. STONE. *Consider the User of Bulletins:* DR. L. O. HOWARD ... 37
Scientific Books:
Eddington on Stars and Atoms: DR. H. T. STETSON ... 41
Special Articles:
The Correlation Between Intelligence and Speed in Conduction of the Nerve Impulse: DR. LEE EDWARD TRAVIS. *A Comparison of Growth Curves of Man and Other Animals:* DR. SAMUEL BRODY. *Progenies from X-rayed Sex Cells of Tobacco:* DR. T. H. GOODSPEED and DR. A. R. OLSON ... 41
Science News ... x

SCIENCE: A Weekly Journal devoted to the Advancement of Science, edited by J. McKeen Cattell and published every Friday by

THE SCIENCE PRESS

New York City: Grand Central Terminal.

Lancaster, Pa. Garrison, N. Y

Annual Subscription, $6.00. Single Copies, 15 Cts.

SCIENCE is the official organ of the American Association for the Advancement of Science. Information regarding membership in the Association may be secured from the office of the permanent secretary, in the Smithsonian Institution Building, Washington, D. C.

Entered as second-class matter July 18, 1923, at the Post Office at Lancaster, Pa., under the Act of March 8, 1879.

GEOLOGY AND THE WORLD AT LARGE[1]

I HAVE no new discovery to announce nor shall I follow the precedent of reviewing the history of geology in part or in whole. Rather I shall ask you to step out of the procession and with me watch it go by. In brief, we shall try to see ourselves as others see us. Frankly, the picture is not flattering. To the world at large geology has taken a back seat. She has lost prestige as compared with other subjects of human thought, and is serving neither herself nor the world as she can and ought. I believe the situation is a challenge to geologists to take stock of where they stand and to again get into the procession in a place commensurate with the large human interest of the subject they represent.

For the past eight years my associations have been mainly and very close with men outside the profession—bankers, merchants, lawyers, judges, manufacturers, bakers, butchers and candlestick-makers. Hundreds of these men call me by my first name and have told me how much they don't know about geology and why.

I live in a town where most of the leading men of all professions are conservative, in theology and otherwise. I do not think that they differ greatly from the leading business and professional men of other towns, and I feel that these men would be vastly enriched in their thinking by a clear knowledge of the larger findings of science in general and of geology in particular.

How many members of your home chamber of commerce or your Rotary or Kiwanis or other service clubs, for example, have any clear idea of geologic time, a conception in which years and centuries sink into insignificance that puts human history in its proper setting, or of the vast geologic changes the earth's surface has undergone or of the story of life's marvelous unfolding up the geologic ages as read in the rocks? My own conclusion is that not one in ten of the big men of my town, the men who own the big stores or manufacturing plants, who dominate its politics, who in a large measure have built and made the town what it is, have more than the vaguest idea

[1] Address of the vice-president and chairman of Section G—Geology, American Association for the Advancement of Science, Nashville, December, 1927.

of these things. They are not real and actual to them. They do not affect their thinking.

More astonishing still I am convinced that the average man of culture of fifty years ago had a better knowledge of these things than the man of culture to-day. Then, every person of culture had some knowledge of geology. It was widely taught in the "academies" of that day, using Dana's "Briefer Story," Steele's "Fourteen Weeks," and other works, and, here in Tennessee, Safford's "Elements of Geology." The fascinating writings of Hayden, Shaler and King, the memories of Lyell, the discussions and disputes of Marsh and Cope, were public property. Geology held a leading place in the museums. Some museums had little else than geologic material, partly because of the activity of Henry Ward in supplying this material. We were a new country with little knowledge of our own mineral resources, and the men who explored this new country and told us of its mineral wealth and earth secrets loomed large in public affairs.

To-day geologic text-books have practically disappeared from high schools and only a small proportion of those who go to college are exposed to this line of knowledge, and I am astonished to find how many of these appear to have missed inoculation and have forgotten about all they knew. Apparently, from what I have gathered from them, our text-books have become so largely a catalogue of facts that the great truths have been lost in the multitude of findings.

Individually most of us are so engrossed in the necessary details of our work that we have all but lost sight of these great truths of which the world at large is blissfully ignorant and of which the world is woefully in need. Our work is no longer spectacular as once it was. It is slow, patient, plodding work, as of the research engineer or surveyor. And when our work does lead out into something interesting or thrilling, we feel that the world at large would not understand, and that by the time we had explained the whole matter so that it would understand the thrill would have worn itself out and become only a shiver. So we content ourselves by telling our fellow workers, conscious that most of them are too busy to read our story after we write it.

The result of all this is that the world at large has lost interest and in large measure even lost track of us. In the field we seldom speak of ourselves as geologists but as mineral surveyors, as that designation is at least partly understood, but not geologists. Geology in the minds of most people is associated only with the finding of mineral deposits, water and fossils. We are often classed with the mineral prospector and in the minds of many have faded out with that picturesque but worthy, if usually impecunious, individual. We hear of great foundations and laboratories for the study of medicine, physics, chemistry, archeology and other sciences, and of expeditions to other lands. We see physics and chemistry and perhaps biology being studied in practically all high schools but what of these have we in geology? A few of our museums feature the bones of giant reptiles. But all too many of them have relegated geology to back rooms and galleries.

So to-day when we are faced with the most stupendous problems facing any science we are handicapped by lack of funds and lack of interest. Geology today is breaking away from its old moorings, whether for better or worse. Great fundamental problems face us. Is isostasy true, and, if so, what are its causes and laws? Do the continents float around at will? Did Mesozoic time begin 25 or 250 million years ago? How came our mountains to be? Is there likely to come another ice age, a state-wide lava flow, a continental flooding, such as has often occurred in the past? All of these problems are being approached from new angles. The very foundations of the deep are being stirred; but the world at large knows little of it, would not understand it if told, and so has little interest and is not inclined to be sympathetic to our call for help.

I said the world at large needs geology. Let me take a single example. Some time ago biology stirred up a pretty rumpus over a little matter called evolution. Unfortunately, evolution was not content to remain simply a theory of the biologist. It insisted on getting mixed up with geology and astronomy, with physics and chemistry, with history and archeology, with philosophy and theology, and right there is where it ran afoul of a very real opposition; for nearly everybody holds some kind of theologic belief and evolution said that much theologic belief failed to fit the facts. Biology, of course, came back with "Here are the facts, see for yourselves." Unfortunately the biologic facts are a little difficult to display. For example, it is hard to show a man his strange embryonic development before he saw daylight and said "Hello, folks." It is difficult to demonstrate to him his vestigial reminders of other days when he was only a monkey, a reptile or a fish. It is difficult to bring home to him the bearing of the facts of geographic distribution.

On the other hand, geology deals with mountains and mastodons and other big things you can see. The slow seaward movement of the land is common knowledge when attention is called to it. The progress of life as revealed in the rocks can be easily shown in museums. Nearly any one can go out and collect fossils. Seashells or shark's teeth in the rocks forming mountain tops compel the thoughtful consideration of any thinking man. Even Mr. Bryan felt impelled to admit that the world was not made in six days. So clear and so wide-spread is geologic evidence that if properly handled it should not be difficult to convince any one, except a certain unnamed person, of the magnitude of geologic time, of the long and involved series of events that has led up to the present shape of our landscapes, of the unfolding progress of life as revealed in the rocks.

It is my personal belief that the world at large needs to know these facts and that if properly presented they will be accepted and that the acceptance will create an open mind toward other great facts. Believing this, are not we geologists in duty bound to give most serious consideration to the problem of how to make these facts a part of the stock of knowledge of the world at large and his wife and children?

How shall we go about it?

First, I suggest we make geology a science. At present geology is hardly more than a collection of facts and a collection of facts is not generally considered to be a science. To be a science facts must lead to hypotheses, theories, laws, by which we guide our action or predicate future results from present causes. Physics and chemistry have a foundation of laws. But what laws can you find in our geologic text-books?

Second, we need to revamp our text-books and teaching. Even though we are not prepared to state laws, our facts are of different orders of value. To-day our text-books are little more than catalogues of facts, all on a dead level. They are like a variety-store window. We need to inject some high lights, some mountains, some foreground and background, to set out our star performers and turn the spotlight on them, having in mind the value of these facts in the after life of the student.

Third, we need to get together on some of our larger facts. When one of us declares our giant reptiles were here six million years ago, and another says sixty million years ago, what is the world at large to think of us? No two text-books to-day use the same major units for a time scale. Most trades are getting together on codes and standards of practice. Are lumbermen and furnace men any more reasonable or fair-minded than we geologists? There is, I find, a wide-spread belief among the younger geologists that business or the church have nothing on geology for conservatism.

Fourth, it is time to distinguish sharply between public and professional papers and reports. We publish, let us say, 3,000 copies of a report for the public at public expense. We may estimate that five hundred of these go to libraries, five hundred reach men who can read them intelligently, leaving two thousand to go to people who can find neither pleasure nor profit in the average geological report. At least that is the reaction I get from talking to many people I meet in the field who have sent for our reports or those of other surveys. Recently I went over the manuscript of a detailed areal report intended to inform the people of the area covered, or others interested, of its geology and mineral resources. I listed about seventy-five words, most of them used many times, that might as well have been written in Hindu so far as conveying any meaning to most of its readers, enough to destroy a large part of the value of the report and to explain why we have difficulty in getting rid of 3,000 copies, while a writer in another science on our same floor can not supply the demand for his books with five editions of 10,000 each.

Fifth, recognizing that the average scientist is not qualified by temperament or otherwise, as will be testified by any lawyer or judge, to make a simple, appealing presentation of scientific facts, let us honor rather than discourage the man, whether scientist or not, who can and will put our findings in popular form. Federal and State Surveys might well make the popularization of geologic facts an important part of their work. The Pennsylvania Survey is at present running carefully prepared articles each month in the State school journal, planning road signs wherever there are geological features on the highway, taking and making opportunities to give popular illustrated talks wherever possible.

Sixth, contact with some of those who have been active in propaganda against science teaching leads me to believe that science herself or rather a very few of her disciples have been primarily responsible for this state of mind. A study of attempts to pass inhibiting or controlled legislation in other lines of work shows invariably a failure on the part of a few of those to be curbed to play the game fairly. So here I believe the irritating cause has been the unguarded speech of a very few people who publicly expressed their private views, ridiculing the religious beliefs of their students or neighbors. I do not propose a gag for such people, but would remind them, recalling that they live in a land in which eighty-five per cent. of the people are conservative, that this country started out with "a decent respect for the opinions of mankind," and that a large proportion of the leading scientists of the country, while they may have exchanged their old theology for a new, find their science no bar to themselves taking an active part in the religious exercises and life of the day.

In conclusion, I believe geology to-day faces the

task of taking the world at large into its confidence and friendship in a very real way, first by simplifying and popularizing or making fully intelligent to the public, all public, but not professional, reports. Second, by rearranging our geologic facts so as to bring into the foreground and limelight the great fundamental truths that all persons should know and recasting our text-books and teaching accordingly. Third, by striving to change geology from a history to a science, by the correlation of our facts into generalizations and, if possible, into definitely stated theories and laws. Fourth, by eliminating as far as possible all differences of interpretation and statement. Fifth, by encouraging the man who can dress our science up so as to attract and hold the interest of the world at large. Sixth, by following the Declaration of Independence in having "a decent respect for the opinions of mankind." That is the challenge. Will we meet it?

George H. Ashley

Harrisburg, Pennsylvania

PURPOSIVE ACTION[1]

It is the purpose of this address to suggest certain directions in which a mechanistic explanation may be sought for the purposive behavior of animals, which has been by some authorities regarded as a unique phenomenon, irreducible to those laws which govern the rest of the universe.

Since I shall have occasion to speak of the motives or drives underlying behavior, it is not inappropriate to say that the drive which lies back of my present purpose is a hearty dislike of the doctrine of emergent evolution, which was so warmly endorsed at the last meeting of this association by Professor Jennings,[2] the retiring chairman of the Zoological Section. This doctrine, as you all know, holds that from time to time something entirely new emerges in the course of evolution. It is considered to be opposed to the doctrine of mechanism, which holds that from the beginning the material universe has been governed by a set of unchanging laws. Now as I read expositions of the doctrine of emergent evolution, it seems to mean either something with which all mechanists will agree, or something which involves the negation of scientific thinking and a return to more primitive modes of thought. First, it may mean that new phenomena make their appearance from time to time: new chemical combinations, new species of living beings. Who would doubt it? This is evolution: there is no need for the distinguishing adjective "emergent." Secondly, it may mean that new fundamental laws of the material universe have been discovered from time to time. Who would doubt this, or that others may yet be discovered which have been operating from the beginning but which our imperfect methods of observation have not previously been able to detect? Thirdly, it may mean that the fundamental laws of the universe modify each other when they enter into new combinations. Who would doubt it, or imagine that we have yet observed all the combinations of those laws which have existed from the beginning? Fourthly, it may mean that from time to time new fundamental laws of the physical universe have come into existence, and may at any time in the present or future do so. Professor Jennings complains that without emergent evolution there is no fun in experimenting. According to the mechanistic theory, he says, "from a sample of the universe we ought to be able to reason out the rest; the experimenters are those of us who can't"; and he goes on to say that this must naturally make the experimenter feel deeply inferior. But what would cheer the experimenter? The thought that he may at any moment observe a new combination and have the fun of showing that it is really reducible to already known laws? The mechanist gets a good deal of enjoyment from such an experience. Or the thought that he may at any moment discover a law which has been in operation always but has hitherto escaped observation? This is a joy for which the mechanist may always hope. Or is the only possible thrill for the experimenter to be derived from the chance that at any moment a new law of nature may *come into existence* and he be there to see? But what ought to discourage an experimenter more finally than such an expectation as this? He is trying to discover a law of nature, but what if at any moment it may be interfered with by a new one that has come into existence? If the universe can not be relied upon to stay on the tracks, why try to find out where the tracks lie? Professor Jennings sees in emergent evolution the only salvation from the dire practical consequences of mechanism. "Mingle," he says, "this perfect doctrine of mechanism with equal parts of the perfect doctrine of natural selection and you get a potion, a cocktail, with a kick that is warranted to knock out ethics and civilization." But if we believe that new laws of nature may at any moment begin to act, in the paralysis of science that would result from the drinking of *this* cocktail, I would give still less for the chances of ethics and civilization.

The mechanist then believes that whatever may be the ultimate truth of the matter, an inclination to

[1] Address of the vice-president and chairman of Section I—Psychology, American Association for the Advancement of Science, Nashville, December, 1927.

[2] Science, 65, 1927, pp. 19–25.

assume emergents in the sense of new forces should be held sternly in check. And it is the object of this paper to suggest how one of the emergents, namely purposive action, may conceivably be reduced to the status of a product of already existing forces.

The vitalist holds that living matter is fundamentally different from lifeless matter, and that its distinguishing characteristic is an emergent, namely purposiveness. As one reflects on the nature of a living body, it does seem to be distinguished from a lifeless body by a tendency to resist and compensate for disturbances of its pattern. It is composed of highly complex molecules, and these whether in living or lifeless bodies are likely to fall apart and disintegrate, thus changing the pattern of the whole. But in a lifeless body this disintegration is balanced by no reconstruction of molecules, while in a living body the pattern is constantly being restored. The actual materials of our bodies are constantly leaving us, but the pattern remains and new materials are forced into the same pattern, which is secured by all manner of devices; moreover, when the pattern can no longer be maintained, by all manner of devices its reappearance in offspring has been ensured. What is this that cares so much about its pattern? No wonder that the vitalist posits emergent entelechies, mysterious agencies that occupy themselves with its preservation. But to the mechanist mysterious agencies are too reminiscent of nature deities, earth spirits, and similar relics of the childhood of human thought to be congenial. And, he asks, is it really true that preservation and restoration of the pattern are peculiar to living matter? The atom also has a tendency to restore its pattern; whenever it loses an electron it makes haste to repair the loss. The mechanist would cling to the faith that the preservations and restorations, even the reproductions, of patterns in living organisms can ultimately be traced to the preservation and restoration of atomic patterns. And if it be said that this is merely to ascribe purpose to the atom, or perhaps to the electron, the mechanist will say, "Well and good; put whatever may be necessary into the beginnings of things, but don't be lavish with emergents during the later processes."

But vitalists in the field of psychology, like Professor McDougall, mean by purposiveness in living organisms more than a mere tendency to restore and reproduce the pattern. Professor McDougall means by purposiveness the organism's anticipation of the results of its action; the end is actually the cause of the action. The organism is not forced by physicochemical laws to preserve and reproduce its pattern; the end to be attained produces the required behavior through a type of causality unknown to lifeless matter.

Now the means by which a living organism maintains its pattern may be divided into molecular activities, such as digestion and respiration, and mass activities such as movements of locomotion, seizing of food, and the like. The former are the province of the physiologist; in the latter, which constitute what is commonly called behavior, the psychologist has an interest, and it is to these that I shall henceforth confine myself.

Purposive behavior, in the sense of behavior objectively adapted to secure the continuance of the individual and the species, may be divided into inherited behavior and learned behavior. (We grant, of course, that the two constantly accompany each other). And it has been customary to include under inherited behavior the simple reflex response to a stimulus and the more complicated responses commonly called instinctive. Now the reflex looks mechanical. It seems, that is, to be dependent rather on the external stimulus plus the animal's physiological state than on any purpose in the animal's mind. And in fact Professor McDougall[3] grants freely that the reflex is mechanical, subject merely to the laws of physiological chemistry. This concession lands the vitalist in certain difficulties from which it takes considerable agility to escape. The first difficulty is that the reflex can be modified by learning, which would seem to obliterate any sharp distinction between it and higher forms of behavior, so that if you grant that the reflex is mechanical you will be put to it to show where mechanism ends and purposiveness begins. This difficulty Professor McDougall meets by asserting that the highly modifiable salivary reflex, for instance, is not a true reflex because it depends on the brain. Only behavior that depends on the brain, we then conclude, is purposive rather than mechanical; it would seem that the emergent "purposiveness" came into existence not with living matter but with the brain. The mechanist may indeed adduce, Professor McDougall says, the case of the frog with brain removed which, if it is prevented from wiping off a drop of acid from its skin with one leg, wipes it off with the other. This conduct looks purposive, but does not depend on the brain. Well, perhaps, Professor McDougall conjectures, in frogs and similar lowly animals purposive action does not depend on the brain.

The second difficulty created for the vitalist by the admission that reflexes are mechanical is that instinctive actions, which on McDougall's theory are manifestations of purposiveness, have been regarded as combinations of reflexes. This view of course must be rejected by the vitalist if the reflex is admitted to be mechanical. Instinctive action, the vitalist holds,

[3] "Outline of Psychology," New York, 1923, pp. 51–56.

is not a chain of reflexes but is guided by the idea of its end, as is shown by the fact that the means taken to secure the end is not mechanically fixed, another means being adopted if one means fails, as in the case of the frog just mentioned. Professor McDougall boldly accepts the consequence of this theory, and asserts that on the first performance of instinctive actions, for example, the first nest-building of a bird, the animal is guided by an inherited mental image of the nest; "the power of thinking of or imagining an object not present to the senses is provided in the form of innate mental structure."[4]

Most of us would hesitate to adopt such a hypothesis, and as a matter of fact F. H. Herrick's[5] careful studies of the instinctive behavior of birds, to which Professor McDougall nowhere alludes, indicate that it looks much more like a series of reflexes than like intelligent purpose. Through first-hand observation Herrick concluded that the series of activities beginning with the spring migration and proceeding through mating, nest-building, egg-laying, care of young in nest, care of young out of nest, and fall migration, is subject to disturbances inconceivable on a purposive theory; for instance, egg-laying sometimes anticipates nest-building, the eggs being laid on the ground, or the migration impulse interrupts the last egg-laying and the young are abandoned. In general when anything interrupts the normal course of instinctive behavior, the dislocated combination of acts that results has much more the aspect of machinery out of order than that of baffled attempts to realize a conscious purpose.

I think we may say that when by "purpose" is meant awareness of the object to be secured, the innate behavior of animals shows no satisfactory evidence of it. But if by purpose we mean merely *persistent striving,* the case is different. There does seem to be in the greater part of animal behavior something persistent, which underlies series of individual acts and unites them by a bond other than that of mere external association. This is shown alike in innate and in learned behavior. One of the most important results of experimental work on animals during the last ten years has been the evidence that animals will not learn without a motive; that a rat will not learn a maze with food in it unless he is hungry; and Szymanski[6] has shown that while various other motives, such as those resulting from uncomfortable surroundings or sex stimulation, will produce learning, a rat will run a given maze only under the influence of the motive that made him learn it. Our mistake as mechanists has been in trying to explain learning as an external linking together of separate acts into a series merely by their repetition. Watson's theory that in learning how to get out of a maze the errors are dropped off not because they involve delay in reaching the goal but because they are less frequently performed than the successful movements is probably the last effort of mechanism in this direction, and it is a failure.

The problem before mechanism in dealing with purpose is not merely to explain the association of transitory acts into series, but to furnish a mechanistic explanation of something that *endures throughout the series.* When in ordinary speech we say that a man has a purpose in what he is doing, we mean that there is something relatively constant throughout his course of action, namely awareness of an end, and when we watch animals engaged in instinctive activities, while their behavior shows that they are not aware of the end, it also shows the presence of something that persists until the end is reached. Can mechanism explain this relatively constant and unchanging factor, or must we make use of entelechies, innate ideas, and other regressions into past modes of thought?

Surveying the physiological possibilities, we find among our bodily processes two types of relatively constant and persistent states, not usually thought of as purposive, and offering no essential obstacle to a mechanistic explanation. The first type comprises internal physiological conditions such as hunger, thirst, fatigue and certain states of the sex organs. The second type includes bodily attitudes, due to the continuous innervation of certain external muscles. Compared to actual movements, both internal physiological states and external bodily attitudes have the character of relative permanence. If we can show that they are involved in purposive action, we shall have a possible mechanistic theory of its essential feature.

The inner physiological states present themselves as the appropriate basis for the motives or drives. The physico-chemical equilibrium of the body is disturbed, either by the lack or by the excess of some important substance. While this condition continues, energy is set free and finds a natural outlet in bodily movement. And movement will continue until the condition ceases, either by restoration of the physiological balance or by the counteracting influence of fatigue. If the external situation is one that has been often encountered, the movements may be adapted either innately or by previous learning to rapid relief of the physiological disturbance, and we

[4] *Op. cit.* p. 202.

[5] *The Popular Science Monthly,* 76, 1910, pp. 532–556, 77, 1910, pp. 82–97, 122–141.

[6] *Pflüger's Archiv,* 171, 1918, p. 374.

say that the animal has acted reflexly, instinctively, or according to habit. If such preformed pathways are not opened, the energy of the physiological state discharges into a wider variety of movements; an animal in a new situation such as a maze runs down all the passages and makes all the turnings possible. Experiments indicate that in maze learning it is the movements nearest the "success" that are earliest learned; that is, while the drive, the persistent physiological state, say, of hunger, becomes associated with all the movements that occur while it lasts, it is most strongly associated with those movements that occur nearest its end. To explain why this should be so, the mechanist can appeal to the established laws of association; the drive will naturally form strongest associations when it is itself strongest, and this of course is when it is nearing its end; further, at the beginning of a repetition of the situation the movements made at the end of the preceding series have the advantage of recency. By the prepotency, thus grounded, of the movements nearest in time to the cessation of the drive, it is possible to explain learning by trial and error; but *only through the influence of the drive* which accompanies the whole series.[7]

Thus with no assumption of conscious awareness of purpose on the animal's part we may hope to explain through the persistent influence of drives the organization of movements into new combinations leading to the cessation of the drive. But what about those cases, common in human behavior, where there *is* awareness of purpose? A man, under the influence of a drive which can not at once be relieved, sometimes works off the impeded energy in random movements as an animal does, but it is his human birthright to think the situation out, guided in his thought by the influence of the *idea* of his goal. This is the climax, the crucial point of the contest between vitalism and mechanism for the explanation of purposive action. Here the idea of the end is actually present, though not continuously present, in consciousness, and not only the idea of the ultimate end, but the idea of means to that end. For this state of affairs the mechanist must conceive a physiological basis capable of being explained on physico-chemical laws.

Why should not the mechanist, who of course holds that a definite nervous process underlies the idea of the end, merely say that this nervous process is the cause of consciously purposive action? Because if we can judge the nervous process underlying ideas from the behavior of ideas themselves, they lack that character of *persistence* which is essential to purposive action. Ideas are essentially transitory: it is impossible for one to endure without change for more than a few seconds. They may recur, but they can not last. Introspective observation of the process of consciously purposive action has shown that the idea of the end to be gained, while present at the outset, may disappear many times during the course of the action or thought without interrupting progress towards the end. The attempt to use the nervous substrate of an idea to explain a coherent series of reactions fails for the same reason that the old mechanistic explanation of learning as an external linking of separate and transitory movements fails: in both cases we must have an underlying process to hold the series together. But in consciously purposive action this underlying process must not only be *persistent,* like the uneasiness of a drive: it must be, so to speak, *constant in direction.*

It was said a little while ago that there are two types of bodily processes which possess that character of relative permanence which is needed for the physical substrate of purposive action: internal bodily states, in which class the drive or motive belongs, and external bodily attitudes.

Now if we watch a man who, when he can not get relief from the influence of a drive by immediate action, begins to think the matter out, we observe that he becomes quiet, that his restlessness ceases. If we are that man, introspection tells us that our quiet is not the quiet of relaxation but that of bodily tenseness, especially in the trunk muscles. Whenever this attitude relaxes, the energy of the drive begins again to escape in random movements; we stop thinking and become restless.[8] For all purposive action there must be a persistent inner physiological state of imbalance, the drive. For purposive *thinking,* we may conjecture that this state must discharge its energy not into immediate action, whether useful or merely random restlessness, but into a quiet, tense bodily attitude. And any idea may become a purpose, the idea of an end, if, being first associated with a drive, it becomes associated with this peculiar, persistent attitude of tense quietness.[9]

Not only does this motor explanation of purposive action seem to me plausible, but I believe we can trace in animal behavior a stage intermediate between the adaptation of acts to ends which occurs by random movements and requires only the persistent influence of the drive, inducing restlessness, and that which occurs by thinking the problem out, under the influ-

[7] M. F. Washburn, "The Animal Mind," 3rd edition, 1926, 329–337.

[8] It was Münsterberg who first suggested in his doctor's thesis, "Die Willenshandlung," that the feeling of activity or effort, the will-consciousness, consists of kinesthetic sensations from our bodily attitude.

[9] M. F. Washburn, "Movement and Mental Imagery," 1916, Chapter 8.

ence of a bodily attitude of quiet tension. Many observers of the behavior of animals in learning a maze have noted that they quickly acquire a bodily orientation towards the center, and tend to correct movements that carry them away from this oriented attitude. Similarly with Hunter's Delayed Reaction apparatus, even when the animals were restrained from going to the correct door for some little time after the signal light had been turned off, they succeeded in doing so by keeping their noses pointed during the delay interval towards the place where the light had been. The original stimulus for this oriented attitude is of course external, the light, or the smell of food in the maze; but the orientation seems to be capable of persisting for some time after the stimulus is gone, and to be revived by associated stimuli, as when a dog entering a room looks under the chair where he left a ball. Following our general custom of deriving our terms for abstract relations from terms meaning spatial relations (as when we speak of "straightening out" a mental puzzle), we use the expression "thought *directed toward a goal.*" May not the steadily tense bodily attitude accompanying directed thought be in some sense a relic of the orientation in lower animals of the entire body towards the stimulus that will bring relief from a drive? In the beginning, while the reflex and tropism were adequate modes of behavior, the drive discharged in a definite direction. As the environment became more complex, the drive discharged into random movements of which those associated with the drive in its last and most intense stages tended to survive and become organized into systems. In this process the drive secured the persistence needed for purposive action, but the definite direction of the tropism was lost. Often, however, in animals, part of the energy of the drive goes into the tendency to maintain and restore a bodily orientation towards the goal; while in man, for whose varied activities general bodily orientation is too confining, directed thinking is sustained by a vestige of this general bodily orientation, the tense quietness of the trunk muscles that may persist even when we turn from one position to another.

In explaining, then, the persistent character of purposive action, the mechanist may substitute for the vitalist's mysterious, emergent entelechy, involving something over and above the ordinary physico-chemical laws, the *drive* as a state of unstable physico-chemical equilibrium, underlying all purposive action, and an attitude of steady contraction of the trunk muscles, into which the energy of the drive may discharge and which accompanies the higher forms of purposive action. These suggestions towards a mechanistic explanation of purposiveness have had to be put concisely and dogmatically because of the limits of my time. If they are highly speculative, they are at least, it seems to me, by virtue of being mechanistic, closer to the spirit of science than the semi-personal and animistic emergents of the vitalist.

MARGARET FLOY WASHBURN
VASSAR COLLEGE

THE COLLECTING OF FOLK SONGS BY PHONOPHOTOGRAPHY[1]

Ear analysis of folk music. The traditional method of the anthropologist in collecting folk or primitive music has been an analysis of the songs by ear, whether taken directly from the lips of a singer or from a phonograph record. This subjective method has many serious limitations.

That the ear is inadequate to describe many of the important elements of music is best indicated by the American Negro vocal embellishments, whose description has baffled the keenest ear. The fast changes of the voice lose their original identity when heard, becoming fused in perception. Another difficulty with a subjective analysis is the bias due to past musical experience which deafens the notator to elements foreign to his own music. For example, the European musician holds that American Negro music belongs to his musical system, while the African analyzes out of the great sound complex reaching his ear so much in common with his own music and so little that is not that he draws a natural but opposite conclusion.

Conventional notation. The conventional symbols which have been used by collectors of folk music were devised as a representation of European music. Consequently to use such symbols neglects those factors which might make a folk music distinctive. In Negro music, that part which is characteristically Negro is not found in the stilted notes on the conventional five-line staff, but rather in the twists and slides between the lines.

Measurable records of music. In the fall of 1925 we undertook a field study of Negro music, but instead of using the cylinder phonograph we substituted a portable phonophotographic camera. The voices of Negroes were photographed on motion picture film, by using an optical lever somewhat on the order of Miller's phonodeik.[2] This photographic method shifted the analysis of folk songs from auditory experience to an objective measurable record of the sound wave.

[1] Presented before the National Academy of Sciences, at Urbana, Illinois, October 18, 1927.

[2] Miller, D. C. "The Science of Musical Sounds." Macmillan, New York, 1916.

Phonophotographic theory. The most strategic approach in a description of folk music is an analysis of the sound wave, because it is the connecting link between the singer and listener. Preceding the sound wave there is a series of events within the organism of the speaker, and following it there is another series within the listener. All these events may be related in a causal series.

What we are calling the speech and music causal series consists of two main segments. The first, or expression, segment consists of a description of the speaking or singing experience, of the neural action occurring at the same time, of the muscular action following, and of the sound-wave resulting. The second, or impression, segment involves a description of the sound-wave, the action of an adequate receptor, together with neural action and auditory experience.

The sound wave overlaps each segment or, taking the causal series as a whole, it occupies a central position. For musical purposes it may best be described in terms of four properties, *viz.*, wave-frequency, wave-amplitude, wave-form and wave-recurrence. Each of these properties of the sound-wave may be converted into related aspects of links either way in the causal series. When paired with attributes of the sound heard, wave-frequency may be converted into pitch, wave-amplitude into intensity, wave-form into timbre, and wave-recurrence into subjective groupings.

The sound wave properties may likewise be converted into aspects of muscular action, which in turn may be translated into aspects of neural action. Frequency, for example, is linked with the length, thickness and tension of the cricothyroid muscle. Much of the pairing remains to be accomplished, but at least the possibility of relating aspects of each link in the causal series is established. The research of the next decade in speech and music will probably be centered on the formulation of laws of relationship of the causal series links.

Once such laws of relationship are established, it will be possible from only a knowledge of the nature of the sound waves of primitive music, not only to understand the action of the ear and the nature of the auditory experience in folk music, but also to go the other way in the causal series and state the muscles and nerves involved and their mode of action. The collector of primitive music then gets a possible description of some of the neurology, anatomy, physiology and psychology in the production and reception of primitive music, when he only photographs the sound-wave.

Pattern notation. It is possible to decipher the code of the sound-wave into the notes, rests and signatures on the conventional five-line staff. The best argument against such a procedure when used alone may be inferred from the notation we have adopted as a representation of speech and music shown in Figure 1.

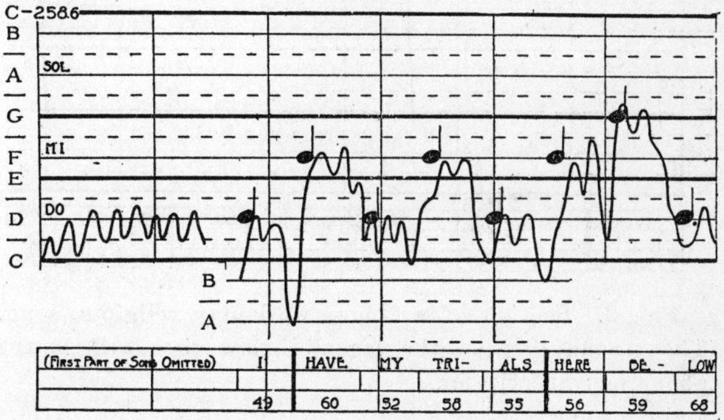

FIG. 1. First part of a Negro spiritual. In the present collection, now in press, there are over thirty folk songs on pattern notation. Leger lines are extended from the staff wherever necessary, in this case the three half steps from B to A inclusive, below the staff proper. The numbers at the bottom of the legend beneath the staff are in terms of .01 sec., representing the duration of a tone.

In this illustration, the graph-curve forms itself into certain definite patterns, which are descriptive of the vocal phenomena of the sound-wave. We are calling this the "pattern notation." The horizontal lines represent a half-step, and the six equal divisions from left to right each have a value of one second. This graph displays only the frequency and recurrence patterns, but wave-energy and wave-form analysis may also be represented.

The distorted and insufficient view of the nature of music revealed by a note-symbol may be seen on the tone "I," Fig. 1. The voice brushes up against the note for a brief time, but the tone begins three half-steps below, and drops rapidly for five half-steps on the release. This type of release is quite common in Negro singing. It seems as if the extended drop releasing "I" were intended to give a running start on the tone following. Then there are the wavy lines at the left of Fig. 1 representing the vibrato, which persist whenever the tone is held for any length of time.

Figure 2 is a sample of a Negro workaday religious song. Here the note-symbol crumbles completely, for many of the tones are entirely intonations. Tones such as *since,* Fig. 2, a glide upward throughout its duration of a quarter-note, suggest that the Negro frequently adds a touch of the dramatic by including speech intonations here and there. The sweeping attacks and releases of tones illustrate how the free-

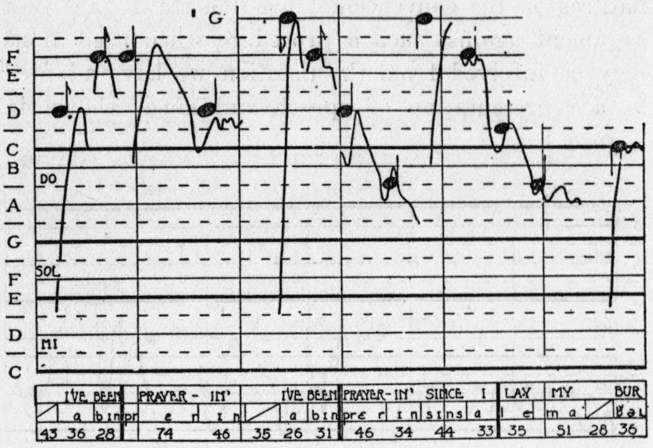

FIG. 2. Section of a Negro workaday religious song. The second line on the legend below the staff is the phonetic transcription.

dom which the Negro enjoys in singing is left intact on the pattern notation.

It is apparent from these examples that no longer need the word "unnotatable" be applied to anything in speech or music.

Negro vocal ornaments. The personal decorations of primitive man are no more tangible than the ornaments of voice, when the latter are brought out by phonophotography. The vocal ornaments may be isolated from a song, classified and placed on exhibit as a particular pattern. With a phonograph record or film to reproduce the music, any one may hear the vocal ornaments which are pictured.

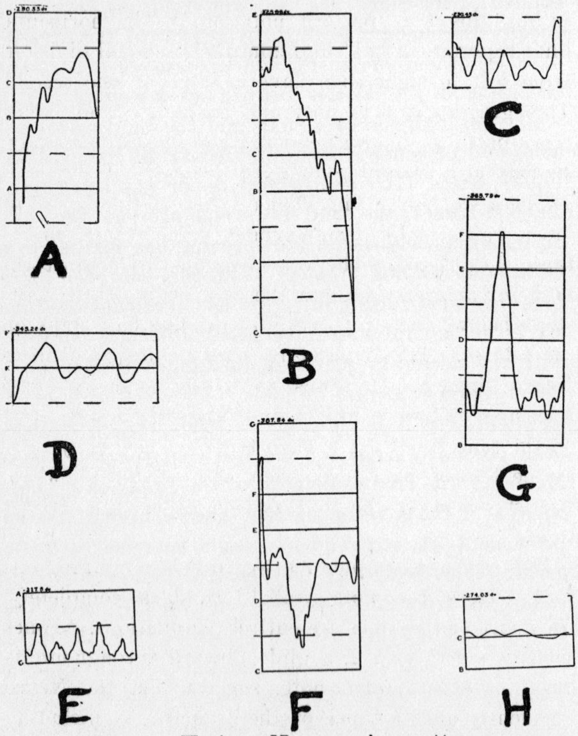

FIG. 3. Various Negro voice patterns.

Such a museum exhibit is presented in Fig. 3. These are close-ups of the pattern notation. *A* represents a Negro attack of a tone, and *B* and *C* releases. The falling intonation at the end of *B* is heard often at the close of a breath-group. The upward flip shown on *C* is not such a frequent pattern, but it is used for variety effect. *D* is a slow quaver, the voice slowly alternating, while *E* is a Negro vibrato. Note the irregularity, for it is characteristic of this pattern among Negroes. The artistic singer much more nearly approaches a smooth curve. *F* shows one variety out of many of the interpolated-tone. The tone is begun and ended on the same pitch and with the same vowel, but a short tone is interpolated somewhere within the limits, sometimes above and sometimes below. *G* is a falsetto-twist, where the voice twists in and out of the falsetto for an instant, giving a peculiar tone coloring. *H* shows an erratic-waver, which is due to the unsteadiness of the vocal cords in holding a tone. There is no definiteness about the wavering as in the case of the vibrato.

Vocal customs. The vocal customs which make one folk music distinctive from another may now be added as a new chapter for the folk-lorist. Some of these customs have been observed by ear, yet even such a factual problem as quarter-tones in various folk music scales is still being debated. By measuring the sound-wave, it is possible to determine all the intervals in given music to a fraction of a vibration, if desired. It follows that the scale of any music existent at the present time may be determined with precision. The interval graph of Fig. 4 is intended

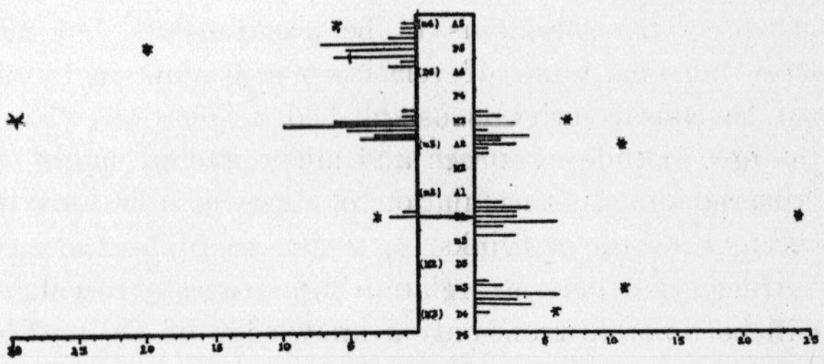

FIG. 4. An interval graph.

to be accessory to the pattern notation, isolating intervals and placing them in compact form for a study of scales.

Another accessory graph, Fig. 5, is the tempo graph. The sudden and expressive speeding up or slowing down of tempo in Negro songs is here illustrated.

Preservation. The many records of folk music lying idle in the museums of America and the *Phonogram Archiven* of Europe in effect are preserv-

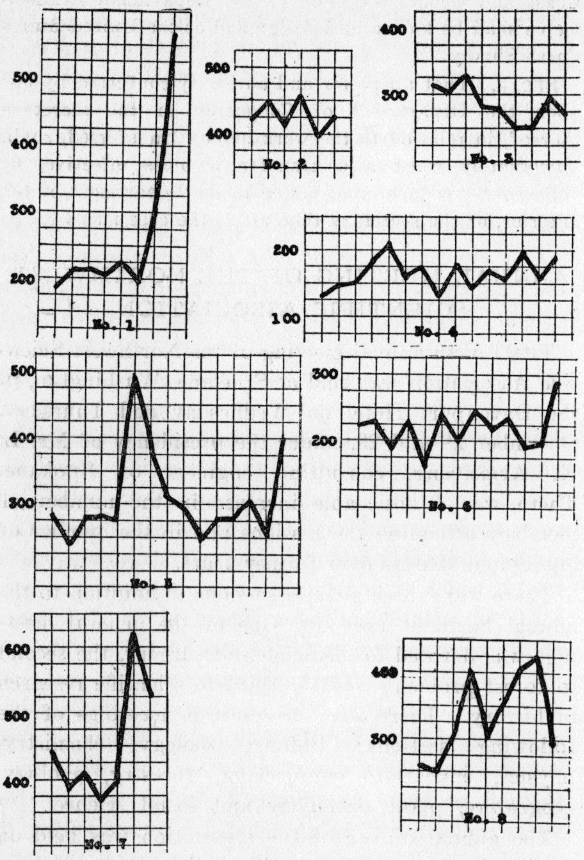

FIG. 5. Some of the tempo graphs of the collection. Vertical values are in seconds, with one square from left to right for each measure in the song.

ing the sound-wave, but not in directly measurable form. The phonophotographic record will not only preserve the sound-wave for measurements, but may use the same waves for auditory reproduction by use of the photoelectric cell.

The cylinder records already collected might be photographed second hand to a profit, now that the announcement of a machine which simplifies the measurements of frequency and recurrence is imminent. There is of course a large error involved in the making of such cylinder records, and the favored method would be to make the record photographic in the original.

MILTON METFESSEL

STATE UNIVERSITY OF IOWA

SCIENTIFIC EVENTS

NEW LABORATORIES FOR THE FACULTY OF MEDICINE AT PARIS

THE Faculty of Medicine of Paris came into possession, in 1920, of a large tract of improved property formerly owned and controlled by the College of Jesuits, rue de Vaugirard, comprising a hectare and a half of land (nearly four acres), which became alienated through the operation of the law pertaining to teaching religious organizations. The property was acquired by the government for 5,500,000 francs and two annuities of 5,000,000 francs each. The Paris correspondent of the *Journal* of the American Medical Association writes that the Faculty of Medicine has decided to establish a hygienic institute and the services of an experimental surgical clinic, under the direction of Professor Pierre Duval. For the latter a gift of the government of Brazil was utilized, which had organized there a model hospital during the war and which turned over to the Faculty of Medicine all its installations and a large amount of material without asking any recompense. But the government has been prevented by the financial crisis from supplying either institution with the 5,000,000 francs promised. Only 1,200,000 francs has been allotted to the surgical clinic. As for the hygienic institute, it still remained, after seven years, in the same condition it was in before. Its director, Professor Léon Bernard, has collected, through various gifts, only 800,000 francs, which has been used for the repairs on these buildings, which had deteriorated owing to their having been neglected over a period of fifteen years. Neither the minister of health nor the city of Paris, nor the general council of the Seine, has sufficient funds, at present, to supply the amount needed, by reason of the creation of overburdensome taxes, which paralyze general activities and yet do not furnish an adequate return, while the high cost of living and the increase of salaries and pensions absorb a large part of the available liquid assets. An anonymous donor has contributed 500,000 francs; the fund into which are paid the levies on gambling, clubs and horse racing has furnished an additional 150,000 francs. With this sum, the buildings that were falling into ruin have been restored and six large laboratories have been built and equipped with the necessary supplies, including suitable quarters for experimental animals. The final results are excellent, but it is claimed that they would not have been possible except for the fact that the Faculty of Medicine was free to dispose of the funds as it chose, whereas if the government had taken charge of the improvements the expenditures might have been twice as great. The architects and contractors granted discounts of from 25 to 40 per cent. on the prices that they demand of the government, which pays their bills only after long delays and innumerable formalities. The new laboratories are intended for the department of physiology, which was very poorly equipped heretofore, and are placed under the direction of Dr. Santenoise. The official dedication took place on November 23, under the chairmanship of the minister of public instruction, although that department did not contribute toward the realization of the project, the actual donor preferring to remain unknown. It is generally assumed, however, that a retired professor of the Faculty of Medicine furnished the funds.

THE PROPOSED TRANSFER OF THE GEODETIC WORK OF THE U. S. COAST AND GEODETIC SURVEY

Bills to authorize the transfer of the geodetic work of the Coast and Geodetic Survey from the Department of Commerce to the Department of the Interior have been introduced into both houses of the Congress. The bill, introduced into the House of Representatives by Mr. Sinnott and referred to the committee on interstate and foreign commerce, follows:

Be it enacted by the Senate and House of Representatives of the United States of America in Congress assembled, that effective sixty days from the approval of this act, and thereafter, the Geological Survey of the Department of the Interior shall be responsible for the execution of geodetic surveys required by the Federal Government in the interior of the United States, including federal, boundary and state surveys, exact levels, triangulation and transverse, the determination of field astronomic positions and variations of latitude, and gravity observations, precise triangulation and leveling in regions subject to earthquakes, and all seismological observations in the United States including the Territories of Alaska and Hawaii.

Sec. 2. That such civilian employees of the Coast and Geodetic Survey, both in Washington and in the field, as may be engaged in work relating to the geodetic and other activities enumerated in Section 1, shall be transferred, without change in classification or compensation, from the Department of Commerce to the Department of the Interior, as the heads of the respective departments may decide: *Provided*, That any commissioned officer now engaged on this work may be detailed by the Secretary of Commerce to duty in the Geological Survey under the direction of the Secretary of the Interior for such period, not exceeding two years from the time when this Act shall take effect, as the Secretary of the Interior may deem advisable, and any officer so detailed shall be entitled to receive the traveling and other allowances authorized by law for the commissioned officers of the Coast and Geodetic Survey.

Sec. 3. The unexpended balances of appropriations, or allotments therefrom, available to the Coast and Geodetic Survey for said activities, including the appropriations for the salaries of the civilian personnel involved, shall be transferred, in such amounts as may be agreed upon by the Secretary of the Interior and the Secretary of Commerce, to the Geological Survey, and shall become available for expenditure under the supervision of the Secretary of the Interior.

Sec. 4. That after this Act becomes effective, the Coast and Geodetic Survey of the Department of Commerce shall be known and designated as the United States Coast Survey.

Sec. 5. That all power and authority conferred by law upon the Department of Commerce, or the secretary thereof, in relation to the work hereby transferred, shall, immediately when said transfer becomes effective, be fully conferred upon and vested in the Department of the Interior, or the secretary thereof, as the case may be.

ANNUAL MEETING OF THE NORTHWEST SCIENTIFIC ASSOCIATION

The fourth annual meeting of the Northwest Scientific Association was held at Spokane, Washington, in the Davenport Hotel on Wednesday and Thursday, December 28 and 29, under the presidency of Mr. L. K. Armstrong, consulting engineer of Spokane. There was a noticeable increase in the number of members attending the sessions and in the number of guests and visitors over former years.

There were three general sessions in addition to the annual business meeting. One of the general meetings was devoted to medicine and surgery, the second to forest problems and the third to scientific research in history. There were also section meetings of the following sections: Botany, zoology, chemistry, physics, education, engineering, forestry, geology, geography, plant pathology and social science.

The annual dinner of the association was held on Wednesday evening in the Elizabethan Room, Davenport Hotel. On this occasion the address of the retiring president, President Chas. H. Clapp, University of Montana, was delivered. His subject was "National Resources and World Problems."

The following officers were elected for the year 1928:

President: Dr. E. A. Bryan, president emeritus of Washington State College, Pullman, Washington.
Vice-president: Dean Ivan C. Crawford, State University, Moscow, Idaho.
Secretary-treasurer: J. W. Hungate, State Normal School, Cheney, Washington.

At the business meeting the report of the committee on facilities for research and publication was adopted. This report carried the recommendation that the association take steps to form a corporation jointly with the Eastern Washington Historical Society, the resulting body to be known as The Northwest Institute of Arts and Science. A committee will be appointed by the incoming president for the purpose of conferring with a committee from the Eastern Washington Historical Society, this committee to report to the association for confirmation of the terms of cooperation. The association also passed a resolution favoring the enactment of the forest research bill now pending in congress.

J. W. HUNGATE,
Secretary-Treasurer

RESOLUTIONS ON THE DEATH OF DR. FRANCIS W. PEABODY

THE following resolutions on the death of Dr. Francis Weld Peabody have been passed by the trustees of the Boston City Hospital:

By the death of Dr. Francis Weld Peabody the Boston City Hospital has lost a distinguished member of its staff. As director of the Thorndike Laboratory, which was established to prove that the study of disease and research into its causes was as necessary a function of a municipal hospital as of one privately endowed, his success has become a part of the hospital's history and the Thorndike Laboratory, under his guidance, has occupied a foremost place among institutions of its kind. His scientific imagination, intellectual capacity, mental balance and persevering zeal brought him fame as an investigator, while his generous encouragement of his assistants and his appreciative support of their efforts created an organization which would reflect credit on any hospital. His brief seven years of service not only demonstrated the wisdom of the experiment, but it founded a tradition whose effect can not be lost. His interest never flagged during his long illness, and through it all he remained the directing force. He never lost his sense of values in his enthusiasm for research, and in his relations with his patient he was preeminently the good physician. He healed when it was possible, but always he comforted. He was an eminent teacher for he sensed the difficulties of his students. Never didactic, he showed them the way to solve their own problems. Meanwhile he instilled the highest ideals of the art of medicine. His life was one of steady growth, and ever widening influence. His attractive personality and forgetfulness of self, his sympathy and understanding helpfulness, bound his colleagues to him with the strongest ties of affection. Young men found in him an inspiration, while the older leaders of the profession, in which he had become a master, saw in him the bearer of the torch which they were laying down. His life must be measured not by the number of his years, but by the record of his accomplishments, and by the heritage of his example. His character combined the strong qualities of his New England ancestry, softened by tolerance and charity, and nowhere was it better shown than in the courage with which for months he faced the inevitable end.

The trustees of the Boston City Hospital, in placing on record their appreciation of the high qualities of the man, and of his work, wish to express their realization of the great loss which the community has suffered. They share the sorrow of the multitude of his friends, and extend to his family their heartfelt sympathy.

THE NINTH INTERNATIONAL CONGRESS OF PSYCHOLOGY

AN International Congress of Psychology will be held at Yale University, New Haven, in the late summer of 1929. After eight European congresses, beginning in Paris in 1889, it has been decided to meet in America, following an invitation extended by the American Psychological Association at the time of the Philadelphia meeting a year ago. This having been accepted by the international committee, plans for the conduct of the congress were drawn up by a committee of the association, and these were finally adopted at the recent Columbus meeting.

The control of the arrangements for the conduct of the meeting has been delegated to a national committee of twenty-one psychologists, eighteen of whom, including the three principal officers, were elected by a nominating committee and a formal ballot from members and associates of the Psychological Association. Three further members were coopted by the elected committee and eighteen of the twenty-one members were present at the meeting for organization at the Ohio State University.

At that time other officers were elected, and the general plans for the congress were considered and in part decided. The possibility of meeting consecutively in Cambridge, New Haven and New York with a visit to Princeton was considered, and the relative advantages of different universities, including Cornell and Chicago. Yale University was selected owing to its convenient location, the social advantages of meeting in a smaller city and the recent notable development of psychology in that institution.

It is hoped that there will be a large attendance of foreign delegates from all parts of the world. Plans have been initiated by which as many exchange and other professorships and lectureships, summer-school positions, etc., as possible will be filled that year by foreign psychologists, and it may be possible to arrange lectures and conferences in different cities. This will have the advantage of increasing appreciation of scientific psychology and in the promotion of international information and good-will, while at the same time assisting to defray the cost of travel for foreign members.

The American Psychological Association now has about 600 members and 200 associates, all of whom are professional psychologists. Election to membership requires an advanced degree or its equivalent, the publication of research work of some consequence and under ordinary circumstances a permanent position in psychology. All members and associates of the association are invited and expected to become members of the congress. Others from North America can become members only by invitation. Invitations will be sent to the leading psychologists of the world and it is hoped that psychological societies in foreign countries will cooperate in the arrangements.

The officers of the congress are:

President: J. McKeen Cattell, New York.
Vice-president: James R. Angell, Yale University.
Secretary: Edwin G. Boring, Harvard University.
Foreign Secretary: Herbert S. Langfeld, Princeton University.
Executive Secretary: Walter S. Hunter, Clark University.
Treasurer: R. S. Woodworth, Columbia University.
Chairman of the Program Committee: Raymond Dodge, Yale University.
Additional Members of the National Committee: John E. Anderson, University of Minnesota; Madison Bentley, University of Illinois; E. A. Bott, University of Toronto; Harvey A. Carr, University of Chicago; Knight Dunlap, The Johns Hopkins University; Samuel W. Fernberger, University of Pennsylvania; William McDougall, Duke University; W. B. Pillsbury, University of Michigan; Carl E. Seashore, University of Iowa; Lewis M. Terman, Stanford University; Edward L. Thorndike, Teachers College, Columbia University; Howard C. Warren, Princeton University; Margaret F. Washburn, Vassar College; Robert M. Yerkes, Yale University.

SCIENTIFIC NOTES AND NEWS

Dr. Charles Greeley Abbot has been appointed secretary of the Smithsonian Institution to fill the vacancy caused by the death of Dr. Charles D. Walcott. Dr. Abbot was appointed assistant director of the institution in 1928, and during the past year has been acting director.

The Perkin medal will be presented to Dr. Irving Langmuir, of the General Electric Co., on January 13 at a joint meeting of the Society of Chemical Industry, Société de Chime Industrielle, American Chemical Society and American Electrochemical Society. Addresses will be made by Dr. E. Hendrick, Dr. W. R. Whitney, Wm. H. Nichols and Dr. Langmuir.

Dr. Simon Flexner, director of the laboratories of the Rockefeller Institute for Medical Research, has been elected an honorary member of the Medical Society of Berlin.

Dr. Hideyo Noguchi, of the Rockefeller Institute, has been elected to membership in the Kaiserlich Leopold Deutsche Akademie der Naturforscher, of Halle.

Dr. Max Wolf, director of Heidelberg Observatory, distinguished especially for his originality and activity in observational astronomy, was elected an honorary member of the American Astronomical Society at its thirty-ninth meeting in New Haven. The constitution of the society permits the election of only one honorary member at each annual meeting. There are but five other living honorary members and the last election was made in 1924.

Dr. Charles D. Marx, professor emeritus of civil engineering at Stanford University, has been elected an honorary member of the American Society of Civil Engineers.

Lloyd E. Jackson and George H. Johnson, senior industrial fellows of Mellon Institute of Industrial Research, University of Pittsburgh, have been elected to honorary membership in the National Association of Dyers and Cleaners.

The Journal of the Washington Academy of Sciences notes that on the occasion of his seventieth birthday, August 13, 1927, the honorary degree of doctor of natural sciences was conferred upon H. Pittier by the University of Lausanne, Switzerland, "to distinguish the merits of his work concerning the natural history of Canton de Vaud (Switzerland) and Latin America and to acknowledge his efforts in the promotion of colonial agriculture."

The court of the University of Wales will confer the honorary degree of LL.D. upon Sir Thomas Lewis, F.R.S., for his distinguished scientific work in medicine, particularly in cardiology; upon Sir Robert Philip, president of the British Medical Association, for his distinguished services to the science and profession of medicine, and upon Dr. H. B. Brackenbury, chairman of the council of the British Medical Association, for his distinguished services to the profession of medicine.

Professor Calmette, subdirector of the Pasteur Institute, has been elected a member of the French Academy of Sciences.

Professor F. Mares, head of the department of physiology of the medical faculty at Prague, recently celebrated his seventieth birthday and is shortly to retire.

The title of emeritus professor of pathology in the University of London has been conferred on Sir Frederick Andrewes, who retired from the university professorship of pathology, tenable at St. Bartholomew's Hospital Medical College, last July.

Dr. Rudolph Matas, who recently retired from the professorship of surgery at Tulane University Medical School, has been made professor emeritus.

Dr. Anson Hayes, who is leaving Iowa State College at the end of the present quarter to become chief chemist of the American Rolling Mills Company, was the guest at a dinner in his honor given by the members of the chemistry faculty on December 19.

Members of the staff of the U. S. Bureau of Dairy Industry gave a dinner in Washington on December

16 in honor of Dr. C. W. Larson, chief of the bureau, who resigned on January 1 to become director of the National Dairy Council with headquarters at Chicago.

DR. FRANK BILLINGS has been elected president of the McCormick Institute for Infectious Diseases, and Dr. James B. Herrick, vice-president. Dr. Ludvig Hektoen is secretary. During the coming year the principal subject for research at the institute will be infantile paralysis.

DR. JAMES G. NEEDHAM, professor of entomology at Cornell University, is chairman of the local committee of the fourth International Congress of Entomology which meets in Ithaca from August 12 to 18, 1928, under the presidency of Dr. L. O. Howard.

DR. FRED H. ALBEE, professor of orthopedic surgery at the New York Postgraduate Medical School, has been elected president of the Pan-American Medical Association for the ensuing year and will soon begin a tour of the Latin-American countries in which the association operates.

DR. EDWARD RAY WEIDLEIN, director of the Mellon Institute of Industrial Research, University of Pittsburgh, was reelected president of the American Institute of Chemical Engineers at the recent St. Louis meeting.

AT the eighteenth annual meeting of the National Committee for Mental Hygiene, New York, on November 10, Dr. Charles P. Emerson, dean of the Indiana University School of Medicine, Indianapolis, was elected president; Drs. Bernard Sachs, New York, and William L. Russell, White Plains, were among the vice-presidents elected, and Dr. William H. Welch, Baltimore, continues as honorary president.

DR. C. R. BALL, senior agronomist in charge of the office of cereal crops and diseases of the U. S. Bureau of Plant Industry, has been elected by the American Society of Agronomy as agronomic adviser to the National Research Council.

AT the annual meeting of the Asociacion de Tecnicos Azucarera de Cuba, H. J. B. Scharnberg was elected vice-president of engineering.

THE council of the Museums and Art Galleries Association of Great Britain has elected Sir Francis G. Ogilvie, chairman of the Geological Survey Board, president for 1927–28, in succession to Mr. J. A. Charlton Deas.

DR. A. A. L. RUTGERS, director of agriculture, industry and commerce in the Netherlands East Indies, has been appointed governor of Surinam (Dutch Guiana).

SIR DAWSON WILLIAMS, who will shortly complete his thirtieth year as editor of the *British Medical Journal,* and who before his appointment to that post in 1898, had for seventeen years been connected with the editorial department, has resigned. Dr. N. G. Horner, who has been assistant editor for the past eleven years, will succeed Sir Dawson Williams as editor.

DR. HUGH POTTER BAKER, who was formerly dean of the College of Forestry at Syracuse University, has been appointed head of a new department of the U. S. Chamber of Commerce which will work with trade organizations.

DR. FRANK E. RICE has resigned as chairman of the department of chemistry at the North Carolina State College to join the Evaporated Milk Association.

B. J. NICHOLS, who has been studying under Professor Svedberg at Upsala under a Swedish-American Fellowship, has returned to this country. He has accepted a position with E. I. du Pont de Nemours & Company in their Wilmington laboratory, where he will be engaged in research in colloids.

PROFESSOR ELIAS T. CLARK, of the forestry department at the University of Washington, is being relieved of some of his work at the university to enable him to serve as supervising logging engineer for several timber companies in the state. The courses Professor Clark is giving at the university at present will remain under his direction.

PROFESSOR JEROME J. MORGAN, assistant professor of chemical engineering in Columbia University, plans to spend the spring months in Europe, leaving in January. He will travel through France, Italy, Germany, England, etc., studying the state of the gas industry and other developments in chemical engineering.

DR. ANGELO GALLARDO, Argentinian foreign minister, who formerly held the chair of zoology at the University of Buenos Aires, has arrived in Berlin as the guest of the German government.

DR. ALFRED ADLER, Vienna, will return to New York to give a series of lectures on psychology from February 14 to March 22.

THE address of the retiring president of the Philosophical Society of Washington, Commander James P. Ault, on "Ocean Surveys—Problems and Developments," was delivered at a meeting of the society held in the Cosmos Club on January 7.

DR. WILLIAM A. WHITE, of Washington, delivered his presidential address to the American Psychoanalytical Society at the Waldorf Hotel on December 27.

DR. HANS ZINSSER, professor of bacteriology and immunology in the Harvard Medical School, addressed the New York Academy of Medicine, January 5, on "The Significance of Bacterial Allergy in Infectious Diseases."

Dr. J. A. Detlefsen, of the University of Pennsylvania, delivered a lecture to the Academy of Stomatology of the Philadelphia County Medical Society on November 30 and to the New York Society of Orthodontists on December 14 on "Hereditary Constitution *vs.* External Conditions in Dental Problems." The data were based on his studies of the dentures of identical twins.

Dr. William J. Mayo, of the Mayo Clinic, Rochester, Minn., will read a paper on splenomegaly and Dr. Alexis Carrel, of the Rockefeller Institute for Medical Research, will show one of his new films dealing with some phases of his researches at the next meeting of the Johns Hopkins Medical Society which will be held in the auditorium of the School of Hygiene and Public Health on January 16.

Dr. Herbert Maule Richards, professor of botany at Barnard College, Columbia University, died on January 9, aged fifty-six years.

Dr. Willis L. Moore, professor of meteorology at George Washington University and formerly chief of the U. S. Weather Bureau, died on December 18, aged seventy-one years.

Dr. J. Homer Wright, assistant professor of pathology at the Harvard Medical School, died on January 3, aged sixty-two years.

Dr. F. S. Luther, president emeritus of Trinity College, and formerly professor of mathematics, died on January 4, aged seventy-eight years.

Dr. Edward V. d'Invilliers, consulting geologist and mining engineer of Philadelphia, died on January 4, aged seventy years.

Federal and state corn borer research programs for 1928 were discussed by agriculturists concerned with the corn borer situation at a conference held at the U. S. Department of Agriculture on January 3. The conference was attended by deans of agricultural colleges, directors of experiment stations and other scientists from 14 states. The program of the department was outlined. The work contemplated falls into six general groups, including: entomology, agricultural engineering, agronomy, animal husbandry, chemistry and soils and agricultural economics.

The annual meeting of the Northeastern Bird Banding Association will be held on January 19, at the University Club, Boston. A field day is planned at Scituate and Cohasset on January 20.

The first annual dinner of the Ringer Society was held on December 10 at Jules Restaurant, London, with Dr. Henry Ellis, in the chair. A large company of guests were present. The president delivered the Ringer oration. The society is named after Sydney Ringer, one of the first clinicians to realize the value of physiology and biochemistry applied to practical medicine, and known by his perfusion experiments with the fluid bearing his name.

The juvenile Christmas lectures at the Royal Institution were delivered by Professor E. N. da C. Andrade on "Engines," commencing on December 29. The general courses of lectures before Easter will begin on Tuesday, January 17, when P. R. Coursey will deliver the first of two lectures on the development of dielectrics for electrical condensers. On Tuesday afternoons there will be six lectures by Professor Julian S. Huxley on the behavior of animals. On Thursday afternoons at the same hour there will be three lectures by Sir William Bragg on Faraday's notebooks; two by Dr. J. J. Fox on optics and chemistry, and two by Group Capt. M. Flack on the physiological aspects of flying. Sir Ernest Rutherford will deliver four lectures on the transformation of matter on Saturday afternoons at three o'clock. The Friday evening meetings will start on January 20, when the discourse will be delivered by Sir William Bragg on photo-electricity. Succeeding discourses will include one (on March 2) on the psychology of the sick, by Sir Farquhar Buzzard, the new Regius professor of medicine at Oxford, and another by the daughter of his predecessor, Miss D. A. E. Garrod, on prehistoric cave art. The discourse on February 3 will be by Professor E. C. C. Baly on photosynthesis, and that on February 17 by the Rev. Dr. E. M. Walker on the university, its ideals and its problems. Other lectures will be given by Professor B. Melvil Jones, Professor E. A. Milne, Sir Ernest Rutherford and others.

Colonel William Cooper Procter, president of the Procter and Gamble Company, has announced a gift of $2,500,000 to the Children's Hospital in Cincinnati, to be used to construct a building to house research work in connection with the hospital and to endow a clinic. The proposed research building, which is expected to cost from $300,000 to $500,000, will accommodate an out-patient clinic, laboratory facilities for research, class rooms and living quarters for research fellows. The endowment will provide an income for the employment of fellows, who will be appointed by the board of trustees of the hospital. The endowment also will provide a budget for clinical investigations, laboratory work, social service studies, child welfare investigations and psychological studies.

PLANS for using an endowment given to Battle Creek College by Mrs. Mary F. Henderson, of Washington, as the basis for a nation-wide race betterment movement were announced by Dr. John H. Kellogg at the close of the Third Race Betterment Conference at Battle Creek, Mich. Mrs. Henderson has given to the institution an endowment of $200,000 and a 4,000-acre farm in Missouri in the interest of race betterment. It is planned to make the college a race betterment institution.

THE grass herbarium of the U. S. National Museum has received from the Institut Botanique, Montpellier, France, through Professor J. Daveau, conservator, a valuable package containing duplicates or fragments of specimens of Paspalum. Among them are a good series of Salzmann's collections of Paspalum from Bahia, Brazil, some of Husnot's from Martinique and other early collections not before represented in the grass herbarium.

THE sum of £100 is being offered by the Royal Society for the Protection of Birds for an invention of a portable apparatus for the detection of small quantities of carbon monoxide in mines, to supersede the use of canaries and small wild birds now forming part of the equipment of rescue brigades. All competing essays should be received by March 31

THE *Nation's Health,* which for a few years has been published in Chicago, has been transferred with its contracts, lists, good-will and other assets to the American Public Health Association to be published with the *American Journal of Public Health.*

UNIVERSITY AND EDUCATIONAL NOTES

THE Carnegie Corporation of New York appropriated $2,000,000 and paid more than $4,000,000 on previous grants for the fiscal year ended on September 30, 1927, in support of colleges, universities and other educational organizations, according to the report of its president, Dr. Frederick P. Keppel, which was recently made public. Of the appropriations $831,500 went for educational studies. "Only $84,-000" was appropriated for libraries, chiefly for the maintenance of library schools. Other grants included $97,600 for adult education, $150,000 for the Carnegie Endowment for International Peace and $500,000 in encouragement of the fine arts.

ON November 8 the city of Cincinnati, by a majority of 31,000, voted for $1,425,000 for its municipal university, the University of Cincinnati. Out of these funds will be constructed an addition to the power plant, library and recitation hall and a new building for the college of education.

DUKE UNIVERSITY has received from Mr. C. C. Dula, president of the Liggett and Myers Tobacco Company, $200,000 to be added to the university's endowment fund.

AN engineering building, which will be erected at a cost of between $250,000 and $500,000, has been donated to Drexel Institute by Cyrus H. K. Curtis, of Philadelphia.

DR. F. A. WOLL has been promoted to be full professor and head of the department of hygiene in the College of the City of New York.

DR. R. F. RUTTAN, director of the department of chemistry at McGill University, and Dr. A. B. MacCallum, head of the department of biochemistry, have resigned. Dr. J. B. Collip, professor of biochemistry at the University of Alberta, has been appointed to succeed Dr. MacCallum.

M. VILLEMIN has been named professor of anatomy at the University of Bordeaux to succeed M. Picqué.

DISCUSSION AND CORRESPONDENCE

ON THE MECHANISM OF ORIENTATION OF ATOMS IN MAGNETIC AND ELECTRIC FIELDS

WHEN atoms possessing magnetic or electric moments are subjected to a field they are supposed to take up definite quantized directions with respect to the field. Experimental confirmation of this view has been made for the magnetic case in the experiments of Gerlach and Stern, but the mechanism by which the orientation takes place presents serious difficulties which may be briefly summarized as follows. In the absence of collisions and radiation the field, of course, can produce only a precession of the atom about the direction of the field. The experiments of Gerlach and Stern, however, show that the atom comes to equilibrium with its moment in definite quantized directions relative to the field and it does this in a time which is less than 10^{-4} sec. Since no collisions are taking place in the beam the only possible method by which the atom can change its energy to become oriented is by the emission or absorption of radiation. But unless the probability of a transition from a non-quantum to a quantum state is very much greater than between two quantum states this process should take something like 10^{10} sec. according to a calculation by Einstein and Ehrenfest.[1]

[1] Einstein and Ehrenfest, *Zeit. für Physik,* 11, 31, 1922.

This difficulty may be avoided if it be supposed that the oven chamber in which the atoms of the beam made their last collision is subjected to a stray field which is parallel to the deflecting field, for it has been shown by experiments with resonance radiation that a small field (of the order of a few gauss) is sufficient to cause complete orientation in the presence of collisions. Although this solution of the difficulty has been ruled out by Stoner on the supposition that the oven chamber was magnetically shielded yet in view of the fact that only small fields are sufficient to produce orientation and since if stray fields were present they would, from the geometry of the apparatus, have been parallel to the deflecting field, it seems that this cause of orientation should be given more weight.

A striking confirmation of the view that the atoms become oriented by stray fields in the oven chamber is provided by the recently published article by E. Wrede[2] on the deflection of beams of electric dipole molecules in a non-homogeneous electric field. In these experiments the oven, where collisions were taking place, was unquestionably field free and the traces produced by the deflected beam shows that the molecules had no definite quantized direction. We have here, then, a case where the field is unable to produce orientation in the absence of collisions.

A further test of the ability of the field to produce orientations might be made by a repetition of the Gerlach and Stern experiment, subjecting the oven chamber to definite magnetic fields. For example, if the oven field were at right angles to the deflecting field the orientations produced during collisions, in the case of atoms with a magnetic moment of but one magneton, would be in such directions that no deflection would be produced unless the deflecting field were able to change the orientation.

Thomas H. Johnson
The Bartol Research Foundation
of the Franklin Institute

[2] E. Wrede, *Zeits. für Physik*, 44, 261, 1927.

THE IDENTITY OF CLEAR CREEK SKULL

Considerable discussion has occurred in regard to the identification of a calvarium found at Clear Creek near Everton, Arkansas, and purchased by Mrs. Bernie Babcock for the Museum of Natural History and Antiquities, Little Rock, Ark. As there has been unusual publicity concerning the age of this skull, it was necessary to obtain its accurate classification. The specimen was examined by Dr. T. Wingate Todd, professor of anatomy, Western Reserve University, and compared with the remarkable collection of models of the important fossil skulls, together with numerous crania of *Homo sapiens* in the Hamann Museum.

The calvarium (Fig. 1) is obviously that of a

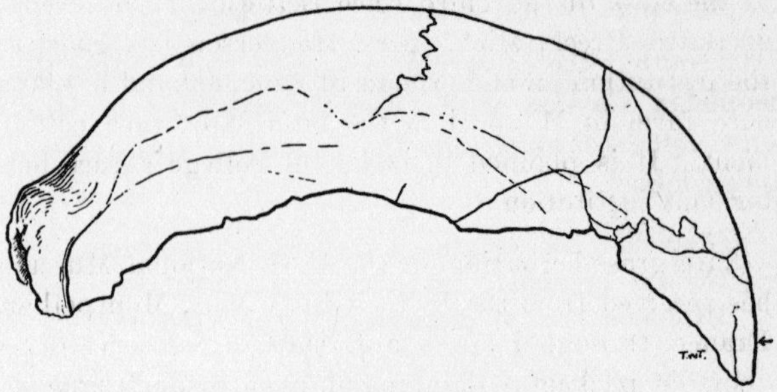

dolicocephalic individual because the cephalic index is approximately 65.4 mm. The large supraorbital ridges proclaim a male, and the union of all vault sutures[1] together with the texture, indicate a man about fifty years of age. The thicknesses of the vault are

Glabellar region	12.5 mm.
Vertical thickness at bregma	7.0 "
Region of lambda	6.5 "
Parietal eminence (approximately)	5.5 "

Compared with corresponding dimensions on the modern male, white cranium, these thicknesses are but slightly greater than those of the average contemporary man.[2]

The supraorbital ridges possess the lozenge characteristics of contemporary dolicocephalic man, whether of white or American Indian stock. There is slight ridging of the sagittal vertex region and slight flattening of the parietal slopes as in primitive

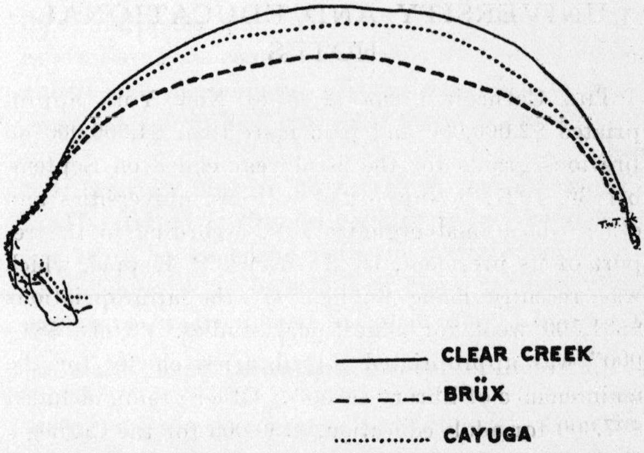

[1] Todd, T. W., and Lyon, D. W., Jr., "Endocranial suture closure; its progress and age relationship, Part 1," *Am. J. Phys. Anthrop.*, 7, 325–384, 1924; and Ectocranial closure in adult males of white stock, Part 2, *Am. J. Phys. Anthrop.*, 8, 23–45, 1925. *Anat. Record*, 27, 245–256, 1924.

[2] Todd, T. W., "Thickness of the male white cranium."

dolicocephalic peoples. The dimensions obtainable are

Glabello-inion length	191.5 mm. (?)
Probable euryon breadth	127.5 "
Minimum frontal diameter	94.0 "

In contour the calvarium resembles very closely the people of Cayuga skull (Fig. 2) presented in Morton's volume,[3] which has the following approximate dimensions:

Glabello-inion length	195.0 mm.
Euryon breadth	127.5 "
Minimum frontal diameter	105.0 "

In our calvarium the frontal bone extends rather further backwards on the vault than in the Cayuga skull.

In Hrdlička's excellent résumé[4] the Rock Bluff cranium discovered in 1866 most closely resembles our specimen. The dimensions of this cranium are

Glabello-inion length	195.0 mm.
Euryon breadth	137.0 "
Minimum frontal diameter	97.0 "

Hrdlička's description fits our skull equally well. Its most noteworthy feature, and that which gives it the appearance of a specimen of low type, is its greatly developed supraorbital ridges. These are not in the form of arcs, however, as in anthropoids and in the human skulls of Spy, Neanderthal, etc., and to a less extent in the two Calaveras specimens, but involve, as general among Indians, only about the median three fifths of the supranasal and supraorbital portions of the frontal bone. They project greatly forward, however.

In comparing the profile of our calvarium with that of Brünn[5] we note that whereas the supraorbital ridges of both are equally pronounced, the Brünn specimen has a lower vault and less prominent forehead.

The calvarium is devoid of organic material, but this may well occur within a century of burial. There is no mineralization or other evidences of great antiquity such as would be indicated by relationship to the Conard Fissure material[6] from northern Arkansas.

[3] Morton, S. G., *Crania Americana*, Phila., Plate 35, 1839.

[4] Hrdlička, A., "Skeletal remains suggesting or attributed to early man in North America." *Forms Bull.* 33, of Smithson. Inst. Bur. Am. Ethnol. 30, 1907.

[5] Schwalbe, G., "Das Schädelfragment von Brüx und verwandte Schädelformen." *Ztschr. f. Morphol. u. Anthrop.*, 9, 81–182, 1906.

[6] Brown, B., "The Conard Fissure; a Pleistocene bone deposit in northern Arkansas," *Manual* American Museum of Natural History, 9, 155–208, 1908.

Mrs. Babcock and the Museum of Natural History and Antiquities are to be congratulated upon the zeal which saved this specimen from oblivion, and, although there is no reasonable doubt of its belonging to an American Indian with a head shaped like that of the notorious Cayuga, its primitive character indicates that we may hope to find other evidence of low grade dolicocephalic people in the locality.

HARVEY S. THATCHER
UNIVERSITY OF ARKANSAS,
SCHOOL OF MEDICINE

BIBLIOGRAPHY OF COLORIMETRY

IN connection with the work of the colorimetry section of the Bureau of Standards and the report of the colorimetry committee of the Optical Society of America, I am desirous of compiling a bibliography of papers and books having direct bearing on colorimetry, spectrophotometry, and color specifications. It is expected that this bibliography will ultimately be published in the Journal of the Optical Society. It will also be of use in replying to frequent inquiries for information on this subject. In the interest of completeness and accuracy, all authors who have contributed to this subject are requested to send me check lists of their papers giving titles and complete journal references.

The following subjects are mentioned as illustrative of the classes of material desired:

1. Color of daylight and artificial sources. (Spectral distribution of energy, color temperature.)
2. Visual psychophysical data. (*E.g.*, visibility of energy, hue discrimination, saturation discrimination, brilliance discrimination, excitations, abnormal color sense.)
3. Theories of color vision.
4. Methods of computing the trilinear coordinates, dominant wave-length, and purity from data on spectral distribution.
5. Spectrophotometric instruments and methods.
6. Spectral transmission of materials.
7. Reflectance of materials.
8. Colorimeters.
9. Systems of color standards.
10. Applications of colorimetry and photometry to chemical analysis.
11. Turbidity and scattering of light.
12. Color nomenclature and terminology.

Reprints will also be of real service and will be gratefully received. I already have a considerable collection of such reprints. They are classified by subjects, and are of great assistance to those engaged in colorimetric research at the Bureau of Standards. This collection has been profitably used not only by regular members of the staff but by temporary research associates and visitors at the bureau. It is desired to keep it up to date and make it as complete as possible. Authors who have reprints available can very effectively assist in the dissemination of information by contributing copies to this collection, since by consulting it workers on a given subject can find together in one place the pertinent literature, the discovery of which would otherwise require diligent and laborious search through many scattered journals on physics, chemistry, psychology, physiology and sundry kinds of technology.

IRWIN G. PRIEST

BUREAU OF STANDARDS,
WASHINGTON, D. C.

NO METEORITE

ON November 12, 1927, newspapers in the Eastern States carried a New York *World* News Service statement that on November 11 a meteor, accompanied by a bolt of lightning, struck at Fairdale, near Montrose, Susquehanna County, Pennsylvania. The lightning set fire to a building and the meteor made holes 12 to 14 inches in diameter in the concrete highway. Of particular interest was the statement that around these holes in the highway was discovered a strange substance that very much resembled bituminous coal.

The Pennsylvania Geological Survey made inquiry through different channels and received a most satisfactory reply and explanation from H. R. Moffitt, district engineer, Pennsylvania Department of Highways, at Scranton. He writes:

> Lightning struck a barn to which an aerial was attached, running thence to the house and down the ground wire and was apparently conducted through the water that covered the ground at this location, to the pavement. The pavement in several places was shattered along the edge about 10 inches in from the edge and about three inches deep, where the concrete was broken out exposing the reinforcing. The total breaks can be repaired with about one gallon of tar and one hundred pounds of stone. The asphalt crack filler, in several places, was blown out and burned and the material resembled soft coal, which I believe gave rise to the newspaper account of the story.

This note is published so that future catalogs of meteorites will not include this one from Fairdale, Pennsylvania.

R. W. STONE

HARRISBURG, PA.

CONSIDER THE USER OF BULLETINS

IN SCIENCE of December 9, Professor R. J. Barnet, under this cleverly worded title, has given some very good advice to those who control the make-up of bulletins. But he might very justifiably have gone further. Those of us who have to consult the technical and non-technical bulletins of the federal government, of the States and of other institutions, often find fault; and as to the librarians, those long-suffering people deserve our very deep sympathy.

Professor Barnet seems especially annoyed by the difficulty he has had in finding the names of the authors of certain American bulletins, and urges very sensibly that these names be displayed uniformly on the cover page or the title page. My first reaction was the reflection: "Well, after all, we do better than the British." I had in mind especially some of the publications of the Board of Agriculture and Fisheries, the authorship of which I have seldom been able to learn. The beautifully illustrated, but anonymous No. 44 of the "Miscellaneous Publications" of this ministry, entitled "Wasps," pleased me so much that, after a very considerable effort, two years in duration, I learned that it was written by that competent entomologist, R. A. Stenton, now of the Parasite Laboratory of the Imperial Bureau of Entomology at Farnham Royal.

But we must not criticize our British friends while we ourselves are open to criticism. We do not follow the advice of our own best people. As long ago as 1919 the Association of Agricultural College Editors formulated recommendations on the very points brought out by Professor Barnet, and yet they have not been followed by all.

Professor Barnet might have pointed out other things. I have been talking them over with Miss Mabel Colcord, the skilled librarian and bibliographer of this bureau, and from our somewhat different viewpoints we have sympathized about several of these other things. How is one to give exact references with the minimum of trouble when such magazines as *The Scientific American* and *The Scientific Monthly* conceal volume and number in their advertising pages? What is one to do about a repaged reprint (See R. H. Rastall, *Nature,* March 20, 1926, page 418)? Then too, why should scientific men from time to time, as they do, send out reprints or preprints carrying only author's name and the title of the article, with no date and no indication of what it is taken from? Why should the division reports from the various British colonies fail to state the country they represent? Why, in bibliographic lists, should translated titles be given without also the title in the language and the wording of the author? In simple justice to the author, it seems that it should be given as he states it. *The Experiment Station Record* of this department fails in this respect. There are other questions of this kind. They have been discussed, most of them, elsewhere and at various times.

I wish to add one last word, on the desirability of printing the name of the author of the species following the scientific plant or animal name. I labored for years to secure this obviously just custom with one important bibliographical publication before the publishers were convinced of its importance.

L. O. HOWARD

BUREAU OF ENTOMOLOGY,
U. S. DEPARTMENT OF AGRICULTURE

SCIENTIFIC BOOKS

Stars and Atoms: A. S. EDDINGTON, Sc.D., F.R.S., Plumian Professor of Astronomy in the University of Cambridge. New Haven: Yale University Press. London: Oxford University Press. pp. 127.

IN "Stars and Atoms" Professor Eddington has given us one of the most valuable and delightful monographs on astronomy that has ever appeared in the literature of science.

The rapid strides of physics and chemistry into the realms of the stars have fairly bewildered students of the older astronomy, and it is a remarkable service which the author has rendered in giving to the general reader, without mathematical details, the essential problems of modern astrophysics. With a sufficiently extensive description of the atom and its ionization that will enable the general reader to picture the mechanism of radiation and radiative temperature, the author portrays the essential make-up of the sun and stars and makes clear the problem of the maintenance of their heat.

When one reads the all too often dogmatic statements concerning recent advances in astronomy, one feels refreshed in finding so great an authority as Dr. Eddington sounding notes of caution while making sharp distinctions between the demonstrable and the speculative.

The saving sense of humor which relieves the dilemma in many an embarrassing scientific situation keeps the reader in friendly terms with the scientist, even in his wildest guesses and in the end fosters a genuine faith and confidence in results of notable significance.

In few books, indeed, does one sense more acutely the true spirit of science in its never-ending quest for divining the nature of things. From the first chapter to the last the reader is carried at almost breathless pace through round after round of astrophysical discovery till he is introduced to matter in all but unbelievable states as it exists in the companion to Sirius.

In his final chapter on stellar evolution, Dr. Eddington makes a strong argument for the annihilation of matter through the radiation of mass, but does not overlook such technical details and perplexities as the simultaneous existence of giant and dwarf stars in coeval clusters, the problem of devising laws for the release of subatomic energy consistent with the demands of astronomical observations and at the same time reconcilable with any satisfactory picture of the annihilation of matter which the student of subatomic activity can postulate.

A lesser scholar than Eddington would not have closed the book with an anticlimax. It is a mark of genius and modesty worthy of a successor to the traditions of Newton that his closing paragraph should read:

> I should like to have closed these lectures by leading up to some great climax. But perhaps it is more in accordance with the conditions of scientific progress that they should fizzle out with a glimpse of the obscurity which marks the frontiers of knowledge I do not apologize for the lameness of the conclusion, for it is not a conclusion. I wish that I could feel confident that it is even a beginning.

H. T. STETSON

SPECIAL ARTICLES

THE CORRELATION BETWEEN INTELLIGENCE AND SPEED IN CONDUCTION OF THE NERVE IMPULSE IN A REFLEX ARC

THE present paper is a preliminary report of a study to determine if there is any relationship between the factors of intelligence and reflex time or speed in conduction of the nerve impulse in a reflex arc.

My work of the last three years as a fellow of the National Research Council has centered around an investigation of the neural processes in stuttering, and there has developed out of this research a refined technique for utilizing action current measurements in functional neuromuscular derangements. In studying certain reflexes during stuttering among patients widely different in intelligence an apparent relationship between reflex time and intelligence or mental ability was noted. These observations were verified on the patellar tendon reflex. Nearly all the excellent work that has been done on this reflex has involved so-called gross reflex time or the time elapsing between the application of the stimulus and the movement of the foot or thickening of the muscle. This gross reflex time probably would not correlate very highly with such mental factors as we wish to study because nine tenths of the time is taken up by movement of the muscles in extending the foot and any factor affecting the central nervous mechanism would be masked. Our technique provides a means of determining the length of time elapsing between the stimulation of the patellar tendon and the production of the action currents in the muscles, which is about one tenth as long as the gross reflex time. In other words, it permits the measurement of speed of conduction in a reflex arc.

We secured a group of forty-four individuals ranging in mental ability from feeble-mindedness to that of very superior university men and gave the Otis test of mental ability, Higher Examination, Form A, which has a reliability coefficient of .921. The correlation between the scores on this test and the reflex times was found to be .87 with a probable error of .024. The bright individual has a short reflex time, while the dull individual has a long reflex time. This high correlation is really astounding inasmuch as we are undoubtedly dealing with an imperfect measure of intelligence. Even if the test scores represented absolute measurements of intelligence we could not expect a higher correlation. We therefore took every precaution to verify our findings both on the instrumental side and on the side of intelligence rating. We looked about for other criteria of alertness or intellectual responsiveness and also for a group of individuals which presented a fairly normal distribution of these mental characteristics. Forty-three university freshmen on whom the University of Iowa qualifying examination scores were available were selected to fulfill the above requirements. This examination aims to measure the ability of a student to do college work. The correlation between the University of Iowa qualifying scores and the reflex time again turned out to be .87 with a probable error of .025. The two correlations being equal is an element of chance. The correspondence between the intelligence ratings and the reflex times was very close, not only for widely separated individuals but for the intermediate subjects as well.

The mean score on the Otis of the forty-four subjects was 53.9 as compared to 53.0 obtained on 2,516 college students reported by Professor Otis. The range of our group was from thirteen to seventy-five as compared to the range of his group, twenty to seventy-five.

The mean score of the forty-three freshmen in the university qualifying examination was 362.0, which is approximately the mean of all freshmen students. The range of our group was the same as that of the entire freshman class inasmuch as every tenth student, which included the highest and the lowest, was selected from a list arranged in the order of percentile rank.

The apparatus finally developed to obtain the reflex time in the knee-jerk consisted of a three-stage, resistance coupled amplifier, a portable, three-element oscillograph, a vacuum-tube oscillator, a mechanical stimulating mechanism and a signal circuit.[1]

The amplifier furnished medium amplification and was exceptionally free from inherent disturbances. The oscillograph is manufactured by the Westinghouse Electric and Manufacturing Company. The element which recorded the action currents was approximately ten times as sensitive as the other two standard vibrator elements which furnish the signal and the time lines. A special photographic unit was devised to replace the one with which the oscillograph was originally equipped. This specially built unit will handle four hundred feet of moving picture film.

The oscillator is a General Radio Company product and was used to furnish a time line of a thousand complete cycles per second. The stimulating mechanism described elsewhere[2] delivered blows of constant intensity and at a uniform rate of six per minute. The signal circuit was actuated by discharging a condenser which had been charged previously.

The electrodes were German silver plates, twenty-seven millimeters in diameter, covered with canton flannel, which was soaked in a saturated saline solution before each experiment. One electrode was placed over the place where the femoral nerve enters the rectus femoris muscle which, according to an unpublished study by Tuttle and MacEwen, is half way between the superior margin of the patella and the anterior superior spine of the ilium. The second electrode was placed peripherally about six inches from the first. Control experiments have shown that the amplifier is stable and able to respond instantaneously to changes in potential impressed on the input.

The subjects were comfortably seated, with the thigh slightly elevated to put some tension on the quadriceps muscles. An explanation of the manner in which the experiment was going to be carried out was given to each subject in order to dispel any fears he might have of being shocked or injured. Care was taken also to select individuals who were not fatigued and who had not been ill recently.

Reflex time is determined in a record by ascertaining the length of time elapsing between the instant of application of the stimulus to the patellar tendon and the arrival of the action currents at the first electrode. Reflex times are read and reported in thousandths of a second. At least eight records were obtained on each subject.

[1] Theodore A. Hunter is to publish elsewhere a technical description of this set up.

[2] Tuttle and Travis. "A Comparative Study of the Extent of the Knee-jerk and the Achilles-jerk." *Am. J. Physiol.* 82, 1927, 147.

All reflex time experiments were made and the records read in ignorance of the results from the intelligence tests. Also fifteen records were selected at random and read by a disinterested person. The agreement between the two readings was practically perfect.

The mean reflex time of the forty-four Otis cases was .0194 seconds. The range was from .0114 to .0268 seconds. The mean reflex time of the forty-three university freshmen was .0197 seconds. The range was from .0154 to .0245 seconds.

Each group gave a fairly normal distribution in reflex time. The great individual differences in reflex time are considered as very important. It varied from 11/1000 to 27/1000 of a second. In other words conduction over a reflex arc in one individual was two and a half times as fast as conduction over the same reflex arc in another individual.

These marked differences in reflex times found in our groups are probably referable to differences in synaptic resistances in the arcs and not to differences in resistance of the nerve trunks. Just how much of the nervous system is involved in the patellar tendon reflex is a debated question, but a recent study by the writer[3] showed that the action current records during the knee-jerk were practically identical with those during voluntary extension of the foot. Both sets of records gave indication of two different rates of discharge, one furnishing the audio or principal frequency of from three hundred to six hundred oscillations per second, and the other, the modulating inaudible frequency of from eight to twelve per second. This slower rate of discharge is probably from the Betz cells in the precentral cortex and would indicate that the higher centers are involved in the knee-jerk. If this is true we are dealing with a considerably greater number of synapses than is commonly thought of in this connection and a larger fraction of the nervous system as well.

Although the individual differences in rate of conduction in the reflex arc we have been studying are great they take on real significance when viewed in connection with the complicated associational paths of the cerebral cortex which probably function in the higher mental processes.

We are here confronted with a new fact—a fact which has become available by the refinement of technique in measurement. It challenges us to reinvestigate all the generally recognized phenomena of this particular reflex. It opens up an unlimited vista of inquiries into the nature of its cause, the conditions under which it varies, and its meaning in psychological and physiological terms. It is conceivable that we are here dealing with a relatively complex reflex arc—perhaps more complex than has been suspected, and it is fair to assume that it is typical of a large number of reflex arcs which constitute an integrated central nervous system. Now, according to the best modern theories of intelligence the cognitive processes may be thought of as hierarchies of reflexes of which the vast majority are perhaps at as low a level in the central nervous system as that of the patellar reflex. If this is true, we have in the type of conduction through the patellar reflex arc a sample of the type of conduction that takes place in all well organized motor life and possibly, as these facts indicate, also the cognitive. Tests of intelligence have always stressed the element of speed and this is perhaps right, because an intelligent response to a complex situation may conceivably be thought of as a prompt response, radiating into a large number of systems. We may think of the central arcs of an individual as having a personal equation, just as we do in a gross way when we observe one man is quick and another is slow in his movements, even in his thought movements.

Whatever the interpretation through further study may prove to be, we have in this concept of the rate of conduction through a central arc, a new approach to the neuro-physiology of intelligence or mental alertness.

LEE EDWARD TRAVIS

UNIVERSITY OF IOWA

[3] Travis, Tuttle and Hunter. "The Tetanic Nature of the Knee-jerk Response in Man." *Am. J. Physiol.* 81, 1927, 670.

A COMPARISON OF GROWTH CURVES OF MAN AND OTHER ANIMALS

IN connection with investigations on the time relations of growth of domestic animals, several charts have been prepared on the growth of man. The purpose of this article is to present four of the most striking, or the most instructive, charts together with a few comments. For a background to this work and for details of technique the reader is referred to a series of Research Bulletins which are being published by the University of Missouri Agricultural Experiment Station (Columbia, Mo.).

Figure 1 represents an equivalence chart for growth of man and animals. It represents growth equivalence only for the phase of growth following puberty. This chart serves to illustrate the fact that the difference between the growth curve of man and that of any other animal under consideration is infinitely greater than the difference between the curves of widely separated species of animals. The growth curve of man is, quantitatively viewed, in a class by itself, unless it is found to be related to the curves of other primates. This figure suggests the following comments:

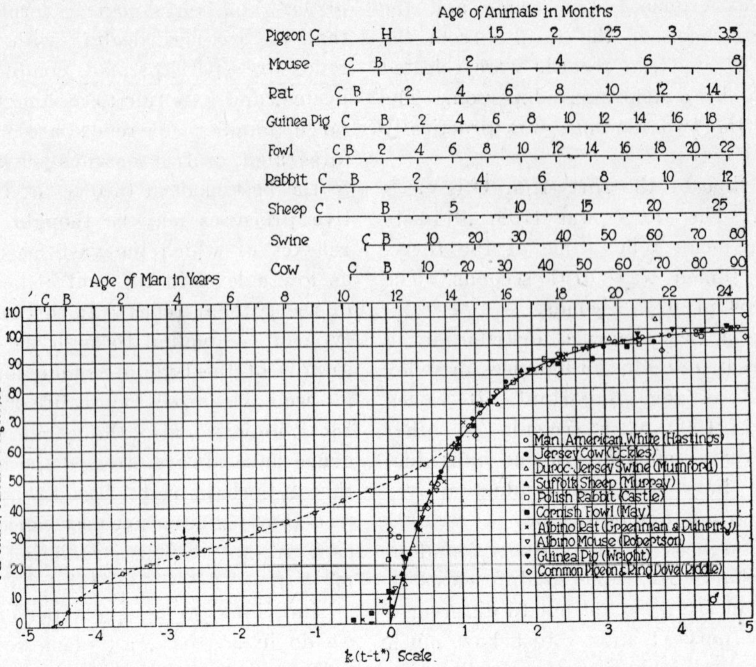

FIG. 1. Growth equivalence during the post-pubertal phase of growth for man and animals. Note that age is counted from birth. For sources of data see Missouri Agricultural Experiment Station Res. Bull. 96 (in press).

1. *The length of the juvenile period.* The length of the juvenile period in man is about 10 years (4 to 14 years). This relatively enormous length of the juvenile period appears to be the most distinguished feature of the growth curve of man.

2. *The position of the pubertal inflection.* In the curve for man, the major inflection (puberty) occurs when the body weight is, roughly, two thirds of the mature weight; in other animals it occurs when the body weight is, roughly, one third of the mature weight.

3. *The post-pubertal phase of growth.* Following the major inflection (puberty) the qualitative course of growth in man and in animals is the same. In both cases the time rates of growth decline by a constant percentage. The numerical value of the percentage decline in the time rates of growth is less, however, in man than in other animals; but the differences are relatively slight. In man it is of the order of 3 per cent. per month; in the sheep, which has the same mature weight as man, it is of the order of 15 per cent. per month. In brief, there are no radical quantitative or qualitative differences between the growth curves for man and other animals during the phase of growth following puberty.

4. *The pre-pubertal phase of growth.* The course of growth during the juvenile, and probably fetal, period of growth is probably qualitatively the same in man and in animals. The time rates of growth tend to increase at a constant percentage rate. There are, however, considerable quantitative differences in this respect. The relatively enormous length of the juvenile period in man as compared to that in animals has

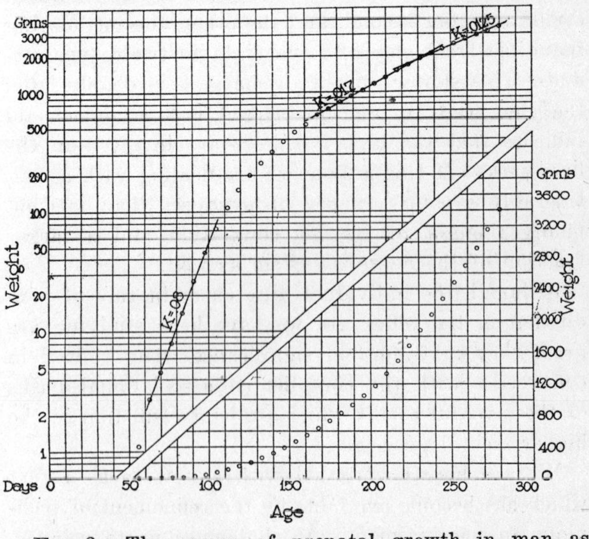

FIG. 2. The course of prenatal growth in man as plotted on arithlog and arithmetic scales. During the third month the rate of growth is about 8 per cent. per day. During the three months preceding birth, the rate of growth varies from 1.7 to 1.3 per cent. per day. The chart was plotted from data published by G. L. Streeter, Carnegie Institution of Washington, Contributions to Embryology, 1920, ix, 143.

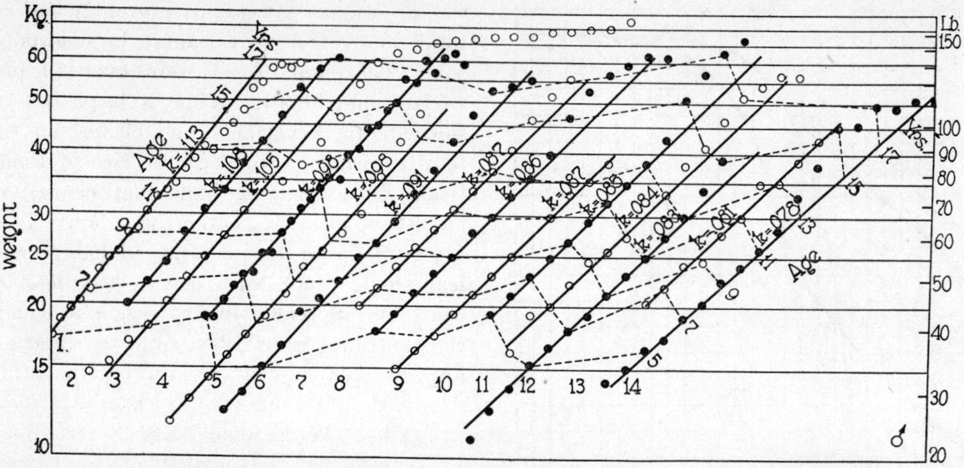

FIG. 3. Chart on an arithlog grid to illustrate the facts that (1) the percentage rate of growth is approximately constant between 4 and 14 years; and (2) that the pubertal acceleration is related to the percentage rate of growth during the earlier phases of the juvenile period. 100 k represents the percentage rate of growth per year. The curves are arranged in a descending order of the values of k. On the left, where the numerical values of k are high, there is no increase in the percentage rate of growth at 12 years; indeed, in curve 1, there is a decrease in the percentage rate at this time. On the right, where the numerical value of k is low, there is a very conspicuous pubertal acceleration. The pubertal acceleration may, therefore, be related to the nutritional condition of the child. For the sources of data see Baldwin, B. T., *The Physical Growth of Children from Birth to Maturity*, Univ. of Iowa Studies in Child Welfare, 1921, 1, 188. Curve 1 represents well-to-do American children (column 1 in Baldwin); curve 2, German (column 106); 3, English (c. 54); 4, American (c. 3); 5, French (c. 76); 6, Italian (c. 122); 7, American (c. 39); 9, English (c. 66); 10, German (c. 79); 11, Russian Jews (c. 120); 12, Japanese (c. 127); 13, Russians (c. 115); 14, Japanese (c. 129). The broken lines on the chart connect the points of the same ages.

already been mentioned. Another difference relates to the percentage rates of growth. In man, the percentage rate of growth during the juvenile period (4 to 14 years) is of the order of 0.03 per cent. per day (10 per cent. per year); in other animals, it is of the order of 3.0 per cent. per day (1,000 per cent. per year).

In the fetal period, too, the percentage rate of growth in man is unusually low. Figure 2 shows it to be of the order of 8 per cent. during the three months preceding birth. In the rat, we have found the rate of growth for nine days preceding birth is of the order of 53 per cent. per day. The difference, however, is not so great as for the juvenile period. Again, it is the juvenile period which, quantitatively considered, is the most conspicuous feature of the growth curve of man as contrasted to the growth curve of animals.

5. *The infantile period.* In addition to the juvenile period, the infantile period in man is conspicuous by its differences from the corresponding segment of the growth curve in animals. It appears to show an inflection similar to the pubertal inflection in the curves of animals; but the inflection proves to be abortive. Sometimes between 2 and 4 years after birth the declining time rates of growth are changed into increasing time rates of growth, and practically constant percentage rates of growth. This constant percentage rate of growth often lasts until 15 years. It is this turn of events which principally differentiates the growth curve of man from that of animal.

6. *The pubertal acceleration.* In children there is often an increase in the percentage rate of growth between the age of 12 and 14 or 15 years. Such an acceleration has not been definitely encountered in the growth curves of domestic animals. This acceleration, however, can not be said to constitute a qualitative genetic difference between the growth curves of man and animals, for it is not a universal feature of the growth curve of man. This pubertal acceleration appears to be related to the percentage rate of growth between 4 and 12 years. If the percentage rate of growth for a given group of children is relatively low during the earlier ages, then there is usually an acceleration between 12 and 15 years; if it is high, there is no acceleration. The pubertal acceleration, when present, appears to be in the nature of compensatory growth for an earlier deficiency. Figure 3 illustrates this statement.

It should be said that growth in length takes place at an approximately constant *time* rate when growth in weight takes place at a constant *percentage* rate (Fig. 4). This is evident from geometrical considerations when growth in length is strictly terminal. It is also evident from physiological considerations; con-

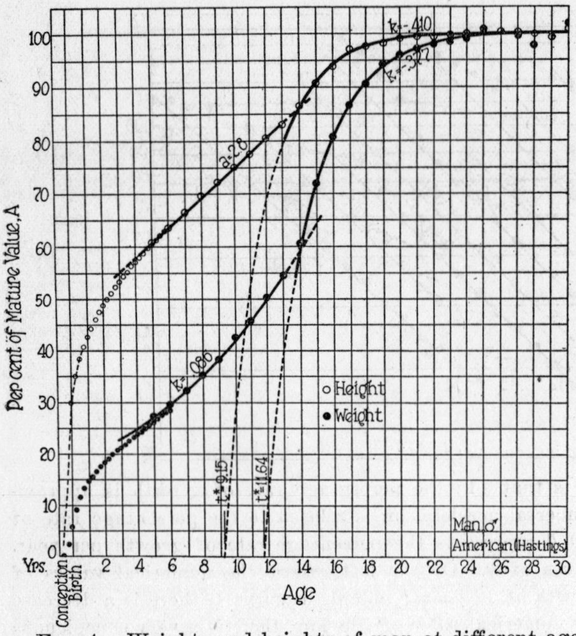

Fig. 4. Weights and heights of man at different ages expressed as percentages of the mature values. While growth in weight between 4 and 14 years takes place at a constant percentage rate (8.6 per cent. per year) growth in height takes place at a constant time rate (2.8 units per year). Data cited by Baldwin.

stant percentage rates of growth in volume and constant time rate of terminal growth both imply that the physiological environment with respect to the growth-limiting process remains constant.

Samuel Brody

Agricultural Experiment Station,
University of Missouri

PROGENIES FROM X-RAYED SEX CELLS OF TOBACCO

In January of this year two greenhouse plants of *Nicotiana tabacum* var. *purpurea* (U. C. B. G. 27014)[1] in full flower were exposed to moderately hard X-rays. Immediately thereafter all open flowers were removed and the remaining buds trimmed to a series of size classes. Within 48 hours all buds except those in which pollen was formed had fallen. In these larger buds the primordia of female sex cells had been set apart and in the majority the megaspore mother cells were in meiotic prophases or divisions. Seed from 7 capsules produced by selfing the flowers from these larger buds have given some 1,000 plants, which began to flower in July.

At the seedling stages the presence of variant plants was apparent. At maturity over 20 per cent. of the total were striking variants; in one population of some 200 plants there were over 70 per cent. of variant individuals. While it is possible roughly to separate these variants into classes on the basis of total external morphology, no two of them are identical. In estimating individual character contrasts an attempted classification has shown 5 flower color types, 8 flower shape types, 6 habit types, and 10 leaf shape types, with many other less obvious but constant differences in expression as compared with the control. Apart from recessive effects which may appear in subsequent generations, the results of hundreds of larger or smaller changes appear in these progenies. With some marked exceptions, fertility in general parallels extent of total variation—the more abnormal, the more sterile. However, only a very few individuals, if any, fail to produce at least a few viable eggs.

Detailed cytological examination of a number of variant plants indicates (a) that they often are $2n = 48$ as in the control—*i.e.*, that the variants are not solely the result of a disturbance of the meiotic distributional mechanism; (b) at diakinesis, P. M. C. may show lack of ability to pair on the part of one or more pairs of chromosomes, indicating that some decided genetic modification has occurred; (c) that occasional production of 2n pollen grains occurs, possibly as a result of failure of cytokinesis in the archesporium; (d) that their somatic tissues may show nuclear and other abnormalities equivalent to those often described as following irradiation of somatic tissues and thus suggesting that these latter effects may be solely the expression of initial nuclear modification and possibly heritable.

Progenies from these populations and from subsequent X-raying of *tabacum* and other *Nicotiana* species are being grown. Special attention is being given to effects of irradiation on mature pollen, since with such material the X-ray technique may be standardized and simplified. Despite the absence of direct evidence of the heritable nature of the effects produced, the extent and character of the variations in hand, the fertility relations displayed and the cytological information obtained suggest that data, in the case of a plant of economic importance, confirming the results of Muller's X-ray experiments, may be forthcoming.

It is interesting that two similar efforts, one on the animal and the other on the plant side, to accelerate evolutionary processes should have been carried on simultaneously.

T. H. Goodspeed
A. R. Olson

University of California

[1] This variety has been grown here in the pure line for many years and has been subjected to genetic and cytological examination in many intra- and interspecific hybrids (*cf. Univ. Calif. Publ. Bot.*, vols. 5 and 11).

SCIENCE

VOL. LXVII JANUARY 20, 1928 No. 1725

CONTENTS

The American Association for the Advancement of Science:
The Inter-Relation of the Medical Sciences: DR. RUFUS COLE 47
Too Little Mathematics—and Too Much: PROFESSOR EDWIN B. WILSON 52
The Importance of Biology for Mankind: DR. W. W. LEPESCHKIN 59
Scientific Events:
The South African Station of the Harvard Observatory; The Battelle Memorial Institute; A Fund for the Study of Colds at the Johns Hopkins University; The New Life Sciences Building at the University of California; A Symposium at the Alfred L. Loomis Laboratory in honor of Professor J. Franck 61
Scientific Notes and News 63
University and Educational Notes 67
Discussion and Correspondence:
The Proposed Transfer of the Geodetic Work of the Coast and Geodetic Survey: DR. GEO. OTIS SMITH. *Unstability at the Absolute Zero of Temperature:* PROFESSOR R. D. KLEEMAN. *The Theory of "Visible Radiation from an Excited Nerve Fiber":* DR. HALLOWELL DAVIS. *The Antiquity of the Deposits in Jacobs Cavern:* VERNON C. ALLISON. *The Mispronunciation of "Data":* R. H. SMITH 67
Scientific Books:
Leriche and Policard on the Physiology and Pathology of the Bone: H. E. JORDAN 70
Scientific Apparatus and Laboratory Methods:
Methods for determining the Color of Objects in Microscopic Mounts: PROFESSOR W. H. DAVIS and F. A. MACLAUGHLIN. *A Modified Erlanger Sphygmomanometer:* A. R. MCLAUGHLIN 71
Special Articles:
Zeolite Beds in the Green River Formation: DR. W. H. BRADLEY. *The Adhesion of Mercury to Glass:* PROFESSOR WILL C. BAKER 73
Science News x

SCIENCE: A Weekly Journal devoted to the Advancement of Science, edited by J. McKeen Cattell and published every Friday by

THE SCIENCE PRESS

New York City: Grand Central Terminal.

Lancaster, Pa. Garrison, N. Y.

Annual Subscription, $6.00. Single Copies, 15 Cts.

SCIENCE is the official organ of the American Association for the Advancement of Science. Information regarding membership in the Association may be secured from the office of the permanent secretary, in the Smithsonian Institution Building, Washington, D. C.

Entered as second-class matter July 18, 1923, at the Post Office at Lancaster, Pa., under the Act of March 8, 1879.

THE INTER-RELATION OF THE MEDICAL SCIENCES[1]

SECTION N of the American Association for the Advancement of Science has for its field the medical sciences. I do not know that in this organization the question what are the medical sciences has ever been raised or discussed. I take it, however, that it is generally assumed that the medical sciences include at least human anatomy and human physiology. At any rate, the workers in these fields find no home in this association except in this section. It is also taken for granted that among the medical sciences are included all the myriad branches of medicine, many of which have sprung into being during recent decades. Recently it has almost seemed that whenever two or three have gathered together to deal with a special medical problem, the suffix o-l-o-g-y has been added to the name of the subject treated, and a new science has been born.

To the practical American there seems to be little value in attempting a rigid classification of the sciences, such as has been attempted by Bacon, Spencer, Karl Pearson and others. Yet any serious consideration of the various sciences and of their interrelations may make us realize how much we take for granted and how illogical in many respects is the present situation.

From its derivation, the term medicine has to do strictly with healing, and the term designates either the agent employed in healing or the branch of knowledge which has to do with the prevention, cure or alleviation of human disease. It is obvious, however, that in spite of this definition medicine has come to mean something much more inclusive than therapeutics. If it does not this section is dealing with the application of science, not science itself, even though various sciences are contributing to it. It is true that the application of knowledge to practical ends neither lessens the importance of that knowledge nor lowers the dignity of him who so uses it. This association, however, is chiefly interested in the pursuit of knowledge, not its application. And in the striving after knowledge, experience has shown that any limitations, such as usefulness, placed upon the results of the searcher seriously handicap him in his

[1] Address of the vice-president and chairman of Section N—Medical Sciences, American Association for the Advancement of Science, Nashville, December, 1927.

effectiveness. The true scientist can not be restricted to the production of results that are immediately useful or even of results that may be useful in the future. Notwithstanding this, we suspect that every scientist, even the most pure, cherishes a secret hope that his results will receive an early application, and the question may even be raised whether every searcher after truth is not stimulated in his endeavors by the consciousness that his contributions are bound in the end to contribute to the well being of mankind. But if scientists have a dogma, it is that the advancement of knowledge can best be accomplished by pursuing it quite independently of any immediate results, and if this association has a slogan, it should be, "Unrestricted Investigation."

For many centuries medicine has suffered from the restrictions implied in the term. At present these may be more imaginary than real, but, at least in the past, these restrictions have exerted an inhibiting influence even on the development of therapeutics itself, and have exerted a still greater inhibition on the growth of knowledge, concerning the real nature of disease in man, and also on knowledge regarding the structure and functions of man in health. These restrictions are partly inherent in the nature of the subject, but to a greater degree they have arisen as a result of the historical development of the organization through which this branch of knowledge has been cultivated.

Man's first interest in disease undoubtedly arose from a desire for relief. When he became conscious of an unusual physical state, usually evidenced by discomfort or "dis-ease," he ascribed it to some supernatural agency, and appealed to the gods for relief. Later he found by chance that through the employment of certain physical agents, pain might be relieved, especially when the abnormal state was the result of some obvious external agency. The priests who were the intermediaries with the gods in relieving the mysterious ailments, also became the healers who applied the less mysterious remedies. Thus originated the healers or physicians, and from the earliest times to the present, physicians have been the custodians of knowledge concerning disease. But physicians have been employed by the sick to heal them, and the physicians therefore could not be entirely disinterested seekers after truth. Under these circumstances, it would not have been remarkable if any seeking for knowledge which physicians undertook, should always have been directed to a search for cure. The Hippocratic Oath expresses lofty moral principles and registers a vow to transmit the knowledge of the art to certain disciples, but it contains not a word about attempting to learn more about disease.

To facilitate the transmission of the curative art to others, schools of medicine were organized, and these later became incorporated in the universities. Knowledge of disease consisted in deductions made from principles, but these principles were based upon the crudest analogies. Even such a state of affairs, however, is eminently satisfying to certain types of the philosophical mind, I will not say to all. It is interesting, if not amusing, to read in the most recent history of medicine, in the introduction written by a philosopher-physician—"And so do we arrive at the paradox—true, as are all genuine paradoxes—that, when in the sixteenth century medicine was, as we should say, less "scientific" than to-day, medicine was indeed, as now it is not, a science in very truth." But for good or ill, and it is difficult for us to be convinced of the evil results, the desire did arise to obtain knowledge about disease which was not deduced from principles, but which was derived from actual first-hand observation. Since little could be known about abnormalities in structure and function until more was known about the normal state, it was only natural that physicians should have been led into the study of anatomy and physiology. It can not be maintained that this knowledge was pursued solely for the sake of curing disease, but the pursuit of this knowledge originated in, and was practically confined to, the medical schools, and the search was almost exclusively conducted by physicians. Vesalius was a physician and even he forsook his study of anatomy for the more lucrative post of physician to Charles V. That Vesalius was a physician and that Harvey was a physician do not detract from their contributions to science. Rather it emphasizes the pride that all members of the medical profession should have in the fact that these men broke away from pursuing an immediately useful object, and attempted to discover Nature's secrets. But in so doing Vesalius and Harvey forsook their field, they entered a new province, they no longer were studying disease, they were no longer studying abnormalities in structure and function; they were studying the normal, the usual. Certain men like Leonardo da Vinci possibly undertook the study of anatomy chiefly to satisfy an insatiable curiosity. But even Leonardo was undoubtedly led to peer beneath the surface, at least partly, through a desire to be better able to depict the human form. Theoretically the study of human anatomy might just as well have been incorporated in the schools of art, but it was not to be, and, from the sixteenth century until to-day, the cultivation of the science of anatomy has occurred almost exclusively in the medical schools. It is only within our own day that those teaching and studying this subject and widening its boundaries, have not at the same time been engaged in applying remedies, healing the sick. True it is that in the halcyon days of the fifteenth and sixteenth and seventeenth centuries the searcher after truth could ramble over the whole field of nature, and pluck flowers wherever he went. The investigator did not have far to go to encounter the unknown, it lay all about him. And very many of the searchers of these centuries were physicians. Paracelsus and his followers, Van Helmont and Stahl, knocking at the door of chemistry, were physicians; Galileo and Gilbert, Copernicus, and numerous others were trained in the art of medicine and many of them practiced it. But whereas physics, at an early day, and chemistry, somewhat later, were divorced from the medical school and were given independent positions in the universities, human anatomy and human physiology retained their incorporation in the medical school, and to this day they have never gained their independence. They are still called medical sciences and have had to bear the burden imposed upon them, by implication at least, of pursuing knowledge for a definite utilitarian purpose. Whatever the situation may be to-day, in the past this burden has too often been more than merely that imposed by implication, it has been a real impediment, sufficient actually to hamper the growth of these sciences. To-day anatomy and physiology are thriving best where they are most free from the restrictions enforced upon them through their inclusion in the medical school. These restrictions are not all associated with the relation of medicine to cure, however. Certain restrictions in the medical school have arisen from the attempt to provide a too rigid and all inclusive curriculum which expresses the antithesis of the university spirit. In England histology or microscopical anatomy is still taught in the department of physiology, to the detriment of anatomy. On the other hand, it must be admitted that in certain medical schools, in this country at least, the attitude is becoming much more liberal. Anatomy is becoming less and less restricted to pure description. We even have professors of physiological anatomy!

What has been said about anatomy and physiology refers to human anatomy and to human physiology. The study of structure and function in what we call the lower animals took a different course. It is to Aristotle that science owes the beginning of zoology, comparative anatomy and embryology. Although Aristotle's father was a physician, and although Aristotle is sometimes spoken of as an Asclepiad, and his enemies accused him of practicing medicine, he took little interest in medicine, and he is said to have produced but one medical work and that one is now lost. As Allbutt says, "Hippocratic physicians accumulated a remarkable series of facts . . . but their work was not, as that of Aristotle, for disinterested science but for practical ends." Ever since Aristotle the study of anatomy, physiology and embryology of animals other than man has not been relegated solely to the medical schools nor been exclusively engaged in by physicians, and this in spite of the fact that these subjects have a very direct relationship to human anatomy and physiology and medicine. Whether this separation from medicine has influenced the growth of these sciences, I do not feel competent to judge, but one may at least say that the followers of these sciences have made distinctly greater contributions to biological theories, and have had more influence in establishing biological principles than have the followers of human anatomy and human physiology.

When physicians became conscious of a desire to extend knowledge, their natural and legitimate field was disease itself. It is true that ever since Hippocrates, physicians had been attempting to describe and classify disease, so far as this could be done by mere observation of symptoms. But, of course, this was but the first step in arriving at any real understanding of disease. It was a long time after the beginning of anatomy before physicians began to make any serious investigation of the abnormalities in structure resulting from disease, at least before morbid anatomy consisted of more than fragmentary observations. It was two hundred years from Vesalius to Morgagni. One may say that only then did physicians begin to be scientists in the modern sense. The high aspirations of pathological anatomy is indicated by the title of Morgagni's monumental work, *De Sedibus et Causis Morborum,* though the title indicates a much greater confidence in the results to be obtained from the mere description of lesions than was justified. At first pathological anatomy was studied and taught by the anatomists, but later, to its great advantage, it became more closely integrated with clinical medicine, that is with the study of the manifestations of disease in the patient during life. As Billroth says, "The new material became vitalized only when the clinical physicians took hold of it and either themselves undertook the dissections or had them performed under their direction." But pathological anatomy, I will not say its followers, became proud, and pathological anatomy became pathology, the science of disease; its votaries became pathologists, and, in this country at least, pathologists they have remained to this day. That this assumption of exclusiveness was justified, no one will claim, for even the most ardent followers of this branch of knowledge must admit that alterations in structure alone can give but a very imperfect conception of disease. If the pathologists, in assuming their new title, were animated by a desire to escape from the restrictions imposed upon medicine by the necessity of obtaining useful results, of promoting cures, no one can blame them. But the separation of pathological anatomy from the study of disease as a whole was neither good for pathological anatomy nor for medicine. Pathological anatomy or pathology, or whatever we call it, is not one of the medical sciences, or a contributory science to medicine. It is a part of medicine itself, unless medicine is to be restricted to the cure of disease. The science of medicine is no more applied pathology than pathological anatomy itself is applied anatomy and histology. The study of pathological anatomy is, or should be, only one of the methods for investigating disease, and the closer it can be interwoven with the other methods the more likely are its results to be of value. The field of pathological anatomy is the study of the effects of disease. To really learn about disease, that is to understand the alterations in function and structure which are exhibited by the abnormal individual, the individual himself must be studied, during life as well as after death, and this study must be combined with an attempt to explain the abnormal phenomena in the light of present knowledge and by the aid of all suitable methods. This is the science of medicine, if such there is, and if there is not such a science there ought to be.

The first and essential step in the pursuit of knowledge concerning disease consists in describing and classifying the phenomena to be studied, and that must be done by observing sick individuals. Disease is not something that exists apart from the patient. Knowledge was long retarded by considering that diseases were entities. Upon the seekers after this kind of knowledge the burdens of utilitarianism bear of necessity more heavily than they do on the followers of anatomy and physiology, or indeed on the votaries of any other science. They can not be entirely escaped. We may study earthquakes, or tides, or the natural attraction of bodies for one another as these phenomena present themselves. Certain phenomena we may reproduce at will. But in the study of disease in man we can not investigate the phenomena with hands off. We must always interfere by attempting to prevent harmful results. Moreover we are powerless to reproduce the phenomena artificially. The science of medicine is not analogous to theology but to demonology, and the restraints of morality, of religion, of conscience will not permit one to study these demons without attempting to cast them out and to destroy them. But one can do both things if he is not controlled entirely by his emotions, or worse by the temptations of self interest, and these are great indeed, but if he is also inspired by curiosity and controlled by reason. The true student of medicine must realize that before disease can be cured it must be understood. And to understand it, it must be studied at the bedside, in the laboratory and at the autopsy table. Clinical medicine, or whatever the study of the more superficial aspects of disease may be called, experimental medicine, pathological anatomy, pathological physiology, are but different aspects of the same thing, the study of disease, the science of medicine. Practical results in the way of cure are bound to follow the development of this science, but these must be the natural outcome, not the objects to be always held in view. Even therapeutics may be pursued in the spirit of a pure science, as witness the growth of pharmacology, which has flourished best and has been most productive when it has attempted to learn, not how to cure patients, but has investigated the action of drugs in producing alterations in function. It thus becomes a matter of emphasis as to whether medicine will be merely an applied science or not.

It must not be assumed, however, that the pursuit of practical ends precludes the advancement of knowledge. The reaction against the Baconian philosophy is not entirely justified. When we are tempted to disparage, let us remember that Bacon's spirit was responsible for the formation of the Royal Society. It would be a rash man who would belittle Pasteur as a scientist, yet most of his work consisted in pursuing very practical ends, and at least one of his two or three fundamental contributions was the direct outcome of an attempt to obtain a utilitarian result. That scientists will obtain useful results goes without saying. That they should not be under any obligations to obtain immediately useful results, and that their work should not be judged by any criterion of utility, experience seems to have shown.

The methods and accumulated results of all sciences must be used in pursuing the science of medicine. That some of these sciences are more closely related to medicine, in their methods and fields of endeavor, than are others is obvious. Biology, comparative anatomy, embryology, bacteriology, protozoology, certain branches of botany, anthropology, human anatomy, human physiology, psychology, and even certain aspects of the social sciences, have many close affiliations with medicine. The methods of the more general and fundamental sciences, mathematics, physics and chemistry become applicable in any science as that science develops, and the degree of development of any branch of science may be tested by the extent to which the fundamental concepts of physics and chemistry may be usefully employed in its pursuit. That biology is ready for such an approach, the development of general physiology bears witness.

That problems of disease may profitably be investigated by the employment of accurate quantitative methods, and be studied in relation to the laws of physics and chemistry, is evidence that the science of medicine already exists and that it has even grown out of its swaddling clothes. But none of these contributing sciences are medical sciences. None of them should be trammeled by serving medicine alone. The only medical science is the science of medicine itself, that is, the science whose field is the study of disease.

Thus far I have not referred to the large number of subjects which, in so far as they receive any scientific treatment at all, are parts of the science of medicine. These are subjects, such as neurology, psychiatry, dermatology, otology, cardiology, angiology, gastro-enterology and so on, *ad infinitum.* On the other hand, there is another group of subjects which are held to be closely related to medicine, but which belong, so far as they belong in any science at all, in some one of the other fundamental sciences. I refer to subjects like histology, cytology, immunology, endocrinology, climatology, radiology and so forth and so on. The multiplicity of these terms illustrates the extent of what we may call growth at the periphery of a science.

It must be admitted that the science of medicine has not reached a high state of development, even such as physiology has attained. And furthermore, we must admit that many of the most important contributions to this science have been made by workers in related fields. Nevertheless, I believe that its greatest advancement will come only when it shall be pursued by men whose primary interest is in disease. Important contributions have been made by clinicians, but only comparatively recently have any considerable number of physicians become conscious of their obligations to contribute to this science, and only still more recently have physicians been given any relief from the burdens of practice which will give them opportunities for studying disease by scientific methods. It is true that many of the contributors to other branches of science also teach, but the practice of medicine is a much more time- and energy-consuming occupation than is teaching.

From the philosophical standpoint, from which the object of all science is but to obtain an interpretation of nature as a whole, it is possible that medicine may be relatively unimportant. It may be, however, that the most important generalizations will proceed not from the study of the normal but from the investigation of the unusual. The object of all science is to reach underlying principles or laws. As Priestly said, "Science is an effort to compress as much knowledge as possible in the smallest compass." And Karl Pearson said, "Nobody believes now that science explains anything; we all look upon it as a short-hand description, as an economy of thought." A great mass of knowledge about the details of disease has been accumulated, and this knowledge is about as accurate as it is in the other domains of biology. This kind of knowledge in recent years has been extending at an enormous rate. Journals devoted to medicine in its various aspects number many hundreds. The science of medicine is developing centrifugally, not centripetally. One important reason for this is that it is so greatly exposed to utilitarian demands. In his efforts to be aware of all the facts the physician has no time for contemplation of their meaning. In his fear of overlooking that which may be of value in prolonging the life of the individual, he fails to discover that which may be of importance for the race. We even lack accurate definitions of disease, injury, recovery, death. Possibly such definitions can never be made. Scientists are not so sanguine as they once were of reducing knowledge of the universe to formulae. But the science of medicine, as all other sciences, demands that efforts be made in this direction. In spite of all that has been said, however, the heterogeneity that exists in the knowledge about disease is no greater than that in some other branches of knowledge, the scientific status of which is never questioned.

Medicine occupies a peculiar position among the sciences. By workers in other fields of science, medicine has been looked upon askance, even disregarded. In most of the classifications of science it is not even mentioned. It is even claimed that there is no such thing as a science of medicine. On the one hand, as medicine, it has been scorned and neglected, and on the other, as the medical sciences, it has been honored and respected, and held to embrace within its borders such important divisions of science as anatomy and physiology, and the name has been used to designate an important section in this association.

Every organization must have a function. There seem in the past to have been some doubts as to what the function of Section N really is. May not one of its functions at least, be the support and promotion of the science of medicine, even though Section N continues to be called the Section of Medical Sciences. On behalf of human anatomy and human physiology, however, although I have no authority to speak for them, I should be glad to see this section called the Section of Human Anatomy, Physiology and Medicine, or the Section of Medicine and Related Sciences.

The support and defense of the science of medicine is needed, the battle is not to be easily won, the result is not certain. Apart from the opposition of those who see in medicine only an art pursued for practical ends, and aside from the inertia, arising from traditional viewpoints, as exhibited in the treatment of medicine in the universities, there is the question that is bound to be raised as to whether the scientific method is, after all, the most effective one for the advancement of knowledge in this particular realm. Great advances have undoubtedly been made in this field through a purely empirical approach. The Nobel prize has just been awarded for a discovery in this field which was not made through what is considered the scientific method. This association believes, however, that the best approach to knowledge is through the gateway of science.

The science of medicine requires workers imbued with the scientific spirit. Opportunities must be available for men who want to learn about disease. These men must be stimulated, and their work given appreciative recognition by workers in better established fields. The bestowal of this recognition and stimulation offers one way in which science may be advanced by this fellowship of scientists.

In what has been said I have merely tried to give expression to what has already been in the minds of most of us. The programs of recent years, and the program of to-day, indicate that the motivating force in this society is the promotion of scientific medicine. Through the efforts of this organization may medicine ever become more scientific, to the great blessing of mankind.

RUFUS COLE

THE ROCKEFELLER INSTITUTE
FOR MEDICAL RESEARCH

TOO LITTLE MATHEMATICS—AND TOO MUCH[1]

IN speaking on a subject like mine of to-night it is necessary to proceed by classification, for what might be too little mathematics for some groups of students could well be too much for others.

First let us consider those who contemplate becoming professional mathematicians. These form a negligible group—negligible in numbers compared with all those who should take some collegiate mathematics, negligible for purposes of instruction because each will go more or less his own precocious way. It is improper for any department selfishly to lay its plan of teaching for the rare Galois or Gauss or Abel, or even for the commoner Richardson or Archibald or Wilson. The future professional who is worth his salt will get along somehow without much of our assistance and possibly even in spite of it. He will follow the courses he wants and make up his deficiencies by private study. The professional knows how to learn, and in mathematics he knows it young. There will be small chance that he have too little mathematics; you may think he can hardly have too much. Herein I should differ with you and maintain that his real danger is "too much." I do not, of course, refer to what he will have learned or may have forgotten by the time he comes to a ripe old age or even by the time he reaches middle life; I am speaking of the future professional mathematician as a student, first collegiate and then graduate. He should not be stuffed with courses until his brain has become a glorified paté de fois gras. That would deaden his originality, doubly diminish his ingenuity, and thus triply hinder his development as a true professional.

Our American university departments sin greatly in the great array of prerequisite specialized courses which they offer and expect their students to take. The aim of any advanced course should be to line out a straight path from relatively elementary work to the research line. When I was in Paris I took a course at the Sorbonne on the dynamical theory of light with Boussinesq. He did not hesitate to take his time to explain that cos $(\pi - x)$ equals $-\cos x$ or to prove some ordinary proposition in solid analytical geometry or to integrate some common differential equation, and yet in 60 lectures he reached material to be found only in his own recent papers. When I asked him why he took the time to prove so many elementary theorems he said that it did the students good to see such propositions demonstrated and that he had a superabundance of time anyhow. Such a course in any one of many fields could be given in our American colleges to seniors who had had three consecutive years of mathematics, if only our teachers had the finesse to give it. A book must be somewhat encyclopedic; a course should be selective, eclectic, for the purpose of helping the student quickly to an original problem upon which he may go to work. You have here at Brown one of the best collegiate departments of mathematics in the United States; you have an able staff; you need not hesitate to offer the doctorate. What you may miss is encyclopedicity, you will for that very reason the more easily make up in the freshness and promptness with which you start on original investigation.

Let us turn from the future professional to the ordinary college man. He may well have too little mathematics, too little for his own future comfort. The college student of inorganic chemistry of 30 years ago who failed to take a good course in calculus has paid heavily for this omission. It has much increased his difficulties in physical chemistry, in the work of van't Hoff and of Nernst, of Lewis

[1] Read before the Mathematical Club of Brown University.

and of Debye. For even longer any one who expected to go on into physics, astronomy or engineering should have had his calculus. To-day the physiologist, the bacteriologist, the biologist, and the student of the public health is reaching problems which require some mathematical insight for their elucidation, and the college student of to-day can scarcely fail to find himself seriously handicapped before middle life if he enters upon any of these fields without a college course in calculus. For many, many years not only arithmetic but algebra and geometry have been regarded as so fundamental in all education both for their own sake and for their uses in other studies that they have been required for entrance to college and have been widely taught even to those who did not plan to go to college. It may to-day safely be said that calculus is for the college student what algebra and geometry are for the high school pupil—of necessity for future use in many a profession, of cultural value for many a student who does not contemplate a profession. So much can not be said of trigonometry—biology, chemistry, physiology, and those branches of business, of medicine and of the public health which depend on statistics hardly use a periodic function; it is the logarithm and exponential which are central. There is small use also for analytic geometry. Graphs we do find everywhere, but the art of deducing theorems by algebraic processes is for the most part special to pure mathematics.

There is real danger that the college student shall have too little mathematics. To-day more are taking too little than too much. Why this serious situation? We may find some light on it if we reflect on the case of the chemist now in middle life. Most likely he took a full year of mathematics in college. Thirty years ago in the great majority of our colleges he had no option but to take it. However he did not learn calculus unless he followed mathematics for two or even three years. In other words we may say that between his algebra of the preparatory school and the method of dealing with variable quantities that he needed there was intercalated by the habits of the mathematical teachers of those days one or two years of work which could at best be of very limited use to him. Conditions are better to-day. We generally get to some calculus in the freshman course. I feel, however, that our collegiate teachers of mathematics could well go somewhat further than they yet have gone in making straight and fair the path of the ordinary student to and through the elements of the calculus both differential and integral.

Now there are two aspects in almost all learning; there is the logical or intellectual side which deals with the meaning of a subject, which is chiefly emphasized in elementary geometry, and the technical or operational side, which is largely placed to the fore in algebra. You may be a first class technician without much understanding of the significance of a subject or you may have a fast intellectual grasp with a negligible technique; you may be a thinker or a doer. These two activities are not entirely antagonistic, to a considerable extent they reinforce each other. In far the greater part of our life we are technicians of one sort or another, we learn how to do certain things. We do not go about learning to walk by first studying our skeletal structure, our musculature, and the laws of the lever. Whenever we need to do something repeatedly with precision we face the problem of developing a technique. The billiard player does not spend his time studying Routh's Rigid Dynamics. He acquires a sort of automatism under voluntary control. We can do the same for factoring or for differentiating. But what is the use; the great majority of us do not take naturally to such pursuits any more than we do to billiards; we have little occasion to use formal mathematics except of the simplest.

It seems to me that one error in much teaching of mathematics for the majority of students is overemphasis on technical processes and correlative underattention to meanings. It is too much mathematics of one sort and too little of another. According to my experience it is very difficult to expect a student to learn good technique and to gain a clear understanding at the same time. I prefer to aim the first general collegiate course at the understanding and to follow this up for those who are to be engineers or mathematicians, physicists or astronomers, and for those who like mathematical operations for their own sake, by a stiff course in technique. Now if you are going to teach or to learn meanings of things, you must not be in a hurry, you must keep your self-possession of mind, you must dwell long on a variety of simple things. What is the problem of learning the calculus so that you may use its ideas in any one of a great variety of applications which may later confront you as chemist or physiologist, as economist or public health officer? You have to get a real understanding of rates and summations, of infinitesimals and infinites, of limits of quotients of two infinitesimals and of sums of an infinite number of infinitesimals. That is about all; it is not much, but it takes time and patience. It requires the avoidance of early generalization. Mathematicians have a fondness for general methods in instruction. They forget that in their own work they almost always use some ingenious special notion and rarely the most general method they know. Not many of us naturally work with E. H. Moore's "General Analysis"! In teaching, one must keep the special to the fore and let the generalization come later as a union in a single view of a variety of specials already known. And in general, one must proceed from the known to the unknown. That is why review is constantly necessary, why the repetition of a demonstration from previous studies is not a waste of time, but actually a time-saver. We do not ourselves readily use that last thing we have learned any more than we use the most general; why expect of our students that which we have learned by experience we may not expect of ourselves? The breathlessness of American life is an index of indigestion. We are stuffed with the latest news, the most recent invention, the newest fad whether of mechanism or of dancing, of science or of sociology. We do not know what they mean, we do not even inquire what are their antecedents from which an inkling of their meaning might be learned. The classics have pretty much vanished from our instruction and science has not yet learned to replace them in poise and in perspective.

Perhaps I might without boring you go somewhat into detail about one way of introducing the few fundamental concepts along which those who need a little mathematical thinking may be led without too much involvement in formal operations. Begin with uniform velocity and its space-time graph of which that velocity is the slope. This is a better definition of slope than through the trigonometric tangent. Follow with uniform acceleration, treating variable velocity in the case of uniform variation as the innate concept that is. Point out the logical and geometrical identity between the relations of uniform acceleration to velocity and time and the relations of uniform velocity to space and time. As much of our fastest thinking is by analogy, it is well to emphasize true analogies. Proceed to deduce by any one of the old fashioned methods the relation between distance and time in uniformly accelerated motion. Then deduce the relation over again by a variation of the argument. Two proofs of one important central theorem which involves the most fundamental of notions give more power and understanding to the student than the proofs of two theorems of which only one is important. Dally over the properties of the quadratic or parabolic space time graph, $s = \frac{1}{2} at^2 + bt$, not so much for the importance of those properties in themselves as for their significance to uniformly accelerated motion. It is remarkable how simply some of the geometry of the parabola develops this way. The fact that any chord of a parabola is parallel to the tangent at the abscissa half way between those of the ends of the chord is but another statement of the proposition that in uniformly accelerated motion the velocity at the mid time of any interval is the mean velocity. That the tangents at the ends of a chord meet on this same mid abscissa means merely that you will cover the same distance whether you move with uniform acceleration or with the initial velocity for half the time and then with the final velocity for the remaining half. So too the fact that the line joining the intersection of two tangents to the mid point of their chord of contact is bisected by the parabola is simple kinematics. All this is helpful for reinforcing the meaning of things fundamental.

When you have reached this point you can hardly resist the temptation of solving the quadrature of the parabola by proving that the curve divides the triangle formed by two tangents and their chord of contact is the ratio 1 : 2. It is a mere corollary obtained by doubling up the construction, and so much simpler than the quadrature of the circle. There is no infinite series to sum; the construction at each step cuts off half as much on the outside as on the inside. And then you have Simpson's Rule. You can take your students back to the quadrature of the circle just for review and to show them how much harder it is. Moreover you have the indefinite quadrature of the parabola, whereas for the indefinite quadrature of the circle you need not merely π but the inverse trigonometric functions. However, you may be strong minded and able to resist this little excursion into quadrature. You could return to uniform velocity to discuss interpolation by proportional parts and then with the aid of uniform acceleration pass on to interpolation to second differences. This latter subject is often, perhaps generally, omitted from mathematical instruction. I have run across more than one candidate for the doctorate who did not know that the condition for safe interpolation with first differences is that the second differences are less than 4. It is true that second differences are not important for themselves; they are, I think, important for the insight they give into the behavior of infinitesimals, and to my mind the infinitesimal is the fundamental thing in calculus. I hold no brief against limits. They are necessary to clear thinking, including clear thinking about infinitesimals. I will not further go into detail, but merely point out that if the teacher has done a good job on uniform and on uniformly accelerated motion and on first and second differences, he is ready for definitions of limits, of infinitesimals, of derivatives and of integrals with the assurance that he has provided kinematical and arithmetic considerations on which those definitions may be cogently illustrated and subsequent developments may be safely built.[2]

My thesis is that if we are to encourage the general student, who ought to be encouraged, to take a little mathematics we should avoid subjects which will be of small use to him and in particular should emphasize ideas and simple applications of the calculus rather than inflict upon him from the start a vast operational technique. We should use simple concrete ingenious special methods instead of setting up general systems of analysis. In short we should consider the student somewhat in the light of our own daily experience properly written down to his present level. We must avoid giving him too much mathematics if we are fairly to expect him to avoid taking too little. According to my experience it is rare in departments of mathematics to hear such questions discussed. Indeed I sometimes think that around universities one seldom hears a discussion of any matter of education, of teaching; there is a lot about administration and about research, both of which I should suppose existed chiefly in the college for their reactions on teaching rather than for themselves. It may be that pedagogic questions are so far settled as no longer to need original and critical thought; at any rate, there is in the vast supply of text books produced by college professors much more of uniformity than in their research, and the uniformity is of a type which suggests a study of other recent and similar texts more than of the history of science, of the method of approach to new subjects, of the great texts of all time.

We have considered together the possibility of too little or of too much mathematics for the future professional and for the general student. Through the exigencies of the institutions in which I have worked, that is through opportunities which have arisen and which it has seemed desirable that I should meet, my course as a teacher has laid successively through modern geometry, mathematical physics, mechanics, aeronautics, physics and now rests in vital statistics. Statistics is peculiarly a subject in which too little or too much mathematics may be used and in which a golden mean is especially necessary to soundness of judgment. When I was in college one might find some astronomer teaching least squares as a method of reducing observations, some physicist lecturing on kinetic theory, some mathematician expounding probability; but statistics was practically unknown to the most varied curriculum. Indeed Yule's text appeared in its first edition only in the year 1899 of my graduation from Harvard. Now everything is changed. There are many courses undergraduate and professional on statistics and a new book comes out almost every other month. What is the intellectual level of these courses and these books? For the most part, so far as I can determine, that level is of the lowest, not comparable with pre-college mathematics or classics, about on a par with manual training. There are presented arrays of tabular material, of methods of calculation and of computation forms, without emphasis on logical analysis, still best represented by the 25-year-old text of Yule, without any substantial introduction to probability and chance, which except for logic gives the only firm foundation upon which to build an understanding of the difficult and treacherous science of statistics. It is as though you should teach applied mechanics without going into mechanics or physics or calculus. It is an exaggerated case of too little mathematics. Of course if our colleges and universities wish to train simple technicians in statistical methods who shall work their arithmometers under the direction of competent statisticians much as draftsmen work under designers, this absence of mathematics and of intellectual attention in statistics may be advantageous. But I take it that no considerable part of the students who follow statistics will be technicians, that each statistical problem which they may meet in after life will require its own formulation prior to any application of technique and will ordinarily be solved, insofar as it is solved, by an exercise of judgment rather than of technique. There is little excuse for not giving a sound theoretical background to statistics; the necessary mathematical technique is minimal. As is pointed out by Fréchet and Hallwachs in their excellent little book, "Probabilité à la Portée de Tous" (probability for everybody), arithmetic and algebra plus a willingness to think hard on knotty points are the requisites; the use of calculus though helpful fairly early can be postponed if unfamiliar to a late stage that is seldom reached in a first course in statistics.

We sometimes see in the press a pronouncement by Nicholas Murray Butler on politics, and again on prohibition. Presumably it was on one of these latter occasions that some scalawag of a compositor is said to have headlined him as Nicholas Murray, butler of Columbia University. What I fear many of us do not see or know are his equally strong trenchant dicta on education. His annual presidential reports are interesting reading and repay study. Let me quote a few detached sentences from the latest:

> Through ignorance the present-day banners of progress are everywhere emblazoned with the names of some of the oldest of humanity's discarded failures. . . . Nor is it in any wise true that all subjects of intellectual interest are of equal value and that the important thing is not what one studies but how he studies it. . . . Just now there is a strong tendency to exalt unduly certain recently devel-

[2] This type of course on the introduction to the calculus could be given in the first semester of the freshman year in forty-five exercises.

oped fields of knowledge which as yet consist almost entirely of futile talk and unproved opinion. . . . The longer one examines programs of study that are now most widely followed, observes the spirit in which school and college teaching is so often carried on, and notes the careful avoidance of anything that makes for genuine scholarship and power of reflective thinking, one is forced to raise the very far-reaching question, whether we have not destroyed the ideal of the liberally educated man and, with it, the liberally educated man himself.

I could quote more, but this is perhaps enough amply to cover what I said earlier about dwelling on the ideas of mathematics in general instruction and what I have just said about the lamentably low intellectual level of most of our courses and texts on statistics. I do not care to have any student making routine arithmetical calculations unless he is mentally equipped to understand the limitations of such methods and the conditions under which such calculations lead to legitimate inferences. Some training of fingers is a necessary accompaniment to the elevating of a brain, but the brain is the important thing for those who would be more than technicians.

Although too little mathematics keeps one from understanding statistics, too much is almost as bad. The mathematician who teaches this or any other applied science is very likely to err on the side of too much. It is a great mistake to think that because one finds his original material in the field of statistics or physics or engineering or physiology, subsequent mathematical analysis must be a contribution to that field—it may be just as pure mathematics as if it had originated as such. Much mathematical statistics has no significant statistical content. Many a memoir on mathematical physics is vacuous of physics. Once late in a course on mathematical physics Willard Gibbs came to set up and discuss the equations of motion of the top. In the course of the work he turned around to us, his face lighting up with a sweet smile, and remarked: There are some who seem to think that the top is chiefly interesting as furnishing exercises in elliptic functions. One branch of statistics where mathematics may easily run wild is in fitting frequency functions. Consider the tables printed in the adjacent column which give the frequency distribution of infant mortality rates for 1918 in I. Cities over 25,000, II. Rural Counties for white infants and III. Rural Counties for colored infants. The data are grouped for convenience. Clearly the rate might within the limits of its range have any value and although you can not have a continuous distribution of a finite number of elements you have here finite samples chosen from theoretical infinite universes and are confronted with the problem of fitting to these data some continuous curves which shall represent as well as may be the dis-

INFANT MORTALITY RATES IN 1918

I. Cities Over 25,000

Rate	Frequency
0– 19	0
20– 39	0
40– 59	1
60– 79	17
80– 99	43
100–119	40
120–139	27
140–159	13
160–179	1
180–199	2
200–219	0
220–239	0
	144

II. Rural Counties, White

Rate	Frequency
0– 19	0
20– 39	9
40– 59	33
60– 79	63
80– 99	64
100–119	38
120–139	16
140–159	8
160–179	2
180–199	0
200–219	1
220–239	0
	234

III. Rural Counties, Colored

Rate	Frequency
0– 19	1
20– 39	1
40– 59	5
60– 79	22
80– 99	19
100–119	42
120–139	37
140–159	30
160–179	19
180–199	17
200–219	10
220–239	12
240–259	8
260–279	4
280–299	2
300–319	1
320–339	0
340–359	0
360–379	1
380–399	0
400–419	1
420–439	0
440–459	1
460–479	1
	234

tributions of the hypothetical universes from which the samples are conceived as drawn.

Let us consider the application to our material of the system of analysis invented by Karl Pearson. The invention was one of great beauty; anybody could be proud of having such an idea. Frequency curves are of three main types: The U-shaped distributions with modes at the two ends, the J-shaped ones with a mode at one end and the skew and symmetric distributions with a mode between the two ends at both of which the distribution sinks to 0. Can frequency curves be reduced to a single system? Pearson's answer is that by and large they can be. His original memoirs should be read, but as an initiation one may more easily read chapter XV of D. C. Jones's "First Course in Statistics." The central idea comes to this: That the various types of curve satisfy the differential equation

$$\frac{dy}{dx} = \frac{y(x+b)}{px^2+qx+r}$$

of which the integrals depend on five parameters (one being a constant of integration) and the types depend on various relations between the four parameters other than the constant of integration. Moreover just as the differential equation $dy/dx = -xy/\sigma^2$ of the normal or Gaussian curve may be obtained from the binomial expansion $(p+q)^n$ so the Pearsonian equation is related to the more general hypergeometrical expansion. It is altogether a magnificent conception. The actual fitting of the frequency function of the appropriate type is made from the values of the first five moments which are:

(1) Zeroth moment. $\Sigma y = N =$ total number of observations.
(2) First moment. $\Sigma yx/N = M =$ the mean value of x.
(3) Second moment. $\Sigma yx^2/N = M^2 + \sigma^2$ gives the standard deviation.
(4) Third moment. $\Sigma y(x-M)^3/N = \sqrt{\beta_1}\,\sigma^3$, related to skewness.
(5) Fourth moment. $\Sigma y(x-M)^4/N = \beta_2\,\sigma^4$, related to kurtosis.

Rules for making the fit and tables to aid in the calculations have been worked out by Pearson. The whole represents a very large amount of work. It may also be stated without much fear of contradiction that even with all the tabular aid provided, fitting some of these types and checking the fit is considerable of a chore.

Is it all worth while? In many cases I am afraid it is not. Howsoever happy I should have been to invent the original conception and to discover how well it worked out, I think that for applications such as the above I should have regretfully abandoned the system as unsatisfactory—as too much mathematics. The three series of infant mortalities have been fitted—I give you the fits taken from the literature. (I do not guarantee them; moreover the scale and the origin are not those of the table, *i.e.*, as they stand they are *not* the equations of the frequency functions—but that is of no moment for the present discussion.)

$$\text{I.}\quad y = 46.5502\left(1+\frac{x}{2.8946}\right)^{4.4296}\left(1-\frac{x}{14.5155}\right)^{22.2126}$$

$$\text{II.}\quad y = 0.005609\left(1+\frac{x^2}{(4.5095)^2}\right)^{-12.5407}\times e^{25.9862\tan^{-1}\frac{x}{4.5095}}$$

$$\text{III.}\quad y = 4.2887\times 10^{27}\,(x-20.9629)^{3.0627}\,x^{-19.9804}$$

Note that although the phenomena, infant mortalities, are of the same sort, the functional types of the frequency distributions are totally different. Moreover the functions are so complicated, taking into consideration not alone the type but also the numerical values, that any ready comparative interpretation of them seems out of the question. (It may be admitted that as mere empirical equations fitting the data they may perhaps be fair; at any rate the calculation involved in comparing them with the original data by Pearson's chi-square test for goodness of fit, is more than I should care to take unless there were some very important good to be had from the work; and finally the fit is obviously so bad at the ends that the X^2-test would probably not be satisfied. I quote the results merely as an example of what I consider to be too much mathematics.)

You may ask how I should treat the data. It is a fair question. But I should have to retort with the question, what do you want to find out from the treatment? Much of our time may be saved from useless exercise of technique if we stop to ask what we are trying to find out and whether there is any expectation that we shall find it out by the application of any technique. But I will waive the question and set to work on the third set. First let us observe that infant mortalities under 20 are unlikely to be of statistical significance among the rural colored population; there are no such values in cities over 25,000 nor among rural whites, and I know of no reasonably large districts in the world where infant mortalities run under 20. Next at the other end of the distribution, mortalities above 400 may be open to suspicion, although there are places in the world, say in India or China, where such figures are not unknown, and maybe the same is true of some negro districts in America. However, we need not worry too much over a bad fit on the ends, and perhaps we shall be as well off anyhow as with equation III. As the distribution contains only positive values of the variable and is skewed toward the origin, the first trial may be made graphically on logarithmic probability paper which has been made familiar to us by Hazen and Whipple.[3] It is seen that the summation curve on this paper is practically straight (Fig. 1). There is evidence that

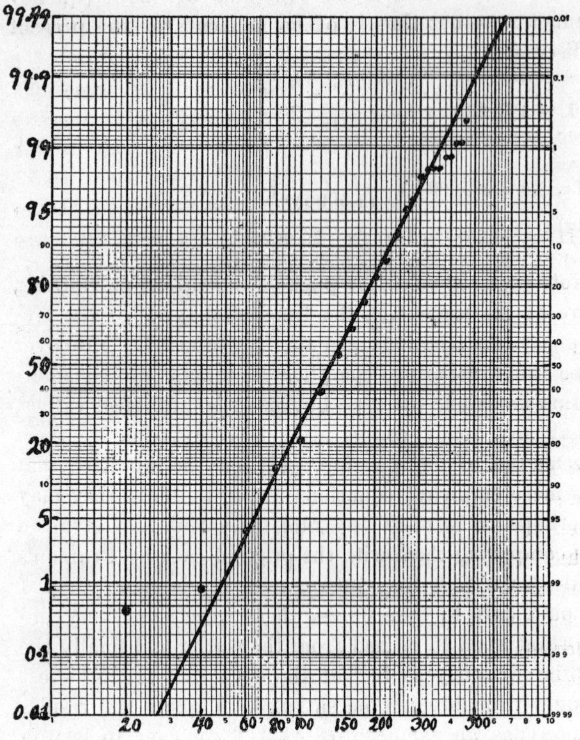

we have too many cases of mortalities under 40 (only 2, to be sure) and over 400; this is in accordance with our suspicions but should not be regarded as confirmation of them. Unless we are in an old field of science with well established fundamental laws, it is not through mathematical developments but by critical analysis of the sources of the data that confirmation of suspicions may be had. The type of frequency function therefore appears to be

$$dy = \frac{234}{\sqrt{2\pi}\,\sigma} e^{[\log(x/x_0)]^2 : 2\sigma^2} \quad d \log x,$$

where dy denotes the number of cases between two neighboring values of the logarithm of the infant mortality, x_0 is the geometric mean or the median of the values of x and σ is the dispersion or standard deviation of the values of log x.

The parameters of the curve may be determined graphically by methods that are well known and simple. For one such determination we have these figures.

Frequency Function of Infant Mortality, 1918; Rural Counties, Colored

Rate	% Less	% Diff.	Freq.	Obs.	Diff.	Diff.^{2}	X^2
20	.00	.00001	0.00234	1	+ 1.0	1.0	(427)
40	.24	.24	.6	1	+ 0.4	.2	.3
60	3.0	2.76	6.4	5	− 1.4	2.0	.3
80	11.3	8.3	19.4	22	+ 2.6	6.8	.3
100	24.8	13.5	31.6	19	−12.6	158.8	5.0
120	39.7	14.9	34.9	42	+ 7.1	50.4	1.5
140	54.0	14.3	33.5	37	+ 3.5	12.2	.4
160	66.3	12.3	28.8	30	+ 1.2	1.4	.0
180	75.5	9.2	21.5	19	− 2.5	6.2	.3
200	82.6	7.1	18.8	17	+ 0.2	.0	.0
220	87.5	4.9	11.5	10	− 1.5	2.2	.2
240	91.3	3.8	9.0	12	+ 3.0	9.0	1.0
260	93.9	2.6	6.1	8	+ 1.9	3.6	.6
280	95.7	1.8	4.3	4	− 0.3	.1	.2
300	97.0	1.3	3.0	2	− 1.0	1.0	.3
340	98.5	1.5	3.5	1	− 2.5	6.2	1.8
380	99.27	.77	1.8	1	− 0.8	.6	.4
420	99.66	.39	.9	1	+ 0.1	.0	.0
460	99.80	.14	.3	1	+ 0.7	.5	1.7
500	99.89	.09	.2	1	+ 0.8	.6	(3.0)
		99.89	234.1	234			$X^2 = 14.3$

The first 6 columns contain, respectively, the rate, the percentage less than that rate, the percentage in the immediate preceding interval of rate, the calculated frequency in that interval, the observed frequency and the differences between the observed and calculated values. The agreement is about all that could be desired. The last two columns give the calculation leading to X^2. The test is vitiated by the very low values of the theoretical frequency in the first single and last double interval; leaving these out we have 18 intervals with $X^2 = 14.3$. This represents a fit so good that chance fluctuations of sampling would produce a worse fit about twice out of three times. Such a correspondence between computed and observed values should be satisfactory and indicate that any more complicated curve such as III above is indeed entirely too much mathematics unless the fit is thereby much improved at the two extremes (as is not the case). The other tables of data can similarly be fitted adequately, I think, on logarithmic probability paper and spare us the annoyance of the complicated Pearsonian equations I and II.

The X^2 test of goodness of fit is due to Pearson and a fine contribution to statistics it was. More recently R. A. Fisher has been over the work and appears to have made some improvements in it and to have given valuable discussions of its application; he also has gone forward with the treatment of the error of the correlation coefficient. Perhaps I may say at this point that, so far as I can judge, R. A. Fisher is to-day the intellectual leader of the biometric school. He is not merely applying the method by rote but is thinking about the problems of statistical analysis in his own right. In his "Statistical Methods for Research Workers" there are several excellent things new with him; the book, however, gives merely

[3] See G. C. Whipple, "Vital Statistics," 2nd Ed., p. 508.

the result; for the detailed reasoning one must consult Fisher's original papers. To Karl Pearson, the great contributor of many important advances in probability and statistics and builder of the science of biometry upon the foundation of Galton, his master, it must be a source of genuine satisfaction, as he nears three score years and ten, to see near at hand so able a disciple as Fisher, an Elisha, who as so often in the history of science, is embroidering, and maybe patching up a bit, the mantle of Elijah ere it falls upon him.

It is interesting to note that the methods of fitting by moments and of estimating goodness of fit by X^2 are logically inconsistent.[4] This may be seen most easily on the zeroth moment which is the total number N of the observations. Let F be the observed frequencies and y the fitted values and let us consider for convenience the actual fit in the intervals tabulated —a discontinuous problem instead of the continuous problems—graduation only instead of graduation plus interpolation.

$$X^2 = \Sigma \frac{(F-y)^2}{y} = \Sigma \frac{F^2}{y} - 2\,\Sigma F + \Sigma y = \Sigma \frac{F^2}{y} - N$$

if we take $\Sigma y = N$. Suppose however that after making this fit we adjust the values of y to new values Z by applying a factor c so that $Z = cy$ and $\Sigma Z = cN$.

$$X^2 = \Sigma \frac{F^2}{Z} - 2\Sigma F + \Sigma Z = \Sigma \frac{F^2}{cy} - 2N + cN$$

The minimum value of X^2_Z will not be given by $c=1$ but, differentiating, by

$$-\left(\Sigma \frac{F^2}{y}\right)\frac{1}{c^2} + N = 0 \quad \text{or by } c = \sqrt{\Sigma \frac{F^2}{Ny}} > 1$$

$$X^2 = N(c^2-1), \qquad X^2_Z = 2N(c-1)$$

The factor c and the change in X^2 are

$$c = \sqrt{1 + X^2/N}, \qquad X^2 - X^2_Z = N(c-1)^2$$

If X^2/N is well below 1, the results simplify to

$$c = 1 + X^2/2N, \qquad X^2 - X^2_Z = X^4/4N$$

and $\Sigma Z = cN$ becomes $N + X^2/2$. In the case above we should have a better fit by taking the total number of observations not as the actual number 234 but as $234 + 7 = 241$, but the improvement in X^2 would not be great. (However, the fit at the two extremes is so bad, small as are the actual numbers of cases, that X^2 if rigorously computed would obtain from the single observation in the 0–19 interval the value 427 which would make c about 1.7 and $X^2 - X^2_Z = 117$ or $X^2_Z = 327$, a great reduction, but still indicative of a very bad fit. Moreover, a change of N from 234 to about 400 is ridiculous, and although X^2 is thereby reduced the fit by any intuitive judgment is far worse.)

From such a simple consideration as this we obtain light on the significance of the X^2 test and yet more upon its limitations which are these: It is not a perfect abstract test but depends on the judgment of the person who uses it in respect both to the details of its arithmetic computation and to its interpretation as a criterion of goodness of fit; it is merely one factor, and a somewhat subjective factor, in aiding the investigator to make up his mind as to whether an attained fit is good enough or not. In the three cases of infant mortalities above mentioned my judgment based largely on graphical evidence and somewhat on a knowledge of the unreliability of the reported figures is that the simple solution I have given is as good as any reasonable person can ask, and this judgment is to my way of thinking not in the slightest called in question, but rather corroborated, by the application of the X^2 test. Many of the criteria of statistics are likewise of this loose character, they are not precisely mathematical truths as statistical criteria no matter how exact they may be as theorems in probability—and no other situation is useful or possible. For this reason I am not interested in a five-figure table of X^2, presumably two significant figures are all that are significant. It is so with many other matters and because it is I prefer that my students should not so much indulge by rote in elaborate but insignificant arithmetic as to form correct judgments by right of sound understanding. It is for this reason that I lament the low intellectual level of books and courses in statistics. It means too much of one kind of mathematics, too little of another kind.

EDWIN B. WILSON
HARVARD SCHOOL OF PUBLIC HEALTH

[4] Puristically speaking. A minimum problem determines its own criteria. Practically, if the fit is efficient (R. A. Fisher), the inconsistency is insignificant. If for simplicity I make so bold as to test the zeroth moment I should perhaps point out that ordinarily the number of observations N is not taken to be a disposable or fittable constant and that the theory of the X^2 test and the tabulated values of X^2 seem to depend somewhat on regarding N as given. Yet in some actuarial practices N is not preserved in the fitted graduation, it is not preserved by the ordinary least squares fit except when the type of fitted function y is of a restricted sort, and there seems to be no reason why a method of fitting appropriate to the theory of sampling might not be developed which should leave N disposable.

THE IMPORTANCE OF BIOLOGY FOR MANKIND[1]

PERMIT me to begin my short address by expressing my great joy to take part in such an important event

[1] Address delivered at the dedication of the new Charles Rebstock Biology Hall of Washington University, St. Louis, November 10, 1927.

for science as the dedication of Rebstock Biology Hall. This event seems to me to be an especially joyful one. I came to this country from Europe only a few weeks ago, where the interest in biological science is abating. The biological laboratories are not frequented in Europe, and one can not dream of founding there new biological institutions, where scientific work could be maintained in a proper manner. It is, therefore, especially joyful that the merits of biology are recognized in this country; and in St. Louis, the name of which has been recently so often repeated by the whole world, a new temple of science arises, devoted to the propagation of biological knowledge.

Biology, including as it does the study of both plants and animals, represents the only basis on which many sciences necessary for mankind are built. In order to avoid the transformation of medicine, agriculture and other applied sciences into quackery and primitive housekeeping their base must be made firm. All success of these sciences depends now only upon the further development of biology. And when their results do not satisfy us sometimes, the cause of this helplessness lies only in an insufficient or not quite correct development of biology. Let us, for instance, regard the cause of the well-known failure to successfully combat such an important and extended disease as cancer.

Our present medical treatment is mostly based on a cardinal principle of biology confirmed by Pasteur, that a spontaneous birth of living beings from dead material is impossible not only in reference to higher organisms but also to bacteria. As many diseases prove to be of a bacterial origin, one supposes usually that all diseases must be produced by microorganisms, though they could not be found in some important and even contagious diseases, as, for instance, in variola or smallpox and scarlet fever. Therefore sometimes cancer is supposed to be produced also by microorganisms. But on the other hand it could only be shown that bacteria can sometimes produce this disease, but it can also be brought about by other organisms and by some poisonous substances. As at the same time some observations have shown that cancer may be hereditary it is very probable that the cause of this disease lies in the organism itself. As is known, cancer consists in an uncommonly luxuriant growth of the epithelic tissue, of the skin, in such a luxuriant growth that the other tissues and even organs are deadened and destroyed thereby. It is evident that we shall only then understand the cause of cancer when we know the phenomena of growth. But what is growth? It is an elementary phenomenon of life, a necessary property of living matter filling those small parts of an organism which are called cells.

It may seem perhaps somewhat incomprehensible that on the occasion of the dedication of a new biological institution a botanist lectures on diseases. But elementary phenomena of life are appropriate to all living cells independently, whether they are plant or animal cells. At the same time only the study of these elementary phenomena of life will permit us to discover the cause of cancer.

I have chosen as an example the case of cancer, but not only this disease, but all the physiological and pathological phenomena of plants and animals depend upon the properties of the living contents of cells. All these processes are carried on in their contents, that is: in protoplasm and nucleus. Therefore in order to direct physiological and pathological processes we must know first of all the properties of protoplasm and nucleus, the properties of living matter.

This thesis has been recognized by a great number of physiologists and physicians, and we see towards the beginning of this century two new branches of biology arise, the so-called cytology and physiology of the cell, which have now hundreds of followers. One of these branches endeavors to study the form and shape of various formations which have been found in the cells of animals or plants. The other branch studies their physical and chemical structure, and physiological properties. Although both these sciences arose not more than 30 years ago, their discoveries are already very important, and it would be no great fault if we predicted that the future of biology will depend upon the progress of these sciences.

More than a hundred years ago chemistry experienced an analogical process of methodical transformation. Thanks to the introduction of quantitative analysis chemistry was able to study the molecules and the change of their structure. The chemistry of substances became the chemistry of molecules and the chemical reactions became quite clear; they proved to be only a consequence of the atomic structure of molecules. The success of the new ideas was so great already at the beginning of the nineteenth century that hundreds of organic and inorganic substances were artificially obtained, and among them such substances as have become so necessary for industry, medicine and agriculture.

Cells play such a part in biology as molecules in chemistry. The atoms are analogous to the formations and structures we find in cells. And since biology studies these formations and structures we could predict its further progress.

But living matter consists of chemical substances. And we see that cell physiology transforms itself by degrees into the chemistry and physics of cells. The chemical composition of the principal substances of living matter is now established, and the following step of the chemistry of cells will be the artificial production of these substances.

The chemical and physical investigations of cells have explained to us the phenomena of diseases and death. The principal substances of living matter have proved to be so very inconstant as to be compared with explosive substances, which explode very easily, that is: they disintegrate into their component parts. They explode by a blow, by heat, by strong light, by the action of various chemical reagents, which react on their component parts. And accordingly the principal substances of living matter could be very easily destroyed by analogical agents: by a blow, by heat, by strong light, by the action of various chemical reagents, which react on their component parts. Therefore the study of explosive substances could help us to learn the properties of living matter. In order to combat against illnesses and diseases we must make the principal substances of living matter constant, so that they would not be so easily destroyed and would not lead living matter and organisms to death. But how can we make them constant? The study of explosive substances shows that the introduction of some chemically indifferent substances, for instance, narcotics, into liquid explosive substances, as for example into nitroglycerin, abolishes their explosive properties. It is sufficient to add only five per cent. of aceton to nitroglycerin to make it quite inexplosive. Accordingly, the introduction of like substances into living matter diminishes its sensibility to injurious influences. But whilst narcotic substances are really indifferent to explosive substances, they are not so in reference to the principal substances of living matter, because these substances contain proteins, which are destroyed by narcotics, and after a short excitement an injurious and dangerous effect is produced and makes living matter more sensible than before. But if we could find such a harmless narcotic substance which would not destroy proteins we could make our living matter constant and in this manner abolish illnesses and diseases. On the other hand, the study of the chemical composition of living matter in bacteria shows that this living matter differs from the living matter of animals and men. We can therefore expect that there are chemical substances which would destroy the principal substances of living matter in bacteria but would not destroy them in man. Therefore the time will certainly come when all harmful bacteria and the diseases produced by them will be expelled from earth forever, and it depends upon us to accelerate the coming of such a time. I am delighted to be able to predict it, and I hope that biology will be able to widen its ways, and to bring near this happy time. The foundation of this new institution proves to me that my hope is not in vain, and that this great country will help biology to display all its manifold powers. Therefore permit me to finish this speech by exclaiming: Long live biology!

W. W. LEPESCHKIN

SCIENTIFIC EVENTS

THE SOUTH AFRICAN STATION OF THE HARVARD OBSERVATORY

WITH the recent purchase of a permanent site on which the South African station of the Harvard Observatory will be erected, the work of erecting the plant has just begun, it is announced by Dr. Harlow Shapley, director of the Harvard Observatory. The site is on top of one of the "kopjes" located outside of the city of Mazelsport, which is fourteen miles from Bloemfontein, Orange Free State, South Africa. Building material, equipment and the instruments which will be used have been arriving in the city since July 1, 1927, when the astronomers first began activities there.

Until the new buildings are completed, the temporary station, which has been operated for some time, will continue to be used. Dr. J. S. Paraskevopoulos, who has been recently appointed assistant professor, and his wife are now in charge of the work of the temporary plant, and two of the four telescopes that are now in Mazelsport, with lenses of ten and eight inches, respectively, are in operation every night.

Cooperating with the Harvard authorities in the erection of the new station, the city of Mazelsport has constructed recently a new highway leading to the top of the hill on which the observatory will be located. When completed, the plant will include a group of buildings consisting of residences, office buildings, laboratories, work shops and garages.

When fully in operation the observatory will house more operating telescopes than any astronomical plant in the world. With three 60-inch telescopes, the observatory will be outclassed in the power of its equipment by only three institutions.

To secure a constant series of photographic plates of the various stars in the Milky Way will be the principal function of the observatory. Studies of these plates, Dr. Shapley states, will have considerable bearing on the knowledge of the size of the universe. The plates will be mailed to the observatory in Cambridge to be studied and filed away in their proper classification.

W. F. Waterfield, of the Cambridge Observatory staff, will leave within a few months to take charge of the final placing of the instruments. Dr. Shapley intends to visit Mazelsport in the future.

THE BATTELLE MEMORIAL INSTITUTE

Announcement of the organization of the Battelle Memorial Institute at Columbus, Ohio, was recently made. The news edition of *Industrial and Engineering Chemistry* gives further particulars. Endowed with a large sum of money from the estate of John Gordon Battelle, his wife and his son, Gordon Battelle, the new institute at once assumes a strong position. A tract of about five acres, opposite the campus of the Ohio State University, has been secured and the construction of the first two buildings, costing about a half million dollars, will be undertaken in the spring. Gerald Wendt, now dean of the school of chemistry and physics at the Pennsylvania State College, has been selected as director, and the organization plans are now under way with the intention of beginning the operations of the institute by the fall of 1928.

The Battelle Memorial Institute has been organized as a corporation, not for profit, in order to perpetuate a trust arising from the joint wills of these three members of the Battelle family. A board of trustees was appointed in the will of Gordon Battelle, one member of which, ex-President Warren G. Harding, has since died. The present board of trustees consists of Joseph H. Frantz, of Columbus, Ohio; Bishop John W. Hamilton, of Washington, D. C., formerly president of the American University; Earl C. Derby, Harry M. Runkle and Gerald B. Fenton, of Columbus, Ohio, and J. Clare Miller, of Ashland, Ky.

Under the terms of the will the institute is to be located in Columbus. The tract now purchased lies on the banks of the Olentangy River and across King Avenue from the campus of the Ohio State University, with a frontage of 300 feet on King Avenue and extending about 1,000 feet southward toward Fifth Avenue. The administration building will face King Avenue and the laboratory buildings will extend southward on Tisdale Street.

While the main object of the institute will be industrial research under the fellowship system, very much as is now the practice at the Mellon Institute, the large income from the funds of the institute itself will be devoted to long-distance industrial research for the broad benefit of American industry and for scientific research. The will provided that any profit arising from the operation of the institute be devoted to charity or to the support of other scientific research.

After an extended inspection trip, in which the chief college and industrial research laboratories in the eastern portion of the United States were studied by the trustees and the director, Otto C. Daret, of Columbus, was designated as architect. The first building will stand as a memorial to the Battelle family and will comprise administrative offices, the library, a large auditorium, a museum, machine shop, stock rooms and a number of laboratory suites. The second building, which will be erected at the same time and will adjoin the administration building, will have individual laboratories on the third floor, but the remaining space, including the basement, first and second floors, will be an engineering shop.

A FUND FOR THE STUDY OF COLDS AT THE JOHNS HOPKINS UNIVERSITY

The Chemical Foundation has made a gift of $195,000 to the school of hygiene and public health of the Johns Hopkins University for the study of "the origin, nature and possible cure of the common cold."

The fund is to be known as "The John J. Abel Fund for Research on the Common Cold" in honor of the professor of pharmacology of the Johns Hopkins School of Medicine, and will provide $25,000 in the first year, $35,000 in the second and $45,000 in the third, fourth and fifth years of the research work.

In his letter announcing the gift Francis P. Garvan, president of the Chemical Foundation, said:

> In asking that the name of your great scientist be connected with this research I am mindful not only of his preeminent position and services in science, but more particularly of his outstanding reputation as the man who, perhaps more than any other living scientist to-day, exemplifies the beneficial application of the science of chemistry to medical problems, which is my abiding interest in such researches as this.

Commenting upon the projected research, Dr. Abel said in part:

> The problem which has been set to our investigation by Mr. Garvan, of the Chemical Foundation, can only be studied by the cooperative efforts of the clinician, the epidemiologist, the bacteriologist, the pathologist, the pharmacologist, the biochemist and the physicist.
>
> Fortunately this spirit of cooperation prevails in the various institutes of the Johns Hopkins University and I am confident that the problem will be attacked with energy, unremitting industry and in a generous spirit of mutual helpfulness by the several investigators into whose hands it will be given.

The research work is to be administered by the following faculty committee: Dr. Lewis H. Weed, dean of the School of Medicine, *chairman;* Dr. William H. Howell, director of the School of Hygiene and Public Health; Dr. Warfield T. Longcope, professor of medicine; Dr. Carroll G. Bull, professor of immunology; Dr. W. H. Frost, professor of epidemiology; Dr. Samuel J. Crowe, professor of laryngology and otology; Dr. Lawrence H. Baker, executive secretary of the medical faculty.

THE NEW LIFE SCIENCES BUILDING AT THE UNIVERSITY OF CALIFORNIA

THIRTEEN departments will be housed by the new Life Sciences Building which is to be erected on the Berkeley campus of the University of California. Floor plans of the building, which is to be 450 by 230 feet, have been prepared and the regents have authorized Supervising Architect George W. Kelham to proceed with the working plans. Construction will start in the spring and the building, it is hoped, will be ready in 1929.

The building will house the following departments: Anatomy, bacteriology, biochemistry, pharmacology, physiology, hygiene, botany, psychology, household science, plant nutrition, zoology, museum of vertebrate zoology and board of health.

The following old wooden buildings will be torn down upon the completion of the new structure: entomology building, Budd hall, plant nutrition, museum of vertebrate zoology, physiology laboratory, hygiene and pathology, botany, botany laboratory, anatomy, psychology, zoology and the public health building.

The new Life Sciences Building, five stories in height, will provide each department with about 60 per cent. more room than it has at present, in all 145,000 square feet of floor space, approximately three acres. It will be in the shape of a hollow rectangle, with the laboratories facing the court inside. An auditorium with seating capacity of 500 will be located at the east end, balanced by the Museum of Vertebrate Zoology at the west end. The classrooms will be grouped at the east end, near the library, but the building itself will have a library of 90,000 volumes. There will be no elevators except those for freight service.

With the completion of the working drawings, plans and specifications, bids will be asked. It is expected the building will cost approximately $1,750,000, the funds to be taken from the $3,000,000 bond issue voted by the people in 1926.

A SYMPOSIUM AT THE ALFRED L. LOOMIS LABORATORY IN HONOR OF PROFESSOR J. FRANCK

THE arrival of Professor J. Franck in this country was made the occasion of a symposium in his honor at the Loomis Laboratory, Tuxedo Park, on January 6. About ninety physicists attended the symposium as the guests of Mr. Alfred L. Loomis. Opportunity was afforded for visiting the laboratory where the various investigations under way were described and illustrated.

The physical research institutions and university laboratories of the east were well represented, the following being among those present:

Dr. Lyman J. Briggs, Bureau of Standards.
Professor Karl T. Compton, Princeton University.
Dr. W. D. Coolidge, General Electric Company.
Professor Bergen Davis, Columbia University.
Dr. C. J. Davisson, Bell Telephone Laboratories.
Dr. Arthur L. Day, Geophysical Laboratory, Washington.
Professor William Duane, Harvard University.
Dr. Gano Dunn, National Research Council.
Professor R. C. Gibbs, Cornell University.
Professor Karl F. Herzfeld, The Johns Hopkins University.
Dr. C. W. Hewlett, General Electric Company.
Professor John C. Hubbard, The Johns Hopkins University.
Dr. Albert W. Hull, General Electric Company.
Professor Edwin Kemble, Harvard University.
Dr. Irving Langmuir, General Electric Company.
Professor F. Wheeler Loomis, New York University.
Professor J. C. McLennan, University of Toronto.
Dr. Howard McClenahan, The Franklin Institute.
Professor Louis W. McKeehan, Yale University.
Professor George B. Pegram, Columbia University.
Captain E. G. Oberlin, Naval Research Laboratory.
Dean Harold Pender, University of Pennsylvania.
Professor F. A. Saunders, Harvard University.
Professor W. F. G. Swann, Bartol Research Foundation.
Professor Oswald Veblen, Princeton University.
Professor H. W. Webb, Columbia University.
Dr. W. R. Whitney, General Electric Company.
Professor Albert P. Wills, Columbia University.
Professor Robert W. Wood, The Johns Hopkins University.

The following papers were presented:

The electrical and optical phenomena connected with the recombination of positive ions and electrons, by PROFESSOR J. FRANCK.

Some new effects in the optical excitation of mercury, by PROFESSOR ROBERT W. WOOD.

Concepts in quantum mechanics, by PROFESSOR W. F. G. SWANN.

Extreme ultra-violet spectra excited by controlled electron impacts, by PROFESSOR KARL T. COMPTON.

The aurora green line, by PROFESSOR G. CARIO.

SCIENTIFIC NOTES AND NEWS

FOR the meeting of the British Association for the Advancement of Science to be held next year in Glasgow from September 5 to 12, under the presidency of Sir William Bragg, the following sectional presidents have been appointed: Section A (mathematical and physical sciences), Professor A. W. Porter; section B (chemistry), Professor E. C. C. Baly; section C (geology), E. B. Bailey; section D (zoology), Professor W. Garstang; section E (geography), Professor J. L. Myres; section G (engineering), Sir William Ellis; section H (anthropology), Sir George Macdonald; section I (physiology), Professor C. Lovatt Evans;

section J (psychology), Professor T. H. Pear; section K (botany), Professor R. H. Yapp; section L (education), Professor A. Smithells; section M (agriculture), Dr. J. S. Gordon. The president of section F (economic science and statistics), has not yet been appointed.

ON February 16, Professor Hugo de Vries will celebrate the eightieth anniversary of his birth. On retiring from his professorship in the University of Amsterdam in 1918 he removed to the small village of Lunteren, Holland, and built for himself a laboratory and an experimental garden for the continuation of his genetical studies on Oenothera. He is still prosecuting these studies with a vigor and effectiveness which excites universal admiration. It is to be hoped that American biological organizations and institutions, biological departments in our universities and numerous personal friends and admirers of Professer de Vries will send appropriate messages to him on this occasion. Messages and resolutions timed to leave the Atlantic seaboard in the first days of February should reach him opportunely.

IN recognition of his thirty-five years as an outstanding teacher in the medical school of the University of Michigan and his international reputation as a pathologist, Dr. Aldred S. Warthin has been the recipient of an honor from his colleagues and former students, in the form of a volume entitled "Contributions to Medical Science." This book of 715 pages includes contributions from sixty-four authors, representing his early colleagues and including one or more representatives from each of his thirty-five successive classes.

THE board of directors of the Geographic Society of Chicago at its last meeting unanimously voted to award its gold medal to Colonel Charles A. Lindbergh. It is planned to present this medal to Colonel Lindbergh at the final meeting for the season in Orchestra Hall on April 24. Commander Richard E. Byrd, a gold medalist of the society, has been invited to come to Chicago to make the address of presentation.

JAMES A. PARSONS, metallurgist for the Dur Iron Company, has received the science award of the Harmon Foundation for his research in aluminum bronze, his discoveries on corrosion testing and his developments in duriron.

DR. WILLIAM RICE, dean of the Tufts College Dental School, will receive the 1928 award of the Rhode Island Dental Society at the semi-centennial convention of the society. The medal will be awarded "for his contribution to dental education, and his leadership and inspiration to the students under his guidance."

DR. HENRY CREW, professor of physics at Northwestern University, was elected president of the American Association of University Professors at its recent meeting in Cincinnati.

A. W. BERRESFORD, electrical engineer, was elected president of the American Engineering Council at the recent meeting held in Washington, D. C.

THE managers of the New York Botanical Garden have elected Henry W. De Forest, chairman of the executive committee of the Southern Pacific Company, president, to succeed Professor F. S. Lee, of Columbia University, who has been president for five years.

C. C. WILLOUGHBY, director of the Peabody Museum at Harvard University, has been made emeritus director. The position of director of the museum has been filled by the appointment of Dr. S. K. Lothrop, formerly research associate in the Museum of the American Indian, New York.

AT the fifty-ninth annual meeting of the trustees of the American Museum of Natural History on January 8, Dr. H. F. Osborn, president-elect of the American Association for the Advancement of Science, was elected president for the twentieth successive year; Mr. Baker, first vice-president, for the fifth year; J. P. Morgan, second vice-president, for the seventeenth year; Mr. Perkins, treasurer, for the second year, and Percy R. Pyne, secretary, for the eighth year. Dr. Osborn has accepted the post of curator-in-chief of the division of mineralogy, geology, geography and astronomy, and he has also accepted the honorary curatorship of the department of geology and paleontology. Dr. G. Clyde Fisher has been made curator of the department of astronomy. The new appointments are: Hawthorne Daniel, curator of the department of printing and publishing and editor of *Natural History;* Miss Francesca R. LaMonte, assistant in ichthyology, and Robert T. Hatt, assistant curator in mammalogy.

DR. ARTHUR PIERSON KELLEY, assistant professor of botany in Rutgers University, will go on February first to the Allegheny Forest Experiment Station, Philadelphia, as associate forest ecologist.

DR. DOUGLAS R. SEMMES, of Richmond, Va., has been appointed to the staff of the Alabama state geological survey.

MORSE SALISBURY, editor of the press bureau of the University of Wisconsin, has been appointed temporarily as chief of the radio service of the U. S. Department of Agriculture pending a new examination. The position has been vacant since the resignation of Sam Pickard to become secretary, and later a member, of the federal radio commission.

DR. B. T. DICKSON, formerly professor of plant pathology in McGill University, arrived in Sydney in November to take up his new duties as senior plant pathologist for the Australian Council for Scientific and Industrial Research.

PROFESSOR OSWALD VEBLEN, Henry B. Fine research professor of mathematics, has been granted a leave of absence for the coming academic year to carry on research work at the University of Oxford. Oxford will send to Princeton for the same period Professor Godfred H. Hardy, Savilian professor of geometry and a foreign member of the National Academy of Sciences.

DR. TAMOH IKEDA, in charge of food control for the bureau of public health of Tokyo, is spending the month of January working under the direction of Professor R. A. Dutcher in the vitamine laboratory of the Pennsylvania State College. Dr. Ikeda is visiting the United States under the auspices of the Rockefeller Foundation.

HARLAN H. ZODTNER, of the Smithsonian Institution, is leaving the United States to spend three years in the Chilean Andes, measuring the sun's radiation, as part of the institution's study of the solar constant. He will relieve H. B. Freeman, present director of the Smithsonian Observatory at Mount Montezuma, near Calama, Chile, who has completed three years in the region.

DR. OSCAR RIDDLE, of the Carnegie Institution, during the latter part of January will deliver a series of lectures at the University of Porto Rico on "Sex, Reproduction and Internal Secretions."

PROFESSOR JAMES FRANCK, of the University of Göttingen, upon his recent arrival in New York was entertained by the departments of physics and chemistry of New York University in the Brevoort Hotel. Dr. Franck delivered a series of lectures at Harvard University during the week of January 9.

DR. NIELS G. HÖRNER, of the Swedish Geological Survey, addressed the geological conference at Harvard University on January 17 on "European Inland Dunes and their Climatic Significance."

DR. HAROLD NORINDER, of the Swedish State Power Organization, will give a lecture at the Franklin Institute on January 26 on "Some Electrophysical Conditions determining Lightning Surges."

THE non-resident lecturer in chemistry at Cornell University under the George Fisher Baker foundation for the second term of the present university year will be Professor George Barger, of the University of Edinburgh, who will lecture upon "Some Applications of Organic Chemistry to Biology." The non-resident lecturer for the first term of the university year 1928–1929 will be Professor Hans Pringsheim, of the University of Berlin, who will lecture upon "The Chemistry of the Monosaccharides and Polysaccharides." The non-resident lecturers are provided with a private research laboratory, and the university extends the privilege of the department of chemistry to visiting chemists who may wish to carry on research under the direction of the lecturers.

DR. CARL F. CORI, from the State Institute for the Study of Malignant Diseases, Buffalo, N. Y., will deliver the third Harvey Society lecture at the New York Academy of Medicine, on Friday evening, January 27. His subject will be "The Influence of Hormones on the Fate of Carbohydrates in the Animal Body."

DR. ALEXANDER WETMORE, assistant secretary of the Smithsonian Institution and retiring president of the Washington Academy of Sciences, gave an address before the 217th meeting of the academy, January 10, on "Prehistoric Ornithology in North America."

PROFESSOR S. R. DETWILER, of Columbia University, lectured to the biological section of the New York Academy of Sciences on January 9, on "Observations on the Growth of Nerves in the Embryo."

A STATUE of the late M. Emile Baudot, the inventor of the telegraph transmission instrument bearing his name, was recently unveiled in the courtyard of the French General Post Office in Paris.

THE Second Church building, now being used to temporarily house the department of zoology of Oberlin College, has been named the Albert A. Wright zoological laboratory, in commemoration of the services to the college of the late Professor A. A. Wright.

A MEETING to commemorate the life and services of the late Charles Doolittle Walcott, secretary of the Smithsonian Institution from 1907 to 1927, will be held in the auditorium of the natural history building on January 24, at 11:00 o'clock. The chancellor of the Smithsonian Institution, the Honorable William H. Taft, Chief Justice of the United States, will preside. Addresses will be delivered by the following representatives of organizations with which Secretary Walcott was actively affiliated: Dr. John C. Merriam, the Carnegie Institution of Washington; Dr. Joseph S. Ames, the National Advisory Committee for Aeronautics; Dr. George Otis Smith, the United States Geological Survey, and Dr. Charles G. Abbot, the National Academy of Sciences.

ALEXANDER E. OUTERBRIDGE, of the William Sellers Company, also lecturer at the University of Pennsylvania, and professor of metallurgy at the Franklin

Institute, died on January 15 at the age of seventy-seven years.

Professor Elmer E. F. Creighton, electrical engineer of the General Electric Co., Schenectady, died on January 13, at the age of forty-nine years.

W. H. Dines, F.R.S., British meteorologist, well known for his explorations of the upper air, died on December 24, aged seventy-two years.

Dr. W. C. F. Newton, research student at the John Innes Horticultural Institution, recently died at the age of thirty-two years. A correspondent writes: "The death of Dr. Newton is deplored by those interested in the development of cytology and genetics. His personality attracted the notice of William Bateson under whose sympathetic directorship he worked several years at the John Innes Horticultural Institution, Merton. He will be remembered for his beautiful study of the chromosomes of *Tulipa* and related genera, and for other work much of which is as yet unpublished."

A joint meeting of the Optical Society of America and The American Physical Society will be held at Columbia University in New York City on February 24 and 25. Special features will include an invited address by Dr. W. F. G. Swann on "Recent Theories of the Atom" and a demonstration of television at the Bell Laboratories.

The annual congress on Medical Education and Medical Licensure and Hospitals will take place in Chicago at Palmer House on February 6, 7 and 8.

The eighth summer term of the American School of Prehistoric Research will open in London on June 28 and close on the Continent the middle of September. Requests for information concerning details of the program and requirements for admission should be addressed to the director, Dr. George Grant MacCurdy, Peabody Museum, New Haven, Conn.

Dr. William Crocker, Dr. Waldemar Lindgren and Dr. A. L. Barrows, of the National Research Council, recently conferred with members of the staff of the Biological Survey in the interest of arranging comprehensive cooperative studies of geological, zoological and botanical problems and other related lines of research, in the Aleutian Islands, Alaska. Effort is being made to enlist in this survey such agencies as the Biological Survey, the Bureau of Plant Industry, the Forest Service, the Geological Survey, the Coast and Geodetic Survey, the Bureau of Fisheries and the Smithsonian Institution.

A royal commission to inquire into and report upon all matters relating to the fishing industry of the Maritime Provinces has been appointed and is holding sittings in all the important fishing centers of the Maritimes, so that those engaged in every branch of the industry will have opportunity to attend its sessions and discuss their problems. Subsequently, at the request of the provincial government of Quebec, which for the past few years has been administering the fisheries in all portions of the province, except in the Magdalen Islands, it was agreed that the scope of the investigation should be extended to the mainland of the Province of Quebec and sittings will be held there when the investigation is completed in the Maritimes.

The council of the British Empire Cancer Campaign is sending invitations to persons and organizations conducting research into cancer to attend the International Convention on Cancer Research next July in London. Receipt of an anonymous gift of $50,000 to the campaign has been announced. The sum of $80,000 also has been set up as a permanent trust by the executors of the estate of William Johnston, of Liverpool. The interest will be applied to cancer research work in Liverpool.

At a special general meeting of the British Institute of Physics held on December 16, and on the recommendation of the board, the Royal Meteorological Society was admitted a participating society of the institute. This is the sixth society to cooperate in the scheme of participation, and an important step is thus taken towards the realization of one of the principal objects of the institute, as expressed at its foundation, namely, to coordinate the work of all existing societies concerned with the science of physics and its applications.

A new meteorological observatory has been ordered by the government of India on the advice of its meteorological director, J. H. Field. It will be built at Poona for special research work, with a view to accurate forecasting of southwest monsoons and will be brought into use the coming summer. About $320,000 has been appropriated for the observatory.

A bequest amounting to about £35,000 has been left by Mr. John Sanderson, manufacturer, of Galashiels, to Edinburgh University for the development of technical and scientific study under the faculty of science.

"The Lasker Foundation for Medical Research" has been established at the University of Chicago with an initial endowment of $1,000,000, the gift of Albert D. Lasker and his wife, Mrs. Flora W. Lasker. Mr. Lasker is former chairman of the United States Shipping Board and head of the Lord and Thomas advertising agency. Research under the spirit of the endowment is to be directed toward establishing the causes, nature, prevention and cure of degenerative diseases. While a definite program has not yet been developed under the foundation, it is said that the first efforts would be made against Bright's disease and heart disease.

ANNOUNCEMENT has been made by the University of Chicago board of trustees of the following subscriptions for the endowment of the Frank Billings Medical Clinic: From Mr. Samuel Insull, $25,000; Mrs. C. K. G. Billings, $10,000; Mr. Charles A. Monroe, $5,000; Miss Margaretta E. Otis, $5,000; Mr. John W. Fowler, $3,000; Mrs. Howard H. Spaulding, $3,000; Mr. John T. Llewellyn, $2,000; Mrs. Theodore Sheldon, $2,000; Mr. Walter S. Brewster, $1,000; Mr. William S. Hay, $1,000; Mr. George M. Reynolds, $1,000; Mr. George E. Scott, $1,000; Mr. and Mrs. William H. Rahmann, $600; Mr. Charles E. Field, $200; Mr. Thomas Meighan, $100, and Mr. R. H. Ritchie, $100. A total of $328,723 has already been received for the fund.

THE research ship *William Scoresby,* after being refitted, has left Portsmouth, England, on another cruise to the Antarctic. She returned from a similar expedition a few months ago. The first port of call will be St. Vincent, and the ship will then proceed by way of Rio de Janeiro and the Falkland Islands to the Antarctic. Commander De La Motte is in charge of the ship, and the trip is expected to last twelve months. The *William Scoresby,* which was built to work in conjunction with Shackleton's *Discovery,* is 180 feet long, of about 700 tons and is equipped with the latest scientific apparatus.

THE late Harry W. Loos has bequeathed a fund amounting to approximately $3,500,000 to Kansas City to be devoted to such charitable, hospital, educational, scientific, literary or research purposes as may be in the public interest.

UNIVERSITY AND EDUCATIONAL NOTES

GEORGE WASHINGTON UNIVERSITY announces receipt of the Isabella King endowment of $30,000 for the establishment of a fellowship or fellowships for special research in biology. The income from this endowment will be available in 1928–29.

DARTMOUTH COLLEGE has received a gift of $300,000 for a new fine arts building from Frank P. Carpenter.

THE National School of Medicine and Pharmacy, Port au Prince, Haiti, recently dedicated its new building. On the first floor are five classrooms, an assembly room, a dental department, a store room and an office for the dean. There are five laboratories on the second floor for the medical sciences. The Rockefeller Foundation made an appropriation of $30,000 for equipment and of another $30,000 for fellowships for men who are to be trained for positions on the faculty of the medical school. These fellowships have been awarded and the physicians are to study in Paris, Strasbourg, Ann Arbor, Boston, New Haven, Chicago, then return to Haiti to become members of the faculty.

AN offer by the joint committee of the Paviors' Company and of the Institution of Municipal and County Engineers to establish a part-time chair of highway engineering in the University of London for post-graduate students has been accepted.

DR. FRANK J. GOODNOW, president of the Johns Hopkins University, has offered his resignation to the board of trustees, to be effective not later than July 1, 1929.

DR. WILMER KRUSEN, director of the department of health and recently elected president of the Philadelphia College of Pharmacy and Science, formally assumed his new duties as president of the school on January 3.

DR. JOSEPH S. CHAMBERLAIN, professor of organic and agricultural chemistry, has been appointed head of the department of chemistry of the Massachusetts Agricultural College. Dr. J. B. Lindsey, formerly head of the department, resigned from this position and is continuing his work as head of the department of plant and animal chemistry of the experiment station, in which work he has been engaged for the past thirty-seven years.

DR. FRANK B. MALLORY, pathologist of the Boston City Hospital, has been appointed professor of pathology at the Harvard Medical School.

DR. E. DAVID FRIEDMAN has been appointed professor of neurology and head of the department at the University and Bellevue Hospital Medical College.

DISCUSSION AND CORRESPONDENCE

THE PROPOSED TRANSFER OF GEODETIC WORK OF THE U. S. COAST AND GEODETIC SURVEY

IN connection with House Resolution 7480, introduced in the House of Representatives by Mr. Sinnott on December 15, 1927, my attention has been called to a circular letter containing unfavorable comments upon this measure, and several scientists interested in our work have written me requesting more specific information. These comments state that the proposed transfer could be justified only on one or more of three suppositions:

First: "That the Coast and Geodetic Survey is not doing the work properly." There is no basis for this supposition. Foreign geodesists allude to the Coast and Geodetic Survey as the foremost geodetic institution in the world, and I concur most heartily in this opinion.

Second: "That the Geological Survey can do the work better." Of course the Geological Survey can not do it better, for we all believe that the work of the Coast Survey is of the very highest quality, but I do believe that the Geological Survey can do it just as well if we can continue to have the cordial cooperation that we have received from the Coast and Geodetic Survey in the past. The circular letter states that the Geological Survey has never done any first order triangulation and traverse and has done no first order leveling for many years. This statement is unfortunate. The facts are that we have done first order triangulation and leveling, but have not done any in recent years because we have felt that it would be a duplication of effort, inasmuch as the Coast Survey was already engaged on similar work. Until recent years the Coast Survey planned a great deal of its first order work to meet our mapping needs, but since the world war it has confined its activities very largely to the program of covering the entire country with these first order arcs or circuits without much attention to the mapping program, except as we have transferred money for specific jobs. Up to recently I think this program has been a wise one, but the adjustment of the western arc of triangulation and a large part of the basic level network have been made and my associates feel that a large part of the first order control work to be executed in the future should be planned to meet the immediate needs of the topographic mapping program.

Third: "That a better theoretical organization can be secured by the transfer." The circular letter states that the Coast and Geodetic Survey is the only purely surveying bureau in the government, while the Geological Survey primarily is concerned with geological investigations. An analysis of our topographic mapping operations during the past seven years will show that only a small percentage of the topographic work has been executed to meet the immediate needs of our geologic program, but that our topographic mapping has been planned rather to meet the general engineering and scientific needs of the country. The circular states that the interior geodetic work has been planned to meet the requirements of the Geological Survey. This is not an entirely correct statement, but if it is true that the primary reason for conducting the interior geodetic work is to provide adequate control for topographic mapping, I am confident that it can be coordinated and performed more expeditiously and economically if it can be administered by the same organization that is charged with the topographic mapping.

I have been informed that the real reason for the circulation of the unfavorable comments is that a number of scientists are concerned with the effect of the proposed transfer upon the results now being secured in the study of earth movements in California, through the cooperation now existing between the Coast and Geodetic Survey and the scientific organizations interested in seismology in California. If the authorization and appropriation for precise triangulation and leveling and seismological observations in regions subject to earthquakes were transferred to the Geological Survey, we should hope to continue to cooperate just as the Coast Survey is now doing. In fact, during the next two years of the program we would probably arrange to have the work continued by personnel detailed from the Coast Survey, as is provided in the bill.

The bill was initiated by the Secretary of Commerce, who several years ago had stated that he would transfer the geodetic work of the Coast Survey to the Geological Survey as soon as he had authority by law. At the hearings before the joint committee on reorganization of the executive departments, both the Secretary of Commerce and the Secretary of the Interior indorsed this proposed transfer.

The present bill was drafted jointly by the two departments and was transmitted to congress with a letter of indorsement signed by the two secretaries. This letter brought out the fact that the primary function of the Coast and Geodetic Survey is to produce nautical charts, while one of the primary functions of the Geological Survey is to produce the standard topographic map of the United States. Geodetic surveys for the control of our coast lines were started by the Coast Survey in the early days of that organization, and later when the need for similar control in the interior of the country was manifest, the Coast Survey extended its geodetic work into the interior. Geodetic control is essential for topographic mapping, and the principal purpose of the geodetic work of the Coast Survey in the interior has been to furnish the control needed by the Geological Survey for its mapping activities. The letter stated that this divided responsibility for the production of the topographic map is fundamentally unsound, and that one agency should be charged with every step in the project.

The proposed bill meets with my hearty approval for the following reasons: The topographic work of the Geological Survey has been planned with the fundamental idea of making as much progress as possible toward the ultimate completion of the mapping program. The interior geodetic work of the Coast Survey has been largely confined to the extension of control to cover the entire country with large arcs or circuits of precise work. Much of this work is being extended over areas already topographically mapped, and such work as the Coast Survey has done in recent years for immediate use in mapping has been actually paid for by transfer of funds from the Geological Survey. While much duplication of effort of the two bureaus has been eliminated through the cordial cooperation that exists, still there is considerable divergence of policies and plans and there is not that degree of coordination which must exist in order that a comprehensive program may be prepared and executed in the most effective way.

Publication of geographic positions and spirit level elevations should be standardized in one organization. The geodetic work should be planned to meet the immediate needs of the mapping program, and often the same geodetic field party should do the precise work and follow immediately with the secondary control now executed by the Geological Survey. A substantial saving of overhead expense in field and office operation and in the procurement and use of equipment would be effected if the transfer were made.

GEO. OTIS SMITH,
Director

UNSTABILITY AT THE ABSOLUTE ZERO OF TEMPERATURE

IT has been shown by the writer (*J. Phy. Chem.*, 31, 747–756 (1927)) that a substance or mixture in the condensed state under its vapor pressure at the absolute zero of temperature T has zero controllable internal energy and entropy. With this as basis the writer has calculated the internal energies of a large number of the elements, which are given in a paper just published (*J. Phy. Chem.*, 31, 1669–1673, 1927). The largest and smallest values obtained were 1,535 and 1,037 cal./mol. for lead and iron respectively. Since G. N. Lewis has already calculated the entropies of these elements, it was possible to calculate also their free energies, the largest and smallest values being $-2{,}791$ and -750 for lead and chromium respectively.

An interesting point presented itself in these investigations. If a substance is lowered in temperature to the absolute zero it may not finally be in a condensed and vaporous phase at zero pressure. A further change at $T=0$ will therefore have to take place before its internal energy is zero. Now it has also been shown by the writer (*J. Phy. Chem.*, 31, 940, (1927)) that the adiabatic of zero entropy corresponds to $T=0$. It follows from this that a change in internal energy at $T=0$ appears as external work. Hence under these conditions a substance will become unstabled at $T=0$ and exert a pressure. On allowing the substance to expand doing external work it will finally end in the condensed state under zero vapor pressure, when its internal energy is zero. It was shown in the paper mentioned that white tin should behave in this manner at $T=0$, and develop while expanding to become stable an average pressure of about 3,000 atmos. Thus certain substances may act like an explosive at or near the absolute zero of temperature.

This result has an interesting astronomical aspect. Dark bodies in interstellar space which are losing more heat than they receive eventually sink in temperature to near the absolute zero, and then may possibly get unstable and explode. This may conceivably happen to our moon some day if it radiates more heat than it receives, and has compounds in its composition possessing this property.

R. D. KLEEMAN
SCHENECTADY, N. Y.

THE THEORY OF "VISIBLE RADIATION FROM AN EXCITED NERVE FIBER"

IN a recent article in SCIENCE,[1] Mrs. Christine Ladd-Franklin gave an exposition of the phenomenon of the reddish-blue arcs and of her interpretation in terms of visible radiation from the excited nerve fiber. A foot-note in this article gives a reference to a paper of mine, and in the same foot-note Mrs. Ladd-Franklin describes an observation of her own and gives her interpretation. To the casual reader it might easily appear that the observation and opinion are quoted from my article. To avoid any such misinterpretation I wish to go on record as disagreeing absolutely with Mrs. Ladd-Franklin's interpretation of the reddish-blue arcs and the other phenomena which she cites, I do not believe that the evidence compels us to assume visible radiation from excited nerve fibers. The explanation set forth by Amberson[2] and others, based on secondary excitation by the action currents of the nerve fibers, seems quite adequate and requires less violent efforts of the imagination.

Mrs. Ladd-Franklin's point concerning the "place coefficient" of the sensation is sound, and we must agree that the secondary excitation is in rod, cone, bipolar cell or ganglia—not in the nerve fiber; but her argument against electrical excitation of one of these elements is unconvincing. Electric stimuli applied to the eye externally may give the sensation of light without a residual image, and this we may

[1] Christine Ladd-Franklin, 1927. SCIENCE, lxvi, 239.

[2] Amberson, W. R., 1924. *Am. Journ. Physiol.*, lxix, 354.

interpret as direct excitation of nerve fibers. This does not prove that an electrical disturbance *localized in the retina,* like a nerve action current, might not stimulate the photosensory mechanism directly.

It is worth noting that the phenomena reported by Nodon[3] of photographic effects from organic substances, which he interprets as due to "radiations" and which Mrs. Ladd-Franklin cites in support of her theory, have long been familiar. The subject has been reviewed by Keenan[4] and the weight of evidence points to the evolution of traces of hydrogen peroxide as the explanation.

HALLOWELL DAVIS

HARVARD MEDICAL SCHOOL

THE ANTIQUITY OF THE DEPOSITS IN JACOBS CAVERN

NELS C. NELSON in SCIENCE, for September 16, 1927, criticizes the article by me on "The Antiquity of the Deposits in Jacobs Cavern," printed in *Am. Mus. Nat. Hist.,* Vol. XIX, Part VI.

Admittedly *not* found in undisturbed strata, the Jacobs Cavern carved "Mastodon" bone must stand or fall upon its own merits. X-ray photographs and specific gravity determinations show this bone to be mineralized; inspection shows that mineralization occurred *after* the carving. Comparative photographs under six definite wave-lengths of light indicate that the bone is old and likewise the carving. Chemical and physical analyses (by experts in these fields) of samples taken in the presence of Mr. Nelson (and their position recorded photographically) show the presence of a second, lower, inhabited layer not examined by Mr. Nelson. The perforation of the carved bone was from both sides; these two holes taper and meet at a slight angle—the shortness and taper of these holes are characteristic of stone drills. The head of the elk-like effigy on the reverse apparently takes advantage of a crack, while the wavy marks on the same side ignore several cracks.

Against these definite data stands the sincere guess of an eminent archeologist.

VERNON C. ALLISON

THE MISPRONUNCIATION OF "DATA"

APROPOS of the controversy concerning the singular and plural usage of "data," may attention be called to the fact that this word is mispronounced much more commonly and with less justification than it is incorrectly used in writings. Probably no other word in the vocabulary of the average scientist is mispronounced more generally. Merely as an example of this fact, the incident mentioned below is noted from the last annual meeting of the Pacific Division of the American Association for the Advancement of Science. The pronunciations "dāta" and "dăta" were used by two different persons on the program at one of the general meetings. In a meeting of the section on entomology one speaker pronounced the word "dāta" another pronounced it "dăta" and a third said "däta." The leading dictionaries including Funk & Wagnall's New Standard and Webster's New International give only one pronunciation, namely, dāta.

In some respects this matter may seem too trivial to be mentioned. However, the student in high school, college and university, and Mr. Average Citizen have come to regard the scientist as one who is peculiarly exact and correct, and this ideal is not enhanced when scientists, in classroom instruction and in public addresses, are careless to the extent of mispronouncing a word that is used so commonly by scientists in general.

R. H. SMITH

UNIVERSITY OF CALIFORNIA

[3] Nodon, A., 1924. *Comptes Rendus,* clxxviii, 1101.

[4] Keenan, G. L., 1926. *Chemical Reviews,* iii, 95.

SCIENTIFIC BOOKS

Les problèmes de la physiologie normale et pathologique de l'os. R. Leriche et A. Policard. Masson et Cie, Paris, 1927.

THIS book of 229 pages, including 23 text figures and an extensive bibliography of 219 titles, is dedicated to the memory of Leopold Ollier, "originator of modern bone physiology." The book represents the fruit of a collaboration extending over a period of ten years. It assembles in a convenient and logical unit much of what had been scattered under separate and joint authorship through various journals since 1909. A new theory of osteogenesis is here developed and firmly based on a large body of data, histological, experimental and radiographic. This theory furnishes a consistent interpretative key for the explanation of certain apparently contradictory facts in normal bone development and regeneration. It explains, moreover, diverse and obscure pathologic condition of bone formation. It reconciles the paradoxical aspects of the current view of osteogenesis which regards the so-called osteoblast, when operating alone, as a bone builder, and when fused in masses, as a bone destroyer or osteoclast.

Osteogenesis is interpreted in essence as a condition of osseous metaplasia of fibrous connective tissue. This is shown to occur in four stages, whether the connective tissue be embryonal, or mature fibrous: a, edematous infiltration; b, multiplication of fibrils; c, conversion of the interstitial fluid into a gelatinous preosseous substance; d, deposition of calcium phosphates and carbonates. These processes are dependent upon humoral and interstitial rather than upon cellular factors.

Osteoblasts are regarded as fibroblasts with only a feeble osteolytic capacity. Their function is to oppose and restrict osseous extension. Cases are cited in which new formation of bone, as disclosed by skiagraph, is unaccompanied by osteoblasts. Conversely, osseous areas in which there is no new formation of bone are covered with osteoblasts of typical epithelioid character. Osteoblasts become secondarily involved in osteogenesis and thus are incorporated as osteocytes. As such they have no osteogenic nor nutrient functions; they are "useless parasites of osseous tissue." However, under the influence of certain pathologic factors they may have their original osteolytic capacity greatly stimulated. Osteolysis also is primarily dependent upon humoral processes. Osteoclasia, by action of osteoclasts, is said to be a relatively minor factor in bone resorption.

The results of experiments with rabbits, involving resections, fractures and transplants, are in accord with the earlier ideas of Havers, Bichat, and Macewen, who regarded the periosteum simply as a structure limiting ossification. The periosteum "blocks osteogenesis." The so-called osteogenetic layer of the periosteum is not a bone-forming tissue; it opposes and restricts the spread of bone. New formation of bone is invariably associated with bone resorption. The formation of callus in the repair of fractures is preceded by resorption of the broken extremities of the bone. Likewise, in the case of bone transplants; the transplant is resorbed before new bone appears. Such resorption supplies the necessary local excess of calcium for the stimulation of the osseous metaplasia. Osseous metaplasia of connective tissue is a reversible process. Bone resorption follows upon increased circulatory activity locally, a condition dependent upon vasomotor control. The authors believe that the results of their investigations open a new chapter in bone pathology, that of bone diseases of vasomotor origin.

H. E. JORDAN

UNIVERSITY OF VIRGINIA

SCIENTIFIC APPARATUS AND LABORATORY METHODS

METHODS FOR DETERMINING THE COLOR OF OBJECTS IN MICROSCOPIC MOUNTS

MICROSCOPISTS who have attempted to determine the color of minute objects in microscopic mounts, such as fungous spores, have felt the need of improved methods.

The method commonly employed for this operation is to observe the object through the microscope, form a mental color image and match this, as soon as possible, with a color on a color chart. However, the color chart is sometimes omitted and an opinion rendered. The results obtained by these methods have been uncertain since an accurate mental color impression of sufficient duration and intensity could not be retained until the observer had made proper comparisons with the standard colors, or his memory of color standards was inaccurate. These difficulties might be overcome if the microscopic object could be projected on a color chart or images of the microscopic object and the color chart observed simultaneously.

Krieger[1] has described a method for determining the color of spore prints made from *Volvaria speciosa Fr.* as a type. However, a good method for determining the colors of spore mounts by microscopic examination remained to be described. The writers have devised methods by which the object in a microscopic mount may be projected and observed simultaneously with those on a chart of standard colors.

In the first method employed by the writers, the apparatus consisted of a microscope equipped with Abbé condenser, camera lucida with drawing board, two table lamps each bearing a 75-watt daylight ground glass bulb, a Ridgway color chart, and a comparing screen which consists of a sheet of gray paper about 8 x 10 inches with a slit 1 x 0.75 inches cut in the center. The color standards were lighted by one of the lamps and the microscope by the other. By properly adjusting the Abbé condenser, the two lamps and the camera lucida, an image of the colored microscopic object was superimposed on the comparing screen beside the slit. While the comparing screen was held stationary, the color standards were moved so that an analogous color showed through the slit. The color standards were further adjusted and proper comparisons made until the slit contained a standard color which matched favorably with that of the microscopic object. By this method, the observer can compare the colors as accurately as his ability will permit. When one type of microscope was used, the microscope was placed on a plane about three inches above the level of the drawing board but when another type was employed, the best results were obtained when this distance was increased to five inches. How-

[1] Krieger, L. C. C. "Observations on the Use of Ridgway's New Color Book. The Color of the Spores of *Volvaria speciosa Fr.*" *Mycologia* 6: No. 1: 29–31. 1914.

ever, the microscope and drawing board may be placed on the same level. The methods of lighting the microscope and chart may also be varied from those already described. Good lighting was obtained with three forty-watt lights; one for lighting the microscope and two for the color chart. When sunlight was employed, it seemed preferable to place the color chart in the bright sunlight, for a short time, and the microscope in a shadow.

In the second method, the apparatus commonly used for making photomicrographs was employed. Working in a darkroom, an image of the microscopic mount was focused on the ground glass of the camera in the usual way. The ground glass was then removed and placed about eight inches back from its natural position and the object refocused. The color standards with the comparing screen were then substituted for the ground glass. The color of the microscopic mount as projected could then be compared with the colors on the color chart by employing methods already described. However, the camera may be removed and an image of the microscopic mount projected on a horizontal surface by aid of a mirror commonly attached to the apparatus for this purpose.

The third method was devised as a laboratory aid in classifying fleshy fungi. Students experienced considerable difficulty in determining the colors of basidiospores, especially those of ochre, brown and rose colors. An eyepiece color comparator was constructed by flowing a negative varnish over a cover glass which could be placed in the tube of an eyepiece to a microscope. Before the varnish had hardened, four narrow parallel bars of transparent water colors were painted across the center. Deep yellow, geranium pink, mahogany brown of the Japanese transparent water colors were employed while India ink supplied the black. The color was more dense on one end of the bar thus giving a comparison of the diluted with the concentrated color. By placing this eyepiece color comparator in the eyepiece of the microscope, its colors and those of the microscopic object could be observed simultaneously and the relative colors of basidiospores determined. The colors on the eyepiece color comparator were standardized by the camera lucida as previously described. Thicker glass for the color comparator was obtained by choosing a microscopic slide of clear, thin white glass and a disc of the desired diameter was cut with shears under water. It seemed inadvisable to place the colors on a microscopic slide or its cover glass.

Finally, the methods described in this article may be successfully employed by one familiar with the use of a camera lucida. Furthermore, the proper lighting of the microscope, photographic apparatus and the color chart insures success when determining the color of microscopic objects by these methods.

W. H. Davis
F. A. MacLaughlin
Massachusetts Agricultural College

A MODIFIED ERLANGER SPHYGMOMANOMETER

About a year ago, when the writer attempted to assemble an Erlanger type recording sphygmomanometer, he was confronted by the impossibility of securing the special rubber bulb used in such apparatus. In casting about for a suitable one, many types of rubber bulbs and finger cots were tried without success until one day, after the cuff had been used for arm plethysmographic apparatus, the cast-off fingers of a rubber glove were tried. The finger of the glove was tied over a disc placed inside a capsule constructed as described (Figures 1 and 2) and served so satisfactorily that the writer thought others might find the apparatus useful.

The center of a ⅞-inch round brass rod was located and a ¼-inch hole was centered and drilled 3/16 inch from the center of the rod. With a lathe a 3/32-inch groove was cut around the circumference of the rod and a 3/16-inch disc cut off. A piece of ¼-inch brass tubing about 2½ inches long was soldered in the hole in the disc. The side and bottom views, respectively, of this disc are shown in figures 1a and 1b.

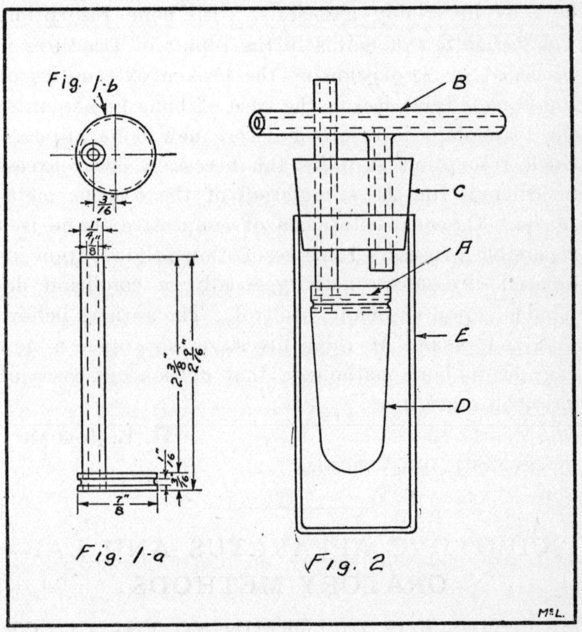

When assembling (see figure 2), the finger of the glove D is slipped over the disc A and tightly tied by means of strong waxed linen thread. The brass tube B is forced through one of the holes in a number 7 rubber stopper C. One arm of the T-tube B is pressed through the other hole in the rubber stopper, and the stopper tightly inserted into a 34 x 90 millimeter homeopathic vial E. By means of a band of thin sheet brass 1½ inch wide the vial, in the inverted position, may be neatly mounted upon a 4 x 4 inch piece of oak board, which will also support the pressure gauge of the sphygmomanometer. The board in turn is supported by a ring stand.

In assembling the completed apparatus the tube leading to the glove finger is connected with the sphygmomanometer pressure system; one tube of the brass T is connected to a compound lever tambour and the other, when provided with a short length of rubber tubing and a pinch cock, serves to control the pressure in the recording system.

The rubber finger was obtained from a Paragold rubber glove, SR702, made by the Seamless Rubber Company, New Haven, Conn. The homeopathic vial is larger than is now regularly catalogued but may be obtained upon special order. Since it is used here as regular equipment, we put it to a variety of uses. It is possible that a smaller disc may be made and a 25 x 70 millimeter vial used.

A. R. MCLAUGHLIN
DEPARTMENT OF PHYSIOLOGY AND PHARMACOLOGY,
MICHIGAN STATE COLLEGE

SPECIAL ARTICLES

ZEOLITE BEDS IN THE GREEN RIVER FORMATION[1]

AT several horizons in the upper half of the Green River formation of Utah and Colorado, an extensive series of Eocene lake beds that contain large deposits of oil shale, there are thin more or less persistent beds resembling sandstone that consist almost wholly of perfect or euhedral crystals of the zeolite mineral, analcite. These crystals differ greatly in size and reach a maximum diameter of nearly 2 millimeters. All are clouded with dust-like inclusions that make them dull gray and opaque. The character of the matrix as well as the proportion of matrix to zeolites differs from bed to bed. Both these factors are significant. In general those beds with relatively few zeolites have a distinctly tuffaceous matrix consisting of silica in the form of the mineral chalcedony in which are embedded many angular fragments and elongate splinters of feldspar and quartz together with laths of biotite and euhedral crystals of orthoclase, apatite and zircon. More rarely they contain good crystals of plagioclase and either hornblende or pyroxene. Clay minerals and carbonates which make up the associated beds are virtually absent. Other zeolite beds contain a very subordinate amount of chalcedonic matrix and if transitional beds between these and the distinctly tuffaceous type had not been found their relation to volcanic ash would have been utterly obscure. In addition to the analcite most of these beds contain a few small crystals of another zeolite mineral, apophyllite. Even some of the analcite crystals contain perfect though minute crystals of apophyllite.

In the summer of 1925 the writer found zeolite beds at one or more horizons at the following localities in Utah: about 700 feet above the base of the Green River formation in the canyon of White River, sec. 27, T. 9 S., R. 25 E., Uintah County and at approximately the same horizon in Hells Hole Canyon, sec. 22, T. 10 S., R. 25 E., also in Uintah County. One of these beds is lenticular and in places exceeds three feet in thickness. In Colorado similar beds were found at several places along White River in the western part of Rio Blanco County and in sec. 26, T. 3 S., R. 99 W., Garfield County.

Besides these crystal beds analcite occurs plentifully also disseminated in many oil shale beds of the Green River formation in Wyoming as well as in Utah and Colorado. Small apophyllite crystals too are scattered through these beds and, like the analcite, the greater number of them are euhedral. Some oil shale strata contain more than 16 per cent. by weight of analcite and others contain 1 or 2 per cent. of apophyllite. In the oil shale the zeolites are associated with numerous euhedral orthoclase crystals, angular quartz fragments and a little volcanic glass in addition to the calcium and magnesium carbonates and clay minerals that are principal constituents of most of the oil shale in this formation.

Field and microscopic study of these two types of zeolite-bearing rock indicates that both minerals formed in place on the lake bottom (or when only shallowly buried in ooze) as a result of interactions between various salts dissolved in the lake water and the dissolution products of volcanic ash that fell into the ancient Green River lakes. Presumably the volcanic material which makes up a really considerable part of the Green River formation came from Eocene volcanoes that were active in or near the San Juan Mountains in Colorado about 200 miles to the southeast.

This almost complete zeolitization of tuffs adds another interesting phase to the broader problem of the alteration of volcanic ash. Its relation to the origin of bentonite, however, is unknown for, so far as the writer is aware, the Green River formation

[1] Published by permission of the director of the U. S. Geological Survey.

contains no bentonite. On the other hand, it contains at least one bed of fairly fresh crystal tuff whose composition is approximately that of the igneous rock andesite. It is altogether likely that careful tracing of these tuffs and zeolite beds will demonstrate that they have an enormous lateral extent, comparable perhaps to bentonite beds. If so they would be of considerable value as precise correlative units.

As these zeolites must have formed at a temperature approximating the mean annual temperature at the earth's surface their occurrence suggests the possibility that the zeolite gels of soils may, under favorable conditions, crystallize into definite minerals. Indeed there appears to be a significant analogy between the occurrence of a natural sodium aluminum silicate gel recently described by Burgess and McGeorge[2] from the alkali soils of Arizona and this occurrence of analcite, a crystalline form of sodium aluminum silicate, in the beds of an ancient alkaline lake. Hence it seems within reason to expect that certain fossil or perhaps even recent alkali soils might contain definitely crystallized zeolites.

A more complete account of these zeolite beds together with the data which led the writer to the conclusions expressed here will be presented later in a report by the U. S. Geological Survey treating the mineralogy of the Green River formation.

W. H. BRADLEY
U. S. GEOLOGICAL SURVEY,
WASHINGTON, D. C.

THE ADHESION OF MERCURY TO GLASS

THE adhesion of *small* drops of mercury to the clean sides of glass vessels is a matter of common laboratory observation. It is seen in partly filled bottles of mercury that have been recently shaken, and it is often noticed in the glass chambers of mercury pumps. Yet larger drops break away leaving the glass "dry."

Observations on the "wetting" of clean surfaces of glasses of special constitution, as evidenced by the *rise* of the mercury meniscus against such surfaces when vertical, have been reported by Schumacher.[1] The observations reported here are of a totally different sort. The glass is that of ordinary laboratory lenses—probably crown glass as the index of refraction in each case was between 1.53 and 1.56. These were cleaned by rubbing the surfaces with a piece of absorbent cotton wet with absolute alcohol. The mercury was singly distilled, and to lessen contamination was transferred from vessel to vessel through a glass siphon that was started by a current of dry air. Before each set of observations the mercury was passed through a paper and cottonwool filter to free it from dust caught on its surface. The observations were made in the open air of the laboratory, so it will be evident that no claim for extreme cleanness of surfaces can be made.

If the surface of a glass lens, cleaned as described above, be brought into contact with a pool of mercury so that the lowest point (the apex) of the glass is say 0.2 mm. below the level of the mercury surface, the air adherent to the glass depresses the mercury in contact with it and holds it out of contact with the glass. After an interval, which may vary from a fraction of a second to several minutes, the fluid pressure seems to drive the air away from the apex of the lens and then, in a flash, a bright mirror spreads over the glass. This may be interrupted by a few small bubbles of imprisoned air. The edge of the mirror surface, or the "circle of extreme contact" of mercury and glass, is well above the general level of the mercury pool—a meniscus being formed at the edge of which the mercury is lifted a millimeter or more. As no reference to this phenomenon could be found in the literature available it was thought worth while to make some quantitative observations on it.

The disposition of apparatus is shown diagrammatically in fig. 1. *A* is the pool of mercury—about 18 cm

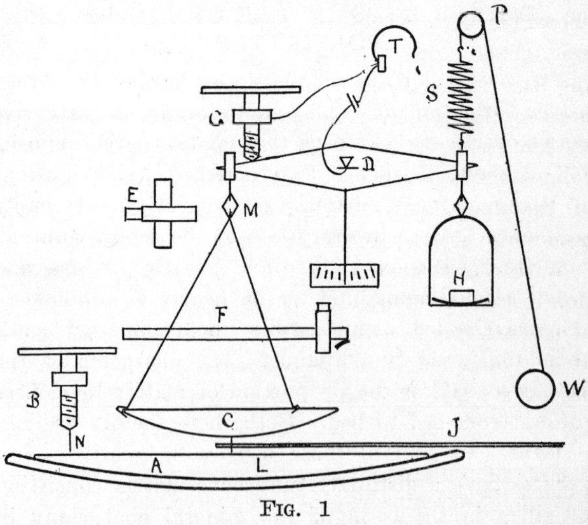

FIG. 1

across—in its shallow glass basin, *B* is a micrometer screw on a fixed stand by which the needle point *N* may be adjusted to contact with the surface of the mercury pool, and by means of which changes in the level of *A* may be followed. *C* is the lens of measured curvature, the lower surface of which is under observation. The lens is held in a frame of steel wires

[2] Burgess, P. S., and McGeorge, W. T., Zeolite formation in soils. SCIENCE, new ser., vol. 64, pp. 652–653, 1926.

[1] *Jour. Amer. Chem. Soc.* Vol. 45, No. 10.

that hangs from one hook of the balance arm *D*. Changes in the level of the lens surface may be measured by observing the displacement of the needle point *M* (rigidly attached to the steel frame) through the reading microscope *E* (scale vertical). The vertical motion of *C* is controlled by the micrometer screw *G* which acts directly on the balance arm *D*. *H* is a counterweight in the second pan of the balance to maintain contact between the balance arm and the point of the screw *G*. *J* is a strip of thin ebonite that carries at its end a "distance piece" *L* formed of 2 mm of the point of a needle. The top of *L* is held against the apex of the lens by the small stiffness of the ebonite strip *J* and the lens is then lowered until the point of *L* comes into contact with the surface of the mercury pool *A*. The reading of the level of the needle point *M* in this position together with the length of the distance piece gives a datum level from which the relative levels of the apex of the lens and the surface of the pool of mercury can be determined, account being taken of changes in the level of the pool itself as revealed by the reading of the screw head at *B*. The level of the pool is of course altered either by the immersion of part of the lens itself or by the drawing up of mercury into the meniscus. Fig. 2

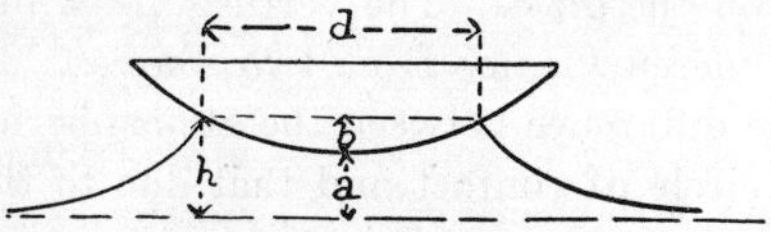

FIG. 2

shows the lens and the mercury meniscus. The diameter of the circle of contact (*d*) is observed *through* the lens by the reading microscope shown with scale horizontal at *F* (fig. 1). From this measurement and the known curvature of the lens the distance *b* (fig. 2) follows from geometry, and this with the distance (*a*) of the apex above the level of the pool gives the maximum lift (*h*) of the mercury in the meniscus.

With plano-convex lenses no correction for refraction in the observed value of the diameter of the circle of contact was necessary. For other lenses the value of *d* is obtained from the observed magnitude by the use of a curve in which the known distances of the points of a pair of micrometer calipers are plotted

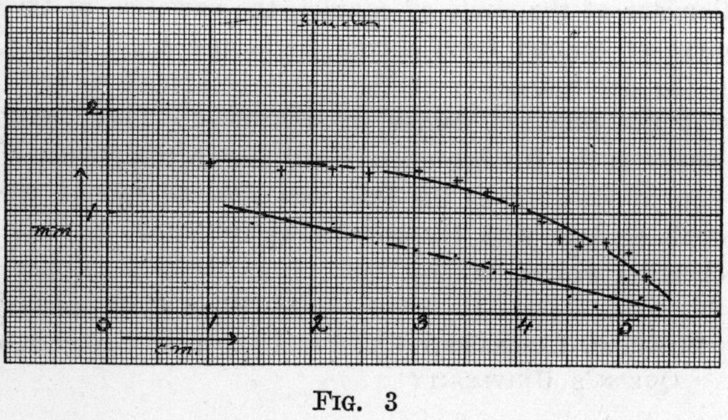

FIG. 3

against their distances as observed through the lens by the microscope *F*, the points being held against the lower surface of the glass.

In all cases within the range available the mercury rose above the level of the pool although the rise was less for circles of contact of larger radius. The rise on gradually lowering the lens into the mercury was always less than the rise found for the same circle of contact on lifting the lens out of the fluid. Fig. 3 shows the values obtained from a plano-convex lantern condenser of radius of curvature 10.41 cm[2]. The abscissae are radii of the circles of contact and the ordinates are the heights of the edge of the mercury meniscus above the general level of the pool. The values plotted in dots were found as the lens was slowly lowered into the mercury, the fluid rising over the clean glass. Those shown in crosses were from measurements made as the lens was gradually lifted, the fluid slipping back over surfaces that had been previously covered with mercury. The curve seems to indicate a vanishing value for *h* just beyond the limit of observation, at a circle of contact of radius 5.75 cm which would lead to an angle of contact for the mercury and lens used of nearly 147°. No test seemed feasible for the electrification of the freshly exposed surfaces, but usually *dry* glass plunged into mercury is strongly electrified on withdrawal. Whether the moisture of the summer air kept the surface sufficiently conducting to discharge it is not known, but the electrical grounding of the mercury pool produced no apparent difference in the results. All the curves obtained are of the same general nature with the one shown in the figure. With all of the lenses, independently of their particular curvature, the lift of the mercury at the edge of the meniscus was about 0.16 cm though with a sample of freshly distilled mercury a lift of 0.200 cm. was once obtained.

A noteworthy feature of the phenomenon was the way the mercury gradually passed from the circle of contact that had just been rendered unstable, by the lifting of the lens, to a new stable circle. Usually it would move fairly quickly and come to rest again within a minute or two; but when the mercury cov-

[2] The radius of curvature was found by rolling calibrated "bicycle balls" of different sizes into contact

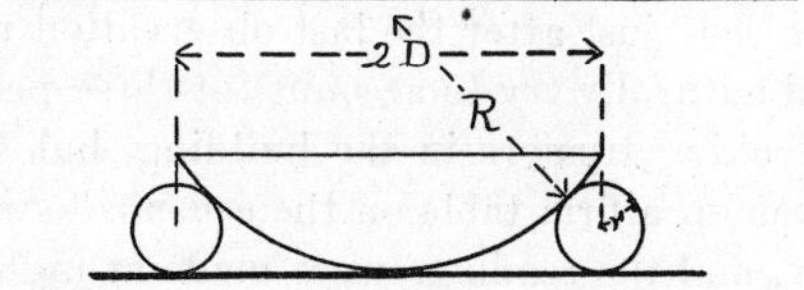

FIG. 4

with the lens as it rested on a flat surface and then measuring the distance from ball to ball with a reading microscope. In Fig. 4 $R = \frac{D^2}{4r}$.

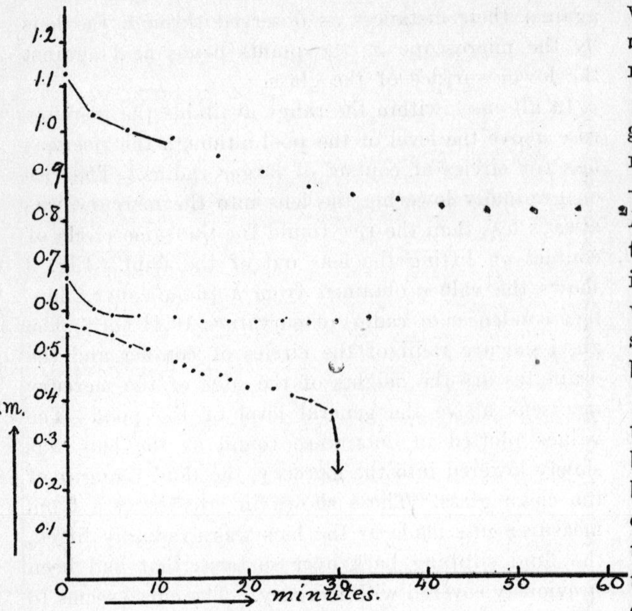

FIG. 5

ered only a small area near the apex of the lens it might be a half an hour or more before the new position was finally reached. Figure 5 shows some typical cases. The ordinates are radii of the circle of contact in cm and the abscissae are times in *minutes* from the first reading of the circle of contact after the lifting of the lens, the level of the lens being unchanged during the series of readings shown in the plot. Those plotted in the upper curve took over an hour to become stable. For the first of the series h was 0.161 cm and for the last 0.155 cm. In the final position the mercury seemed to be in a state of abnormal adhesion to the glass ("stuck") for a careful lifting of the lens through 0.003 cm did not alter the radius of the circle of adhesion, and this seemed *quite stable* at the increased height above the mercury pool. Another lift of 0.005 cm, however, started a rapid shrinking of the radius that led to the breaking of the meniscus in a few seconds. The middle curve is a record of the attaining of stability from a circle of radius smaller than that of the upper curve. The lowest line of dots shows a case where the contraction of the circle reached the point where it rapidly became more and more unstable, leading to the breaking of the meniscus just after the last observation plotted. One would naturally try to account for these peculiarities by invoking tremors in the building, but the apparatus was on a firm table on the cement floor of the laboratory, and the readings were made at night when the observer was alone in the building. Usually, as noted in connection with the upper curve of figure 5, after the circle had attained a stable position the lens might be lifted from 0.001 to 0.002 cm before the edge would be "pulled away from its moorings" to recommence its slipping over the glass to a new position of rest.

To measure the force exerted by the mercury on the glass the following additions were made to the apparatus. A light spiral spring S—from a Jolly balance —was attached to the second balance hook of the arm D (Fig. 1) and from its upper end a string ran over the pulley P to the small winch W. By means of this it was possible to exert small but definite forces upwards on the pan H until the contact between the screw point of G and the balance arm just broke, the break being indicated by the telephone circuit T.

The meniscus being formed, the winch was slowly turned until the contact at the point of G was just broken. The balance arm was then in equilibrium between the forces exerted by the mercury and those exerted by the masses suspended from the hooks and the force set up by the spring S. The screw G was then raised out of the way, the position of the pointer of the balance was noted, the levels and diameter of the circle of contact read, then the meniscus was broken and the change in the masses on the pan of the balance to restore equilibrium at the same pointer reading gave a measure of the force exerted by the mercury on the glass. The vertical force on the lens from the mercury came from two sources. First, that due to the difference between the atmospheric pressure over the circle of contact and that due to the smaller pressure of the mercury in contact with the glass. Second, there was the vertical part of the force due to the surface tension of the mercury around the circumference of the circle of contact. A series of measurements was made for different circles of contact and for different lenses, all of which led to the magnitudes to be expected from the known constants of mercury. These observations were of no use as determinations of the surface tension of mercury for the following reasons: (1) The value for the surface tension comes from the difference between the observed equilibriating force and the force due to the difference of pressures as noted above, and, except for the smallest circles of contact, these are too nearly of the same magnitude to give their difference much value. (2) Owing to the great density of mercury errors in the diameter of the circle of contact, the variation of the curve of contact from a true circle and small errors in the determination of the levels combined to prevent the required degree of exactness. Then, too, there was the further uncertainty due to the phenomenon of sticking as the lens was lowered enough to break contact with the control screw before the observation was made.

WILL C. BAKER

PHYSICAL LABORATORY,
QUEEN'S UNIVERSITY

SPECIAL ISSUE CONTAINING GENERAL REPORTS OF THE SECOND NASHVILLE MEETING OF THE AMERICAN ASSOCIATION FOR THE ADVANCEMENT OF SCIENCE AND ASSOCIATED SOCIETIES. EDITED BY BURTON E. LIVINGSTON, PERMANENT SECRETARY

SCIENCE

VOL. LXVII JANUARY 27, 1928 No. 1726

CONTENTS

The American Association for the Advancement of Science:
- *General Reports of the Nashville Meeting* 77
- *The Council Roll* 85
- *The Roll of the Executive Committee* 88
- *Legislative and Executive Proceedings* 88
- *Resolutions on the Public Welfare* 91
- *The Annual Conference of Section and Society Secretaries* 91
- *Report of the Treasurer* 91
- *Financial Report of the Permanent Secretary* 93
- *Report of the Committee on the Place of Science in Education* 95
- *Grants for Research* 96
- *Officers for 1928* 97
- *Future Annual Meetings* 98
- *Special Notes* 99

Scientific Events:
New Buildings for the Physical Sciences at the University of Chicago; The Pure Science Fund at Princeton University; The U. S. Coast and Geodetic Survey; The Institute of Chemistry 99

Scientific Notes and News 101

University and Educational Notes 103

Discussion and Correspondence:
Ovarian Secretion and Tumor Incidence: DR. LEO LOEB. *Laws relating to Mathematical Operations:* PROFESSOR G. A. MILLER. *Soil Science Publication in Russia:* DR. J. S. JOFFE 104

Scientific Books:
Dakin's Elements of General Zoology: DR. HUBERT LYMAN CLARK 105

Scientific Apparatus and Laboratory Methods:
A Convenient Device for Plant Solution-Culture Work: DR. FREDERICK S. HAMMETT. *A Method for Cutting Glass Tubing:* HERMAN E. SEEMANN 106

Special Articles:
Reflection of Light from the Surfaces of Leaves: PROFESSOR CHARLES A. SHULL 107

Science News x

SCIENCE: A Weekly Journal devoted to the Advancement of Science, edited by J. McKeen Cattell and published every Friday by

THE SCIENCE PRESS

New York City: Grand Central Terminal.
Lancaster, Pa. Garrison, N. Y.
Annual Subscription, $6.00. Single Copies, 15 Cts.

SCIENCE is the official organ of the American Association for the Advancement of Science. Information regarding membership in the Association may be secured from the office of the permanent secretary, in the Smithsonian Institution Building, Washington, D. C.

Entered as second-class matter July 18, 1923, at the Post Office at Lancaster, Pa., under the Act of March 8, 1879.

THE AMERICAN ASSOCIATION FOR THE ADVANCEMENT OF SCIENCE

GENERAL REPORTS OF THE SECOND NASHVILLE MEETING OF THE AMERICAN ASSOCIATION FOR THE ADVANCEMENT OF SCIENCE AND ASSOCIATED SOCIETIES

GENERAL FEATURES

IN convocation week, from December 26 to December 31, was held at Nashville, Tennessee, the eighty-fourth meeting of the American Association for the Advancement of Science, the annual meeting for the association year 1927–28. This was the second Nashville meeting, the association having met in that city once before, in August, 1877. The sessions of the association and the associated societies were well accommodated mainly in the buildings of Vanderbilt University, the George Peabody College for Teachers and the Ward-Belmont College for Women.

President A. A. Noyes, eminent leader in chemical research and in chemical instruction, director of the Gates Chemical Laboratory of the California Institute of Technology, Pasadena, presided at the meeting and took part in many sessions. The retiring president, Dr. L. H. Bailey, well-known author and editor of articles and standard books on botany, horticulture and rural life, was unable to be present, because of convalescence from a serious illness, but he sent a note of greeting, which was read at the opening session.

Fourteen sections of the American Association appeared in the program of this meeting and thirty-five independent organizations of science workers met with the association. Most of these are officially *associated,* and the majority are officially *affiliated* with the association. Their names will be shown in the reports on the sessions of sections and societies, in the next following issue of SCIENCE.

ATTENDANCE, SESSIONS AND PAPERS

One thousand six hundred and sixty-two persons were registered at the second Nashville meeting. While this registration is not so large as that for some other recent annual meetings, it and other features are indicative of very widespread interest and mark this meeting as very successful. For the sake of comparison, the registration records of the last eight meetings are shown below:

Third Chicago Meeting (Dec., 1920), 2,413.
Second Toronto Meeting (Dec., 1921), 1,832.
Fourth Boston Meeting (Dec., 1922), 2,339.
Third Cincinnati Meeting (Dec., 1923), 2,211.
Fifth Washington Meeting (Dec., 1924), 4,206.
Kansas City Meeting (Dec., 1925), 1,931.
Fifth Philadelphia Meeting (Dec., 1926), 3,181.
Second Nashville Meeting (Dec., 1927), 1,662.

It is certain that the number of persons actually in attendance was considerably larger than is indicated by the registration record, for many local people and some from away failed to register.

The residence distribution of those who registered at Nashville is shown by the accompanying list.

Registration at Nashville by States and Provinces

Alabama	41
Arizona	5
Arkansas	23
Australia	1
California	31
Colorado	7
Connecticut	19
Cuba	1
Delaware	5
District of Columbia	79
England	2
Florida	34
France	1
Georgia	40
Illinois	156
Indiana	57
Iowa	54
Kansas	33
Kentucky	38
Louisiana	43
Maine	3
Manitoba	3
Maryland	25
Massachusetts	38
Mexico	2
Michigan	59
Minnesota	27
Mississippi	29
Missouri	61
Montana	1
Nebraska	14
New Hampshire	3
New Jersey	17
New Mexico	1
New York	126
North Carolina	47
North Dakota	5
Ohio	111
Oklahoma	17
Ontario	11
Oregon	1
Pennsylvania	61
Porto Rico	3
Quebec	2
Rhode Island	9
Saskatchewan	2
South Carolina	19
South Dakota	1
Sweden	1
Nashville	67
Tennessee (outside of Nashville)	76
Texas	41
Utah	3
Vermont	3
Virginia	30
Washington	8
West Virginia	14
Wisconsin	48
Wyoming	3
Total	1,662

Altogether there were one hundred and sixty-three scientific sessions held at Nashville. Omitting about fifty papers presented by title only, 1,141 papers and addresses were delivered. There were thirty-one luncheons, dinners, smokers, etc., all well attended.

MEETING PLACES AND FACILITIES

The general hotel headquarters were at the Andrew Jackson Hotel, which very generously placed many complimentary rooms at the disposal of the association. Other hotels were headquarters for societies. About four hundred persons were lodged very conveniently and inexpensively in dormitories of the George Peabody College for Teachers and the Ward-Belmont College for Women and the hotel headquarters for some societies were in those dormitories, which were made specially available for this purpose. Meals and luncheons were served at the cafeterias of Wesley Hall and Kissam Hall, Vanderbilt University, at the cafeteria of the George Peabody College, at the dining room of the Ward-Belmont College for Women, and at the cafeteria of the Southern Y. M. C. A. Graduate School.

The registration offices (in charge of Mr. Sam Woodley, executive assistant, of the Washington office of the association), the news office (in charge of Mr. Austin H. Clark, news manager) and the general science exhibition (in charge of Major H. S. Kimberly, exhibition manager) were all in the lobbies of the Andrew Jackson Hotel.

A total number of twenty-three lanterns and twenty-two daylight screens were very kindly loaned by the Bausch and Lomb Optical Co., of Rochester, N. Y. The association hereby expresses to that firm its very appreciative thanks for this great help.

The Nashville educational institutions were very generous in helping to make this meeting a success. Rooms for the sessions were placed at the disposal of the association by Vanderbilt University, the George Peabody College for Women, the Southern Y. M. C. A. Graduate School and the Scarritt College for Christian Workers. To all these institutions the association and the associated organizations are very grateful.

The Nashville Chamber of Commerce was very generous to this convention and a large degree of credit and appreciative thanks for the very successful outcome are due to the indefatigable personal interest and industry of Mr. W. N. Porter, convention secretary of that organization.

Dr. W. S. Leathers, professor of medicine and public health, Vanderbilt Medical School, was general chairman of the Nashville committees. He devoted himself with great efficiency and tact to the very complicated preparations throughout many months before the meeting opened. To his able general oversight and foresight in this work the association and the associated societies owe very much indeed.

Mr. John W. Barton, vice-president of the Ward-Belmont School, was very active as chairman of the committee on general arrangements and of the committee on finance and the results of his very generous and efficient services were much in evidence throughout the meeting. To him the association and all who attended are very grateful indeed.

All the members of the several local committees and the representatives for the several sections of the association, whose names are shown below, joined in the great cooperative work that made the second Nashville meeting so very satisfactory; to them is here expressed the hearty gratitude of the association and of all who attended this meeting.

LOCAL COMMITTEES FOR THE SECOND NASHVILLE MEETING

General Chairman of Nashville Committees

W. S. Leathers, M.D., professor of preventive medicine and public health, Vanderbilt Medical School.

Committee on Arrangements

John W. Barton, *chairman*, vice-president of Ward-Belmont School.
J. A. Webb, *secretary*, professor of chemistry, George Peabody College.
L. C. Glenn, professor of geology, Vanderbilt University.
G. Canby Robinson, dean and professor of medicine, Vanderbilt Medical School.
J. T. McGill, professor emeritus of organic chemistry, Vanderbilt University.
A. E. Parkins, professor of geography, George Peabody College.
W. N. Porter, convention secretary of the Nashville Chamber of Commerce.
J. M. Breckenridge, professor of chemistry, Vanderbilt University.
G. R. Mayfield, associate professor of German, Vanderbilt University.
A. F. Ganier, assistant engineer, N. C. and St. Louis Railroad.
H. H. Shoulders, president of the Nashville Academy of Medicine.
E. L. Bishop, state health commissioner of Tennessee.
A. W. Wright, assistant professor of pathology, Vanderbilt Medical School.
H. C. Weber, superintendent of the Nashville Public Schools.

Committee on Finance

John W. Barton, *chairman*
Henry E. Colton
Charles M. McCabe

Committee on Meeting Places

A. E. Parkins, *chairman*
F. J. Lewis
R. E. Baber
W. H. Hollinshead
W. D. Strayhorn

Committee on Hotels and Housing

W. N. Porter, *chairman*
Lee J. Loventhal
S. J. Garrison

Committee on Exhibition

J. M. Breckenridge, *chairman*
F. B. Dresslar
E. W. Goodpasture

Committee on Local Transportation

A. F. Ganier, *chairman*
J. P. W. Brown
W. F. Pond

Committee on Publicity and Non-technical Lectures

G. R. Mayfield, *chairman*
H. A. Webb
T. J. Horner
T. H. Alexander
J. S. Stahlman, Jr.

Committee on Entertainment

A. W. Wright, *chairman*
C. P. Connell
Mrs. A. B. Benedict
W. W. Carpenter
T. Graham Hall
Thomas E. Jones

Local Representatives for Sections of the Association

Section A (Mathematics): C. M. Sarratt
Section B (Physics): C. R. Fountain
Section C (Chemistry): L. J. Bircher
Section D (Astronomy): James McClure
Section E (Geology and Geography): L. C. Glenn
Section F (Zoological Sciences): E. E. Reinke
Section G (Botanical Sciences): J. M. Shaver
Section H (Anthropology): W. D. Weatherford
Section I (Psychology): Joseph Peterson
Section K (Social and Economic Sciences): C. B. Duncan
Section L (Historical and Philological Sciences): H. C. Sanborn
Section M (Engineering): W. H. Schuerman
Section N (Medical Sciences): P. D. Lamson
Section O (Agriculture): K. C. Davis
Section Q (Education): S. J. Phelps
For Organizations not related to Any Particular Section: C. P. Connell

OFFICIAL REPRESENTATION AT THE NASHVILLE MEETING

Cards of invitation were sent out, as usual, asking research institutions and laboratories and scientific organizations to name representatives for the meeting. Following are the names of those that did so: University of Arizona; University of California; Stanford University; University of Denver; Wesleyan University; Carnegie Institution of Washington; Federal Horticultural Board; National Research Council; Smithsonian Institution; U. S. Department of Agriculture; U. S. Coast and Geodetic Survey; U. S. Bureau of Entomology; U. S. Public Health Service; U. S. Weather Bureau; War Department; Northwestern University; Drake University; Iowa State College; University of Kentucky; Clark University; Harvard University; Wellesley College; Worcester Polytechnic Institute; University of Michigan; University of Minnesota; St. Louis University; Washington University; New Jersey Agricultural Experiment Station; American Museum of Natural History; Brooklyn Botanic Garden; College of the City of New York; Cooper Union; University of Rochester; Rockefeller Institute for Medical Research; Case School of Applied Science; Marietta College; Oberlin College; Ohio Wesleyan University; Western Reserve University; Haverford College; Mellon Institute of Industrial Research; University of Pittsburgh; Brown University; University of Texas; West Virginia University; Eastman Kodak Company, Rochester, N. Y.; B. F. Goodrich Company, Akron, Ohio; Incandescent Lamp Department of General Electric Co., Nela Park, Cleveland, Ohio; Leeds & Northrup Company, Philadelphia, Pa.; Western Electric Company, New York, N. Y.

Many other organizations and institutions were unofficially represented at the meeting, and it is probable that some official representatives failed to register as such.

THE PRELIMINARY ANNOUNCEMENT AND THE GENERAL PROGRAM

The preliminary announcement of the Nashville meeting appeared in SCIENCE for December 2, 1927, occupying about seventeen pages of that issue, which was sent to all members of the association. It contained the usual preliminary information about the meeting, including statements about the many section and society programs. The latter statements were based on material supplied by the section and society secretaries.

The secretaries also supplied the manuscripts for their programs as these appeared in the general program of the meeting and most of the manuscripts were at hand by December 15. The editing and printing of the general program, a book of over 130 pages, was again in the hands of the program editor, Dr. Sam F. Trelease, of Columbia University. Dr. Trelease and Mrs. Trelease went to Nashville and devoted themselves, day and night, to this work from December 15 to the time the book was finished, on the day before Christmas. This is a very difficult kind of material from the editorial viewpoint, a large proportion of the composition being classified headings and subheads, technical words and phrases and personal names. Our hearty thanks are again due to Dr. and Mrs. Trelease, and also to the botanical department of Columbia University, of which he is a member, which made it possible, as in recent years, for the program editor to devote so much time to the general program during more than a month just preceding the meeting.

A new feature of the general program this year is a fourteen-page index of names of persons reading papers or delivering addresses, an index of about 1,200 entries. This index, which represents about fifteen hours of practically uninterrupted labor on the part of the editor and Mrs. Trelease—for it could not be prepared till page proofs of the book were available and no minute could then be lost—is an exceedingly valuable feature of the general program, which was used and appreciated by every one.

Sixteen pages of advertising—of books and apparatus for science work—are included in the Nashville program, the income from which helped to pay the cost of printing the book. The hearty cooperation of the advertising firms is greatly appreciated. Their names are shown below. An E following a name indicates that the firm thus designated had an exhibit in the general exhibition.

American Association for Medical Progress, Inc. (E), 370 Seventh Avenue, New York, N. Y.
Baker and Co., Inc., 54 Austin St., Newark, N. J.
Bausch and Lomb Optical Co. (E), Rochester, N. Y.
Brooklyn Botanic Garden, 1000 Washington Ave., Brooklyn, N. Y.
Eastman Kodak Co., Rochester, N. Y.
General Biological Supply House (E), 761 East 69th Place, Chicago, Ill.
General Radio Co., 30 State St., Cambridge, Mass.
Kny-Scheerer Corporation of America, 10 West 25th St., New York, N. Y.
Lancaster Press, Inc., Lancaster, Pa.
E. Leitz, Inc. (E), 60 East 10th St., New York, N. Y.
Mallinckrodt Chemical Works, St. Louis, Mo.
Open Court Publishing Co., 337 E. Chicago Ave., Chicago, Ill.
Thermal Syndicate, Ltd., 58 Schenectady Ave., Brooklyn, N. Y.
Triarch Botanical Products (E), Botanical Laboratory, University of Pennsylvania, Philadelphia, Pa.
University of Chicago Press (E), 5750 Ellis Ave., Chicago, Ill.
Victor Talking Machine Co. (E), Camden, N. J.
John Wiley and Sons, Inc., 440 Fourth Ave., New York, N. Y.
Williams and Wilkins Co., Mt. Royal and Guilford Aves., Baltimore, Md.

The typographical and artistic excellence of the general program are largely due to the very fine work of the Cullom and Ghertner Co., of Nashville, who cooperated very cordially with the program editor in every respect.

REDUCED RAILWAY FARES

Reduced railway rates, on the certificate plan, were available for those who attended this meeting, as has been true of recent meetings. The money-saving to those who took advantage of this arrangement amounted to one fourth of the regular railway fare; that is, the reduced rate for the round trip was one and one half times the regular one-way fare. The total number of railway certificates validated at Nashville was 1,057. They represented an aggregate of $25,701.18 for the one-way trips to Nashville and an aggregate of half of that amount, or $12,850.59, for the return trips. The total amount saved through the availability of the reduced rates was therefore $12,850.59, which amounts to an average saving per person of $12.15. This constitutes a very tangible service accomplished by the association for its members and for the members of the organization meeting with it.

THE SCIENCE EXHIBITION

The general science exhibition was arranged in the lobby of the Andrew Jackson Hotel, where the registration and the news offices were also located. The general exhibition was in charge of the exhibition manager, Major H. S. Kimberly, who was ably assisted by the local committee on exhibition, the chairman of which was Professor J. M. Breckenridge, of Vanderbilt University. The management of the Andrew Jackson Hotel, in charge of Mr. Turney M. Cunningham, was very helpful and cooperated cordially in this as well as in other features of the arrangements. The displays of the exhibitors were intensely interesting to all present and the exhibition played a very important part as the main social center of the meeting.

The following is a list of the firms and organizations that occupied booths. The names of those that also had advertising space in the general program are each followed by an A.

American Association for Medical Progress (A), New York, N. Y.
Bausch and Lomb Optical Co. (A), Rochester, N. Y.
P. Blakiston's Son and Co., Philadelphia, Pa.
Central Scientific Co., Chicago, Ill.
Coleman and Bell Co., Norwood, Ohio.
Denoyer-Geppert Co., Chicago, Ill.
General Biological Supply House (A), Chicago, Ill.
General Electric Co., Schenectady, N. Y.
La Motte Chemical Products Co., Baltimore, Md.
Leeds and Northrup Co., Philadelphia, Pa.
E. Leitz, Inc. (A), New York, N. Y.
Southern Biological Supply Co., Inc., New Orleans, La.
Spencer Lens Co., Buffalo, N. Y.
Triarch Botanical Products (A), Philadelphia, Pa.
University of Chicago Press (A), Chicago, Ill.
University of North Carolina Press, Chapel Hill, N. Car.
Victor Talking Machine Co. (A), Camden, N. J.
Weston Electrical Instrument Corporation, Newark, N. J.

An exhibit of photographs of the region of the Great Smoky Mountains was interesting to those who like the out-of-doors. It was contributed by the Knoxville Chamber of Commerce. Several fine exhibits by the special scientific societies were housed at the Southern Y. M. C. A. Graduate School. It is unfortunate that we have not yet reached the time when these special exhibitions by scientific societies can be given adequate notice in the general program and in these reports. Information concerning them seems always to be inadequate for more than mere mention. We shall continue to try to secure good accounts of them in time for printing in the programs of future meetings.

THE FIFTH AWARD OF THE AMERICAN ASSOCIATION PRIZE

The American Association prize of $1,000 is awarded annually to the author of a notable contribution to the advancement of science given at the annual meeting. The funds are generously supplied by a member who wishes his name withheld. Nominations for the Nashville prize were received from the secretaries of the sections and societies and the award was made by the committee on prize award and announced through the news service Friday evening.

The winner of the prize is this year Dr. H. J. Muller, professor of zoology in the University of Texas, for his outstanding contribution entitled "Effects of X-Radiation on Genes and Chromosomes," which was presented before the Joint Genetics Sections of the American Society of Zoologists and the Botanical Society of America, in the Wednesday-morning session. The following abstract of Dr. Muller's paper has been contributed by him, having been sent from Austin, Texas, by air mail.

"The Effects of X-Radiation on Genes and Chromosomes."

(*Abstract*)

This paper reported the author's experiments of the past fifteen months on the hereditary effects on X-rays applied to the fruit fly, *Drosophila melanogaster*. By means of special courses, the discrimination of mutations in individual genes from genetic recombinations of various sorts (due to segregation, non-disjunction, etc.), was facilitated, and lethal as well as visible changes were rendered detectable. Results in the second and later generations, based on several thousand cultures, showed that gene mutations had occurred in the most heavily treated germ cells at about 150 times the frequency of those in the controls, derived from the same source, while in germ cells less heavily treated the result was intermediate. Germ cells in all stages studied were susceptible to the effect: these included oögonia, ova, spermatozoa shortly before fertilization, and spermatozoa when rayed either in the male or in the female receptacles six or more days prior to fertilization.

The induced mutations resembled spontaneous ones, inasmuch as: (1) The great majority were lethal; of the rest most, but not all, reduced viability or fertility. (2) Recessives greatly outnumbered definite dominants. (3) Many of the visible effects were relatively inconspicuous. (4) Though "new" mutations were somewhat more frequent, there were also numerous repetitions of familiar mutations. (5) All regions of the chromatin were affected, but the induced mutations were more densely distributed in those regions of the linkage map in which more spontaneous mutations have occurred. (6) Multiple allelomorphism occurred. (7) So also did reverse mutation of genes already mutant when treated. The two latter facts argue against the effects always being complete losses or inactivations. (8) Though point-mutations were the rule, there was an occasional "line-mutation" involving a row of neighboring genes, as if by an electron that had passed parallel to the chromonema. (9) The vast majority of the treated genes, both mutant and normal-seeming, remained stable in their inheritance throughout succeeding generations, though at least one case of an "eversporting" condition arose.

Evidence was secured (by making use of non-disjunction) that only one of the two identical genes, or allelomorphs, present in a diploid cell, is caused to mutate at a time. The effect on a given gene, in a haploid germ cell, is "fractional," in that only a fraction of the resulting embryo will receive mutant gene material, the remainder being of normal gene content. Since there is no evidence of an indiscriminate intermingling of the mutant and normal tissues thereby arising, it becomes unlikely that the gene is compounded of many interchangeable members. This is also evidenced by the stability of treated genes in heredity.

Besides gene mutations, frequent rearrangements of gene order—involving inversions, translocations, duplications, etc., of chromosome sections—were found, by genetic evidence, to be produced by X-rays. These provided information concerning various questions. For example, cytological verification of two such cases yielded direct evidence for the physical validity of the linkage maps and of the corollary theory of crossing-over.

H. J. MULLER

JANUARY 8, 1928.

The committee on award this year was composed of the members named below:

Robert J. Terry, *chairman*, professor of anatomy, Washington University, St. Louis, Mo.

L. J. Cole, professor of genetics, University of Wisconsin, Madison, Wis.

William Duane, professor of biophysics, Harvard University, Cambridge, Mass.

G. Canby Robinson, professor of medicine, Vanderbilt University, Nashville, Tenn.

Charles Schuchert, professor of paleontology, Yale University, New Haven, Conn.

To these gentlemen is here expressed the gratitude of the association for their efficient service in this important and delicate part of the association's work.

The complete list of winners of the American Association prize is as follows:

(1) The Cincinnati award, January, 1924. L. E. Dickson, for contributions to the theory of numbers.

(2) The Washington award, January, 1925. Divided equally between Dr. Edwin P. Hubble, for con-

tributions on spiral nebulae, and Dr. L. R. Cleveland, for contributions on the physiology of termites and their intestinal protozoa.

(3) The Kansas City award, January, 1926. Dr. Dayton C. Miller, for contributions on the ether-drift experiment.

(4) The Philadelphia award, January, 1927. Dr. George D. Birkhoff, for mathematical criticism of some physical theories.

(5) The Nashville award, January, 1928. H. J. Muller, for contributions on the influence of X-rays on genes and chromosomes.

Special attention should be called to the purpose for which the prizes are awarded; that is, to stimulate interest in high-class contributions at the annual meetings and to encourage the presentation of the best American scientific work on these occasions. The more noteworthy advances made during the year in every field of knowledge should always be presented at the annual meeting. It is the hope of the donor of the American Association prize that it may serve each year as a concrete and tangible aid to some American science worker, enabling him to go further along his chosen line.

THE NEWS SERVICE AT NASHVILLE

(*Report by Austin H. Clark, News Manager*)

The outstanding feature of the Nashville meeting as compared with previous meetings was the increased interest on the part of the press, an interest which was clearly demonstrated by the high standing in their profession of all the representatives of newspapers, magazines and publishers of books who were in attendance. This increased interest in the proceedings was accompanied by a remarkable increase in the general appreciation of scientific work and a determination to present science to the people in a thoroughly dignified way. Certain aspects of science in the recent past have given rise in Tennessee to a considerable amount of controversy, and it might have been expected that at this meeting the local papers would seize the opportunity of reviving the discussion. Nothing of the sort occurred. On the contrary, the local papers handled a delicate situation in such a masterly way as to give a new broader meaning to the phrases southern courtesy and southern hospitality.

The gentlemen who reported the meeting for the daily papers were the following:

John L. Cooley, science editor, Associated Press.
W. M. Darling, Associated Press, Nashville.
Watson Davis, Science Service.
David Dietz, science editor, Scripps-Howard papers; also representing the NEA Service.
Richard FitzGerald, Jr., Nashville *Tennessean.*
William S. Howland, Nashville *Tennessean;* also representing the United Press and the *Christian Science Monitor.*
Coleman B. Jones, science editor, Associated Press.
Stanley Johnson, Nashville *Banner.*
Waldemar Kaempffert, science editor, New York *Times.*
Allen Shoenfield, Detroit *News.*
E. B. Stahlman, Jr., Nashville *Banner.*
Frank Thone, Science Service.

Of the scientific magazines *Popular Mechanics,* Chicago, was represented by Mr. J. Earle Miller, and *Science* and the *Scientific Monthly* were represented by Professor J. McKeen Cattell and Mr. Jaques Cattell. Mr. Frank Parker Stockbridge examined the material presented at the meeting, with a view to preparing a series of feature articles.

It is worthy of special mention that for the first time the Associated Press was represented by its science editors, and the New York *Times* was also represented by its science editor.

For the first time publishers of scientific books were prominently in evidence. There were present, to look over the situation and to make contracts, Mr. Edward M. Crane, president of the D. Van Nostrand Company, New York; Mr. Robert S. Gill, secretary-treasurer of the Williams and Wilkins Company, Baltimore, and Mr. Charles C. Thomas, of Springfield, Illinois.

The success of the news service at the Nashville meeting was due in no small degree to the energy and ability of the local committee on publicity, of which the chairman was Professor George R. Mayfield, of Vanderbilt University. Professor Mayfield not only handled the preliminary announcements and arrangements for the news service in a very effective way but also throughout the meeting he was daily in touch with the news office, materially assisting the work of the news manager.

The plan of handling the abstracts sent in was the same as that adopted at the Philadelphia meeting last year (see SCIENCE for January 28, 1927, pages 80–81). There were received by the news service altogether 415 abstracts and papers. Of these thirty-seven were mimeographed and the remainder were classified as follows: A, 27; B, 32; C, 91; D, 184; it was not found necessary to mark any of them X this year. No less than forty-four abstracts were received after the papers had been read; because of their lateness these could not be used by the news service. The number of abstracts received was smaller than the number received last year, but this fact in no way represents a falling off of interest in the news service, nor does it indicate any decline in the value of the material presented. The difference is entirely accounted for by the fact that the authors of many highly technical papers, which would be quite unintelligible to the layman, refrained from submitting abstracts.

Thanks to the energy and foresight of Professor Mayfield and to the able assistance of Dr. Frank Thone, an unusually comprehensive radio program was offered in connection with the meeting, which was arranged by the association and Science Service jointly. The talks were as follows:

Friday evening, December 23, Station WSM.—"The Meeting of the American Association for the Advancement of Science at Nashville." Professor George R. Mayfield, Vanderbilt University.

Tuesday evening, December 27, Station WSM.—"Photographing the Planets." Dr. Robert G. Aitken, Lick Observatory.

Wednesday evening, December 28, Station WSM.—"New Miracles with X-rays." Professor Winterton C. Curtis, University of Missouri.

Wednesday evening, December 28, Station WSM.—"The Natural History of Children." Dr. William E. Ritter, president of Science Service.

Thursday evening, December 29, Station WSM.—"The Sea." Austin H. Clark, Smithsonian Institution.

Thursday evening, December 29, Station WBAW.—"Wild Life in Louisiana." Percy Viosca, Jr., state biologist of Louisiana.

Friday evening, December 30, Station WSM.—"Floods of the Mississippi from a Meteorological Standpoint." Dr. Harry C. Frankenfield, U. S. Weather Bureau.

THE GENERAL AND COMPLIMENTARY PROGRAMS

There were nine general sessions of the association at Nashville, and four evening lectures especially arranged for the students and the general public of the city.

The opening session, on Monday evening, December 26, was held in the auditorium of Nashville's beautiful and imposing War-Memorial Building. The convention was opened by Dr. W. S. Leathers, general chairman of the local committees on preliminary arrangements, who introduced Dr. James H. Kirkland, chancellor of Vanderbilt University, and Judge Grafton Green, chief justice of the Supreme Bench of Tennessee. Dr. Kirkland welcomed the scientists on behalf of the educational and scientific institutions of Nashville. Judge Green extended to them the welcome of the state of Tennessee and the city of Nashville.

The chair was then taken by Dr. Arthur A. Noyes of the California Institute of Technology, president of the American Association. In reply to the addresses of welcome, Dr. Noyes delivered an address which will be printed in the next issue of SCIENCE.

The main address of the opening session of the annual meeting is regularly given by the retiring president of the association, who was this year Dr. L. H. Bailey, of Ithaca, N. Y., eminent authority and writer in botanical science, horticulture and rural life and editor of many most useful books of reference. Dr. Bailey was unfortunately unable to be present at Nashville, because of convalescence from a serious illness, but a note from him was read by Dr. W. J. Humphreys, general secretary of the association.

The opening session was completed by an invited lecture on the Mayan remains in Yucatan and Guatemala, by Dr. Sylvanus G. Morley, of the Carnegie Institution of Washington, who gave a fascinating account of his recent excavations. Beautiful and instructive lantern slides were shown.

The general reception followed the opening session. It was held in the Andrew Jackson Hotel and was well attended. Refreshments were served and very enjoyable entertainment was furnished by the Fisk University Singers. These are selected from among the students of Fisk University, of Nashville, the oldest college of liberal arts for Negroes in America. They preserve the unique, simple, spiritual character of the old Negro folk-songs and melodies of the old South. The local committee on entertainment, the chairman of which was Professor A. W. Wright, of Vanderbilt Medical School, merit the thanks of all who attended the reception, which was unusually enjoyable and successful.

For the first time in the history of the annual meetings of the American Association a reception was given Monday evening to Negroes interested in science, by Fisk University, which has been mentioned just above. For this special feature the association is indebted to Dr. Thomas E. Jones, president of Fisk University.

The second general session, Tuesday evening, in the auditorium of the War-Memorial Building, was held jointly, according to custom, with the Society of the Sigma Xi. The sixth annual Sigma Xi Lecture was given on this occasion, by Dr. Clarence Cook Little, president of the University of Michigan, eminent authority and student in the field of genetics and eugenics. The title of his address was "Opportunities for Research in Mammalian Genetics." The lecturer emphasized the great need for intensive research on mammalian genetics, pointing out the certain applications of the results of such research in the improvement of domestic animals and in physiological and psychological genetics as related to human pathology and medicine.

"The Distribution of Scientific Knowledge" was the topic of a symposium occupying both forenoon and afternoon on Wednesday. The several speakers represented the points of view of the investigator, the journal editor, the book publisher, the writer of scientific feature articles, the press syndicates and the editor of a metropolitan newspaper.

The fifth Josiah Willard Gibbs Lecture of the American Mathematical Society was delivered at a general session on Wednesday afternoon at 4:30. In this session, as in recent years, the association joined with the American Mathematical Society, under the auspices of which the Gibbs lecture is given. The lecturer this year was Professor Ernest W. Brown, eminent mathematician and astronomer, of Yale University. Professor Brown's subject was "Resonance in the Solar System."

"Edward Emerson Barnard, his Life and Work" was the subject of an illustrated lecture by Dr. Robert G. Aitken, of the Lick Observatory, given at the general session Wednesday evening, in the auditorium of the War-Memorial Building. This was the retiring vice-presidential address for Section D (Astronomy). Edward Emerson Barnard was a son of Nashville. Born in this city in 1857, Barnard was graduated from Vanderbilt University in 1886. He made many very valuable contributions to astronomy and was a leader and authority in his field. He died in 1923.

Two general sessions occurred on Thursday afternoon, one presenting a symposium on the "Economic Relations of Science Workers" and the other a symposium on "Aquiculture." The former of these was under the auspices of the association's Committee of One Hundred on Scientific Research, of which Dr. Rodney H. True, of the University of Pennsylvania, is secretary. At this symposium President Noyes gave the opening address, which was followed by papers on the "Relation of Research to Wealth Increase," by Harrison E. Howe; "Comparative Salary Scales of Trained Men," by Rodney H. True; and "Family Budgets of University Faculty Members," by Jessica B. Peixotto. A discussion followed.

The symposium on Aquiculture was arranged under the auspices of the Committee on Aquiculture, recently organized through the National Research Council. The program was in charge of Dr. Robert E. Coker, of the University of North Carolina. Several important papers on various aspects of marine biology were presented. The Committee on Aquiculture invites the counsel and cooperation of those interested in hydrobiological research or in the practical development of aquiculture. It is hoped that botanists, zoologists, geologists, chemists, meteorologists, engineers, economists and others may cooperate to promote the utilization of water areas for the culture of fishes, water birds, crustacea, pearl mussels, fur-bearing mammals, aquatic and swamp plants, etc.

The Thursday evening session was devoted to a lecture on "Science and the Newspapers," by Dr. William E. Ritter, president of Science Service. One of Dr. Ritter's main thoughts in this lecture is expressed as follows: "Science and journalism are both very powerful influences in modern civilization, but they have developed independently in large measure and they are sometimes more or less antagonistic. A study of the work of such men as Benjamin Franklin and Thomas Jefferson, who combined scientific research with ardent support of the newspapers and who mightily influenced our material development, leads to the thought that closer cooperation is needed between the scientists and the journalists."

An illustrated lecture on "Slow-Motion Pictures of Sounds and their Bearing on Speech and the Psychology of Audition" was given at the Friday evening symposium, by Professor Mark H. Liddell, of Purdue University. He presented some of the results of his recent studies on the physics of the sounds of human speech, in which new and highly refined physical methods have been employed. Records of sound waves were shown and different kinds of sounds and noises were produced and compared.

Four non-technical lectures were arranged for the week of the meeting, complimentary to the people of Nashville, including school and college students. These were well attended. The speakers and their topics were as follows:

Tuesday evening. Dr. William M. Mann, director of the National Zoological Park, Washington, D. C. "Collecting Wild Animals for Our National Zoo," with motion pictures.

Wednesday evening. Dr. C. E. K. Mees, director of the research laboratory of the Eastman Kodak Co., Rochester, N. Y. "Production of a Photographic Image," with lantern slides and motion pictures.

Thursday evening. F. R. Moulton, of Chicago. "Science and Civilization."

Friday evening. Mr. Arthur Sterry Coggeshall, curator of education in the Carnegie Museum, Pittsburgh. "Turning Back the Clock Ten Million Years, an account of the Age of Dinosaurs," with slides and motion pictures.

Seven radio talks were given, as shown in the preceding section.

THE COUNCIL ROLL AT NASHVILLE

The affairs of the association are entirely in the charge of the council, which consists of the president, the fifteen vice-presidents, the treasurer, the general secretary, the permanent secretary, the fifteen section secretaries, the council representatives of the affiliated societies and state academies, the eight elected council members and those members of the executive committee who are not otherwise members of the council.

Past presidents of the association and the presidents of the divisions and local branches are officially invited to attend council sessions. The council meets only at the annual meetings of the association. Four sessions were held at Nashville.

The complete roll of the council for the eighty-fourth meeting is shown below, arranged alphabetically. Each member's name is followed by an italic phrase, showing his status in the council. The record of attendance at the four Nashville sessions is shown by numerals that precede the members' names, these numbers representing, respectively, the sessions on Monday, Tuesday, Wednesday, and Thursday, December 26 to December 29. Thus, the numerals 2 and 3 before a name indicate that the member whose name is so marked was present at the Tuesday and Wednesday sessions but was absent from the other sessions. Each member's record of attendance was submitted to him by mail before this list was prepared, with the request that needed corrections be made, but it is possible that a few errors may still require correction. In such cases the permanent secretary's office should be promptly informed. A few substitutes took the places of members who could not come to Nashville, and these are named and so indicated in the list.

MEMBERS AND INVITED GUESTS OF THE COUNCIL FOR THE SECOND NASHVILLE MEETING, WITH NOTES AS TO THEIR STATUS AND RECORDS OF THEIR ATTENDANCE

(*Prepared by Sam F. Trelease, secretary of the council.*)

Adams, Roger, *Vice-President for Section C.*
Adams, Walter S., *Vice-President for Section C.*
2, 3 Aitken, Robert G., *Rep. Astronom. Soc. Pacific.*
Aldrich, J. M., *Rep. Entomol. Soc. Amer.* (H. E. Ewing, substitute for the Nashville meeting.)
1, 2, 3, 4 Alexander, William H., *Rep. Ohio Acad. Science.*
Anderson, John E., *Rep. Amer. Psychol. Assoc.* (S. C. Garrison, substitute for the Nashville meeting.)
3, 4 Archibald, R. C., *Secretary of Section A.*
1 Ashley, George H., *Rep. Pennsylvania Acad. Science.*
Bailey, L. H., *Past President (1926) and Rep. Bot. Soc. Amer.*
1, 2, 3, 4 Bakke, A. L., *Rep. Honor Soc. Phi Kappa Phi.*
3, 4 Ball, C. R., *Rep. Honor Soc. Phi Kappa Phi.*
Barnes, Harry Elmer, *Vice-President for Section L.*
Barr, A. S., *Secretary of Section Q.*
2, 4 Bartlett, Harley Harris, *Rep. Amer. Soc. Naturalists.*
Bergey, David H., *Rep. Soc. Amer. Bacteriologists.* (H. M. Weeter, substitute for the Nashville meeting.)
Berkey, Charles P., *Rep. Geol. Soc. Amer.*
1 Bishop, E. L., *Rep. Amer. Public Health Assoc.*
Bloom, Lansing B., *President of the Southwestern Division.*
Boose, M. C., *Rep. Amer. Ceramic Soc.*
Boring, Edwin G., *Rep. Amer. Psychol. Assoc.*
Bowman, Isaiah, *Rep. Amer. Geographical Soc.*
Brasch, Frederick E., *Secretary of Section L.*
1, 2, 3, 4 Breckenridge, J. M., *Rep. Amer. Chem. Soc.*
Breed, Robert S., *Rep. Soc. Amer. Bacteriologists.* (H. N. Parker, substitute for the Nashville meeting.)
1 Brown, Harold, *Rep. Amer. Soc. Parasitologists.* (Substitute for M. C. Hall.)
2, 3 Brown, P. E., *Secretary of Section O.*
Buchanan, H. E., *Rep. New Orleans Acad. Sciences.* (Substitute for H. W. Moseley.)
2, 3, 4 Budington, Robert A., *Rep. Amer. Soc. Naturalists.*
1, 2, 3, 4 Cairns, W. D., *Rep. Math. Assoc. Amer.*
Cajori, Florian, *Rep. History Science Soc.*
2, 3 Caldwell, Otis W., *Rep. National Education Assoc.*
3, 4 Call, L. E., *Vice-President for Section O.*
Campbell, W. W., *Past President (1915).*
1, 2 Cattell, J. McKeen, *Exec. Comm. Member and Past President (1924).*
Chamberlin, T. C., *Past President (1908).*
Clinton, G. P., *Rep. Amer. Phytopathol. Soc.*
Coates, Charles E., *Rep. Amer. Oil Chemists' Soc.*
1, 2, 3, 4 Cole, Fay-Cooper, *Secretary of Section H.*
3, 4 Cole, Leon J., *Rep. Amer. Genetic Assoc.*
2, 3, 4 Collingwood, Harris, *Rep. Soc. Amer. Foresters.*
Compton, Arthur H., *Vice-President for Section B.*
Compton, Karl T., *Rep. Amer. Physical Soc. and Optical Soc. Amer.*
Coulter, John Merle, *Rep. Amer. Assoc. Univ. Professors and Past President (1918).*
3 Courtis, Stuart A., *Rep. Nat. Soc. Coll. Teachers Education.*
Crittenden, E. C., *Rep. Illuminating Engineering Soc.*
3, 4 Crocker, William, *Vice-President for Section G.*
1, 2, 3 Cunningham, Bert, *Rep. North Carolina Acad. Science.*
Curtis, W. C., *Rep. Amer. Soc. Zoologists.* (Substitute for H. V. Neal.)
3 Curtiss, Ralph H., *Rep. Amer. Astronom. Soc.*
Dains, F. B., *Rep. History Science Soc.*
3, 4 Dean, George A., *Rep. Amer. Assoc. Econ. Entomol.*
Dellinger, J. H., *Rep. Inst. Radio Engineers.*
Dice, Lee R., *Rep. Amer. Soc. Mammalogists.*
Dickson, L. E., *Elected Member.*
2, 3, 4 Dietrichson, Gerhard, *Secretary of Section C.*
Dorsey, Maxwell Jay, *Rep. Amer. Soc. Horticultural Science.*
4 Downing, E. R., *Rep. Nat. Education Assoc.* (Substitute for O. W. Caldwell.)
Dresden, Arnold, *Rep. Amer. Math. Soc.*
3, 4 Drushel, J. Andrew, *Rep. Amer. Nature-Study Soc.*
1 Dunlap, Knight, *Vice-President for Section I.*
Dunn, Gano, *Rep. Amer. Inst. Electrical Engineers.*
1, 2 Eaton, S. V., *Rep. Amer. Soc. Plant Physiologists.* (Substitute for R. P. Hibbard.)
Ellery, Edward, *Rep. Sigma Xi.*
1, 2, 3, 4 Enders, Howard E., *Rep. Indiana Acad. Science.*
Estabrook, Arthur H., *Rep. Eugenics Research Assoc.*
4 Ewing, H. E., *Rep. Entomol. Soc. Amer.* (Substitute for J. M. Aldrich.)
Faig, John T., *Rep. Amer. Soc. Mechanical Engineers.*
1, 2, 3, 4 Fairchild, H. L., *Exec. Comm. Member.*
3, 4 Fenneman, N. M., *Rep. Assoc. Amer. Geographers.*
Flexner, Simon, *Past President (1919).*

3 Flint, W. P., *Rep. Illinois Acad. Science.*
Focke, T. M., *Rep. Math. Assoc. Amer.*
3 Fort, Tomlinson, *Rep. Amer. Math. Soc.*
1, 2, 3 Fox, Philip, *Secretary of Section D and Rep. Amer. Astronom. Soc.*
1, 2, 3 Freeman, Frank N., *Secretary of Section I and Rep. Nat. Soc. Study of Education.*
Garber, R. J., *Rep. Amer. Soc. Agronomy.* (M. M. Hoover, substitute for the Nashville meeting.)
1, 2, 3, 4 Gardner, Wright A., *Rep. Alabama Acad. Science.*
Garrison, S. C., *Rep. Amer. Psychol. Assoc.* (Substitute for John E. Anderson.)
Gates, Arthur I., *Vice-President for Section Q.*
Giddings, N. J., *Rep. West Virginia Acad. Science.*
1 Glenn, Leonidas C., *Rep. Amer. Inst. Mining and Metallurgical Engineers.* (Substitute for G. R. Mansfield and for David White.)
2, 3, 4 Goldforb, A. J., *Secretary of Section N and Rep. Soc. Exp. Biology and Medicine.*
Good, E. S., *Rep. Amer. Soc. Animal Production.* (Substitute for E. W. Sheets.)
Goode, J. Paul, *Rep. Assoc. Amer. Geographers.*
2, 3, 4 Guthe, C. E., *Rep. Amer. Anthropol. Assoc.*
Guy, J. Sam, *Rep. Georgia Acad. Science.* (T. H. McHatton, substitute for the Nashville meeting.)
Hall, M. C., *Rep. Amer. Soc. Parasitologists.* (Harold Brown, substitute for the Nashville meeting.)
3, 4 Hargitt, Geo. T., *Secretary of Section F.*
1, 2, 3, 4 Harnly, Henry J., *Rep. Kansas Acad. Science.*
Harper, Robert Almer, *Rep. Torrey Bot. Club.* (A. B. Stout, substitute for the Nashville meeting.)
Harris, J. Arthur, *Rep. Torrey Bot. Club.*
Harshberger, John W., *Rep. Ecol. Soc. Amer.*
Hartwell, Burt L., *Rep. Amer. Soc. Agronomy.* (Forman T. McLean, substitute for the Nashville meeting.)
2, 4 Heck, N. H., *Secretary of Section M.*
Hedrick, William A., *Rep. Amer. Fed. Teachers of Math. and Nat. Sciences.*
2, 3, 4 Herrick, Glenn W., *Rep. Amer. Assoc. Econ. Entomol.*
Hess, Alfred F., *Rep. Soc. Exp. Biology and Medicine.*
Hibbard, R. P., *Rep. Amer. Soc. Plant Physiologists.* (S. V. Eaton and C. A. Shull, substitutes for the Nashville meeting.)
3, 4 Hoover, M. M., *Rep. Alabama Acad. Science.* (Substitute for R. J. Garber.)
2, 3, 4 Howard, L. O., *Elected Member and Past President (1920).*
4 Hughes, A. L., *Secretary of Section B.*
1, 2, 3, 4 Humphreys, W. J., *General Secretary of the Association and Rep. Amer. Meteorol. Soc.*
4 Jackson, Dunham, *Vice-President for Section A.*
Joerg, W. L. G., *Rep. Amer. Geographical Soc.*
Jones, Lauder W., *Rep. Amer. Chem. Soc.*
Jordan, David Starr, *Past President (1909).*
3, 4 Juday, Chancey, *Rep. Wisconsin Acad. Sciences.*
Keith, Arthur, *Rep. Geol. Soc. Amer.*
Kellogg, Vernon, *Exec. Comm. Member.*
Kemp, W. W., *Rep. Nat. Soc. Coll. Teachers Education.*
Kober, George M., *Rep. Amer. Medical Assoc.*
Koch, Julius A., *Rep. Amer. Pharmaceutical Assoc.*
Kofoid, Charles A., *President of the Pacific Division.*
Laughlin, H. H., *Rep. Eugenics Research Assoc.*
Leathers, W. S., *Vice-President for Section K and rep. Amer. Public Health Assoc.*
Leighty, C. E., *Rep. Amer. Genetic Assoc.*
2, 3, 4 Lewis, I. F., *Rep. Bot. Soc. Amer.*
Lidbury, F. A., *Rep. Amer. Electrochem. Soc.*
1, 2, 3, 4 Livingston, Burton E., *Permanent Secretary of the Association.*
3, 4 Lloyd, Francis E., *Rep. Amer. Soc. Plant Physiologists.*
Loomis, F. B., *Rep. Paleontological Soc. Amer.*
2, 3, 4 Lutz, Frank Eugene, *Rep. Amer. Soc. Zoologists.*
1, 3, 4 Lyon, Marcus Ward, Jr., *Rep. Amer. Soc. Mammalogists.*
MacDougal, D. T., *Elected Member.*
1, 2, 4 Macelwane, James B., *Rep. Seismol. Soc. Amer.*
Mansfield, G. R., *Secretary of Section E.* (Leonidas C. Glenn, substitute for the Nashville meeting.)
McClung, C. E., *Vice-President for Section F.*
1, 2, 3, 4 McGill, John T., *Rep. Tennessee Acad. Science.*
1, 2, 4 McHatton, T. H., *Rep. Georgia Acad. Science.* (Substitute for J. Sam Guy.)
2 McLean, Forman T., *Rep. Amer. Soc. Agronomy.* (Substitute for Burt L. Hartwell.)
McMurrich, J. Playfair, *Rep. Amer. Assoc. Anatomists, and Past President (1922).*
Merriam, John C., *Elected Member.*
3, 4 Metcalf, Clell Lee, *Rep. Entomol. Soc. Amer.*
3, 4 Metcalf, Z. P., *Rep. Amer. Microscopical Soc.*
Michelson, A. A., *Past President (1910).*
3, 4 Michelson, Truman, *Rep. Amer. Anthropol. Assoc.*
1, 3, 4 Middleton, Austin R., *Rep. Kentucky Acad. Science.*
1, 2, 3, 4 Miller, E. C. L., *Rep. Amer. Electrochem. Soc.*
Mitchell, S. A., *Rep. Amer. Assoc. Univ. Professors.*
Moore, E. H., *Past President (1921).*
1, 2, 3, 4 Morehouse, D. W., *Rep. Iowa Acad. Science.*
Moseley, H. W., *Rep. New Orleans Acad. Sciences.* (H. E. Buchanan, substitute for the Nashville meeting.)
2, 3, 4 Moulton, F. R., *Exec. Comm. Member and Rep. Sigma Xi.*
Neal, H. V., *Rep. Amer. Soc. Zoologists.* (W. C. Curtis, substitute for the Nashville meeting.)
Nicholas, Francis C., *Rep. Maryland Acad. Sciences.*
Nichols, E. L., *Past President (1907).*
1, 3, 4 Noyes, A. A., *President of the Association.*
1, 2, 3 Noyes, W. A., *Exec. Comm. Member.*
1, 3 O'Kane, Walter C., *Rep. New Hampshire Acad. Science.*
3 Okkelberg, Peter, *Rep. Michigan Acad. Science.*
Oldfather, W. A., *Elected Member.*
1, 2, 3, 4 Osburn, Raymond C., *Rep. Ecol. Soc. Amer.*
Parker, H. N., *Rep. Soc. Amer. Bacteriologists.* (Substitute for Robert S. Breed.)
1, 2 Patterson, Herbert, *Rep. Oklahoma Acad. Science.*
Piersol, George M., *Rep. Amer. Medical Assoc.*
Pratt, Joseph H., *Rep. Amer. Soc. Civil Engineers.*
Pupin, M. I., *Exec. Comm. Member, Rep. Amer. Inst. Electrical Engineers, and Past President (1925).*
Reddick, Donald, *Rep. Amer. Phytopath. Soc.*
Richards, C. R., *Rep. Amer. Soc. Mechanical Engineers.*
Richards, Theodore W., *Past President (1917).*
Richtmyer, F. K., *Rep. Optical Soc. Amer.*
Robinson, G. Canby, *Vice-President for Section N.*
3, 4 Salter, R. M., *Rep. Amer. Soc. Agronomy.*

1 Sanders, George E., *Rep. Canadian Soc. Tech. Agriculturists.*
4 Sapir, Edward, *Rep. Linguistic Soc. Amer.*
Sauveur, Albert, *Rep. Amer. Inst. Mining and Metallurgical Engineers.*
Schroeder, E. C., *Rep. Amer. Veterinary Med. Assoc.*
4 Schuchert, Charles, *Vice-President for Section E.*
Senior, H. D., *Rep. Amer. Assoc. Anatomists.*
Sharp, Clayton H., *Rep. Illuminating Engineering Soc.*
Sheets, E. W., *Rep. Amer. Soc. Animal Production.* (E. S. Good, substitute for the Nashville meeting.)
1, 3, 4 Shull, C. A., *Rep. Amer. Soc. Plant Physiologists.* (Substitute for R. P. Hibbard.)
Stewart, G. W., *Elected Member.*
4 Stout, A. B., *Rep. Torrey Bot. Club.* (Substitute for R. A. Harper.)
Studebaker, J. W., *Rep. National Education Assoc.*
4 Talbot, A. N., *Vice-President for Section M.*
1, 2, 3, 4 Terry, R. J., *Vice-President for Section H.*
Townley, S. D., *Rep. Seismol. Soc. Amer.*
1, 2, 3, 4 Trelease, Sam F., *Secretary of Section G.*
4 True, Rodney H., *Elected Member.*
3, 4 Van Cleave, H. J., *Rep. Amer. Microscopical Soc.*
Van Horn, Frank R., *Rep. Mineralogical Soc. Amer.*
1 Waddell, John A. L., *Rep. Amer. Soc. Civil Engineers.*
1, 2, 3, 4 Ward, Henry B., *Exec. Comm. Member.*
Warwick, C. L., *Rep. Amer. Soc. Testing Materials.*
Weaver, John Ernst, *Rep. Nebraska Acad. Science.*
Webb, Harold W., *Rep. Amer. Physical Soc.*
Weeter, H. M., *Rep. Soc. Amer. Bacteriologists.* (Substitute for David H. Bergey.)
Welch, William H., *Past President (1906).*
Whipple, Guy M., *Rep. Nat. Soc. Study of Education.*
White, David, *Elected Member and Rep. Paleontological Soc. Amer.* (Leonidas C. Glenn, substitute for the Nashville meeting.)
Wilson, Edmund B., *Past President (1913).*
Wilson, Edwin B., *Exec. Comm. Member.*
Wirt, John L., *Treasurer of the Association.*

THE ROLL OF THE EXECUTIVE COMMITTEE AT NASHVILLE*

The executive committee held sessions on Monday, Tuesday and Wednesday mornings. The first session was in the Andrew Jackson Hotel, while the others were in the council room in the Industrial Arts Building, George Peabody College for Teachers. Following is the roll of the committee. The numbers preceding each name indicate the sessions at which the member was present, as in the case of the council roll above. The number in parenthesis after each name denotes the calendar year at the end of which the member's term of office was to expire. Dr. H. L. Fairchild and Dr. W. A. Noyes automatically retired from the committee at the end of this Nashville meeting, and Dr. John Johnston, U. S. Steel Corporation, New York City, and Dr. David R. Curtiss, Northwestern University, were elected as their successors.

* The number in parenthesis denotes the year at the end of which the member's term of office was to expire.

1, 2 J. McKeen Cattell (1930), *chairman,* Garrison-on-Hudson, N. Y.
1, 3 A. A. Noyes (1927), president of the association, Pasadena, Calif.
1, 2 W. J. Humphreys (1928), general secretary of the association, Washington, D. C.
1, 2, 3 Burton E. Livingston (1928), permanent secretary of the association, Baltimore, Md., and Washington, D. C.
1, 2, 3 H. L. Fairchild (1927), Rochester, N. Y.
Vernon Kellogg (1928), Washington, D. C.
3 F. R. Moulton (1929), Chicago, Ill.
1, 3 W. A. Noyes (1927), Urbana, Ill.
M. I. Pupin (1929), New York City.
1, 2, 3 H. B. Ward (1930), Urbana, Ill.
Edwin B. Wilson (1928), Boston, Mass.

LEGISLATIVE AND EXECUTIVE PROCEEDINGS AT NASHVILLE

The executive committee of the council met in the Andrew Jackson Hotel on Monday morning, December 26, and held two other sessions, in the council room, Industrial Arts Building, George Peabody College for Teachers, on Tuesday and Wednesday mornings, following the council sessions. The council met at the Andrew Jackson Hotel on Monday afternoon, December 26, and in the council room on Tuesday, Wednesday and Thursday mornings. No business was transacted at any of the general sessions at Nashville. The following paragraphs summarize the business proceedings at this meeting:

(1) The council minutes of December 31, 1926, and of December 26, 27 and 28, 1927, were read and approved by the council.

(2) The audited report of the treasurer for the fiscal year ending September 30, 1927, was accepted by the council and ordered to be printed in SCIENCE in the usual manner. It appears elsewhere in this issue of SCIENCE.

(3) The audited financial report of the permanent secretary, for the association year ending September 30, 1927, was accepted and ordered printed in SCIENCE. It also appears elsewhere in the present issue.

(4) The following appropriations were made from the treasurer's funds available for the current year:

For journal subscriptions for 418 life members	$1,254.00
For life-membership fees of three emeritus life members, on account of the Jane M. Smith Fund for this special purpose	300.00
For rental of treasurer's safety-deposit box	20.00
For grants for research, to be allotted by the Committee on Grants	3,000.00
To the Naples Zoological Station	500.00
To the Annual Tables of Physical and Chemical Constants	200.00

To these should be added an appropriation of $100 to the National Conference on Outdoor Recreation, authorized by the executive committee at its recent autumn meeting and now reported to the council, and the total of appropriations from the treasurer's funds for the current year therefore amounts to $5,374. There remains an unappropriated balance of treasurer's funds available for the current year, amounting to $1,411.45. It is possible that about $1,200 of this balance may be appropriated for the use of the Committee of One Hundred on Scientific Research, but that matter is left in the hands of the executive committee, with power, because no report and proposed budget for the Committee of One Hundred was received in time for action at Nashville.

(5) The following members were elected to emeritus life membership according to the provisions of the will of the late Jane M. Smith:

Frank A. Gooch (joined in 1876, elected to fellowship in 1880), 291 Edwards St., New Haven, Conn. A.B., Harvard, 1872; A.M., Ph.D., 1877; Ph.D., Vienna, 1875–76; honorary A.M., Yale, 1887. Professor of chemistry and director of the Kent Chemical Laboratory, Yale University, 1885–1918; emeritus professor since 1918.

Alfred Springer (joined in 1875, elected to fellowship in 1880), 312 East 2nd St., Cincinnati, Ohio. Ph.D., Heidelberg, 1872; secretary, Section C, 1882; assistant general secretary, 1883; general secretary, 1884; vice-president for Section C, 1892.

Warren Upham (joined in 1876, elected to fellowship in 1880), Minnesota Historical Society, St. Paul, Minn. A.B., Dartmouth, 1871; honorary A.M., Dartmouth, 1894; Sc.D., Dartmouth, 1906. Has held positions with the New Hampshire Geological Survey, the Minnesota Geological Survey, the U. S. Geological Survey and the Western Reserve Historical Society. Archeologist of the Minnesota Historical Society since 1914.

(6) The council established a committee to look into the question of securing American funds for the Naples Zoological Station, the committee to consist of Edmund B. Wilson, Henry B. Ward and a third member named by these two.

(7) The council expressed its great appreciation of the very valuable services rendered by Dr. Sam F. Trelease, program editor, and by Mrs. Trelease. Special mention was made of the complete index of speakers' names, which this year, for the first time, is part of the general program. Day and night for two weeks preceding the opening of the meeting Doctor and Mrs. Trelease devoted themselves to the very arduous task of getting the program printed on time. The book was completed Saturday, December 24. An honorarium of $200 was voted to the program editor on account of his efficient work on the Nashville general program.

(8) Eighty fellows were elected by the council, distributed among the several sections as follows:

Section A (Mathematics)	1	Section I (Psychology)	1
Section C (Chemistry)	3	Section M (Engineering)	22
Section E (Geology and Geography)	2	Section N (Medical Sciences)	11
Section G (Botanical Sciences)	35	Section O (Agriculture)	5

(9) By action of the council the newly formed Colorado-Wyoming Academy of Science was officially affiliated with the American Association, with the financial provision that both an academy allowance and a division allowance are not to be paid for the same member in any case.

(10) The executive committee was authorized by the council to arrange, in connection with each annual meeting of the association, an academy conference and the council approved of the following named officers of the conference for the current year: Chairman, William H. Alexander, U. S. Weather Bureau, Columbus, Ohio; secretary, Howard E. Enders, Purdue University, LaFayette, Ind.

(11) The permanent secretary was asked to make a study of the problem of the extra journals (*The Scientific Monthly* and the *Science News-Letter*), with the advice and assistance of Dr. Cattell and Dr. Kellogg, and to present at a later meeting of the executive committee suggestions for improvements in arrangements for these journals.

(12) A special telegram was sent to the secretary of each associated organization meeting at this time elsewhere than in Nashville, inviting the organization to hold sessions at the New York meeting next year.

(13) It was voted by the council that men of science from outside of the United States and Canada who are members of scientific associations in their own countries are to be appointed honorary associates if they attend an annual meeting of the American Association, the associate fee and the registration fee being remitted in such cases.

(14) Resignations were presented, and accepted by the council, from the section secretaries named below, the reason for the resignation being, in all three cases, the press of other work: Raymond C. Archibald, secretary of Section A (Mathematics); Frederick E. Brasch, secretary of Section L (Historical and Philological Sciences); A. J. Goldforb, secretary of Section N (Medical Sciences).

(15) It was voted that the spring meeting of the executive committee of the council shall regularly occur at Washington, D. C., on the Sunday preceding the spring meeting of the National Academy of Sciences.

(16) The executive committee appointed Arthur A. Noyes a committee of one to consider possible improvements in the procedure for awarding the American Association prize and to send to the permanent secretary at an early date suggestions for such possible improvements.

(17) On recommendation by the executive committee, the council voted that the annual meeting of December, 1929, is to be held at Des Moines, Iowa, on invitation of Drake University and the Des Moines Chamber of Commerce.

(18) The executive committee instructed the permanent secretary to study and report on the possibilities of holding the meeting of December, 1930, in Montreal. That meeting has been tentatively set for Cleveland, but no definite arrangements have yet been made and the committee noted the desirability of holding an annual meeting in Canada in the near future.

(19) The executive committee named a special committee, consisting of J. McK. Cattell, Burton E. Livingston and Sam F. Trelease, to decide upon the general-headquarters hotel for the New York meeting next year.

(20) The executive committee voted that the registration fee for the New York meeting shall be two dollars, one dollar being remitted to members in good standing of the American Association for the Advancement of Science.

(21) The council adopted a resolution favoring the maintenance of the highest standards in the system of the national parks of the United States. This resolution appears elsewhere in this issue of SCIENCE.

(22) The council adopted a resolution favoring the establishment of wild-life experiment stations in the United States. This resolution appears elsewhere in this issue of SCIENCE.

(23) The following resolution was adopted by the council:

Resolved: That the American Association for the Advancement of Science approves of the project, brought to its attention by Dr. Gregory D. Walcott, for the publication of source-books in the history of science, and names a committee of three to cooperate with the advisory board for this project, the members of the committee to be Gregory D. Walcott, Edwin G. Conklin and Harlow Shapley.

(24) A report of the Committee on the Place of Science in Education was presented to the council, a summary of which appears elsewhere in this issue of SCIENCE. The report was accepted and the council authorized the committee to publish a more complete report, which is being prepared, this publication to be financed without drawing on association funds other than those specially designated for the use of the Committee on the Place of Science in Education.

(25) The council authorized the Committee on Place of Science in Education to proceed with its plans for a comprehensive and cooperative study of educational systems and for the development of a council of science teachers, it being understood that these projects are to be financed without drawing on association funds other than those specially designated for the use of the Committee on the Place of Science in Education.

(26) The council named a committee of four to investigate and report on the relation of existing tariff laws in the United States to scientific research, the committee to consist of Edward B. Mathews, Johns Hopkins University; Austin H. Clark, Smithsonian Institution; William A. Noyes, University of Illinois; and Frederick E. Wright, Geophysical Laboratory, Washington, D. C.

(27) The council named a committee of four to investigate and report on the project, suggested by Mr. Joseph L. Wheeler, of supplying to libraries and the general public lists of recommended books on science, the committee to consist of Joseph L. Wheeler, Enoch Pratt Library, Baltimore; Edward W. Berry, Johns Hopkins University; Burton E. Livingston, Johns Hopkins University; and Robert B. Sosman, Carnegie Institution of Washington.

(28) The council unanimously elected Dr. Henry Fairfield Osborn, president of the Museum of Natural History, New York City, as president of the American Association for the Advancement of Science.

(29) On nominations received in the regular way from the respective section committees, the association vice-presidents for the following named sections were unanimously elected for the ensuing year: Section A (Mathematics), Raymond C. Archibald; Section B (Physics), P. W. Bridgman; Section C (Chemistry), C. E. K. Mees; Section D (Astronomy), J. S. Plaskett; Section E (Geology and Geography), Frank Leverett; Section F (Zoological Sciences), M. F. Guyer; Section G (Botanical Sciences), Charles E. Allen; Section H (Anthropology), Fay-Cooper Cole; Section I (Psychology), Howard C. Warren; Section M (Engineering), Robert Lemuel Sackett; Section O (Agriculture), C. A. Mooers; Section Q (Education), Truman L. Kelley.

(30) On nominations received from the respective section committees, the council unanimously elected the three section secretaries named below, their terms of office to expire at the end of the New York meeting next year: Secretary of Section A (Mathematics), Charles N. Moore; secretary of Section N (Medical Sciences), James Harold Austin; secretary of Section H (Anthropology), C. H. Danforth. The secretaries of Sections A and N had resigned, as noted above, and the election of a secretary of Section H was made necessary by the election of Dr. Fay-Cooper Cole (who has been secretary) as vice-president for the section.

(31) On nominations presented by a nominating committee, the council unanimously elected two members of the council, two members of the executive committee, two members of the committee on grants and one member of the finance committee, in accordance with provisions of the Constitution, the terms of office of these to expire at the end of December, 1931. The names of those elected are as follows:

Elected council members: Arthur H. Compton, University of Chicago, and Austin H. Clark, Smithsonian Institution. These succeed W. A. Oldfather and G. W. Stewart, whose terms expired at the end of this meeting.

Members of executive committee: John Johnston, U. S. Steel Corporation, New York City, and David R. Curtiss, Northwestern University. These succeed H. L. Fairchild and W. A. Noyes, whose terms expired at the end of this meeting.

Members of the Committee on Grants: Walter S. Adams (representing astronomy), Mount Wilson Observatory, and Karl F. Kellerman (representing botanical sciences), U. S. Department of Agriculture. These succeed A. Hrdlička and B. M. Davis, whose terms expired at the end of this meeting.

Member of the Finance Committee, Arthur L. Day, Geophysical Laboratory, Washington, D. C., who was elected to succeed himself.

(32) The council unanimously nominated Dr. J. McK. Cattell to succeed himself as representative of the American Association in the board of trustees of Science Service.

(33) The next meeting of the executive committee will occur at the Cosmos Club, in Washington, on Sunday, April 22, 1928. The next meeting of the council will occur at New York on Thursday, December 27, 1928.

RESOLUTIONS BEARING ON THE PUBLIC WELFARE ADOPTED BY THE COUNCIL AT NASHVILLE, DECEMBER 28, 1927

A Resolution on the Maintenance of the Highest Standards in the System of the National Parks of the United States.

Resolved: That the American Association for the Advancement of Science

(1) Approves the creation of those national parks only which meet the highest standards of the system, namely, which are wholly or almost wholly areas of original, unmodified natural conditions, each a unique example of its landscape or geologic type in the country; and

(2) Declares that, as the only reservational system for preservation of the primitive and majestic in nature, the protection inviolate of the system of national parks demands extraordinary watchfulness and care; and

(3) Recognizes that, by reason of its peculiar limitations and conditions, the system of national parks possesses facilities for popular education in nature and for inspiration, which have incalculable value to individuals and the nation.

A Resolution Favoring the Establishment of Wild-Life Experiment Stations in the United States.

Resolved: That the American Association for the Advancement of Science recommends the establishment of wild-life experiment stations for the better conservation, development and utilization of the wild-life resources of our national parks and forests, such stations to be established and supported by federal, state or private agencies or some combination of these.

THE ANNUAL CONFERENCE OF SECTION AND SOCIETY SECRETARIES

(*Based on minutes furnished by Geo. T. Hargitt, Secretary of the Nashville Conference*)

The secretaries of the sections and of the associated societies meeting with the American Association at Nashville, together with the members of the executive committee of the association council, the executive assistant and the news manager, held the annual secretaries' conference at the Andrew Jackson Hotel on the evening of Friday, December 30, following a complimentary dinner provided by the association for this occasion. There were twenty-two in attendance, but a few left early because they were returning home that night. Many questions of the management of the association and of the relation of the association to the associated organizations were discussed and the conference was even more satisfactory and profitable than any of the earlier ones. The custom of holding this conference in connection with the annual meeting each year, inaugurated at the second Toronto meeting, in December, 1921, is now well established. It furnishes opportunity for bringing together those who have to do with the organization and work of the association, especially in relation to the associated organizations. Dr. Geo. T. Hargitt, secretary for Section F (Zoological sciences), served as secretary of the secretaries' conference. He was requested to prepare a program of topics for discussion at the New York conference next year, by means of correspondence with the other members. The secretaries' conference thus becomes, in a sense, perpetual, and continues throughout the year. Further notes concerning its problems are to be published in SCIENCE from time to time.

The secretaries' conference adopted the following resolutions of appreciation.

(1) *Resolved:* That the secretaries' conference at Nashville requests the permanent secretary to express to President A. A. Noyes the appreciative thanks of the association and the associated societies for the fine and efficient manner in which he has presided at the council sessions and at general sessions of the association at Nashville and has performed the other duties of his office as president.

(2) *Resolved:* That the secretaries' conference at Nashville requests the permanent secretary to convey to the institutions of Nashville that have so generously taken part in making this meeting such a pronounced success, an expression of the grateful appreciation of the association and the associated organizations.

(3) *Resolved:* That the conference of association and society secretaries asks the permanent secretary to express the gratitude of the association and of the associated organizations to the members of the local committees on arrangements for this meeting, without whose very efficient preliminary work the meeting could not have occurred.

(4) *Resolved:* That the conference of association and society secretaries asks the permanent secretary to thank heartily the editors of the local newspapers and the press representatives from away who covered the Nashville meeting, for the very excellent and extensive publicity given to this meeting.

REPORT OF THE TREASURER FOR 1926–27

In accordance with the provision of Article III, Section 6, of the By-Laws, the treasurer respectfully submits herewith the following report for the fiscal year ending September 30, 1927.

Collections from all sources during the year amounted to $31,874.78. Included in the amount are the following items:

Payment of a mortgage held by the association on a real estate loan	$20,000.00
Additional donation to the Prize Fund by the original donor, thus guaranteeing the Prize Award for the next five years	3,000.00
Sixteen Life Membership fees, increasing the endowment fund by a like amount	1,600.00

Disbursements made in accordance with direction of the council and executive committee amount, in the aggregate, to $6,366.18, including the $1,000 Prize awarded to Dr. George D. Birkhoff at the fifth Philadelphia meeting.

A reserve fund of $4,364.08 was established in conformity with a resolution adopted by the council December 27, 1926.

The total amount of funds of the association, consisting of contributions received from Richard T. Colburn, W. Hudson Stephens, Friends of Association, Sustaining and Life Memberships, Jane M. Smith and Prize Fund, is $159,075.01.

The details of receipts, disbursements and disposition of funds are shown in the following itemized statements.

Respectfully submitted,
(*Signed*) John L. Wirt,
Treasurer.

Washington, D. C.
October 1, 1927.

CASH STATEMENT

October 1, 1926–September 30, 1927

Receipts

1926 Oct. 1	Balance from last report		$ 12,242.47
	Redemption of mortgage		20,000.00
	Addition to Prize fund		3,000.00
	Revertments (credited to reserve fund):		
	Moyer S. Fleisher grant	$ 200.00	
	W. F. G. Swann grant	196.00	
	Accumulated interest purchased	93.33	489.33
	16 life-membership fees		1,600.00
	Interest on Jane M. Smith fund	300.00	
	Interest on mortgage	1,020.00	
	Interest on other securities	4,983.42	
	Interest on bank balance	482.03	6,785.45
			$44,117.25

Disbursements

Grants for 1927, allotted by Committee on Grants:		
William H. Cole	$ 150.00	
Henry B. Collins, Jr.	350.00	
Bruce Fink	300.00	
Jacob Kunz	200.00	
Ann Morgan	150.00	
Knight H. Dunlap	300.00	
J. G. Frayne	150.00	
S. O. Mast	300.00	
J. G. Frayne	150.00	2,050.00
Allotments by council or executive committee:		
Naples Zoological Station	$ 500.00	
International Annual Tables	200.00	
Concilium Bibliographicum	200.00	
Committee of One Hundred	551.18	
Thomas Barbour (for Barro Colorado Laboratory)	300.00	1,751.18
Philadelphia Prize (George D. Birkhoff)		1,000.00
Three emeritus life memberships (Jane M. Smith fund)		300.00
415 Journal subscriptions for life members		1,245.00
Safe-deposit box for securities		20.00
		6,366.18
Cash in bank		37,751.07
		$44,117.25

BALANCE SHEET, SEPTEMBER 30, 1927

Assets

Investments:		
Endowment and reserve funds	$121,323.94	
Cash awaiting investment	25,516.80	$146,840.74
Current assets:		
Income account, cash available	7,234.27	
Prize fund	5,000.00	12,234.27
		$159,075.01

Liabilities

Endowment and reserve funds:		
General:		
W. Hudson Stephens	$ 4,381.21	
Richard T. Colburn	85,586.45	
Friends of Association	3,559.00	
Sustaining-membership fees	6,000.00	
Life-membership fees	37,950.00	
Jane M. Smith fund	5,000.00	
Reserve fund	4,364.08	146,840.74
Current Liabilities:		
Balance of $1,000 appropriated for Committee of One Hundred	448.82	
Prize fund	5,000.00	5,448.82
Accumulated income, unappropriated (cash in bank)		6,785.45
		$159,075.01

AUDITOR'S REPORT

I certify that I have audited the accounts of the treasurer of the American Association for the Advancement of Science for the period October 1, 1926, to September 30, 1927. The securities representing the investments of the association, as listed in the treasurer's report to the council, have been exhibited and verified with the exception of the Pittsburgh, Shawmut & Northern bonds, which were represented by a certificate of deposit, and $10,500 worth of U. S. Second Liberty Loan bonds, which had been deposited for redemption and were represented by a receipt. The income from all investments was duly accounted for. The financial statements accompanying the report of the treasurer were in accord with the books of the association and correctly summarized the accounts.

(*Signed*) Robert B. Sosman,
Auditor.

Washington, D. C.,
November 22, 1927.

NOTES ON THE TREASURER'S REPORT

The permanent secretary calls attention to the fact that, omitting the Jane M. Smith fund for emeritus life membership (which has a capital of $5,000 and draws interest at the rate of 6 per cent.), the average rate of interest received for the fiscal year 1926–27 is 4.77 per cent. The income for the year may be classified, according to the several funds in the treasury, as follows:

W. Hudson Stephens fund	$ 209.13
Richard T. Colburn fund	4,085.04
"Friends of Association" fund	169.79
Sustaining-membership fees (living members)	143.22
Sustaining-membership fees (deceased members)	143.22
Life-membership fees (living members)	1,317.38
Life-membership fees (deceased members)	417.67
Jane M. Smith fund	300.00
Total income available for use in 1927–28	$6,785.45

Of the last amount, $5,374.00 has now been appropriated (see "Proceedings at Nashville," above), leaving a balance available for further appropriations this year amounting to $1,411.45. The treasurer's reserve amounts to $4,364.08, available for emergencies.

FINANCIAL REPORT OF THE PERMANENT SECRETARY FOR THE FISCAL YEAR 1926–27

(October 1, 1926, to September 30, 1927)

Dr.

To balance from last account:		
*Publication fund	$ 1,000.00	
*Special fund for Committee on Place of Science in Education	848.93	
*Emergency fund	5,000.00	
*Available for general purposes	2,025.68	$ 8,874.61
To receipts from membership dues:		
Annual dues previous to 1926	$ 80.00	
Annual dues for 1926	715.00	
Annual dues for 1927	67,527.77	
Annual dues for 1928	720.50	
Entrance fees	655.00	
Life-membership fees	1,600.00	71,298.27
To other general receipts:		
Life-membership Journal subscriptions (from the treasurer)	$ 1,245.00	
Interest on bank accounts	649.03	
Contribution from member	25.00	
Sale of Proceedings volume	293.75	
Miscellaneous receipts	332.60	
Overpayments, etc.	255.72	2,801.10
To special journal subscriptions:		
SCIENCE and *Scientific Monthly*	$ 2,509.38	
Science News-Letter	8,022.00	10,531.38
To receipts from members for Agassiz Bust fund		1,310.00
To receipts from treasurer for Committee of One Hundred		551.18
To receipts for Joint Committee on Promotion of Research in Colleges:		
From A. A. A. S. Committee of One Hundred	$ 300.00	
From National Research Council, Division of Educational Relations	100.00	
From American Council on Education	100.00	500.00
Bank interest on special fund for Committee on Place of Science in Education		33.96
Philadelphia Meeting:		
Fund raised by local committee	$ 4,027.25	
Registration fees	1,303.00	
Sale of programs	10.50	
Sale of advertising space in program	425.00	
Exhibition:		
Receipts from exhibitors	3,591.50	
Donations	500.00	9,857.25
Nashville Exhibition:		
Receipts from exhibitors		868.97
		$106,626.72

Cr.

By subscriptions to official journal		$ 42,610.75
By Division, Local Branch, and Academy allowances:		
Pacific Division	$ 1,613.00	
Southwestern Division	264.00	
State College (Pa.) Local Branch	14.25	
Affiliated state academies	1,195.50	3,086.75
By expenses, General Secretary		4.75
By expenses, Washington Office:		
Salaries	$12,330.96	
Office and addressograph supplies	307.96	
Printing and stationery	1,528.32	
Telephone and telegraph	159.91	
Postage, correspondence and billing	1,805.98	
Exchange	26.09	
Express, freight and drayage	47.73	
Notary fees	1.00	
Furniture and equipment	525.54	
Miscellaneous expense	328.93	17,062.42
By Circularization		2,314.72
By miscellaneous expenses:		
Life-membership fees (to treasurer)	$ 1,600.00	
Refunds of overpayments, etc.	255.72	
Contribution of American Institute of Sacred Literature	55.00	
Travel expenses	1,377.00	
Section expenses	658.87	
Annual meeting (Philadelphia):		
Preliminary announcement $ 555.84		
Program (printing) 2,085.00		

Report	874.27		
Popular lectures	305.10		
Exhibition	3,841.50		
General expenses:			
At Washington	1,421.99		
At Philadelphia	2,987.15	12,070.85	
Annual meeting (Nashville):			
Exhibition	$ 890.93		
General expenses (Washington office)	95.54	986.47	17,003.91
By expenses, Committee of One Hundred			551.18
Agassiz Bust fund:			
Total fund collected, paid to Hall of Fame		$ 1,310.00	
Expenses, circularizing members for Agassiz Bust fund		362.33	1,672.33
By expenditures Joint Committee on Promotion of Research in Colleges			269.84
By special subscriptions:			
SCIENCE and *Scientific Monthly*		2,499.00	
Science News-Letter		8,022.00	10,521.00
Total expenditures			95,097.65
By new balance:			
Checking account (American Security & Trust Co.)		21.14	
*Publication fund		2,000.00	
*Special fund for Committee on Place of Science in Education		882.89	
*Special fund for Joint Committee for Promotion of Research in Colleges		230.16	
*Emergency fund		5,000.00	
*Available for general purposes		3,394.88	11,529.07
			$106,626.72

(*Signed*) BURTON E. LIVINGSTON,
Permanent Secretary.

AUDITOR'S REPORT

As auditor for the association for the year 1926–27, I have employed Mr. W. R. Gallaher, an accountant at the Interstate Commerce Commission, to go over the accounts of the permanent secretary for the year ending September 30, 1927. He makes the following report:

"This is to certify that I have examined the receipts and disbursements in currency, checks, etc., of the permanent secretary's office of the American Association for the Advancement of Science for the twelve months ending September 30, 1927, and have found the records correctly kept. Proper vouchers were shown for all disbursements.
(*Signed*) W. R. GALLAHER,
Accountant."

I have reason to believe that Mr. Gallaher is an experienced and reliable accountant and that the above statement is a dependable report on the state of the accounts that were audited.

Very truly yours,
(*Signed*) ROBERT B. SOSMAN,
Auditor.

Washington, D. C.,
November 21, 1927.

* Funds designated by an asterisk are all in the Savings Department of the Federal-American National Bank, of Washington.

NOTES ON THE PERMANENT SECRETARY'S FINANCIAL REPORT

The permanent secretary adds the following notes on his financial report for the fiscal year 1926–27, which may be of interest.

The publication fund is a reserve for the publication of the Proceedings volume, containing the Summarized Proceedings and the Directory of Members, which appears every four years. The most recent volume was published in December, 1925, and the next one is to appear in the fall of 1929. It will include the accounts of the fifth New York meeting and will carry the membership record forward to about June, 1929. From the general income is set aside each year the sum of $1,000 for the publication fund, which amounted to $2,000 on September 30, 1927. The emergency fund is simply a reserve for emergencies; it is available for general purposes and is maintained at $5,000 in the absence of emergencies.

Receipts from annual-membership dues and entrance fees paid by new members amounted to $69,698.27 for the year 1926–27. Life-membership fees are all turned over to the treasurer at the end of each year and the treasurer pays annually to the permanent secretary's office a sum amounting to three dollars for each living sustaining or life member, which covers the cost of the regular journal subscriptions for these members. The amount thus received from the treasurer in 1926–27 was $1,245.00. This amount may be added to the income from annual dues and entrance fees, giving $70,943.27 as the total receipts on account of all memberships throughout the year in question.

It is interesting to observe, from the notes on the treasurer's report, that the income from the invested fees of living sustaining and life members for 1926–27 is shown as $143.22 + $1,317.58, or $1,460.60, which exceeds by $215.60 the cost ($1,245.00) of the journal subscriptions for these members. At the present time the income from the fees of living sustaining and life members is therefore a little more than sufficient to care for their journal subscriptions. Indeed, these subscriptions were this year more than cared for by the income ($1,317.38) from the fees of living life members alone.

Payments for the special journal subscriptions for the *Scientific Monthly* and the *Science News-Letter* (at three dollars each) are all turned over to the respective publishers of the journals and the work of handling these is a definite contribution from the association toward the support of the journals and toward the popularization of science. About eight per cent. of the new members joining between October 1 and December 20, 1927, subscribed for one or the other of the extra journals and these are equally distributed between the two journals, four per cent. to each. For the same period 2,796 subscriptions were received from old members for one or the other of the extra journals, two thirds of these being for the *News-Letter* and one third for the *Monthly*.

The Agassiz Bust fund ($1,310) was raised by personal subscriptions from members of the biological and geological sections. The cost of circularization for this fund amounted to $362.33, which was not charged against the fund, consequently the association actually contributed this amount. The fund itself ($1,310) has been transmitted to the Hall of Fame, New York University, as a contribution from members of the American Association toward the cost of a bust of Louis Agassiz, which is to be unveiled in the Hall of Fame probably next May.

The accounts for the expenses of the Philadelphia meeting are not as complete as they should be, for no final report has been received from the local committee for that meeting, but they are presumably nearly correct as shown in the permanent secretary's report, where the total extra expense on account of that meeting appears as $8,229.35, omitting the cost of the exhibition. Aside from exhibition receipts, the income from the meeting was $1,303.00 from registration fees and $435.50 from advertising and sale of the program, or $1,738.50 in all, leaving a deficit for that meeting amounting to $8,229.35—$1,738.50, or $6,490.85. Of this deficit $4,027.25 is shown to have been covered by locally raised funds, and consequently the real deficit for the Philadelphia meeting was $2,463.60, paid from the current funds of the permanent secretary's office.

The annual exhibition at Philadelphia is shown by the report to have cost $3,841.50 and the gross income therefrom is shown to have been $4,091.50, with a net income of $250.00. An advance fund of $500 had been appropriated for initial expenses of the exhibition, of which only $250 had been expended, and this expenditure was offset by the net gain. Therefore the exhibition was really a source of neither gain nor loss.

For the year considered the association paid $42,610.75 for membership journal subscriptions and $17,062.42 for the regular expenses of the Washington office and it contributed $3,086.75 toward the expenses of its divisions and local branch and of the affiliated academies of science. It is interesting to note that the amount contributed to divisions, branch and academies is a little larger than the appropriation ($3,000) for individual grants for research, derived from the treasurer's funds.

At the beginning of the year 1926–27 there was available for general purposes $2,025.68 in the permanent secretary's hands. At the end of the year this balance is shown as $3,416.02 ($21.14 in the checking account and $3,394.88 in the savings account), the gain being $1,390.34, or about 2 per cent. of the total income on account of all memberships for the year.

REPORT OF THE COMMITTEE ON THE PLACE OF SCIENCE IN EDUCATION

Following is the summary report of the Committee on the Place of Science in Education (Dr. Otis W. Caldwell, *chairman*), which was accepted by the council at its session on December 29. In connection with this summary report, the reader is referred to paragraphs 24 and 25 of the section on "Legislative and Executive Proceedings," in this issue of SCIENCE.

REPORT

The Committee on the Place of Science in Education has prepared a report for the council which it now submits. This report summarizes the work of the committee up to the present time. The committee has considered the whole subject of the relations and uses of science, of which science teaching in schools and colleges is but a part. Outlines and suggestions have been published as the work progressed, these resulting in much correspondence and in local conferences, and the conclusions are included in the report.

The committee also reports that a more complete statement of its work is nearly ready for publication, and requests authorization to proceed with publication when that statement is completed. The manuscript will consist of about fifty typed pages. It should be published in such a way as to secure wide circulation. It is expected that special funds will be secured by the committee to cover the cost of publication.

Three further needs have become recognized by the committee, through its conferences. To meet these needs the council is requested to approve the following recommendations:

(a) That some organization of national scope, such as the United States Bureau of Education, or the Research Division of the National Education Association, be asked by this committee to undertake a comprehensive and intensive study of the situations, tendencies and needs of science instruction in educational systems.

(b) That the services of a field secretary be secured, to work with existing agencies, to distribute information on research in science education, to stimulate further research, to operate as a sort of clearing-house agent and to continue the organizing of new groups of science teachers, writers for popularization of science, etc. This field secretary should work under the guidance of the Committee on the Place of Science in Education, or under the guidance of a national council of science teachers as soon as such a council is formed.

(c) That a national council of science teachers be organized to advance science teaching, to increase public appreciation of science and to secure for science teachers increased facilities and a wider usefulness. The services of a field secretary would be very useful in the organization of such a council.

(*Signed*) OTIS W. CALDWELL,
Chairman.

GRANTS FOR RESEARCH, FOR 1928

An appropriation of $3,000 was made by the council at Nashville for individual grants in aid of scientific research, to be allotted to applicants by the Committee on Grants for Research. Fifty-six applications were received and considered in the regular way by the committee. The sums requested amounted, on the whole, to $18,500. Since only $3,000 was available for this allotment, it follows that a very large number of applicants must be disappointed. This fact should not be allowed to discourage applications for future years, however, for the committee feels that better selections are possible when the number and amounts of the applications greatly exceed the possibilities for actual grants. Members who have research projects suitable for grants from the association should not hesitate to make application.

Applications are made on special blanks, obtainable from the Washington office of the association, and they may be sent in at any time. Allotments are made only at the time of the annual meeting. In recent years the amount of a single grant has not exceeded $500 and most of the grants are for smaller sums. This year the largest grant is for $350.

The chairman of the Committee on Grants for Research has reported the following allotments of funds for 1928, all of the council's appropriation for this purpose being thus used up. The list is arranged according to the several fields of science represented.

Physics

James W. Broxon, University of Colorado, Boulder, Colo. For studying pressure variation of the natural ionization in gases at high pressures $350

A. L. Hughes, Washington University, St. Louis, Mo. For studying ionization and photoelectric effects with polarized light 150

Astronomy

Heber D. Curtis, Allegheny Observatory, Pittsburgh, Pa. For completion of large special comparator for parallax and proper motion investigations on the extensive stock of plates which have been taken with the Thaw Photographic Refractor at Allegheny Observatory 300

Geology and Paleontology

Seismological Society of America (S. D. Townley, Treasurer, Stanford University, Calif.). For investigation of earthquakes occurring on the Pacific Coast of the United States 200

Ferdinand Canu, 18 Rue de Peintre Lebrun, Versailles, France. For studying the Bryozoan fauna of the Galapagos Islands 150

Zoology

Phineas W. Whiting, Bussey Institution, Boston, Mass. For genetic work with the parasitic wasp, Habrobracon, especially in relation to sex-determination and parthenogenesis 150

Winterton C. Curtis, University of Missouri, Columbia, Mo. For studying effects of irradiation upon regeneration 300

Henry H. Collins, 916 Adelaide St., Pittsburgh, Pa. For investigation of the effects of inter-specific gonad transplantation upon the development of specific characters in ontogeny and in regeneration, in certain urodele amphibia, together with incidental studies of life histories and geographic variations 200

Botany

William R. Maxon, U. S. National Museum, Washington, D. C. For preparation of manuscript for a volume describing the pteridophyta of Jamaica, to be published as one of the series now issuing from the British Museum (Natural History), "Flora of Jamaica," by Fawcett and Rendle 300

Joyce Hedrick, 106 E. Spring St., Oxford, Ohio. For continuing research of Dr. Bruce Fink on "The Lichen Flora of the United States" 200

Anthropology

Henry B. Collins, Jr., U. S. National Museum, Washington, D. C. For archeological research at ancient village sites in northern Alaska, particularly on St. Lawrence Island, for the purpose of tracing ancient migrations in the vicinity of Bering Strait 300

Physiology and Medicine

Elery R. Becker, Iowa State College, Ames, Iowa. For investigation of the physiological rôle in their host of the protozoa which inhabit the rumen and reticulum of normal, healthy ruminants 300

Roy L. Moodie, 1021 11th St., Santa Monica, Calif. For the study of surgery in pre-Columbian Peru 100

GENERAL OFFICERS OF THE ASSOCIATION FOR 1928

The president and the vice-presidents for any year automatically become the retiring president and the retiring vice-presidents for the following year. Consequently this list shows the names of the president and vice-presidents for 1927 as well as for 1928. Dr. L. H. Bailey, of Ithaca, N. Y., was retiring president for 1927. The section secretaries are elected for a four-year term, expiring at the end of 1928, but the secretaries of Sections A, H, L and N found it necessary to resign at the Nashville meeting. For Sections A, H and N their successors were elected for a term of one year.

President

Henry Fairfield Osborn, American Museum of Natural History, New York, N. Y.

Retiring President

Arthur A. Noyes, California Institute of Technology, Pasadena, Calif.

Vice-Presidents, Retiring Vice-Presidents and Secretaries of the Sections

Section A (Mathematics):

Vice-president, Raymond C. Archibald, Brown University, Providence, R. I.

Retiring Vice-president, Dunham Jackson, University of Minnesota, Minneapolis, Minn.

Secretary, Charles N. Moore, University of Cincinnati, Cincinnati, Ohio. (To succeed Raymond C. Archibald, resigned.)

Section B (Physics):

Vice-president, P. W. Bridgman, Harvard University, Cambridge, Mass.

Retiring Vice-president, Arthur H. Compton, University of Chicago, Chicago, Ill.

Secretary, A. L. Hughes, Washington University, St. Louis, Mo.

Section C (Chemistry):

Vice-president, C. E. K. Mees, Eastman Kodak Co., Rochester, N. Y.

Retiring Vice-president, Roger Adams, University of Illinois, Urbana, Ill.

Secretary, Gerhard Dietrichson, Massachusetts Institute of Technology, Cambridge, Mass.

Section D (Astronomy):

Vice-president, J. S. Plaskett, Dominion Astrophysical Observatory, Victoria, B. C., Canada.

Retiring Vice-president, Walter S. Adams, Mt. Wilson Observatory, Pasadena, Calif.

Secretary, Philip Fox, Dearborn Observatory, Northwestern University, Evanston, Ill.

Section E (Geology and Geography):

Vice-president, Frank Leverett, University of Michigan, Ann Arbor, Mich.

Retiring Vice-president, Charles Schuchert, Yale University, New Haven, Conn.

Secretary, G. R. Mansfield, U. S. Geological Survey, Washington, D. C.

Section F (Zoological Science):

Vice-president, M. F. Guyer, University of Wisconsin, Madison, Wis.

Retiring Vice-president, C. E. McClung, University of Pennsylvania, Philadelphia, Pa.

Secretary, Geo. T. Hargitt, Syracuse University, Syracuse, N. Y.

Section G (Botanical Sciences):

Vice-president, C. E. Allen, University of Wisconsin, Madison, Wis.

Retiring Vice-president, William Crocker, Boyce Thompson Institute for Plant Research, Yonkers, N. Y.

Secretary, Sam F. Trelease, Columbia University, New York, N. Y.

Section H (Anthropology):

Vice-president, Fay-Cooper Cole, University of Chicago, Chicago, Ill.

Retiring Vice-president, R. J. Terry, Washington University, St. Louis, Mo.

Secretary, Charles H. Danforth, Stanford University, Calif. (To succeed Fay-Cooper Cole, resigned.)

Section I (Psychology):

Vice-president, Howard C. Warren, Princeton University, Princeton, N. J.

Retiring Vice-president, Knight Dunlap, Johns Hopkins University, Baltimore, Md.

Secretary, Frank N. Freeman, University of Chicago, Chicago, Ill.

Section K (Social and Economic Sciences):

This section is not organized at present.

Section L (Historical and Philological Sciences):

This section is not organized at present.

Section M (Engineering):

Vice-president, Robert Lemuel Sackett, Pennsylvania State College, State College, Pa.

Retiring Vice-president, A. N. Talbot, University of Illinois, Urbana, Ill.

Secretary, N. H. Heck, U. S. Coast and Geodetic Survey, Washington, D. C.

Section N (Medical Sciences):

Vice-president, A. J. Goldforb, College of the City of New York, New York, N. Y.

Retiring Vice-president, G. Canby Robinson, Vanderbilt University, Nashville, Tenn.

Secretary, James Harold Austin, University of Pennsylvania, Philadelphia, Pa. (To succeed A. J. Goldforb, resigned.)

Section O (Agriculture):

Vice-president, C. A. Mooers, University of Tennessee, Knoxville, Tenn.

Retiring Vice-president, L. E. Call, Kansas State Agricultural College, Manhattan, Kans.

Secretary, P. E. Brown, Iowa State College, Ames, Iowa.

Section Q (Education):

Vice-president, Truman L. Kelley, Stanford University, Calif.

Retiring Vice-president, Arthur I. Gates, Teachers College, Columbia University, New York, N. Y.

Secretary, A. S. Barr, University of Wisconsin, Madison, Wis.

Permanent Secretary

Burton E. Livingston, Johns Hopkins University, Baltimore, Md. (Association mail address: Smithsonian Institution Building, Washington, D. C.)

General Secretary

W. J. Humphreys, U. S. Weather Bureau, Washington, D. C.

Treasurer

John L. Wirt, Carnegie Institution of Washington, Washington, D. C.

Secretary of the Council and Program Editor

Sam L. Trelease, Columbia University, New York, N. Y.

Executive Assistant

Sam Woodley, Smithsonian Institution Building, Washington, D. C.

Auditor

R. B. Sosman, Geophysical Laboratory, Carnegie Institution of Washington, Washington, D. C.

News Manager

Austin H. Clark, U. S. National Museum, Washington, D. C.

Manager of Exhibition

H. S. Kimberly, Smithsonian Institution Building, Washington, D. C.

The Council

The council for 1928 consists of the newly-elected president, the general secretary, the permanent secretary, the treasurer, the vice-presidents, the section secretaries, all members of the executive committee not otherwise members of the council, the representatives of the affiliated organizations, and the eight elected council members named below.[1]

Austin H. Clark (1931), U. S. National Museum, Washington, D. C.

Arthur H. Compton (1931), University of Chicago, Chicago, Ill.

L. E. Dickson (1930), University of Chicago, Chicago, Ill.

David White (1930), U. S. Geological Survey, Washington, D. C.

John C. Merriam (1929), Carnegie Institution of Washington, Washington, D. C.

Rodney H. True (1929), University of Pennsylvania, Philadelphia, Pa.

L. O. Howard (1928), U. S. Department of Agriculture, Washington, D. C.

D. T. MacDougal (1928), Desert Laboratory, Tucson, Ariz.

(The first two names replace those of W. A. Oldfather and G. W. Stewart, whose terms expired at the end of 1927.)

The Executive Committee

The executive committee consists of the newly-elected president, the general secretary, the permanent secretary, and the eight elected members named below.[2]

David R. Curtiss (1931), Northwestern University, Evanston, Ill.

John Johnston (1931), U. S. Steel Corporation, New York, N. Y.

J. McKeen Cattell (1930) (*chairman*), Garrison-on-Hudson, N. Y.

Henry B. Ward (1930), University of Illinois, Urbana, Ill.

F. R. Moulton (1929), 327 S. La Salle St., Chicago, Ill.

M. I. Pupin (1929), Columbia University, New York, N. Y.

Vernon Kellogg (1928), National Research Council, Washington, D. C.

Edwin B. Wilson (1928), Harvard School of Public Health, Boston, Mass.

(The first two names replace those of H. L. Fairchild and W. A. Noyes, whose terms expired at the end of 1927.)

The Committee on Grants for Research[2]

Walter S. Adams (1931) (for Astronomy), Mt. Wilson Observatory, Pasadena, Calif.

Karl F. Kellerman (1931) (for Botany), Bureau of Plant Industry, Washington, D. C.

W. Lash Miller (1930) (for Chemistry), 8 Hawthorne Ave., Toronto, Ont., Canada.

Oswald Veblen (1930) (for Mathematics), Princeton University, Princeton, N. J.

L. G. Hoxton (1929) (for Physics), University of Virginia, University, Va.

Vernon Kellogg (1929) (for Zoology), National Research Council, Washington, D. C.

Joseph Erlanger (1928) (for Physiology), Washington University School of Medicine, St. Louis, Mo.

Nevin M. Fenneman (1928) (for Geology), University of Cincinnati, Cincinnati, Ohio.

(The first two names replace those of B. M. Davis and A. Hrdlička, whose terms expired at the end of 1927.)

FUTURE ANNUAL MEETINGS

The American Association meets annually in convocation week, the dates for the meetings being determined by a rule adopted by the council. When New Year's day falls on Thursday, Friday or Saturday the meeting period is the week (Monday to Saturday, inclusive) in which New Year's day occurs. When New Year's day falls on Sundays the meeting period is

[1] The number in parentheses denotes the year at the end of which the member's term of office is to expire.

[2] The number in parentheses denotes the year at the end of which the member's term of office is to expire.

the preceding week. And when New Year's day falls on Monday, Tuesday or Wednesday the meeting opens on December 27 and continues through January 2. Plans of individuals and societies may thus be made years in advance. It requires just twenty-eight years to complete the cycle of dates and days. Dates and meeting places for the next five annual meetings are shown below.

1928–29 (New York): Thursday, December 27, 1928, to Wednesday, January 2, 1929.

1929–30 (Des Moines): Friday, December 27, 1929, to Thursday, January 2, 1930.

1930–31 (probably Cleveland or Montreal): Monday, December 29, 1930, to Saturday, January 3, 1931.

1931–32 (probably New Orleans): Monday, December 28, 1931, to Saturday, January 2, 1932.

1932–33 (Chicago): Monday, December 26, to Saturday, December 31, 1932.

SPECIAL NOTES

(1) This issue of SCIENCE contains only the general reports on the second Nashville meeting. Reports of the sessions of sections and societies are to appear in the next following issue, for February 3.

(2) The journal subscriptions of members for 1927 who have not yet enrolled for 1928 are to be continued to include the issue of SCIENCE for February 3. Dues for 1928 that have not been paid earlier should be paid now; otherwise the journal subscriptions can not be continued longer.

(3) All who are interested in the advancement of science and education should belong to the American Association. New members are received at any time. Information about the organization and work of the association and about the responsibilities and privileges of membership therein may be secured at any time from the permanent secretary who is to be addressed at the Washington office of the American Association for the Advancement of Science, Smithsonian Institution Building, Washington, D. C.

SCIENTIFIC EVENTS

NEW BUILDING FOR THE PHYSICAL SCIENCES AT THE UNIVERSITY OF CHICAGO

ANNOUNCEMENT of a new building for physics, mathematics and astronomy was made on January 12 by President Max Mason, of the University of Chicago, at the annual dinner of the trustees to the faculty.

A gift from Mr. Bernard A. Eckhart, president of the B. A. Eckhart Milling Co., has been added to a fund already available and has made it possible for the university to proceed with a building on a scale adequate to the needs of these three important departments rather than a building of limited possibilities. "In recognition of Mr. Eckhart's benefaction, the building will be known as the 'Bernard A. Eckhart laboratory.'"

The laboratory will be erected to the east of Ryerson physical laboratory. Charles Z. Klander, well-known Philadelphia architect, is now engaged in drafting plans for the laboratory, and has already submitted sketches for a structure of Gothic design in harmony with the university's style of architecture.

Ryerson physical laboratory, given the University of Chicago thirty-four years ago by Martin A. Ryerson in honor of his father, is now inadequate to the needs of the three departments, which have been among the most productive in the university. Most of the activities of the astronomy department, however, are centered in the university's Yerkes Observatory at Williams Bay, Wis.

A correspondent writes: "The physics department at Chicago is distinguished, the only three awards of the Nobel prize in physics to America having been made to University of Chicago men, Albert A. Michelson, Arthur H. Compton and Robert Millikan, now head of the Norman Bridge Laboratory of Pasadena, California. In the mathematics department, Professors E. H. Moore, Gilbert A. Bliss, Herbert E. Slaught and Leonard E. Dickson are among the leading mathematicians of the country."

THE PURE SCIENCE RESEARCH FUND AT PRINCETON UNIVERSITY

PRESIDENT JOHN GRIER HIBBEN has announced that, in consideration of the fact that Princeton University has already received in cash more than a million dollars toward its three-million dollar pure-science research fund, the General Education Board has granted the university for the coming year the interest on half its conditional gift of one million dollars.

The gift of the General Education Board of one million dollars was contingent on the university raising the other two million dollars from other sources. The grant for the coming year amounts to $25,000, representing five per cent. interest on half of the conditional gift. $1,461,000 has already been pledged toward the $2,000,000 which Princeton University must raise, of which $1,133,945 has been paid.

President Hibben has made the following statement regarding the fund:

The funds already received for pure science research have enabled the trustees to appoint five research professors who, with the cooperation of other professors in their departments, graduate students and National Research Fellows and International Research Fellows, are carrying on research in science to a degree unprecedented in Princeton.

In the mathematics department a group of research students comprising six National Research Fellows and two International Research Fellows—one a privat-docent at Berlin and the other a professor from Russia—are engaged in research in analysis situs and differential geometry, the chief fields of research of our mathematicians.

In the chemistry department the number of men engaged in research is 30 per cent. greater than last year. A considerable number of the investigators in chemistry are engaged in catalytic studies. They include a research associate from Sweden, an International Research Fellow from Berlin, one National Research Fellow, a visiting professor on leave from India, a visiting fellow from Oxford and several graduate students.

Investigators in the department of physics are cooperating with those in the department of chemistry in a combined attack on problems of excited atoms, dielectrics and the electrical properties of molecules. Important spectroscopic work is also being done in collaboration with the department of astronomy. Twenty-four men are conducting experiments in physics, including nine members of the regular staff, nine graduate students, three National Research Fellows, one International Research Fellow from Göttingen, one Procter Fellow from Cambridge University, England, and one fellow each from the research laboratories of the General Electric Company and the Westinghouse Company.

In the department of biology, researches on heredity and mutation in plants, on the localization of developmental materials and processes in animal eggs, on the origin of the vascular system in vertebrates, on the morphology and physiology of bioluminescence and the biochemistry of photosynthesis are being conducted by twelve members of the staff and graduate students.

RESOLUTION REGARDING THE U. S. COAST AND GEODETIC SURVEY

THE following resolution, prepared with the authority of the council of the Geological Society of America, was adopted by the society assembled in annual meeting at Cleveland, on December 30, 1927.

WHEREAS, Housebill No. 7480 to transfer the geodetic, seismologic and related services of the U. S. Coast and Geodetic Survey to the U. S. Geological Survey is before the committee on interstate and foreign commerce of the house and has been presented in the senate, and

WHEREAS, The proposed transfer, if effected, would materially change the status of the specified scientific research which is of great importance to science and to the people of the United States, and

WHEREAS, The proposed administrative change would disrupt the Coast and Geodetic Survey and would terminate the activity of that organization in lines of research in which it has long been engaged and in which it has won the respect and confidence of the scientific world among all nations;

Therefore, be it resolved, That it is the sense of this society that the proposed transfer should be made only after thorough consideration by competent scientific authority and in accordance with the recommendations which that authority may make; and

That to this end we recommend that the proposed legislation be referred to the National Academy of Sciences for appropriate action, and further that copies of this resolution shall be forwarded to the committees of the House and Senate having charge of the respective bills.

BAILEY WILLIS,
EDWARD B. MATHEWS,
Committee

THE SECOND SESSION OF THE INSTITUTE OF CHEMISTRY

THE second session of the Institute of Chemistry of the American Chemical Society will be held in Evanston, Illinois, from July 23 to August 18. Every effort is being made to arrange the lectures and conferences of the institute in such a way as to offer a unique service to chemists both industrial and academic. The committee in charge of the institute consists of N. E. Gordon, chairman of the A. C. S. committee on chemical education, University of Maryland; B. S. Hopkins, chairman of the division of chemical education, A. C. S., University of Illinois; H. E. Howe, editor, *Industrial and Engineering Chemistry* and head of the A. C. S. news service, Washington, D. C.; C. E. K. Mees, Eastman Kodak Company; S. W. Parr, president of the American Chemical Society, University of Illinois; C. L. Parsons, secretary of the American Chemical Society, Washington, D. C.; C. M. A. Stine, E. I. du Pont de Nemours and Company; G. L. Wendt, Pennsylvania State College; F. C. Whitmore, National Research Council; W. R. Whitney, General Electric Company, and F. W. Willard, Western Electric Company. The executive secretary will be C. D. Hurd, Northwestern University, Evanston, Illinois.

Following is a tentative list of subjects for conferences for the Institute of Chemistry. Suggestions and criticisms should be sent to F. C. Whitmore, National Research Council, Washington, D. C. There will be 28 conferences, arranged at times when two and a half hours will be available for each. Thus, several conferences will be devoted to the same subject if it seems important enough to warrant this.

One group of subjects will deal with the help which chemistry can give for the better utilization of raw materials:

Agricultural products
Coal

Petroleum
Metals
Animal products

Only certain aspects of these subjects can be covered. In addition, certain miscellaneous subjects have been suggested for conferences:

Chemotherapy
Disposal of municipal wastes
Rubber
Science and national defense
Chemistry life processes
Synthetic "raw" materials
Antioxidants
Cellulose

Suggestions are needed regarding the special phases of these topics which can best be treated and regarding the best men to lead the discussions. Conferences will not be limited to the subjects listed above.

SCIENTIFIC NOTES AND NEWS

DR. HUGH S. TAYLOR, David D. Jones professor of research chemistry at Princeton University, has been awarded the Nichols medal by the New York section of the American Chemical Society. Presentation of the medal will be made at a meeting of the section on March 9, when Dr. Taylor will speak on "Catalysis as an Inspiration of Fundamental Research."

DR. LOUIS B. WILSON, director of the Mayo Foundation, has been elected an honorary member of the Royal Society of Medicine at Rome.

DR. JOSEPH EASTMAN SHEEHAN, of New York, was decorated with the Order of Alphonso XII by the personal physician of the king of Spain, January 3, in recognition of his work in plastic surgery.

AT the Christmas meeting of the American Psychological Association in Columbus, Ohio, a dinner was given by twenty-five psychologists for Professor Margaret F. Washburn, of Vassar College. Professors Bentley, of Illinois; Langfeld, of Princeton; Yerkes, of Yale; Pillsbury, of Michigan, and Mull, of Sweetbriar, spoke and Professor Warren, of Princeton, presented to Miss Washburn a volume of studies in her honor. The dedication of the volume reads as follows: "To Margaret Floy Washburn, teacher, editor, author, scientist, twenty-five years professor of psychology at Vassar College, the editor of *The American Journal of Psychology,* on completing thirty-three years of distinguished service to psychology, this volume is dedicated by her colleagues."

THE following officers for 1928 have been elected by the Washington Academy of Sciences: *President,* Robert B. Sosman, Geophysical Laboratory; *Non-Resident Vice-presidents,* B. W. Evermann, Museum of the Academy of Sciences, San Francisco, Calif., J. G. Lipman, Agricultural Experiment Station, New Brunswick, N. J.; *Corresponding Secretary,* L. B. Tuckerman, Bureau of Standards; *Recording Secretary,* W. D. Lambert, Coast and Geodetic Survey; *Treasurer,* R. L. Faris, Coast and Geodetic Survey.

AT the annual meeting of the Mineralogical Society of America held at the Case School of Applied Science from December 29 to 31, the following officers were elected: *President,* Esper S. Larsen, Harvard University; *Vice-president,* Lazard Cahn, Colorado Springs, Colorado; *Secretary,* Frank R. Van Horn, Case School of Applied Science; *Treasurer,* Alexander H. Phillips, Princeton University; *Editor,* Walter F. Hunt, University of Michigan; *Councillor 1928–1931,* Ellis Thomson, University of Toronto.

DR. DOUGLAS W. JOHNSON, professor of physiography at Columbia University, has been elected president of the Association of American Geographers.

DR. CARL L. MCDONALD has been elected president of the Academy of Medicine of Cleveland for the ensuing year.

DR. EMERY R. HAYHURST, professor of hygiene in the Ohio State University College of Medicine, Columbus, has been made chairman of the national committee of the United States for the Fifth International Medical Congress for Industrial Accidents and Occupational Diseases to be held in Budapest in September, 1928.

ON December 31, when the resignation of Dr. C. W. Larson as chief of the Bureau of Dairy Industry became effective, Secretary Jardine designated Dr. L. A. Rogers, senior bacteriologist of the bureau, as acting chief of the bureau, effective January 1, to serve until further notice. Dr. Rogers is in charge of the dairy research laboratories of the bureau.

S. B. HASKELL, director of the Massachusetts Experiment Station, resigned on December 15 to take a position with the agricultural department of a synthetic nitrogen products corporation.

CHARLES MERVYN SLAGG, chief of the tobacco division for the Department of Agriculture, Dominion of Canada, with headquarters at Ottawa, has resigned his commission to become director of tobacco investigations for the commonwealth of Australia. After visiting tobacco investigation stations in Massachusetts, Connecticut, Virginia and Wisconsin, he will sail from the Pacific coast to Melbourne, where his headquarters will be stationed.

DR. WILLIAM CROCKER, director of the Boyce

Thompson Institute for Plant Research at Yonkers, New York, will take up his four months' residence in Washington, D. C., beginning February 1, to complete his service as chairman of the division of agriculture and biology of the National Research Council. Dr. Crocker will be available for consultation at the institute on the 1st and 15th of each month during this absence.

Dr. John K. Small, head curator of the museums and herbarium of the New York Botanical Garden, has been granted leave of absence for a period of several weeks so that he may cooperate with Thomas A. Edison in his rubber investigations. Dr. Small left for southern Florida on January 17.

Dr. Howard A. Kelly, professor emeritus at the Johns Hopkins University, Baltimore, delivered the Hunterian oration before the Hunterian Society in London on January 16. This is the second successive time the honor has fallen to an American physician, the last Hunterian address having been delivered by Dr. John M. T. Finney, of Baltimore.

Dr. C. W. Kanolt, research physicist of the U. S. Bureau of Mines, gave an address on January 17 before the University of Pittsburgh chapter of the Sigma Xi on "The Production of Extremely Low Temperatures."

On January 7, Dr. H. F. Moore, research professor of engineering materials, University of Illinois, delivered an address to the Royal Canadian Institute, on the subject "Fatigue of Metals."

John B. Taylor, consulting engineer of the General Electric Co., will address the Franklin Institute on February 2, on "Making Sound Visible and Light Audible."

The seventh series of Beaumont lectures which are under the auspices of the Wayne County Medical Society, Detroit, was given by Dr. George Draper, assistant professor of clinical medicine, Columbia University College of Physicians and Surgeons, on January 23 and 24, on (1) "Human Constitution; What It means and How to study It"; (2) "The Patient and His Physician," and (3) "The Sex Factor in Total Personality."

E. C. Andrews, state geologist of New South Wales, gave a public lecture on January 6 at the University of Cincinnati on "Broken Hill, a Romance of Australian Mining." The lecture was under the auspices of the Bag and Hammer Student Geological Society. Dr. Andrews also addressed the faculty and students of the department of geology on "Problems of Australian Geology."

Dr. Corneille Heymans, professor of pharmacology of the faculty of medicine of the University of Ghent, spoke on "Contributions to the Physiology and Pharmacology of the Cardio-Inhibitory and Respiratory Centers," at Stanford University on December 7.

Major-General George Washington Goethals, the distinguished engineer, died on January 21, aged seventy years.

Dr. James Campbell Todd, professor of pathology at the University of Colorado school of medicine since 1911, died on January 6, aged fifty-four years.

Dr. Julius Grinker, professor of nervous and mental diseases at the medical school of Northwestern University, died on January 11, aged sixty years.

Joseph Francis O'Byrne, professor of descriptive geometry at the Colorado School of Mines, died on December 22.

Dr. Willard Parker Ward, of Savannah, Georgia, known for his work on the metallurgy of manganese, died on January 17, aged eighty-two years.

The British Medical Journal states that the late Mr. W. Thelwall Thomas, of Liverpool, who died last September, has bequeathed £5,000 each to the University of Liverpool, to endow a fellowship in surgical pathology; the Royal College of Surgeons of England, and the Royal Medical Benevolent Fund for pensions for medical men and their widows. He has also given £1,000 to the Liverpool Medical Institution for the annual purchase of books of reference or journals. He directed that his house in Rodney Street should be used as chambers for medical men so long as the executors shall think fit; the portrait in oils of himself he bequeathed to the University of Liverpool.

President W. W. Campbell, of the University of California, announced on December 12 that among other scholarships available, a Sheffield Sanborn scholarship of $325 for a student in the school of medicine; also gifts of $450 for a study of the relation of the intestinal flora to disease; of $100 by Dr. Curle Latimer Callander in support of the Callander surgical and topographic anatomy fund; of $200 for the use of the Hooper Foundation, and of $100 by Dr. Theodore C. Lawson, Oakland, as partial repayment of a scholarship awarded him in 1919.

The French correspondent of the *Journal* of the American Medical Association writes that the mayor of Lyons has been informed that the Rockefeller Foundation will guarantee to the University of Lyons, for the purchase of sites and for the construction of buildings to be used by the faculté de médecine et de pharmacie, the sum of 41,206,000 francs ($1,648,240), on condition that the sum of 15,000,000 francs is supplied from other sources or furnished by the government of France. Accordingly, the president of the cabinet, in agreement with the minister of public instruction, has allotted 12,000,000 francs, payable in three annual sums. There remains only 3,000,000 francs to be guaranteed. Furthermore, 100,000,000 francs is required to complete the Grange-Blanche Hospital. That is the part that is to be undertaken by the city of Lyons. The new buildings of the faculté de médecine are to be erected in the vicinity of the Grange-Blanche Hospital, so that there may be an intimate association with the hospital clinics.

THE first allotment under the Rollin D. Salisbury memorial research fund of the University of Chicago has been made to Professor J Harlen Bretz, of the department of geology, for the continuance of his studies of the "scablands" of Washington formed by the scouring action of floods flowing from the glaciers at the close of the last glacial period.

ACCORDING to the *Journal* of the American Medical Association a conference on pellagra called by the governor of Arkansas on December 6 was attended by about 400 persons; in opening the meeting, the governor reviewed the work that had been done since the Mississippi flood last spring by Arkansas physicians and those from other states who came to help, and urged full cooperation between all forces of the state for the control and prevention of pellagra. Dr. Joseph Goldberger, U. S. Public Health Service, Washington, D. C., who addressed the conference, stated that the records for 1927 indicate a considerable increase in the deaths of persons from pellagra in Arkansas. The number for the last year, it is said, will total between 600 and 700.

THE Federal Radio Commission has authorized the General Electric Company, Schenectady, N. Y., to erect an experimental station in Oakland, Calif., with 10,000 watts power and wave-length of 10 to 40 meters, for "the development of improved methods of facsimile transmission and television." Construction will start immediately. It is expected the station will be completed by March 1. The visual images will be transmitted by wireless, using at first both continuous and interrupted waves.

THE Geological Survey of Denmark will celebrate its fortieth anniversary in June next year by a series of excursions and meetings to which foreign geologists are to be invited. Before the meeting to be held in Copenhagen, two simultaneous four-day excursions will be arranged (June 21–24): to Bornholm, which forms part of the Baltic Shield and is of great petrological, stratigraphical and tectonic interest; or, alternatively, to Moën and South Sjælland, where remarkable dislocations in the Senonian white chalk can be compared with the undisturbed formations. The meeting itself (June 25–28) will be devoted to lectures and discussions on the general geology of Denmark and to visits to the celebrated museums of Copenhagen. After the meeting an eleven-day excursion (June 29–July 9) will enable visiting geologists to study a wide range of glacial phenomena in north-west Sjælland, Fyn, Langeland and Jylland. Further particulars relating to the detailed program, accommodations and charges will be provided in a later circular.

THE Paris correspondent of the London *Times* writes that the French government has decided to undertake an official investigation of the agriculture of the country. During the latter half of the last century reports were compiled by the Ministry of Agriculture every ten years, in which information in regard to the nature and size of agricultural properties, the distribution of crops in different parts of France, the methods of cultivation, the use of fertilizers, etc., were set out in statistical form. The last of these reports was issued in 1892. Since then no detailed and comprehensive survey of French agriculture has been taken. The only official statistics issued relate to the yield of crops and numbers of sheep, cattle and horses and these are admittedly based on insufficient data. A minor consideration in deciding the government to make the survey without delay is that the International Agricultural Institute, which has its seat in Rome, and of which France is a member, has asked for information with a view to compiling a report on agriculture throughout the whole world. This information the French government would be unable to supply unless the survey were made.

UNIVERSITY AND EDUCATIONAL NOTES

BY the will of the late Dr. Morris Herzstein, one of the prominent physicians of San Francisco, Stanford University is to receive $100,000 for a chair of biology.

ON February 23 the new building of the Philadelphia College of Pharmacy and Science will be dedicated. The formal dedicatory exercises will be presided over by Dr. Wilmer Krusen, who was recently installed as president of the college.

IT is reported that Dr. Gregorio Amo, of California, will give shares of his oil holding to the amount of about $1,700,000 for the establishment of a fund to permit foreign students to study at the Central University of Spain. Dr. Amo also presented King Alfonso with $400,000 to be used in the creation of a university city.

TRUSTEES of Western Reserve University have voted

to offer the chair of medicine, left vacant by the death of Dr. Charles F. Hoover, to Dr. Cyrus Cressy Sturgis, now professor of medicine in the University of Michigan and director of its research hospital.

JOHN WILSON, assistant chief geologist for the Pan-American Oil Company, has been appointed assistant professor of geophysics at the Colorado School of Mines.

AT the Harvard Medical School, Dr. William E. Ladd has been appointed assistant professor of surgery, Dr. Robert M. Green, assistant professor of applied anatomy, and Dr. Edward P. Richardson, John Homans professor of surgery.

DR. MILO HELLMAN, research associate in physical anthropology at the American Museum of Natural History, has been appointed professor of comparative dental morphology at the New York University College of Dentistry.

DISCUSSION AND CORRESPONDENCE

OVARIAN SECRETION AND TUMOR INCIDENCE

IN an article under this title which appeared in SCIENCE for December 16, 1927, Dr. William S. Murray reports on experiments in which he analyzed the effect of ovarian hormones on the incidence of mammary cancer in mice. In this connection he refers to the historical development of this problem as follows: "It has been known for some time that the internal secretions of the ovaries play an important part in the physiological condition of females during and after the gestation period. That the influence of these hormones has also a direct effect upon the ability of mice to combat the growth of neoplasms has been demonstrated by Dr. L. O. Strong (1922) in his work upon transplanted tumors. Dr. Leo Loeb has "also" (quotation marks added by the writer) published a brief note on the effects of castration and enforced non-breeding on tumor incidence. More recently (1927) Dr. Carl F. Cori has published a very interesting paper on the results of castration and ovarian transplantation in mice."

This statement tends to create an erroneous impression as to the development of our knowledge of this problem. Instead of having "also published a brief note," I have published in addition to this brief note two extensive papers containing detailed data on this question. The first of these appeared as the first article in Volume I of the *American Journal of Cancer Research,* January, 1916, p. 1. The second appeared in the *Journal of Medical Research,* September, 1919, p. 477. In these papers I gave the first experimental proof that internal secretions may play an important rôle in the origin of tumors. I showed that there is a definite quantitative relationship between the time during which the ovarian hormones have had a chance to act on the mammary gland and the incidence of mammary cancer. This I proved through castration carried on in mice at different ages. I also showed that prevention of breeding lowers the incidence of cancer but not to the same degree as castration at an early period of sexual maturity. I furthermore attempted to produce mammary cancer in male mice through transplantation of ovaries without succeeding in this attempt. Dr. Cori also was unsuccessful in similar experiments, while Dr. Murray succeeded in obtaining a positive result in 4 out of 210 operated male mice, therefore in less than 2 per cent. of his animals.

Since my first complete article on this problem appeared, I have repeatedly in various papers discussed the theoretical importance of this question in the etiology of cancer. I may also add that it was only possible for the writer to undertake the study of this problem, because I had for many years previously studied the rôle of heredity in the etiology of cancer in investigations based on the conviction that heredity in cancer can only be satisfactorily analyzed, if different families of mice are bred separately under identical environmental conditions. Accordingly in cooperation with Miss A. E. C. Lathrop, I was able to obtain strains of mice with definitely known inherited cancer incidence which differed in the case of different strains. Thus we could prove the quantitative interaction between hereditary factors and factors founded on the inner environment of organisms. Furthermore I had occasion to point out that there are indications that a similar quantitative interaction exists also between hereditary factors and outer environmental factors. The question as to the effect of various glands with inner secretion on the growth of transplanted tumors is a problem of an entirely different character and experiments of this kind can throw no light on the rôle of hormones in the origin of cancer.

LEO LOEB

DEPARTMENT OF PATHOLOGY,
WASHINGTON UNIVERSITY
SCHOOL OF MEDICINE

LAWS RELATING TO MATHEMATICAL OPERATIONS

ONE of the most fundamental differences between the mathematics which preceded the nineteenth century and the mathematics of to-day is the fact that we now lay much more stress on certain laws which govern many of our mathematical operations. Among these are those now known even by the student of elementary algebra as the commutative law and the distributive law. While attention was called to these laws in what is commonly regarded as the most influential mathematical text-book ever written, *viz.*, the "Elements of Euclid," very little stress was laid on them before the nineteenth century. As evidence of this fact we may note that modern mathematical historians have as yet furnished no instance where a special name was given to either of these laws before 1814 when a French writer, F. J. Servois, gave them their present names.

Another fundamental law which is now commonly explained in our text-books on elementary algebra is the associate law. It is well known that this law plays a prominent rôle in the modern subject known as the theory of abstract groups and that no one has as yet given an instance where a special name was assigned to it before W. R. Hamilton introduced its present name, about thirty years after F. J. Servois had introduced the names of the two laws noted above. It is known that A. M. Legendre directed attention to this law in 1798 and proved its validity as regards the multiplication of positive integers, but no one seems to have thus far noted any instance of its earlier explicit use. Its implicit use is very old since it is involved in the rule that the volume of a rectangular parallelopiped is equal to the product of three concurrent edges.

The history of these fundamental laws relating to the entire domain of mathematics, from the most elementary subjects to the most advanced, exhibits the slowness with which mathematical concepts sometimes gained their present positions in the literature. In particular, the attitude of mind which accords to the theory of groups a somewhat prominent position in the mathematics of to-day can perhaps be best explained by noting the growing stress placed on the laws which underlie very ancient mathematical operations. At any rate such profound changes relating to scientific questions should be of general interest even if it can not be foreseen whether they will be permanent. It is also possible that wide publicity relating to the present stage of our knowledge along these lines may lead to additions thereto.

G. A. MILLER

UNIVERSITY OF ILLINOIS

SOIL SCIENCE PUBLICATION IN RUSSIA

DR. A. YARILOV, editor of the Russian journals on soil science, "Bulletin Pochvoveda" and "Pochvovedenie" (Moscow, U. S. S. R., Vozdvizhenka 5, Gosplan) writes that beginning with the year 1928 the journals will publish papers in the original languages as submitted. He invites American colleagues to make use of these journals and in that way establish closer contact between soil science workers of the United States and Russia.

J. S. JOFFE

N. J. EXPERIMENT STATION.
NEW BRUNSWICK, N. J.

SCIENTIFIC BOOKS

The Elements of General Zoology. A Guide to the Study of Animal Biology, correlating Function and Structure with notes on practical exercises. By WILLIAM J. DAKIN, D.Sc., F. Z. S., professor of Zoology in the University of Liverpool. Oxford University Press, London: Humphrey Milford, 1927.

METHODS of teaching zoology are as numerous as the teachers but they group themselves naturally in three classes, those stressing structure, those emphasizing function and those magnifying habits and life histories. Professor Dakin's method is obviously the second as shown by his sub-title, and hence the morphologist, as well as the natural historian, has to make a very conscious effort to form a fair opinion of the real merits of the book. Were it entitled, "The Elements of Animal Physiology," its contents and purpose would be much better indicated. It is somewhat irritating to find animal physiology arrogating to itself the title of zoology. No one wishes to deny the vast importance of function, not merely as the concomitant but even as the "explanation" (in large part at any rate) of structure, but it is after all only a portion of the field of zoology. Some physiologists are poor zoologists because of a deficient knowledge of morphology, a complete ignorance of taxonomy, and a total indifference to habits and life histories. The real zoologist is the man who is interested in animals as living organisms whose structures, relationships, and natural history are vitally important—not the man who looks on them solely as machines.

Aside from this objection to Professor Dakin's title, the main criticism of his book has to do with omissions. Naturally any attempt to deal with the whole animal kingdom in one volume, even if only function is considered, necessitates omissions both numerous and important. The success of the writer must be judged in part by what he excludes, as well as by what he includes. Some of the omissions from the present volume are, to say the least, surprising. The most considerable perhaps is the complete omission of echinoderms—the phylum is mentioned on page 5 as one of "the most important phyla" in the animal kingdom (ten are given) but no further reference is made to it. The striking features of the skeleton, the unique method of excretion, the equally unique means of adhesion and locomotion and the surprising metamorphosis from extraordinary larval forms are all alike ignored. Another striking case is that of the cephalopods, whose unusual modes of locomotion, remarkable means of concealment when in retreat, and highly developed eyes, surely demand at least a reference. On page 298, the statement occurs: "The most complicated eye in the Mollusca is found in the scallop"—one wonders just what is meant by "complicated" and why the cephalopod eye is overlooked. Omission of many other extraordinary structures, functions and activities among invertebrates might be cited but lack of space forbids. Among the vertebrates we find no reference to the shell and skeleton of turtles, only a trivial allusion to the locomotion of snakes, no reference to the nest-building and egg-laying of birds, and no reference to animal voices, not even the singing of birds. It would of course, be foolish, and unfair to Professor Dakin, to extend indefinitely this list of omissions, but the point the reviewer wishes to emphasize is that too much is overlooked or ignored to justify calling this book "The Elements of General Zoology."

That there is much of value in the volume is beyond question. The text is clear, the illustrations and diagrams good and the marginal subtitles are helpful. There is a brief introduction of 8 pages, followed by Section I "An Introduction to the Protozoa." The 25 pages thus used form one of the most satisfactory chapters in the book. Just enough of classification is introduced to hold together the facts and the student who really masters this account will have a coherent idea of the Protozoa. Section II, "The Study of the Biology of the Multicellular Animals" occupies over 400 pages and suffers from the attempt to omit everything in the nature of a classification. It is not necessary to enumerate here all the chapters or to discuss their contents. The general arrangement is that of the usual text-book on physiology—nutrition, respiration, blood and its circulation, locomotion, nervous system and sense organs, excretion and reproduction. A chapter on the animal skeleton precedes that on locomotion, while another on the cell is intercalated between locomotion and the nervous system—just why at this point it is hard to see. Chapters on life histories, on the fresh-water pond as an animal community, on symbiosis, parasites, disease and bacteria and on the animal as a whole, make up the remainder of this section. A dozen of the chapters end in suggestions for "Practical Work," experimental studies and observations by the students themselves. The discussion of the animal as a whole leads to a brief account of some of the aspects of heredity and evolution, and the relation of biology as a study, to human life. The book ends with 35 pages of general instructions for laboratory work, a brief appendix, and a not very satisfactory index of four pages. The student who really masters the contents of Section II will have an admirable idea of animal physiology, but his ideas of structure will undoubtedly be more or less confused and he will know almost nothing of the animal kingdom.

HUBERT LYMAN CLARK
MUSEUM OF COMPARATIVE ZOOLOGY,
CAMBRIDGE, MASS.

SCIENTIFIC APPARATUS AND LABORATORY METHODS

A CONVENIENT DEVICE FOR PLANT SOLUTION-CULTURE WORK

THE paraffin-impregnated corks commonly used as supports for the seedlings in plant solution-culture investigation present certain disadvantages which I have attempted to eliminate by substituting perforated paraffin discs supported on glass rods of appropriate design.

Two hundred cc. of hot water are measured into a 250 cc. Pyrex beaker which is placed on a hot-plate. To this is added ten grams of paraffin m.p. 52–56° C. When the latter is melted the beaker is removed from the hot-plate. When the paraffin disc has solidified by cooling, it is loosened with a thin-bladed knife and removed from the beaker. The diameter is lessened by paring off a millimeter or two from the circumference so that the disc fits loosely within the beaker in which the cultures are to be made.

The glass supports are made from 4 mm. rod. This is cut into 15 cm. lengths and marked off accurately at 2.5, 5.0, 10.0, and 12.5 cm. with a blue pencil. Right-angle bends are carefully made at these points using an iron block 2.5 cm. high as mold, and the small but hot flame of the micro-burner for heating. The complete support has this shape.

Four notches are cut in the paraffin disc so that it rests easily on the two supports hanging from the

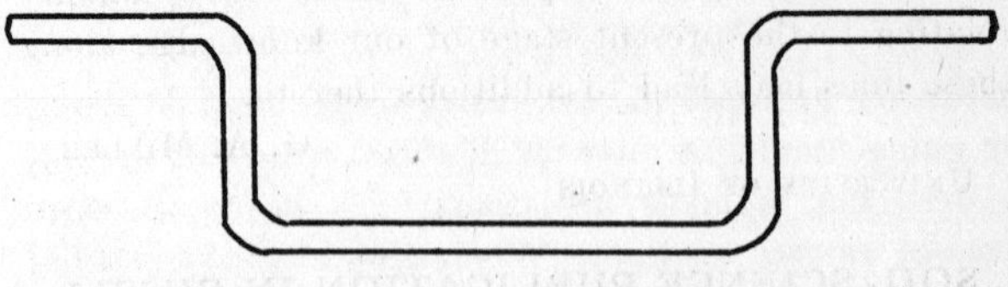

edge within the beaker. When the discs and supports are properly made the former present a plane surface parallel with the surface of the culture solution which can be of any desired distance from the disc. Then the convenient number of holes is made in the paraffin disc through which the roots come in contact with the culture solution. These holes are made of any desired diameter by means of appropriately selected cork-borers. In order to prevent cracking of the disc it is necessary that the cork-borer be hot. I have found that immersion of the instrument in hot water does this best. So heated, a little well-like curbing is formed around the hole which serves nicely to keep the seedling raised from the flat upper surface of the disc.

It will be at once evident that this device is capable of any modification necessary to suit the individual need. It also allows of easy adjustment of depth of culture solution and degree to which the roots are immersed therein. Its convenience will be apparent to those who have wrestled as I have with the un-plastic cork.

FREDERICK S. HAMMETT
RESEARCH INSTITUTION OF THE
LANKENAU HOSPITAL,
PHILADELPHIA, PA.

A METHOD FOR CUTTING GLASS TUBING

THE accompanying figure illustrates a method which has been found to be successful for cutting heavy glass tubing. A piece of bare, soft-drawn copper wire "W" is wrapped once around the tube "T" and fastened to the work bench. A mixture of carborundum powder and glycerine makes a convenient grinding compound. A to and fro motion of the glass in a direction parallel to the plane of the figure produces relative motion between the wire and glass and the carborundum is thus carried around. The glass should occasionally be turned so as to make a cut of uniform depth. In case it is

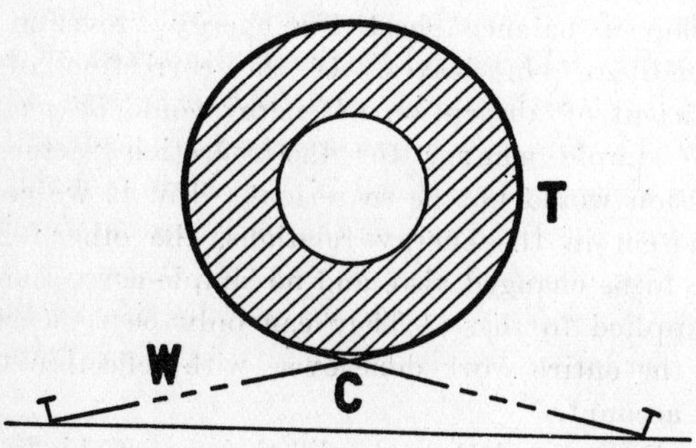

necessary to locate the cut exactly some kind of clamp or guide should be used until a groove is started. If a deep cut is made the point "C" where the wire crosses causes binding. When this stage is reached it is well to mount the tube in a lathe and hold the wire in the groove using only one half of a turn. (Be sure to protect the lathe from the compound.) New wire should replace the old frequently to avoid binding when the new is used.

The author's first use of the method was in cutting a Pyrex tube having an outside diameter of 4.4 centimeters and 1.2 centimeter walls. Number 80 carborundum powder was used, first with Number 18 wire and then with Number 20. The cutting time was about three hours. Finer wire and powder would be better for smaller or more delicate pieces.

The method has the advantages of simplicity, small breakage risk and freedom from strains introduced by methods using heat. It is particularly useful in cutting short lengths of tubing.

HERMAN E. SEEMANN
DEPARTMENT OF PHYSICS,
CORNELL UNIVERSITY

SPECIAL ARTICLES

REFLECTION OF LIGHT FROM THE SURFACES OF LEAVES

THE classical studies of Brown and Escombe[1] on the interchange of energy between the leaf and its environment form our only important sources of information as to the quantitative income and outgo of energy during the processes of photosynthesis, transpiration and thermal emissivity. They measured the solar radiation with much care, determined the coefficient of absorption of energy by the leaf, measured the amount of energy expended in the various forms of internal work, and the gain and loss of energy during positive or negative thermal emissivity at the leaf surface. From these various determinations they attempted to construct a balance sheet of the energy income and outgo of the leaf.

Careful consideration of their work makes it obvious that their figures, which account for 100 per cent. of the energy inflow in terms of work and transmission, can not be as accurate as they appear to be at first glance. The most patent error is one to which they referred, but neglected because they thought it was a small error. This is the reflection of light from the leaf surface, which, they say, with perpendicular incidence "must be very small in amount." The reflected light was allowed to enter, as an error, into the calculation of the coefficient of absorption, which is therefore too large.

During the last two years many measurements of the reflection of light from leaf surfaces have been made by means of the Keuffel and Esser direct reading spectrophotometer. This instrument is designed to measure the percentage of reflection at an angle of 90° to the surface of the leaf when the incident light falls upon the leaf from almost every possible angle. By means of a wheel, carrying a wave-length

[1] Brown, Horace T., and Escombe, F. "Researches on some of the Physiological Processes of Green Leaves with Special Reference to the Interchange of Energy between the Leaf and its Surroundings." *Proc. Royal Soc.* London B. 76: 29–111. 1905.

TABLE I

PERCENTAGE OF 90° REFLECTION OF BRIGHT DIFFUSED LIGHT FROM THE SURFACES OF LEAVES

Species	Wave Lengths in mμ														
	430	440	460	480	500	520	540	560	580	600	620	640	660	680	700
Syringa vulgaris															
Upper surface	3.0	3.5	4.5	4.5	4.5	5.0	6.0	6.5	6.0	5.5	5.0	5.0	4.0	3.5	3.0
Lower surface	8.5	8.0	8.5	9.0	10.0	12.0	16.0	16.0	14.0	13.0	12.0	11.0	8.0	8.0	8.0
Morus rubra															
Upper surface	4.0	4.5	5.5	5.5	5.5	6.5	8.5	8.5	7.0	5.5	5.0	5.0	5.0	5.0	4.0
Lower surface	7.5	8.0	8.0	9.0	10.0	12.5	14.0	15.0	13.0	11.0	10.0	10.0	9.0	7.5	10.0
Populus alba															
Upper surface	6.5	7.5	9.0	10.0	12.0	14.0	19.0	20.0	16.5	13.0	12.0	12.0	10.5	10.0	8.5
Lower surface	50.0	50.0	50.0	50.0	50.0	51.0	50.0	52.0	53.0	51.0	52.0	51.0	50.0	51.0	50.0
Psedera quinquefolia, autumn crimson															
Upper surface	5.0	4.5	4.5	5.0	5.5	6.0	7.0	6.5	7.0	9.0	12.0	13.0	12.0	8.0	17.0
Lower surface	9.0	11.0	13.0	14.0	14.0	17.0	19.5	21.5	22.5	24.0	26.0	28.0	22.0	18.0	28.0
Betula alba, autumn yellow															
Upper surface	5.0	6.0	6.0	7.0	8.0	16.0	24.0	30.0	33.0	35.0	37.0	39.0	42.0	38.0	32.0
Lower surface	11.0	12.0	12.0	13.0	15.0	23.0	26.0	30.0	32.0	33.0	33.0	34.0	39.0	36.0	35.0

scale, the constant deviation prism of the spectrometer may be adjusted to throw light of any desired wave-length into the comparison telescope. It is possible, therefore, to measure the percentage of reflection in each portion of the spectrum from 430 mμ to 700 mμ. The measurements were made at about 20 mμ intervals across the spectrum, for many different kinds of leaves, chosen for variation in color, texture, and quality of surface. The accompanying Table I presents a few of the measurements.

From the measurements presented, it is seen that the greatest reflection in green leaves usually falls at about 540 to 560 mμ, and in the darkest green leaves like those of *Syringa vulgaris,* the reflection is a little over 6 per cent. in this region of the spectrum. In lighter green leaves, as in *Populus alba,* the reflection is much greater, 20 per cent. at 560 mμ. The under surface of the leaf of *P. alba* is very hairy and white. The reflection from this surface was about the same across the entire spectrum as would be expected in a gray color, and accounted for fully 50 per cent. of the incident light.

In autumn colored leaves, such as the crimson leaves of *Psedera quinquefolia* and the brilliant yellow leaves of the white birch, *Betula alba,* the greatest reflection naturally occurs in the brighter regions of the spectrum, at 640 and 660 mμ. The upper surface reflection of *Psedera* leaves is low in comparison with the reflection from *Betula* leaves. The latter in autumn brilliancy reflect over 40 per cent. of the incident light, the former about 13 per cent. Many other measurements have been made with similar results. These will be published in detail elsewhere.

The results indicate that we are not justified in omitting reflection as a factor when we attempt to develop a balance sheet for energy "revenue and expenditure" of leaves. If the correction of the coefficient of absorption of energy could be made in some simple manner for the reflection factor, the omission would not be so serious. But if we correct this item in the energy relations, the other figures have to be changed also, and no simple correction can be applied to these. They can only be remeasured, and the entire work done over, with reflection taken into account.

As Brown and Escombe did their work chiefly with the leaves of one species, *Catalpa bignonioides,* it is certain that many leaves differ from this species in mass per square centimeter of surface. This difference will also disturb the calculated balance of energy with special reference to thermal emissivity. The energy relations of leaves are therefore in need of reinvestigation, and the balance sheet of energy should be constructed on the basis of a more critical study of all the energy factors involved, and on the basis of a study of a number of leaf types.

CHARLES A. SHULL

UNIVERSITY OF CHICAGO

SPECIAL ISSUE CONTAINING REPORTS OF THE SESSIONS OF SECTIONS AND SOCIETIES AT THE SECOND NASHVILLE MEETING OF THE AMERICAN ASSOCIATION FOR THE ADVANCEMENT OF SCIENCE AND ASSOCIATED SOCIETIES. EDITED BY BURTON E. LIVINGSTON, PERMANENT SECRETARY

SCIENCE

VOL. LXVII FEBRUARY 3, 1928 No. 1727

CONTENTS

The American Association for the Advancement of Science:

The Response to the Addresses of Welcome at the Opening Session at Nashville: PRESIDENT A. A. NOYES ... 109

The Newly Elected President: B. E. L. ... 111

Reports of Sessions of Sections and Societies at the Second Nashville Meeting ... 113

Special Notes ... 131

Scientific Events:

National Research Fellows at Princeton University; Presentation of the Nichols Medal to Professor Hugh S. Taylor; Medal Presentations to General Carty and Dr. Coolidge ... 132

Scientific Notes and News ... 133

University and Educational Notes ... 135

Discussion and Correspondence:

Discovery of Further Hominid Remains of Lower Quaternary Age from the Chou Kou Tien Deposit: DR. DAVIDSON BLACK. *An Instance of the Increase of Malaria by Civilization:* DR. L. O. HOWARD. *The Scientific Men of Harvard and Columbia:* DR. J. MCKEEN CATTELL ... 135

Reports:

Address of the President of the Australasian Association for the Advancement of Science ... 138

Special Articles:

Nutritional Anemia on Whole Milk Diets and its Correction with the Ash of Beef Liver: J. WADDELL, C. A. ELVEHJEM, H. STEENBOCK and E. B. HART ... 139

Societies and Academies:

The Geological Society of America: PROFESSOR CHARLES P. BERKEY. *Indiana Academy of Science:* HARRY F. DIETZ ... 140

Science News ... x

SCIENCE: A Weekly Journal devoted to the Advancement of Science, edited by J. McKeen Cattell and published every Friday by

THE SCIENCE PRESS

New York City: Grand Central Terminal.

Lancaster, Pa. Garrison, N. Y.

Annual Subscription, $6.00. Single Copies, 15 Cts.

SCIENCE is the official organ of the American Association for the Advancement of Science. Information regarding membership in the Association may be secured from the office of the permanent secretary, in the Smithsonian Institution Building, Washington, D. C.

Entered as second-class matter July 18, 1923, at the Post Office at Lancaster, Pa., under the Act of March 8, 1879.

THE AMERICAN ASSOCIATION FOR THE ADVANCEMENT OF SCIENCE

THE RESPONSE TO THE ADDRESSES OF WELCOME AT THE OPENING SESSION AT NASHVILLE

(*By President A. A. Noyes*)

In response to your welcomes I would say at the start we are heartily glad to be here! And this for various reasons: First of all, we look forward to enjoying the famed hospitality of the South in this, one of its leading cities, and to becoming acquainted with its people. But more important still is the hope that our visit here may in some small measure contribute to the already active scientific and educational development of this section of the country. One of your distinguished writers, Professor Mims, has recently described for us "The Advancing South"; and most important among its many advances is, as he rightly emphasizes, that of its intellectual life. The purpose of this association is the advancement of science in its broadest sense; and it is glad to meet again in the South for the reason that conditions are now clearly propitious for a rapid extension of scientific activities here.

I desire especially to reciprocate Dr. Kirkland's greetings from the educational institutions of this state, and to thank them for their cordial welcome. The present success of these institutions affords the best assurance that this state will play its part in the larger development of science which is to take place during the next decades in this country and especially in the South.

It might be desirable on the occasion of this fifty-year anniversary of the former Nashville meeting, to review in broadest outlines the advance of the sciences during the last half-century; but this would be more suitable for the substantial address of a retiring president than for the short responses which I am making to your kind welcomes. I may, however, briefly refer to certain pronounced changes in the viewpoints of scientific investigators.

About forty years ago the physical sciences, physics and chemistry, seemed to have reached a nearly stationary condition, as exemplified by the oft-quoted remark of an eminent physicist that the future advances of physics were to consist in adding another decimal place to the known values of natural constants—which reminds me of the remark of a distinguished scientist who, when asked why he did such work, replied, "I guess I am like the Irishman that said, 'When I see a head, I hit it,' so when I see an inexact constant I go at it." Moreover, scientists in those fields were becoming over-conservative in the scientific use of the imagination. Thus the philosopher-scientists Mach and Ostwald in Germany urged that the primary aim of science is a representation of natural phenomena without the aid of hypothesis. Then in 1886–87 burst into the realm of chemistry the general theory of solutions of van't Hoff, the ionic hypothesis of Arrhenius, and the development of these theories by Nernst and others; and a new branch of chemistry, physical chemistry, came into being. In physics during the last decade of the nineteenth century the discoveries of X-rays by Roentgen, of radioactivity by Becquerel and the Curies, and of the phenomena of gaseous conduction by J. J. Thomson, opened the way for a most extraordinary development of physical science—that of modern sub-atomic or electronic physics. Physicists became eager, optimistic, imaginative; and volumes of exciting discoveries poured out of the laboratories of the world. Relativity, non-Euclidean geometry, and non-Newtonian mechanics appeared on the scene. The exactness under all conditions of the most fundamental laws of physics was questioned and reexamined. Energy came onto the stage, and matter took a back seat. A less mechanistic conception of natural phenomena arose.

In the meantime in the biological sciences the existence of evolution as a fundamental phenomenon of life was established by converging evidence from paleontology, embryology, genetics, and comparative anatomy, with a certainty comparable with that of the Copernican conception of the solar system. While even less can be said to-day of the processes by which evolution takes place than was thought to be known fifty years ago, the facts that evolution has been going on and that many animal and plant types have gone through definite stages of development can only be doubted by an individual who like an ostrich buries his head in the sand out of a vague dread that he may see something shocking.

These advances in the physical and biological sciences have greatly influenced the philosophic and religious thinking of the scientific man; for it is a great mistake to think the tendency of advancing science is towards materialism. Just the opposite. The repeated discoveries of new and unexpected types of phenomena in the physical world make us realize more than ever the limitations of our understanding, and lead us to feel with Tennyson that "as knowledge grows from more to more, will more of reverence in us dwell." And we like to repeat to ourselves the words of a poet-scientist of England (Whetham):

We scatter the mists that enclose us
The seas are ours and the lands,
The quivering ether knows us
And carries our quick commands.
From the blaze of the sun's bright glory
We sift cach ray of light;
We steal from the stars their story
Across the dark space of night.

But beyond the bright search-lights of science,
Out of sight of the windows of sense,
Old riddles still bid us defiance
Old questions of why and whence.
There fail all sure means of trial
And end all the pathways we've trod
Where man by belief or denial
Is weaving the purpose of God.

Moreover, the fuller establishment of evolution as a principle of life, and the implication of that principle that man in his present state may be "the herald of a higher race," give us a system of ethics which makes us charitable to the failings of our fellow men and eager to work for the further development of our race; also a religious viewpoint which leads us, more than any static ready-made universe could do, "to reverently ponder the ways of God." To us the process of evolution becomes the most striking manifestation in all nature of the underlying power "which passeth all understanding"—a view so finely expressed in the well-known words of another poet:

A first-mist and a planet,
A crystal and a cell,
A jelly-fish and a saurian,
And caves where the cave-men dwell,
Then, a sense of law and beauty
And a face turned from the clod;
Some call it Evolution,
And others call it God.

We are delighted to receive also the welcome from the civic interests of this state; for science needs the aid of the intelligent men engaged in other professions and in industry and commerce. There are few things more promising for the advancement of science in this country than the whole-hearted way in which leading men of affairs are interesting themselves in the promotion of research. And most significant is the fact that this interest applies not so much to research in its application to their own industries (shown by the establishment of great research laboratories, such as those of General Electric Company, American Telegraph and Telephone Company, the du Pont Company, and many others), as to fundamental research in pure science.

The last year has afforded a striking instance of this—the only one I have time to mention. The National Academy of Sciences, a sister organization of this association, realizing that America, in proportion to its wealth and population, is not contributing anything like its share to the advancement of science, and believing that this is largely due to very inadequate financial support of the investigators of this country, undertook to secure from our larger corporations a fund of $20,000,000 for the promotion of research in all the varied branches of pure science. It was clearly seen that the first step in such a campaign must be to get the aid of prominent men of affairs, whose support would carry weight with our industrial leaders. The first remarkable thing was that there was no difficulty whatever in securing this support. Herbert Hoover, in spite of his many obligations, accepted the chairmanship of the board of trustees of the fund; and such men as Elihu Root, Charles Hughes, Andrew Mellon, Owen Young, John W. Davis, Edward House, J. J. Carty, and Gano Dunn became members of the board and have for the most part taken an active part in its work. The second remarkable thing was that there was no need of convincing either these men or the leaders of industry consulted that the fund should be used for research in science itself rather than in its industrial applications. They saw that the latter was a field of research that should be prosecuted by the industries themselves within their own establishments—not by universities or endowed research institutions. They realized too, as Professor Tyndall said in substance fifty years ago in his lectures in New York, that "just as the stream dwindles when the fount dries, so surely will technical developments lose all vitality when they cease to be nourished by new scientific discoveries." Scientific discovery "puts not only money into the pockets of individuals, but millions into the exchequers of nations," yet even greater are its intellectual and spiritual contributions to the welfare of mankind.

Well, the campaign was undertaken under these favorable auspices, and is now progressing satisfactorily. Already a considerable sum payable through a period of ten years has been secured, and the prospects are good for more.

But it is not alone on the financial side that science needs the support of the intelligent people of any community. While *science* has through daily experience come to be universally recognized as vitally important, yet it is often not realized that science does not "just grow"—that it arises from *research*, and that research is a sensitive plant which will grow successfully only from carefully selected seeds—the best brains of the nation; and which must be protected against the frost of dogmatic intolerance, against the drought of administrative routine, against the flood of modern mass education, against overforcing through the impatient demands of practical men, and against the blights of poverty and social neglect. Research will come to its own in any community only when its members, in the words of Pasteur, regard their research laboratories as their temples.

THE NEWLY-ELECTED PRESIDENT OF THE AMERICAN ASSOCIATION

ALL who are interested in the advancement of science in America and in the world at large must be deeply gratified by the election of Henry Fairfield Osborn as president of the American Association for the Advancement of Science. This is the highest honor that can come to an American worker in science from his colleagues, and Professor Osborn's work is surely an excellent example of the finest endeavor for which the American Association stands. Primarily a vertebrate paleontologist his influence for advancement has been much broader than that field. His work has been remarkably effective in many lines of scientific thought. He is well known as a research worker, author, educator and administrator.

The president-elect was born at Fairfield, Connecticut, on August 8, 1857, the son of William Henry and Virginia Reed (Sturges) Osborn. On the paternal side he is descended from the Osborns of Salem, Massachusetts, of the colonial period. On the maternal side his descent is from Nathan Gold and Andrew Ward, of the time of the Revolution, and from Rev. Ebenezer Pemberton, one of the three founders of Princeton College. His maternal grandfather was Jonathan Sturges, who was president of the New York Chamber of Commerce. His father was a founder and for many years president of the Illinois Central Railroad.

Educated at the Columbia Grammar School and Lyons Collegiate Institute, of New York City, and at Princeton College, Osborn received the A.B. degree in 1880. He was greatly influenced by President McCosh in philosophy and by Professor Arnold Guyot in geology. His field work in paleontology began immediately after graduation, for he took part in geological expeditions to Colorado and Wyoming in 1877 and 1878. In 1878–79 he took courses in anatomy and histology at the College of Physicians and Surgeons and at Bellevue Medical College, in New York City. In the year 1879–80 he studied embryology at Cambridge University, under Francis Balfour, and comparative anatomy in London, under Thomas Henry Huxley. He also spent some time in Germany. Having held the first E. M. Biological

Fellowship at Princeton for the years 1880–83, he was appointed assistant professor of natural science at that institution in 1881, and professor of comparative anatomy in 1883, where he remained seven years.

Professor Osborn was called to Columbia University in 1890 to the Da Costa chair of biology. Here he organized the zoological department, instituted scientific expeditions and started the Columbia Biological Series of publications, which he edited for a number of years. In 1894 he served on the administrative board of publications and as a trustee of Columbia University Press. From 1892 to 1895 he was dean of the faculty of Pure Science at Columbia University. He retired from active teaching in 1910, but since then has remained in Columbia as research professor of zoology.

The new president's career in university work has been amply adequate for very great eminence, but he has also won the position of dean of American museum organizers and administrators. Throughout the last nine years of his Columbia period he served as curator of the department of vertebrate paleontology in the American Museum of Natural History, New York City. In the last named year he withdrew from the active curatorship and he has since then been honorary curator. To research, writing, editing and the administration of the museum he has devoted the last thirty-seven years. He was assistant to the president from 1899 to 1901 (when he inaugurated the present internal organization of the museum and started the museum journal and the memoir series of publications), trustee and vice-president from 1901 to 1908, and he has been president of the Board of Trustees since the death of President Jesup in 1908.

As curator in vertebrate paleontology, President Osborn led in the organization of many expeditions that went out from the American Museum in search of vertebrate fossils, largely to the regions made famous by the pioneer work of Leidy, Cope and Marsh. He was a member of the exploration parties of 1893, 1897, 1903, 1906, 1907, 1908, 1909 and 1910 and he has also accompanied some expeditions of later years. In 1907 the expedition to the Fayûm, in Egypt, secured, among many other valuable finds, fossils representing two very early stages in the evolution of the elephant and led to the Memoir on the Proboscidea now in press. His earlier prediction that Africa is to be considered as the original homeland of this great mammal appears to have been fully confirmed.

During the administration of President Osborn have occurred remarkable advances in paleontological technique at the American Museum of Natural History, and great improvements in the teaching value of the exhibits, through attractive grouping and posing. In his museum period has been assembled what is said to be the most extensive collection of vertebrate fossils in existence, notably the collections of fossil horses and of fossil proboscideans representing geological times from the Tertiary forward. These fossil collections have become a standard of excellence. The president has continually encouraged and stimulated research and the distribution of knowledge of natural history in the City of New York. His many and important contributions to public education were the reason for his receiving the Roosevelt Medal of Honor, presented by President Harding in 1923.

Professor Osborn has also a fine record of research achievement in the U. S. Geological Survey, to which he was appointed, as vertebrate paleontologist, in 1900. He was promoted to the rank of senior geologist in 1924. In this connection he is bringing out his greatest research contribution, a monograph on "The Titanotheres of Ancient Wyoming, Dakota and Nebraska," which is now in press.

As chairman of the executive committee of the New York Zoological Society (1896–1903, 1907–1909), Dr. Osborn organized and established the administrative and scientific work of the society and supervised details of the plans for the splendid facilities of the New York Zoological Park. He was vice-president of the Zoological Society in 1897 and president from 1909 to 1923. As a mark of its appreciation of his long-continued interest and devotion, the New York Zoological Society has elected him to honorary presidency for life.

In 1906 Professor Osborn was elected to the secretaryship of the Smithsonian Institution, held to be the most honored scientific post in the United States, but he was obliged to decline. He has held the presidency and other responsible offices in many American scientific and educational organizations. He is a member of the National Academy of Sciences and the American Philosophical Society and an associate fellow of the American Academy of Arts and Sciences. His name is on the rolls of a very large number of learned organizations, both American and foreign. He has received many medals of honor and numerous honorary degrees.

The president-elect became a member of the American Association for the Advancement of Science in 1881, being elected to fellowship in 1883. He became a life member in 1917. He is shown, on the cards of the Washington office, as specially interested in Sections E (Geology and Geography), and F (Zoological Sciences). He was vice-president (for Section E) in 1892 and has served the association in various other capacities from time to time. His scientific record and his leading position in affairs that interest scientific workers make Professor Osborn an excellent choice to represent the work and ideals of the American Association.

Professor Osborn's publications are many and in many fields. According to available information he has published seven scientific memoirs, eleven books and over seven hundred papers. He edited "A Naturalist in the Bahamas" (1910), a memorial to Dr. John I. Northrup, and "Fifty Years of Princeton, '77" (1927). The following are the titles of his books: "From the Greeks to Darwin" (1894), "Evolution of Mammalian Molar Teeth" (1907), "The Age of Mammals" (1910), "Huxley and Education" (1910), "Men of the Old Stone Age" (1915), "Origin and Evolution of Life" (1917), "Impressions of Great Naturalists" (1924), "The Earth Speaks to Bryan" (1925), "Evolution and Religion in Education" (1926), "Creative Education in School, College, University and Museum" (1927), "Man Rises to Parnassus" (1927). A survey of his published papers shows 14 on geology, 35 on zoology, 24 on comparative anatomy, 3 on eugenics, 30 on anthropology, 77 on evolution, 285 on paleontology, 52 on education, 5 on psychology, 80 on biographic subjects, 52 on administrative subjects and 36 in other fields.—B. E. L.

REPORTS OF THE SESSIONS OF SECTIONS AND SOCIETIES AT THE SECOND NASHVILLE MEETING

THE general reports of the second Nashville meeting have been published in SCIENCE for January 27. The present issue is mainly devoted to special reports of the sessions of the several sections and of the societies that took part in that meeting. Almost all reports from section or society secretaries were in hand by January 14. These have been edited and assembled for the following pages.

The permanent secretary is very grateful to the secretaries of the sections and societies for their hearty cooperation in this work, especially for the promptness with which the reports have been received this year. The material here presented is classified according to the sections of the association, after the manner of the arrangement of the general program of the meeting. It is to be noted that the days of the week mentioned are those from Monday, December 26, to Saturday, December 31, 1927.

SECTION A (MATHEMATICS)

Vice-president and chairman, R. C. Archibald; *retiring vice-president,* Dunham Jackson; *secretary,* C. N. Moore, University of Cincinnati, Cincinnati, Ohio. With the section met the American Mathematical Society (*president,* Virgil Snyder; *secretary,* R. G. D. Richardson, Brown University, Providence, R. I.) and the Mathematical Association of America (*president,* W. B. Ford; *secretary,* W. D. Cairns, Oberlin, Ohio).

(*Report from R. C. Archibald*)

Section A held a joint session Thursday afternoon with the two affiliated organizations. Professors Jackson and Ford presided, and three papers were presented: the first by Professor E. V. Huntington, of Harvard University, retiring chairman of the section; the second by Professor Dunham Jackson, retiring president of the Mathematical Association of America, and the third by Professor Arnold Dresden, of Swarthmore College, representing the American Mathematical Society.—Professor Huntington gave a non-technical account of "The Notion of Probable Error in Elementary Statistics." This address was published in SCIENCE for December 30, 1927.

Professor Jackson spoke on "The Human Significance of Mathematics." It was contended that the significance of advanced mathematical study in human society is more profound than an analysis of the immediate applicability of current research would indicate. Mathematics is of great benefit in promoting the habit of exact thinking, in some at any rate, of those who have experience of it. The universality and permanence of mathematical truth make a profound appeal to the constructive imagination and constitute a bond of common experience between thinking men of all times and places. Since mathematical knowledge as we possess it is a product of human thinking, the process of acquiring it contributes materially to the comprehension of the manner of working of the human intelligence and of the extent to which reliance can be placed on the results of its free play. And since our knowledge comes only in restricted measure from the discoveries of the great leaders in the science, and very largely from the collective experience of the race, every serious student, whether personally engaged in research or not, may feel that he contributes something to the completeness of the structure. This paper is to be published in *The American Mathematical Monthly*.

Professor Dresden's paper dealt with "Some Philosophic Aspects of Mathematics." Discussions of the foundations of mathematics occasioned by recent work of Brouwer, Hilbert and others led to the consideration of certain questions which bear on the essential character of the subject; *viz.,* the meaning of "existence" in mathematics, and the basis for confidence in the validity of its conclusions. In its essential aspects, mathematics has no strictly objective basis, but is, in a very definite sense, subjective and temporal; belief in the validity of mathematical conclusions rests upon respected successful verifications made in the applications of mathematics.

The American Mathematical Society held sessions for the presentation of seventy-two papers on Wednesday morning and afternoon and Thursday morning. There were in attendance 138 members, a number that compares favorably with 188, the number who attended the Philadelphia meeting last year, the largest in the history of the society. There were also in attendance fifty-two non-members. At the first session Professor James Pierpont, of Yale University, gave an interesting address on "Mathematical Rigor, Past and Present," in which were rapidly reviewed some of the main features of the development of standards of rigor in analysis since the invention of the calculus by Newton and Leibnitz. Not until the days of Cauchy, Gauss, Abel and Dirichlet did analysts employ reasoning relative to infinite processes which resembles that of to-day. Improvement in rigor has in the main been brought about by discovering possibilities whose existence had not been suspected and which rendered a good part of former proofs unsatisfactory. The next step taken to give mathematical reasoning more strength is due to Weierstrass. Until his time geometric notions were freely admitted in analytic proof. But the discovery of continuous functions without derivatives made manifest the wide gap which existed between geometric notions and their analytic formulation. Weierstrass was thus led to place all analysis on a purely arithmetic foundation. His name has been a synonym of mathematical rigor for fifty years. There has now arisen a school inaugurated by Kronecker and continued in one form or another by Poincaré, Borel, Weyl and Brouwer, who call themselves finitists, empiricists or intuitionalists. These aim to introduce a far more exalted type of rigor than has hitherto been deemed necessary, which if carried through will require a rebuilding of present analysis from the ground up. This movement is hotly challenged by the formalist school, whose protagonist is Hilbert. Time alone will settle the controversy. This address is to be published in the *Bulletin of the American Mathematical Society*.—The fifth Josiah Willard Gibbs lecture of the American Mathematical Society, on "Resonance in the Solar System," was delivered at the general session Wednesday afternoon, by Professor E. W. Brown, of Yale University. The lecturer developed certain consequences of resonance phenomena amongst the periods of revolution of planets and satellites. By means of the analogy to the motion of a frictionless pendulum under a periodic disturbance, the indeterminate nature of the problem of three or more bodies over long periods of time was emphasized. Two principal conclusions were drawn: (1) that any actual system like the solar system was in a continual state of development, owing to gravitational action alone; (2) that speculations into the remote past or remote future of such a system were more likely to be valid if reached by probability methods than if attempted by exact analysis. The address will appear in the *Bulletin of the American Mathematical Society*. The society elected Professor J. W. Young, of Dartmouth College, and Professor H. L. Rietz, of the University of Iowa, as vice-presidents for two years. Professor J. L. Coolidge, of Harvard University, was appointed to represent the society in the National Research Council for three years from July 1, 1928.

The Mathematical Association of America held its twelfth annual meeting on Friday morning and afternoon, when seven papers were presented. President Ford presided. The following elections were announced: Professor A. J. Kempner, of the University of Colorado, and Professor F. D. Murnaghan, of the Johns Hopkins University, as vice-presidents for one year; Professors Archibald, Eisenhart, Lane and Rietz, as trustees for a term of three years.—On Thursday a very successful dinner for the mathematicians was held at the Ward-Belmont School.

SECTION B (PHYSICS)

Vice-president and chairman, A. H. Compton; *retiring vice-president,* W. Duane; *secretary,* A. L. Hughes, Washington University, St. Louis, Mo. With Section B met the American Physical Society (*president,* K. T. Compton; *secretary,* H. W. Webb, Columbia University, New York City) and the American Meteorological Society (*president,* C. F. Marvin; *secretary,* Charles F. Brooks, Clark University, Worcester, Mass.).

(*Reports from A. L. Hughes and Charles F. Brooks*)

Section B and the American Physical Society held meetings on Wednesday, Thursday and Friday. Nearly one hundred members of the section attended the meetings. The address of the retiring vice-president, Professor W. Duane, of Harvard University, was given on Wednesday afternoon, on "The General Radiation." Beginning with a rapid recapitulation of the main facts known about the general radiation in X-rays, the speaker pointed out how some of them receive a natural theoretical interpretation while others can not as yet be accounted for on any theory. He then went on to describe his investigations on the general radiation from matter in the gaseous state. Professor Duane finds that the distribution of the general radiation from a gas differs considerably from that from a solid in that the energy is more concentrated towards the short wave-length limit. Theory has at present no explanation to offer for this result. Pro fessor Duane's address will be published later in Science. The address of the retiring vice-president was followed by a lecture by Dr. C. J. Davisson, of the Bell Telephone Laboratories, on "Diffraction of Electrons by a Crystal of Nickel." One of the most perplexing phenomena in physics is that radiation in some effects behaves exactly as though it were waves in a continuous medium, while in others it behaves like a torrent of tiny particles traveling with the velocity of light. Hitherto, the electron has been satisfactorily accounted for by supposing it to be a tiny material particle. Dr. Davisson and Dr. Germer have found, however, that when electrons impinge on a suitable metallic crystal surface they reemerge in definite directions, exactly as though they were X-rays of proper wave-length falling on the crystal. This behavior can not be explained at all on the supposition that the electron is a tiny material particle. The great significance of these results is that they show, for the first time, that the electron behaves in some phenomena just like a wave, while in others, it behaves like a particle. These discoveries are to be regarded as among the most fundamental of recent years.

The American Physical Society had a program occupying five half days. Fifty-three papers were communicated. On Wednesday Professor K. T. Compton, president of the American Physical Society, gave the presidential address on "Recent Studies of Electrical Discharges in Gases." He described briefly the principal features of the electrical discharge in gases, outlined various theories which had been proposed and pointed out the difficulties which bar the way to the application of the theories to actual conditions, except in specially selected, simple cases. He then proceeded to describe recent advances in this field (many of which have come from Professor Compton's own laboratory) and showed how we have now a much improved understanding of the various types of discharge and of the causes of the transitions between them.—On Thursday evening a very successful dinner was held, attended by over one hundred persons. The Nashville meeting will be remembered with pleasure by all who attended because of the unusually excellent arrangements for the physicists at the Ward-Belmont College.

The American Meteorological Society joined with Section E (Geology and Geography) and the Association of American Geographers in a symposium on "Problems of the Mississippi River," which occurred Thursday morning. About 150 persons attended. Five of the eight papers were on meteorological subjects. Four Weather Bureau flood forecasters, Frankenfield, Williamson, Barron and Cline, presented the fundamentals of flood causation and flood prediction in the Mississippi Valley, while Brooks, on behalf of Bangs and himself, gave a weather-map discussion of the great rainfall of April, 1927, to which was due the unusual magnitude of the recent flood. Special tribute was given to Dr. I. M. Cline, on account of his surpassing public service in the Louisiana region of the flood. The prime importance of the rainfall in the middle and lower parts of the Mississippi Basin and the relative insignificance of all other factors were emphasized and a plea was made for a thorough-going meteorological investigation of great rain periods and their antecedents.—A session was devoted to local climatological studies. Another was on winds. A third was largely on storms, but included papers on radio, and on the correlation periodogram.—Of special import to Tennessee was the Tennessee Weather Service session and luncheon on Friday, organized by Fergusson, Nunn and Williamson, all of them Tennessee meteorologists. A group of the cooperative observers of the state joined with many Weather Bureau officials and others to talk over affairs of mutual interest and the session was presided over by Professor C. F. Marvin, chief of the U. S. Weather Bureau and president of the American Meteorological Society. Mrs. Ross Woods, who maintains the long-record station at Palmetto, Tennessee, brilliantly addressed the group on "Duties and Experiences of a Cooperative Observer" and other observers spoke informally. The luncheon proved a most enjoyable occasion, with Roscoe Nunn as toastmaster.—William J. Humphreys was elected president and Edward Alden Beales vice-president for two years, while Willis Ray Gregg and Charles F. Brooks were continued as treasurer and secretary, respectively. The one-hundred-dollar prize of the Meisinger Aerological Research Fund was announced for award at the end of 1928. Resolutions were adopted (1) thanking the George Peabody College for Teachers for the excellent facilities of this meeting, (2) urging increased government appropriations for the *Monthly Weather Review* and (3) requesting an appropriation of $25,000 from Congress for a special investigation of ocean meteorology in relation to floods in the Mississippi and other rivers.

SECTION C (CHEMISTRY)

Vice-president and chairman, Roger Adams; retiring vice-president, Lauder W. Jones; secretary, Gerhard Dietrichson, Massachusetts Institute of Technology, Cambridge, Mass.

(*Report from Gerhard Dietrichson*)

Section C held meetings on Tuesday, Wednesday and Thursday. On Wednesday morning it joined with Section N (Medical Sciences) in a symposium on "Some Contributions of Other Sciences to Medicine," an account of which will be found in the report of Section N. Section C held four other sessions. Professor Lauder W. Jones, of Princeton University, delivered the retiring vice-presidential address Tuesday afternoon, on "A Glimpse at Chemistry Here and Abroad." Having traveled extensively throughout Europe during the past two years, Professor Jones discussed some interesting comparisons of post-war conditions. He stated that the situation in many of the university laboratories, especially outside of Germany, is still disappointing but that it is gradually improving. European research institutions are somewhat more favorably situated. In an address entitled "Valence and the Electronic Theory," Professor W. A. Noyes, of the University of Illinois, reviewed the historical development of valence conceptions, leading up to the modern electronic theory, discussing in this connection his own notable contributions in connection with nitrogen trichloride and hypochlorous acid. As a result of the illness of Dean James Kendall, of New York University, his paper on "Separations by the Ionic-Migration Method" was read by the secretary of the section. In this paper Dean Kendall first told about his attempted separation of isotopes, which has not yet been accomplished. The separation of the constituents of other mixtures has been very successful, however. Among these may be mentioned the rare earths, radium and barium, and the alkaloids. Professor Harry B. Weiser, of Rice Institute, presented a paper entitled "Ionic Antagonisms in Colloid Systems." Through a study of the precipitating action of various electrolytes on inorganic colloids such as arsenic trisulphide and copper ferrocyanide, Professor Weiser has attempted to formulate the mechanism of the antagonistic effect of salt pairs. On the basis of his formulations he has proposed an explanation of the permeability of cell membranes. There were eleven shorter papers, some by members of the Vanderbilt University Medical School. These papers, as well as those presented at the joint session, showed clearly the increasingly close relation between some phases of medical and chemical research.

SECTION D (ASTRONOMY)

Vice-president and chairman, Walter A. Adams; *retiring vice-president,* Robert G. Aitken; *secretary,* Philip Fox, Northwestern University, Evanston, Ill.

(*Report from Philip Fox*)

The American Astronomical Society did not meet with Section D this year, and the attendance at the section session was therefore small. Two very successful sessions were held, however, one jointly with the Tennessee Academy of Science, and the general session of Wednesday evening was arranged by Section D. A report on the preparation of the extension of Burnham's Catalogue of Double Stars was given by Robert G. Aitken. The speaker outlined the form the publication will take, showing sample pages. The manuscript is ready through eight hours of right ascension and funds are available for printing as soon as the work is finished. Dinsmore Alter gave results of the application of correlation periodogram to the analysis of sun-spot data, expressing some doubt of the existence of a true period, but stating that, if such exists, 11.46 years seems to represent it most closely. C. T. Elvey compared the relative intensities of the Green Nebular Lines N_1 and N_2, finding that the intensity ratio of N_1 to N_2 was equal to 2.76, for the cases studied. R. H. Curtiss reported on the Lamont expedition to South Africa. He stated that the Blömfontein station would be ready to start the double star survey on the southern sky early in January. It is with deep regret that we realize that death interceded to prevent Professor W. J. Hussey from completing this great work, which he so effectively planned. A second paper by R. H. Curtiss was a review of the early years of stellar spectroscopy and the growth of the idea of spectral classification. The final paper, by C. C. Wylie, gave an illustrated account of the circumstances connected with the fall and finding of the Tilden Meteorite. (See SCIENCE, November 11, 1927, p. 451.)—The Wednesday afternoon session, held with the Tennessee Academy of Science, was commemorative of Edward Emerson Barnard, perhaps the most illustrious man of science native of Nashville. (See report of Tennessee Academy, in this issue of SCIENCE.)—At the general session Wednesday evening was delivered the address of the retiring vice-president of Section D, on "Edward Emerson Barnard, His Life and Works," by Robert G. Aitken.

SECTION E (GEOLOGY AND GEOGRAPHY)

Vice-president and Chairman, Charles Schuchert; *secretary,* G. R. Mansfield, U. S. Geological Survey, Washington, D. C. With the section met the Association of American Geographers (*president,* M. R. Campbell; *secretary,* Charles C. Colby, University of Chicago), and the National Council of Geography Teachers (*president,* R. G. Buzzard; *secretary,* George J. Miller, State Teachers College, Mankato, Minn.)

(*Reports from G. R. Mansfield, Charles C. Colby and George J. Miller*)

Although the Geological Society of America met at

Cleveland this year, yet the Nashville meeting of Section E brought together an interested group of about forty. A number in attendance at Nashville went later to the Cleveland meeting. Section E joined with the Association of American Geographers in a dinner Wednesday evening and with the American Meteorological Society and the Association of American Geographers in a session Thursday morning. Independent sessions of Section E were held Tuesday morning and afternoon and Wednesday morning. Nineteen papers were presented. Tuesday, the principal day of the meeting, was devoted to a symposium on the Mesozoic-Cenozoic stratigraphy of the Gulf States. At the morning session six state geologists displayed maps of their respective states and described the formations of Mesozoic and Cenozoic age. Professor Charles Schuchert, who presided, gave a paper on the paleogeography of North America during the Triassic and Jurassic, which served as a setting for the afternoon papers. L. W. Stephenson gave two papers, both of which were notable for their clarity and able presentation. The first served as an introduction to the paleontologic group and dealt with the major marine transgressions and regressions and with the structural features of the coastal plain. The second described the Upper Cretaceous or Gulf series and was illustrated by an elaborate correlation chart. A paper by F. B. Plummer and H. J. Plummer on the Midway correlations on the basis of the foraminifera was also noteworthy. It showed how serviceable a close and detailed study of these minute forms may prove in the identification of certain strata or horizons. On Tuesday evening a smoker was held at which the maps used during the symposium were on display and served as the basis of protracted and animated discussion. At the session Wednesday morning Austin F. Rogers contributed a noteworthy mineralogical study of the origin of the brown rock phosphate of Tennessee. C. Wythe Cook showed that the Hornerstown (greensand) marl and the Vincentown sand of New Jersey, long considered as belonging to the Upper Cretaceous, are really of Eocene age. G. R. Mansfield summarized the results of a long program of research by members of the U. S. Geological Survey in the Rocky Mountains of southeastern Idaho. At the joint dinner Wednesday evening Dr. G. H. Ashley delivered the address of the retiring vice-president for Section E, on "Geology and the World at Large." This paper was published in SCIENCE for January 13.

The Association of American Geographers held sessions from Wednesday to Saturday. A most successful feature of this meeting was the field trip on Friday, a field study of the Highland Plain and the Cumberland Plateau, of the Nashville Basin. Each of the two communities studied was traversed by a well-chosen route, by means of automobile buses. A mimeographed log showing the principal characteristics of each area helped very greatly in promoting discussion.—The Association of Geographers joined Section E and the Meteorological Society in a joint symposium Thursday morning, on "Problems of the Mississippi River." The meteorological conditions that cause floods in the river and the régime of the river during last spring's floods were treated in a series of scholarly papers by H. C. Frankenfield, R. M. Williamson, and W. E. Barron (all of the U. S. Weather Bureau), and C. F. Brooks, of Clark University. I. M. Cline, of the New Orleans station of the U. S. Weather Bureau, showed that the floods of last spring were predicted well in advance of their occurrence. William H. Haas, of Northwestern University, pointed out that any lengthening by the enlargement of meanders or by the extension of the "passes" into the Gulf would consequently result in a new and higher base level being imposed on the old, and the levees would have to be raised from time to time indefinitely. Conversely, any shortening of the route by which the river reaches the gulf would automatically bring on a new adjustment, with base level lower than the present, which would practically eliminate the necessity of further levee construction.

The five regular half-day sessions were notable for the general excellence of the papers and for active and discriminating discussion. Taken as an inventory of the trend and progress of American productive scholarship in geography, the papers given at Nashville show that the wave of interest in detailed, quantitative studies of small areas, which appeared a few years ago, is bringing highly meritorious results, and that rapid progress is being made in method and technique, both as to performance in the field and in the presentation of the results of field work. A paper by Preston E. James, of the University of Michigan, on "The Blackstone Valley of Massachusetts and Rhode Island," was particularly noteworthy for the effectiveness of its technique; the paper by Robert S. Platt, of the University of Chicago, on "A Field Study of an Iron Range Community: Republic, Michigan," was remarkable for its closely knit organization; and the contribution of Glenn T. Trewartha, fellow of the Guggenheim Foundation, on "A Regional Study in Eastern Shizuoka Prefecture, Japan," illustrated very well how technique and method devised for work in this country may be efficiently employed in a land where the language barrier presents maximum difficulty. Further evidence of current interest in the study of unit areas was furnished by a report of progress on an experiment in cooperative field work being made by Wallace W. Atwood, W. Elmer Ekblaw, Clarence F. Jones and Charles F. Brooks, all of Clark University.—As in recent years the Association of Geographers joined Section E at the dinner for geologists and geographers. On that occasion was given the retiring vice-presidential address for Section E, by G. H. Ashley, on "Geology and the World at Large," and the presidential address for the Association of American Geographers, by M. R. Campbell, on "Geographic Terminology." Dr. Ashley's address has appeared in SCIENCE for January 13, 1928.

The Nashville meeting was unusually pleasant. The members were lodged in the comfortable dormitories of the George Peabody College for Teachers and the college cafeteria was kept open for their use. The sessions were held in the Social Religious Building of that institution and each afternoon those in attendance were the guests at tea of the department of geography.—The officers for 1928 are: *President,* Douglas W. Johnson, Columbia University; *vice-president,* W. L. G. Joerg, American Geographical Society; *secretary,* Chas. C. Colby, University of Chicago; *treasurer,* V. C. Finch, University of Wisconsin.

The National Council of Geography Teachers met on Tuesday and Wednesday, with a program that presented two distinctive features in the field of educational geography. Organizing geographical courses in teacher-training institutions was the theme of the first session, with special reference to the problem of giving adequate training in subject-matter, at the same time retaining a professional viewpoint. A summary of this important discussion will appear in the *Journal of Geography.* Another important topic was the significance of field studies in teacher training. The presidential address, by R. G. Buzzard, of the Illinois State Normal University, Normal, Ill., dealt with this phase of the work. Systematic field study is now being done in a number of the teachers' colleges of the country and plans for expansion are being matured. Mr. L. O. Packard, of the Teachers College of the City of Boston, was elected president for the ensuing year.

SECTION F (ZOOLOGICAL SCIENCES)

Vice-president and chairman, C. E. McClung; *retiring vice-president,* Winterton C. Curtis; *secretary,* Geo. T. Hargitt, Syracuse University, Syracuse, N. Y. The following-named organizations met with the section: The American Society of Zoologists (*president,* S. J. Holmes; *secretary,* D. E. Minnich, University of Minnesota, Minneapolis, Minn.), the Entomological Society of America (*president,* F. E. Lutz; *secretary,* J. J. Davis, Purdue University, Lafayette, Ind.), the American Association of Economic Entomologists (*president,* R. W. Harned; *secretary,* C. W. Collins, Melrose Highlands, Mass.), the American Society of Parasitologists (*president,* R. P. Strong; *secretary,* W. W. Cort, the Johns Hopkins University, School of Hygiene and Public Health, Baltimore, Md.) and the Wilson Ornithological Club (*president,* Lynds Jones; *secretary,* Howard K. Gloyd, Kansas State College, Manhattan, Kan.).

(*Reports from Geo. T. Hargitt, D. E. Minnich, J. J. Davis, C. W. Collins and W. W. Cort*)

A very successful and enthusiastic meeting of the many groups of zoologists associated with Section F was held at Nashville. The sessions were in rooms of the new Medical School of Vanderbilt University and thanks are due those who made the very satisfactory arrangements, as well as to the Medical School. Many papers were presented by informal demonstration rather than by formal reading, a method which added greatly to the interest and value of the contributions. All papers contributed by members of Section F were placed in the program of the American Society of Zoologists. Professor Winterton C. Curtis, of the University of Missouri, the retiring vice-president for the section, gave his retiring vice-presidential address, entitled "Old Problems and a New Technique," at the zoological dinner Thursday evening. He reviewed the older methods of investigation and pointed out their advantages and limitations. He then outlined the newer method and technique of irradiation by X-rays, showing the delicacy and specificity of this technique. The opinion was expressed that this newer approach offered a far more delicate method for the analysis of biological factors and a more promising field of experimentation than are offered by any of the older methods. This interesting and valuable address is to be printed in SCIENCE.

The American Society of Zoologists held sessions for the formal reading of papers on Wednesday, Thursday and Friday mornings and Thursday afternoon. Forty-five papers were read, exclusive of those on joint programs. These were distributed as follows: general and comparative physiology, 30; protozoology, 2; comparative anatomy, 4; cytology, 4; embryology, 5. The sessions were well attended, the attendance frequently running well over one hundred. On Wednesday afternoon the program was given over to informal demonstrations and exhibits, about thirty papers being presented in this manner. This session was particularly successful, as attested by large attendance and enthusiastic comments. On Wednesday evening a large group attended the Biological Smoker, which was held in the Alumni Memorial Building of Vanderbilt University. The program closed at noon on Friday.

The Entomological Society of America held its twenty-second annual meeting on Tuesday and Wednesday, twenty-five unusually interesting papers being presented. One afternoon was devoted to an interesting symposium on "The Physiology of Insects." The papers on the general program dealt with every phase of entomology. R. H. Painter, of Kansas State Agricultural College, gave the results of a study of the method and nature of chinch bug feeding punctures and showed the relation of this study to the problem of resistant and susceptible varieties of plants. T. J. Headlee, of the New Jersey Agricultural Experiment Station, showed the practical possibilities of using the thermal constant in timing spray treatments for the codling moth. R. W. Leiby, of the North Carolina State Department of Agriculture, reported the structure of the intestine of the cotton boll-weevil and the abnormal pathology of cells of the intestine following feeding upon cotton foliage dusted with calcium arsenate. C. H. Kennedy, of Ohio State University, gave interesting results of a study of the origin and dispersal of the strong-flying, river dragon-flies (Macromia), presenting evidence that these dragon-flies originate in the Mississippi Valley and spread through Alaska and into Asia, Europe, Australia and South Africa.—The annual public address of the society was given this year by Dr. H. T. Fernald, of Massachusetts Agricultural College, on "Insects, the People and the State." The meetings were well attended, with from sixty to one hundred or more present at each session. Officers for the coming year were elected as follows: *President*, E. O. Essig; *secretary-treasurer*, J. J. Davis, Purdue University, Lafayette, Indiana.

The American Association of Economic Entomologists met from Tuesday to Friday, attendance being unexpectedly good, with more than two hundred present.—At the meeting of the Section of Plant Quarantine and Inspection (*chairman*, J. H. Montgomery; *secretary*, W. B. Wood) S. B. Fracker, of Washington, D. C., acted as secretary in the absence of Mr. Wood. In his address as chairman, J. H. Montgomery emphasized the importance of quarantine activities. Reports of the Central, Southern and Western Plant Boards and of the National Plant Board showed these organizations to be functioning in the direction of increased efficiency and uniformity. Introducing a symposium on the activities of the Federal Horticultural Board, Dr. C. L. Marlatt described "Recent Developments in Federal Plant Quarantine Work," emphasizing the control operations against the Mexican fruit-worm and the cotton pink-bollworm. Other papers dealt with the pink-bollworm and the Thurberia weevil, Narcissus inspection, the Mexican fruitworm, Pacific port inspection and pear-blight eradication. After a round-table discussion, during which developments in the Japanese-beetle and gipsy-moth problems were discussed informally, L. S. McLaine was elected chairman and S. B. Fracker secretary for 1928.—The Section of Apiculture (*chairman*, F. E. Millen; *secretary*, G. M. Bentley, Knoxville, Tenn.) held its session Tuesday afternoon and evening. No session of this section has ever been more successful in either interest or attendance. The chairman of this section for 1928 is H. F. Wilson and E. N. Cory (College Park, Md.) is secretary.—The Cotton States Branch held a joint session with the main organization Thursday afternoon, at which papers dealing with entomological problems in the South, including those related to the cotton boll-weevil, were presented. The general program opened Wednesday afternoon, with a business session. Reports of various committees were read, these being followed by the address of President R. W. Harned, entitled "Entomology in the Southern States." The speaker gave a most interesting compilation of the development of entomology in the South, showing that interest in entomology in those states ranks almost as high as California and some of the more populous Eastern states. There were six papers on the European corn-borer, which attracted much attention, with lively discussion following their presentation. There was a symposium on insecticides, where four entomologists reviewed briefly the development in this field to date. Nine papers under the heading "Insecticides and Appliances" were read, which covered in a large measure the interesting developments of the past year in this field. Two outstanding papers were presented at this session on "The Preparation of a Special Light Sodium Fluosilicate" and on "The Preparation of Special Calcium Arsenates containing less than 40 per cent. of Arsenic as As_2O_5," and the uses of these materials as boll-weevil poisons, by Captain H. W. Walker, of the Chemical Warfare Service. There were discussions of entomological problems related to truck, cereal, forage and field crops, forest and shade trees and ornamental plants, deciduous fruits, bulbs, greenhouse crops and tropical and sub-tropical plants. New data were presented on the codling moth. On Wednesday evening the seventh annual entomologists' dinner was held in honor of Dr. L. O. Howard, for thirty-three years chief of the U. S. Bureau of Entomology. Two hundred and forty-nine members and guests attended this dinner. Dr. H. A. Morgan, president of the University of Tennessee, acted as toastmaster. The occasion was one of the most pleasing that the Entomological Association has enjoyed at its annual conventions. Dr. C. L. Marlatt, the present chief of the U. S. Bureau of Entomology, paid tribute to the work of Dr. Howard and Dr. Howard responded in a most fitting manner, also showing many slides and giving sidelights on his contacts with European entomologists. Dr. F. E. Lutz spoke on "Unapplied Entomology." Entertainment was furnished by local talent. The Extension Entomologists and Insect Pest Survey held a meeting Tuesday evening at the Hotel Hermitage, which was well attended. Professor W. B. Herms, of the University of California, was elected president; J. E. Graf, of the U. S. Bureau of Entomology, was elected vice-president and C. W. Collins (Melrose Highlands, Mass.) continues as secretary of the association.

The American Society of Parasitologists held its third annual meeting from Tuesday to Friday, with about fifty members present. One of the outstanding features of the program was the address of the retiring president, Dr. R. P. Strong, entitled "Some Parasitic Infections Observed in Equatorial Africa during 1926 and 1927." Dr. Strong gave a survey of some of the findings of his African expedition. In addition to the contributed papers, a symposium on the teaching of parasitology and a program of invited papers on medical parasitology were held. Great interest in teaching problems was in evidence. The discussion brought out the fact that one of the greatest needs of teachers of this subject is more adequate information on methods of obtaining material, and a very large number of practical suggestions along this line were brought out both in the papers themselves and in the discussion.

The invited papers on medical parasitology were of unusual interest. J. F. Kessel reported experiments in which he was able to infect various animals with certain of the intestinal protozoa of man, and suggested that host specificity is not as rigid in many parasitic protozoa as has been usually believed. P. D. Lamson, of the Medical School of Vanderbilt University, summed up the recent advances made by his group on carbon-tetrachloride poisoning, including the extremely important finding that the toxicity of this drug is related in a definite way to calcium deficiency. A. C. Chandler gave an illuminating analysis of the methods and results of his recent epidemiologic studies on hookworm disease in India, in which it has been shown that in only a few places is the intensity of the infestation with hookworm sufficient to make this disease a real public-health problem.

For the first time a number of the papers on the contributed program were presented by demonstrations, which proved to be very successful. An extensive demonstration on creeping eruption, a disease produced by the wanderings of the larvae of the canine hookworm (*Ancylostoma braziliensis*) in the human skin, was given by W. E. Dove and attracted a great deal of attention. The demonstration period gave an opportunity for a social hour, at which tea was served. A total of forty-five contributed papers were listed on the program, fourteen in protozoology, twenty-three in helminthology, four in medical entomology and four in general parasitology. More than half of the papers were related to parasites of man or of domesticated animals. An unusually large number of interesting and important contributions were made, only a very few of which can be mentioned here. There were three papers by G. W. Hunter, L. J. Thomas and H. E. Essex, respectively, which gave important new light on tapeworm life cycles. In two papers L. R. Cleveland first showed how to separate a trichinomonas of man from bacteria and then gave results of experiments on its growth in pure cultures of various microorganisms. These studies appear to open up a new field of possibilities in cultural studies of parasitic protozoa. In a very interesting and challenging paper on "The Economic Importance of Veterinary Parasitology," M. C. Hall pointed out how tremendous is the economic loss due to parasites of domesticated animals. Abstracts of the contributed papers appeared in the December number of the *Journal of Parasitology,* sent to all the members of the society. The following officers were elected for 1928: *President,* C. A. Kofoid; *vice-president,* R. W. Hegner; *secretary-treasurer,* W. W. Cort.

The Wilson Ornithological Club met with the section, but no report of its sessions has been received.

SECTION G (BOTANICAL SCIENCES)

Vice-president and chairman, William Crocker; *retiring vice-president,* Benjamin M. Duggar; *secretary,* Sam F. Trelease, Columbia University, New York City. The following named organizations met with the section: The Botanical Society of America (*president,* H. H. Bartlett; *secretary,* Arthur J. Eames, Cornell University, Ithaca, N. Y.), the American Phytopathological Society (*president,* M. F. Barrus; *secretary,* R. J. Haskell, U. S. Bureau of Plant Industry, Washington, D. C.) and the American Society of Plant Physiologists (*president,* Charles A. Shull; *secretary,* Scott V. Eaton, University of Chicago, Chicago, Ill.).

(*Reports from Sam F. Trelease, Arthur J. Eames, Paul B. Sears, C. W. Dodge, S. C. Brooks, F. J. Schneiderhan, J. F. Adams and Scott V. Eaton*)

As in recent years, Section G arranged a single session of invited papers of general interest, held jointly with its constituent societies on Wednesday afternoon. Dr. B. M. Duggar gave the vice-presidential address on "Recent Viewpoints and Evidence tending to characterize the Agencies of Typical Mosaics." Dr. Chas. F. Hottes spoke on "Chromidia in Plant Cells." (These are fragments of chromatin lying freely in the cell, not massed into a nucleus.) Dr. W. W. Lepeschkin read a paper on "The Effect of Alcohol on the Turgor Pressure of Spirogyra." Dr. E. C. Stakman spoke on "Epidemiology of *Puccinia graminis*." Dr. A. B. Stout read an address on "Dichogamy in Flowering Plants." These were all very valuable contributions, but inadequate space prevents giving more than their titles here.

The Botanical Society of America, with a registered attendance of 218, held a successful meeting from December 27 to 31. The usual dinner for all botanists was held jointly with the American Society of Naturalists. The retiring president of the Botanical Society, L. H. Bailey, was unfortunately prevented by illness from delivering the presidential address, and President H. H. Bartlett related some of his experiences while living and collecting in Sumatra during the past year. President-Elect A. H. R. Buller spoke briefly.—Officers of the Botanical Society were elected as follows: *President,* A. H. Reginald Buller; *vice-president,* Irving W. Bailey; *council representatives,* H. H. Bartlett and I. F. Lewis; *corresponding members,* Abbé G. Bresadola, S. Ikeno, C. H. Ostenfeld, O. Rosenberg and R. von Wettstein. The following paragraphs summarize the reports of the four sections of the Botanical Society:

The General Section (*chairman,* G. P. Burns; *secretary,* Paul B. Sears) met on Wednesday, Thursday and Friday, with well-attended sessions and a program of twenty-six papers. Researches were reported in both descriptive and experimental morphology, and in cytology, genetics, physiology, paleobotany, taxonomy, ecology and technique. One session was devoted to a discussion of the teaching of botany. Of outstanding interest was the presentation of points of view that are being developed in the teaching of general botany at Chicago, Missouri and Wellesley. Gilbert M. Smith was elected *chairman,* and Paul B. Sears, *secretary* for the ensuing year.

The Mycological Section (*chairman,* W. C. Coker; *secretary,* C. W. Dodge) held two sessions with papers on cytological, morphological and physiological researches on fungi. The first session was devoted to general papers and phycomycetes. C. L. Porter reported on the effect of varying hydrogen-ion concentration and temperature upon a large number of pathogenic fungi. W. C. Coker discussed the occurrence of a large number of water-moulds in the soil. At the second session, W. J. Bach and F. A. Wolf discussed the cause of Citrus melanose. H. H. Whetzel discussed in great detail the relationships between fungi of the *Botrytis cinerea* group and Sclerotinia. C. W. Dodge discussed the morphology, phylogeny and taxonomy of the higher Plectascales. Structures resembling sexual organs were reported for Mesophellia and the systematic position of this genus was definitely determined as in the Ascomycetes instead of the Basidiomycetes. J. N. Couch discussed the structure and development of tropical species of Septobasidium, reporting germination of basidiospores.—At the joint session of the Mycological Section of the Botanical Society with the American Phytopathological Society, A. H. R. Buller discussed the growth of the mycelium of *Armillaria mellea* in relation to luminosity. J. H. Craigie reported an investigation upon sex in the rusts, in which it was found that *Puccinia graminis* is heterothallic. (See report of Phytopathological Society, below.) J. J. Taubenhaus and L. J. Pessin discussed the hydrogen-ion toleration of *Phymatotrichum omnivorum* in relation to possible control of this disease. B. O. Dodge reported on the morphology and cytology of fertile hybrid perithecia from crossing *Neurospora sitophila* and *N. tetrasperma.*

The Physiological Section (*chairman,* C. O. Appleman; *secretary-treasurer,* S. C. Brooks) held three scientific sessions, of which one was a round-table discussion on "Mineral Nutrition," and two were for the reading of twenty-five original papers. Paper mulch, by maintaining superior soil conditions and controlling weeds, will perhaps lead to radical changes in truck-crop cultivation. Lewis H. Flint reported on several years of field trials of paper mulch, with gratifying increases in yield. Adelia McCrea reported significant increases in both yield and drug potency of *Digitalis purpurea,* which in the seed bed had been grown under a special glass transmitting sunlight ultra-violet. Eloise Gerry described the effects of fire on wood structure and on yield of resin in long-leaf pine and also reported preliminary studies on the production of heptane by *Pinus Jeffreyi.*—On the theoretical side, a paper by D. T. MacDougal, J. B. Overton and G. M. Smith presented evidence for the existence in woody stems of continuous vascular air connections, and provoked much discussion of both methods and conclusions. The discussion was further stimulated by A. F. Hemenway's paper on the rate of sap flow in desert plants, as measured by the spread of introduced dyes. O. L. Sponsler and W. H. Dore explained, with the aid of space models, the arrangement of atoms and molecules in ramie cellulose, and the train of argument by which the structure of the individual C_6 units and their relative positions were deduced. W. E. Burge and collaborators showed that the intake of dextrose, levulose and galactose by Spirogyra is parallel to the utilization of these substances by Paramoecium and higher animals, in that it is increased by insulin and by optically active as opposed to optically inactive amino-acids.—The round-table discussion of mineral nutrition was introduced by D. R. Hoagland, and various phases of the subject were treated by J. S. McHargue, E. S. Johnston, F. W. Parker, W. J. Robbins, W. E. Tottingham and S. C. Brooks. Spirited discussion ensued, centering particularly about the effects of boron, the effects of light and the definition of terms.

The Systematic Section (*chairman,* C. C. Deam; *secretary,* F. T. McFarland) held two sessions. The Wednesday morning session was given over to the reading of six papers dealing with problems of classification, distribution and education in taxonomy. The Thursday morning session was taken up by an informal discussion of the flora of the Mississippi Valley.

The American Phytopathological Society held its eighteenth annual meeting from Tuesday to Friday. The attendance was about 175 and the arrangements were the best in recent years. It was generally remarked that the small daylight screen used this year for slide projection was quite unsatisfactory to a large part of the audience; larger screens are greatly needed.—Sixty-five new members were added to the roll, the total membership being now 750. Officers for 1928 were elected as follows: *President,* H. P. Barss; *vice-president,* F. D. Heald; *councilor,* F. D. Fromme. —The program contained ninety papers, twenty-nine more than last year's program. Four were given in joint session with Section G and twelve with the Mycological Section of the Botanical Society. The remaining papers may be classified according to subjects, as follows: crown gall, 10; potato and vegetable diseases, 11; cereal and forage diseases, 11; fruit diseases, 9; tobacco diseases, 8; mosaic diseases, 8; diseases of ornamentals, 7; sweet-potato diseases, 3, and miscellaneous papers given before the Southern Division of the Society, 7.—The dinner was attended by 169 persons. The principal speaker was Watson Davis, of Science Service. A quartette of typical Tennessee darkies crooned soft southern melodies and negro spirituals in a most effective manner, giving a background of unflagging interest. The reincarnation of Charles Darwin, in the person of F. D. Fromme, in a haunted atmosphere with a metaphysical accent, was another feature of the dinner. The dinner program was shorter and better than usual, an innovation that was greatly approved.

The causes and control of overgrowths and hairy root in nursery stock were dealt with by seven speakers. Wound overgrowth and crown gall of apple occurring in England, France and Holland were reported on by A. J. Riker.—Francis O. Holmes discussed technique for comparing various concentrations of tobacco-mosaic virus.—The importance of strict sanitation in propagating tobacco, for the control of true tobacco mosaic, was emphasized by W. D. Valleau and E. M. Johnson.—Tobacco ringspot was shown to be a virus capable of infecting a wide range of plants, by S. A. Wingard and F. D. Fromme, who succeeded in infecting plants of nineteen genera, representing eleven families.—Treating undelinted cotton seed with fungicidal dusts was reported to be economical by N. C. Woodroof.—C. R. Orton discussed the effect of disinfectants on the germination of seeds kept in storage for indefinite periods, reporting that the organic mercury dusts did not decrease germination, but increased it in many cases after storage periods of from one to three years.—The effectiveness of organic and inorganic mercury compounds for the control of large and small brown-patch of turf have again been confirmed by the studies of John Monteith, Jr., and A. S. Dahl.—New physiologic forms of *Tilletia tritici* may be the explanation for the gradual increase of the wheat disease in America, especially in Kansas, Virginia and Pennsylvania, according to E. G. Gaines.—Two new dust treatments for oat smuts were reported by J. D. Sayre and R. C. Thomas. The fungicidal base used was formaldehyde and iodine.—J. Johnson found that the properties of the potato rugose-mosaic virus are quite different from those of certain other potato viruses studied, such as leaf-rolling mosaic and spot necrosis.—S. P. Doolittle and M. N. Walker presented evidence to show that the aphis transmission of cucumber mosaic results from the virus being carried into the plant tissues on the proboscis of the insect and that the minute amount of the virus thus carried is exhausted during the first feeding period.—Further studies on the black root-rot of apple caused by *Xylaria mali* nom. nov., show that the fungus is also actively parasitic on Norway maple and Mahaleb cherry.—E. E. Wilson presented data which further emphasize the relationships of the time of leaf-fall to the maturity of ascospores of *Venturia inaequalis.* Additional studies on certain phases of this important apple disease were presented by G. W. Keitt with E. E. Wilson and J. M. Hamilton.—The toxic constituent of sulphur fungicides, according to H. C. Young and Robert Williams, is pentathionic acid. When sulphur was freed of its pentathionic acid and then placed in Van Tieghem cells it was not toxic to spores of *Sclerotinia cinerea.* A simple test for pentathionic acid was described.

Probably the most noteworthy contribution of the meeting was a paper by J. H. Craigie on the heterothallism of the rust fungi. Investigations of sex in these fungi have shown that *Puccinia graminis* and *P. helianthi* are heterothallic. The sporidia are of two kinds, designated plus and minus. A plus sporidium gives rise to a plus mycelium and a set of pycnia that produce plus pycnospores. A minus sporidium gives rise to a minus mycelium and a set of pycnia that produce minus pycnospores. When a plus and a minus sporidium are sown close together on a leaf, the plus and minus mycelia resulting therefrom intermingle and produce diploid aecia. When plus pycnospores are brought into contact with a minus pycnium, or minus pycnospores with a plus pycnium, diploid aecia are produced, within a few days of transfer, on the under side of the pustule receiving the pycnospores. The pycnium is to be regarded not as a spermagonium, producing non-functional spermatia, but as an active organ which develops either plus or minus pycnospores and attracts flies, by means of which pycnospores of one sex are carried to pycnia of another sex.

The American Society of Plant Physiologists met from December 27 to 30. A dinner for all plant physiologists was held Wednesday evening, at the Chamber of Commerce, in commemoration of the 250th anniversary of the birth of Stephen Hales. President Charles A. Shull delivered a very interesting address at that time, on the life and work of Hales, with illustrations by means of lantern slides taken from Hales's famous book, "Vegetable Staticks." Dr. Burton E. Livingston followed with an address announcing the establishment of the Stephen Hales Prize Fund by the society. He emphasized the importance of this, the first fund to be established for a prize in plant physiology. The first award of the Stephen Hales Prize is to be made at the New York meeting next December. Finally, the election of the second Charles Reid Barnes Life Member of the American Society of Plant Physiologists was announced by Professor F. M. Andrews, chairman of the committee on that honorary membership. This honor is conferred for outstanding research in plant physiology. It was this year conferred on Professor F. E. Lloyd, of McGill University, Montreal.—Reports of committees at the business meetings indicated encouraging progress in many directions. President Shull called attention to the present excellent financial condition of *Plant Physiology* (the official journal of the society), which is already established as successful in every way. A unanimous vote of thanks was extended by the society to President Shull for his indefatigable efforts on behalf of the society since its organization. Dr. S. V. Eaton, secretary of the society, reported a large increase in membership during the year.—For the first time, arrangements were successfully made this year by which conflicts were completely avoided between the sessions of the Society of Plant Physiologists and those of the Physiological Section of the Botanical Society, to the great gratification of all.

The papers presented at Nashville were varied and generally of great excellence. F. M. Andrews, of Indiana University, described the opening of crocus and tulip flowers in response to temperature increase of a single degree or less.—W. E. Tottingham and H. Lowsma, of the University of Wisconsin, reported that chemical analyses of wheat plants, grown respectively in red-yellow, green-violet and ultra-violet light, showed highest nitrate assimilation and protein synthesis in the green-violet region.—Charles A. Shull, of the University of Chicago, described a quantitative study of the reflection of light from leaf surfaces. Reflection was found to be most complete for green light and low for red and blue light.—J. D. Sayre, of Ohio State University, found that light of wave-length greater than 680 $\mu\mu$ was ineffective in chlorophyll formation in many species of crop plants. —D. R. Hoagland, A. R. Davis and P. L. Hibbard, of the University of California, discussed the influence of one ion on the absorption of another by Nitella in dilute solutions.—S. Dunn and A. L. Bakke, of Iowa State College, showed that the amount of dye taken up by the wood of different species could not generally be directly correlated with their known hardiness.

The joint session of the society with Section G and the other affiliated societies is reported elsewhere. The valuable and spirited discussion before the Physiological Section of the Botanical Society on Thursday morning, on the mineral nutrition of plants, was followed in the afternoon by an equally interesting symposium before the Society of Plant Physiologists, on "What Needs to be Done Next in Plant Physiology?" C. B. Lipman, of the University of California, in a paper read by D. R. Hoagland, emphasized, among other things, a need for reform in the teaching of botany in laboratory and classroom. B. E. Livingston, of the Johns Hopkins University, drew attention to the present need for studies on the plant as a whole, especially in relation to its environment, and the need for further data on the interrelation of influential conditions, their mutual effects and their ranges of influence. D. T. MacDougal, of the Carnegie Institution of Washington, emphasized the great present need for work on photosynthesis, permeability, the dynamics of colloids and environmental influences on growth. E. J. Kraus, of the University of Chicago, urged that more attempts be made to correlate as yet isolated biological phenomena and pleaded for greater mutual understanding among physiological workers as well as for unremitting efforts in all phases of research.

At the final session on Friday morning occurred the first public showing of a motion-picture film on the "Physiology of Gametes in the Conjugatae," by F. E. Lloyd, of McGill University. This film vividly portrayed great activity in the protoplasm of conjugating cells and demonstrated the importance of vacuoles in the process.—A. R. Davis and D. R. Hoagland, of the University of California, described a simple apparatus for controlling the atmospheric environment of plants grown in culture solutions. It was found possible to predict plant yields and to duplicate results. —A progress report on chemical composition in relation to growth and reproductive responses in apple trees was made by Walter Thomas, of Pennsylvania State College, in which certain deficiency indices were described.—F. T. McLean and B. E. Gilbert, of Rhode Island Agricultural Experiment Station, presented results of studies on aluminum toxicity.—G. J. Peirce, of Stanford University, presented further observations on the behavior of algae found in brines, suggesting that these organisms may possibly be regarded as indicators of molecular drift toward regions of crystallization.—Moisture content, foliar transpiring power, and wilting, in relation to curing of hay, were described by A. L. Bakke and E. R. Henson, of Iowa State College, who found that differences between hay cured in the windrow and in the swath were smallest when the evaporation conditions were most intense.—H. L. Van de Sande-Bakhuyzen, of Stanford University, outlined a new theory of growth, permeability and correlation, based principally on hydration phenomena.

ORGANIZATIONS RELATED TO BOTH SECTIONS F AND G

(*Reports from E. W. Sinnott, George D. Fuller, H. J. Van Cleave, L. C. Dunn and Elmer Roberts*)

The American Society of Naturalists (*president*, C. E. McClung; *secretary*, L. J. Cole, University of Wisconsin, Madison, Wisconsin) presented on Friday afternoon a symposium on "Temperature and Life." The speakers emphasized not only the great importance of temperature in all vital activities but also the complexities of its various effects and the many difficulties which confront the physiologist in separating the influence of temperature from those of other factors in the environment. The speakers were as follows: M. H. Jacobs, Royal N. Chapman, James G. Dickson, Chas. F. Hottes and H. L. Shantz. The annual dinner of the society was held jointly with the Botanical Society of America on Friday evening.

The Ecological Society of America (*president*, C. Juday; *secretary*, A. O. Weese, University of Oklahoma, Norman, Okla.) met on Wednesday, Thursday and Friday. There were three general sessions, an invitation program in charge of the president of the society, and joint sessions with the Botanical Society and with the Society of Zoologists. Business sessions were also held daily and an informal dinner was held on Wednesday evening. The presidential address was given by Dr. Juday, at the morning session on Thursday. It was entitled "Chemical and Biological Studies of Some Lakes in Northwestern Wisconsin." A notable feature of the meeting was an invitation program Wednesday afternoon, consisting of seven papers. Four of these dealt with the inter-reactions of various classes of organisms. S. A. Waksman discussed the question of "Forest Humus, a Problem in Soil Microbiology." Elias Melin reviewed the present state of our knowledge of the "Mycorrhizal Fungi of Forest Soils and Their Relation to Tree Growth." The ecological relations of the root systems of forest trees were also discussed in papers by W. B. McDougall and J. E. Weaver. "The Present Status of Our Knowledge of the Ecology of Protozoa of the Soil" was presented by C. E. Skinner and the "Bioecology of Forest and Range" was dealt with in a paper by Walter P. Taylor and W. C. McGinnies. A. G. Vestal discussed the "Forest of the San Francisco Region in Relation to Chaparral and Grassland," and G. A. Pearson's paper was on the "Measurement of Physical Factors as an Aid to Silviculture."—The society confirmed the action of its president and his associates in forming the Ecological Society of America, Incorporated, under the laws of the State of Wisconsin. Simultaneously with incorporation a new class of membership was established, "Sustaining Members," whose dues are $10.00 per year. The extra funds obtained from such memberships are to be used in the publication of the results of research. The following officers were elected: *President*, H. L. Shantz; *secretary-treasurer*, A. O. Weese, University of Oklahoma, Norman, Okla.

The American Microscopical Society (*president*, Z. P. Metcalf; *secretary*, H. J. Van Cleave, University of Illinois, Urbana, Illinois) held its forty-sixth annual meeting on Wednesday. The following officers were elected: *President*, P. S. Welch; *secretary*, H. J. Van Cleave. The custodian of the Spencer-Tolles Fund, Professor Henry B. Ward, reported that the fund now has properties valued at more than $12,500. Grants from this fund for the encouragement and support of original investigations are available to members of the society. The report of the treasurer shows a balance of $1,378.90 in the general fund. The secretary called attention to the fact that sixty new members have been admitted during the year, approximately two hundred having been added during the three years of his term of office.

The Genetics Sections of the American Society of Zoologists and the Botanical Society of America (*chairman,* R. A. Emerson; *secretary-treasurer,* L. C. Dunn, Storrs, Conn.) held well attended sessions on Wednesday, Thursday and Friday. The reading of papers occupied three mornings, one afternoon was devoted to demonstrations and on one afternoon the sections met jointly with the Geneticists Interested in Agriculture for a symposium on "Irregularities of Chromosome Behavior in Relation to Plant and Animal Improvement." Forty contributions were offered, twenty-four of them being read at the formal sessions.—Five of the papers read, one of the demonstrations and one of the papers given by title only, dealt with the effect of X-rays on plants and animals. Chief interest centered in the recent attempts to alter the course of inheritance and the frequency of mutation by treatment with X-rays. The most extensive experiments on this question were reported in detail by H. J. Muller, whose paper (for which the American Association Prize was awarded this year) is abstracted in the section on the Prize. By use of a special technique for measuring the frequency of mutations in *Drosophila melanogaster* he obtained results indicating that the application of sublethal doses of X-rays to sperm was followed by a large increase in the mutation rate of treated, as compared with control, cultures. The mutation rate in some treated cultures was estimated at 15,000 times the normal rate. F. B. Hanson, working in Dr. Muller's laboratory at the University of Texas, reported on the direct effect of X-rays on the productivity and sex ratios of Drosophila and reported also the appearance of many mutations in the X-rayed cultures. From the botanical side L. J. Stadler reported on the occurrence of new endosperm characters that apparently had arisen by mutation in maize ears X-rayed at the time of fertilization. The same investigator presented evidence for the occurrence of mutations in seedlings from treated barley seeds. T. H. Goodspeed and A. R. Olson reported that many variant types had been found in the progeny of X-rayed Nicotiana plants, and gave evidence of a considerable degree of chromosome irregularity following the treatment.—A direct effect of X-rays on colored mice was reported by R. T. Hance.—Four papers dealt with disease resistance. Two showed the inheritance of resistance to specific diseases in chickens.—C. H. Danforth reported that skin grafted from one young chicken to another assumed during growth the characters of the donor in respect to feather color and pattern but assumed the characters of the host in respect to sex and growth rate.—The following officers were elected for 1928: *Chairman,* H. J. Muller; *society representative,* O. E. White.

The Geneticists Interested in Agriculture held their eighth annual meeting jointly with the Genetics Sections of the Botanical Society and the Society of Zoologists on Thursday afternoon, with about one hundred and twenty-five persons in attendance. The program consisted of a symposium on "Irregularities of Chromosome Behavior in Relation to Plant and Animal Improvement," and a talk by Dr. L. C. Dunn on "Genetics in Europe." A. F. Blakeslee discussed irregularities of chromosome behavior in plants, drawing largely upon his work with Datura and pointing out that in many forms various combinations may be produced by breeding and preserved by vegetative reproduction. H. J. Muller emphasized the fact that most of the causes of irregularities in animals were either lethal in effect or produced sterility or other abnormal conditions; consequently little opportunity for animal improvement could be expected from this source. Following the symposium L. C. Dunn spoke briefly of research in genetics in Great Britain, Germany and Russia. Dr. C. M. Woodworth, of the Illinois Experiment Station, Urbana, Ill., was elected chairman.

SECTION H (ANTHROPOLOGY)

Vice-president and chairman, R. J. Terry; *retiring vice-president,* R. Bennett Bean; *secretary,* Fay-Cooper Cole, University of Chicago, Chicago, Ill.

(*Report from Fay-Cooper Cole*)

Section H held its sessions on Tuesday, Wednesday and Thursday. Since the Anthropological Association was holding its sessions elsewhere the attendance was small, but interest was keen and ample time was allowed for the discussion of papers. The first day was given over to problems relating to individual and race changes, which are of equal interest to physical anthropologists and students of the social sciences. A way must be devised to take the place of laboratory methods used in general biology. Investigations carried on in families which make up the various groups under question was favored.—The second day was devoted to archeology. Among the papers read, that dealing with the excavations of Beloit College in Northern Africa was of special interest. The sites excavated indicate an extensive culture of Aurignacian date, while the skeletal material appears to show a type of mankind varying somewhat from the dominant groups in Europe at that time. A lively discussion followed the presentation of evidence of three finds of relics of man associated with remains of Pleistocene mammalia by Dr. Oliver Hay.—On Thursday the members of the section were conducted, by Professor P. E. Cox, state archeologist of Tennessee, to an extensive series of Indian mounds about thirty miles from Nashville. The anthropology dinner was held Tuesday evening.

SECTION I (PSYCHOLOGY)

Vice-president and chairman, Knight Dunlap; *retiring vice-president,* Margaret Floy Washburn; *secretary,* Frank N. Freeman, University of Chicago, Chicago, Ill.

(*Report from Frank N. Freeman*)

An important feature of the program of Section I at the Nashville meeting was a joint session with the Southern Society for Philosophy and Psychology. This society holds its regular annual meeting in the spring, but this year it joined officially with Section I for one session. Several papers were contributed by members of the Southern Society and the session at which they were given was perhaps the most interesting of the meeting.—According to custom, Section I joined with Section Q for one session.—In her retiring vice-presidential address Dr. Margaret Floy Washburn presented an able argument in support of the mechanistic conception of animal behavior as contrasted with the vitalistic theory of emergent evolution. Dr. Washburn's address has appeared in SCIENCE for January 13.—The chairman of the section for the next year is Dr. H. C. Warren, and the newly elected section committeeman is Dr. M. Bentley.

SECTION K (SOCIAL AND ECONOMIC SCIENCES)

Vice-president and chairman, W. S. Leathers; *retiring vice-president,* Joseph H. Willits. The Metric Association (*president,* George F. Kunz; *secretary,* Howard Richards, 156 Fifth Ave., New York City) is the only one of the associated organizations that took part in the Nashville meeting.

(*Report from Howard Richards*)

Section K held no sessions at Nashville. It is hoped that some of the associated societies of this section will hold sessions or contribute programs for the great New York meeting next year. While it seems to be clear that the natural and exact sciences (which virtually make up the field of the American Association at present) and the social and economic sciences have very much in common and that these two groups of investigators have much to gain from some contact with each other, yet it is not generally customary for the two groups to meet at the same time and place. It follows that the session of this section in recent years have not generally enjoyed the atmosphere of research and discussion that characterizes the sessions of most of the other sections. The association is hopeful that workers in the social and economic sciences may be willing to join with it, at least at some annual meetings, in order that the research aspect of these great and important lines of study may from time to time be adequately represented along with the natural and exact sciences. The executive committee of the association will be glad to receive the benefit of suggestions from men of science who are interested in this general project, which is as important as it seems to be difficult.

The Metric Association held its eleventh anniversary meeting on Thursday, with an industrial conference in the morning and an engineers' conference and an educational conference in the afternoon. There were also a Weight and Measure Luncheon and the usual Metric Dinner. Seven metric advocates of Nashville institutions made a strong showing. A steady trend toward complete metric usage was reported.

SECTION L (HISTORICAL AND PHILOLOGICAL SCIENCES)

Section L is not yet organized. In recent years special committees on the history of science and on philology or linguistic science have arranged programs for the annual meetings. For the Nashville meeting no program was arranged on the history of science, which is now being adequately developed by the affiliated History of Science Society, and that society did not meet with the association this year. At the request of the executive committee of the association a session on linguistic science was arranged for this meeting by the newly-formed Linguistic Society of America, which is affiliated. A brief report on this session follows:

(*Report from Leonard Bloomfield*)

The session on linguistic science was held Friday afternoon with a small but interested group. Discussion was lively. Professor G. M. Bolling, of Ohio State University, presided. There were two papers on general linguistics. Professor E. Sapir (University of Chicago) reported on an association experiment in which a meaning was arbitrarily assigned to a vocal form, this form then altered by small steps, the observer being asked to state the meanings he associated with the altered forms. The results showed a high correlation between specific changes of form and of meaning. Professor Bolling read a paper discussing the postulate that phonetic laws have no exceptions; he pointed out the origin of the postulate's wording in a dispute of fifty years ago, and showed that under a tenable definition of the terms "law" and "exception" or under a modern rewording, the postulate is necessary for the science of language—a necessity which exemplifies the close connection of linguistics with natural science. Two papers dealt with problems of Algonquian study. Professor Truman Michelson (Bureau of American Ethnology) discussed the historical changes owing to which the

Arapaho language to-day diverges from other Algonquian, and pointed out the importance of the alternation of certain sounds in Central Algonquian. Professor Leonard Bloomfield (University of Chicago) presented certain forms of Swampy Cree which confirm a reconstruction that had hitherto depended on purely theoretical prediction. In the field of Indo-European Professor W. Petersen (University of Florida) discussed the Latin vi-perfect as an example of the irradiation of a formal element. Linguistic borrowing, as exemplified by loans from American English into the Hungarian spoken in America, was discussed in a paper by Professor F. R. Preveden (DePauw University).

SECTION M (ENGINEERING)

Vice-president and chairman, A. N. Talbot; *retiring vice-president,* C. R. Richards; *secretary,* N. H. Heck, U. S. Coast and Geodetic Survey, Washington, D. C.

(*Report from N. H. Heck*)

Section M met on Wednesday. The program of the morning session was arranged by the Engineering Association of Nashville. An afternoon session and a dinner were held jointly with Section C, the dinner being under the auspices of the Engineering Association of Nashville. The morning program included papers dealing with subjects of general interest but with special local appeal.—Wilbur A. Nelson, Virginia state geologist, discussed methods of developing the natural resources of Tennessee. Methods now in use by successful state geological surveys were described and new methods were suggested.—Major John F. Conklin, U. S. A., discussed the power possibilities of the Cumberland drainage area. The paper showed that the development of power will aid in flood control, while, with proper precautions, it will not interfere with the use of the river for navigation.—C. N. Bass, Tennessee highway commissioner, showed that Tennessee, by an improved highway system, has erased sectional lines and greatly aided progress. Travel in the United States by automobile, expressed in passenger miles, was 2.5 times as great in 1926 as by train. The congestion problem leads to much study.—George C. Fischer, Nashville smoke inspector, discussed smoke abatement in Nashville. Abatement of smoke was undertaken in 1926, by education, inspection, instruction and recommendation. The use of coke helped a great deal and the adoption of underfeed stokers with down-draft boilers has been effective.—C. R. Fountain, of the George Peabody College, on behalf of the institute of Radio Engineers, gave a paper on the contribution of radio to engineering. By animated motion pictures he showed the behavior of the electrons in radio tubes, etc., and pointed out that radio is a stimulus to youth to study engineering sciences, this being probably its greatest contribution to engineering.—At the afternoon session the address of the retiring vice-president for Section M, Dr. C. R. Richards, on the functions of Section M, was read in his absence. Section M, it is thought, should attempt to bridge the gap between the engineer and the fundamental scientist, furnishing opportunity for the engineer to voice his scientific needs and announce his achievements in adapting science to industry, and for the scientist to forecast the application of new theories and important discoveries. The publication of the results of such discussions should be provided for in some way and this need is an important problem before the section and the association. The main aim should be to establish a bond of interest and sympathy between engineers and scientists. Discussion followed and the project to make effective some of Dr. Richard's recommendations was referred to the section committee of Section M.—N. H. Heck discussed the earthquake situation in the Mississippi Valley, advancing several theories to account for the occurrence of mid-continental earthquakes, the processes of erosion and sedimentation being given important weight. Since no one knows whether or not a future great earthquake is now preparing, the need for scientific investigation is obvious. The plan of Dr. James B. Macelwane, S. J., for seismograph observations, triangulation and precise levels was described. Engineers should not only support this investigation but should keep in touch with work of the same sort being done elsewhere.—John A. L. Waddell presented a remarkable conception of a proposed national institute, to follow the lines of "L'Institut de France," but on a much larger scale. It was suggested that Section M might initiate action in establishing such an institute. After considerable discussion this matter was referred to the section committee, with instructions to make recommendations at the New York meeting.—Professor Thorndyke Saville, of the University of North Carolina, was unable to attend the meeting but sent a paper, "Water-power Development and the Interconnected Transmission Systems of the Southeast." By means of the most extensive system of interconnected power stations in the world, power may be relayed from Muscle Shoals and other Alabama water-power stations to the Virginia coal fields and steam-power generated at the mines might be sent in the reverse direction. Great additions will be necessary in the near future, about 60 per cent. of which will come from hydroelectric developments, the rest coming from steam plants. Great need for a comprehensive investigation of the hydrographic phenomena of all the streams of this system was pointed out.

The address at the dinner was given by H. F. Moore, of the University of Illinois, on the "Mechanics of Materials: a Contribution of Applied Science to Pure Science." The theory of the mechanical failure of solids and the limits of reliability of the theory of elasticity are being worked out in engineering laboratories, and in the future the development of the mechanics of wave stress will probably be demanded. Intellectual aloofness from practical application and self-satisfied contempt of theory are alike marks of a narrow mind. The highway between pure science and applied science is not a one-way street.

SECTION N (MEDICAL SCIENCES)

Vice-president and chairman, G. Canby Robinson; *retiring vice-president,* Rufus I. Cole; *secretary,* A. J. Goldforb, College of the City of New York, N. Y.

(*Report from A. J. Goldforb*)

The Nashville program of Section N included subjects in anthropology, biochemistry, physiology, medicine, public health, parasitology, pathology and pharmacology. There was a program of invited papers and two joint sessions, with Section C (Chemistry) and with the American Public Health Association.—Dr. Rufus I. Cole, director of the Hospital of the Rockefeller Institute, in his retiring vice-presidential address (see SCIENCE for January 20, page 47) emphasized medical science and the sciences related to it. Dr. Aleš Hrdlička, of the U. S. National Museum, discussed the contributions of anthropology to medicine, and *vice versa.* He urged that a chair of anthropology be established in each medical school.—Dr. E. C. Kendall, of the Mayo Foundation, reviewed the problem of biological oxidations, discussing the contributions of chemists and biologists on this fundamental problem of the internal processes of organisms. He pointed out significant results in this field, the calorigenic relationships, the nature of intermediary metabolism, the influence of food accessories on metabolism, the oxidation influence of hormones, with a running commentary on problems still to be solved.—The recent dramatic development of our knowledge of anemia was reviewed by Dr. G. H. Whipple, of Rochester University Medical School, whose pioneer work led to the discovery of the etiology of pernicious anemia. Grains, vegetables and fish are least effective in stimulating hemoglobin regeneration, while leafy vegetables, meats and certain fruits are more effective. Liver is most effective.—Dr. Alfred F. Hess, of New York University and Bellevue Medical College, outlined the contributions of chemistry, physics and pathology to the solution of the problem of rickets, giving a cogently reasoned analysis of the influence of ultra-violet rays upon bone formation and on chemical substances in the superficial tissues of animals and plants. The effect of such diverse treatments as those of cod-liver oil and light upon normal bone formation were discussed and it was emphasized how specific are the effective wave-lengths and the substances involved and how minute is the quantity that transforms a rachitic animal into a healthy one.

The afternoon session was devoted to important medical problems of particular significance in the South. Colonel A. M. Stimson, of the U. S. Public Health Service, discussed the control of malaria and the extent to which its eradication may be evaluated in terms of money.—Dr. C. C. Bass, of Tulane University Medical School, reviewed the contributions of parasitology to medical science. He outlined cooperative work by workers in these two fields, in the eradication of hookworm, bubonic plague, malaria, etc., and pointed out the necessity of studying the protozoa of the intestine, of the mouth and of the vagina. It was suggested that pellagra may be due not merely to diet deficiencies but to insect hosts as well.—Dr. R. S. Cunningham, of Vanderbilt University Medical School, gave an analysis of tissue reactions to tubercle bacilli.—Dr. E. W. Goodpasture, of Vanderbilt University Medical School, gave the results of a study on a virus disease of poultry, which disclosed bodies that seem to be of great significance in the theory of virus disease in general.

SECTION O (AGRICULTURE)

Vice-president and chairman, L. E. Call; *retiring vice-president,* C. F. Marbut; *secretary,* P. E. Brown, Iowa State College, Ames, Iowa. The American Society of Agronomy contributed to the program of one session and the following named societies associated with the section held sessions of their own: the American Society of Horticultural Science (*president,* E. J. Kraus; *secretary,* C. P. Close, College Park, Md.), the Potato Association of America (*president,* H. C. Moore; *secretary,* Walter M. Peacock, U. S. Department of Agriculture) and the Crop Protection Institute (*chairman,* W. C. O'Kane; *secretary,* Paul Moore, National Research Council, Washington, D. C.).

(*Reports from P. E. Brown, C. P. Close and Paul Moore*)

A joint session with the American Society of Agronomy and the Association of Economic Entomologists dealt with "The Corn-borer Situation." The papers emphasized the need of cooperation in corn-borer research and brought out recent developments in the entomological, agronomic and mechanical aspects of this problem. At the annual dinner of Section O and the associated societies was given the retiring vice-presidential address of Dr. C. F. Marbut, on "A Hitherto Neglected Factor in the Agricultural Situation."

The American Society for Horticultural Science held its annual meeting Tuesday to Thursday, with an attendance that surpassed the record. Some of the points brought out are indicated below. Yields of thirteen or fourteen tons of tomatoes per acre were reported for the varieties Marglobe, Columbia, Norton and Norduke, grown in Indiana.—It was found that the dry-matter content of tomato fruits varied inversely with the soil-moisture content.—Removal of apical buds of young tomato plants delayed production of first fruits about a week. Periodically leaf-pruned tomato plants in soil cultures with a liberal supply of nitrogen showed carbohydrate-nitrogen ratios that varied inversely with severity of pruning which was also true when similar plants were systematically root pruned.—Vitamin A in green asparagus fed to white rats at Michigan State College maintained good health, while rats fed blanched tips lost weight and died.—In Kansas in 1926 and 1927 it was found, with the Worden grape, that there was so little correlation between cane length or cane diameter and crop production that careful selection of canes as to size at time of pruning is not necessary. Peach fruit buds showed negative correlation between length of shoot and carbohydrate content; with high nitrogen content long shoots are produced and carbohydrates are used in growth, but with low nitrogen content little growth occurs and carbohydrates accumulate.—Fall-grown cabbage plants that are to flower in the spring show enlargement of stem apex in fall and winter, the flower-stalk primordium being differentiated about February 1; branches and flowers emerge about April 1.—Sweet-corn varieties with high percentage of translucent endosperm were of higher quality than others; as were also those with low percentage of pericarp and very little starchy endosperm; while high percentage of starchy endosperm is usually associated with low quality.—The haploid chromosome number in pollen mother cells is, in general, 8 for sweet cherries and 16 for sour and Duke varieties; abnormal chromosome behavior is associated with a high degree of pollen sterility in Duke varieties, and to a lesser extent in certain sour varieties. Attention was given to the occurrence of polycary in the microspores of sweet varieties.—Catalase activity of apple blossom buds in autumn varies but little with the vigor of the trees. No direct relationship was found between catalase activity and bud size.—From studies on ether extracts of year-old tissue of mature Jonathan apple trees it was found that the percentage of fat at the tops of shoots increased in April and decreased in early May.—Apple scions grafted on piece roots change the root character to that typical of the scion variety; variability of trees in the nursery row appears to be due principally to the manner in which the grafts were made and to differences in the scions while the use of seedlings as stocks seems to have little influence.—Hardening or blackening of the calyx end of the pear fruit seems related to the root stock used, being most often found on trees propagated on *Pyrus serotima, Pyrus ussuriensis* and Kieffer, but occurring only rarely on *Pyrus communis* or quince stocks.

The Potato Association of America met Wednesday, Thursday and Friday, this being its fourteenth annual meeting, but no report of the session has been received.

The Crop Protection Institute held its annual meeting on Tuesday evening, with a dinner at the Hermitage Hotel. The secretary-treasurer reported excellent progress; there are prospects for some endowment and the institute should be incorporated. Nearly $75,000 has been available in the last eighteen months and nearly $50,000 has been expended. Fifteen investigators were employed in projects. The chairman mentioned some of the projects now being worked on and emphasized the great advantage of the present cooperative plans, by which many institutions contribute to the same project. For example, the project on crown gall, under the chairmanship of Dr. R. E. Melhus, enjoys the cooperation of the U. S. Department of Agriculture, the University of Minnesota, Iowa State College and many nurserymen. Among the other projects are those of oil sprays, cattle repellants, oil emulsions, fineness of sprays and organic compounds of mercury and thallium as treatments against insects in stored grain. A promising series of poisons is being developed, derived from furfuramid, and a study of substances derived from oxidation of oils has been begun. Work is being carried on in fifteen states. Suggestions and constructive criticism is invited.

SECTION Q (EDUCATION)

Vice-president and chairman, Arthur I. Gates; *retiring vice-president,* Melvin H. Haggerty; *secretary,* A. S. Barr, University of Wisconsin, Madison, Wis.

(*Report from A. S. Barr*)

Section Q met on Monday, Tuesday and Wednesday. One session dealt with experimental study of teaching, one with educational psychology (a joint session with section I), two sessions with matters of school administration and two with miscellaneous researches. The retiring vice-presidential addresses for Sections I and Q were given Tuesday evening at a joint meeting of the two sections with the Phi Delta Kappa Fraternity.

Retiring vice-president M. E. Haggerty spoke on "The Improvement of College Instruction." Pointing out that much present criticism of college instruction was ill-founded, he reviewed some problems peculiar to American colleges and universities: namely, those related to need for new objectives, curriculum construction, personnel management, improvement of examinations and marking systems, better teaching and the training of college teachers. Dr. Margaret Floy Washburn, retiring vice-president for Section I, gave a clear and vigorous paper on "Purposive Action," which has appeared in SCIENCE for January 13. In the discussions on the experimental study of teaching, led by H. L. Donovan (Peabody College), it was pointed out that about eight hundred thousand persons are employed in teaching, a third as many as in all other professions. Considering the rapid turn-over in the teaching profession, its training load is twice that of all other professions combined. Frank N. Freeman (University of Chicago) reviewed the contributions of educational psychology to the development of teaching procedures.

Seven papers on a variety of subjects were read at the joint session of Sections I and Q. Bird T. Baldwin (Iowa Child-Welfare Station) reported on a three-year study of the growth of elementary school children. Some of his results are: A marked overlapping of scores is found in all grades; the median increments on composite scores for boys and girls in the three years show insignificant sex differences; a pupil's future score can be predicted with fair accuracy from his previous score or scores, the difference between the actual score and the estimated score being approximately a half-year's educational growth. —A. S. Courtis (University of Michigan) proposed a new measure of teaching ability, based on the change of rate of growth in the children taught; his paper is to appear in *School and Society*.

Ten papers treated of the various aspects of school administration. G. D. Strayer (Columbia University) reviewed progress made in making school administration more scientific; P. C. Packer (University of Iowa) spoke on the function of the university school of education; N. L. Engelhardt (Columbia University) summarized researches on school buildings; H. F. Clark (Indiana University) read a brilliant paper on public school finance in the light of modern economic theory, pointing out, among many other things, that although it is usually assumed that schooling increases the income of the individual, yet a study of the earnings of groups of equal ability, the members of which have gone to school different lengths of time, does not support this assumption. Attention to economic theory might show advantages for planning the educational system in terms of the number of people that can be used in each of the occupations and professions.

Twelve papers were read in the two sessions devoted to a discussion of current research. Data gathered by W. C. Ruediger (George Washington University) from about six hundred college students show that 35 per cent. never had a course in physics, while the corresponding percentages for other subjects are as follows: Chemistry, 32; zoology, 59; physiology, 39; history and appreciation of art, 64; ancient history, 11; European history, 23. F. P. O'Brien (University of Kansas) concluded that colleges are successful neither in attracting nor in holding the mentally fit; 53 per cent. of those whose mental scores had placed them in the upper half of the range of high-school graduates do not apply for entrance to any institution of higher learning and the students eliminated (more than half of whom left in the first year) are not inferior. O. W. Caldwell (Columbia University) described the new educational internship of the Lincoln Institute of School Experimentation as a means of training experimental workers. Lentz (Washington University) presented new tests of sex interest. Many other interesting, important and stimulating contributions were made.

ORGANIZATIONS NOT SPECIALLY RELATED TO ANY PARTICULAR SECTION

In addition to those already named, the following organizations held sessions at the Nashville meeting: The Society of the Sigma Xi (*president,* F. R. Moulton; *secretary,* Edward Ellery, Union College, Schenectady, N. Y.), the American Nature-Study Society (*president,* George R. Green; *secretary,* E. Laurence Palmer, State College, Pennsylvania), the Tennessee Academy of Science (*president,* W. S. Leathers; *secretary-treasurer,* John T. McGill, Vanderbilt University, Nashville, Tenn.), the Gamma Alpha Graduate Scientific Fraternity (*president,* Richard Hartshorne; *secretary,* Sidney M. Cadwell, 561 W. 58th St., New York City), the Honor Society of Phi Kappa Phi (*president,* L. H. Pammel; *secretary,* C. H. Gordon, University of Tennessee, Knoxville, Tenn.), and the Sigma Delta Epsilon Graduate Women's Scientific Fraternity (*president,* Julia A. Colpitts; *secretary,* Amy G. McKeel, Cornell University, Ithaca, N. Y.).

(*Reports from Edward Ellery, John T. McGill, Sidney M. Cadwell, R. M. Peterson and Amy G. McKeel*)

The Society of the Sigma Xi held its twenty-eighth convention on Tuesday. Reports were made by the officers and charters were voted for chapters at the University of Maryland, Lehigh University, University of Illinois College of Medicine, and Kansas State Agricultural College. Officers were elected as follows: *President,* Vernon Kellogg; *secretary,* Edward Ellery; *treasurer,* George B. Pegram. The annual dinner was followed by the Sixth Annual Sigma Xi Lecture, delivered at the Tuesday evening general session of the association, by President Clarence Cook Little, of the University of Michigan, who spoke on "Some Opportunities for Research in Mammalian Genetics."

The American Nature-Study Society met on Tuesday and Wednesday. No report has been received.

The Tennessee Academy of Science, officially affiliated with the American Association, on Monday afternoon joined Section D in a session devoted to reminiscences of the late Edward Emerson Barnard, a native of Nashville. The latter session was opened by Judge Robert Ewing, chairman of the Board of Trustees of Watkins Institute, Nashville, who was a member of the reception committee for the first Nashville meeting, fifty years ago. J. W. Braid, chemist-photographer and instrument maker, spoke of Barnard's first work with Van Stavoren, photographer and portrait painter, his enthusiasm for astronomy, his use of an old spyglass as his first telescope, etc. P. R. Calvert, who was intimately associated with Barnard for eight years in the gallery of R. Poole, successor to Van Stavoren, told the story of Barnard's introduction to Simon Newcomb in the State Capitol at the meeting of the American Association in Nashville in 1877. Barnard joined the association at that meeting. Olin H. Lambeth told of Barnard's exceptional admission to the university as a special student, and at the same time as assistant instructor in astronomy. Robert G. Aitken, Philip Fox and D. W. Morehouse gave interesting accounts of their association with Barnard at the Lick and Yerkes observatories. The session closed with a tribute to Barnard by Miss Mary R. Calvert, his niece and his secretary and assistant for many years at the Yerkes Observatory. Since Barnard's death she has carried to completion his last great work, the "Atlas of Selected Portions of the Milky Way," recently published by the Carnegie Institution of Washington. A collection of photographs, medals and other Barnardiana was on exhibition during the meeting.

The Gamma Alpha Graduate Scientific Fraternity held a dinner Thursday evening, at which Dr. William Crocker, of the Boyce Thompson Institute for Plant Research, spoke on "A Pan-American University in Porto Rico: a Great Move for International Peace." The projected university would be affiliated with the other graduate schools at the University of Porto Rico. Porto Rico is the best common meeting ground for the Spanish and English cultures of the western hemisphere, which among other things makes the island very well suited for an international educational project.

The Honor Society of Phi Kappa Phi held its tenth general convention on Tuesday evening and Wednesday. There was an active discussion of concrete methods for the encouragement of scholarship in educational institutions. Favorable action was taken on a petition for a chapter at Parsons College, Fairfield, Iowa. Officers were elected as follows: *President,* R. C. Gibbs; *secretary,* C. H. Gordon.

The Sigma Delta Epsilon Graduate Women's Scientific Fraternity held its annual convention following a breakfast on Wednesday morning. The breakfast was open to all women interested in science and was attended by fifty-seven women, representing twenty-eight institutions. Dr. Frances Wick, of Vassar College, spoke on "Some Reflections upon Invisible Radiations and Their Effects," and her talk was much appreciated by physicists and biologists alike.

SPECIAL NOTES

(1) This issue of SCIENCE contains the reports of the sessions of sections and societies at Nashville. The general reports of the meeting have appeared in the preceding issue, for January 27.

(2) Copies of the issue for January 27 may be had free from the permanent secretary's office, Smithsonian Institution Building, Washington, D. C., so long as the supply lasts.

(3) Members who were enrolled for the year 1927 but who have not yet sent in their dues for 1928 are asked to do so now; otherwise the journal subscriptions can not be continued longer.

(4) All who are interested in the advancement of science and education should belong to the American Association. New members are received at any time. Information about the organization and work of the association and about the responsibilities and privileges of membership therein may be secured at any time from the permanent secretary's Washington office, Smithsonian Institution Building, Washington, D. C.

SCIENTIFIC EVENTS

NATIONAL RESEARCH FELLOWS AT PRINCETON UNIVERSITY

DEAN ANDREW FLEMING WEST, of the Princeton Graduate Schools, writes in his report to President John Grier Hibben:

Since the World War provision has been made for appointing specially qualified persons as National Research Fellows in mathematics, physics and chemistry. Up to the present time there have been 188 graduates of American universities appointed to these fellowships. The following table shows all the universities which have trained ten or more of these fellows and have received ten or more of them for advanced study after their appointment.

PLACE OF GRADUATE TRAINING

1. Princeton University	22
2. University of Chicago	21
3. University of California	13
4. Yale University	13
5. Harvard University	12
6. University of Wisconsin	12
7. The Johns Hopkins University	11

REGISTERED AS NATIONAL RESEARCH FELLOWS AT

1. Harvard University	41
2. Princeton University	32
3. California Institute of Technology	30
4. University of Chicago	28
5. University of California	13
6. Yale University	11

It thus appears that Princeton heads the list in the number of National Research Fellows trained and comes second in the number of National Research Fellows registered for advanced study. We could hardly ask for a more striking proof of the wisdom of the policy of limited enrolment and strict standards of admission to our Graduate School.

PRESENTATION OF THE NICHOLS MEDAL TO PROFESSOR HUGH S. TAYLOR

AWARD of the Nichols medal for 1928 to Professor Hugh S. Taylor, head of the department of chemistry in Princeton University, already noted in SCIENCE, was announced on January 18 by the New York section of the American Chemical Society.

The award, determined by "the research published during the current year which in the opinion of the jury is most original and stimulative to further research," will be formally conferred upon Professor Taylor at a national gathering of chemists in Rumford Hall, New York City, on March 9, when he will deliver an address on "Catalysis as an Inspiration of Fundamental Research."

Other speakers will include Professor James Kendall, head of the department of chemistry in New York University, and Professor Wilder D. Bancroft, of Cornell University. The medal was established in 1903 by Dr. William B. Nichols, a charter member of the American Chemical Society, to encourage original research in chemistry.

The jury of award consisted of Professor Arthur W. Thomas, Columbia University, chairman; D. H. Killeffer, secretary of the New York Section; Dr. B. T. Brooks, consulting chemist; Dr. C. E. Davis, chief chemist of the National Biscuit Company, and Dean Kendall.

Dr. Taylor was appointed professor of physical chemistry at Princeton in 1922, and occupied this position until last year, when he was appointed to the newly created research professorship of chemistry. This chair was contributed by Miss Gwethalyn Jones, of Chicago, in memory of her father, David B. Jones, a graduate of Princeton, and as part of the newly organized endowment for scientific research in Princeton University.

MEDAL PRESENTATIONS TO GENERAL CARTY AND DR. COOLIDGE

THE John Fritz medal, which was awarded to General John J. Carty in November, 1927, and the Edison medal, which was awarded to Dr. William D. Coolidge in December, 1927, will both be presented to the medalists at a meeting to be held in the Engineering Auditorium, New York City, on February 15, in connection with the annual winter convention of the American Institute of Electrical Engineers. Members of the engineering profession and other friends of the medalists are invited to attend.

The presentation ceremonies will include an address by Dr. Michael I. Pupin, who will outline the achievements of Dr. Coolidge, the presentation of the Edison medal by President Gherardi, of the American Institute of Electrical Engineers, and the response of the medalist; the announcement of the John Fritz medal award by Chairman J. V. W. Reynders, of the board of award, an outline of the achievements of General Carty by Bancroft Gherardi, the presentation of the John Fritz medal by Robert Ridgway, chairman of the board when the award was made, and the response of General Carty.

The John Fritz medal was awarded to General Carty "for pioneer achievement in telephone engineering and in the development of scientific research in the telephone art. The award was made unanimously by a board composed of sixteen representatives of the American national societies of civil, mining, mechanical and electrical engineers, having an aggregate membership of 57,000.

This medal is awarded not oftener than once a year for notable scientific or industrial achievement.

It is a memorial to John Fritz, late of Bethlehem, Pennsylvania, long a leader in the iron and steel industry of America.

The Edison medal was awarded to Dr. William D. Coolidge "for his contributions to the incandescent electric lighting and the X-ray arts." This award was made unanimously by the Edison medal committee, consisting of twenty-four members of the American Institute of Electrical Engineers.

SCIENTIFIC NOTES AND NEWS

DR. THEODORE W. RICHARDS, director of the Gibbs memorial laboratory at Harvard University, has been elected a corresponding member of the French Academy of Sciences, in the section of chemistry.

DR. SIMON FLEXNER, director of the Rockefeller Institute for Medical Research, has been elected an honorary member of the Vienna Microbiological Society.

THE Royal Photographic Society, London, has awarded the Progress Medal, the highest honor the society can bestow, to Dr. S. E. Sheppard, of the Kodak Research Laboratories.

PROFESSOR E. W. BROWN, professor of mathematics in Yale University, has been elected an associate of the Royal Academy of Belgium. M. Armand Renier, director of the geological services of Belgium, and Professor Lucien Hauman, professor of botany in the University of Brussels, have been elected *correspondents* of the academy.

THE gold medal of the Royal Astronomical Society has been awarded to Professor R. A. Sample, astronomer-royal for Scotland, for his theory of the four great satellites of Jupiter. Jackson-Gwilt bronze medals have been awarded to Dr. W. H. Stevenson for his work on faint variable stars and Herschel instruments, and to W. Reid, of Cape Town, for his discovery of six new comets.

PROFESSOR SERGIUS VON OLDENBURG, president of the Russian Academy at Leningrad, has been made a corresponding member of the Prussian Academy of Sciences.

PROFESSOR EMIL ABDERHALDEN, of the University of Halle, Professor Ludolf von Krehl, of the University of Heidelberg, and Professor Georg Rost, of the University of Freiburg, have been made honorary members of the Academy of Medicine of Rome.

DR. J. WALTER FEWKES retired as chief of the U. S. Bureau of American Ethnology on January 15. Dr. Fewkes was appointed ethnologist in the bureau in 1895 and chief of the bureau on March 1, 1918. His retirement will allow him to complete manuscripts on certain field researches already accomplished, and he will at the same time continue to cooperate in the work of the bureau.

CHARLES C. WILLOUGHBY, who retires as director of the Peabody Museum of American Archeology and Ethnology at Harvard University next September, has been made director emeritus.

AT a recent meeting of the trustees of the Academy of Natural Sciences of Philadelphia, Mr. William Procter, of Bar Harbor, Maine, was elected research associate in marine biology. Mr. Procter has organized and is conducting a biological survey of the Mount Desert Region, Maine. A well-equipped marine laboratory located at Corfield, Bar Harbor, Maine, has just been completed where he, with a scientific staff of five men, will continue during the summer months the work begun two years ago in temporary quarters.

J. ERIC THOMPSON, of the Field Museum of Natural History, has left for British Honduras, as the head of an expedition which will investigate the civilization of the ancient Maya Indians.

PROFESSOR W. L. BRAGG, Langworthy professor of physics at the University of Manchester, England, will give a series of lectures on "Crystal Physics" at the Massachusetts Institute of Technology. The course of thirty lectures will start on February 7 and will be given Tuesday, Wednesday, Thursday and Friday afternoons at 4 o'clock.

DR. LEON W. COLLET, professor of geology and paleontology, University of Geneva, Switzerland, gave a lecture on "The Formation of the Alps" at the American Museum of Natural History on January 27.

SIR ARTHUR NEWSHOLME, formerly principal medical officer, local government board for England and Wales, will lecture on the evenings of January 25 and 26 at the University of California on "Dying Diseases" and "The Good Samaritan up to date." Sir Arthur was formerly a visiting professor at the Johns Hopkins University School of Hygiene and Public Health, Baltimore.

UNDER the auspices of the recently established Mead-Swing foundation, Professor Herbert S. Jennings, of the Johns Hopkins University, recently gave two lectures at Oberlin College, as follows: January 12, "Biological Fallacies and Human Affairs," and January 13, "What can We Hope from Eugenics?"

THE New York Academy of Medicine conducted a symposium on graduate medical education on January 19; the speakers were Drs. Louis B. Wilson, Mayo Foundation; Ludwig Kast, New York, and John E. Jennings, Brooklyn.

DR. GEORGE F. KAY, state geologist of Iowa, gave

an illustrated lecture to the staff and graduate students of the department of geology of the University of Chicago, on January 16. The subject was "The Present Status of the Glacial Studies in Iowa."

DR. W. J. HUMPHREYS, of the U. S. Weather Bureau, gave an illustrated lecture on "Clouds and Cloud Splendors" to the Sigma Xi of the University of Kentucky, on January 19.

DR. WALLACE OSGOOD FENN, professor of physiology at the University of Rochester, will deliver the fourth Harvey Society lecture at the New York Academy of Medicine, on February 10. His subject will be "The Metabolism of Nerves."

THE memory of Dr. Albert J. Ochsner is honored by the American College of Surgeons which has established on Ochsner memorial foundation for clinical research. Three months after Dr. Ochsner's death in July, 1925, the board of regents of the college of surgeons established the memorial fund with a grant of $100,000 and the appointment of a committee to secure an additional $900,000. It was announced at the recent meeting of the college in Madison that the fund now has reached $300,000.

THE University of California at Los Angeles will move, as has already been announced, to a new site on the hills overlooking the Pacific, west of Los Angeles. The main classroom building is to be called Josiah Royce Hall, and is to contain a complete collection of Royce's writings as a memorial to him. A correspondent writes: "In view of the fact that Royce was so frequent a contributor to the pages of SCIENCE, I have thought that the journal might like to call attention to this commemoration. The Royce collection, when completed, will offer to the student a fuller and more intimate access to the thought of Royce than exists elsewhere. The department of philosophy is responsible for the completing of the collection. Any information regarding the existence of works, addresses or articles by Royce now out of print would be of great assistance."

WILLIAM C. MILLS, curator of the department of archeology of Ohio State University, died on January 17, aged sixty-eight years.

DR. ANNA MORSE STARR, associate professor of botany at Mount Holyoke College, recently died at the age of sixty years.

FREDERICK LEROY SARGENT, of Cambridge, Mass., at one time professor of botany at the University of Wisconsin, and associated with the Harvard Botanical Museum, died on January 16, at the age of sixty-four years.

PROFESSOR GEORG FENDLER, until recently chemical director of the new research institute for foodstuffs in Berlin, recently died, aged fifty-four years.

THE annual meeting of the British Association for the Advancement of Science will be held in South Africa in 1929.

THE second meeting of executives of the chemical industries will be held in Washington, D. C., on February 16, under the auspices of the U. S. Department of Commerce.

THE city of Moscow has appropriated $150,000 for a planetarium to demonstrate to the people how the solar system functions. The planetarium, identical with the one in Berlin, has been ordered from the Zeiss Optical Company, Jena.

A FELLOWSHIP for investigating the effects of ethylene in low concentrations in the air and in foods upon animal metabolism, and the acceleration of enzyme action by ethylene has been instituted at the University of Minnesota by the Eli Lilly Co., manufacturing chemists. The holder of the fellowship, Elmer T. Ceder, is working under cooperation between the department of pharmacology under Dr. A. D. Hirschfelder and the section of plant physiology of the Minnesota Agricultural Experiment Station with Dr. R. B. Harvey.

THE committee in charge of the Institute of Chemistry of the American Chemical Society is anxious to get the best films on chemical and related subjects for presentation at the Institute of Chemistry which meets in Evanston, Illinois, from July 23 to August 18, 1928, Those who have seen unusually good films are asked to write the chairman of the committee, Frank C. Whitmore, National Research Council, Washington, D. C., or the executive secretary, Charles D. Hurd, Northwestern University, Evanston, Illinois.

THE Boyce Thompson Institute for Plant Research, Inc., has completed arrangements to provide for the future welfare of its employees. A program of cooperative retirement and death benefit has become effective through contract with the Metropolitan Life Insurance Company. Upon presenting this to the employees, 98 per cent. of those who were eligible applied for membership. Under the retirement provisions, an employee who retires at the age of 65 will receive a life income. The amount of this income will depend on the salary and the number of years of service at the institute. It is found that this averages 2 per cent. of the salary for every year of service. The death benefit provision ranges from $1,000 to $3,000. In case an employee is disabled before rendering 5 years of service, the death benefit is payable in installments. In case the disability occurs after 5 or more years of service a disability pension is payable for life. Another helpful provision is that the subscribing employees are also entitled to the service of a visiting nurse furnished free of cost by the insurance company.

THE survey made by the Social Science Research Council of the rural sociology research in progress in the United States in the year 1926–27 showed that $400,000 was being expended on 86 projects. Of this total, $175,000 was being expended by land-grant colleges and agricultural experiment stations in 21 of the states. The $400,000 total was almost exclusive of all sums spent by federal bureaus.

THE records of the Great Lakes Ornithological Club have recently been given to the Royal Ontario Museum of Zoology, Toronto. These records cover the period from May, 1905, to December, 1927, and include observations on the occurrence and abundance of birds both migrant and resident at Point Pelee, Ontario. This area is of special interest for two reasons. Extending into Lake Erie as it does it serves as a sort of funnel through which migrations are concentrated, and, being the most southern mainland point in Canada, some birds typical of more southern regions are found as residents of Canada only at this point.

ACCORDING to the Experiment Station *Record*, provision was made by the last Alabama legislature for five substations to be known as the Tennessee Valley, the Sand Mountain, the Black Belt, the Wire Grass and the Gulf Coast Substations. Two of these substations are to be established prior to September 30, 1928, and the remainder during the following year. An appropriation of $25,000 was made for buildings and equipment for each substation and $12,000 each for maintenance and operation. The act requires the donation of not less than 200 acres of representative soil for each substation.

ON November 8 the steamer *Halcyon*, of the U. S. Bureau of Fisheries, was sold at Woods Hole, Mass. The *Halcyon* is a wooden vessel 108 feet 6 inches long, over all, with a 22-foot beam and 10-foot draft, built in 1917. Her cost, including equipment, was $44,000. The vessel was well built but of unusual design, being planned originally for both the collection of seed lobsters along the Maine coast and offshore investigations. After the acquisition by the bureau of the *Albatross II*, the need for the *Halcyon* ceased.

SPONSORED by King Albert and the leading industrialists and financiers of Belgium, a move has been started for the establishment of a permanent museum and laboratory for scientific research. It will probably be situated in Brussels. It is hoped to develop the projected museum and laboratory into a center of study where all nations would exhibit their scientific equipment. The first of the exhibitions would be held in 1930.

UNIVERSITY AND EDUCATIONAL NOTES

A. P. GIANNINI has placed his 1927 income, as president of the Bancitaly Corporation, at the disposal of the University of California. Under the terms of the gift, $1,000,000 will go toward the establishment of the Giannini Foundation of Agricultural Economics and $500,000 will be used for erection of a building on the university campus in Berkeley, dedicated to ways and means of improving the economic condition of farmers, dairy and livestock men and fruit growers in California.

DR. JOHN GOODRICH CLARK, who was chief gynecologist at the University of Pennsylvania when he died last May, left an estate of over $1,000,000, a large part of which will go to the university.

LARS G. ROMELL, of the Swedish Forest Experiment Station at Stockholm, has been appointed to the Charles Lathrop Pack research professorship in forest soils at Cornell University and will take up his duties about April 1. The establishment of this professorship, said to be the first of its kind in an American university, has been made possible by the recently announced endowment of $130,000 for the chair, together with important additional gifts for its operating funds, from the Charles Lathrop Pack forestry trust.

PROFESSOR LEON BRILLOUIN, of the Collège de France, has been appointed acting professor of theoretical physics in the University of Wisconsin for the second semester of the academic year 1927–28.

DR. JESSE PERRY ROWE, professor of geology at the University of Montana, has been appointed visiting professor of geology at Princeton University for the academic year 1928–29.

DR. HERBERT SPENCER HARNED, professor of physical chemistry at the University of Pennsylvania, has been appointed professor of the same subject at Yale University.

DISCUSSION AND CORRESPONDENCE

DISCOVERY OF FURTHER HOMINID REMAINS OF LOWER QUATERNARY AGE FROM THE CHOU KOU TIEN DEPOSIT

AT a meeting of the Geological Society of China held on December 2, 1927, announcement was made of the discovery of a lower molar hominid tooth in the cave deposit at Chou Kou Tien near Peking. The new specimen was obtained close to the site from which the first hominid teeth from this locality were recovered and in the same stratum of the deposit. (V. this Journal, Dec. 17, 1926, p. 586.) This deposit, which at first was thought to be Upper Pliocene, is now known to be basal Lower Quaternary in age (very early Pleistocene). The find was made on October 16 by Dr. Birger Bohlin, paleontologist attached to the Geological Survey of China. Mr. C. Li, geologist from the survey, and Dr. Bohlin have been in charge of the extensive excavations on this important site which have been carried on during the past season by the Geological Survey in cooperation with the department of anatomy of the Peking Union Medical College.

The tooth is a relatively unworn and perfectly preserved left lower permanent molar, having incompletely formed root tips and evidently from an individual in the stage of development represented by that of an eight-year-old modern European child. The general morphology of this specimen leaves no room for doubt as to its hominid status and it evidently was derived from the same jaw as that from which came the lower premolar tooth discovered last year by Dr. O. Zdansky. A full description of the latter specimen and of the associated worn upper molar has been published this year by Dr. Zdansky. (*v. Bull. Geol. Soc. China,* Vol. V, No. 3.)

Evidence of a convincing nature points to a close mutual relationship between the two individuals, adult and immature, represented by the teeth recovered from the Chou Kou Tien deposit. The newly discovered specimen displays in the details of its morphology a number of interesting and unique characters, sufficient it is believed to justify the proposal of a new hominid genus *Sinanthropus,* to be represented by this material. A complete and fully illustrated report on this new specimen is now in press and will be published early in December in Series D, *Palaeontologia Sinica,* Vol. VII, Fasc. 1.

DAVIDSON BLACK

DEPARTMENT OF ANATOMY,
PEKING UNION MEDICAL COLLEGE,
PEKING, CHINA
NOVEMBER 24, 1927

AN INSTANCE OF THE INCREASE OF MALARIA BY CIVILIZATION

IN 1910, in the *Atti Soc. per gli Studii della Malaria* (Rome), the writer published an article about the apparently paradoxical situation that results in the gradual disappearance of malaria following the settlement of a new country and its reappearance as the result of a dense civilization. The perfectly obvious reasons for this were detailed in the article.

Just now a new and striking instance comes to my eye in an important paper, just received, entitled "Report of an Investigation of a Malaria Epidemic in Solo (Dutch East Indies), 1926," by S. L. Brug and Dr. E. W. Walch (Batavia, 1927).

It seems that in the old days a part of the city of Solo (150,000 inhabitants) was from time to time inundated during the wet monsoon. The Dutch authorities diked one side of the city and constructed a storm-water canal on the other. This storm-water canal is flushed at regular intervals during the wet monsoon, and during the dry monsoon carries comparatively little water. Pools form in the corrugated bottom and others are made by the digging of sand for cement used in making houses. Formerly the town seems to have been comparatively free from malaria, but towards the end of 1925 this disease began rapidly to increase, with a high mortality, reaching a climax in January, 1926.

Although, of course, there were other breeding places of Anopheles, the portions of the city most affected were along the storm-water canal which had not been flushed for an abnormally long time. It is reasonably supposed that the Anopheles carriers bred in the storm canal pools, and that the normalization of the water of the canal at all times in the future is plainly indicated.

L. O. HOWARD

WASHINGTON,
JANUARY 7

THE SCIENTIFIC MEN OF HARVARD AND OF COLUMBIA

IN my statistical study of the distribution of American men of science, printed in the fourth edition of the "Biographical Directory of American Men of Science" (December, 1927) and in abstract in SCIENCE (November 25, 1927), it is stated that of 1,176 leading scientific men of the United States, Harvard has 89.5 and Columbia 46.5 (the fraction referring to a part time or emeritus position), whereas in 1906 of the leading 1,000 scientific men Harvard had 66.5 and Columbia 60. It is also shown that when the men are weighted by objective methods (the situation being substantially the same when they are only counted) Harvard stands first among universities in seven of the twelve sciences, second in three and third in one, whereas Columbia stands first in only one science and in no other has a rank among all institutions higher than fifth.

While not mentioned in the book, it may be noted that the disparity between the two universities is greatly increased by the circumstance that Harvard has 1,088 officers of instruction, Columbia, 2,075.

Harvard has one scientific man of high standing for 121 students, Columbia one such man for 693 students, part time students being in both cases included. Harvard has one member of the National Academy of Sciences for 31 teachers, Columbia one member for 172.5 teachers. Exactly one third of the Columbia members (who are more than one fourth of all members of the academy in these subjects) are in departments of which I was once head and were brought to the university by me long before they had been elected to membership in the academy.

A letter has been received from a distinguished officer of Columbia University in reference to these statistics, stating that it is proposed to see "what information you had to go on for the statement that is so entertaining. . . . It will be great sport." It has even been intimated that my figures are influenced by personal prejudice, which brings to mind a more or less relevant academic anecdote. After a professor of dermatology had been called to a German university, it was rumored among the students that it was because the professor of pathology had been cured by him of a serious disease. At the first opportunity the professor of pathology addressed his class, indignantly explaining that no German professor would in such a matter be influenced by personal considerations, and adding, "It is true that Dr. X treated me for ——, but he could not cure me."

As a matter of fact the selection of the scientific men for my statistical work is entirely impersonal. This is obvious from the published descriptions of the methods used, but it should be emphasized, for I have had not only many letters (one from a Harvard professor on the day that this is written, accusing me of awarding a star to a man because he had been appointed to a professorship at Columbia!), but also visits asking that stars be assigned, and they have even been added to the sketches when the printed proofs were returned. The final vote was from 1,196 of the 1,572 leading scientific men of the country and my only part was to be one of 66 who voted for the psychologists.

As the relative position assigned by the statistics to Harvard and Columbia in zoology has been especially questioned, it may be desirable to consider it from another aspect. The names of individuals in my statistical work have not been used by me, though this has been done by others, for they are available to any one who checks over the some 13,500 names in the book. We have, however, in the membership of the National Academy of Sciences a criterion which while less exact still has high validity for purposes of comparison.

MEMBERS OF THE NATIONAL ACADEMY OF SCIENCES

HARVARD	COLUMBIA
Zoological Sciences	
W. B. Cannon	G. N. Calkins
W. E. Castle	T. H. Morgan
W. T. Councilman	Edmund B. Wilson
Harvey Cushing	
William Duane	
Otto Folin	
L. J. Henderson	
Reid Hunt	
E. L. Mark	
G. H. Parker	
Richard P. Strong	
W. M. Wheeler	
Edwin B. Wilson	
Hans Zinsser	
Botany	
E. M. East	R. A. Harper
B. L. Robinson	
Roland Thaxter	
Geology	
R. A. Daly	C. P. Berkey
W. M. Davis	
Mathematical and Physical Sciences	
S. I. Bailey	M. T. Bogert
Gregory P. Baxter	Edward Kasner
George D. Birkhoff	M. I. Pupin
P. W. Bridgman	
Edwin H. Hall	
C. L. Jackson	
A. E. Kennelly	
E. P. Kohler	
A. B. Lamb	
Theodore Lyman	
Arthur Michael	
William F. Osgood	
G. W. Pierce	
Th. W. Richards	
Frederick A. Saunders	
Albert Sauveur	
Harlow Shapley	
George F. Swain	
Psychology and Anthropology	
	Franz Boas
	John Dewey
	Edward L. Thorndike
	R. S. Woodworth

Zoology is in fact next to psychology the strongest scientific department at Columbia and its strength is emphasized by the possession of the two most distinguished zoologists of the United States. It is indeed overemphasized by this circumstance as one of them (now over seventy-one years of age) will soon retire and the other will soon pass to the new heaven for good Americans in southern California.

In my classification the zoologists of the American Museum were assigned to it and the zoologists of the

Carnegie Institution to it, and this should be taken into consideration. But it may also be noted that Harvard University and the Massachusetts Institute of Technology have close relations and if the projected union had been formed, the strength of the institution would have been 109.5, in place of the 89.5 assigned to Harvard.

The members of the National Academy of Sciences in the zoological sciences who are at Harvard and Columbia are printed here, biophysics, biochemistry and vital statistics being included. In order to show the exact situation the lists of members of the academy are given also for the other sciences.

This information is printed not in order to exalt Harvard, but rather in the interest of Columbia. The economic evolution of the modern world should now establish the greatest of universities in New York City. If Columbia can not become worthy of this position, it must be the work of the state and the city.

During the ten years of Seth Low's administration many distinguished professors were called to Columbia and it attained a rank nearly equal to Harvard, the number of leading scientific men in the two universities then being 60 and 66.5. During the last twenty-five years Columbia has been losing ground, not only in the sciences but also in other fields. President Butler himself remarks in his annual report for 1925 that Columbia University can not replace "older scholars of distinction and large achievement" because "a choice must be made from a larger or smaller group of mediocrities." This situation is in part due to the attitude expressed by a prominent trustee who wrote[1] in 1921: "It is very difficult to discharge professors once employed. They make common cause and howl about academic freedom. We have had trouble along this line in Columbia, where they taught sedition and disloyalty, and that enabled us to get rid of eight or ten at the time."

Trustees and administrative officers must learn that the greatness of a university is not in building, nor in endowment, nor in number of students, but in men and in the freedom and the opportunity given to them.

J. McKeen Cattell

REPORTS

ADDRESS OF THE PRESIDENT OF THE AUSTRALASIAN ASSOCIATION FOR THE ADVANCEMENT OF SCIENCE

In his presidential address to the Australasian Association for the Advancement of Science at Hobart, on January 16, 1928, Mr. R. H. Cambage referred to the great need for the further application of science to primary production. This, he said, embraced such fundamental utilities as the production of grain, fruit, butter, wool and meat, and he stated that it was a matter for satisfaction that the Commonwealth and State Governments, as well as private bodies, were showing increased appreciation of the value of science to these problems.

He mentioned that a few years ago a thorough knowledge of dairy bacteriology and its application to the production of butter had resulted in increasing the output of first grade butter in New South Wales from 48 to 96 per cent.

When referring to wheat he said: "It is difficult to find anything among the primary products of Australia which owes more to science than wheat production. This is a matter of national concern, and it is most comforting to know that the great pioneering work carried out by William James Farrer is not only being continued at departmental experiment farms and universities, but with most progressive results. New and better drought and rust-resisting varieties of wheat and other grain are being produced, and experiments are being made for the purpose of breeding rust and flag-smut-resisting plants which will also have other good characters."

Mr. Cambage referred to the action of the pastoralists in arranging for the Australian Pastoral Research Trust to receive a contribution at the rate of two shillings a bale of the 1927 wool-clip, with the hope of raising £200,000, for scientific research in connection with the industry. This action he regards as a most definite advance in Australia in the recognition of the benefits of science.

He commended the recent action of the Federal Government in inviting five leading pastoralists to act as a committee to enquire into the conditions of the pastoral industry in Australia, and advise on the best methods of conserving the national wealth represented by the industry. It provides, he stated, further evidence that the authorities concerned are quite alive to the necessity of abandoning the old happy-go-lucky methods of trusting to chance in regard to seasons, but rather look for the introduction of some reasonable scheme of insurance that may have for its object the avoidance of excessive losses rather than the making of enormous profits.

He concluded the first portion of his address by saying that it is the desire of the Australasian Association for the Advancement of Science, which includes New Zealand, to inspire and stimulate a science sense in the public mind, and this, he thought, could best be done by demonstrating how the principles of

[1] "A Barton Hepburn: His Life and Service to his Time." By Joseph Bucklin Bishop. New York, 1923. Page 293.

pure science may be applied successfully to familiar economic problems.

In the second part of his address Mr. Cambage discussed the "Origin and Development of Portion of the Australian Flora." He summarized the position as follows:

There appear to be more genera common to Africa and the eastern half of Australia only than to Africa and the western half of Australia only, so that evidence of a direct land connection between these two countries is meager. It is thought that many genera which are common to Africa and Australia have reached these countries from the same source in the north, and have then developed in response to environment.

From available evidence it would seem that, at least since Cretaceous time, the northern hemisphere has had a greater land mass than the southern, and, as a result, there has been more room for plant development in the north than in the south. Probably the Pleistocene and even earlier glacial periods have been instrumental in permitting many genera to pulsate across the tropics from temperate northern regions, and in the process, and after arrival in the south, there have been much radiation, development and evolution. Although there probably has been more migration to Australia from the north, there is evidence in some cases of secondary radiation from the south, especially in the genus *Eucalyptus*.

It seems undoubted that some genera common to Australia and New Zealand have reached both countries from the north, some species coming down the east coast of Australia, while others have gone by way of New Caledonia and adjoining islands to New Zealand. Except for a land connection between northeastern Australia and islands to the north, perhaps as late as Pliocene time, Australia has long been isolated from the rest of the world. There appears to be more evidence in favor of a former land connection between Antarctica and South America, and perhaps New Zealand and Australia, than between Africa and Antarctica.

Studies of the many changes which have taken place in the history of the world's flora, of its adaptability to environment, its response to changes of climate and soil, its ability to overcome many adverse conditions, all combine to impress one with the conviction that the marvelous act of creation not only embodies the initial giving of life, but also provided inherent power and initiative for the necessary development and evolution required for the persistence of that life, in harmony with its varying surroundings and dominating influences.

SPECIAL ARTICLES

NUTRITIONAL ANEMIA ON WHOLE MILK DIETS AND ITS CORRECTION WITH THE ASH OF BEEF LIVER

IN an earlier article[1] we published data showing that experimental anemia in rabbits induced by the feeding of a whole milk—Fe_2O_3 diet could be corrected by the addition of the *ash* of lettuce or of cabbage. In the case of animal tissues, both dried liver and dried "spleen-marrow" were found to be potent if fed at a level of 2 gms. per animal per day as a supplement to the whole milk—Fe_2O_3. The daily administration of the *ash* of 2 gms. of dried "spleen-marrow" delayed the onset of anemia to some extent, but appeared inefficient over a long period of time.

This paper deals with experiments on the use of the *ash* of beef liver as a corrective or preventative of nutritional anemia. Rats were used as the experimental animal. They were selected at 50–60 gms. in weight and placed on screens with whole milk as the sole diet. They were weighed weekly and hemoglobin determinations made periodically by the Newcomer method. When the hemoglobin readings had reached 6–8 gms. per 100 cc. of blood, and the evidence was sufficient that the animal had become anemic but not beyond the possibility of response, the use of the experimental ration was begun. The animals were then fed on screens in separate cages and individually. The normal hemoglobin content of rat's blood may be taken at 12–14 gms. per 100 cc. of blood. After the animal was placed on the experimental diet weekly weighings and periodic determinations of the hemoglobin were continued.

In experimental anemia induced by whole milk feeding there is iron starvation as one of the factors in operation. To determine how effective additions of iron salts may be in the correction of this anemia $FeCl_3$ was prepared from standard iron wire of highest purity. Two gms. of iron wire were dissolved in dilute HNO_3, the solution of ferric nitrate evaporated to dryness, taken up in excess of HCl, the iron precipitated with NH_4OH, filtered and washed thoroughly until free from chlorides. The precipitate was then dissolved in the theoretical amount of HCl necessary to convert the Fe to $FeCl_3$. In order to obtain complete solution of the $FeCl_3$ an excess of .42 gms. of HCl was added and the solution made to a volume, 1 cc. of which equaled 1.0 mg. of Fe. The $FeCl_3$ was fed at a level of 0.5 mgs. of Fe per animal per day without a resultant correction of the anemia.

We next turn to beef liver and beef liver *ash*. This material was dried at 65° C. over a period of 6–7 days and then ground to a fine powder. In certain experiments the dried liver was fed directly by suspending it in the whole milk. Iron determination on the dried liver showed that it was necessary to feed daily

[1] E. B. Hart, C. A. Elvehjem, J. Waddell, R. C. Herrin, *J. Biol. Chem.* 1927, LXXII 299. Iron in Nutrition. IV. Nutritional Anemia on Whole Milk Diets and its correction with the Ash of Certain Plant and Animal Tissues or with Soluble Iron Salts.

1.72 gms. of this material in order to introduce 0.5 mgs. of iron—a quantity exactly equivalent to the iron fed as $FeCl_3$. In addition the ash of the dried beef liver was prepared by incinerating the material in porcelain dishes in an electric furnace at 650°–750° C. After incineration to an ash the ash was digested in strong HCl for six hours at room temperature, diluted with water and the insoluble residue filtered off. The filtrate was evaporated almost to dryness, taken up with water, and diluted to a volume, 1 cc. of which was equivalent to 1.0 mg. of Fe. This solution was not perfectly clear.

This HCl extract of liver ash was fed to anemic rats at a level which introduced 0.5 mgs. of Fe daily. It was administered by directly stirring it into a portion of the daily allowance of whole milk. The results from the use of these materials in contrast with the $FeCl_3$ from iron wire were indeed very striking and showed unmistakably that 0.5 mgs. of iron from these sources is distinctly potent in restoring to normal the hemoglobin content of the blood of anemic rats. The detailed data which led us to the above conclusions, together with a further analysis of this problem, will be published later. At this time we only wish to re-emphasize the fact that nutritional anemia induced by a whole-milk diet is an inorganic deficiency and that the *ash* of liver as well as the *ash* of certain plant materials is a potent source of the correctives.

J. WADDELL
C. A. ELVEHJEM
H. STEENBOCK
E. B. HART

THE LABORATORY OF AGRICULTURAL CHEMISTRY,
UNIVERSITY OF WISCONSIN

SOCIETIES AND ACADEMIES

THE GEOLOGICAL SOCIETY OF AMERICA

AT the annual meeting of the Geological Society of America, held in Cleveland, December 29, 30 and 31, 1927, the following officers were elected for the year 1928:

President: Bailey Willis, Stanford University.
First Vice-president: Alfred C. Lane, Tufts College.
Second Vice-president: William H. Collins, Geological Survey of Canada.
Third Vice-president: August F. Foerste, Dayton, Ohio.
Fourth Vice-president: Esper S. Larsen, Harvard University.
Secretary: Charles P. Berkey, Columbia University.
Treasurer: Edward B. Mathews, The Johns Hopkins University.
Editor: Joseph Stanley-Brown, New York, N. Y.
Councilors (1928–1930): George R. Mansfield, United States Geological Survey; William E. Wrather, Dallas, Texas.

Thirty-one fellows were also elected, bringing the total membership to 559.

The Cleveland meeting had the largest attendance in the history of the society, with a registration of 374. One hundred and eight titles of papers were listed on the program, and four general addresses were delivered. Abstracts of all papers presented had been printed and distributed in advance of the meeting.

The Penrose medal, given for outstanding achievement in geologic science, was presented to Prof. Thomas Chrowder Chamberlin, of Chicago.

The annual meeting of 1928 will be held in New York City.

CHARLES P. BERKEY,
Secretary

INDIANA ACADEMY OF SCIENCE

THE Indiana Academy of Science held its 43rd annual meeting at the University of Notre Dame, Notre Dame, Indiana, on December 1, 2 and 3, 1927.

The officers in this meeting were as follows: *President,* Frank B. Wade, Indianapolis; *Vice-president,* F. J. Breeze, Muncie; *Secretary,* Ray C. Friesner, Indianapolis; *Asst. Secretary,* W. P. Morgan, Indianapolis; *Treasurer,* M. W. Lyon, Jr., South Bend; *Editor,* John J. Davis, Lafayette; *Press Secretary,* Harry F. Dietz, Indianapolis.

The meetings of the academy proper were preceded by the annual informal meeting of the entomologists of Indiana on December 1. At the regular meetings of the academy the number of papers presented in the various sections were as follows: general, 6; bacteriology, physiology and hygiene, 6; botany, 27; chemistry, mathematics and physics, 35; geology and geography, 18, and zoology, 16.

The annual public lecture was given by Dr. Wilfred H. Osgood, curator of zoology, Field Museum of Natural History, Chicago, who spoke on "Nature and Man in Abyssinia," illustrating his lecture with motion and still pictures.

The officers elected for the ensuing year were: *President,* E. G. Mahin, Notre Dame University, Notre Dame; *Vice-president,* W. N. Hess, DePauw University, Greencastle; *Secretary,* Ray C. Friesner, Butler College, Indianapolis; *Asst. Secretary,* W. P. Morgan, Indiana Central University, Indianapolis; *Treasurer,* M. W. Lyon, Jr., South Bend; *Editor,* John J. Davis, Purdue University, Lafayette; *Press Secretary,* Harry F. Dietz, Department of Conservation, Indianapolis.

HARRY F. DIETZ,
Press Secretary

SCIENCE

Vol. LXVII FEBRUARY 10, 1928 No. 1728

CONTENTS

American Association for the Advancement of Science:
Old Problems and A New Technique: Professor Winterton C. Curtis ... 141
Spaces of Statistics and their Metrization: Dr. Harold Hotelling ... 149
Paul Heinrich von Groth: Professor Edward H. Kraus ... 150
Scientific Events:
The Ella Sachs Plotz Foundation for the Advancement of Scientific Investigation; The Journal of the Swedish Forestry Society; Statement regarding the Dismissal of the Health Commissioner of Chicago; The Report of the Delegate of the Botanical Society of America to the Third Pan-Pacific Congress ... 152
Scientific Notes and News ... 154
University and Educational Notes ... 158
Discussion and Correspondence:
Alexandrovsk Biological Station: R. B. Harvey. *The Etiology of European Foulbrood of Bees:* Dr. A. G. Lochhead. *Concerning Man's Antiquity at Frederick, Oklahoma:* Dr. Leslie Spier. *"Exit the Tentamen, But . . . " What?:* Dr. W. J. Holland. *Visible Radiation from Excited Nerve Fiber Again:* Dr. Christine Ladd-Franklin ... 158
Quotations:
Genesis and Evolution ... 162
Separations by the Ionic Migration Method: Professor James Kendall ... 163
Scientific Apparatus and Laboratory Methods:
Determining Soil Moisture by Methyl Alcohol: Professor George J. Bouyoucos. *A Convenient Method of measuring Quantities of Chloroplast Pigments:* Howard B. Sprague ... 167
Special Articles:
The Isolation and Function of Phosphocreatine: Dr. Cyrus H. Fiske and Y. Subbarow ... 169
Science News ... x

SCIENCE: A Weekly Journal devoted to the Advancement of Science, edited by J. McKeen Cattell and published every Friday by

THE SCIENCE PRESS

New York City: Grand Central Terminal.

Lancaster, Pa. Garrison, N. Y.

Annual Subscription, $6.00. Single Copies, 15 Cts.

SCIENCE is the official organ of the American Association for the Advancement of Science. Information regarding membership in the Association may be secured from the office of the permanent secretary, in the Smithsonian Institution Building, Washington, D. C.

Entered as second-class matter July 18, 1923, at the Post Office at Lancaster, Pa., under the Act of March 8, 1879.

OLD PROBLEMS AND A NEW TECHNIQUE[1]

It is a truism to say that new instruments and new modes of technique may be as productive of advances in science as generalizations that point the way for many investigations. The telescope, the photographic plate and the spectroscope in astronomy, the chromometer and the thermometer in physics, the balance in chemistry, the microscope and the microtome in biology are trite examples of instruments and related technical processes so commonly used that their importance is forgotten. During the past twenty-five years, the string-galvanometer and methods of determining small amounts of gases in blood and other fluids of the body have been productive of great advances in physiology; while instruments for micro-dissection, and methods of staining, like those with hæmatoxylin, have made possible a flood of investigations.[2] The Greeks failed in

[1] Address of the retiring Vice-president and Chairman of Section F, American Association for the Advancement of Science, read at the Zoologists dinner, Nashville, December 29, 1927.

[2] The advent of such methods is sometimes vividly remembered by those who lived through the period. Recalling that I had once heard my former teacher, Professor S. F. Clarke, of Williams College, speak of the coming of ribbon sections in the early eighties of the last century and knowing that two other veteran American Zoologists, E. B. Wilson and E. L. Mark, were students abroad at this period, I inquired of these individuals. Each has contributed items of interest, but the statement by Professor Wilson is the most comprehensive. He says: "I first became acquainted with the ribbon method of section-cutting at the laboratory in Cambridge just after its discovery by Caldwell in 1882, and as I had very recently completed a research which involved the laborious cutting of great numbers of small eggs, one by one, and mounting the sections singly, you can imagine the surprise and pleasure with which I saw them reeled off wholesale by the ribbon method. As it happened I was, I think, the first person to introduce this method in Germany, having taken it over to Leuckart's laboratory in the early winter of the same year, and I have never forgotten the astonishment with which the operation was viewed by the group working there at the time. It was at first employed simply by the old method of cutting by hand with a razor on a flat-topped glass plate secured to a table, and was only a little later extended to the Thoma sliding microtome. It seemed to me then, and still seems to me, to be one of the most important steps

science as much through technical limitations as through their political collapse. In physical science, for example, they lacked accurate and convenient instruments for the recording of time and temperature, but more particularly they lacked methods of computation. One can appreciate the difficulties of such simple arithmetical processes as multiplication and division by Roman numerals, but the technique of the Roman system was less cumbersome than that used by the Greeks. The advent of the Arabic system, with its decimal point and with zero as a "placeholder," marked a new era for the natural sciences as well as for mathematics. I have thus referred to familiar advances of science through instruments and methods, because I believe the biological sciences have now at hand a technique that is not fully appreciated, although its importance has been demonstrated. I refer to the technique of *irradiation.*

The discovery of X-rays by Röntgen (1895) and of radium by the Curies (1898) was soon followed by applications in the medical field to diagnosis of gross features like skeletal fractures, and, when the "selective" action of the rays was discovered, to the treatment of malignant growths. That the more general possibilities in medicine were appreciated by Röntgen is shown by the fact that his original communication was made before a medical society and his first account published in a medical journal. These early applications were marked by sacrifice, since neither the danger to the operator nor the present modes of protection were known at the outset. Sterilization, burns, and even death were the lot of more than one radiologist, and patients no doubt suffered. But the present effectiveness of irradiation in the treatment of certain cancers is worth more than these earlier costs. Subsequent extensions of the method and of X-ray photography in clinical medicine are familiar. No hospital is complete, no physician's or dentist's service adequate unless X-ray diagnosis is available.

In correlation with the initial extensions in medical science, the interest of biologists was aroused, and during the first decade of the century certain general investigations were undertaken. Bohn ('03), Willcock ('04), and others conducted experiments upon the effects of radium and of X-rays in lower organisms. Gager ('08), exposed *Enothera* to radium and obtained changes that resembled mutations. The effects of irradiation upon the tissues and embryos of higher vertebrates were likewise examined in exploratory investigations. The "selective" action of the rays, in destroying certain types of cells, was studied by medical workers, and, later, the "differential" action of different wave-lengths. The existence of a "latent period" between irradiation and tissue changes was established. Within the cell, it was seen that the nucleus, and particularly the chromatin, was most susceptible to radium and to the X-radiations. There was, however, no such extension of radiology in the general biological field as occurred during the second decade of the century in the field of medicine. Interest in other lines, the war, and failure to obtain results that promised returns of general importance were no doubt responsible. While our medical colleagues went forward in the use of the X-rays in diagnosis and therapeutics, if not in research, biologists lagged behind. In like manner, ultra-violet irradiation began to be utilized in medical practice during the second decade of the century, without attaining a corresponding importance in biology.

My own interest in the technique of irradiation was aroused by a renewal of earlier studies upon the cellular changes during regeneration in planarians. In the regeneration of *Planaria maculata,* after reproduction by fission, it had been observed that cells called "formative cells" were the active units. These formative cells have relatively large nuclei and spindle-shaped cell bodies sometimes with extended processes. They divide by mitosis and seem capable of migration through the mesodermal syncytium or parenchyma. At the time of regeneration they are the only important source of new tissue. If my interpretations are correct, they form ectodermal, endodermal and mesodermal cells, nervous tissue, and special organs like eyes and pharynx. Moreover, they give rise to the germ cells when reproductive organs are formed. During the later stages of embryonic development similar cells are abundant in the mesodermal region. It seems, therefore, that the formative cells constitute a "meristem," which is the source of new cells during growth and regeneration, which has descended without modification from similar cells in the embryo, and which is the path of descent for the germ-plasm. These conclusions have been confirmed with minor exceptions by other investigators, and recently checked in *Planaria agilis,* another spe-

in the technique of microscopical anatomy, and especially of embryology. I do not know when the staining of sections on the slide was first introduced, but it certainly was prior, I think, to the discovery of the ribbon method; if I remember rightly it began with the use of shellac as the means of fixing sections to the slide, some time before the invention of the albumen method by Paul Mayer. It might interest you to know that I still have my old series of sections of the Renilla eggs cut singly, I think in 1881, forty-six years ago. I am obliged to confess that, from the modern point of view, they are rotten sections, but it cost blood to make them at the time.''

cies with powers of fission and regeneration similar to those of *P. maculata*.

Not all planarians regenerate as effectively as do *Planaria maculata* and *P. agilis*. In returning to the problem of regeneration during recent years, my interest was centered upon the relative abundance of formative cells in different species in relation to their respective powers of regeneration. It is a familiar fact to workers with planarians that some species have almost no power of regeneration. Such planarians are in marked contrast with species like *Planaria maculata* and *P. agilis,* which regenerate rapidly and completely. Other species of planarians have what one may call the "capacity" to regenerate, but only at a slower "rate." One may thus speak of the *power of regeneration* as including *capacity* and *rate*. A species like *Planaria maculata* or *P. agilis* has great capacity and a high rate, while *Dendrocœlum lacteum* has little capacity and a slow rate. *Phagocata gracilis* has the capacity, but the regeneration proceeds at a slower rate than it does in *Planaria agilis* or *P. maculata*.[3] To check these facts of general observation, experiments upon the relative powers of regeneration in these three genera (*Planaria, Phagocata* and *Dendrocœlum*) were undertaken, with results that confirmed what was known from more superficial examination.

With these differences in regenerative power established, the numbers and activities of the formative cells in the non-regenerating species, *Dendrocœlum lacteum,* were examined for comparison with *Planaria maculata* and *P. agilis.* This was done by making counts of these cells in measured areas. Although it was recognized that such counts could not be made without a large margin of error, it seemed that a quantitative statement might thus be obtained that would have more value than general terms like "few" and "many." As a result of such counts it was estimated that *Planaria maculata* possessed about 44 formative cells per unit area, and *Dendrocœlum lacteum* about 9, a difference that is in accordance with the powers of regeneration in the two species. It was therefore possible to make the declaration that the *power of regeneration is correlated with the number of formative cells.* If I may descend to a colloquialism—"show me the formative cells of a planarian and I will tell you approximately its power of regeneration, or show me its power of regeneration and I will tell you the relative numbers of its formative cells." The observations confirmed the conclusions regarding the rôle of formative cells in the regeneration of species like *P. maculata* and *P. agilis,* since it was shown that a species like *Dendrocœlum lacteum* with very few of these cells had scant power of regeneration.

At this point it seemed that confirmations might be obtained by further comparisons between regenerating and non-regenerating species, but that more direct evidence could not be obtained by the methods that had been employed. A more satisfactory test would be to destroy the formative cells and thus transform a planarian capable of regeneration into one incapable of such changes. The formative cells appeared to be undifferentiated and embryonic. If undifferentiated cells could be killed in higher animals by irradiation, it seemed that they might be killed by this means in planarians; and once they were killed it should be impossible for the individual to regenerate. Such experiments were tried with *Planaria agilis* (*cf.* Figs. 1–4). When a sufficient exposure was used (approximately 12 skin-units in clinical terminology) no regeneration occurred, although the worms remained alive without external signs of abnormality in structure or function for some time beyond the twelve-day period during which regeneration was completed in the controls of these experiments. When these irradiated worms were sectioned it was found that the formative cells were so reduced in numbers, if not all destroyed, that there seemed to be none remaining in many of the specimens. The mesodermal region was thus changed from its characteristic appearance in *Planaria agilis* to the appearance seen in *Dendrocœlum lacteum* in which there are few formative cells and in which there is scant power of regeneration. Lesser exposures to X-rays partially checked the regeneration and the numbers of formative cells were noticeably reduced. In an experiment with radium, in which an exposure about equivalent to that with the X-radiations was used, regeneration was inhibited in a similar manner.

Unfortunately, it has not been possible to keep the irradiated worms alive for an extended period. At the end of three weeks, or about one week after regeneration is complete in controls, the X-rayed individuals begin to show abnormalities of structure and function. Death ensues about four weeks after the irradiation. It is hoped that further experiments will give worms which can not regenerate, in which formative cells can not be found, and which can be kept alive in a normal state for longer periods. One could then eliminate the possibility that it is the destruction of something else in the planarian, upon which the formative cells are dependent, that is responsible for the check upon regeneration and that disappearance of the formative cells is merely the

[3] *Phagocata gracilis* is not so favorable for this purpose because of its multiple pharynges, but *Dendrocœlum lacteum* is a perfect illustration of scant power of regeneration as compared with a species like *Planaria maculata.*

Inhibition of Regeneration in Planarians by X-rays and Destruction of Formative Cells

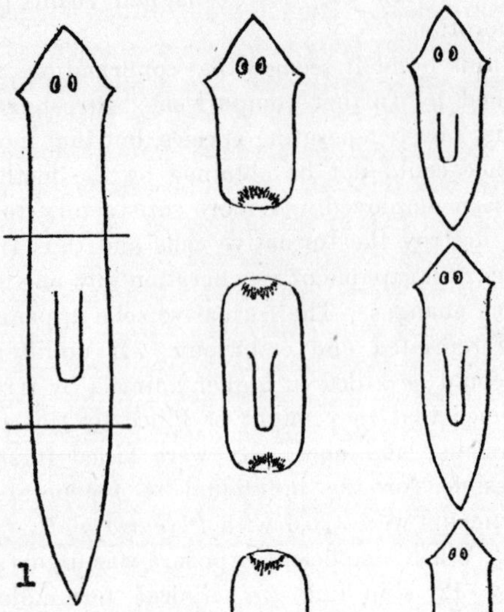

FIG. 1

Planaria agilis

Normal regeneration — 1 day — 12 days

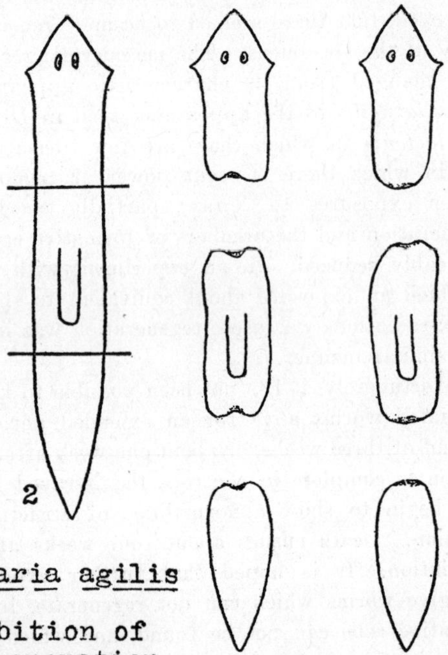

FIG. 2

Planaria agilis

Inhibition of regeneration by X-rays — 1 day — 12 days

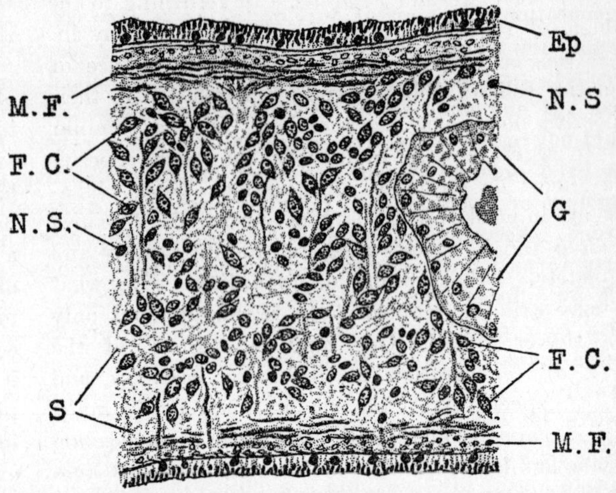

FIG. 3 Planaria agilis

Section showing the numerous formative cells in the mesodermal region of the normal worm

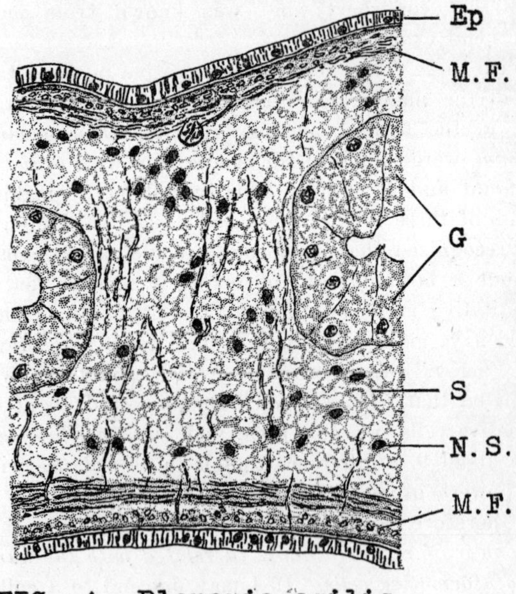

FIG. 4 Planaria agilis

Section showing destruction of formative cells by X-rays. The mesodermal syncytium, with its small, dense nuclei, the gut, and other structures are still normal in appearance

Ep, epithelium; F. C., formative cells; G, branch of gut; M. F., muscle fibers; N. S., nuclei of mesodermal syncytium; S, mesodermal syncytium. (Drawn by Wiley Crawford.)

first step in a series of degenerative changes that end in death of the individual. The formative cells may be the "indicators" and not the ultimate factors in regeneration. In view of our limited knowledge concerning the manner in which radiations produce their effects in protoplasm, this possibility must be considered. If one could secure irradiated planarians that could not regenerate and possessed no formative cells, but lived indefinitely with no other abnormalities in structure or functions, this possibility might be disregarded. According to the hypothesis that the new parts formed during growth and regeneration come only by differentiation of formative cells and that the germ cells of the planarian have a similar origin, such a planarian would be unable to reproduce either sexually or asexually and it would be incapable of growth by increase in the number of its cells. It would be an interesting animal. What would be its expectation of life? Would it exhibit senescence and rejuvenescence, if there are such phenomena in planarians? Would it eventually acquire new formative cells and become capable of regeneration? Would it have an axial gradient? A technique that gave such results would enable us to attack the problem of differentiation as it has not been attacked before.

In testing the formative-cell hypothesis as extended to other animals, experiments with X-rays have been conducted upon sponges and cœlenterates. It has been shown that regeneration can be completely inhibited in the hydroid *Tubularia crocea,* as reported at these meetings. An initial experiment with hydra has been likewise successful. The histological changes involved in these cases among the cœlenterates have not yet been ascertained. The experiments with sponges have not yet given significant results.

Proceeding to other illustrations of applications of the technique of irradiation: Regeneration is an aspect of development. What promise does such a technique hold for students of development in general? That much remains before we shall have reached a satisfactory understanding of ontogeny has been recently set forth in a masterful way by F. R. Lillie ('27), in an essay entitled "The Gene and the Ontogenetic Process." In speaking of the process of embryonic segregation, Lillie says: "We have no present working hypothesis of this most fundamental aspect of the life history." Workers in embryology, therefore, admit that they have reached a point of "diminishing returns" by sectioning and staining, by microdissection, and that even the talisman of physicochemical explanation has failed in its older methods. New technical methods are needed to carry us much farther and enable us to formulate new hypotheses.

There has been, as yet, no great progress, although enough has been accomplished to show possibilities by the technique of irradiation. Working with the ultraviolet radiations, Just has produced Nereis larvæ with nuclei that contain 70 chromosomes instead of the normal 28. Here the maturation divisions go on without polar-body formation so that the sperm nucleus unites with four egg nuclei instead of with one; each egg nucleus as well as that of the sperm has the haploid number of chromosomes—14, thus giving the total of 70. These larvæ produced by irradiation live in the laboratory as long as the controls. Ultra-violet radiations also change the original polarity of Nereis eggs and embryos. Eggs exposed before insemination show the site at which the egg is "hit" by the rays, since there is a blister at this place in the cortex. The first cleavage plane always passes through this area. As the eggs are not oriented for exposure to the rays, any region may be affected, the animal pole, vegetal, or any point in the infinite number between. Hence there is an alteration of polarity. The larval worms show a definitely localized area of injury which can be traced back to this original injury by the rays. The method of irradiation has also been used in various studies of artificial parthenogenesis and cross-activation that have sought to determine the rôle of maternal and paternal pronuclei and of the egg cytoplasm (*cf.* G. Hertwig, '13). While the results have not been revolutionary, it has been shown that irradiation furnishes a means of destroying parts of eggs, particularly the nucleus, in a way that can hardly be approached by mechanical operations. Moreover, it can be used effectively upon eggs *en masse* and without the toilsome procedure of operating with varying success upon each individual cell. In general, these results that have been obtained by irradiation as a technique of research within the field of embryology promise a method by which one may hope to destroy or derange parts of cells and embryos, without injury to the whole, in a manner that makes the finest mechanical operations crude by comparison. With such a technique, important advances may be expected in a renewed attack upon ontogenetic problems.

Turning to another field, Mavor, in studies conducted since 1920, has confirmed the selective action of X-rays upon undifferentiated tissues and upon germ cells in *Drosophila.* The resistance to lethal doses of the rays remains the same during the larval period; but increases markedly during pupation, when the adult parts are being differentiated, until it reaches a new level of stability in the imago. The most susceptible period in the germ-cell cycle is the growth period of primary oöcytes and spermatocytes in *Drosophila* as in other forms. Upon the basis of this underlying phenomenon of selective action by the rays, Mavor has produced non-disjunction in which the eggs either lacked the sex chromosome or possessed two sex chromosomes. Eggs having two sex chromosomes, when fertilized by a Y-bearing sperm, produced exceptional females which in turn produced exceptional daughters and thus propagated the condition brought about by the irradiation. There is, therefore, in this effect of X-rays on germ cells a very clear case of an external agent which modifies the mechanism of inheritance in such a way that a permanent effect is produced. In like manner Mavor has effected by use of X-radiations a reduction of the crossover value in the left half of the first or sex chromosome by X-rays, and an increase of the crossover value in the middle region of the second chromosome. He has also produced gynandromorphs from X-rayed mothers, presumably by elimination of the sex choromosome after fertilization. It is further interesting, as shown by X-raying the anterior and posterior halves of pupæ, that these effects upon the germ cells are not produced when a part of the fly not containing the germ cells is treated. That is, the effects probably occur only when the germ cells are subjected to irradiation and not through any influence transferred from irradiated body cells to the germ cells. It thus appears from the work of Mavor that X-radiations can modify the mechanism of inheritance, through chromosomal changes, in such a manner that permanent effects are produced and transmitted through successive generations without lethal abnormalities. The germ-plasm is changed, but not by the method of the Lamarckians.

The recent work of Muller upon *Drosophila* is widely known. Muller considers the changes he has produced by X-rays truly mutational and not to be confused with the well-known effects of the rays upon the distribution of the chromatin, like non-disjunction and non-inherited crossover modifications. Briefly, he finds that exposure of the sperm to relatively heavy doses of X-rays induces the occurrence of true "gene mutations" in a high proportion of the germ cells. The nature of the crosses was such as to be much more favorable for the detection of mutations in the X-chromosomes than in the other chromosomes, so that most of the mutant genes dealt with were sex-linked; there was, however, ample proof that mutations were occurring similarly throughout the chromatin. When the heaviest treatment was given to the sperm, about a seventh of the offspring that hatched and bred contained individually detectable mutations in their treated X-chromosome. Estimates of the mutations presumably produced in all the chromosomes indicate that the heavier irradiation had caused a rise of about fifteen thousand per cent. in the mutation rate over that in the untreated germ cells. Lighter irradiation produced the gene mutations in lesser numbers. "The visible mutations caused by raying were found to be similar, in their general characteristics, to those previously detected in non-rayed material in the extensive observations on visible mutations in *Drosophila* carried out by Bridges and others." Mutations already familiar, like "white eye," "miniature wing," and "forked bristles," were obtained, and also mutations of a sort not exactly like any seen previously. Muller, therefore, concludes that: "many of the changes produced by X-rays are of just the same kind as the 'gene mutations' which are obtained, with so much greater rarity, without such treatment, and which we believe furnish the building blocks for evolution." He also finds many inherited disturbances in the crossover frequency. In confirmation of these results, Hanson, who has been studying the effects of irradiation upon the sex-ratio of *Drosophila,* has obtained what he considers gene mutations as well as mutations that are seemingly due to chromosomal changes.

It thus appears that two types of genetic modification may be produced in *Drosophila* by the X-radiations—an aberrant distribution of chromosomes and hence new combinations of characters, and gene mutations. In confirmation of these findings in an animal, Stadler reports the production of both types of mutation in plants. In corn, irregular distribution of chromosomes occurs with a certain low frequency in the early cell divisions in endosperm development. This results in mosaic seeds, in which a portion of the endosperm lacks one or more chromosomes. The frequency of occurrence of this phenomenon has been increased about thirty-fold by X-ray treatment at the time of fertilization. Again, in young seedlings of barley Stadler has produced gene mutations by similar irradiation. In this instance the possibility that the gene mutations may in reality be the result of an irregular segregation has been eliminated. These mutations reported in barley are induced in somatic cells, from each of which a self-fertilizing inflorescence is later derived. Each mutant, therefore, segregates in the progeny of a single head, and its absence in the progeny of other heads of the same plant proves that the change occurred in the ontogeny of the plants irradiated. Several viable and morphologically distinct recessive types of such gene mutations have occurred in the progeny of the plants thus subjected to irradiation. To these studies by Mavor, Muller, and Stadler may be added the recent work of Gager and Blakeslee upon *Datura,* which shows irregularities of chromosomal behavior as a result of X-irradiation and which suggests gene mutations and other intrachromosomal changes. The results reported by Goodspeed and Olson upon tobacco plants seem to be in this category, since they do not clearly indicate gene mutations.

From the theoretical standpoint, the chief interest of such results within the field of genetics lies in their bearing upon the problem of the composition and behavior of chromosomes and genes, and thus upon the mechanism of heredity, variation, and evolution. From the practical standpoint, any technique that will induce abundant mutations presents opportunities for the production of improved breeds of domesticated animals and plants beyond anything dreamed of by the slow method of selecting what nature offers. To secure mutations that he desired, Burbank raised plants by the millions, discarding the ninety-and-nines. The advantage of more frequent mutations is obvious. On the medical side, these results, as Muller explains, point to dangers in the practice of temporary sterilization by irradiation. Return of fertility after irradiation does not mean that the germ cells are again normal, since mutations may have been induced that will appear in descendants with disastrous consequences.

Fully developed as well as latent genetic characters may be changed by irradiation. As part of a general program dealing with the biological effects of X-rays, Hance and Murphy have found that following certain exposures the colored hair of agouti mice drops out and after four or five weeks is replaced by white hair. Thus, in an adult animal, a character that is known to be inherited according to the Mendelian law can be changed by the X-radiations. The change seems permanent, as it has persisted for more than twelve months without modification. Speculating upon the causes of such an effect, Hance suspects destruction at its source of the enzyme tryosinase, the color activator, and hence failure of the oxidation of the color base, tryosin. At first what seem to be colorless tryosin granules are recognizable in the hairs, but later the hairs are without such granules and thus resemble the hairs of a normal albino. Nevertheless, "a permanent change has been produced in a mature genetic character by means of X-rays. It is believed that this change is the result of the inhibition or actual killing of the part of the cell concerned with the manufacture of the enzyme needed in the production of color. Since the new color, or rather lack of color, is permanent, it follows that the alteration is passed on to the cells that replace the ones that first encountered the X-rays."

A most interesting attack upon the entire problem of irradiation is being undertaken at the University of Cincinnati, under the leadership of Dean Herman Schneider and Professor George Sperti. The organization of this research is such that individuals in all the related fields, such as physics, chemistry, mathematics, bacteriology, zoology, and physiology, work in intimate association and with mutual support in a laboratory organized for basic investigations. By means of more accurate filters than have been previously used, these investigators have determined critical wave lengths at which chemical dissociation is produced in certain inorganic compounds, and in certain enzymes. They have also determined a wave length at which death occurs in many species of bacteria, and in a variety of the lower animals. Working with ultra-violet radiations, they find, for example, that all bacteria, thus far subject to investigation, are killed when a certain wave length (about 2900 A°) is reached. These particular results have been turned to practical advantage by patenting methods of sterilization for commercial products, the royalties from which are to be used in support of subsequent investigations. A specific example is that of an enzyme that was placed on the market for bread-making, but proved unusable because of bacterial contamination. To kill the bacteria by heat would have destroyed the enzyme, to kill them by antiseptics was not possible in a food product. When the problem was presented to the group at Cincinnati, the solution that suggested itself was to use a wave length that would kill the bacteria, but not destroy the enzyme, since it had been found that the lethal wave length differed in the two instances. The attempt was successful and I understand that the enzyme, minus the troublesome bacteria, is now in use.

To consider more general aspects of the problems open to attack by this new technique, one may distinguish between the obvious morphological and physiological effects produced by irradiation, in destruction of cells and modification of functions, and *how these effects are produced,* that is, the nature of the action of radiations upon protoplasm. The histological and cytological effects can usually be determined with no great difficulty. If one merely attempts destruction of certain parts in order to determine their rôle in development, as with the formative cells of planarians, one may leave the question of how these effects are brought about to investigators whose competence lies within the physico-chemical field. But the problem of how the changes are produced commands attention, because of its intrinsic interest and because it is likely to give clues to physiological processes that have eluded our understanding. This indeed may be the more important item in the end. Most investigators have used the methods of the morphologist. It is clear, however, that disturbances which effect changes that can be directly observed in cells are likely to be of a rather gross nature and that the more delicate functions of cells can not be adequately determined by such methods. Perhaps the studies upon the effects of irradiation in *Drosophila,* spectacular though they are from the standpoint of heredity, will prove more important as a means of detecting physiological changes, too subtle for other modes of demonstration, than as a means of changing genetic constitution. Such studies provide a means of analyzing the effects of X-rays on cells. They show how X-rays may produce a permanent change in a cell without altering its vitality. A method of experimentation has been developed indicating lines of further investigation which may help toward a clear understanding of the exact physical and chemical changes produced by X-rays in living protoplasm, and so of hidden physiological processes. This physiological aspect of the problem can not be elaborated within the limits of the present discussion, but it may be cited as an important field of investigation that is opened by the method of irradiation.

From the morphological standpoint, intensive study should now be directed to the changes produced within the cell. It was formerly believed that the cell was most sensitive during the period of mitosis. It still seems that chromatin is particularly susceptible to radiations, but it now appears that cells are most susceptible during the period just preceding mitosis. Thus, Mohr ('19) has shown, in his classic experiments with radium upon the locust, *Decticus,* that the primary spermatocytes and oöcytes are most sensitive during the growth period, although the cells may be easily affected during the maturation divisions. Working with cells from chick embryos under soft X-rays in tissue-cultures, Strangeways and Oakley ('23) have shown that the cell phases are affected in the following order: first the prophase; next, the later phase of mitosis; and last the inter-division phases of the cell cycle, although many of these "fully formed cells" remain normal in appearance even after prolonged exposure. These investigators have also demonstrated a latent period of about 15 to 20 minutes before the effects upon the cells can be recognized. It appears, however, that the changes produced by the radiations are not specific, since they resemble those in cells growing in unfavorable or in modified media. With lesser exposures, mitosis could be checked, but was resumed after a time if the cultures were returned to the incubator. Although the nucleus and particularly the chromosomes seem most sensitive to irradiation, the cytoplasm is also affected as Packard ('16) and others have shown. It even seems that one can distinguish between a primary effect upon the nucleus, as seen in the mitosis immediately following, and a secondary effect that occurs first in the cytoplasm although it is more apparent in the nuclear changes that it eventually produces (G. Hertwig, '20 and A. Politzer, '25). Between these two effects there may be a period of seemingly normal nuclear division (Stein, '26).

The study of physical and chemical changes within cells is subject to great limitations as compared with the study of such changes in non-living bodies. Methods of chemical analysis and synthesis have only limited applications, since they kill cells at the outset wherever they are applied effectively. Evidence from staining is subject to similar limitations. Microdissection supplements these methods, but has its own disadvantages. By such means, we "know in part and we prophesy in part" when we attempt "to prove all things" concerning cell activities. Results like those obtained by the group at Cincinnati, in destroying specific chemical compounds by specific wave lengths, suggest that it may be possible to destroy visible substances within nucleus or cytoplasm without lethal injury to the cell and thus identify their chemical nature. Such a method may lead to results undreamed of in our present philosophy of cell physiology. Consider what might be done with the problems related to the cytoplasm by such a technique. Results no less remarkable seem to have been accomplished in the nucleus without lethal injury to the cell.

We are thus confronted by the fundamental physiological problem, *the nature of the effects of radiations upon the cell.* Of this we know relatively little, although one can by irradiation change the nature of cells without lethal injury, as the geneticists have done; or completely destroy one type of cell without apparent injury to other types in the same organism, as in the familiar cancer therapy and as I have done in experiments with planarians. The only effect of the absorption of X-rays by an atom that physicists recognize is the expulsion of a high-speed electron. This must be the starting point in any purely physicochemical theory of the action of X-rays upon protoplasm. The problem is one for the biophysicist. If he can solve it, we may hope for notable advances in our knowledge of cellular physiology.

Problems that demand immediate investigation, if biologists would make full use of the X-rays and other radiations as an instrument of research, are: the exact measurement of exposures, the cause of the latent period, the "differential" action of diverse wave-lengths, and whether light exposures actually have the stimulating effects that have been claimed. Fields of biological investigation that seem most vulnerable to an immediate attack by this technique of irradiation are: morphogenesis, heredity, and the physiological effects of radiations.

Belief that the method of irradiation presents alluring possibilities as a tool of biological investigation therefore seems justified by results already accomplished. It is possible by use of radiations to destroy certain types of cells, as though by a surgical operation of surpassing delicacy. We can also reach within the cell and effect changes, particularly in the nucleus. It seems that we can even change the genes and thus inheritance. Most important of all, irradiation promises clues to basic physiological processes. In medicine it has found many applications. It may assume equal importance in the breeding of domesticated plants and animals. In the general field of biological science it offers a new technique before which old problems may fall.

WINTERTON C. CURTIS
UNIVERSITY OF MISSOURI

SPACES OF STATISTICS AND THEIR METRIZATION[1]

WE may generalize the ordinary statistical graph by considering an n-dimensional space in which each coordinate represents a statistical variate. How much arbitrariness is there in the choice of a particular coordinate system? In many familiar cases almost any change of coordinates is meaningless; geometry can then hope to throw but little light on the problem, compared to that which it supplies for physical problems, in which such transformations as those of the Euclidean group are held not to change the nature of the case. But certain situations arise in which real invariant properties exist for rather extended groups of transformations.

One of these cases is in economics. Let p_1, p_2, . . . , p_n be the prices of n commodities; and with these prices ruling, let q_1, q_2, . ., q_n be the respective quantities that can be sold. Now the same market situation can be expressed otherwise by giving the commodities different definitions; *e.g.,* a certain quantity of iron and wood will make a certain number of Fords and a certain number of garages; if we know the equations of transformation we have the same information given by either pair of quantities. Wheat of different grades can be, and is, mixed in different ways to meet the grading systems in different countries. We can readily prove that under these transformations in the manifold of prices, quantity is a covariant vector. Dually, in the manifold of quantities price is a covariant vector.

Another example is in biology. If an individual be regarded as fully specified by the dimensions of n organs he is, by definition, a point in a space of n dimensions. A species is a cluster of points, and may be typified by its center of gravity. Coordinates may be transformed by changing the methods of measurement; thus we may give the height of a man's shoulder and the length of his arm, or we may give the height of his hanging hand and the length of his arm.

But in all this no invariant distance element has appeared. We are impelled to look about for some quadratic form, preferably a quadratic differential form, of statistical significance.

Now a quadratic form of overshadowing importance is found in the exponent of the normal law of probability in n variables. The various reasons for adopting this law are strongest when the deviations of which the quadratic form is a function are small, and so it is natural to take it as a quadratic differential form.

The idea of random migration has received much mathematical consideration by Karl Pearson, Lord Rayleigh and others. It may be applied to particles in a biological n-space to discuss evolution. A son differs from his father in n ways; if these deviations are all independent and have equal dispersions, the probability of a set of deviations $\delta x_1, \ldots, \delta x_n$ is proportional to e^{-T}, where T is a constant multiple of $\delta x_1^2 + \delta x_2^2 + \ldots + \delta x_n^2$, and so may be said to define the *distance* from father to son. If the deviations are not independent, product terms $\delta x_i \; \delta x_j$ appear in T. If finally the dispersions and degrees of interdependence of the δx's depend on the x's we have the quadratic differential form with variable coefficients, and therefore a Riemannian geometry. That the dispersions do in fact vary with the size is evident by considering the difference in centimeters in the length of a pair of twin elephants, and then comparing this with the variability in length in a litter of mice. It may safely be assumed that the intercorrelations, for a given species, may also vary with size and shape.

In this way we obtain a metrical space, in general curved, as a matrix for possible organisms. A species, represented by a swarm of particles, diffuses gradually by an accumulation of small changes in a manner analogous to the conduction of heat in this curved space. It would eventually become so diversified as to supply the naturalist with every conceivable kind of specimen were it not for the effect of selection. This may be pictured as a system of heat "sinks," of refrigerated localities, spread here and there to trap and annihilate unwary individuals. On the whole the losses due to the sinks are of course made good by natural increase.

The center of gravity of a swarm of individuals may be taken to represent the species. Suppose that we have a collection of fossils which shows us the location of this point at each of two times a million years apart; it is desired to know its most probable positions at intermediate times. If we have no

[1] Presented to the American Mathematical Society, September 9, 1927.

"sinks," no selective action, then the most likely path is a geodesic. If we do have "sinks" they act as propulsive forces and we encounter the following generalization of the theory of differential equations. At each point, instead of having a definite direction of motion assigned, as by differential equations, we have a pencil of directions (or an (n–1)-parameter family of directions) with a function, which will be a normal error function, giving the probability that the direction of motion will lie between any assigned limits. This enables us to assign to the curves joining two points a distribution of a species of probability. For fixed end points the selection of the most probable curve is a problem in the calculus of variations. If g_{ij} is the fundamental tensor and φ_i a vector giving the most probable direction we shall in fact minimize

$$\int_{t_1}^{t_2} \sum_{i,j=1}^{n} g_{ij}(\dot{x}_i - \varphi_i)(\dot{x}_j - \varphi_j)\, dt,$$

where $\dot{x}_i = dx_i/dt$.

The minimizing equations for the integral may be interpreted as the differential equations of a dynamical system. Indeed we may consider the most probable path as the trajectory of a particle shooting through the curved space under a field of force. However, the form of the integral shows that the force will in general depend upon the direction of motion, as with an electrical charge moving in a magnetic field.

The derivation of the criterion that the integral shall be minimized is a simple generalization of a derivation in the article on "Differential Equations subject to Error, and Population Estimates,"[2] in which I use the same considerations in their simplest form to obtain estimates of intercensal populations. That was in one dimension, but it may readily be generalized by considering a system of variables having correlated changes, such as the population of a city, the number of children in its schools, the number of telephones and so on. The leading difficulty in applications of this kind is to arrive at the tensor g_{ij}.

There is nothing to prevent empirical determination from measurements of parents and offspring of the fundamental biological tensor giving the distance element which we have defined. In fact all the measurements which have been made in the study of heredity may be regarded as steps in this enterprise. As a sufficient accumulation of data makes the hypothesis of flatness untenable we shall be driven to look for some other kind of space, as simple as is possible without contradicting the data. A space which in some sense or other has constant curvature will be wanted as a second approximation, and mathematicians will be asked to supply equations of suitable type, with parameters for biological workers to determine empirically and check by tests of goodness of fit.

This problem which biology is approaching has already been faced by physics. The hypothesis of Euclidean space-time as a matrix of physical events served adequately for several centuries; but more refined measurements have required its modification. Mathematical physics has been grappling with the problem of supplying as simple a statement as possible of the properties of the world-order without contradicting known facts. Such a statement is indeed what we call an explanation. It is altogether likely that the considerations of simplicity which led Einstein to his cosmological equations may some day cause the same equations to appear as the foundation of biology.

HAROLD HOTELLING

STANFORD UNIVERSITY,
CALIFORNIA

[2] *Journal of the American Statistical Association*, September, 1927, pp. 283–314.

PAUL HEINRICH VON GROTH

IT is with deep regret that we record the death of Professor Paul Heinrich von Groth in Munich, Germany, on December 2, 1927. With the passing of Professor Groth the Mineralogical Society of America has lost one of its most distinguished honorary life fellows, the science of mineralogy one of its greatest leaders and the world of science a courageous pioneer, an ardent investigator, an energetic and efficient author and editor and an inspiring teacher.

Paul Heinrich von Groth was born on June 23, 1843, at Magdeburg, Germany. His father was a portrait painter. The training for his life's work Professor Groth obtained at the school of mines in Freiberg, at the college of engineering in Dresden and at the University of Berlin, at which institutions he spent the years 1862 to 1870. The degree of doctor of philosophy was conferred upon him by the University of Berlin in 1868.

From 1870 to 1872 Professor Groth was a member of the teaching staffs of the Technische Hochschule in Charlottenburg and of the University of Berlin. When the University of Strassburg was being reorganized, shortly after the close of the Franco-Prussian war, Groth was called to the chair of mineralogy, for he had already acquired a splendid reputation as an investigator of great promise, especially in the field of chemical crystallography, to the development of which he subsequently contributed so extensively.

Groth held the professorship at Strassburg from

1872 to 1883. During this period he not only supervised the construction of a new laboratory, which set a very high standard for that time, and completely reorganized the mineral collections, but he also carried on extensive researches and published a long list of papers. Moreover, it was while at Strassburg that Groth began his notable career as an author and editor, for during that period he wrote two text-books and a guide to the mineral collections and founded the *Zeitschrift für Kristallographie und Mineralogie.*

Thus, in 1874, the first edition of his "Tabellarische Übersicht der Mineralien" was published, which later appeared in four German editions and in 1904 was translated into French. Two years later, in 1876, his "Physikalische Kristallographie und Einleitung in die Kenntnis der wichtigen Substanzen" appeared. This soon became the standard text in the field of physical crystallography, and later passed through four German editions. In 1910 this important text-book was made more directly available to English-reading students, when portions of it were translated into English by Jackson. The third book to be written by Groth while at Strassburg was the excellent guide to the mineral collections of the university, published in 1878.

As already indicated, the *Zeitschrift für Kristallographie und Mineralogie* was founded by Groth. It was first issued in 1877. As sole editor Groth published 52 volumes of the *Zeitschrift* and three more as joint editor with Professor E. Kaiser, making a total of 55 volumes during the years 1877 to 1920. As is well known, since 1921 the *Zeitschrift* has been under the editorship of Professor P. Niggli, of the University of Zürich. Upon the occasion of Groth's eightieth birthday, in 1923, the 58th volume was issued as a Groth Festschrift, and contained 32 papers by his friends and former students.

In 1883 Professor Groth was called to the University of Munich as the successor to Professor Franz von Kobell. His tremendous energy was at once transferred to that institution, and he soon reorganized the instruction in mineralogy and installed in new quarters the extensive royal Bavarian mineral collections, of which he was made custodian. Under Groth's leadership the Mineralogisches Institut of the University of Munich became one of the chief centers for crystallographic and mineralogical study, advanced students being attracted from all over the world, particularly from the United States.

During his professorship at Munich Professor Groth stimulated and supervised many investigations dealing with various phases of crystallography and mineralogy. He also continued to write text and reference books and 13 additional volumes were placed to his credit, of which only the following will be mentioned: "Grundriss der Edelstein-Kunde" (1887), the monumental work on "Chemische Kristallographie" in six volumes (1904 to 1919), "Elemente der physikalischen und chemischen Kristallographie" (1921), and "Die Entwickelungsgeschichte der mineralogischen Wissenschaften" (1926). The last book was published after his retirement from active teaching and when he had all but lost his eyesight.

Professor Groth's contributions to the mineralogical sciences were widely and most favorably recognized for he was elected to honorary membership in many learned societies. Since he had had many students from the United States and Canada it, indeed, was fitting that he should have been elected an honorary life fellow of the Mineralogical Society of America in 1926. Prominent universities also gladly testified to Professor Groth's preeminent position among the world's leading scientists of his period, the Universities of Cambridge and Geneva having conferred upon him the honorary degree of doctor of science and the University of Prague that of doctor of philosophy.

Professor Groth's activities were so varied and many of his contributions so fundamental and far-reaching that they exercised a profound influence not only upon the development of mineralogy but also upon certain phases of chemistry and physics. Accordingly many of his views on morphotrophy and isomorphism and on chemical crystallography in general have become firmly embodied in chemical literature. Furthermore, the remarkable advances in our knowledge of crystal structure as the result of the development of X-ray analysis, dating from 1912, are in large measure due to Groth's long and enthusiastic advocacy of the point system theory of crystal structure.

Until the very last Professor Groth was keenly interested in American mineralogy. In 1893 he came to the United States and served as a member of the jury of awards for the division of Mines and Minerals of the World's Exposition held in Chicago that year. While in this country he visited some of our leading universities, museums and mining and mineral localities.

In March, 1926, I was privileged to visit Professor Groth twice in his home in Munich. Although he was then in his eighty-third year and nearly blind, he displayed the same enthusiasm for his beloved science and still retained the alertness of mind that had attracted so many students to him and inspired them to achievement. At that time he eagerly inquired about his friends and former students in this country and Canada.

During the 60 years of Groth's activity, crystallography has passed by various stages of development from the list of the more or less descriptive sciences to that of the exact sciences permitting of precise measurements. To this advance Professor Groth and his many students contributed in no small measure.

EDWARD H. KRAUS

UNIVERSITY OF MICHIGAN

SCIENTIFIC EVENTS

THE ELLA SACHS PLOTZ FOUNDATION FOR THE ADVANCEMENT OF SCIENTIFIC INVESTIGATION

DURING the fourth year of the Ella Sachs Plotz Foundation for the Advancement of Scientific Investigation the total number of grants made was twenty-four. Seventeen of the new grants were made to scientists in countries outside of the United States. In the four years of its existence the foundation has made fifty-five grants and investigators have been aided in the United States, Great Britain, France, Germany, Austria, Hungary, Switzerland, Italy, Sweden, Esthonia and Czechoslovakia.

The list of investigators and of the researches which have been aided in the current year is as follows:

Dr. William deB. MacNider, University of North Carolina Medical School, $500 a year for two years for further studies on experimental nephritis.

Dr. W. W. Swanson, University of Minnesota, $500 for an investigation of the osmotic pressure of the plasma proteins in nephritis.

Professor Dr. W. Weichardt, Erlangen, $250 for an investigation on a scientific basis for nonspecific therapy.

Professor Dr. W. Schlayer, Berlin, $250 for a study of the exchange of various substances, including indican and uric acid, from the tissues to the blood.

Dr. Leo Hess, Vienna, $200 for a study of the biology of jaundice.

Dr. Hermann Sternberg, Vienna, $250 for physiological, pharmacological, histological and pathological investigations of the respiratory tract, particularly as concerns hay-fever, asthma and vasomotor rhinitis.

Dr. David Scherf, Vienna, $250 for animal experiments on arrhythmia of the heart.

Dr. Alfred Neumann, Vienna, $280 for a study of the chemical and biological characteristics of the granules of leucocytes.

Dr. Leon Asher, Berne, $250 for a study of the mechanism of the so-called autonomic poisons or drugs.

Professor O. Loewi, Graz, $500 for researches on the mechanism of insulin effect and diabetes.

Professor Dr. Ernst Loewenstein, Vienna, $1,000 for a study of the chemotherapy of infectious diseases, especially of tuberculosis.

Dr. Waldemar Gohs, Vienna, $279 for researches on bacteriophage.

Professor Maurizio Ascoli, Catania, $1,000 for research on the prevention of Malta fever.

Dr. R. Wartenberg, Freiburg, $200 for continuation of encephalographic and myelographic studies.

Dr. Andrea Andreen Svedberg, Stockholm, $550 for research on intermediary metabolism of carbohydrates with special reference to diabetes in dogs and men.

Dr. Robert Chambers, Cornell University Medical School, $750 for a study of the reaction of protoplasm under various physiological, pathological and pharmacological conditions.

Dr. Charles Hruska, Ivanovice, $500 for a study of immunity in anthrax.

Professor Leon Blum, Strasbourg, $1,000 for researches on nephritis and study of the therapeutics resulting from them.

Dr. Erwin Becher, Munich, $300 for investigations in uremia.

Dr. Henry G. Barbour and Dr. R. Glenn Spurling, University of Louisville School of Medicine, $750 for investigations on the prevention of fluid loss from the circulation.

Dr. M. S. Dooley, University of Syracuse, $700 for studies on the direct and indirect effects of drugs, including anesthetics, upon the medullary centers.

Dr. Ernst Weichmann, Cologne, $250 for a study of permeability of cells.

Thorndike Memorial Laboratory, Boston City Hospital, $500 a year in recognition of Dr. Peabody's services.

Dr. James E. Dawson, Edinburgh, $250 a year for two years (made in 1926) for investigation on the pathology of the breast.

THE JOURNAL OF THE SWEDISH FORESTRY SOCIETY

WITH the volume of 1927 *The Journal of the Swedish Forestry Society* (Svenska Skogsvardsföreningens Tidskrift) completes its 25th year. During the last quarter century it has taken a leading place among the technical forestry journals of the world, and the growing interest during the past decade for Swedish forestry has been due no little to the excellence of this publication in presenting the results of research to the world. Recognizing the increasing international interest in forestry, and forest research in particular, the editors announce the following new policy, beginning with the 1927 volume:

1. The journal will be devoted exclusively to reports of scientific forest investigations and papers on forest policy and forest economics. Book reviews will be included, but all notices, etc., of local interest only will be published in the popular bimonthly organ "Skogen" ("The Forest").

2. All articles will be accompanied by full résumés in French, German or English.

3. Papers of more general international interest will be published *in extenso* in one of these languages.

In embarking on this policy, the editors are following the custom of other scientific journals of international appeal. In view of the changes which now enable the journal to address itself to a wider reading public, it is earnestly hoped that American foresters, ecologists, pathologists, entomologists and research workers in other branches of biological science will give the publication their hearty support.

The editor-in-chief is Professor Henrik Hesselman, in charge of the natural science division of the Swedish Institute of Experimental Forestry (Statens Skogsförsöksanstalt), and was chairman of the section on forest soils at the International Congress of Soil Sciences at Washington in 1927. The assistant editor is Erik Lundh, secretary of the Swedish Forestry Society and docent at the Forest School.

The journal will be published in four large parts each year, two before and two after the summer. Owing to the fact that the reports of the experiment station (Meddelanden fran Statens Skogsförsöksanstalt) are published by the society, arrangement can be made to have them accompany the journal as supplements. Both publications are printed in large, readable type on heavy glazed paper, and are profusely illustrated with many clear illustrations, graphs, tables, etc. Colored plates are frequently included. The journal thus offers a very attractive medium for publication, and it is to be hoped that American investigators may be interested in submitting manuscripts. The undersigned has consented to act as American representative, and will be glad to answer inquiries regarding subscriptions and advertising, and forward material submitted for publication. A limited supply of sample copies of the last volumes of the "Tidskrift" and "Meddelanden" are available and will be sent on request to organizations and individuals interested.

HENRY I. BALDWIN

BERLIN, NEW HAMPSHIRE

STATEMENT REGARDING THE DISMISSAL OF THE HEALTH COMMISSIONER OF CHICAGO

FOLLOWING the dismissal of Dr. Herman N. Bundesen, former health commissioner of Chicago, and his replacement by Mayor Thompson's personal physician, a surgeon with no public health training, a public statement has been issued by many prominent men in public health work in the United States, protesting against the influence of politics affecting the public health and welfare of the people at large. Not only has Dr. Bundesen been eliminated from Chicago's health department, but also his principal assistants, J. C. Geiger, M.D., deputy health commissioner; Arthur E. Gorman, chief sanitary engineer, and I. S. Falk, Ph.D., director of surveys.

The statement reads:

The undersigned workers in the field of American public health desire to express an emphatic protest against the action of the Mayor of the City of Chicago in replacing Dr. Herman N. Bundesen, the health officer of that city, by a physician who, whatever his personal standing, is without apparent qualifications or experience to fit himself for the discharge of the serious duties of the office in question.

Permanence of tenure for competent health officials is an absolutely essential factor in the protection of the public against preventable disease; and the case in question seems particularly flagrant in view of the extraordinary record of Dr. Bundesen, whose brilliant services have aroused nation-wide admiration. Sacrifice of the lives of citizens of Chicago to political exploitation and personal whims is more than a local matter, since unsanitary conditions in one community may react upon an entire continent.

The action of the mayor of Chicago strikes a blow at the most fundamental principles of good government. It should meet with prompt and vigorous rebuke from all people of Chicago who care for the reputation of their city and it should stimulate citizens everywhere to see that city charters are amended so as to make such interference with good health administration impossible in their own communities.

The statement is signed by twenty-three men eminent in the field of public health including: Dr. A. C. Abbott, director, School of Hygiene and Public Health, University of Pennsylvania; Dr. Charles V. Chapin, superintendent of health, Providence; Dr. Haven Emerson, professor of public health administration, Columbia University; Dr. Livingston Farrand, president, Cornell University; Dr. Allen W. Freeman, professor of public health administration, the Johns Hopkins University; Dr. Louis I. Harris, commissioner of health, New York City; Dr. William H. Howell, director, School of Hygiene and Public Health, the Johns Hopkins University; Dr. William H. Park, director, bureau of laboratories, Department of Health, New York City; Dr. Ray Lyman Wilbur, president, Leland Stanford University, and Dr. C.-E. A. Winslow, professor of public health, Yale University.

REPORT OF THE DELEGATE OF THE BOTANICAL SOCIETY OF AMERICA TO THE THIRD PAN-PACIFIC CONGRESS

THE following is the report of the delegate of the Botanical Society of America to the third Pan-Pacific Congress:

TO THE SECRETARY,
BOTANICAL SOCIETY OF AMERICA.

It is desired that what follows may be considered to be a brief and informal report of the delegate of the

Botanical Society of America to the Third Pan-Pacific Science Congress held at Tokyo, Japan, whose scientific formal program extended from October 30 to November 11, 1926, but whose more extended excursions began October 18 and continued until November 19. During the whole of this considerable period, the delegates participating (together with their accompanying families) were regarded as the guests of the local committees and all living and traveling expenses provided for out of funds at their disposal. Your delegate joins the other foreign delegates in feeling that no form of words is adequate for the expression of their appreciation of the wonderful hospitality of the Japanese Government and its official representatives and of the marvelous executive ability and extreme courtesy of its citizens of both high and low degree. The management of the complicated detail of the scientific, social and travel program is beyond ordinary expression of sincere and genuine praise.

The particular general achievement of the congress was the effecting of a permanent organization to perpetuate its work and continue its ideals. The "*Pacific Science Association*" came into being at the closing general session, the units being the National Research Councils, or other outstanding scientific body, of each Pacific unit of territory. A constitution and by-laws were adopted and Java was selected for the next meeting with 1929 as the year for reassembling.

The principal measures of botanical interest instituted or sanctioned by the proceedings of the congress are:

(1) The representation of biology on the Committee for Oceanographic Research;
(2) The inclusion of endemism and migration with reference to the insular floras (and faunas) of the Pacific Ocean;
(3) Geological and paleontological evidence as to the shores of the Pacific in divisions of Tertiary time (this having relation to existence or non-existence of land bridges);
(4) The botanical point of view as preeminent in the investigation of the coral reefs of the Pacific Ocean;
(5) The resolution calling for the setting aside of localities of particular botanical interest, and
(6) The resolution urging the Chilean Government to take measures looking towards the protection of the peculiar floral features of the Juan Fernandez Islands.

Your delegate attended a luncheon given by the Botanical Society of Tokyo to visiting botanists, delivered three papers, *viz.*—"Endemism and Migration with Particular Reference to the Floras of the Pacific Islands," "Coral Reef Problems in the Pacific and Indian Oceans" and "A Botanical Point of View of Coral Reef Theories, with Especial Relation to the Coral Reefs of the Pacific Ocean." He also proposed a resolution to institute a committee to be composed of biologists, oceanographers and geologists to outline the problems connected with the origin and growth of the coral reefs of the Pacific Ocean and to suggest methods of investigation for their solution. This resolution was adopted by the congress.

Respectfully submitted,
(Signed) W. A. Setchell,
Delegate

The following resolution was adopted by the society at the recent Nashville meeting.

The Botanical Society of America wishes to express, through Professor Sakurai, its deep appreciation of the unusually successful conduct of the Third Pan-Pacific Science Congress convened at Tokyo in October and November, 1926; and to thank the Imperial Japanese Government for making possible a meeting of such significance for scientific and international cooperation. It wishes also particularly to thank the Botanical Society of Tokyo, the Botanical Institutes of the Imperial University of Tokyo, and the other scientific organizations of Japan for the assistance generously extended to the American delegates and for their delightful hospitality throughout the extended period before and after the meetings of the congress, during which they traveled and studied in Japan.

SCIENTIFIC NOTES AND NEWS

Dr. Hendrik Lorenz, professor of mathematical physics at Leyden, died on February 25, at the age of twenty-five years.

The Faraday medal "for notable scientific or industrial achievement in electrical engineering or for conspicuous service rendered to the advancement of electrical science" has been awarded by the Institution of Electrical Engineers, London, to J. A. Fleming, F.R.S., formerly professor of electrical engineering in the University of London.

The council of the Geological Society has made the following awards: Wollaston Medal to Dr. D. H. Scott, lately honorary keeper of the Jodrell laboratory, Royal Botanic Gardens, Kew, in recognition of the value of his researches in fossil botany; Murchison Medal to Dr. J. J. Sederholm, director of the Geological Commission of Finland, in recognition of his researches in petrology, especially of the granites and gneisses of the pre-Cambrian complex of Fennoscandia; a Lyell medal to Professor S. H. Reynolds, C. Wills, professor of geology in the University of Bristol, in recognition of the value of his researches in the stratigraphy of the Paleozoic rocks, and in vertebrate paleontology; a second Lyell medal to Dr. W. D. Lang, keeper of the department of geology in the British Museum, for his researches in stratigraphy and paleontology, especially with reference to the Bryozoa; the Wollaston donation fund to Mr. James Wright, for his researches on the Crinoidea of the

Carboniferous Limestone of Scotland; the Murchison geological fund to Dr. George Slater, in recognition of the value of his researches in glaciology; and the Lyell geological fund to Mr. Ben Lightfoot, for his researches on the economic geology of Southern Rhodesia.

THE list of British New Year honors includes, as reported in *Nature,* the names of the following men of science and others associated with scientific work. *Baronet:* Major-General Sir Richard Havelock Charles, sergeant surgeon to the king, a past president of the Royal Society of Tropical Medicine and Hygiene. *K.C.V.O.*: Sir Frank Baines, until lately Director of Works, H. M. Office of Works. *Knights:* Professor Jahangir Cooverjee Coyajee, professor of political economy and philosophy in the Presidency College at Calcutta; F. G. Hallett, secretary of the joint examining board, Royal College of Physicians of London and Royal College of Surgeons of England; Brigadier-General H. B. Hartley, fellow and tutor of Balliol College, Oxford, and member of the chemical warfare committee; Dr. E. H. Pascoe, director of the Geological Survey of India; Principal C. Grant Robertson, vice-chancellor and principal of the University of Birmingham; Dr. T. E. Stanton, superintendent of the engineering department, National Physical Laboratory; A. E. Aspinall, secretary of the Imperial College of Tropical Agriculture, Trinidad. *C.M.G.:* Major R. G. Archibald, director of the Wellcome Research Laboratories, Khartum; Mr. O. T. Faulkner, director of agriculture, Nigeria.

THE King of Spain has conferred the grand cross of the order of civil merit on Dr. Aldo Castellani, director of tropical medicine at the Ross Institute and Hospital, London, now lecturing at Tulane University, in recognition of his investigations into tropical diseases. Dr. Castellani recently visited Madrid at the invitation of the Spanish government to lecture on the subject of malaria. The King of England has conferred the rank of honorary knight commander of the Order of St. Michael and St. George upon Dr. Castellani.

HERBERT HOOVER, secretary of commerce, has been awarded the gold medal of the American Institute of Mining and Metallurgical Engineers for "achievement in mining."

DR. ALEXANDER WETMORE, assistant secretary of the Smithsonian Institution, has been elected a corresponding member of the Zoological Society of London.

THE Woman's Medical College of Pennsylvania announced in connection with the recent celebration of the ninety-first birthday of Dr. William W. Keen that a chair of surgery will be named in his honor in the new college to be built at the Falls of the Schuylkill. The sum of $100,000 will be raised to endow the chair. Dr. Keen was for several years professor of surgery at the Woman's Medical College.

ON November 21, 1927, at the psychology laboratory of Stanford University, a dinner was held in commemoration of Dr. Frank Angell's seventieth birthday and of the thirty-fifth year since the founding of the Stanford Laboratory. Dr. Angell took this occasion to recount his Leipzig experiences with the late Professor E. B. Titchener and to describe incidents connected with the establishing of the psychology departments both at Cornell and at Stanford. A portrait of Dr. Angell was unveiled and presented to the psychology laboratory at this time. The chairman of the occasion was Dr. Catharine Cox Miles.

PROFESSOR ARTHUR H. COMPTON, recent Nobel prize winner, was guest of honor at a faculty dinner at the University of Chicago on January 12.

ALEXANDER SILVERMAN, head of the department of chemistry at the University of Pittsburgh, was tendered a dinner by the students and faculty of Bryn Mawr College on January 12, following which he delivered an illustrated lecture on "Glass: One of Man's Blessings."

THE following officers of the Botanical Society of America were elected at the Nashville meeting: *President,* A. H. R. Buller, of the University of Manitoba; *Vice-president,* I. W. Bailey, of Harvard University. Corresponding members of the society were elected as follows: Abbé Giacomo Bresadola, Professor Seiichiro Ikeno, Professor C. H. Ostenfeld, Professor Otto Rosenberg and Professor Richard von Wettstein.

AT the annual meeting of the Anthropological Society of Washington on January 17, the following officers were elected to serve for the current year of 1928: *President,* Dr. Charles L. G. Anderson; *Vice-president,* Frank H. Roberts, Jr.; *Secretary,* Dr. John M. Cooper; *Treasurer,* Henry B. Collins, Jr.

AT the annual meeting of the American Association for the Study of Allergy in Washington, D. C., Dr. Harry S. Bernton, Washington, D. C., was elected *president;* Dr. Richard A. Kern, Philadelphia, *vice-president,* and Dr. Albert H. Rowe, Oakland, Calif., *secretary-treasurer.* The next meeting of the association will be at Minneapolis on June 11.

DAVID F. JONES, Watertown, S. D., has been elected president of the American Pharmaceutical Association and will be installed at the next annual meeting.

PROFESSOR D. D. JACKSON, head of the department of chemical engineering at Columbia University, has accepted the chairmanship of the coordinating committee, which is in charge of the coming visit of English chemists and chemical engineers, members and guests of the Society of Chemical Industry.

Professor Wilder D. Bancroft, of the department of chemistry at Cornell University, has been appointed a member of the advisory committee of the cancer research fund of the University of Pennsylvania.

C. A. Brautlecht, head of the department of chemistry and chemical engineering at the University of Maine, has been elected chairman of the Northeastern division of the American Pulp and Paper Mill Superintendents Association.

William Procter, research associate of the Academy of Natural Sciences of Philadelphia, has been elected to serve on the board of managers of the Wistar Institute to fill the vacancy caused by the death of Mr. George Vaux, Jr.

The Smithsonian Institution has awarded the Walter Rathbone Bacon research fellowship for the years 1928–1930 to Dr. Paul Bartsch, curator of mollusks in the U. S. National Museum. Dr. Bartsch will make use of the award to collect material for the completion of a monograph he has long had under way on the land shells of the West Indies.

At the American Museum of Natural History Clifford H. Pope has been promoted from assistant to assistant curator of herpetology; Dr. Chester A. Reeds, curator of invertebrate paleontology, has had his title changed to curator of geology and invertebrate paleontology, and John Treadwell Nichols, assistant curator of recent fishes, has been made curator of recent fishes.

Dr. David Fairchild, senior agricultural explorer in charge of the office of foreign plant introduction, U. S. Bureau of Plant Industry, relinquished charge of that office on January 5, and Knowles A. Ryerson assumed the direction of the office. Dr. Fairchild will continue as senior agricultural explorer and will act as adviser and consulting specialist in matters pertaining to research problems in foreign-plant introduction.

Philip G. Colin has resigned from the Rockefeller Institute for Medical Research to take a position with the Tidewater Oil Company, Bayonne, N. J.

Louis E. Dawson has resigned his position in the carbohydrate laboratory, U. S. Bureau of Chemistry and Soils, to take a position in the research department of H. O. Wilbur & Sons, manufacturers of cocoa and chocolates, Philadelphia, Pa.

Dr. N. L. Britton, director of the New York Botanical Garden, recently went to Porto Rico to continue the botanical and horticultural studies of West Indian plants.

Dr. J. W. Gidley, of the division of vertebrate paleontology in the U. S. National Museum, will leave shortly for Melbourne, Florida, where he expects to spend about two months in securing data on Pleistocene vertebrates.

Asher Hobson, permanent United States delegate to the International Institute of Agriculture at Rome, sailed for Europe on January 4. He will be located at Geneva, Switzerland, where he will gather research material in the development of a study which he has under way dealing with the institute.

Dr. F. F. Nord, of the Physiological Institute, Berlin, who worked during 1926–27 in the division of agricultural biochemistry at the University of Minnesota, addressed on his way home the Pan-Pacific Research Institute at Honolulu and delivered lectures at the Imperial University of Kyoto, the Indian Chemical Society at Calcutta and at the Universities of Patna, Benares and Allahabad.

The next series of Lane medical lectures will be given in October, 1928, by Professor F. d'Herelle, directeur du service bacteriologique du Conseil Sanitaire, Maritime et Quarantinaire at Alexandria, Egypt. The program has not been decided upon, but the lectures will probably cover filterable viruses and the bacteriophage. Dr. Walter Straub, professor of pharmacology at the University of Munich, has consented to give the Lane medical lectures in 1929. The course will probably be given in April.

Professor H. Kramers, of the University of Utrecht, will lecture at the University of Michigan during the coming summer session (June 15 to August 30). He will lecture twice a week on "Wave Mechanics" and twice a week on "Survey of Recent Work in the Quantum Theory." Courses will also be given by Drs. Uhlenbeck and Goudsmit, recently of the University of Leyden, supplementing those of Professor Kramers.

Dr. H. H. Gran, professor of botany in the University of Oslo, Oslo, Norway, will offer a course in marine diatoms at the Puget Sound Biological Station, Friday Harbor, Washington, during the session beginning on June 18.

Dr. Wade Hampton Frost, professor of epidemiology in the School of Hygiene and Public Health at the Johns Hopkins University, gave the Cutter lectures on preventive medicine at the Harvard Medical School on February 2 and 3. The subjects of the lectures were "Infection, Immunity and Disease in the

Epidemiology of Diphtheria" and "Some Conceptions of Epidemics in General."

DR. OSCAR RIDDLE, of the Carnegie Station for Experimental Evolution, Cold Spring Harbor, New York, delivered a series of six lectures during the month of January at the School of Tropical Medicine of the University of Porto Rico, San Juan, on "The Internal Secretions in Evolution and Reproduction" and "Control and Transformation of Sex in Animals."

DR. HERBERT E. IVES, of the Bell Telephone Laboratories, will address the Franklin Institute on February 15 on "Television."

DR. EDWIN HUBBLE, astronomer in the Mount Wilson Observatory, will give a lecture on February 20 in San Francisco under the auspices of the Astronomical Society of the Pacific. Dr. Hubble will speak on "The Exploration of Space."

DR. FRANCIS G. BENEDICT, director of the Nutrition Laboratory of the Carnegie Institution of Washington, gave an address at Mount Holyoke College, South Hadley, Massachusetts, on "The Heat Production of Humans and Animals and Factors Affecting it," on January 21.

DR. COLIN G. FINK, of Columbia University, gave an illustrated address on "Recent Advances in Electrochemistry" at the meeting of the American Institute of Electrical Engineers held at Waterbury, on January 24. On February 3 Dr. Fink lectured before the McGill chapter of Sigma Xi and on February 15 he will lecture to the chemical students of Yale University, on the subject "Corrosion, its Cause and Prevention."

DR. W. F. G. SWANN, director of the Bartol Research Foundation, Philadelphia, read a paper on "Theories of the Atom," before the American Philosophical Society on February 3.

A TABLET in memory of Sir William Osler was unveiled by the Hamilton Medical Society, on December 28, 1927, near his former home in Dundas, Ontario.

DR. ERNEST C. SCHROEDER died on January 24, at Bethesda, Md., where he was superintendent of the Experiment Station of the Bureau of Animal Industry, United States Department of Agriculture. During his forty years of public service Dr. Schroeder made important contributions to the knowledge of animal diseases.

DR. OWEN F. BURGER, plant pathologist of the Florida Agricultural Experiment Station, died on January 26, from injuries received in an automobile collision. Dr. Burger was forty-three years of age.

EDWARD MALLINCKRODT, president of the Mallinckrodt Chemical Works, died on February 3, aged eighty-three years. Mr. Mallinckrodt has given more than $1,000,000 to scientific education and to hospitals. The largest single item was $500,000 to Harvard for a building to house the department of chemistry.

BRADSHAW HALL SWALES, honorary assistant curator of the division of birds in the U. S. National Museum, died on January 23, in his fifty-fourth year.

CHARLES W. MEAD, honorary curator of Peruvian archeology on the scientific staff of the American Museum of Natural History, died on February 3 at the age of eighty-two years.

DR. JOHANNES FIBIGER, professor of pathological anatomy at the University of Copenhagen, who was awarded the Nobel prize last October for his work on cancer, died on January 31.

A CORRESPONDENT writes of Dr. Chase Palmer, who died in San Francisco at the age of seventy-one years on November 18, 1927, as follows: For the past few years Dr. Palmer had been engaged in research and consulting work on chemical problems with special reference to the occurrence and recovery of petroleum. His undergraduate work was begun at Princeton and continued at the Johns Hopkins, where he received the degrees of A.B. in 1879 and Ph.D. in 1882. Dr. Palmer was engaged in teaching for a number of years, doing research work as time permitted. From 1907 he was almost entirely occupied with research with the United States Geological Survey till 1919 and with the Southern Pacific Company till 1921. His later publications were largely on geochemical studies of ore deposition and enrichment and on the geochemistry of waters, with special reference to the relations between natural waters and petroleum. His work on oil-field waters has been of much practical value in the production of oil.

AT the next meeting of the Columbia University chapter of the Sigma Xi, to be held in the new Chandler laboratories on February 16, Dr. H. C. Sherman will describe the research activities of the department of chemistry and Dr. Thomas B. Freas will explain the arrangement and equipment of the laboratories and at the conclusion of his talk will conduct a tour of inspection through the building.

THE Science League of America, Inc., has arranged with Station KFRC, one of the largest broadcasting stations on the Pacific Coast, to give a series of radio talks on evolution, by the president of the Science League, Maynard Shipley. These talks will be given on alternate Thursday afternoons, at 4 o'clock, the last one having been on February 2 on "What Evolution means to you."

The following series of lectures will be given at the New York Botanical Garden on Saturday afternoons at 3:30: February 4, "Important Tropical Fruits," Dr. H. A. Gleason; February 11, "Yellowstone Park's Trees, Flowers and Wonders," Dr. Henry R. Rose; February 25, "California Gardens," Miss Hilda Loines; March 3, "Rambles of a Naturalist among the Indians," Dr. Clyde Fisher; March 10, "Plant Hybrids: How they are produced and their Uses," Dr. A. B. Stout; March 17, "Botanizing in Trinidad," Dr. Tracy E. Hazen; March 24, "Florida," Dr. J. H. Barnhart, and March 31, "The Present Status of Evolution," Professor John M. Coulter.

UNIVERSITY AND EDUCATIONAL NOTES

A donation of $128,000 to Columbia University by the alumni of the College of Physicians and Surgeons to found a professorship in pathology at the medical school has been announced by Dr. Francis Carter Wood, as spokesman for the alumni. The money will be held in trust by the university until it reaches the sum of $200,000. The professorship will be called the Francis Delafield professorship, in honor of the founder of the pathology laboratory at the College of Physicians and Surgeons.

A gift of $1,650,000 for the erection of four residence halls for women students at Cornell University has been announced by Dr. Livingston Farrand. The name of the donor was withheld by request.

Ground has been broken for the $750,000 institute of pathology at Western Reserve University. The building is a gift of the Rockefeller Foundation.

The publication of the report of Charles F. Adams, treasurer of Harvard University, shows that the total endowment of Harvard, exclusive of land and buildings used for educational purposes, is now more than $82,000,000.

At the University of New Hampshire, a separate graduate school under its own director has been established. Although no director has been officially chosen to head the new division of the state university, it has been intimated that Dr. Hermon Slobin, head of the department of mathematics, would fill the position.

Dr. James Buell Munn, assistant dean of Washington Square College of New York University, has been elected dean of the college. Dr. Munn will succeed Dr. John R. Turner, who recently was elected president of West Virginia University.

Drs. Marion Arthur Blankenhorn and Roy Wesley Scott, now associate professors of medicine at Western Reserve University, have been promoted to the rank of clinical professor.

Associate Professor J. B. Reynolds, of Lehigh University, has been promoted to a full professorship of mathematics and theoretical mechanics.

Ralph G. Meeder, assistant professor of biology at Hamilton College, has been appointed instructor of biology at Wesleyan University, Connecticut.

Professor Arthur Hutchinson, F.R.S., professor of mineralogy and fellow of Pembroke College, has been elected master of Pembroke College in succession to the late Dr. W. S. Hadley.

Professor James Henry Dible has been appointed professor of pathology and bacteriology in the Welsh National School of Medicine.

DISCUSSION AND CORRESPONDENCE

ALEXANDROVSK BIOLOGICAL STATION

For biologists who have an interest in the low temperature relationships of organisms, probably no station is better situated than the one at Alexandrovsk at the mouth of the fjord by which the Kola River empties into the Arctic Sea. The faunal materials available at this station are brought into the arctic by the warm waters of the Gulf Stream. Many of the forms are in great abundance and easily obtainable. They have an interesting relationship to the fluctuating currents of the Gulf Stream. Owing to the changes in position of the four divisions of this current there is much fluctuation in the temperature, salinity, acidity and other ecological factors in this portion of the Arctic Sea.

The station is well established, having been in operation for twenty-eight years. The four major buildings are well situated immediately at the water's edge. Good housing space is available for 120 regular students who spend part of the summer months at Alexandrovsk, and for the 150–200 students who visit the station for a few days. There is usually a staff of 25–30 instructors, research workers, and specialists in residence. The director, Dr. G. A. Kluger, has made special arrangements for the entertainment of foreign scientists. Usually there are several persons in residence who can speak any of the principal languages.

The instruction at the station is excellent in comparative zoological anatomy. This phase of the work is under the direction of Dr. Nicholas Tanaseiichock with three assistants and three preparators. In the division of physiology Dr. Kreps was working on the effects of the acidity and salinity of the water on the distribution of the organisms. Interesting work was in progress on intracellular digestion in medusae. In plant physiology Mlle. Vera Bersook was working on the rate of photosynthesis in algae.

The physiological work is greatly aided by a very complete hydrographic survey which has been in progress for several years. The station by motor ship sends expeditions on a triangular course of survey to 76° N. Lat. in February, May, August and November of each year.

Botanical instruction under Mlle. Titiana Voblikoff is concerned mainly with the classification and distribution of algae and lichens. There is a substation branch in the Hibini Mountains where collections of plants other than the arctic flora may be made.

Research is in progress through the whole year. The Arctic does not freeze in this region, owing to the warm waters of the Gulf Stream and owing to the action of a 13-foot tide. The main portion of the instructional work is given to three parties of students, each party spending five or six weeks in residence at Alexandrovsk.

The station publishes a series of reports in addition to journal articles. These may be had in exchange.

R. B. HARVEY
UNIVERSITY OF CAMBRIDGE,
CAMBRIDGE, ENGLAND

THE ETIOLOGY OF EUROPEAN FOUL-BROOD OF BEES

THE attention of the writer has been directed to a communication from Denis R. A. Wharton appearing in SCIENCE, November 11, 1927, similar to one published in *Nature,* August 27, 1927, dealing with the cause of the disease of bee larvae commonly known as European Foul-brood, and the possible rôle of *B. alvei* (Cheshire and Cheyne) as an etiological factor. The article in question is based on data obtained, in part, by Mr. Wharton while temporary assistant under the writer's direction in the Division of Bacteriology, Central Experimental Farm, Ottawa, the publication being unauthorized, and, in the opinion of the writer, somewhat premature, particularly in view of the desirability of a thorough preliminary verification of the results obtained.

The organism isolated from diseased brood, which in pure culture was found to be capable of transmitting the disease, appeared to be closely related to, if not identical with, *Streptococcus apis* described by Maassen[1] but capable of considerable morphological variation showing types which are impossible to distinguish microscopically from what is commonly called *B. pluton* (White)[2] which is usually stated to be the exciting cause of the disease. The claim of White, however, may be said to be based on indirect evidence, on the basis of microscopical and inoculation tests with impure cultures, *B. pluton* apparently not having been obtained in pure culture. The similarity of certain stages of *Str. apis* in pure culture with the appearance of *B. pluton* in diseased material raises doubts as to whether the latter can be said to exist at all.

In obtaining the organism in pure culture from the comb containing larvae dead of foul-brood, a preliminary enrichment medium appears essential. Our most recent experiments have shown the most suitable substrate yet employed to be one containing peptone 1 per cent., K_2HPO_4 0.05 per cent., honey 1 per cent., yeast 1 per cent. and agar 0.15 per cent., slightly acid ($pH = 6.2$ approx.) A preponderance of the *"pluton"* form over *B. alvei* or other "secondary invaders" in the raw material is desirable if the coccus form is to be readily established. After two or three transfers the organism may be readily obtained in pure culture by regular plating methods.

Respecting the rôle played by *B. alvei,* experiments on the life-cycle of this organism are still in progress. Results so far obtained indicate that *B. alvei* is to be regarded as more than a secondary invader as is now usually stated. Depending on the nature of the substrate, upon the period and temperature of incubation, this organism exhibits a pronounced polymorphism which indicates that the typical rod forms and endospores most commonly encountered are but stages in the life history of the organism. The development of coccoid forms of *B. alvei* is particularly pertinent to the question of the etiology of European Foul-brood. Recent experiments were made with a culture of *B. alvei* which had been kept for over two years with occasional transfers on nutrient agar and nutrient dextrose agar. On these media as well as on solid substrates containing yeast, endospore formation is prompt, and further morphological changes are seldom. On a medium composed of peptone 1 per cent., K_2HPO_4 0.05 per cent., dextrose 0.5 per cent., saccharose 0.5 per cent., agar 1.5 per cent. ($pH = 6.8$), the type of growth is very different, being more transparent in character and endospore formation much lessened, being even absent on repeated transfers. After establishment of *B. alvei* on this substrate, subsequent plate cultures kept at room temperature for 3 to 5 weeks have repeatedly given rise to coccoid forms which in morphology and group

[1] Maassen, A. "Zur Aetiologie der sogenannten Faulbrut der Honigbienen." *Arb. aus d. Kaiserl. biol. Anst. f. Land. u. Forstw.* Bd. VI, Heft. 1, 53–70. 1908.

[2] White, G. F. "The cause of European Foul-brood." *U. S. D. A. Bur. Ent. Circ.* 157. 1912.

arrangement can not be distinguished microscopically from the forms which were found to be capable of transmitting the disease. So far attempts to stabilize this coccoid form of *B. alvei* have been unsuccessful, its separation by replating having resulted either in a return to the original rod type or a failure to grow on the medium employed. These difficulties in connection with the stabilization of new forms have been already emphasized by Löhnis and Smith.[3] These authors have shown the possibility of stabilizing coccoid cells from *Azotobacter,* while Cunningham and Jenkins[4] have obtained a coccus from cultures of *B. amylobacter* (A. M. et. Bredemann). That a similar stabilization of a coccoid form of *B. alvei* is feasible, is reasonable to presume, and its accomplishment would lend support to the hypothesis regarding the identity of *B. alvei* with the organism responsible for the infection in foul-brood, and furnish interesting light regarding the relationship of developmental phases of pathogenic bacteria to virulence. With all work concerned with etiology and pleomorphism, however, too much emphasis can not be laid upon the necessity for repeated confirmation of results. The writer would have preferred to withhold even this preliminary communication which is given reluctantly in view of the outlined circumstances.

A. G. Lochhead
Division of Bacteriology,
Central Experimental Farm,
Ottawa, Canada

CONCERNING MAN'S ANTIQUITY AT FREDERICK, OKLAHOMA

Among the several recent reports of evidences of Pleistocene man in America, the case of Frederick, Oklahoma, must be received with caution. In 1926 the owner of a fossil-bearing gravel pit at this place unearthed several artifacts. The site was first examined and reported by J. D. Figgins, H. J. Cook and O. P. Hay,[1] and later by C. N. Gould, C. E. Decker and the writer.

The gravel pit has been sunk into a stratum of gravel and sand which caps a ridge a half mile wide and several miles in length. The stratum is from ten to twenty-five feet deep and lies on beds of Permian age. The ridge is the highest point for some miles around, the red beds falling away to the Red River. All observers are agreed that the gravel bed is of Pleistocene age; the presumption being that it was deposited in a valley bottom, subsequent erosion of the surrounding areas having left it in its present high position.

The artifacts are two arrowheads or blades and five possible metates or mealing slabs. According to Mr. Holloman, the owner, one blade was from the very bottom of the gravel, he having picked it up from loose material at the foot of the pit face as it was torn down by workmen. The second was at a somewhat higher level, four to eight feet. Mr. Holloman stated that he scratched this artifact from the face of the pit with his fingers. The slabs, identified as metates by Mr. Figgins, were taken from a level of a foot or two above the blades. All observers are agreed on the honesty of Mr. Holloman's representations.

Figgins, Cook and Hay concluded that the human artifacts are original constituents of this Pleistocene gravel bed as it was first laid down. Before this verdict becomes generally accepted, I should like to broach several problems.

No scientific man has seen the gravels in the immediate vicinity of the spot where the finds were made. These were all found within a short distance of one another, near the center of the gravel pit which now extends over several acres. We do not know the original position of the surface at this point with respect to the artifacts. The deposit is considerably eroded. There is the possibility that these artifacts lay on the surface of a depression, were subsequently covered by wash, and have only a specious claim to the antiquity of the near-by fossils.

As against this possibility is the fact that I was told that no artifacts have been found on the surface in the vicinity. On the other hand, it is quite possible that they may yet be found. The ridge presents the only body of suitable material for flaking blades for miles around and at the same time affords a wide view of the surrounding country.

The artifacts themselves are equivocal. The blades are clearly artifacts, resembling modern Indian forms, but the metates are questionable. It is difficult to decide from Mr. Figgins' illustrations whether the slabs were fabricated, and I have not seen the originals. They may be water-worn boulders. While at the time Mr. Figgins wrote that no other stones of a similar nature had been found, our party saw several slabs, clearly water-worn, which suggests the possibility that some of them had been selected as metates because of their close resemblance to such forms.

[3] Löhnis, F., and Smith, N. R. "Studies upon the lifecycles of the bacteria—Part II: Life history of Azotobacter." *Jour. Agr. Res.* 23, 401–432. 1923.

[4] Cunningham, A., and Jenkins, H. "Studies on *Bacillus amylobacter* A. M. et Bredemann." *Jour. Agr. Sci.* 17, 109–117. 1927.

[1] J. D. Figgins, "The Antiquity of Man in America" (Natural History, 27, 1927, 229–239). Harold J. Cook, "New Geological and Paleontological Evidence bearing on the Antiquity of Mankind in America" (*loc. cit.*, 240–247). Oliver P. Hay, "Early Man in America" (*Science News-Letter*, 12, 1927, 215–216).

More important than these conjectures, which are at best only possibilities, is the incongruity of the find with all we know of man's cultural history.

First with respect to the metates; among living peoples these are in use only by those who are cereal-raisers or who are in contact with them. For example, in North America grinding slabs are used only by the corn-raising Southwestern Indians and their seed-gathering neighbors of the Basin-Plateau region. Indeed the use of the metate may not be of remote date even in this area, and all Americanists are agreed that cereal-raising is not one of the original constituents of Indian culture. In the Old World also cultivation is a Neolithic art, that is, of geologically Recent provenience.

The blades are likewise of European Neolithic type, or at best of Solutrean technique (from the middle or close to the fourth glaciation).

Yet Dr. Hay has it that this deposit is of early Pleistocene age. The fossil animals include "a primitive elephant, a mastodon, two species of camels, two species of ground-sloths, a glyptodon and three or four species of horses, one very large, one pony-like. . . . As to the animals, I hold that they are characteristic of the first interglacial stage (the Aftonian) of the Pleistocene."

If Dr. Hay is right, and I have no reason to doubt his identification, we are confronted by an unusual situation. Artifacts which would be identified by an archeologist as Recent (or terminal Pleistocene) are held to be of the same age as an early Pleistocene fauna. This incongruity seems not to have occurred to Dr. Hay.

Is there any warrant to support this from what we know of the course of human events elsewhere? I think not. The earliest definitely human remains from the Old World (*H. heidelbergensis*) date from the second interglacial or the first. The Frederick deposit may antedate this. The earliest human artifacts (Chellean or Pre-Chellean) date from the middle or close of the third interglacial. These are quite roughly made in contrast to the well chipped Frederick blades. The zoological evidence conforms. Most authorities are agreed on man's anthropoid ancestry. The anthropoids are Old World forms; there are no known anthropoid prototypes of man in America.[2]

It seems to me that the onus of proof rests with those who hold that Neolithic implements are congruous with an Aftonian age. I am doubtful that the mass of cultural and zoological evidence to the contrary now available will be set at naught.

LESLIE SPIER
UNIVERSITY OF OKLAHOMA

[2] The case of *Hesperopithecus*, a single tooth of Tertiary age from Nebraska, seems disposed of by W. K. Gregory's recent determination of it as pertaining to an extinct peccary (SCIENCE, n.s., 66, 579–581).

"EXIT THE TENTAMEN, BUT . . ." WHAT?

UNDER the above caption, minus the last word, my esteemed friend, Mr. Wm. T. M. Forbes, in the issue of SCIENCE for October 28, 1927, undertook to reply to an article from my pen published in the same journal, July 1, 1927, entitled "Exit Hübner's Tentamen." Mr. Forbes addresses numerous questions to me. At one point he says: "What would Dr. Holland do about it?" To all of his numerous queries I shall give appropriate answers elsewhere in a journal more strictly devoted to the technical nomenclature of entomology, and shall in that article show how greatly Mr. Forbes, and others, who hold with him, have misunderstood the writings of Hübner, and his tentative system of classification. There is only one point upon which I wish to touch in this brief paper.

Mr. Forbes at the end of his paper says: "In bringing in the *Verzeichniss,* Dr. Holland does not mention that ten years had intervened and that in the meantime Hübner had used all the Tentamen names of butterflies as generic (as the first names of binomials) also many of the moths. This fact completely invalidates his argument."

Passing by the implication that I was making an "argument" in a matter which in my judgment is not open to argument, and was simply stating obvious truths, this allegation of Mr. Forbes awoke my utter astonishment. I am familiar with every page and line which Hübner gave to the world. Mr. Forbes's statement seemed to me most amazing. Accordingly I wrote to him inquiring upon what he based his sweeping statement that from 1806 to 1816 Hübner had used "binomials" in his nomenclature of the butterflies. Mr. Forbes has kindly replied to my inquiry and informs me that he based his assertion upon the legends of the plates in Vol. I of the *Sammlung exotischer Schmetterlinge.* Mr. Forbes's answer still more amazes me. Any one, who takes the trouble to look at these plates from a corner of one eye, can instantly see that the legends are all *trinomial,* and not *binomial,* as Mr. Forbes says. Mr. Forbes is under an illusion. *Three* is *not* equal to *two,* as *twice four* is not equal to *five.* Hübner in the legends of these plates was consistently true to the "System" he had adopted. On these plates he gives 1, the name of the *Stirps;* 2, the name of the *familia;* 3, the name of the *Gattung* (species). Not once does he employ a generic name, either in his sense, or ours. Mr. Forbes is wholly in error.

As Mr. Forbes's premise is false, and contrary to facts, his conclusion is equally false. His "argument" involves the logical error of *petitio principii.* It is *not true* that Hübner used "binomials" during the period mentioned by Mr. Forbes, and it can only be by sophistry, which flies in the face of Hübner's own usage and explicit and oft-repeated statements, that it can be made to even seem that he used "binomials" in the period indicated. He came to use binomials at a later date, and finally toward the end of his life adopted the "binomial system of nomenclature," as we know it to-day. The legends of the plates in Vol. I of the *Sammlung exotischer Schmetterlinge* are *not* binomial, they are *absolutely* trinomial. I squarely take issue with Mr. Forbes on this point.

My motive for writing the foregoing lines is to simply let any reader of Science, who may have read my article of July 1 and Mr. Forbes's reply, understand that I am in thorough disagreement with him. I do not wish silence on my part in these columns to be construed as assent.

W. J. Holland

Carnegie Museum

VISIBLE RADIATION FROM EXCITED NERVE FIBER AGAIN

The phenomenon of the "Reddish Blue Arcs and the Reddish Blue Glow of the Retina" is a very remarkable one—especially when it is exhibited (as I exhibit it) in a dark room before a whole audience at once. All are agreed that one is seeing entoptically certain optic nerve fibers on the surface of the retina —but why are they visible? I have given reasons for believing that they are emitting physical light—and this has required no "violent efforts of the imagination," as Dr. Davis[1] supposes that it has done—one has only to remember that nerve, when excited, gives out heat, and that heat is, objectively, the same thing as light. It happens that a physicist has just stated this explicitly: "The experimental evidence for thinking that light is a form of energy and *that radiant heat is of exactly the same nature as light* is overwhelming."[2] (Italics mine.) But may the cause be (Gertz) a secondary stimulation of some organ-fibers, ganglia, bipolar cells, or rods and cones—by means of action currents? There is a residual image, so nothing but rods or cones can be concerned—they alone contain the highly specific light-sensitive substance which furnishes a residual image. An electric current sent in from the outside gives visual sensations but with no residual image; "this does not prove, however," says Dr. Davis, "that an electrical disturbance *localized in the retina* (italics his) might not stimulate the photosensory mechanism directly." Now a current from the outside might conceivably have attacked the optic nerve only after it has left the eyeball, but that it actually runs along the fibers on the surface of the retina is proved by the fact that structural details of the retina are marked out by it—for instance, at certain intensities the blind spot will be seen to be of a different color from the rest of the field. Since this is the case, it is inconceivable that an action current generated *within* the nerve fiber should play any different rôle from one that comes into it from a battery on the outside. It follows that nothing but physical light attacks the photosensory mechanism.

My theory has now been beautifully confirmed by Deane B. Judd, of the Bureau of Standards (*American Journal of Psychology*, October, 1927).

Christine Ladd-Franklin

1 Science, 1928, LXVII, 69.

2 Crew, Henry, 1927, "General Physics," 319–320.

QUOTATIONS

GENESIS AND EVOLUTION

There will be no more monkeying in the public schools with the Mosaic account of creation as recorded in the book of Genesis, if Representative Hobbs's bill to prohibit it finds favor with his fellow members of the General Assembly and is approved by the Governor. Mr. Hobbs, who is the accredited representative of the sovereign legislative district composed of Wolf and Powell Counties, has introduced a bill to prohibit the teaching in the public schools of the state any theory of evolution that conflicts with his understanding of the sacred texts of Holy Writ.

Statesman Hobbs has eight children, whose simple faith in the Hebraic account of creation he would protect with the strong arm of the law. Many earnest, honest sticklers for the letter of the law will approve and applaud this zealous guarding by the Wolf-Powell statesman of the faith once delivered to the saints. Why should the great Commonwealth of Kentucky trail behind progressive states like Tennessee and Texas in this matter of protecting its youth against this threatening heresy? Was not the Grecian Socrates put to death for corrupting the faith of the youth in his time, respecting the virtues of the gods? Was not Galileo severely punished by the Hobbs law of his age for contradicting the Biblical teaching about the solar system?

Representative Hobbs serves well his state in seeking to call a halt on these venturesome modern school teachers. They have already poisoned the minds of a mighty multitude with the false doctrines that the earth is round, that the planets revolve around the sun, that this earth instead of being the sum and center of the universe is but a sand grain on the limitless shores of creation and, instead of being only six thousand years old, has been revolving through space for untold ages. What about these idle fellows who spend their nights, not in honest sleep, but in peering through great telescopes into the starry heavens, or instead of reading the story of creation, so beautifully told in the book of Genesis, go reading the riddle of the rocks in a vain effort to controvert Moses' account of the beginning of things?

This revolutionary evolution theory is gaining alarming headway, and unless something is done about it right away there is no telling what may happen. And popular education is doing it. Woodrow Wilson, the greatest educator of his time, when asked his opinion of evolution said: "I take it no educated man questions the established fact of organic evolution." The schools and universities are to blame for the spread of this dangerous doctrine, and if statesman Hobbs would insure the rising generation against this corrupting teaching he should introduce a bill abolishing all public and private schools. The uneducated man accepts what he has been told by mother and the preacher; asking no questions. But as soon as the child appears in school, he begins to ask a reason for things. Oh, for a return of the simple faith in witches and ghosts and horse shoes and rabbit feet, a flat earth and a revolving sun, etc., and no questions asked. Lawmaker Hobbs is Kentucky's hope for this happy return of the good old days, but, alas! it is to be feared that he is casting his pearl before swine in that sceptic bunch at Frankfort.—*Kentucky Republican.*

SEPARATIONS BY THE IONIC MIGRATION METHOD

The development of the ionic migration method for effecting difficult separations has been described in a number of articles appearing in the *Proceedings of the National Academy of Sciences*[1] and in the *Journal of the American Chemical Society.*[2] This series of investigations, carried out at Columbia University between 1920 and 1926 and continued at New York University since the latter date, has now given results of interest in several quite diverse fields. The presentation of an informal summary and the correlation of the results obtained are the purposes of this paper.

The work was started as an attempt to devise a practicable method for the separation of isotopes. Other investigators had succeeded in obtaining, at best, only a very slight degree of separation of isotopic elements into their various atomic species after heroic expenditures of time and labor by other methods, and it appeared that there did exist the possibility here of obtaining a quick and decisive result. The situation with regard to ionic mobility may be explained very briefly. A long-standing controversy has been waged on this property; one school insisting that ionic mobility is fundamentally dependent upon ionic volume, another being equally confident that it is fundamentally dependent upon ionic mass. The results available in the literature for homologous series of organic anions and cations have been utilized by both parties to give their respective points; but, since we have no definite knowledge as to what amount of solvent accompanies any ion in its journey towards an electrode and since it is the *total mass* or *total volume* of the ion and of its accompanying solvent envelope which must be taken into account, such data obviously offer us no means for definitely determining the problem.

The discovery that isotopes possess *equal atomic volumes,* made by Soddy and Richards in 1914,[3] first put us in a position to impose a crucial test, for isotopic ions necessarily *differ in mass.* If mass is influential, therefore, it should be possible to obtain a separation of isotopes by taking advantage of the fact that the lighter ion will migrate more rapidly than the heavier. This idea of an "isotopic race," however, can not be carried out experimentally as simply as it might seem at first sight. Ions do not compete under the influence of the electric current in the manner of a track meet, unless we extend our experiences to include a continuous relay race. We can not start all of our ions at one point and obtain a separation by noting when those of a certain species have passed a given goal, for there must be maintained a steady supply all the way from one electrode to another in order for the current to pass, and it will not help us much if a faster ion hurries ahead of its slower neighbor, since it will merely find itself in the company of other slower ions which happened to start a little in advance. By a modification of the experimental procedure, nevertheless, our "isotopic race" may be converted into a "parade" which can be suitably regulated.

The apparatus used is shown in the accompanying diagram, and its applicability may be illustrated by a condensed description of the technique employed in the case of chlorine.

An agar-agar gel A containing sodium chloride is inserted as a short middle section in a long horizontal tube of pyrex glass, one and a half inches in internal diameter. On one side of the chloride gel is added a gel B containing sodium hydroxide; on the other side a gel C containing sodium acetate. The ends of the tube

[1] *Proc. Nat. Acad. Sci.*, 9, 75, 1923; 10, 458, 1924; 11, 393, 1925.

[2] *Jour. Amer. Chem. Soc.*, 48, 2619 and 3114, 1926.

[3] Aston, "Isotopes," 17, 1922 (Arnold and Co.).

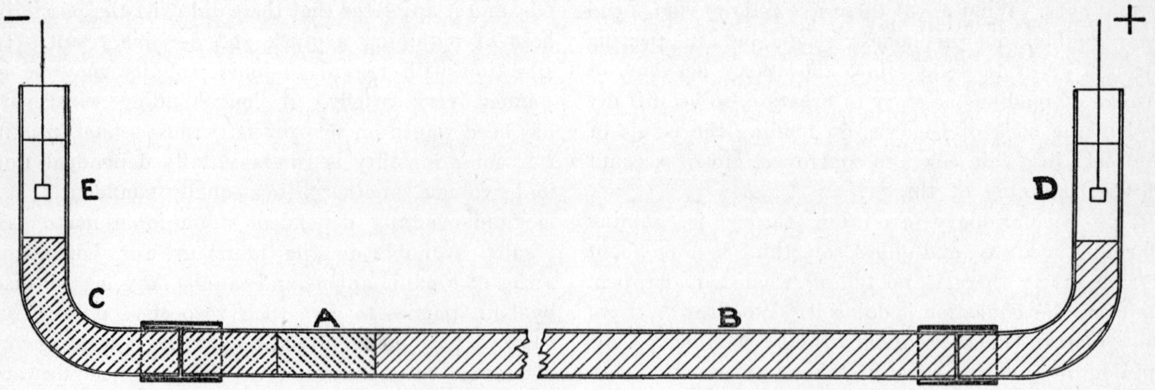

FIG. 1

are connected with right-angled pyrex bends of the same diameter, and the gels continue well up into these bends, as in the diagram. Above the hydroxide gel, after it has set, is poured concentrated sodium hydroxide solution D, and above the acetate gel a solution E of sodium acetate in concentrated acetic acid. Platinum electrodes are placed in these two solutions, and a current is passed through the tube, the electrode in D being made the anode and the electrode in E the cathode. The heating effect of the current upon the gel may be minimized by submerging the tube in a long trough filled with running tap-water.

At the beginning of the run, the boundary surfaces between the various sections of the gel are perfectly sharp. When the current is turned on, the boundaries move toward the anode. Inasmuch as there is a faster-moving ion in front of the chloride ion, and a slower-moving ion behind it, admixture of the salts is absolutely prohibited and the boundaries remain distinct throughout the whole experiment. In order to maintain the width of the chloride section approximately constant, it is well to arrange the concentrations of the various salts in their respective gels in accordance with the transference numbers of their anions. Even if this is not done, however, the boundary concentrations soon automatically adjust themselves to the required ratios. Care must be taken that the solution around the cathode always contains sufficient excess of acetic acid to neutralize the sodium hydroxide that is there formed.

The rate at which the boundaries move depends upon the potential drop between the electrodes, the length of the tube, and the concentrations of the solutions. In actual practice, the horizontal tube is made up of three three-foot sections, connected by rubber bands, and the current is regulated (100 to 500 volts) so that the boundaries advance about 12 to 18 inches a day. When the front chloride boundary has almost reached the end of the tube, the apparatus is taken apart. The two rear sections are discarded, two new sections filled with hydroxide gel are inserted in front of the chloride, and new bends are fitted on as before. The chloride ions are now forced to migrate into these two new sections, and the whole procedure is repeated until they have progressed through about 100 feet of the gel. The chloride gel is then removed from the tube and immediately cut up into strips about 1 cm. in width.

If, now, the isotopic chloride ions with atomic masses 35 and 37, respectively, possess significantly different mobilities, the front segments of the gel will contain only the faster-moving and the rear segments only the slower-moving isotope. Preliminary experiments in which a mixture of two sodium salts with anions of known mobilities was substituted for the middle sodium chloride section fully demonstrated this point. Thus when a mixture of sodium iodide and sodium thiocyanate was employed and the boundary was moved only a few feet, the front segments were found to contain only sodium iodide and the rear segments only sodium thiocyanate. The observed lag of the slower ion was almost exactly equal to that calculated from the difference in mobilities. In this particular case, the difference is approximately 16 per cent. In subsequent experiments this difference was narrowed by choosing other suitable pairs of ions; *e.g.*, barium and calcium, barium and strontium, and iodide and chloride. The differences in mobilities are here reduced to 8 per cent., 5 per cent., and 1 per cent., respectively, and the results obtained showed that the method could be depended upon to provide a very considerable degree of separation even at the lowest limit tested.

It was highly disappointing, therefore, to be forced to admit from the results of all our experiments with isotopic ions that no significant separation could ever be detected. The only conclusion that can logically be drawn is that the mobilities of isotopic ions are well within 1 per cent. of equality and that those workers are substantially justified who contend that volume is the decisive factor in determining ionic mobilities. More recent theoretical advances, it must be added, support this view, although the matter is still not absolutely settled.[4]

Experimental difficulties encountered in connection with this work on isotopes can not be discussed in full

[4] Jette, *Phil. Mag.*, 3, 58 (1927).

detail here, but mention may be made in passing, of two points. One was the impossibility of determining whether any separation was proceeding within a section except by interrupting its progress irretrievably through segmentation and analysis. In other words, there was no way of telling in advance if a run of 100 feet was any more advantageous than a run of 10 feet, or whether a run of 500 feet should be preferred. It was proposed by one assistant to solve this difficulty by incorporating with the material under examination a small amount of a substance containing a colored ion with a mobility *intermediate* between those of the two isotopes. The end of an experiment would then be automatically announced by the appearance of a thin colored strip in the center of the section, the gel in front of this strip containing only the faster isotope and the gel in the rear of it only the slower. Unfortunately, no colored ion with the properties required has yet been discovered. A second difficulty consisted in fixing the exact position of the boundaries during a run. Slight changes in the color of the agar-agar gel induced by the different salts present, or slight differences in the refractive index of the various sections were sometimes sufficiently good indications, but the much larger variations in their electrical resistance offered, in general, more dependable assistance. The approximate position of a boundary could frequently be determined merely by lifting the apparatus from the water trough for a few minutes, running the hand along the tube and noting the place at which a temperature gradient became evident. Finally, more exact information was obtained by fusing two short platinum wires through the glass at suitable points on the tubes and establishing the passage of a boundary past these points by noting when an abrupt change occurred in the electrical resistance of the gel between them.

Although all the work on isotopes, as has been stated, led to no successful separations, yet the positive results obtained in the test experiments on known mixtures did inspire the hope that the ionic migration method might, after all, prove of practical service in the separation of more familiar materials which are ordinarily obtained by the chemist in a pure state only with extreme difficulty. The most important instance of this type is furnished by the family of the rare earth metals. The group of elements known as the rare earths comprises the elements of atomic number 57 to 71 inclusive, and yttrium with atomic number 39. These elements are distinguished by such extraordinary alikeness in chemical and most physical properties, due to the identical arrangements of their two outer shells of electrons, that they actually approach isotopes in similarity. It is necessary, in practice, to take advantage of slight differences in solubility observed for corresponding salts and to resolve a given mixture into its components by a long series of fractional crystallizations or precipitations, ranging in number from several hundred to many thousand according to the elements present and the degree of purity desired. These operations are so laborious and time-consuming that chemically pure samples of individual rare earth compounds are practically unknown, save on the shelves of a few skilled workers in the field of atomic weights. The "rareness" of the rare earths is due not so much to the lack of abundance of their ores in nature as to the lack of a simple method for their separation.

Little is known of the relative mobilities of the rare earth cations in aqueous solution, but ionic volume and hydration variations within the group may be expected to cause differences in ionic mobilities which will, in most cases, exceed one per cent., so that a ready analysis of a given mixture into its pure components should be, in general, feasible. The experiments described below furnish, in fact, two instances of the successful separation of typical binary rare earth mixtures by the ionic migration method.

The first separation attempted was upon a mixture of yttrium and erbium, kindly furnished by Professor James, of the University of New Hampshire. Potassium was used as a preceding faster ion and trivalent chromium as a following slower ion. Not only could the position of the rear boundary be more conveniently followed in this particular case because of the color of the chromic solution, but it was also found possible to observe the actual progress of the separation within the rare earth section in a very simple way by means of a small direct-vision hand spectroscope. The majority of the rare earths give solutions with characteristic absorption spectra and, by noting the increase or decrease in intensity of the most prominent lines in various parts of a section, the experimenter could immediately detect any change in composition in the whole length of the section without interrupting the run. Here yttrium rapidly accumulated in the front half of the section and erbium was relegated to the rear. After a run of fourteen days, during which the boundaries moved two meters, an almost perfect separation had been effected.

The next mixture tested consisted of neodymium and praseodymium, two elements which are so nearly alike that their first differentiation by Otto von Welsbach still forms one of the triumphs of technique in this difficult field. Neodymium salts exhibit a purple solution in water, however, while praseodymium salts give a green solution. A beautiful crystal of neodymium nitrate and an equally fine specimen of praseodymium sulphate were secured from the

Chandler chemical museum of Columbia University and the careful work of several years was deranged in a few minutes by mixing these two salts to obtain a solution with an intermediate neutral tint. With this solution as a central section and with the same arrangement as in the preceding experiment, it required only a few days' migration to disclose the fact that the front portion of the section was becoming distinctly green and the rear portion purplish. Observation by means of the spectroscope simultaneously showed that the characteristic absorption lines of praseodymium were becoming more pronounced in the front section and fading out in the rear, with the opposite behavior for the neodymium. At the end of ten days, substantially complete separation had been accomplished.

Experiments with other mixtures of rare earths showed that, while complete separation could not be secured in every case, yet in most mixtures the mobilities of the ions were sufficiently divergent to compel a very rapid concentration of one particular component in the front or in the rear section. The method may, therefore, be considered as a general new method for obtaining pure samples of the rare earth elements with the expenditure of much less time and trouble than is required by the classical method of fractional crystallization. Professor Hopkins, of the University of Illinois, is, it may be mentioned, at present attempting to utilize the ionic migration method for the more rapid concentration of illinium (the last member of the rare earth family, discovered by him in 1925) from the neodymium and samarium residues in which minute traces of it exist.

Important industrial uses for the rare earth elements will undoubtedly be discovered as soon as more convenient means for their isolation are developed. Aluminum remained a chemical curiosity until this same end was achieved, and while the later members of the aluminum family may not duplicate the successful career of their brilliant brother, yet it would indeed be strange if nature had omitted to endow them, alone of all the elements, with no properties of service to mankind.

The success of the experiments with rare earths suggested that the method might be applicable to the separation of radium from barium. The concentration of radium from the barium residues of carnotite ores at present involves a very tedious series of fractional crystallizations, and, since it had already been found that barium could be separated from the other elements of the alkaline earth family by the method here under discussion, it appeared very probable that a similar separation from radium, the last member of this same family, could also be accomplished. Samples of barium residues containing known amounts of radium and of mesothorium (an isotope of radium) were obtained and, after a few days' migration, the sections were segmented and their radioactivity examined. It was found that the radioactive components of each mixture tested accumulated very rapidly in the front part of the section. The ease of the separation in this case is so striking as to suggest that the ionic migration method may come into technical use for the concentration of radium in barium residues.

An attempt to separate hafnium and zirconium did not lead to such conclusive results. Hafnium exists to the extent of several per cent. in all zirconium ores, and the similarity in properties is so pronounced that the actual discovery of hafnium was not definitely established until 1923. A sample of hafnium-rich zirconium oxide was kindly furnished us by Professor Hevesy. The elements were not amenable to separation by the ionic migration method in the form of positive ions, owing to hydrolysis, and only after considerable search was a suitable negative complex ion discovered in the form of a complex oxalate. After long migration, analysis showed a very slight accumulation of hafnium in the rear of the section, the mobilities of the complex anions being evidently so close together as to render a complete separation impracticable.

The results in an entirely different field have been of better promise. Many of the alkaloids particularly useful for medicinal purposes are derived from natural sources as mixtures of several individual members which can be separated by the ordinary methods of organic chemistry only with great difficulty. The alkaloids, however, are weak bases which form soluble hydrochlorides, and the mobilities of the cations of these salts are not identical. It should, consequently, be possible to obtain a pure sample of an especially valuable alkaloid from the mixture of similar materials with which it naturally occurs by use of the ionic migration method, and several preliminary experiments indicate that the method is indeed applicable in a majority of cases. Details will appear in a forthcoming communication.

Several other lines of research are also being followed. A very interesting case is the search for the missing element number 87. This element, from its position in the periodic system, should be a highly radioactive alkali metal. Just as radium is found associated with barium, so this missing element might be expected to occur in nature with other members of the alkali metal group. Now it is a very significant fact that the only elements of low atomic weight which exhibit radioactivity are potassium and rubidium. Two alternative explanations have been advanced, the first being the obvious suggestion that the radioactivity is due to an infinitesimal trace of the missing alkali element, the second being that it is due to some unstable isotope of the commoner alkali metal. Without going into details, it may be stated that each alternative has, at present, more experimental facts in its disfavor than in its favor, and a third entirely novel explanation is by no means excluded. The present method appears to furnish some hope of advancing our solution of this question for if, by migration of a potassium or rubidium salt, it should be found that the radioactivity was concentrating in the very front or in the very rear of the section, then the isotopic explanation would presumably fall into the discard and further investigation might very conceivably justify the announcement of the discovery of the missing element.

The experiments thus far completed on potassium have not given any final results. It is true that no noticeable concentration of the radio-activity in either the front or the rear has been obtained, but this can quite plausibly be ascribed to the fact that the mobility of the unknown alkali metal ion is substantially the same in aqueous solution as that of potassium ion. The heavier members of the alkali metal group, indeed, all have ionic mobilities in water which are substantially identical within the limits of experimental error. In methyl alcohol solution, however, it has been shown that the mobilities differ very markedly and consequently it may be expected that the addition of some methyl alcohol to the aqueous gel will stagger the values sufficiently to enable a separation to be secured if any unknown alkali metal is present. This point is being tested experimentally at the present time.

Finally, the possibility is being investigated of the applicability of the method to the separation of organic isomers of various types. More complex biochemical problems, such as the concentration or isolation of specific proteins or even of vitamins from natural sources, are probably also open to attack by the ionic migration method, but the experimental technique in such cases has not yet been worked out in detail.

JAMES KENDALL

NEW YORK UNIVERSITY

SCIENTIFIC APPARATUS AND LABORATORY METHODS

DETERMINING SOIL MOISTURE RAPIDLY AND ACCURATELY BY METHYL ALCOHOL

IN a former communication (this Journal, April 5, 1927) the use of alcohol was proposed as a basis for a very rapid means of determining the moisture content of soils and possibly of other materials. The form of alcohol that was then suggested was ethyl alcohol. In order to ascertain whether there are other liquids that would be more satisfactory than ethyl alcohol, an investigation has been conducted in which a large number of liquids have been examined. It has been discovered that of all the liquids studied, methyl alcohol seems to be the most satisfactory, as it is the most powerful dehydrating agent. Indeed, this form of alcohol seems to be able to replace or reduce the moisture content of soils down to practically the absolutely dry basis, as will be readily seen from the data below.

	Percentage of water recovered from water added to oven dry soils. Per cent.
Sand	100.05
Loam	100.03
Clay	99.99
Muck	99.01
Silica gel	99.30

The directions for executing a moisture determination by methyl alcohol are the same as those already published (this Journal, April 15, 1927) for ethyl alcohol. There are five points in the procedure, however, that one must always pay special attention to. These are first, the soil must be stirred with a strong rod and reduced to the particle state so the alcohol can come into intimate contact with the entire soil mass. Second, the liquid must be always filtered. Third, great care must be taken to prevent evaporation. The latter can be mainly accomplished by keeping the funnel covered during filtering. Fourth, the temperature of the liquids should always be recorded and reduced to the same basis. And fifth, in calibrating the hydrometer, the specific gravity of the absolute alcohol should be taken under controlled temperature. Allowing the alcohol to stand in running tap-water, to attain the temperature of the latter is sufficient.

It is advisable to use absolute methyl alcohol.

In case of soils containing more than 50 per cent. of moisture, such as muck and peats, only about 10 grams of soil should be used to 50 cc of alcohol.

GEORGE J. BOUYOUCOS

MICHIGAN AGRICULTURAL EXPERIMENT STATION

A CONVENIENT METHOD OF MEASURING QUANTITIES OF CHLOROPLAST PIGMENTS

ALTHOUGH the photosynthetic mechanism in the leaves of plants has long attracted the attention of workers in science, the relation between quantities of chloroplast pigments and growth has scarcely been touched. Apparently, the chief difficulty has been the lack of a rapid and fairly accurate method which did not require a great outlay of chemical equipment.

Willstätter and his coworkers devised a simple method of extracting and purifying these pigments, and estimated the quantities colorimetrically. They used solutions of potassium dichromate as color standards for carotin and xanthophyll, having previously evaluated the standards in terms of the pigment in question. The chlorophylls (a plus b) were estimated quantitatively by saponifying the chlorophylls with methyl alcoholic potash to form chlorophyllins. These solutions of chlorophyllins were taken up in water and then measured colorimetrically, using as standards, solutions made up from a known quantity of pure chlorophyll which had been similarly transformed to chlorophyllins. These colorimetric methods are not then measured colorimetrically, using as standards are not chemically stable and (2) because the tint of potassium dichromate solutions is not identical with that of carotinoid solutions, therefore, giving variable results.

Willstätter's method of extraction and separation of the chloroplast pigments has been given in detail by Stiles.[1] Recently Dr. F. M. Schertz, of the United States Department of Agriculture, has modified Willstätter's method, and kindly made the revised method available to the writer for certain investigations on the relations between chloroplast pigments and growth in maize. Dr. Schertz's method, which is simple and adequate for the study of problems of this nature, is now in the press.

The quantitative estimation of the pigments after extraction and separation has also been investigated by Schertz.[2, 3]. He finds the spectrophotometric analysis of solutions a more accurate method than the use of Lovibond slides in a colorimeter. However, the spectrophotometer is an expensive instrument and available to a very limited number of workers.

Since early in 1925 the writer has been using a method of estimating chloroplast pigments in solution which has given consistently good results, is simple, inexpensive and within the reach of the ordinary research laboratory. The amounts of the respective pigments are determined by comparing with artificial color standards of identical tint making use of a Duboscq colorimeter.

The chlorophylls (a plus b) were obtained in the form of aqueous solutions of the chlorophyllins (a plus b which are green by transmitted light. A color standard which matches the tint of the mixture of chlorophyllins obtained from maize was prepared by making 0.3 cc of a one half per cent. aqueous solution of Malachite Green and 11.2 cc of a one half per cent. aqueous solution of Napthol Yellow (Martius yellow) upto 5,500 cc with distilled water. The concentration of color in this standard is the equivalent of 10.708 milligrams of pure chlorophyll (supplied by Dr. Schertz) saponified to chlorophyllins and diluted with water to make 1 liter.

The carotin color standard was made by adding 3.4 cc of a one half per cent. aqueous solution of Napthol Yellow and 0.5 cc of a one half per cent. aqueous solution of Orange G. crystals to 1 liter of distilled water. The tint of this standard is identical with that of pure carotin dissolved in petrol ether and is the equivalent in concentration with carotin solutions containing 1.890 mgms of carotin per liter of solvent.

The xanthophyll color standard was made by adding 2.8 cc of a one half per cent. aqueous solution of napthol yellow to 1 liter of distilled water. The tint is identical with that of pure xanthophyll dissolved in petrol ether and is the equivalent in concentration of 1.537 mgms of xanthophyll per liter of solvent.

Evaluation of the carotinoids was accomplished by making readings of solutions of the pigments in the colorimeter in terms of their respective standards, and also making readings of the solutions in the König-Marten's spectrophotometer at the Bureau of Standards at Washington through the courtesy of that bureau and with the assistance of Dr. Schertz.

There appear to be several advantages in using these artificial color standards for quantitative estimation of the chloroplast pigments: (1) The materials and equipment are inexpensive and are therefore within the reach of a large number of workers in science. (2) The method is fairly accurate, because the tint of the standards is practically identical with that of the pigment solutions, and delicate readings may be made in the colorimeter by varying the volume of the solutions in question. (3) The method is rapid; readings may be made as soon as purification is complete, thus eliminating the large errors caused by decomposition of the pigments in manipulation. (4) The one half per cent. aqueous solutions of the dyes keep for many months (20 by test) without deterioration. 10 grams of each of the dyes, solutions of which have been evaluated in terms of the pigments, should be sufficient for a period of years.

[1] Stiles, Walter, "Photosynthesis. The assimilation of carbon by green plants," London, 1925.

[2] Schertz, F. M., "The quantitative determination of carotin by means of the spectrophotometer and the colorimeter," *Jour. Agr. Research* 26 (1923), p. 383.

[3] Schertz, F. M., "The quantitative determination of xanthophyll by means of the spectrophotometer and the colorimeter," *Jour. Agr. Research* 30 (1925), p. 253.

Different lots of the same dyes may vary in purity, and therefore each new lot should be evaluated in terms of solutions of pigments of known concentrations. The color standards fade slowly when exposed to light and should be made up fresh from the one half per cent. aqueous solutions every few weeks. The one half per cent. solutions should be discarded if they become turbid or if sediments appear.

Full details regarding the preparation and use of these color standards, as well as the results of the studies on relations between chloroplast pigments and growth of maize, will be published in the near future.

HOWARD B. SPRAGUE
COLLEGE OF AGRICULTURE,
RUTGERS UNIVERSITY,
NEW BRUNSWICK, N. J.

SPECIAL ARTICLES

THE ISOLATION AND FUNCTION OF PHOSPHOCREATINE

I. ISOLATION

IN a previous communication[1] we have offered indirect proof of the presence in voluntary muscle of a compound containing one molecule each of creatine and phosphoric acid. The amount of this substance in muscle is considerable (0.4 to 0.5 per cent.); in fact it (and not free creatine) is the principal "extractive" as long as the muscle has not been stimulated or otherwise disturbed. During muscular contraction the compound undergoes hydrolysis, and the same change occurs outside the body under the influence of an enzyme in the muscle or of acid, whereas resynthesis takes place when fatigued muscle is permitted to recover.

At the time of our first report, the leading evidence for the existence of a creatine-phosphoric acid compound depended upon its separation from free creatine by precipitation with copper in very slightly alkaline solution. Under all the conditions enumerated above the precipitate so formed contains creatine and a peculiarly unstable form of phosphoric acid in equimolecular proportions, excepting when—in consequence of stimulation or some other cause—complete hydrolysis of the substance has occurred, and then the copper precipitate is free from both the named constituents. In view of the quantitative nature of the evidence, and of the variety of conditions under which the test has been applied, a different explanation of the results described is hardly possible, and we felt no hesitation therefore in stating that such a compound actually exists. The precise nature of the substance, however—in particular the question whether it contains anything besides creatine and phosphoric acid—can hardly be settled with certainty except by its isolation in the pure state.

Within a few days of the publication of the paper mentioned, we succeeded in isolating a barium salt in crystalline form, but the method of preparation was unsatisfactory and the yields were very poor. After many variations of the original procedure had been tried, the conclusion was finally forced upon us that the use of barium for this purpose is successful only when preceded by a series of preliminary separations (with other metals) in the course of which a large amount of material is lost. By using calcium in place of barium, however, most of the phosphocreatine in protein-free muscle filtrates can readily be separated, in a crystalline condition, from all the other organic phosphoric acid compounds present, but in order to remove these impurities without hydrolysis of the desired product it must be crystallized from alkaline solution. Under these circumstances the result is not a single substance. It contains both secondary and tertiary salts, and (partly because carbonate is present) the carbon content is too high. To obtain the pure secondary salt, having the composition required by theory, special measures must be taken, for this salt in aqueous solution is acid and therefore unstable. The final product crystallizes in spherulites, and has the composition $C_4H_8O_5N_3PCa.4H_2O$. The most probable structure of the new substance is hence the following:

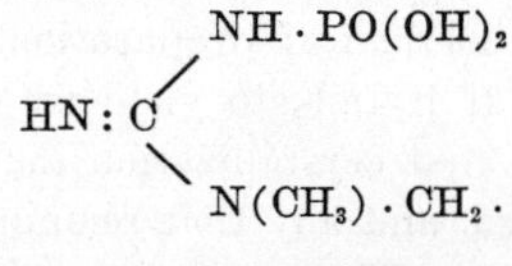

and its most characteristic chemical property, *viz.*, marked instability in acid solution, is in fact characteristic also of the few other known compounds which contain the group $-NH.PO(OH)_2$. This is the first substance containing phosphorus attached to nitrogen to be isolated from natural sources, and the instability of the phosphamic group marks it as one of considerable biological importance, as will be seen in the next section. The details of preparation will be published elsewhere.

II. FUNCTION

In spite of much investigation, the function of creatine in muscle has remained as much a mystery as it was at the time of the discovery of this substance 97 years ago. Having found that most of the creatine in normal resting muscle is combined with phosphoric acid, and that the compound is destroyed during contraction at a rate which rivals that of glycogenolysis and lactic acid production, we naturally anticipated

[1] C. H. Fiske and Y. Subbarow, SCIENCE, Vol. 65 (403)—1927.

that some light might at last be thrown on this time-honored question. Among the possibilities which suggest themselves is a change in hydrogen ion concentration accompanying the hydrolysis of phosphocreatine, and either augmenting or opposing the increase in acidity associated with the formation of lactic acid. The determination of the direction and magnitude of this effect becomes therefore a matter of some consequence.

From experiments with a preparation of the crystalline calcium salt which we had in our possession several months ago it was evident that hydrolysis in slightly acid solution resulted in a very marked decrease in acidity. This was one of the preparations to which we have referred in the first section as being a mixture of two salts, containing too much carbon, consequently the presence of organic impurities which might account for the observed effect could not be excluded. Moreover, the existence of a special neutralizing mechanism has been denied on the ground that muscle acquires the same pH whether lactic acid is produced within it as a result of stimulation or whether the same amount of lactic acid is added artificially to a muscle suspension in which enzyme action has presumably been stopped.[2] For this reason, and because of the importance of the question in relation to the chain events occurring during muscular contraction, we regarded our observations as uncertain until they could be confirmed with material that was analytically pure. While engaged in collecting a fresh supply of phosphocreatine for this and other uses we found that our first method of preparation could not be relied upon, for if it fails to yield an essentially pure product on the first crystallization the substance is largely decomposed, and any that remains intact is less pure than before. The consequence is that the confirmation of our earlier results has been delayed still further through the necessity of developing an entirely new process free from this element of risk.

The second dissociation constant (k_2') of phosphocreatine, determined by the titration of a 0.005 M solution of the pure secondary calcium salt with acid, is about 2.5×10^{-5}, or roughly 250 times as great as the second constant of o-phosphoric acid at the same ionic strength. This result, which is presumably to be attributed to the "unmasking" of the carboxyl group, establishes the function of phosphocreatine in muscle—or one function, since there may be others—as that of neutralizing a considerable part of the lactic acid formed during muscular contraction.

The other dissociation constants have not been determined, but on the addition of alkali to a solution of the secondary salt no marked evidence of buffer action appears until well beyond the turning point of phenolphthalein. It follows that the third constant is much less than 10^{-7}, so in resting muscle,—which according to the most recent evidence[2] is practically neutral—phosphocreatine exists wholly as the secondary salt.

Calculations based on these facts show that the hydrolysis of phosprocreatine (taking an average figure of 0.45 per cent. for the amount in resting cat muscle) liberates sufficient base under optimum conditions (pH 6)[3] to neutralize the lactic acid formed up to a concentration of about 0.23 per cent.[4] Approximately half of this amount of lactic acid, moreover, can be neutralized at pH 7, *i.e.*, without the development of any acidity at all. Since the lactic acid maximum for complete fatigue, at least in isolated frog muscle, is 0.4–0.5 per cent. (or even more under special circumstances), it appears that this new mechanism is peculiarly designed for the neutralization of the lactic acid formed in muscular exercise of moderate intensity. Finally, it should be noted that the occurrence in contracting muscle of a reaction by which fixed base is set free necessarily detracts to some extent from the importance of protein[5] in the neutralizing process. The hydrolysis of phosphocreatine seems now to be the principal factor permitting contraction to take place to a limited extent without the appearance of fatigue, if it is true—as has been claimed[2]—that the main restriction on muscular performance is the accumulation of acid in the cells.[6]

Cyrus H. Fiske,
Y. Subbarow

Biochemical Laboratory,
Harvard Medical School

[2] O. Meyerhof and K. Lohmann, *Biochem. Z.*, Vol. 168 (128)—1926.

[3] *I.e.*, the maximum amount of base is released (in dilute solution) at pH 6, which is roughly the acidity of completely fatigued muscle.[2]

[4] This figure is necessarily a rough one, including as it does the supposed "physiological minimum" (0.06 per cent. lactic acid) for mammalian muscle (W. M. Fletcher, *J. Physiol.*, Vol. 47 (361)—1913; G. Embden, E. Schmitz, and P. Meincke, *Z. Physiol. Chem.*, Vol. 113 (10)—1921).

[5] O. Meyerhof, *Arch. ges. Physiol.*, Vol. 195 (22)—1922.

[6] The existence in muscle of a special device for neutralizing acid raises a number of interesting questions which can not be answered without further experimental data. For example, judging from some recent observations made by Meyerhof and Lohmann (Naturwissenschaften, Vol. 15 (670)—1927), the hydrolysis of phosphocreatine in brief periods of stimulation proceeds more rapidly than the production of lactic acid. This is difficult to reconcile with the prevailing view that contraction is a response to increased acidity, but further investigation may show that the inconsistency is only an apparent one.

SCIENCE

VOL. LXVII FEBRUARY 17, 1928 No. 1729

CONTENTS

Wellesley College and the Development of Botanical Education in America: DR. C. STUART GAGER 171
Neurology and the Teaching of Medicine: DR. FOSTER KENNEDY 178
The Celebration of the Centenary of Marcelin Berthelot: DR. ATHERTON SEIDELL 180
Scientific Events:
An International Convention on Cancer Research; The Proposed Pan-American Geodetic Institute; New Building for the Yale School of Medicine; The 1929 Budget of the U. S. Department of Agriculture 185
Scientific Notes and News 187
University and Educational Notes 191
Discussion and Correspondence:
Applied Geophysics: PROFESSOR A. S. EVE. *The Multiple Origin of Tumors:* PROFESSOR H. E. EGGERS. *The Cuticula of Nematodes:* DR. THOMAS B. MAGATH. *An Unusual Atmospheric Phenomenon:* BOYD W. BARTLETT. *Psycho-endocrinology:* DR. LOUIS BERMAN 192
Quotations:
State Academies of Science 195
Reports:
Resolutions Adopted by the International Geodetic and Geophysical Union: CH. LALLEMAND 196
Scientific Apparatus and Laboratory Methods:
Infiltrating Pig Embryos with Paraffin: T. L. MALUMPHY 197
Special Articles:
The Anatomy of the Corium: DR. O. V. BATSON. *The Dialysis of Pituitary Extracts:* DR. OLIVER KAMM 198
Science News x

SCIENCE: A Weekly Journal devoted to the Advancement of Science, edited by J. McKeen Cattell and published every Friday by

THE SCIENCE PRESS

New York City: Grand Central Terminal.

Lancaster, Pa. Garrison, N. Y.

Annual Subscription, $6.00. Single Copies, 15 Cts.

SCIENCE is the official organ of the American Association for the Advancement of Science. Information regarding membership in the Association may be secured from the office of the permanent secretary, in the Smithsonian Institution Building, Washington, D. C.

Entered as second-class matter July 18, 1923, at the Post Office at Lancaster, Pa., under the Act of March 3, 1879.

WELLESLEY COLLEGE AND THE DEVELOPMENT OF BOTANICAL EDUCATION IN AMERICA[1]

IT is an honor for one to be assigned any part, however minor, in the exercises for which we have assembled to-day, and I am not insensible to the high honor of being invited to give the address this evening. The most significant distinction between man and the rest of creation is his intellect, and the most important matter that can ever concern us is the advancement and diffusion of knowledge. We are met this afternoon to dedicate a beautiful building to these uses.

I have been fortunate in knowing something of this building from the time when it existed only as a need, then as a dream, then through all the various stages of plans in mind, blue prints, bids and contracts, disappointments and delays which mark the construction of every building worth having—and now the welcome stage of a dream come true.

I had almost said, "the final" stage of a dream come true; but that would have implied a misunderstanding of the entire situation, for the completion of this building bears somewhat the same relation to the department of botany of Wellesley as the graduation of students from college bears to their life work—it is only a commencement. True it is not, if I may use a pleonasm, an initial beginning, but it marks the beginning of bigger and better things, not only for botany in Wellesley, but for botany in America, for whatever facilitates better work in any discipline, anywhere, is a benefit to all.

What has gone into this building? Brick and mortar, of course, as those can testify who have watched it rise from day to day. But more than brick and mortar. Aspirations and ideals, hopes and wishes, ability in planning, impatience at delays, discouragements vanquished by zeal and persistence, a determination to have the best in order that the best may be accomplished; love, devotion and sacrifice—the building is fairly held together by these imponderables more firmly than by beams and concrete.

I would like to emphasize, if I may, the comparison of this occasion to a college commencement, for just as commencement day has been preceded by years of activity and accomplishment that justify the final diploma, so this building has been preceded by years

[1] Address delivered at the dedication of the new Botany Building, Wellesley College, November 4, 1927.

of splendid accomplishment (in the study and teaching of botany) that fully justify it. In his "Address on University Education," delivered at the opening of the Johns Hopkins University in 1876, Huxley spoke as follows:

> I would say that whenever you do build, get an honest bricklayer, and make him build you just such rooms as you really want, leaving ample space for expansion. And a century hence, when the Baltimore and Ohio shares are at one thousand premium, and you have endowed all the professors you need and built all the laboratories that are wanted, and have the best museum and finest library that can be imagined; then, if you have a few hundred thousand dollars you don't know what to do with, send for an architect and tell him to put up a façade.

One could not truthfully say that all of the conditions laid down by Huxley as justifying a beautiful building have been here fulfilled, but enough of them have been met fully to justify this building.

It is true that Pasteur's early laboratory was an unhealthy cellar, that radium was discovered in an old shed, and that much of the world's scientific work has been poorly and inadequately housed, but there is no argument in all that. Men have attained the highest levels of religious experience in groves and tents, but I have never heard it argued that religion ever suffered by the building of beautiful temples, although such temples may at times have sheltered a worship wholly unworthy of shrine and worshipers.

If education and science are among the most important activities of the human race, they are worthy of being housed in as suitable and beautiful buildings as may be thought justified for business or religion. Beautiful architecture, like beauty in any form, is worth promoting for its own sake. Why should not beautiful buildings be planned for science and education?

I have referred to the gradual development here of the work for which this building is intended. Wellesley College was opened in 1875, at a period when botanical instruction in American liberal arts colleges was the exception rather than the rule, and when professors of botany were almost as scarce as blue roses. Asa Gray had studied and taught botany to the glory of Harvard College since 1842, but with the title "professor of natural history." He retired, two years before Wellesley College was opened, to devote himself to the herbarium and botanical research, leaving George Lincoln Goodale as professor of plant physiology and W. G. Farlow as assistant professor of botany.

At this time there were several men in medical schools teaching the specialized branch of botany known as materia medica, but so far as I can ascertain, there were (besides Farlow's at Harvard) only five chairs with the title "professor of botany," and only two more with the title "professor of botany and"—some other science, thus: Professors of botany: Edward Tuckerman, at Amherst, 1858; Daniel Cady Eaton, at Yale, 1864; William James Beal, at Michigan Agricultural College, 1870; Charles Edwin Bessey, at Iowa Agricultural College, 1870, and Sarah A. Oren, at Purdue University, 1875. Miss Oren was preceded in Purdue by John Hussy, who was professor of botany from 1875–1876. The other two were Albert Nelson Prentiss, professor of botany, arboriculture and horticulture at Cornell University, 1868, and Thomas Jonathan Burrill, professor of botany and horticulture at the University of Illinois, 1870.[2]

The botanists, Sereno Watson and Alphonso Wood, also flourished at about this time, but, so far as I can ascertain, not as professors of botany.

From the above information it will be seen that Wellesley was in the front rank of pioneers in America in the establishment of her chair of botany in 1878, and was probably the first woman's college in the world to have a separate chair. It is of special interest for us here that the establishment of a "school of botany" at Wellesley was a cherished hope of the founder, Mr. Durant.

It is perhaps not surprising to find this early attention to botany in a woman's college, for it is a venerable notion that botany is pre-eminently a study for women. Thus, as early as 1796, Jean Jacques Rousseau entitled his one botanical book, "Letters on the elements of botany addressed to a lady." In this book he stated his conviction that, "the study of nature abates the taste for frivolous amusements, prevents the tumult of the passions, and provides the mind with a nourishment which is salutary, by filling it with an object most worthy of its contemplations."

We should not fail to mention in this connection the splendid pioneer work in botanical teaching in the early years of the Troy Female Seminary (now known as the Emma Willard School). This school was founded in 1821, and as early as 1829 there was published (at Hartford, Connecticut) the first of several editions of "Familiar Lectures on Botany" for the use of higher schools and academies, by Mrs. Almira H. Lincoln, vice-principal of the seminary and teacher of botany there. The author states in her

[2] I am indebted to Dr. John Hendley Barnhart for the larger part of these data, but I have not made a sufficiently thorough search of the records to feel sure that I may not have omitted some professorship of botany established or filled in 1875. The years given above for each name are the years when the incumbents were appointed.

preface that the book was the outgrowth of some years of instruction of large classes in botany. We may infer, therefore, that botanical instruction was organized at the Troy Female Seminary at least prior to 1829, and over thirty years before the establishment (in 1858) of the first chair of botany in an American college.[3]

I believe that no botanist giving this address could resist the temptation to quote from Mrs. Lincoln's book:

> The study of botany seems peculiarly adapted to females; the objects of its investigation are beautiful and delicate; its pursuit leading to exercise in the open air is conducive to health and cheerfulness. Botany is not a sedentary study which can be acquired in the library; but the objects of the science are scattered over the surface of the earth, along the banks of winding brooks, on the borders of precipices, the sides of mountains, and the depths of the forest.

This would seem to imply that the early botanical work of the Troy Female Seminary was largely of the nature of what is now known as ecology, and one may picture classes of females, far huskier than we usually associate with that epoch, climbing steep banks and mountains, and pushing their way through the underbrush of dense forests in search of specimens and knowledge. The picture is not over-drawn, for in the catalogue of 1844–45 the "Report of the Committee of Examination" of the school, reads, in part, as follows:

> The class in botany we consider especially deserving of praise. We could not only judge of their proficiency by their familiarity with their text-book, but their knowledge was put to a practical test by the actual analysis of plants and flowers. This they did with a fluency and accuracy that gave most conclusive evidence of their own diligence and their teacher's faithfulness. Each young lady had an herbarium in which were pressed and tastefully arranged from 100–300 specimens, all labelled according to their classes, orders, genera and species. These have all been collected and arranged during the term, and mostly in the immediate vicinity of Troy, at no greater distance than would suffice for a morning walk or an afternoon ramble. In climbing hills and threading woods and valleys in search of flowers, the young ladies together with instruction have gathered strength, health and beauty.
>
> The study of botany seems to be peculiarly appropriate for women. Her skilful and tasteful hands find a pleasing task in the cultivation of flowers. Wherever we see the windows filled with the most beautiful flowers, native and exotic, the columbine trailing its vines over the portico, the garden walk fringed with violets, and shaded with roses, we there recognize the finger of woman, and look for the abode of neatness, order, cheerfulness and virtue. In all ages flowers have been made the objects of her care and the emblems of her purity and beauty.

Here we have an early expression in America, of the notion, once more prevalent than now, that botany is essentially a study for females. No misconception ever died harder; it is not dead yet, but like most erroneous ideas, it persists only among persons whose information does not entitle them to hold any opinion on the subject.

But from the above quotation, the fact emerges that instruction in botany was given by a woman in one of the first schools for women to be established in America.

As early as 1873 courses in botany (Gray's Botany) were given at Mount Holyoke Female Seminary by Miss Henrietta Edgecomb Hooker,[4] but Mount Holyoke was not chartered as a college until twenty years later. Without investigating the matter further, I hazard the guess that the courses given by Mrs. Lincoln at Troy were the first (or one of the first) courses in botany to be given by a woman in any country. In harmony with this fine tradition, Article VI of the By-Laws of Wellesley College states that the college shall provide instruction in botany. The first professor of botany, Susan Maria Hallowell, was at first professor of natural history—from 1875 to 1878. In 1878 she became professor of botany, and the college calendar for 1877–8, under the heading "Instruction in botany," outlines the subject-matter to be covered, and contains the following paragraph:

> Students are encouraged to make independent observations and self reliant researches; and, avoiding hasty inferences from partial data, to form judgments of things noted, and correctly describe the results of their observations. To secure this end, they are instructed in the best methods of study and observation.

That is a rather remarkable statement, considering the year in which it was published, and is evidence that Wellesley College was one of the pioneers not only in having a separate department of botany, but in emphasizing that something should be acquired by the study of botany besides information about plants, and in introducing the laboratory method of instruction in undergraduate courses.

Harvard appears to have been (in 1872) the first American college to introduce laboratory work in undergraduate instruction in botany. The following year Professor Charles E. Bessey required laboratory

[3] The Catalogue of the Troy Female Seminary for 1839–40 specifies an additional special charge of three dollars a term for students taking botany. This appears to be one of the early instances in America (if not the earliest) of a laboratory fee in botany.

[4] Her name appeared in the *Thirty-ninth Annual Catalogue (1875–76)* as Miss Etta E. Hooker.

work in the undergraduate courses at the Iowa Agricultural College, at Ames, without knowing that this had been done the year before at Harvard. Wellesley, therefore, was among the very first colleges in the world to adopt in undergraduate botanical instruction the only rational method of education in any science.

Appleton's "American Cyclopaedia," edition of 1881, in the article "Wellesley College," states that:

> The grounds comprise 300 acres, including a greenhouse, from which the students are supplied with flowers for their botanical researches.

Further on, in the same article, we read that,

> Wellesley College was established to give young women opportunities for a collegiate education fully equal to those provided for young men. It is arranged for collegiate methods of instruction only, and *for courses of difficult study.*

From the italic words it is evident that botany was no snap; but in the presence of my contemporaries—both students and teachers—I will not dwell on the continuity of this reputation, so splendidly maintained from the beginning until the present moment.

This period should not be passed over without a word of appreciation of the substantial pioneer work of Professor Hallowell, so fittingly commemorated during the current year by the endowment of the Susan M. Hallowell chair of botany.

I am still full of the enthusiasm engendered by my visit one year ago through the botanic garden and arboretum of Wellesley College. What a magnificent opportunity would have been lost if a portion of this beautiful campus had not been set apart for a botanic garden! The opportunity amounted to an obligation; the plan is admirable, and the present accomplishment a matter for congratulation, not only to the department of botany, but to the college as a whole, to the local community and to the botanical world.

When one contemplates the unique educational values of museums and botanic gardens, it seems strange indeed that they have, in America at least, almost without exception, developed independently of colleges and universities. In the old world, botanic gardens commonly developed as adjuncts to university botanical instruction—as at Pisa, Genoa, Amsterdam, Oxford, Cambridge and elsewhere; but even in the old world the outstanding botanic gardens developed as institutions wholly or largely independent of colleges, as, for example, the Chelsea Physic Garden, the Jardin des Plantes and the gardens at Berlin, Kew and Buitenzorg. In America the botanic garden of John Bartram (Philadelphia, about 1730), the Elgin Botanic Garden of Dr. David Hosack (New York, about 1801), the new California Botanic Garden (established this year), and the Missouri, New York and Brooklyn gardens, all developed as independent institutions, although affiliations have been established between the last three and local universities. Among university and college botanic gardens may be mentioned those at Harvard, the University of Pennsylvania, the Johns Hopkins University, Michigan Agricultural College, and more recently those at the University of Michigan and Stanford University. Among women's colleges the botanic gardens of Smith and Mount Holyoke are perhaps most widely known.

One of the best wishes I can give for Wellesley College is the early and vigorous development of its botanic garden and arboretum, and the organization of its courses of instruction in a way to make the fullest use of them.

Out of his wisdom and wealth, Aristotle endowed (at Athens) the first botanic garden of which we have record. From that day to the establishment of the Brooklyn Botanic Garden in 1910, the endowers of botanic gardens appear to have been men. The fashion of women benefactors, set by Brooklyn, soon began to spread. In 1914 Miss Susan Minns, of Boston, a student (together with Miss Hallowell) of Agassiz and of Gray, made a contribution of $50,000 toward the construetion of a new botany building. This fund had increased to $80,000 by the time the new building was begun. In 1921 Mrs. Cordenio A. Severance (after the death of her husband) generously doubled an endowment fund which Mr. and Mrs. Severance had previously given for the botanic garden, now known as the Alexandra Botanic Garden, in memory of their daughter, the total endowment being $30,000.

In 1923 Mrs. Robert Shaw, of Wellesley, gave to the college a substantial fund in memory of her father as an endowment for the Horatio Hollis Hunnewell Arboretum, and additional funds for the initial work of development. In June of this year (1927), Miss Minns made another liberal gift of $11,000 as an endowment fund for the Hallowell Memorial Library, wisely specifying that the income from this fund is to supplement, but not to replace, the annual appropriation from other college funds for the botanical library. Mention should also be made of the recent generous gift of Dr. John Farwell of $100,000, to establish, in memory of his wife, the Ruby Frances Howe Farwell chair of botany.

To announce these facts here and now is taking coals to Newcastle, but to one who, like the speaker, has devoted much of his time and effort for a number of years endeavoring to secure more nearly adequate funds for botanical science, it is a source of gratification and pride to proclaim such benefactions as these.

Lest any one may feel that I am wandering from the dedication of the new building, let me emphasize the fact that a botanic garden is indispensable for the highest accomplishment in the work for which this building is intended.

The Elgin Botanic Garden, to which I referred a moment ago, was one of the earliest botanic gardens in America. It was established and maintained by Dr. David Hosack immediately after his appointment, in 1795, as the successor to Dr. Samuel L. Mitchill, the first professor of botany in Columbia College. In a pamphlet on "The establishment and progress of the Elgin Botanic Garden (New York, 1811), Dr. Hosack quotes from the *Transactions* of the New York State Agricultural Society for 1794, as follows:

> The establishment of a garden is nearly [i.e., closely] connected with the professorship of botany under the college, and the lectures on that branch must be always very lame and defective without one.

Then, referring to his appointment as professor of botany, he continues:

> I now readily perceive that an abstract account of the principles of these sciences (botany and materia medica), as taught by books, coloured engravings, or even with the advantages of an herbarium must necessarily be very imperfect and unsatisfactory, when compared with the examination of living plants, growing in their proper soils, with the advantages of culture; that a study, in itself both highly useful and agreeable, was necessarily rendered uninviting from the manner in which its principles were illustrated, and that a botanical establishment was indispensably necessary in order to teach this branch of medical science with complete effect.

After endeavoring to teach botany for two years and a half without a botanic garden, Dr. Hosack, in November, 1797, presented a memorial to the president and board of trustees of Columbia College, urging them to provide a botanic garden. "Since I have had the honour of an appointment to this professorship," he said, "it has been to me a source of great regret that the want of a *Botanical Garden,* and an extensive Botanical Library, have prevented that advancement in the interests of the institution which might reasonably have been expected."

In these quotations we find not only the germ of the once famous Elgin Botanic Garden, but one of the earliest expressions in America of the great importance of a botanic garden for the most effective teaching of botany.

It were possible, to be sure, to lay out this or any other college campus purely from the standpoint of beautiful landscape effect without any regard whatever for the botanical affinities of the trees and shrubs, or the accomplishment of any but esthetic results. And beauty, of itself, is educative. But there is a type of beauty often lost sight of by artists (or by those who are merely artists), which consists in the perfect adaptation of a thing to its uses (such, for example, as the perfection of the floral mechanism of orchids to secure insect pollination), or the utilization of a thing to the full extent of its capacities (such, for example, as the playing of an organ by a master). One who comprehends the morphology of an orchid flower can see in it immeasurably more beauty than one who sees it only as a pleasing combination of color and form. So a college campus, laid out as a botanic garden without sacrificing its landscape effects may serve science and art and education. It possesses a manifold beauty because it serves a multiplicity of ends. And it would seem almost incredible that an educational institution should not be keenly interested to make its campus (as well as its buildings) yield the fullest possible educational returns.

But what *is* the purpose of this building? "For the teaching of botany," you say. Emphatically, no! It will be used for that, but its purpose is education through botany. One of the greatest of modern fallacies is the idea that students go to college primarily to learn. (I am told that this fallacy now has few adherents in the student bodies themselves!) This idea underlies all the present-day talk about vocational training in our colleges. Four years of college should contribute toward fitting graduates to follow successfully some vocation, but the chief purpose of our undergraduate liberal arts college is to educate; education and learning or training are not synonymous.

Just as the purpose of the college is to educate, so the ultimate purpose of every course of instruction in every subject should be the education of those who pursue the subject. To learn about plants is one thing; education through botany is quite a different matter, a more serious matter, a vastly more important matter. How completely this conception of the function of botany in college instruction was recognized in Professor Hallowell's 1878 announcement, quoted above! This department of botany and this college may well be proud of that statement.

I shall not vie with Spencer and Huxley and others in attempting to define education, but it is a self-evident truth (except to those who lose sight of it!) that one may be a walking cyclopedia of information about plants, and yet, every time he writes, or enters into conversation, or passes judgment (so-called), or states his opinion, or evaluates issues, or discloses his taste, or reveals his understanding (or the lack of it) of the relation of botanical knowledge to knowledge as a whole, and its significance in the history of civilization and in modern life, he may reveal a lack of education more clearly than he reveals his knowledge of plants.

If this building is to be devoted only to teaching people botany, the money could have been better expended; if it is to be devoted to education through botany, the money could not have been spent to better purpose.

What are the educational values to be derived by the study of botany? In the first place, the student will learn whether or not botany is his major interest in life. This is the most important and most vital question to be answered by the four undergraduate years of college. "What is my major life interest?" Not until this question is satisfactorily answered can the most effective education even begin.

I had the pleasure of teaching beginning botany for about ten years, and after a few preliminary years, while I was learning much more than I was teaching, I began to say to the students, at the last meeting of the class, something like this:

I know perfectly well that some of you are delighted beyond words that this is the last meeting of the class, and that you will never take another botany course, nor read another book on botany, nor ever again glance at a plant except as an object of beauty, so long as you live, if you can avoid it. If you have discovered that this is your attitude toward botany, you could not have made a more vital discovery. The next most important thing for you to find out is this: "What subject does appeal to you more than any other, so that you shall want to elect all of it you are allowed to in college, and devote the best of yourself to its pursuit thereafter."

Some of you have discovered that, until you began the study of botany, you were never really interested in anything before. You thought you had been interested, but you find you were mistaken. Your keenest regret is that the course is over, and you mean to elect all you have time for in college, to specialize in some branch of botanical science for your major post-graduate study, and to devote your life to the study and teaching of botany. You, too, are to be congratulated, not because you have discovered that botany is your life interest, but because you have discovered what your major interest in life is.

More surprised classes I never saw than those who listened to that statement. Congratulations from the "Prof" that they find they do not like his subject! One who is merely giving instruction in botany could never see his work from that angle; one who teaches botany as an educational discipline could never see it from any other. The former always regards his introductory course merely as a preparation for advanced courses; the latter regards it as an introduction of a developing mind to a new realm of thought, which may or may not make a strong appeal. But a course planned with the latter thought in mind should and will serve as one of the best possible preparations for advanced courses, should his students wish to elect them.

In common with other sciences, botany when properly taught is also peculiarly fitted for teaching people *how* to acquire knowledge and *how* to think. As I have emphasized elsewhere, the great lesson to be learned from the recent science-and-theology flare-up is that most people do not know *how* to think. They hold firmly to opinions and cherish prejudices, but they have not the most elementary conception of how a scientist proceeds in the acquisition of knowledge and the formulation of general notions and principles.

Again the ramifications of botany into other sciences, and into non-scientific disciplines, such as history, art, religion, social customs, commerce, literature, and others, qualify it to be, if one desires, a central motive in a program of education. For example:

The most widely disseminated of all human races has, for several thousand years, celebrated a feast with unleavened bread because its ancesters, on one of their famous racial migrations set out on their journey so hastily that they forgot to take with them a supply of tiny microscopic plants, without which bread is unleavened. An entire nation of American Indians has developed its culture around the Indian corn or Maize as a motive. The culture of another group centers around the acorn.[5] The cultivation of plants marks the beginning of fixed habitations, an absolutely essential condition for the development of civilization. The growing of cultivated plants is the foundation of industry and commerce. One can not follow out the botany of the objects in any living-room without being brought into contact with nearly every continent and nearly every clime. For botany is more than morphology and physiology, taxonomy and ecology, anatomy and cytology. The study of botany and the history of botany would afford as liberal an education as the study of any "five-foot shelf of books," and would afford certain educational results that could never be obtained by the reading of any number of lineal feet of printed matter.

Why is it that the history of botany (and of other sciences, for that matter) is so seldom taught in our colleges? What an educational opportunity is being missed! To one who knows the fascinating interest of the subject, its cultural value, the importance of its lessons for everyday thinking and judging, and the flood of light which it throws on modern science

[5] Two interesting rooms in the Brooklyn Museum are devoted to exhibits illustrating these two types of primitive culture.

and other departments of thought, the general neglect of the history of science in our educational programs is difficult to understand. In the Wellesley College *Calendar* for 1926–1927 courses of instruction are listed in 27 disciplines, of which 18 are non-scientific and 8 scientific. With the exception of Logic and Psychology, Philosophy, Reading and Speaking, and Spanish, courses in the history of the various subjects are offered in all the non-scientific disciplines, varying in proportion from 9 historical courses out of 11 in Art to one historical course out of 45 in Physical Education. In Mathematics one course out of 18 is historical. The department of History offers courses in almost every aspect of human activity, but no course in the history of science. However, such courses belong properly under the various sciences.

In the eight natural and physical sciences, historical courses are offered only in astronomy.

These data are assembled from the Wellesley College Catalog, not with any thought of criticism, but merely as the most appropriate concrete example (on this occasion) of a condition which is almost universal in American collegiate education.

The fact emerges that our colleges are neglecting one of the most valuable aspects of human thought and endeavor, and science is needlessly impoverishing itself as an educational discipline. Will Wellesley College not wish to be one of the leaders in correcting this educational defect, just as it was a leader in its early years in the introduction of laboratory work, and in other aspects of higher education?

Not more than fifty years ago, when science was only an entering wedge in the college curriculum, the protagonists of the older disciplines were accustomed to speak of the classics and other non-scientific studies as "the humanities" in contrast to the sciences, which were not then recognized as possessing humanistic values. But in 1919 Sir William Osler, Regius Professor of Medicine at Oxford, delivered his presidential address before the Classical Association. In this address on "The Old Humanities and the New Sciences," Osler elaborated the humanistic value of scientific studies in a program of education. "Our wonder at the extent and variety of the knowledge demanded by the school of *Literae Humaniores,*" says Sir William, "pales before the gasping astonishment of what is not there. Now and again a hint, a reference, a recognition, but the moving forces which have made the modern world are simply ignored. Yet they are all Hellenic, all part and parcel of the humanities in the true sense, and all of prime importance in modern education."

Possibly, as Osler suggests, the elimination of most of the science from the classical curriculum is due to the fact that the intellectual treasures of Greece and Rome were transmitted to us through ecclesiastical conduits and sieves, and only that was allowed to pass which was considered of interest and importance. Whatever the explanation, the classical student is incredulous (if not indifferent) when told that Aristotle founded the first botanic garden of which there is record, that he endowed it in his will, and that he was primarily a biologist. Those of us who prepared for our scientific careers by four or more years of classical studies in the last quarter of the nineteenth century learned almost everything of Theophrastus, a pupil of Aristotle's, *except* that he was, in the judgment of some writers, the founder of modern botany, and the director of the botanic garden established at Athens by Aristotle.

I refer to these facts because they emphasize in a striking way that, if we follow out the history of such a science as botany, we are taken straight to the heart of the old humanities; the cleavage between the sciences and the humanities vanishes—the sciences become humanities.

Says a recent writer in the English periodical, *Nature:*

"As a medium of culture, the history of scientific discovery opens up to the imagination vistas of man's endeavor which place it in the front rank of humanistic studies. *But,*" he continues," we doubt, however, whether much of the science teaching in schools, either primary or secondary, could be regarded as science for citizenship instead of science for specialists, and we should welcome a movement which would broaden its scope and change its character."

Here is the great opportunity for the liberal arts colleges, such as Wellesley, to regard the purpose of most of their courses to be primarily the *education* of their students, not the training of specialists. There is perhaps no greater need in our nation to-day than men of broad, scholarly education, whether or not they possess in addition the technical training fitting them for some profession.[6]

And now I have tried your powers of endurance and courtesy to the very limit, with scarcely a word about research. In the back of my own mind research has been taken for granted as the indispensable foundation and inspiration of teaching. How can one teach who isn't a student? He could only hear recitations—or, what is worse, give lectures—when he ought to be inspiring others to study. If one wishes to get a real thrill, let him discover a new fact or principle. We are all familiar with the classic story

[6] The educational importance of the history of science is emphasized in Paper No. 8 of the Report by the Adult Education Committee of the Board of Education, entitled, ''Natural Science in Adult Education,'' London, 1927.

of Archimedes, running fresh from his bath through the streets of Syracuse, shouting "*Eureka, eureka,*" in his joy at having discovered the principle of specific gravity. We are told that Newton was so overcome with emotion, when he saw that his calculations on gravitation were confirming his hypothesis, that he could hardly hold the pencil to finish the equations. When Pasteur showed Biot how to make dextro-tartaric and laevo-tartaric acid, Biot exclaimed, "My dear boy, I have loved the sciences so much all my life that what you show me makes my heart thump." When Davy discovered the metal potassium he danced about his laboratory in high glee, and was too excited to continue his experiments.

The best thing I can wish for this building is that its laboratories may be the scene of many heart thumps (over science!), and of many ecstatic dances (over the discovery of truth!).

Wellesley is a college, but that is no reason why the teaching which is, perhaps, its main function, should not rest upon the solid foundation of research in progress. It is a truism that nothing is more wholesome for a college nor more stimulating to a student than an atmosphere of research penetrating laboratories and classrooms and campus. Nothing could be more unfortunate, from the standpoint of education, than to have a student, after four years of undergraduate residence, leave a college with the impression that any department of knowledge, and in particular, any science, is static—a finished product.

It was Frederick the Great who said: "The greatest and noblest pleasure which men can have in this world is to discover new truths; and the next is to shake off old prejudices." What a wonderful privilege to be able to study and teach! What a fine thing it is to provide a building and equipment devoted to the advancement of sciencc and of cducation through science!

I congratulate this Department of Botany, I congratulate Wellesley College, I congratulate the botanical and educational world on this splendid opportunity and the correspondingly great responsibility.

C. STUART GAGER
BROOKLYN BOTANIC GARDEN

NEUROLOGY AND THE TEACHING OF MEDICINE[1]

To be the orator of the day on an occasion as important as this is to feel at once uplifted and cast down; by the honor one is raised, and by the sense of inferiority one is made to realize that indeed one is much lower than the angels. Graduates in the humanities, you, our new friends, are Freshmen in medicine—some of you have come because throughout your life you have been shapen in medicine, you have felt a driving urge which bade you examine the living things around you, be interested in the vagaries of the people you knew—may be, however, some have chosen this arduous trade because their fathers before them plied it and they count on his name and favor as aid and comfort for the hard launching in a not entirely appreciative world. A handicap this almost —for the spirit of practice comes only from within; an aptitude, a power to learn, may be inherited but to try to follow exactly the steps of one's father is perhaps to court the fate of Icarus. The wings with subtly-blended wax fastened on his shoulders were those which his father Daedalus had fashioned and by them he had been borne aloft. These wings lifted the ambitious Icarus, but the sun, you remember, melted the wax and he fell into the Aegean Sea—so the adventure and attrition of Practice may be the solvent of such wings; for it is the man himself, his sure selection of essentials, his ready grasp of problems, the skill of his hands, his humor, his instinct for the problems of others rather than his own, his love of the weakness of humanity as well as its strength; his pity for frail, great-brained, great-hearted, things like ourselves caught in the wheels and hammers of biological law. These are inborn and can not be transferred by will or directed in action—and they are the very stuff of happy and useful living. Those men who have a call for medicine have these qualities or most of them, but to those who doubt themselves—and who does not?—we would say that hard work will bring greater results here unaided by great brilliance of intellect than in any other profession.

Do you remember how Lydgate found that he must go doctoring—this in George Eliot's novel "Middlemarch":

> One vacation, a wet day sent him to the small home-library, to hunt once more for a book which might have some freshness for him; in vain! unless indeed he took down a dusty row of volumes with grey paper backs and dingy labels—the volumes of an old Cyclopedia which he had never disturbed. The page he opened on was under the head of anatomy and the first passage that drew his eyes was on the valves of the heart. He was not much acquainted with valves of any sort but he knew that valvae were folding doors, and through this crevice came a sudden light startling him with his first vivid notion of finely adapted mechanism in the human frame. The moment of vocation had come, and before he got down from his chair, the world was made

[1] An address at the opening of session, September, 1927, Cornell University Medical College, New York City.

new to him by a presentment of endless processes filling the vast spaces planked out of his sight by that wordy ignorance which he had supposed to be knowledge. From that hour, Lydgate felt the growth of an intellectual passion.

Again we read of him—showing that this passion touched—as it must touch—his feelings as his mind.

His scientific interest soon took the form of a professional enthusiasm. He carried to his studies in London, Edinburgh and Paris, the conviction that the medical profession as it might be was the finest in the world; presenting the most perfect interchange between science and art; offering the most direct alliance between intellectual conquest and the social good. Lydgate's nature demanded this combination; he was an emotional creature, with a flesh and blood sense of fellowship which withstood all the abstractions of special study. He cared not only for "cases" but for John and Elizabeth, especially Elizabeth.

It was my good fortune as a recent graduate in medicine to come into close contact with some of the greatest minds in English neurology—and many of them like Ferrier, Gowers and Hughlings Jackson, with the later brilliant aid of Victor Horsley, had been notable builders of our science in the latter part of the last century. It is not easy for us to realize that when they began their work, knowledge of the functions of the brain and spinal cord was very little greater than had obtained since Grecian and Roman times. Their labors were crowned with marvelous results in the course of fifty years—but their work was necessarily of the nature of adventurous engineers—they gathered the materials for the building, they collected the stones and cement; Jackson, of whom it was said that his guess was worth ten men's facts, might be described as an architect of flying buttresses', Ferrier dug foundations, fortified the true walls of Jackson's theories and dynamited weak fabrications—Gowers writing the "Bible of Clinical Neurology" in inimitable prose when still under forty-five wore down his health and added not much to his fortune by the erection of mighty arches and the giving of form and meaning to the whole. Not all the work of their hands remained standing—here a pillar and there a weak foundation has crumbled and worn down, but on the whole we have a good home over our heads, to be builded higher and stronger by succeeding generations. In the nature of things, however, these men had to be collectors—anatomical facts cemented by meager physiology—they had to catalogue and classify new diseases and give names to symptoms and habitations to observed phenomena. They had always to be collecting and listing and ordering new specimens, and their interests lay naturally with those specimens most easily recognized as being different from normal—and such specimens were the end products of disease. We are now less interested in states of advanced deterioration and more concerned with the earliest departures from smooth working. We have come to understand how meagerly we know the normal and how necessary it is to grasp the infinite variety of natural regular processes in the organism. Problems in the natural history of disease are now more engrossing than the disease itself—we are more concerned for instance with the pathways of infection of the central nervous system than we are in neat descriptions of hopelessly paralyzed muscles resulting therefrom. This digging after roots deep in the ground is tough unproductive looking work—we have almost lost interest in the flowers and shrubs on the surface—and, for a while, less spectacular results may be available for show. This search for prime causes has also changed or rather better adjusted our value as a single specialty—added knowledge has revealed our unity with general medicine—we are discontented with labeling a disease "subacute combined sclerosis of the spinal cord"—we must find out its affiliations with pernicious anemia and with antecedent gall-bladder disorder. Epilepsy has ceased to be a diagnosis and has become a damning verdict—we must try to find the toxic factors which give rise to epileptic phenomena, which is now looked on as but congeries of symptoms produced by other agents.

This change from the static to the dynamic viewpoint makes cells on biochemistry, endocrinology, psychology and, as ever, on anatomy and physiology. These sciences, too, must in their turn be made more dynamic, more vital, more human. Twenty years ago, descriptive anatomy and amphibian physiology were the total vogue—much progress has been made since then—but there is still a divorce between the so-called pure sciences and medicine and surgery. The student of physiology should *as such* be familiar with normal heart sounds, with the normal fundus of the eye, with the appearance of the vocal cords in action—he may know the oculo-motor nerve of the eye, but what has he seen of convergence, accommodation or pupillary reactions? In short, there should be more physiology in the wards, and more humanity in the laboratory and the dissecting room. The normal must be made manifest, handled, seen, recognized, understood, before the abnormal can be appreciated—we must know truth before we know error—and we must know that there is no absolute in either. Was it not jesting Pilate, two thousand years ago, asked what is truth and did not stay for an answer? But he referred to ethics, not muscles and nerve tracts—and truth of function *can* be reached if a student study muscles in action, then dissect them, and *about the same time* be shown them paralyzed by both a lower and upper motor neuron lesion. The X-ray department can be used to supplement physiological demonstration of digestion and heart mechanism. The instruments of clinical precision should be familiar and usable long before they are employed to detect the presence of disease.

The ophthalmoscope, the stethoscope, the laryngoscope, the otoscope, the blood-pressure apparatus, give up physiological secrets which must be mastered before those of medicine can be comprehended. Neurological cases often afford better examples of normal and abnormal function than any animal experiment in a laboratory—and coordinated education can make readily available all such material for students of the basic sciences.

The undergraduate in medicine then would have more time in the hospital to learn the very difficult art of history taking; the probing of the earliest manifestation of disease; he would grow more easy in the handling of his human charges—he would in short be more valuable in the search after first causes—more able to play his part in the open mobile warfare of the present day medicine and less of a static cataloguing agent in the trench warfare of the past. We don't yet know if man is energy or a machine. We compromise between the ideas of Plato and Aristotle and call him a transformer of power. His nervous system is three dimensional—and some of us suspect it may yet be four! Dreams though compounded of past experiences may be shot through with aspiration; the discontent of man with himself and his works forever scourging him upward can not yet be seen with stains of gold and silver, though we know some of the defects of structure which forbid the expression and perhaps existence of such torturing impulses. The study of the brain tells the tale of our painful climbing from the depths, of the building and controlling our powers of perception and adaptation—and may be from these neuronic origins spring man's nobility and lyric ecstasy as well. You will learn in this university something of the substantial workings of human powers and processes, their continuity with those of all living creatures, and, may be, you will find that control of human breedings must precede betterment in human brains.

We bid you welcome as our comrades to carry on the torch given us by our teachers—the torch that lets us see clearly—Man, half brute, half angel, most wonderfully made in mechanism, whose spirit denies the universe itself as boundary.

FOSTER KENNEDY

CORNELL UNIVERSITY MEDICAL COLLEGE

THE CELEBRATION OF THE CENTENARY OF MARCELIN BERTHELOT[1]

ONE of the axioms frequently expressed by Marcelin Berthelot is that "Science is essentially a collective endeavor and owes its progress to the efforts of a multitude of workers in all periods and of all nationalities, who by common agreement are associated in the search for truth and its application to the improvement of the conditions of man." A more succinct expression of this idea is that "Science reveals the persistence and the necessity of human collaboration. It impresses our heart and spirit with the vivifying notion of solidarity."

He advocated repeatedly the advantages to the progress of science of cordial relations among scientists and a mutual appreciation of the efforts of each. It was this precept which stimulated the common generous spirit exhibited at this first gathering in so many years of the chemists of all nations.

The organizers of the celebration desired that it should not be simply a passing ceremony without beneficial consequences. They wished to honor the memory of Berthelot in a manner which would prepetuate his ideals of service and the promotion of more friendly relations between all chemists. It was believed that the most fitting monument to him would be a house of chemistry which would serve as a meeting place not only for the chemists of France but for those of every country.

It was realized that an invitation to all nations to participate in its accomplishment would give to each a more personal interest in the enterprise. Furthermore, it was desired that those who might enjoy the benefits of the undertaking should regard themselves as constituent members and not as invited guests. This broad-minded point of view is more clearly appreciated when one considers the difference between an invitation to make use of the facilities provided by an organization and an offer of the privileges of membership in it.

Invitations were, therefore, addressed to all countries of the world to unite with France in celebrating the one hundredth anniversary of the birth of Marcelin Berthelot and to contribute any sum they might desire towards erecting a memorial to him in the form of an international house of chemistry. This invitation was accepted in the spirit in which it was sent by practically every nation and the ceremonies which I wish briefly to describe were held in Paris on October 24–26 last.

It is fitting, however, that attention should first be

[1] Address delivered before the meeting of the Chemical Society of Washington, January 12, 1928.

directed to the thoroughness with which the celebration was planned. The Berthelot committee was formed a year or more in advance and the leading men of science and of the government accepted prominent places on it. There are probably few countries in the world where science is so highly appreciated as in France and the most complete support that a nation could give such a movement was obtained.

The French subscription to the undertaking was officially opened at a ceremony held at the Sorbonne on May 5. At that time representatives of the leading scientific and other national organizations pledged the support of each to the undertaking. Shortly thereafter the central committee began issuing regular bulletins to the press reporting the subscriptions received. The total grew gradually from a few million francs to more than ten millions and at the time of the ceremonies in October it had reached fifteen and a half millions, of which nearly seven had been received from countries other than France.

Those who have aided in preparing for national meetings know something of the difficulties which are encountered. The impossibility of correctly estimating in advance the number likely to be present is very much greater in the case of an international gathering. Furthermore, the misunderstanding resulting from difference in customs in different countries are much more pronounced, and the consequence of any possible neglect of attention to a guest is far more serious than to a fellow countryman. Hence, one can readily imagine the exceptional qualifications the Berthelot committee was called upon to exhibit. That they succeeded admirably in their efforts is certainly the consensus of opinion of all who were fortunate enough to be present.

The opening function was a reception in the salons of the Sorbonne. Here one met previous acquaintances and quickly made new ones. The following day the delegates were invited to visit, at the École de Pharmacie, a collection of mementoes of Berthelot. Here was assembled the apparatus used by him in some of his most notable investigations, his manuscripts, note books and in general all kinds of souvenirs of his scientific activity.

From the École de Pharmacie every one proceeded to the Collège de France to visit the laboratory occupied by Berthelot during the last years of his life. Here the delegates were welcomed by M. Croiset, the administrator of the Collège de France. Since the laboratory and lecture hall were too small to contain the hundreds who were present the speakers addressed the assembly from a stand erected in the court yard. M Croiset said, "You have come to the Collège de France like pilgrims of the middle ages came to sanctuaries renowned by the virtues of a patron saint. As pilgrims of modern science you come to this house which has listened to the teachings of Marcelin Berthelot and which has been the witness of his fruitful meditations. You come both to render homage to a grand memory and to be inspired by a great example. The life of Berthelot is one on which it is particularly profitable to meditate." In continuing the speaker pointed out that Berthelot knew how greatly the exchange of ideas, intellectual collaboration and communications between scientists contribute to the development of the spirit of peace and friendship which is the guarantee of real progress.

Following M. Croiset, Professor Schlenck, director of the Chemical Institute of the University of Berlin, responded in the name of the German delegation. It should be remarked that Germany accepted in a very cordial manner the invitation to participate in the celebration and sent twelve of its leading chemists. Among these may be mentioned Nernst, Haber, Willstätter, Neuberg, Bodenstein, Wieland, Markwald, Huttig and others whose names I failed to note. Professor Schlenck, speaking for the first time in France since the war, said that "Genius has its own roads which are indeed those of natural science and philosophy and all lead to the same end which is the ennobling of humanity. This high aim is the object of all the sciences. It makes of the scientists of all lands the priests of the same temple and should unite them more ideally than any other human interest. This is why I see in the sciences a basis particularly favorable for the mutual understanding of peoples and for the profound comprehension of the soul of each. The genius of Berthelot has had an incontestable influence in this direction and it is for this reason particularly that the German delegation renders special homage to his memory."

Following Professor Schlenck, our own Professor Bogert spoke in the name of all other foreign delegates. He said, "We are here as at the table of our older brother. The scientists of all countries are united thus as members of the same family and their only rivalry should be to do more and better work. Scientists have often been reproached for being a little detached from terrestrial things. However, it is in their work that the material and ideal unite and often the most complicated problems are solved in the most elementary manner. The straight route followed by Berthelot does not deviate far from the throne of God."

The large gathering then paid a visit to the laboratory, which will celebrate in three years the four hundredth anniversary of its founding. The amphitheater where Berthelot taught is an incomplete semi-circle with benches without backs rising in tiers. The wormholed stairs give and squeak at each step. According to present-day standards the laboratory is far from adequate for its purpose, but M. Moureu and his staff and students numbering about twenty still use it for research of a very high type. Like so many long-established laboratories in European countries the inspiration of historical associations compensates for the lack of modern conveniences.

After the visit to the laboratory, Dr. Baker, president of the Chemical Society of London, placed a wreath at the base of the statue of Berthelot which stands in front of the Collège de France.

There next followed the dedication of a tablet erected on the house in the rue Saint Martin where Berthelot lived from 1852–1861. The house, not far away, where he was born on October 25, 1827, had been demolished in city improvements and could not receive the distinction now paid to this later abode of the great scientist.

In the afternoon the city of Paris joined in the general homage paid to Berthelot by means of a reception held in the great halls of the Hotel de Ville. The addresses there emphasized the gratitude of the city to one of its most illustrious children. Son of a Parisian, born in the shadow of the city hall and passing his entire life in Paris, made it particularly fitting that the city should honor his memory.

In the evening there was held the most solemn function of all. This was the ceremony in the grand amphitheater of the Sorbonne, at which the contributions of Berthelot to science were extolled and the engrossed addresses of appreciation brought by the delegates from the learned institutions of the world were formally handed to M. Painlevé, the president of the Berthelot committee.

One half of the main central portion of the hall was occupied by the delegates from France and the other by those from foreign countries. The larger number were in their academic robes and wore their decorations. The various brilliant colors of these, the uniforms and glistening helmets of the municipal guard, the striking green costumes of the members of the academies, the elegant dresses of the ladies in the galleries and the flowers, flags and decorations, of which the central feature was a magnificent bust of Berthelot, all combined to make a wonderful scene. At nine o'clock, to the strains of the "Marseillaise," President Doumergue, of France, and his staff entered and took seats immediately in front of the estrade.

M. Painlevé first called upon M. Charles Moureu, who is the successor of Berthelot in the chair of chemistry at the Collège de France. He described in a most beautiful manner the chemical work of Berthelot. Tributes were then paid to Berthelot by M. Georges Lecomte, director of the French Academy; M. Lacroix, perpetual secretary of the Academy of Science; M. Wéry, president of the Academy of Agriculture, and M. Glay, president of the Academy of Medicine. Attention was especially directed to Berthelot's conception of science as a collective endeavor, an endless chain of which each one forges a link.

M. Hozda, Minister of Public Instruction of Czecho-Slovakia, next spoke in the name of the foreign delegations. In concluding his brilliant address he said, "From age to age France has emitted an enormous quantity of light, the reflection of which is seen on the faces of all nations. To this it should be added that the hearts of all nations radiate towards France the warmth of their admiration and appreciation."

After the music which followed the address of M. Hozda the list of the names of delegates who were bearers of addresses from the learned institutions of the world was read. These were called according to the alphabetical order of the names of each country and unexpectedly began with Abyssinia, Afghanistan, Algeria and later others, which one did not expect to find associated with the rest of the world in honoring a great chemist. When the name of the United States was reached addresses were carried forward for the American Chemical Society by Dr. Bogert, for the Washington Academy of Sciences by Dr. Tisdale, for Princeton University by Dr. Trowbridge, for Harvard University by Dr. James H. Woods, for the Mellon Institute by Dr. Weidlein and for the Johns Hopkins University by myself. There was indeed a very long procession and many brought voluminous testimonials and unusual marks of their esteem.

When the last bearer of an address had given it into the hands of M. Painlevé, he expressed in a most beautiful manner the thanks of France and of French science to the sixty nations for their collaboration in paying honor to Berthelot. In continuing, he said, the organizers of the centenary celebration in desiring to prolong the work and hopes of the grand departed have requested the aid of all the world in a humane enterprise, the erection of a house of chemistry, open to investigators of all countries and of all origins, where all might assemble and discuss freely their doctrines and find there collected the documents pertaining to every chemical question which might engage their attention.

In response to criticisms that had no doubt been brought to his attention, he said:

Have I need to rectify certain interpretations, certain misunderstandings which this generous project has provoked? Has one not accused the initiators of pretending to impose upon the development of chemistry a sort of domination which will be exercised by the medium of the center thus created? Ah! in what brain of an infant could have been born this ambition of greatness, which would have been the laughing stock of the scientific world if ever it had been conceived? The activity of the Maison de la Chimie will be more modest and otherwise fruitful. It will permit the doctrines, the theories, the schools the most diverse and the farthest separated, to know each other and to mix together for the greatest good of all, instead of inclosing themselves in an isolation resulting from ignorance and pride.

The Maison de la Chimie will respond to the noble ideal of solidarity and will be at the same time a factor in scientific progress and the bringing together of peoples. It will recall to those who may forget, that chemistry is not a destructive force but a benefactress. Consecrated to the science which received so vigorous an impulse from him and to which he devoted his life, erected under his shield, the Maison de la Chimie will bear at its summit the name of Marcelin Berthelot. It is an honor of which he was worthy, and of a grander one he did not dream.

The next morning at 10 o'clock a commemorative ceremony was held at the Pantheon. This magnificent building is the hall of fame of France and in it are interred the ashes of Marcelin Berthelot and his wife. Two addresses were given. The first of these was by the Prime Minister of France, M. Raymond Poincaré, who is also a distinguished mathematician and a member of the institute. This address exhibited a detailed knowledge of Berthelot's works, which would have done credit to a chemist. I regret that there is not time to quote it all because it exposes even more clearly than has been done by many of the chemists who have attempted it the brilliant researches of Berthelot. The portion referring to the Maison de la Chimie is, however, particularly beautiful and is as follows:

In this Maison which we are going to erect in honor and for the benefit of chemistry, the scientists of all lands will meet and learn to know each other better. They will find there a fireside where future civilization will be elaborated. To the science which they will there serve together they will open each day a larger field of experiences. They will demand of it an increase of the productivity of the soil, the amelioration of the conditions of agriculture and enrichment of the countryside. They will command it to make nutrition more healthful and normal, they will make of it an auxiliary of medicine and pharmacy, the councilor of therapeutics and of the clinic, the enlightened collaborator of public hygiene. They will enlarge its industrial mission, open the factories to it, assign to it the task of remaking and coloring textiles, of composing essences and carburants, of augmenting the general prosperity by the multiplication of indispensable products.

Many times it has come to me, I confess, to celebrate the disinterested character of science and even to extol research where all thought of practical application is eliminated. I am aware that there is nothing more beautiful than the continued effort of a scientist who pursues the truth, without personal preoccupation and who expects nothing from science but the satisfaction of cultivating it. But a scientist has also the duty of being a citizen in his country and a man in humanity. He should not withdraw himself from the society which surrounds him. He should not turn from those who suffer and who hope. The Maison de la Chimie will have its windows on the people in the street and will not shut its doors either to misery or to suffering. It will not be the abode of silence and of solitary thought; it will be the great workshop of life, of action, and of progress.

The other address was given by M. Gallardo, the Minister of Foreign Affairs of the Argentine Republic, who responded in the name of the foreign delegations. He extolled in the highest terms Berthelot's contributions to science and his noble character.

The ceremonies were interspersed with music and the entire setting and decorations, consisting of a large background bearing the name of Berthelot and flanked by two great illuminated torches, were most impressive. On leaving the Pantheon the delegates were transported in large motor cars to Versailles, where a banquet of 1,200 covers was held in the hall of battles of the palace and presided over by M. Herriot, Minister of Public Instruction in France.

The response in the name of the foreign delegates was here given by Professor Amé Pictet, of Switzerland. He expressed the gratitude felt by all towards French chemists and their government for the invitation to participate in the magnificent undertaking in honor of Berthelot. He expressed the sense of obligation universally felt for the benefactions which have come to all from the work of Berthelot. He called attention particularly to the fact that Berthelot had never drawn any personal benefit from his numerous discoveries. He likened Berthelot to a powerful lamp, such as is erected in large cities at the intersection of streets, in such a manner that each of the different arteries and those who live and work or pass through them may be benefitted by the light given out. "This is the rôle which Marcelin Berthelot has played in the great city of chemists. By the side, however, of the precious light there is a little free space, large enough that one has dreamed of constructing there a house, of which the corner-stone will be laid to-morrow. A better location could not have been chosen. Placed thus in full light, situated at the extremity of the roads which converge toward it, this house will be seen by all. By all the arteries which lead to it will arrive the materials needed for its construction and later there will arrive those who will occupy this sanctuary of science." Professor Pictet emphasized particularly that all countries had responded to the appeal of French science and that the assemblage was truly international. This he considered a capital point and a precious guarantee of the future of our science. He concluded by saying, "I come in the name of all the foreign delegates to express to you our hopes for the success and prosperity of the future Maison de la Chimie."

M. Herriot then delivered a discourse which was frequently interrupted by the heartiest applause. He mentioned that of all the works of Berthelot, the most beautiful, without doubt, was his life. It abounded in seductive pictures. He referred to the comradeship between Berthelot and Renan, the great French writer and philosopher. His address described the work of Berthelot in the most poetical manner. It is remarkable that a person so occupied with the affairs of state as M. Herriot could have such a profound knowledge and appreciation of science. One of the most striking of his remarks was, "We thank him with respect for having proclaimed and demonstrated the candid sovereignty of the intelligence."

After the banquet the palace and gardens of Versailles were visited by the delegates and the grand fountains made to play especially for their pleasure.

In the evening the delegates were entertained at a gala performance at the opera.

The third day of the ceremonies, Wednesday, October 26, began at 10 o'clock with the laying of the corner-stone of the Maison de la Chimie.

The site which has been donated by the French government consists of a triangle bounded by the Avenue du President Wilson, the Avenue d'Jena and the Gardens of the Trocadero. The magnificent equestrian statue of George Washington is at the intersection of the two broad avenues. The beautiful Place des États Unis is a short distance away and the palatial new embassy purchased by the United States is directly across the Avenue d'Jena from the site. In the matter of the choice of a location a more delicate attention to the United States could not have been shown. The site is one of the most beautiful in the world and it is certain that the magnificent building to be erected on it will constitute a monument to chemistry such as has not hitherto been conceived.

The ceremonies were dignified and impressive. The first address was that of M. Donat Agache, president of the Société de Chimie industrielle, who spoke in the name of the French subscribers. He emphasized particularly the profoundly useful character of the undertaking. He pointed out that "In constructing the Maison de la Chimie, France sought no kind of hegemony, even scientific, but by the mutual aid and human collaboration in the domain of science wishes to realize the dream of Berthelot, that all the chemists of the world should unite their efforts and work to ameliorate the conditions of living, that their discoveries should lighten the physical efforts of work in the fields, the mines and factories, that their science would not again seek to produce toxic gases or horrible explosives; the chemistry of war, which if we do not take care might destroy civilization itself; but the pacific bodies: fertilizers, colors, fats, rubber, oils, fuels, all of which produced in abundance would make life more comfortable."

The next speaker was M. Zumeta, Minister to France from Venezuela, who spoke in the name of the foreign subscribers. Among the thoughts to which he gave expression was that "We take part in the laying of this first stone of a monument which is erected by the peoples of the earth, as an arch of alliance and as a fireside for investigators of all nations interested in the secrets of matter and desirous of unraveling them for the elevation, the glory and happiness of the human race." He also pointed out that the great thinker who is the object of this commemoration condensed in the most happy synthesis of his life the thought that "The triumph of science is to assure to men the maximum of morality and of happiness."

M. Ernst Cohen, president of the International Union of Pure and Applied Chemistry, said, "We other foreign chemists have been profoundly touched by these ceremonies. We will return to our countries persuaded that science is an endeavor essentially collective." He then translated into several languages the words of Berthelot expressing this idea, and terminated by the hope that this noble thought of a French scientist might be engraved in our souls as well as on the façade of the Maison de la Chimie.

M. Jean Gérard, secretary of the Berthelot committee, then read the list of subscriptions received from 41 countries, showing a total of 15,538,940 francs.

M. Herriot in his final remarks thanked the donors and mentioned that international conciliations founded on science are in the image of those which Berthelot wished to see realized for the happiness of men. Chemistry, he said, is an all-powerful science which even encircles the mystery of life. The advancement of chemistry is not an academic divertisement but the affirmation of the profound ties which unite peoples. He pointed out that this reunion in its simplicity marks a date in the history of humanity. It is an act of faith.

Those present then gathered around the block of stone which was to be the first of the Maison de la Chimie and M. Herriot carefully sealed in it the iron box containing the manuscripts which, as said by a writer in one of the newspapers of Paris, would show to future generations that there was an hour when men swore to love each other.

Following the laying of the corner-stone the delegates were invited to Chantilly for luncheon and a visit to the magnificent Chateau which is now the property of the Institute of France. The ceremonies were brought to a close by a reception in the evening at the Elysée Palace tendered by M. Doumergue, the President of France.

In conclusion I regret to mention that the pleasure of the American delegates in their participation in the ceremonies was marred somewhat by the action which had been taken in September by the Council of the American Chemical Society in regard to the Maison de la Chimie. Although this was evidently based upon a misunderstanding, it was rightly regarded as an unjust criticism of the project. The mistaken basis of that action was undoubtedly a confusion in the minds of some between the proposed International Office of Chemistry and the Maison de la Chimie. The two are not identical.

Although from the American point of view there may be worthy arguments against participation in an international office of chemistry, there can certainly be no just criticism of the kind of Maison de la Chimie which is to be erected in honor of Marcelin Berthelot. This, as repeatedly emphasized by its sponsors and many friends, is a beneficent enterprise having for its object the advancement of chemistry and the promotion of good-will between the nations of the world.

ATHERTON SEIDELL

HYGIENIC LABORATORY,
WASHINGTON, D. C.

SCIENTIFIC EVENTS

AN INTERNATIONAL CONVENTION ON CANCER RESEARCH

AT the quarterly meeting of the grand council of the British Empire Cancer Campaign, held on January 10, under the presidency of Sir John Bland-Sutton, it was announced that an International Convention on Cancer Research was being convened for next July in London, and that the Royal Society of Medicine had placed their headquarters at the disposal of the British Empire Cancer Campaign for the purposes of the meetings of the convention. Sir J. Bland-Sutton, past-president of the Royal College of Surgeons and vice-chairman of the campaign, has been appointed president of the convention.

The London *Times* reports that the convention committee, charged with the arrangements, informed the grand council that the work of the convention would be divided into the following sections: Pathological, diagnosis, medical treatment, surgical treatment, radiological treatment and public health and statistics. Chairmen had been appointed for some of these sections: Sir Thomas Horder, with Sir William Willcox as vice-chairman, of diagnosis section; Professor Lazarus-Barlow, pathological section; Sir Charles Gordon-Watson, surgical treatment section; Professor Sidney Russ, with Dr. Robert Knox as vice-chairman, radiological treatment section, and Lieutenant-Colonel F. E. Fremantle, public health and statistics section.

Invitations are being sent to all parts of the world to those whose names are closely associated with modern research into the cancer problem, and all the universities and medical schools of the United Kingdom will be invited to send delegates to the convention. The chairman of the convention committee, Mr. J. P. Lockhart-Mummery, reported that Sir Richard Garton, chairman of the finance committee, was making a generous donation towards the expenses of the convention and that no part of the campaign's funds would be used in connection with it.

Sir Richard Garton, in submitting the report of the finance committee, announced that a trust fund had been created by the executors of the late Mr. William Johnston, of Liverpool, to be known as "the Aileen Congreve Memorial Fund," which amounted to a sum of £18,147. Of this amount £16,000 will become a permanent trust, the interest on it being applied to cancer research work in Liverpool, through the scientific committee set up in connection with the Lancashire, Cheshire and North Wales Council of the British Empire Cancer Campaign, now in process of formation. The chairman of the finance committee also reported that an anonymous donation of £10,000 had been received by the campaign through Sir Basil Mayhew, auditor to the campaign, and that the interest on such fund would be available for the general research work fund of the campaign.

THE PROPOSED PAN-AMERICAN GEODETIC INSTITUTE

THE Mexican delegation to the Pan-American Conference has submitted a plan for the organization of a Pan-American Geodetic Institute.

In a review of the history of the science of geography the Mexican delegation introduced a report prepared by the department of agriculture and public works of the government of Mexico in which great emphasis is placed on the fact that the existing world geographical institution, known as the International Council of Investigators, does not suffice for solution of the localized problems of America.

Functions of the proposed institute, the location of which is to be later decided by the nations, are detailed as follows:

1. The coordination, distribution and propagation of geographical studies in American states.

2. It shall serve as an organization of cooperation among the geographical institutes of America, in order to facilitate the study of geographical problems.

3. It shall carry out and coordinate investigations call-

ing for the cooperation of several countries and control of scientific investigations.

4. It shall be entrusted with the publication of all reports ordered by the American states.

5. It shall participate in the study of frontiers, in order to facilitate the acceptance of the natural nature of a geographical character and serve as an intermediary between American states for a better understanding between them.

6. It shall be in charge of the formation of an archive comprising maps of the entire American continent, classified by countries as well as by libraries, containing all the geographical works published by American states.

The plan was later approved by the Pan-American conference in plenary session. It proposes an ambitious central organization in an American capital to be chosen by lot, with affiliated organizations in all new world republics contributing to its store of knowledge.

Each government would appoint one member who shall have been an active geographer in the service of his country. The number of votes appertaining to each delegate and the quotas due from each country for the maintenance of the institute would both be computed on the basis of population of each republic compared to the total population of all the nations represented.

NEW BUILDING FOR THE YALE SCHOOL OF MEDICINE

PLANS for a new building for the Yale School of Medicine, costing $1,250,000 and consisting of an addition to the Anthony N. Brady memorial laboratory, have been announced at the university. The entire cost will be met by the General Education Board.

The construction began several months ago and it is now expected that the building will be completed by the beginning of the next school year. The total capacity is 1,600,000 cubic feet, which is 20 per cent. larger than the Sterling Hall of Medicine, which was built a few years ago.

The new building, at the corner of Cedar Street and Congress Avenue, is joined with the administration building of the New Haven General Hospital by a covered archway. Together with the existing wing of the Anthony N. Brady laboratory, built in 1917, the new building has a total cubic capacity of 2,200,000 cubic feet.

The ground floor of the Brady laboratory, which will be the entrance floor for students and workers in the new building, will be given over to locker and rest rooms. The first floor of the Brady laboratory will be occupied by the school of nursing for its administrative offices and classrooms.

The ground floor of the new Cedar Street wing, as well as that of the Congress Avenue wing, will be devoted to technical procedures essential for the work in the laboratory. Among these are the surgical pathology activities and a large well-equipped photographic establishment.

The first floor of the new wing on Cedar Street, as well as on Congress Avenue, and the second floor of the Congress Avenue wing are to be occupied by pathology. The whole of the second floor of the Cedar Street wing will be occupied by the department of public health, headed by Professor C.-E. A. Winslow. On the third floor of both the old and new wings on Cedar Street and the whole of the Congress Avenue wing on this floor will be located all of the university's activities in bacteriology.

The fourth floor of the Cedar Street wing contains a dormitory suite for the use of the staff in pathology and bacteriology, so that these men may be available at all times, not only to conduct time-consuming investigations, but also for emergency service, which their particular departments are frequently called upon to render.

THE 1929 BUDGET OF THE U. S. DEPARTMENT OF AGRICULTURE

THE budget for the fiscal year 1929, transmitted by the president to congress on December 7, recommends total appropriations of $142,753,229 for the work of the U. S. Department of Agriculture for all purposes, including $77,500,000 for road construction. Items for which increases are allowed total $3,714,679, this figure being offset by reductions in other items aggregating $824,439. The budget recommends that $150,000 of the balance remaining from the $10,000,000 corn-borer control fund, provided by the act of February 23, 1927, be made available for a special research program designed to assist in meeting the situation arising out of the corn-borer infestation. Including the special fund for research in relation to the corn-borer situation, about $1,300,000 of the increases included in the budget is for research work by the Department of Agriculture.

An increase of $480,000 is recommended in the funds authorized by the Purnell Act for payments to the state experiment stations for agricultural research, or $10,000 additional for each of the 48 states, making a total of $3,840,000 to be available during 1929 for this purpose under the Hatch, Adams and Purnell Acts. An increase of $41,256 is recommended for extending the research work of the Bureau of Dairy Industry. Increases in several of the subappropriations of the Bureau of Animal Industry, aggregating $120,620, are recommended to provide for adjustments in the compensation of field veterinarians. A net increase of $495,180 is included for forestry, including $200,000 for cooperation with states in fire suppression on state and privately owned timberlands, under the terms of the Clarke-McNary reforestation act. For effectively meeting the menace to the southern fruit industry presented by the occurrence of the Mexican fruit worm in Texas, the budget includes $34,100 for researches on this insect and $100,000 for control operations. An increase of $68,220 is included for developing and extending the agricultural outlook work, including researches on the fundamental economic principles underlying production and marketing, with a view to adjusting production to probable demand for farm products. For further developing the cooperative marketing work of the department an increase of $39,560 is provided. To further carry out the provisions of the act of March 3, 1927, authorizing the collection of statistics of the grade and staple length of cotton, an increase of $335,000 is included. An additional $34,820 is recommended for strengthening the port and border inspection in connection with the plant quarantine act, and $50,000 is provided for the control of pink bollworm of cotton in Arizona and New Mexico. For enforcing the milk import act of February 15, 1927, and the caustic poison act of March 4, 1927, $50,000 and $25,000, respectively, are recommended.

The budget recommends the creation of a unit in the department to be known as the plant quarantine and control administration, and the consolidation thereunder of all the regulatory and control activities affecting plants and plant products now conducted under the Federal Horticultural Board, the Bureau of Entomology and, to a slight extent, the Bureau of Plant Industry. The Bureau of Entomology, thus relieved from regulatory and control duties, will confine its activities to insect research projects, which present many pressing problems requiring attention, the solution of which, it is believed, will be materially advanced under the new arrangement.

SCIENTIFIC NOTES AND NEWS

THE great Dutch mathematical physicist, Hendrik Antoon Lorentz, born in 1853 and appointed professor in the University of Leyden in 1878, died, according to a cablegram from Holland, on February 5. The death of Professor Lorentz was reported by cable to the newspapers as the issue of SCIENCE for last week was going to press and unfortunate errors in the notice were reproduced, the proof not having been read by the editor.

THE American Society of Swedish Engineers has presented to Dr. E. F. W. Alexanderson, consulting engineer of the General Electric Company, the John Ericsson Medal for achievement in electrical engineering. The presentation was made at a dinner in Brooklyn on February 11.

PROFESSOR WILLIAM BERRYMAN SCOTT, oldest active professor in Princeton University, celebrated his seventieth birthday on February 12. In recognition of Dr. Scott's service to education and particularly to geological research, a dinner was given to him at the Nassau Club. Dr. Henry Fairfield Osborn, a former associate of Professor Scott at Princeton, was chairman of the committee which arranged for the dinner.

PROFESSOR WHEELER P. DAVEY, vice-dean of the school of chemistry and physics at the Pennsylvania State College, has been elected a fellow of the Institute of Physics of London.

THE Cameron Prize, awarded by the University of Edinburgh to a person who, in the course of the five years immediately preceding, has made any highly important and valuable addition to practical therapeutics, has been awarded to Professor C. Levaditi, of the Pasteur Institute, Paris, for his work on the chemotherapy of syphilis and his other contributions to our knowledge of microbiology.

THE Reale Accademia dei Lincei has elected Professor Giovanni Georgi, of the University of Cagliari, a correspondent in the section of mechanics, and Professor N. E. Nörlund, of the University of Copenhagen, a foreign member in the section of mathematics.

AT the recent quarterly meeting of the council of the Royal College of Veterinary Surgeons, the diploma of honorary associate was conferred on Sir John McFadyean, late principal and dean of the Royal Veterinary College, London.

A GOLD medal has been awarded by the school of industrial art of the Pennsylvania Museum to Nicola D'Ascenzo, worker in stained glass. The presentation was made on the fiftieth anniversary of the founding of the school. This is the first year that the medal has been offered.

PREVIOUS to his recent return to the United States from China, Dr. Henry S. Houghton, dean of the State University of Iowa College of Medicine, was decorated with the Order of Chia Ho Chang for outstanding service in medical work in China. Dr. Houghton was presented at this time with a silver bowl inscribed with the names of the staff of the Peking Union Medical College, with which he had been connected for about nine years.

PROFESSOR ROSWELL C. GIBBS, professor of physics at Cornell University, has been elected president of Phi Kappa Phi, national honorary scholastic society.

Dr. Bashford Dean, professor of zoology in Columbia University and professor of fine arts in New York University, has resigned his curatorship of the department of arms and armor of the Metropolitan Museum of Art and has been elected a trustee to fill the vacancy caused by the death of Harry Payne Whitney.

Dr. George R. Minot, professor of clinical medicine at Harvard University, has been chosen to succeed the late Dr. Francis W. Peabody as director of the Thorndike Research Laboratory of the Boston City Hospital.

Edmund Heller, formerly on the staff of the Field Museum of Natural History, of Chicago, has been appointed director of the Milwaukee Zoological Park.

Carl Richter has been appointed curator of zoology at the Chamberlain Memorial Museum, Three Oaks, Michigan.

George A. Olson, agricultural director of The Gypsum Industries, Chicago, has resigned. Previous to going to Chicago, Mr. Olson was in charge of chemistry at the Washington Agricultural Experiment Station.

Arthur W. Gray has resigned as physicist of the Calco Chemical Company to become vice-president and director of research of Dielectric Products, Inc.

Dr. A. W. Miller, for the last ten years chief of the field-inspection division of the U. S. Bureau of Animal Industry, has been selected by Secretary Jardine to fill the position recently made vacant by the resignation of John T. Caine, 3rd, who was chief of the packers and stockyards division of the bureau.

Dr. Ethel Drever Simpson, of the Cornell Medical College in Ithaca, who has been granted a National Research Fellowship in Medicine, is the daughter of the late Sutherland Simpson, professor of physiology in Cornell University, and is to continue the researches she began with her father under the direction of Dr. John Tait, professor of physiology in McGill University, Montreal.

Nature states that, in consequence of the increased activity in oil-field investigation in Australia, and following the appointment of Dr. W. G. Woolnough as commonwealth geological adviser, the services of Mr. Frederick Chapman, of the British National Museum, have been lent to the commonwealth for a year as government paleontologist.

Sir James Colquhoun Irvine, principal and vice-chancellor of the University of St. Andrews, Scotland, has accepted an invitation to take a leading part in the Institute of Chemistry of the American Chemical Society which meets in Evanston, Illinois, from July 23 to August 18, 1928. Sir James was the principal European guest at the chemical sessions of the Institute of Politics at Williamstown in 1926, when the idea of an Institute of Chemistry was first conceived.

Professor Constantin Carathéodory, of the University of Munich, who is visiting the United States as the first visiting lecturer of the American Mathematical Society, has completed a series of lectures at a number of American universities. Professor Carathéodory is now in residence at Harvard University. Arrangements for additional lectures will be announced later.

Dr. Paul Alexandroff, of Moscow, and Dr. Heinze Hopf, of Berlin, have been granted International Education Board fellowships for 1927–28, for the purpose of becoming acquainted with the work of American mathematicians in the field of analysis situs. They are studying at Princeton and Harvard.

Dr. D. C. Carpenter, associate in research chemistry at the New York State Agricultural Station, has been granted a year's leave of absence for study in the laboratory of Dr. T. Svedberg, at the University of Upsala. Dr. Carpenter is traveling under the auspices of the International Education Board, and will visit laboratories in Copenhagen, Berlin, Leipzig, Halle, Stuttgart, Munich and Vienna.

Professor Thomas F. Cooke, of the department of physics of the University of Buffalo, and Mrs. Cooke sailed on January 21 from New York for the Mediterranean. They will spend the remainder of the year in study and travel in Europe.

Dr. Wm. H. Taliaferro, professor of parasitology in the University of Chicago, arrived in San Juan, Porto Rico, on January 9, where he will be the guest of the University of Porto Rico, until his return to the United States about April 1. He will give a course in protozoology at the school of tropical medicine, San Juan, and will carry on immunological studies in malaria and other parasitic diseases.

Dr. Mary W. Calkins, professor of psychology in Wellesley College, during December gave two lectures at Bedford College, University of London, on "Conceptions of Meaning" and "The Nature and Types of Value." Dr. Calkins also read a paper before the British Psychological Society on "Self Psychology."

Professor Paul Walden, of the University of Rostock, gave a lecture at Harvard University, February 8, on "The Walden Inversion."

Dr. Dayton C. Miller, professor of physics in the Case School of Applied Science, addressed the Washington Academy of Sciences, February 16, on "Photographing and Analyzing Sound Waves."

According to *Popular Astronomy*, Professor Frederick Slocum, director of the Van Vleck Observatory, has accepted an invitation this year to give the lectures which have become an annual feature for the people in Miami, Florida. The lectures are given under the auspices of the Southern Cross Observatory.

DR. BAILEY WILLIS, president of the Geological Society of America, lectured at Ohio State University on February 3 on the subject "Earthquakes." The lecture was under the joint auspices of the graduate school and the society of the Sigma Xi. In the afternoon Dr. Willis spoke before the seminar of the department of geology on "Some Aspects of the Earth's Dynamics."

DR. JOHN C. HEMMETER, professor of clinical medicine in the Johns Hopkins University, spoke at a meeting of the History of Ideas Club, Baltimore, on February 14 on "The Prerequisites to a Philosophy of History."

L. J. R. HOLST, vice-president of Brock and Weymouth, Inc., Philadelphia, will lecture before the Franklin Institute on February 23 on "Topography from the Air."

DR. HENRY LAURENS, professor of physiology in Tulane University, lectured before the chapters of Sigma Xi at the University of Missouri and the University of Kansas recently on "The Physiological Action of Radiant Energy."

PROFESSOR LAWRENCE J. HENDERSON, of the department of physiology at Harvard University, delivered an address before the Royal Canadian Institute, Toronto, January 28, on the subject "Physical Chemistry of the Blood."

THE presidential address of Dr. Eugene L. Opie, before the Pathological Society of Philadelphia, was given on January 12, on "Experimental Production of Leukemia and Related Conditions."

DR. TOBIAS DANTZIG, professor of mathematics at the University of Maryland, is conducting a course in advanced mathematics for physicists and chemists at the U. S. Bureau of Standards during the present academic year.

DR. ROSS A. GORTNER, head of the department of biochemistry at the University of Minnesota, recently delivered a series of four lectures under the auspices of the graduate school and the plant institute at the Ohio State University. The subjects follow: "Proteins in the Lyotropic Series," "Colloid Chemistry in Relation to Vital Phenomena," "Certain Electrokinetic Properties of Colloid Systems and Their Influence on Colloid Behavior," and "Chemical Problems Involved in Flour Strength."

DR. ALEŠ HRDLIČKA, of the U. S. National Museum, Washington, D. C., lectured in Chicago on January 24, before the Chicago Chapter of the Sigma Xi, on "The Glacial Age and its Relation to Man"; on January 25 and 26 at the University of Chicago, on "Origin and Evolution of Man in the Light of the Latest Knowledge" and "The Lessons of Human Evolution"; on January 27 before the downtown science group on "Human Evolution—Past, Present and Future."

THE Portland Academy of Medicine has recently been addressed by Dr. Corneille Heymans, University of Ghent, upon "Contributions to the Physiology and Pharmacology of the Vagus and Respiratory Centers," by Dr. T. Wingate Todd, Western Reserve University, concerning "The Bowels of the Profession," by Dr. Arthur L. Bloomfield, of Stanford University, upon his "Observations on the Composition of the Gastric Juice and the Mechanism of its Secretion," and by Dr. Moritz Weber, of the Hooper Foundation for Medical Research, on "Osteodystrophia Fibrosa: Clinical and Pathological Aspects, Etiology and Experimental Reproduction."

DR. E. SCHRÖDINGER, who recently visited the United States, is to lecture in London on wave mechanics at the invitation of the Royal Institution. It has been arranged provisionally that the lectures shall be given on March 5, 7, 12 and 14.

ON November 21, 1927, the memory of Reginald Somers Cocks, who for twenty years occupied the Richardson chair of botany at Tulane University, was honored when a bronze tablet was unveiled in the botany laboratory in the science building.

DR. WILLIAM C. L. EGLIN, vice-president of the Philadelphia Electric Company and president of the Franklin Institute, died on February 7, aged fifty-eight years.

DR. GEORGE ERIC SIMPSON, of the department of physiological chemistry at the University of Pennsylvania, died on December 23 at the age of thirty-nine years.

PROFESSOR JAMES LOCKE, at one time professor of chemistry at the Massachusetts Institute of Technology, died on February 11 at the age of fifty-eight years.

MRS. FLORA WAMBAUGH PATTERSON, formerly mycologist in charge of the pathological collections, U. S. Bureau of Plant Industry, died on February 5, aged eighty-one years. Mrs. Patterson retired from the bureau in 1923 after a period of twenty-seven years.

William Wallace Payne, of the observatory of the National Watch Company, Elgin, Ill., and founder of *Popular Astronomy*, died on January 29, aged ninety-one years.

Dr. Truman W. Brophy, well-known oral surgeon of Chicago, died on February 4, in his eightieth year.

Nature announces the deaths of Sir Dyce Duckworth, formerly president of the Clinical Society of London from 1891 until 1893 and foreign correspondent of the Paris Academy of Medicine, on January 20, aged eighty-seven years; Surgeon Rear-Admiral Sir Percy Bassett-Smith, a past president of the Royal Society of Tropical Medicine and Hygiene, on December 29 at the age of sixty-six years, and Professor C. Diener, professor of paleontology in the University of Vienna, well known as the editor of the "Fossilium Catalogus," on January 6, aged sixty-five years.

The Helminthological Society of Washington has passed the following minute: "The Helminthological Society learns with profound regret of the death of Professor Francesco Saverio Monticelli, a foreign corresponding member of this society since 1911. His election among the first group of twenty foreign parasitologists was a recognition of his distinguished achievements, now extending over forty years. He has joined the illustrious group of Blanchard, Ijima, Linstow, Looss, Luehe, Manson, Parona and Shipley, elected at the same time and now passed away. His work remains as the scientist's most fitting memorial and will long perpetuate his memory. This society laments his passing while at the same time it pays tribute to his worth and accomplishments. No better monument could a man have than that posterity remember his as a life well spent in the advancement of human knowledge."

The nineteenth annual meeting of the Paleontological Society held at Cleveland, Ohio, from December 29 to 31, had the largest attendance and the largest election of new members in its history, making the total number of members in this affiliated branch of the Geological Society of America now 322. Twenty-one papers were delivered and the presidential address by Professor W. A. Parks on "Some Reflections on Paleontology" was given in joint session with the Geological Society of America. The following officers were elected for the year 1928: *President,* A. F. Foerste, Dayton, Ohio; *first vice-president,* M. G. Mehl, Columbia, Missouri; *second vice-president,* E. R. Cumings, Bloomington, Indiana; *third vice-president,* G. R. Wieland, New Haven, Conn.; *secretaary,* R. S. Bassler, Washington, D. C.; *treasurer,* Carl O. Dunbar, New Haven, Conn.; *editor,* Walter Granger, New York City.

The 226th meeting of the northeastern section of the American Chemical Society was held on February 10, in Boston. The meeting was devoted to a discussion of the measurement of hydrogen ion concentration. Dr. William M. Clark, professor of physiological chemistry, the Johns Hopkins Medical School, read a paper on "Oxidation and Reduction," and gave an account of his studies of oxidation-reduction equilibrium in systems of dyes made by the potentiometer. Dr. W. A. Taylor, president of the LaMotte Chemical Products Company, Baltimore, Md., discussed the colorimetric method of "Hydrogen Ion Control in Industrial Processes," illustrating by experiments based on a color method devised by himself and his associates.

The spring meeting of the American Society of Mechanical Engineers is to be held in Pittsburgh from May 14 to 17. The technical program has been completed and the manuscripts for the papers are expected to be in hand by March 1 so that they may be printed and distributed in advance of the meeting. Special sessions will be devoted to the iron and steel industry, the glass industry and the ceramics industry. In addition, the fuels, power, materials handling, machine shop practice, railroad and hydraulics divisions will sponsor sessions. There will be another group of sessions centering around the division of applied mechanics and the special research committee of mechanical springs.

Electrical engineers in New York and London planned to hold a joint meeting on February 16 through the use of two-way radio communication across the Atlantic. Programs of the American Institute of Electrical Engineers and the British Institute of Electrical Engineers were to be exchanged. The American Institute opened its meeting in New York on February 13.

The invitation extended by the University of Virginia to the eastern section of the Seismological Society of America to hold their third annual meeting at that institution has been accepted by the executive committee on behalf of the section. The exact date has not been arranged.

The Aristogenic Association, an organization which has for its purpose the extension of human life, and the development of leaders, with a view to improving the human race in the future, met for the first time on February 2, at the Union Club, New York, as guests of William S. Moore. Dr. C. Ward Crampton was chairman of the meeting. Among those who spoke were Professor James T. Shotwell and George Haven Putnam.

THE fifteenth International Geological Congress will be held in South Africa in 1929, and the date of the inaugural meeting in Pretoria is to be during the fortnight following July 29. The special subjects provisionally proposed for discussion are: (*a*) magmatic differentiation; (*b*) pre-Pleistocene glacial periods; and (*c*) the stratigraphy, paleontology, and world distribution of the Karroo system.

GENERAL UMBERTO NOBILE, designer, constructor and pilot of the airship *Norge,* in which the expedition of Captain Raoul Amundsen, Lincoln Ellsworth and General Nobile voyaged from Spitzbergen to Alaska over the North Pole in 1926, has left for Germany and Russia to make final arrangements with the governments of those countries for the Italian airship expedition with which he proposes to make scientific studies in the polar regions this summer. It is reported that with the exception of mechanics the crew will be composed entirely of scientific men, who will take the observations which are the object of the expedition.

ACCORDING to the Tokio correspondent of *Industrial and Engineering Chemistry,* more than five thousand engineers attended the first general meeting of the Kogakkai (the Engineering Society) on November 3 at the Tokyo Imperial University. The Kogakkai is made up of twelve technical societies, including those relating to mining, iron and steel, civil engineering, ordnance and explosives, shipbuilding, architecture, chemical industry, hygienic industry, electrical engineering, telegraphy and telephony, illuminating engineering and mechanical engineering. M. Okochi, head of the Institute of Physical and Chemical Research, gave an address on the fundamental industries. He selected the precision mechanical and the dye-stuff industries as types. Addresses were given on the recent advances in twelve important industries by the representatives of the related societies. Y. Oshima, president of the Society of Chemical Industry, Japan, told of the recent progress of chemical industry in Japan. On the two following days, sectional meetings of each society were held and about one hundred and sixty papers were read, fourteen being those of the Society of Chemical Industry. Six popular lectures and one radio broadcasting were given. Factories and laboratories were open for inspection by attending members. The International Engineering Congress will be held in Tokyo in October, 1929, under the auspices of the Kogakkai. The congress proposes to discuss various engineering problems for the promotion of international cooperation in the study of the engineering science in all its branches.

ACCORDING to press reports the offer by the General Education Board of the Rockefeller Foundation of $1,250,000 to aid the University of Minnesota in establishing a medical center on condition that the city of Minneapolis build a general hospital adjacent to the university was definitely rejected on January 5, at a joint meeting of the public welfare committee of the city council and the committee of twenty-three representing the board of regents, the public welfare board, and the Hennepin County Medical Society.

THE *Journal* of the American Medical Association states that an allotment of $2,000 has been made by the U. S. Treasury Department of the public health service for the preparation of an exhibit to be used at the International Exhibition at Seville, Spain, that will be held in October, 1928. The U. S. Government is participating in this exposition, and all of the government departments and bureaus will be represented. The exhibit of the public health service that is being prepared includes the subjects of smallpox vaccination, venereal diseases, tularemia, safe water and other miscellaneous items.

IN connection with the seventy-fifth annual meeting of the American Society of Civil Engineers it was announced that Charles E. Fowler, consulting engineer of New York, had given the society a trust fund for the granting of annual awards and prizes for engineering work, the awards to be bestowed in memory of the donor's late mother.

UNIVERSITY AND EDUCATIONAL NOTES

EIGHT fellowships worth from $4,000 to $9,000 a year will be established at the New York Orthopedic Dispensary and Hospital from the income of a gift of more than $1,000,000 from the residuary estate of Mrs. John Innes Kane. Mrs. Kane's will made bequests of approximately $4,000,000, including two $500,000 gifts to Columbia University, and directed the executors to distribute the residuary estate among such groups as she might select during her own lifetime.

A GIFT of $2,500,000 for the study of Oriental art has been made by the estate of the late Charles M. Hall, of Oberlin, who acquired $45,000,000 by a process of refining aluminum, which he devised. An institution in Peking will be endowed under the direction of Harvard University and the University of Peking.

FIRE destroyed the main building of Villanova College, Philadelphia, on January 28, and seriously damaged the monastery, with a loss estimated at $2,000,000. The chemical, physical and biological laboratories were a total loss.

IT is announced that the Cleveland Clinic Foundation will receive the $400,000 estate of the late Frank Billings on the death of his widow.

ST. LUKE'S HOSPITAL and Washington University, St. Louis, are named in the will of Edward Mallinckrodt, chemical manufacturer, as preferred recipients of his estate, estimated at several millions, all of which he left to charity and education.

THE board of regents of the University of Michigan has authorized the establishment at the university of a department of graduate medicine, and has asked Dr. James D. Bruce to undertake its organization.

DR. WILER PENFIELD, assistant professor of surgery at Columbia University and neurological surgeon at the Presbyterian Hospital, has been appointed professor of neurological surgery at McGill University.

DR. JOHN C. FORBES has been appointed clinical chemist for the three hospitals of the Medical College of Virginia. Dr. William B. Porter, professor of medicine, has instituted the new clinical chemistry laboratory with Dr. Sidney S. Negus, professor of chemistry, assisting in the details involved.

DR. JOHN A. MCGEOCH, of Washington University, has been appointed acting professor of psychology for the summer session of 1928 at the University of North Dakota.

DR. A. K. MACBETH, reader in chemistry at the University of Durham, has been appointed to the Angas chair of chemistry in the University of Adelaide.

PROFESSOR JACOB, of the University of Toulouse, has been appointed professor of geology at the University of Paris.

PROFESSOR FOSSE, of Lille, has been appointed to take the place of the late Professor Simon in the department of chemistry at the National Museum of Natural History at Paris.

DISCUSSION AND CORRESPONDENCE

APPLIED GEOPHYSICS

AT the present time that subject which may be termed pure geophysics is making, in some directions, rapid progress owing to the practical applications of geophysics to underground exploration. A financial magnate exclaimed to the writer in two consecutive sentences, "It is impossible to know what is underground," and "Any one who could tell what was underground would be worth millions upon millions." I assured him that neither of these extreme views was true, and reminded him of X-rays, and of radio or wireless and of their successes in revealing the unseen. An electro-magnetic explanation left him cold and weary, for finance, like government, is often in the hands of men extraordinarily ignorant of the world in which they live. They are, however, usually experts in arithmetic and human nature!

The geophysical methods employed are divided naturally into two groups. In the northern mining regions magnetic, electrical and electromagnetic methods prevail, and these regions are often hilly, rocky, mountainous. In the southern or Gulf of Mexico region, which is often flat, the underground irregularities—such as the salt domes on the flanks or tops of which oil is often found—are sought for with seismic, gravitational, magnetic and recently with electrical methods.

For the guidance of those who are looking for further information the following references will be helpful. We are promised at an early date a translation into English of Ambronn's excellent treatise[1] on geophysics. This is to be written up to date by the author, and to include a full bibliography. Most of our readers will already have read, with pleasure and interest, the recent report[2] of Dr. Mason, president of Chicago University, which summarizes his investigations in field and laboratory during the last four years. There is also a large five-volume treatise, four parts of which have appeared, "Lehrbuch der Geophysik," by Professor B. Gutenberg (Gebrüder Borntraeger, Berlin).

The U. S. Bureau of Mines at Washington has recently issued a small bulletin, Technical Paper 420, which gives a brief and concise summary, primarily intended for mining men, of the principles and methods and apparatus available. It may be noted that in fig. 17 a battery appears to be giving an alternating current, owing to the omission from the diagram of a commutator which is, however, clearly mentioned in the text. Further criticism is not given here because the present writer and his colleague, Dr. D. A. Keys, are the authors.

As regards electrical and electromagnetic methods it may now be fairly claimed that these have stood well the preliminary tests, and that next they must face the fiery ordeal of achieving their actual purpose of discovering, in a useful manner, the conductors which are below the earth, and of discerning, as far as possible, their size, shape, depth and nature. This is a searching demand! Some ore bodies, such as zinc blende, do not conduct better than the rocks surrounding them, and thus evade detection. Underground water may conduct sufficiently well to simulate an ore body, thus deceiving an enthusiast who would not

1 "Methoden der Angewandten Geophysik," Dr. Richard Ambronn, Göttingen. (Theodor Steinkopff, Dresden and Leipzig.)

2 "Physical Exploration for Ores," Dr. Max Mason. (Physical Exploration Corp., 111 Broadway, N. Y.)

be fooled by surface water. A thin rich vein of worthless pyrites might prove an exciting discovery to a geophysicist, while the mine manager would view it with cold disdain.

The fact, however, remains beyond a doubt that good conductors can be located underground by several different electrical and electromagnetic methods, while they could not be detected by magnetic methods, and that suitable schemes may, and probably will, prove to be of great service alike to mining men and to geologists.

In games like golf and billiards, and in the more serious hazards of war by land or by sea, as much, or truly much more, depends on the man than upon the clubs, cue, weapons and ships—on the material things which he has at his disposal. For the expert and skilful man will insist on using to the utmost the very best, and on its maintenance at the very best. So too in geophysics a torsion balance, or a magnetometer, does not make a survey. These things are subsidiary to the skill and intelligence of the man who uses them, who understands their possibilities and limitations, who interprets their readings wisely. Since these things are true, the greatest country or state will always be that which develops most properly the real intelligence of its children and youth—always the sole greatest asset of any people.

To return to our main subject—geophysical prospectors sometimes claim too much, mine managers often expect too much. Disappointment leads them to join the scoffers. That is not the road to progress! There must be mutual confidence and cooperation between managers, engineers, geologists and physicists. So far none of them has proved infallible; all have to play the game of "blindman's buff" or "hoodman blind." All have to search with all the scientific aids possible. Diamond drills can not be used over the whole face of the earth. The day may come when the geologist will go before, and the geophysicists will follow after, next come the engineers with diamond drill, and behind them all the other men who, with joy and singing, will gather up most of the dollars.

A. S. EVE

McGILL UNIVERSITY

THE MULTIPLE ORIGIN OF TUMORS

PARTLY from clinical observation, partly from the intensive experimental work on neoplastic disease which has been carried on during the last quarter century, we now know of a considerable number of means by which tumors, particularly malignant tumors, may be artificially induced. These come under several distinct categories.

First, certain chemical irritants may induce them with some regularity. Coal tar applied to the skin over long periods of time, or injected into the tissues; indol; various arsenic compounds; and—a matter here of clinical observation—various aniline products—all have the effect of stimulating tissues to malignant hyperplasia, in some cases at least preceded by a period of benign overgrowth.

Second, physical irritation, best manifested by long applications of the X-ray, has the same effect. Third, embryonal tissues introduced into the adult animal may in certain circumstances develop into malignant tumor; best, perhaps, when to the effect of transplantation is added the element of chemical irritation, as by coal tar or indol. Fourth, malignant tumors may develop, as shown by Maud Slye, purely on the basis of hereditary factors. We may have malignant tumors induced by certain nematode parasites, acting in a manner as yet not fully determined. And finally, rather recently it has been shown by Blumenthal and his coworkers that in a certain proportion of human cancers *B. tumefaciens* may be isolated from the outskirts of the tumor. This, grown in pure culture and inoculated into plants and certain animals, may cause what to all appearances are tumors in them. In the case of the animal inoculations, sections show a fairly definite picture of malignant neoplastic growth, and on transfer to other animals of the same species the new growths behave like typical inoculable tumors. Of some significance in this connection is the fact that the organisms disappear in the later stages of the tumor, and in those resulting from transfer.

Instead of being in ignorance of the causative factor of neoplastic growth, we are really in a position of embarrassment at having too many possible causes, and the real problem in connection with the etiology of tumors would appear to lie in the reconciling of these to a single common factor. That there is such a common factor can not be questioned; the entire picture of neoplastic disease, both benign and malignant, is too definite to permit doubt on that score. As a matter of fact, the nature of that factor is shown in the histology of all tumors—it lies in their common possession of the property of more or less unrestricted growth—absolutely unrestricted in the case of the more malignant ones.

Viewed in this light, neoplastic proliferation must then be considered as a common type of reaction to a variety of causes—a reaction characterized by the more or less complete suppression of the usual normal balanced cellular activities with a corresponding accentuation of the single activity of cellular multiplication. In the sense of being a reaction to injury, tumor development would then be simply a special type of inflammatory phenomenon—one which is shown originally by the single cell or group of cells, as a result of which it loses its normal environmental inhibitions and becomes capable of free and unlimited growth.

If this view is right, then neoplasms, and especially malignant neoplasms, must be regarded as tissues which in response to a number of different irritants react by showing a release from the normal growth gradients which ordinarily regulate body structure. The real problem of cancer then becomes a study of these gradients, and from the therapeutic standpoint their reestablishment when once lost or the prevention of their loss. The present line of study, largely devoted to the determination of the character of these irritants, will of course always be a matter of importance, but of secondary rather than primary grade.

Some of our therapeutic measures in the control of cancer are already directed to the former end. The use of radium and the X-ray, for instance, is essentially an effort to accomplish two things which tend toward a reestablishment of lost gradient—the inhibition through destruction—at best usually partial—of the unrestricted cell division, plus the stimulation of connective tissue growth to the point where this more nearly equals the proliferation rate of the tumor cells.

It would seem no longer correct to speculate as to the "cause of cancer." We would seem to have reached the point where it is necessary to recognize that there are a number of distinct causes, related only in the sense that they produce a common effect. Neoplasms then constitute an entity in the same sense that acute inflammation is an entity—a single type of reaction brought about by a variety of causes—and like that, an inflammatory process in that it is a reaction to injury.

To prove this experimentally aside from the finding of a still greater number of causative factors will be a difficult matter. One possible means would lie in the establishment of immunity, as to *B. tumefaciens*, and the demonstration that this immunity did not protect against other causes of cancer, as for instance, coal tar.

H. E. EGGERS

UNIVERSITY OF NEBRASKA
COLLEGE OF MEDICINE

THE CUTICULA OF NEMATODES

IN an abstract published in the December, 1927, number of *The Journal of Parasitology*, on "The Cuticula of the Neamathelminthes," Justus F. Mueller states that he has found the cuticula of Gordius and Macracanthoyhynchus to be chemically homogeneous and that of Ascaris to be separated into two chemically distinct substances. All four substances are proteins of albuminoid character, none related to chitin. The three substances found in Ascaris and Gordius are fairly similar, while that of the acanthocephala is different. He states that he does not agree with me (*Camallanus americanus*, nov. spec. *Trans. Amer. Microsc. Soc.*, 1919, 38: 49–170) in calling the substance in Ascaris cornein, and states I was in error because of incorrectly translating Reichard.

Since the abstract does not call attention to the point I was attempting to make in my study, it would leave in the minds of those not familiar with the facts an incorrect idea. In the first place my error, for which I apologize, was due to my misconstruing the force of the subtitles of Reichard's paper; I thought at that time the heading "Cornein" was intended to refer to the cuticula of worms and my error was not one of translation. The whole purpose of my contribution was to show that the cuticula of nematodes was not chitin but was a protein of albuminoid nature. In this I am glad to see that Mueller agrees. Cornein is also an albuminoid. I had been taught and had read in many commonly used texts, in the article written on nematoda for the Encyclopedia Britannica by Shipley and Beddard and in articles on nematodes by such men as Ransom, Hall and Ward that the cuticula of nematodes was chitinous. Indeed some zoologists, as proof of the supposed relation of worms and arthropods, stated that both had chitinous covering. As pointed out in my paper, Leuckart was undoubtedly responsible for the misconception, although he knew that the two coverings were fundamentally different. In spite of the fact that men as far back as Lassaigne (1843) pointed out the difference in the cuticula of Ascaris and the chitin described by Odier, authors still referred to the covering of nematodes as chitinous. My study was undertaken to show conclusively the differences in the structures. I concluded that the cuticula of nematodes was composed of a protein of the albuminoid type, closely related to connective and supportive tissue and unrelated to chitin. In this I carried on further the work of Reichard and agreed with him in his work, but incorrectly stated that he called the substance cornein.

Mueller states that he has for the first time correctly analyzed this material, basing his statement on the fact that he analyzed the two parts separately, unless he means to imply that the actual analysis of all other authors was erroneous. The former statement depends on the point of view. By his own statement the two parts form the cuticula; therefore to analyze them together would certainly constitute a true analysis of the cuticula, just as, in analyzing the liver or spleen, one does not separate them into their many components. Reichard called attention to certain physical and chemical differences in two layers of Ascaris and I described four layers for Camallanus. Others have subdivided the cuticula of nematodes into different layers, and in partly dried material one is often able to strip off several layers. Mueller's statement that the cuticular layers of Ascaris are "fairly similar" leads me to hope that his analysis may be regarded as in a general way confirming my own.

It is interesting to note that Ward states in his chapter on Parasitic Worms (Ward and Whipple, "Fresh Water Biology") in discussing the cuticula of nematodes that "it has been correctly designated as cornein by Reichard." Since no reference to my incorrect statement is made in this text book it may be inferred that Ward also was misled by the subtitles.

THOMAS B. MAGATH

MAYO CLINIC,
ROCHESTER, MINNESOTA

AN UNUSUAL ATMOSPHERIC PHENOMENON

ON the morning of December 14 a rather unusual atmospheric phenomenon, the so-called circumzenithal arc, was observed at Brunswick, Me. It had the form of a bright rainbow-like arc about 90 degrees in extent with its center of curvature approximately at the zenith. The colors were much more clearly defined than in the ordinary rainbow, the red being at the outer edge of the arc and the violet at the inner. The arc extended in azimuth roughly from west to south. When the phenomenon first appeared the sun was at an altitude of some 20 degrees, and the edge of the arc at about 70 degrees. The arc remained visible for about half an hour. The weather at the time was clearing, and low lying fog clouds moving from north to south partially obscured the sun although blue sky was visible near the zenith. The surface temperature was slightly above freezing.

The phenomenon just described while rare is not unknown. It may be explained by the refraction of the sun's rays in passing through columnar snow crystals with tabular caps, the crystals acting as right prisms. A detailed explanation of the circumzenithal arc is given by Humphreys in "Physics of the Air," p. 511. The striking feature of this particular occurrence of it was its duration. As generally observed it has lasted only about five minutes, while in this instance it was distinctly visible for a full half hour.

BOYD W. BARTLETT

BOWDOIN COLLEGE

PSYCHO-ENDOCRINOLOGY

NEW words are sometimes as important events in history of science as new discoveries. For the word means the crystallization of a new concept. And the crystallization of a new concept means the attainment of one of the ideals of science: the correlation of the relationships of hitherto unrelated observations and findings. Such new concepts are valuable not only for classification of the activities of the worker in science in the past, but also for orientation towards the problems and methods of the future.

Accumulating information during the past fifty years has pointed to an importance of the endocrine glands for the problems of the science of psychology. Whether that science be looked upon as the study and control of consciousness or whether it be looked upon as the study and control of the behavior of an organism as a whole reacting to an environment makes no difference. From either viewpoint, evidence has accumulated that the endocrine glands, modifying conditions in the organism in general and in the nervous system in particular, are of the utmost significance for the data of psychology.

It is time I think an attempt was made to collect under the rubric of a single name the results of various individual investigations in the fields of psychology, biochemistry and medicine, where they will be collectively available to the research worker. I propose the word "psycho-endocrinology" as the name for that branch of science which deals with the relation of the endocrine glands to mental activities and processes, as well as to behavior, including the individual characteristics in health and disease, summarized in the term personality.

LOUIS BERMAN

QUOTATIONS

STATE ACADEMIES OF SCIENCE

THE American Association for the Advancement of Science has now in affiliation with it the academies of science of twenty-two states. As an organization this association and its affiliated organizations are not much given to talking of themselves. The report of the activities and progress of the state academies as told in an address of the president of the New Hampshire Academy and published in SCIENCE would indicate that they have a position of importance in creating an interest in scientific achievements and disseminating valuable scientific information. The name of the association might suggest an exclusive gathering of college professors and scientists. While it has in its own membership and that of the affiliated organizations men of learning and attainments in scientific research at the same time it has members who may never have spent an hour in a scientific laboratory, whose part in the organization is that of individuals of the ever-increasing number in this country who are interested in science and who find in one or more of its branches, as the report says, an avocation or a hobby distinct from their ordinary life routine.

The first of the associated organizations dates back to 1853, when the New Orleans Academy of Science, now known as the Louisiana Academy, was formed. It was not until the period from 1866 to 1870 that the number of academies had reached four. This number had increased to twenty by 1924, when the Alabama Academy was formed. The youngest of the affiliated organizations is the South Carolina Academy, which became a member of the association in October of this year. The credit of being the pioneer in this field should perhaps belong to the Maryland Academy of Science, originally formed in 1797.

Besides the associated organizations in the eastern and southern states there are a Pacific division and a southwestern division of the American Association. It is an evidence of the national interest in scientific studies that there are academies of science in all the Pacific Coast states, with which are affiliated other scientific organizations in the Rocky Mountain states, British Columbia, Alaska and the Hawaiian and Philippine Islands, and that in the southwest there is an affiliation of similar organizations covering the states of Arizona, New Mexico, Colorado, the two bordering Mexican states of Sonora and Chihuahua and the state of Texas west of the Pecos.

The number of members enrolled in the academies varies widely; the New Orleans Academy has about fifty members, while the Maryland and Indiana academies have about 800. There is apparently no hard and fast rule regarding the qualifications for members. The New Orleans society is limited to research workers, which may account for its small membership. In fourteen of the academies any one "interested in science," "interested in the progress of science" or "interested in scientific work" may become an active member. Georgia requires five years of recognized scientific work or some notable contribution to science. New Hampshire asks for proficiency "in some branch of science," North Carolina wants active interest in the promotion of science and Maryland stands out in requiring, besides an interest in science, "a desire for self-improvement and a desire to help others." Most of the state academies apparently interpret the term science to cover "most of the field of classified knowledge and orderly thinking."

The work which the academies have undertaken or accomplished varied largely with the demands which the different states have made upon the organizations. In a general way all have endeavored to arouse interest in scientific matters, publish papers primarily for non-scientific readers, present non-technical lectures, encourage scientific research among graduate students and foster higher standards of scientific work. Some of the academies have sought to make collections of scientific literature that might not otherwise be accessible to students. The New Hampshire Academy financed from its own funds the publication of Professor J. W. Goldthwait's valuable "Handbook of the Geology of New Hampshire." The Maryland Academy has its own building, which it opens to the use of the scientist. Eight of the state academies have libraries of their own; the library of Kansas contains 4,000 volumes on research, Indiana has 6,000 volumes and Wisconsin offers the student several thousand books on modern attainments besides 700 exchanges of publications from all parts of the world. The inference which the president of the New Hampshire Academy draws from his study of scientific advance in the last few years is that "the state academies have been and are very valuable, not only to the members but also to the progress of science and education in general and consequently to the public at large."—*New York Sun.*

REPORTS

RESOLUTIONS ADOPTED BY THE INTERNATIONAL GEODETIC AND GEOPHYSICAL UNION[1]

I. In view of the decision unanimously adopted, June 29, 1926, by the International Research Council at its general meeting at Brussels, according to which the contribution to be paid by each of the adhering countries is to be henceforth calculated in gold francs, the sum originally adopted as the unit of contribution, in each union, to be at the same time reduced in a proportion included between a third and a fifth of the present figure;

Considering that, for the International Geodetic and Geophysical Union, the unit of contribution has been until that time fixed at 2,600 French paper francs, which, in the beginning of 1919, were equivalent to about 1,800 gold francs:

The General Assembly unanimously proposes to replace provisionally, beginning with 1928, this amount by a round sum of 900 gold francs and invites its bureau to bring this resolution to the attention of the International Research Council and of the national committees of the various associated countries.

II. In view of the desire expressed by the American National Committee of Geodesy and Geophysics to have, in the future, the International Geodetic and Geophysical Union and the International Astronomical Union hold their meetings the same year at an interval of only a few weeks and in cities not too

[1] Resolutions adopted by the third general assembly of the International Geodetic and Geophysical Union held at Prague, Czecho-Slovakia, September 3 to 10, 1927. Translated from the French by H. D. Harridan, Department of Terrestrial Magnetism of the Carnegie Institution of Washington.

distant from each other so as to facilitate attendance at these meetings by scientific men interested in the work of both unions;

The General Assembly of the International Geodetic and Geophysical Union invites its bureau to enter into correspondence with the Bureau of the International Astronomical Union for the purpose of carrying out, if possible, the proposal in question.

III. The assembly reelects unanimously, as president of the union, M. Charles Lallemand, whose term of office, according to article 6 of the statutes, had expired.

IV. On the proposal of the Section of Geodesy:

The General Assembly recommends that the governments possessing a submarine fleet undertake, as soon as possible, gravity determinations on board submarines by the new method of Vening-Meinesz—such determinations being of the greatest interest to geodesy.

V. On the proposals of the Section of Seismology:

(1) The General Assembly recommends that seismological installations be made in the following regions:

(a) In the northern part of Spain and in the Balearic Islands to complete the réseau of Spanish stations.

(b) In New Caledonia and Tahiti to complete the réseau of the French colonies.

(2) At the request of the American Committee of Geodesy and Geophysics, the General Assembly recommends that, wherever it may be possible, observations and studies be made, in common, on the ocean deeps and on their relations with the bottom-relief, with gravity anomalies, and with depth of seismic centers.

VI. On the proposals of the Section of Meteorology:

(1) The General Assembly notes with satisfaction that the published tables of observations made in the upper atmosphere contain results from tropical stations and from stations in the Southern Hemisphere, in particular wind and temperature soundings at Hongkong and wind soundings at Colombo and Dewa in the Island of Ceylon, at seven stations in Brazil, at Pretoria in South Africa, at Melbourne in Australia, and at Apia in the South Pacific; it recommends that this work be continued and developed through international cooperation.

(2) The General Assembly further recommends that, as far as possible, copies of the minutes of the section be made available to meteorologists desirous of carrying out investigations and that a list of persons to whom these minutes should be sent be drawn up by the national committees.

VII. On the proposals of the Section of Oceanography:

(1) The General Assembly approves the creation of a permanent mixed commission organized with the cooperation of the sections of seismology and volcanology for the purpose of collecting all the documents of use for the study of the phenomenon of bores.

(2) The General Assembly approves the creation of a permanent mixed commission organized with the cooperation of the Section of Meteorology for the purpose of studying the influence of polar ice on climates, especially in the Southern Hemisphere.

VIII. On the proposals of the Section of Volcanology:

(1) The General Assembly, considering that studies of the thermal gradient of the earth are not only of interest to pure science, but also to industrial applications, recommends that the Italian government kindly intrust to its National Research Council the mission of undertaking such investigations on the volcanoes of Italy and especially on Vesuvius.

(2) In view of the importance to science which is offered by the state of the extinct volcanoes and the lavas of the Aegean Sea, the General Assembly recommends that the petrological laboratory of the University of Athens continue its systematic studies of this subject.

(3) At the request of Professor Ktenas, of the Academy of Athens, it recommends that the new volcano in the Kamenis Islands of the Santorin Archipelago, the eruption of which began August 11, 1925, keep the name of the great geologist Fouqué.

(4) In view of the international interest presented by the measurement of the speed of propagation of longitudinal and transversal waves in solid and fluid magmas near the point of fusion, it recommends that such measurements be undertaken by countries having active volcanoes in their territory and in that of their colonies.

CH. LALLEMAND,
President of the Geodetic and Geophysical Union

H. G. LYONS,
Secretary-General

SCIENTIFIC APPARATUS AND LABORATORY METHODS

INFILTRATING PIG EMBRYOS WITH PARAFFIN

AFTER much experimentation in our laboratories with various methods for infiltrating pig embryos with paraffin, we have found the method described below as the most satisfactory and one never failing to give the desired results.

When the embryos have been thoroughly dehydrated they are cleared in oil of cedar or origanum. They should remain in the clearer for one hour after sinking to the bottom of the container to insure thorough clearing. The embryos are then removed and washed in xylol for ten minutes to prepare them for subsequent treatment by removing the oil which adheres. Next, the embryos are placed in a solution of paraffin-xylol. The most satisfactory solution is prepared by dissolving at ordinary room temperature 24 grams of paraffin in 100 cc of xylol. It is well to have this solution prepared a few days in advance to prevent delay. The amount of solution used should be three or four times the bulk of the embryos. The embryos are left in this solution from two to six days depending on their size. (See Schema at end.) After removing the embryos dip them once or twice in xylol, then place them in melted paraffin and put in oven. The melting-point of the paraffin should not exceed 52 degrees Centigrade nor should the temperature of the oven. At the end of fifteen minutes the paraffin is poured off and fresh-melted paraffin put on. This procedure should be repeated at least three times. At the end of forty-five minutes it is wise to smell of the embryos to make certain that all the xylol has been removed. If the slightest trace of xylol is detected change the paraffin a fourth time. All the xylol must be removed, otherwise the imbedding paraffin will crystallize and great difficulty will be experienced in sectioning.

It is a well-known fact that heat is detrimental to all tissue, even adult tissue, not to mention its effect upon embryonic. In infiltrating tissue it is most essential to submit it to heat for the shortest time possible. Heat shrinks, hardens and distorts tissue, thereby rendering it worthless. We have found pig embryos to shrink from 1/16 to 1/4 their natural size when submitted to heat for as short a period as two hours at 52 degrees Centigrade. The tissue shrinks and hardens so rapidly that it is impossible for the paraffin to penetrate and as a consequence imperfect infiltration results, particularly in those parts of the embryo where shrinkage is the greatest. In sectioning, the parts not infiltrated crumble and fall out. This is invariably the case with the liver of the embryo. The liver is very compact, the interstices minute and the shrinkage great. By using a paraffin-xylol solution a sufficient amount of paraffin penetrates the tissues so that when the embryo is placed in the melted paraffin and put in the oven, the paraffin, which has already penetrated the embryo from the paraffin-xylol solution, melts and by capillary action rapidly draws in the fresh paraffin and forces the xylol out in less than one hour. The maximum shrinkage in pig embryos takes place after the first ninety minutes in the oven.

An objection which might be raised against the use of paraffin-xylol is that tissue left in xylol for many hours becomes brittle and brittleness is as ruinous to tissue as heat. This objection is true when xylol is used as the clearer—but when cedar oil or oil of origanum is used as the clearer the embryos may remain in paraffin-xylol for a week without becoming brittle.

Below is a Schema which shows the relative amount of time necessary for embryos of various sizes to remain in the paraffin-xylol solution in order that they may be thoroughly infiltrated after being in the oven from 45 to not more than 60 minutes.

SCHEMA

Size of Embryo	Length of Time Embryo is in Solution of Paraffin-Xylol
7 mm. to 10 mm.	48 hours
11 mm. to 15 mm.	54 hours
16 mm. to 20 mm.	65 hours
21 mm. to 24 mm.	77 hours
25 mm. to 29 mm.	88 hours
30 mm. to 34 mm.	95 hours
35 mm. to 39 mm.	104 hours
40 mm. to 45 mm.	110 hours
46 mm. to 50 mm.	119 hours

T. L. MALUMPHY

HOLY CROSS COLLEGE,
WORCESTER, MASS.

SPECIAL ARTICLES

THE ANATOMY OF THE CORIUM

IT was pointed out by Dupuytren[1] in 1836 that a round, pointed awl thrust into the human skin produced not round openings but linear slits. This property of the corium was very fully studied by K. Langer in 1861.[2] From the work of Langer it is evident that in the human there are very definite directions in which these cleavages take place and that these directions are constant for an anatomical part. Nussbaum[3] and Burkard[4] have studied these cleavage lines in the human foetus and have shown the changes that take place during development.

[1] Quoted by K. Langer.

[2] Langer, K. "Über die Spaltbarkeit der Cutis." *Sitz. berichte d. K. akad. d. Wissenschaften S.* 19 Bd. 44, 1862.

[3] Nussbaum, Ilse. "Über die Spaltungsrichtung Menschlicher Embryonen." Inaug-Diss. Berlin, 1923.

[4] Burkard, Otto. "Über die Hautspaltbarkeit Menschlicher Embryonen." *Arch. f. Anat. u. Physiol. Anat. Abt.* S. 13, 1903.

The correlation between these cleavage lines in the human and the direction of the supporting fibers in the tela subcutanea was reported by me before the American Association of Anatomists in Nashville in 1927.[5] On the basis of earlier experimental work (Batson and Zinninger[6]) which shows that tension physiologically applied produces connective tissue fibers in the direction of the pull, it was postulated that the manner of distribution of the retinacula cutis and the anatomy of the more extensive deposits of fibrous tissue, now going under the name of various fascias, together with the connective tissue fibers of the corium responsible for the cleavages (earlier studied by von Langer) were the result of the tension placed upon these structures by their own weight, and by the weight of associated structures (*i.e.*, capital hair, mammae and genitalia). Naturally both the circumferential and linear growth of the parts covered by the skin must not be overlooked as a source of tension. This growth factor is significant in studying the direction of fibers and cleavages in the developing organism. Skin muscles likewise play their part.

It has been found that the "splitability" of the corium may be studied after it has been detached from the underlying structures, and this has made possible the gathering of much additional information on the human and opened up the possibility of the study of the detached animal skin. These split-like cleavages have been produced in the corium of the following: the dog-fish, the frog, the dog, the pig and the chimpanzee. It would appear that if the arrangement of the corium fibers were due to functional factors, that the direction of these cleavages should have a direct relationship to the posture of the animal. Further with the knowledge of the habits of any form it should be possible to foretell the directions of the principal cleavages in that comparative form. Parenthetically it might be added that these cleavages in addition to being present in the skin and mucous membranes may be demonstrated in the serous membranes of the body, vessels, periosteum, dura mater, cartilages and in the capsules of parenchymatous organs as well. The specific study of these ramifications of the problem are now in progress in this laboratory. The lines of cleavage in the corium of the dog which have been more specifically studied do not resemble the human but correspond to what would be supposed, considering the postural habit of the animal. This correlation strengthens the previously proposed idea that the anatomy of the corium was developed through function. The wide variety of animals showing cleavage lines in the corium can leave no doubt that this property of the corium is common to all animals.

Leather, that is tanned corium, shows this same property. The cleavages may be at any angle to the furrows of the animal's skin or to the "grain" of the leather. Laboratory tests show that leather is stronger in the direction parallel to the direction of the cleavage. This idea negates a common one that an area of leather has its strength uniform in all directions. This finding applied to the manufacture of leather articles should secure the maximum of strength and a greater uniformity of product.

Studies of the microscopic anatomy of the corium responsible for these splits occurring in a longitudinal direction are now under way. Three possibilities suggest themselves as explanations; 1. More connective tissue fibers in the direction of tension. 2. Greater length of connective tissue fibers in the direction of tension and 3. Difference in character of the fibers running in the direction of tension. The first notion, *i.e.*, that the cleavages are due to a greater number of connective tissue fibers lying in that direction seems the most probable.

O. V. BATSON
UNIVERSITY OF CINCINNATI

[5] Batson, O. V. "The Anatomy of the Tela subcutanea." *Anatomical Record*, p. 4, Vol. 35. 1927.

[6] Batson, O. V., and Zinninger, M. M. "The Experimental Production of Annular Ligaments, as an Example of the Influence of Function upon the Differentiation of Connective Tissue." *Bull. Johns Hopkins Hospital*, p. 124, Vol. XXXVIII, 1926.

THE DIALYSIS OF PITUITARY EXTRACTS

THE physiologically active material contained in extracts of the posterior lobe of the pituitary gland diffuses readily through the ordinary dialyzing membranes.[1] The rate of dialysis suggests that the active principle (or principles) is considerably more complex than adrenalin, but somewhat simpler than insulin or the parathyroid hormone.

In a preliminary report[2] I compared the relative rate of dialysis of pituitrin with that of a compound of known molecular weight (adrenalin) and suggested 600 as the approximate molecular magnitude of the pituitary principle. This early work appeared deficient because it relied only upon the pressor assay method but the actual laboratory results have now been verified and are presented below.

In the meantime an excellent report[3] on the dialysis of pituitary extracts has been published by Smith and

[1] *J. Physiol. 25*, 87 (1899); *Am. J. Pharm. 86*, 291 (1914); *Biochem. J. 9*, 307 (1915); *Brit. Med. J.* I, 502 (1900); *Proc. Roy. Soc.* (London), B. *77*, 571 (1906); *J. Pharmacol. 15*, 81 (1920).

[2] Washington Meeting, Amer. Chem. Soc., April, 1924.

[3] *J. Pharmacol. 24*, 391 (1924).

McClosky, of the U. S. Hygienic Laboratory, and these workers have applied both the pressor and oxytocic assay methods. They found that the two types of activity show identical diffusion rates, thus suggesting the presence of a single hormone.

Smith and McClosky have so adequately described the technique of preparing and using collodion membranes for this dialysis work that further experimental details are unnecessary. The only variation in the present work consisted in the use of a volume of solvent outside of the membrane exactly equal to that contained inside and provision for uniform stirring. The collodion membrane, cast in the form of a large-size test-tube, was suspended in a glass cylinder of such diameter that the liquid level inside was exactly equal to that outside.

In the following experiments the active material was dissolved in one fourth per cent. aqueous acetic acid and dialyzed against acetic acid of the same strength. At the beginning of the experiment the outside concentration was, of course, 0 per cent. The maximum per cent. attainable in the outside chamber (50 per cent.), obviously was not attained since the experiment was not run to final equilibrium. Samples were withdrawn for assay usually at 15, 30, 60 and 120 minute intervals and subjected to assay. The experiments were conducted at a temperature of 25° C.

EXPERIMENT I

Dialysis of Pituitrin

Assay by Pressor Method

Time	Concentration Inside	Concentration Outside
0 min.	100 per cent.	0 per cent.
30 "	......	12 per cent.
60 "	......	20 per cent.
180 "	50–60 per cent.	40 per cent.

In all cases the potency of the pituitary solutions is expressed in terms of the U. S. P. standard. The potency of adrenalin is expressed in terms of 1:1000 adrenalin solution.

In order to rule out the error due to variations in permeability of the collodion membranes, the adrenalin was dialyzed through the same membrane used in the first experiment and with the following results:

EXPERIMENT II

Adrenalin Dialysis

Time	Concentration Inside	Concentration Outside
0 min.	100 per cent.	0 per cent.
15 "	......	13 per cent.
30 "	......	22 per cent.
60 "	60 per cent.	35 per cent.

From the above figures it is apparent that adrenalin dialyzes twice as rapidly as does the pressor principle of pituitary extracts and if the laws of diffusion of gases are applicable to the dialysis of these complex substances through collodion membranes one might conclude provisionally that the pituitary principle is approximately four times as complex, from the standpoint of molecular magnitude, as is adrenalin.

In the following two experiments a different membrane was used and also a more concentrated pituitary solution. The samples were assayed by both the pressor and oxytocic methods.

EXPERIMENT III

Dialysis of the Pressor Activity

Time	Concentration Inside	Concentration Outside
0 min.	400 per cent.	0 per cent.
15 "	......	40 per cent.
30 "	......	80 per cent.
60 "	......	100 per cent.
120 "	250 per cent.	160 per cent.

EXPERIMENT IV

Dialysis of the Oxytocic Activity

Time	Concentration Inside	Concentration Outside
0 min.	480 per cent.	0 per cent.
15 "	......	70 per cent.
30 "	......	100 per cent.
60 "		120 per cent.
120 "	325 per cent.	175 per cent.

Although the above results are not as uniform as the physical chemist might expect in a quantitative experiment, it must be remembered that the results are all based upon physiological assays on animals and are actually within the accuracy of the experimental methods. For this physiological work I am greatly indebted to Messrs. L. W. Rowe and E. P. Bugbee.

The results of experiments III and IV verify the claim that the pressor and oxytocic activities dialyze at practically uniform rates and agree with the assumption that a single active principle is responsible for both types of physiological activity. Indirect evidence of this kind, however, is not final and we must still consider the possibility of two active principles that are similar not merely in chemical constitution but also in molecular magnitude.

The molecular weight of the active principle (or principles) may be considered as approximately 600 until direct measurements are available.

OLIVER KAMM

CHEMICAL RESEARCH DEPARTMENT,
PARKE, DAVIS AND CO.,
DETROIT, MICHIGAN

SCIENCE

VOL. LXVII FEBRUARY 24, 1928 No. 1730

CONTENTS

Atomic Hydrogen as an Aid to Industrial Research: DR. IRVING LANGMUIR 201

James Campbell Todd: DR. E. R. MUGRAGE 208

Scientific Events:
The Arnold Arboretum; Gifts to the College of Physicians and Surgeons by the Alumni Association; Radio Broadcasts of Twice-daily Weather Reports; Dinner in Honor of Dr. L. O. Howard 209

Scientific Notes and News 211

University and Educational Notes 215

Discussion and Correspondence:
The Ichnology of Texas: DR. ROY L. MOODIE. *Fossil Tracks on the North Rim of the Grand Canyon:* CHARLES W. GILMORE and GLENN E. STURDEVANT. *Corm Rot of Gladiolus:* LUCIA MCCULLOCH and DR. CHARLES THOM. *Undulant Fever in America:* DR. FREDERICK W. SHAW. *Are Salt Solutions Musical?* DR. O. C. MAGISTAD. *Banana Stowaways:* DR. L. A. ADAMS. *On the Velocity of Sound:* DR. P. I. WOLD and GEORGE R. STIBITZ..... 215

Scientific Books:
Stanford's The Story of Nathaniel Bowditch: DR. H. T. STETSON 218

Reports:
American School of Prehistoric Research: PROFESSOR GEORGE GRANT MACCURDY 219

Special Articles:
On the Distribution of Critical Temperature for Spawning and for Ciliary Activity in Bivalve Molluscs: PROFESSOR THURLOW C. NELSON. *Starvation Ketosis of the Primates:* DR. THEODORE E. FRIEDEMANN 220

Science News x

SCIENCE: A Weekly Journal devoted to the Advancement of Science, edited by J. McKeen Cattell and published every Friday by

THE SCIENCE PRESS

New York City: Grand Central Terminal.

Lancaster, Pa. Garrison, N. Y.

Annual Subscription, $6.00. Single Copies, 15 Cts.

SCIENCE is the official organ of the American Association for the Advancement of Science. Information regarding membership in the Association may be secured from the office of the permanent secretary, in the Smithsonian Institution Building, Washington, D. C.

Entered as second-class matter July 18, 1923, at the Post Office at Lancaster, Pa., under the Act of March 8, 1879.

ATOMIC HYDROGEN AS AN AID TO INDUSTRIAL RESEARCH[1]

IT is difficult for me to express adequately my appreciation of the honor you have conferred upon me through the award of this beautiful medal. I wish to thank you and also my other friends, Hendrick and Whitney, for the kind, although exaggerated words spoken about me.

I am sure that those of you who know Whitney well, or in fact all you who have just heard him speak, will understand that this medal should properly be regarded as a second award to him. The work for which this medal is now given was made possible by the remarkable inspiration and guidance which only Whitney can give.

Although I am a chemist by training, my work during recent years has been mostly in physics. The chemical work I have done has been largely purely scientific, started, at least, without thoughts of practical applications. Thus when I received notice of the action of the Perkin Medal Committee, while I was in Italy a few months ago, it puzzled me that I should have been chosen, especially when I considered that the medal is given for work in applied chemistry. I can assure you that I am not guilty of any deep laid plan to secure this medal. It came to me as a complete surprise—a surprise similar to those I have experienced when I have first realized that some purely scientific observations that I had made were capable of industrial applications.

On returning home from abroad, and finding that the committee had made the award mainly for my work on atomic hydrogen and its applications to welding, I was at first inclined to choose as a subject for this address an account of other work on atomic hydrogen completed more than ten years ago, but which I have neglected to publish except in such abbreviated form that it is nearly useless. Since one of the objects of the Perkin Medal is to stimulate research, it would seem particularly fitting that this award should thus lead directly to the publication of the results of investigations which would otherwise largely be lost.

[1] Address given on the occasion of the presentation of the Perkin medal, on January 13, at a joint meeting of the Society of Chemical Industry, Société de Chimie Industrielle, American Chemical Society and American Electrochemical Society.

The work that I refer to was experimental work extending over more than a year, on the kinetics of the interaction between hydrogen and oxygen at low pressures in contact with a hot tungsten filament. At temperatures below 1600°K the oxygen oxidizes the tungsten exactly as though no hydrogen were present, but an adsorbed monatomic film of oxygen poisons the filament so that the hydrogen can not be dissociated into atoms as it would be if there were no such film. The hydrogen is incapable of interacting directly with this adsorbed oxygen. However, after the oxygen has been used up by this reaction and gradual evaporation of the film has exposed a few tungsten atoms on the surface of the filament, the hydrogen suddenly and almost instantly removes the rest of the oxygen in the film and thus permits the dissociation of the remaining hydrogen. Without the hydrogen, the oxygen film would not evaporate appreciably. These experiments prove that the interaction between oxygen and hydrogen on tungsten takes place only between adjacent adsorbed atoms—a kind of flank attack. A direct action between the oxygen and hydrogen does not occur. These phenomena are clearly identical in character with the electro-chemical phenomena of passivity—a subject which has not been well understood.

This work, however, as you see, is pure physical chemistry, and so is not really a suitable subject for this address. I trust, however, that this award will stimulate research equally well by leading me to publish this material in its proper place at an early date.

Somewhat over a year ago I read a paper before the American Chemical Society on atomic hydrogen and its application to the welding of metals. Although the industrial applications of this process are developing rapidly, I have not been particularly closely associated with this recent progress, and therefore do not feel qualified to address you on this subject.

I believe the primary object of the Perkin Medal is to do honor to the memory of Sir William Perkin, that pioneer who devoted himself to pure scientific research after having led in the industrial applications of research for fifteen years. This object is best attained by encouraging the kind of research that he valued so highly. The medal should thus be regarded not as a reward for accomplishment nor as a prize to stimulate competition in research, but rather as a means of directing attention to the value of research and to the methods of research that are most productive. Having this in mind, I am going to tell you, although somewhat reluctantly, the history of some of my own work, in so far as it illustrates a method of industrial research that has proved valuable.

Two Types of Industrial Research

The leaders of industries are frequently conscious of the need of improvement in their processes and even of the need of new discoveries or inventions which will extend their activities.

It is thus logical and often extremely profitable to organize research laboratories to solve specific problems. Efficiency requires that the director shall assign to each worker a carefully planned program. Experiments which do not logically fit in with this program are to be discouraged.

This type of industrial research, which should often be called engineering rather than research, has frequently been very successful in solving specific problems, but usually along lines already foreseen.

This method, however, has serious limitations. Directors are rare who can foresee the solutions sufficiently well to plan out a good campaign of attack in advance. Then, too, the best type of research man does not like to be told too definitely what must be the objects of his experiments. To him scientific curiosity is usually a greater incentive than the hope of commercially useful results. Fortunately, however, with proper encouragement, this curiosity itself is a guide that may lead to fundamental discoveries, and thus may solve the specific problems in still better ways than could have been reached by a direct attack; or may lead to valuable by-products in the form of new lines of activity for the industrial organization.

Of course no industrial laboratory should neglect the possibilities of the first and older method of organized industrial research. I wish, however, to dwell this evening upon the merits of the second method in which pure science or scientific curiosity is the guide.

The History of the Gas-Filled Lamp

I first entered the research laboratory of the General Electric Company in the summer of 1909, expecting in the fall to return to Stevens Institute, where I had been teaching chemistry. Instead of assigning me to any definite work, Dr. Whitney suggested that I spend several days in the various rooms of the laboratory, becoming familiar with the work that was being done by the different men. He asked me to let him know what I found of most interest as a problem for the summer vacation.

A large part of the laboratory staff was busily engaged in the development of drawn tungsten wire made by the then new Coolidge process. A serious difficulty was being experienced in overcoming the "off-setting" of the filaments, a kind of brittleness which appeared only when the lamps were run on alternating current. Out of a large number of samples of wire, three had accidentally been produced which gave lamps that ran as well with alternating as with direct current, but it was not known just what had made these wires so good. It seemed to me that there was one factor that had not been considered, that is, that the off-setting might possibly be due to impurities in the wire in the form of gases. I therefore suggested to Dr. Whitney that I should like to heat various samples of wire in high vacuum and measure the quantities of gas obtained in each case.

In looking through the laboratory I had been particularly impressed with the remarkably good methods that were used for exhausting lamps. These methods were, I thought, far better than those known to scientific research workers. My desire to become more familiar with these methods was undoubtedly one of the factors that led me to select for my first research an investigation of the gas content of wires.

After starting the measurements that I had planned, I found that the filaments gave off surprisingly large quantities of gas. Within a couple of weeks I realized that something was entirely wrong with my apparatus, because from a small filament in a couple of days I obtained a quantity of gas which had, at atmospheric pressure, a volume 7,000 times that of the filament from which it appeared to have come; and even then there was no indication that this gas evolution was going to stop. It is true that in the literature, for example in J. J. Thomson's book on the "Conduction of Electricity Through Gases," one found many statements that metals in vacuum give off gases almost indefinitely, and that it is impossible to free metals from gas by heating. Still I thought that 7,000 times its own volume of gas was an entirely unreasonable amount to obtain from a filament. I spent most of the summer in trying to find where this gas came from, and never did investigate the different samples of wire to see how much gas they contained. How much more logical it would have been if I had dropped the work as soon as I found that I should not be able to get useful information on the "off-setting" problem by the method that I had adopted.

What I really learned during that summer was that glass surfaces which had not been heated a long time in vacuum slowly give off water vapor, and this reacts with a tungsten filament to produce hydrogen, and also that vaseline on a ground glass joint in the vacuum system gives off hydrocarbon vapor, which produces hydrogen and carbon monoxide.

To me, however, that summer's work was so interesting that I dreaded to return to the comparative monotony of teaching, and gladly accepted Dr. Whitney's offer to continue at work in the laboratory. No definite program of work was laid down. I was given first one assistant and then others to continue experiments on the sources of gas within vacuum apparatus, and a study of the effects produced by the introduction of various gases into tungsten filament lamps. The truth is that I was merely curious about the mysterious phenomena that occur in these lamps. Dr. Whitney had previously found that gases have a habit of disappearing in lamps, and no one knew where they went to, so I wanted to introduce each different kind of gas that I could lay my hands on into a lamp with a tungsten filament and find out definitely what happened to that gas.

It was the universal opinion among the lamp engineers with whom I came in contact that if only a much better vacuum could be produced in a lamp, a better lamp would result. Dr. Whitney particularly believed that every effort should be made to improve the vacuum, for all laboratory experience seemed to indicate that this was the hopeful line of attack on the problem of a better lamp. I felt, however, that I really didn't know how to produce a better vacuum, and instead, proposed to study the bad effects of gases by putting gases in the lamp. I hoped that in this way I would become so familiar with these effects of gas that I could extrapolate to zero gas pressure, and thus predict, without really trying it, how good the lamp would be if we could produce a perfect vacuum.

I should like to add here parenthetically, that this principle of research is one which I have found extremely useful on many occasions. When it is suspected that some useful result is to be obtained by avoiding certain undesired factors, but it is found that these factors are very difficult to avoid, then it is a good plan to increase deliberately each of these factors in turn so as to exaggerate their bad effects, and thus become so familiar with them that one can determine whether it is really worth while avoiding them. For example, if you have in lamps a vacuum as good as you know how to produce, but suspect that the lamps would be better if you had a vacuum say 100 times as good, it may be the best policy, instead of attempting to devise methods of improving the vacuum, to spoil the vacuum deliberately in known ways, and you may then find either that no improvement in vacuum is needed, or may find just how much better the vacuum needs to be.

During these first few years, while I was thus having such a good time satisfying my curiosity, and publishing various scientific papers on chemical reactions at low pressures, I frequently wondered whether it was quite fair that I should spend my whole time in an industrial organization on such purely scientific work, for I confess I didn't see what applications could be made of it, nor did I even have any applications in mind. Several times I talked the matter over with Dr. Whitney, saying that I could not tell where this work was going to lead us. He replied, however, that it was not necessary, as far as he was concerned, that it should lead anywhere. He would like to see me continue working along any fundamental lines that would give us more information in regard to the phenomena taking place in incandescent lamps, and that I should feel perfectly free to go ahead on any such lines that seemed of interest to me. For nearly three years I worked in this way with several assistants before any real application was made of any of the work that I had done.

In adopting this broad-minded attitude Dr. Whitney, I believe, showed himself to be a real pioneer in the new type of modern industrial research.

For my study of the effect of gases, I had to devise new types of vacuum apparatus. I needed particularly to be able to analyze the small quantities of gas that existed in the tungsten lamp. With some of this special apparatus I was able to make a practically complete quantitative analysis of an amount of gas which would occupy about 1 cubic millimeter at atmospheric pressure. In this sample of gas we could determine the percentages of oxygen, hydrogen, nitrogen, carbon dioxide, carbon monoxide and the inert gases.

In regard to the fate of the different gases which I introduced into the lamp bulb, I found that no two gases acted alike. Oxygen attacked the filament and formed tungstic oxide WO_3. That seemed simple enough, but I found that the kinetics of the reaction presented many features of considerable scientific interest.

In studying the effect of hydrogen, very peculiar phenomena were observed. A limited amount of hydrogen disappeared and became adsorbed on the bulb where it remained in a chemically active form, capable of reacting with oxygen at room temperature, even long after the tungsten filament had been allowed to cool. This suggested hydrogen atoms and seemed to confirm some conclusions that I had already drawn from observations on the heat losses from tungsten filaments in hydrogen at atmospheric pressure. In making squirted tungsten filaments and sometimes in cleaning the drawn wire, filaments were heated in this manner in hydrogen. Because of the fact that tungsten filaments melt at a temperature more than 1500° higher than platinum, it had seemed to me that tungsten furnishes a tool of particular value for the scientific study of phenomena in gases at high temperatures. From my work on lamps I knew approximately the relation between the resistance of tungsten wire and its temperature, and could thus use a tungsten wire as a kind of resistance thermometer. By connecting a voltmeter and an ammeter to the tungsten filament which was being heated in hydrogen, I could determine the temperature from the resistance and also find the heat loss from the filament in watts. I wanted to see if anything abnormal happened when the temperature was raised to the extremes which were only possible with tungsten.

The results greatly interested me, for they showed that the energy loss through the gas, which increased in proportion to the square of the temperature up to about 1800°K, increased at a much higher rate above that, until at the highest temperatures the energy varied in proportion to about the fifth power of the temperature. This result could be explained if the hydrogen at high temperatures were dissociated into atoms. The diffusion of the hydrogen atoms from the filament, and their recombination at a distance from it would cause an enormous increase in heat conduction. After publishing these preliminary results, I was naturally much interested in getting any other information I could in regard to the properties of these hydrogen atoms. A very large number of experiments, extending over several years, were thus made in this study of atomic hydrogen. Nearly all of these experiments would have seemed quite useless, or even foolish, to a man who was making a direct and logical attack on the problem of improving tungsten lamps.

When nitrogen at low pressure was introduced into a bulb containing a tungsten filament at extremely high temperatures, such as 2800°K, the nitrogen disappeared at a rate which was independent of its pressure—in other words, here was a case of a reaction of zeroth order. This suggested that the reaction velocity was limited by the rate at which the tungsten evaporated from the filament. To check this hypothesis the rate of loss of weight of filaments at various temperatures was measured in good vacuum. This rate varied with the temperature in accordance with known thermodynamic laws, and since the rate per unit area was independent of the size of the filament, it was concluded that the loss of weight was really due to evaporation and not to chemical action of residual gases or to electric currents that passed from the filament to the surrounding space.

A comparison of the rate of disappearance of nitrogen with the loss of weight in the filament showed that one molecule of nitrogen disappeared for every atom of tungsten that evaporated. A brown compound WN_2 was formed which deposited on the bulb and decomposed when water vapor was introduced, forming ammonia gas.

From time to time the question kept arising—how good would a lamp be if it had a perfect vacuum; and now, from studies of the character I have described,

I began to have an answer. Hydrogen, oxygen, nitrogen, carbon monoxide, and in fact every gas that I introduced, with the exception of water vapor, did not produce blackening of the lamp bulb. The serious blackening that occurred with only small amounts of water vapor depended upon a cyclic reaction in which atomic hydrogen played an essential part. The water vapor molecules coming in contact with the hot filament produce a volatile oxide of tungsten, and the hydrogen is liberated in atomic form. The volatile oxide deposits on the bulb where it is reduced to the metallic state by the atomic hydrogen, while the water vapor produced returns to the filament, and causes the action to be repeated indefinitely. Thus a minute quantity of water vapor may cause a relatively enormous amount of tungsten to be carried to the bulb.

The question then arose whether the traces of water vapor, which might still exist in a well-exhausted lamp, were responsible for the blackening which limited the life or the efficiency of many of these lamps. We made some tests in which well-made lamps were kept completely immersed in liquid air during their life so that there could be no possibility of water vapor coming in contact with the filament. The rate of blackening, however, was exactly the same as if no liquid air had been used.

Having thus proved that the blackening of a well-made lamp was solely due to evaporation, I could conclude with certainty that the life of the lamp would not be appreciably improved even if we could produce a perfect vacuum.

Early in 1911 Mr. William Stanley, one of the pioneers in the electrical industry, felt that our company should do more fundamental work in connection with heating devices. Since I had become interested in the theory of heat losses from filaments in gases, I was glad to do work along these lines, so that I undertook to direct a small laboratory at Pittsfield, Mass., at which I spent about two days a week. Besides studying the heat losses from plane surfaces at various temperatures, I measured the heat losses from wires of various sizes in air at different temperatures, working at first with platinum wires, and was able to develop a theory of the heat losses which enabled me to calculate the loss from a wire of any size at any temperature in any gas, assuming however that the gas did not dissociate at high temperatures.

Having now a definite theoretical basis on which to calculate the normal loss by convection, I was able to prove that the abnormal rate of heat loss which I had previously observed with tungsten filaments at high temperatures in hydrogen was due to actual dissociation, and in fact I was thus able to calculate the heat of dissociation and the degree of dissociation at different temperatures.

However, to make sure of these conclusions, I wished to make measurements of the heat losses in gases which could not possibly dissociate, and therefore undertook experiments with heated tungsten wires in mercury vapor at atmospheric pressure. A little later I made experiments with nitrogen to see if this gas dissociated at high temperatures but found that it did not do so. In both of these gases the filaments could be maintained at temperatures close to the melting point for a far longer time than they could be if heated in vacuum at the same temperature. Thus the rate of evaporation was greatly decreased by the gas, many of the evaporating tungsten atoms being brought back to the filament after striking the gas molecules.

By this time I was familiar with all the harmful effects which gas can produce in contact with filaments and knew under what conditions these bad effects could be avoided. Particularly I realized the importance of avoiding even almost infinitesimal traces of water vapor. Thus, when I found a marked effect of mercury vapor and nitrogen in reducing the rate of evaporation, it occurred to me that it might be possible to operate a tungsten filament in gas at atmospheric pressure and obtain a long useful life. Of course, it would be necessary to raise the temperature far above that at which the filament could be operated in vacuum so as to compensate for the serious loss in efficiency due to convection, by the improved efficiency resulting from the rise in filament temperature. Whether or not the increased rate of evaporation, due to this increase in temperature, would more than offset the decrease in the rate due to the gas, was a matter that could only be tested by experiment.

In connection with the studies of the heat losses from filaments of various diameters at incandescent temperatures, I had found that the heat loss increased only very slowly with the diameter, so that the loss per unit area from a small filament was enormously greater than from a large filament. Calculations showed that it was hopeless to get practical lamps with filaments in nitrogen, if these filaments were of very small diameter. For example, a filament one mil in diameter, which corresponds to an ordinary 25 watt lamp, if run in nitrogen at atmospheric pressure would consume 4.8 watts per candle at a temperature of 2,400° K, which would give 1 watt per candle with a filament in vacuum. This great loss in efficiency is due to the cooling effect of gas. To bring back the efficiency of the gas-filled lamp to that of the vacuum lamp, it would be necessary to raise the temperature from 2,400 to 3,000° K, which would have caused a 2,000-fold increase in the rate of evaporation, and such an increase could certainly not be compensated for by the effect of the gas in retarding the evaporation.

With filaments of much larger diameter, however, the effect of the gas in decreasing the efficiency was not nearly so marked. We therefore constructed lamps having filaments of large diameter in the form of a single loop and filled these lamps with nitrogen at atmospheric pressure. We ran these lamps with a filament temperature so high that in spite of the gas the efficiency corresponded to about 0.8 watt per candle, instead of the usual 1 watt per candle at which we tested our vacuum lamps. We were disappointed to find that these lamps blackened much more rapidly than vacuum lamps of similar efficiency, so that the total useful life of the lamp was short.

This result, which is what most lamp engineers would have expected, seemed to indicate that the necessary rise in temperature to offset the heat losses by the gas increased the evaporation by more than the amount of the reduction in evaporation due to the gas. If I had not previously become so familiar with the behavior of various gases, this discouraging result might easily have stopped further experimenting in this direction. However, I noticed that the bulb had *blackened* during the short life of the lamp whereas from my knowledge of the interaction of tungsten and nitrogen I had expected a deposit of a clear brown color. I felt that the black deposit, therefore, could mean only one thing—water vapor, notwithstanding the fact that to avoid this water vapor we had taken precautions which were greater, I believe, than had ever been used before for the preparation of moisture-free gases and glass surfaces. We were thus led to take still greater precautions and use still larger bulbs so that the glass surfaces could not become overheated by the convection currents in the gas that rose from the filament. We were then soon able to make lamps having a life of over 1,000 hours with an efficiency about 30–40 per cent. better than could have been obtained with filaments in vacuum.

As I look back upon these experiments I feel that we were very fortunate at that time in not having had at our disposal a supply of argon gas. From theoretical reasons I had concluded that argon should be better than nitrogen, and if I had had argon I should therefore probably have tried it first. If these lamps had blackened, because of traces of water vapor, I would naturally have attributed this to the increase in evaporation caused by the high temperature, and would have had no reason for suspecting that water vapor was the cause of the trouble, for, of course, in argon a brown deposit would not be expected in any case.

The lamps that we were able to make in this way, with an improved efficiency, were limited to those which took a current of 5 amperes or more, so that the method was not applicable for 110-volt lamps with less than 500 watts. Some time later, however, it occurred to me that the benefits derived from the large diameter of the filament could be obtained with one of smaller diameter by coiling the filament in the form of a helix, bringing the turns of the helix very close together. In this way, and by the use of improved tungsten filaments that do not sag so readily at high temperatures, and by using argon instead of nitrogen, it has gradually been possible to construct gas-filled lamps which are better than vacuum lamps down to wattages of about 40 or 50 watts. These smaller lamps, although not much better in efficiency than the vacuum lamp, have the advantage of giving a much whiter light. In the case of the larger lamps, the use of the gas filling together with the special construction of the lamp more than doubles the efficiency.

The invention of the gas-filled lamp is thus nearly a direct result of experiments made for the purpose of studying atomic hydrogen. I had no other object in view when I first heated tungsten filaments in gases at atmospheric pressure.

Even at the time that I made these experiments at higher pressures, they would have seemed to me useless if my *prime object* had been to improve the tungsten lamp.

I hope I have made clear to you the important rôle that properly encouraged scientific curiosity can have in industrial research. This illustration that I have given is not at all exceptional. I could have given any one of several others equally well.

Many industrial laboratories have followed Dr. Whitney's lead in devoting a fairly large fraction of their activities to these rather purely scientific researches. Certain men at least are not expected to be responsible for practical applications, but are freely allowed to make fundamental scientific investigations. The type of man who does this work best can usually be attracted only to those industrial laboratories that have adopted this policy.

However, I do not believe that this second method of research is growing in popularity solely because it is found to be profitable. I feel rather that most of our leaders in industrial research are eager to adopt this method, in so far as economic factors may permit, because they realize the debt that modern industry owes to the pure science of the past and because the modern conceptions of service and the growing *esprit de corps* of American industry help make them glad of any opportunity to contribute to scientific knowledge. I know personally that such motives as these have guided Dr. Whitney in the leadership he has taken.

I believe in the near future there will be a much increased demand for men with scientific training who are capable of doing more independent thinking.

Better Education Needed

Our schools and universities devote so much effort to imparting information to students that they almost neglect the far more important function of teaching the student how to get for himself what knowledge of any subject he may need. Even in grammar school, children are crammed with more information on arbitrarily selected subjects than even the average well educated adult can retain.

Of course students should be taught the fundamental principles of mathematics and of various sciences, as well as of other subjects, but much of the knowledge of data upon which these principles depend and other necessary information should be obtained by the efforts of the student through experimentation and individual reading.

As I look back on my own school and college days, it seems to me that the things of most value were learned spontaneously through interest aroused by a good teacher, while the required work was usually comparatively uninteresting. The university student should have leisure for some independent work and opportunities for continuing his interest in hobbies of various kinds which he should have had long before he entered college. I realize that it is difficult so to arouse the student's interest that he will spend the added leisure in these ways rather than in spending still more on the bleachers cheering the football team in their practice games. But a well planned effort is worthwhile.

The importance of arousing even a young boy's interest in independent work can hardly be overemphasized. My real interest in science was derived from my brother Arthur, who encouraged me to have a workshop at the age of 9, and later a laboratory when I was only 12.

I can illustrate my father's influence in stimulating independence by the following incident. When I was 12 I climbed one or two Swiss mountains of moderate height with my older brother Arthur. Soon after Arthur had to go to Heidelberg to arrange for his studies, thus leaving me with my mother and younger brother at a hotel in the Rhone Valley. I had become so enthusiastic over mountain climbing that I wished to climb everything in sight, but the dangers of Alpine climbing were such that my mother did not dare let me go alone. When my father arrived for a week-end visit from Paris, he consented to allow me to climb alone any mountain I liked if I would promise to do it in accord with the following three rules: (1) I must stay on a distinct trail; (2) I must use the same trail going and returning; (3) I must make certain of returning at 6 o'clock by allowing as much time for descending as for ascending. Before these rules went into effect, however, I had to prove that I could and would make such sketches, maps and notes of the trails used for the ascent that I could always return by the same route. I thus climbed several mountains about 7,000 feet high, often requiring several days of repeated effort before I could discover a route that led to the top. Perhaps it is this experience which makes me even to-day always wish to find my own way rather than be told the way.

Until I was fourteen I always hated school and did poorly at it. At a small boarding school in the suburbs of Paris, however, being an American and having a friend who was influential with the head of the school, I was freed from much of the absurdly rigorous discipline to which the French boys were subjected. Thus, I could spend time alone in the school laboratory and was encouraged by one of the teachers to learn to use logarithms and solve problems in trigonometry, subjects not required by the curriculum.

I have been fortunate in having many wonderful teachers. Three of them have been recipients of this Perkin Medal. Whittaker and Chandler were my teachers at Columbia and Whitney during the last eighteen years. Professor R. S. Woodward, at Columbia, in connection with his courses in mechanics, was extremely stimulating and encouraged me to choose and solve my own problems for class work instead of those required in the regular course.

I should like to see spontaneous work of this kind take a much more prominent part in our educational system—at least for students who have more than average ability.

The Value of Hobbies

Very great benefit may be derived from hobbies. Probably each person should have several of them. Just recently I met a small boy, only six years old, who had an overpowering, wide-eyed enthusiasm for collecting insects. He weighed each one of them within a milligram, and then, after desiccating them thoroughly over calcium chloride, weighed them again. Many elaborate notes and even correspondence resulted. I am afraid our universities, with their dormitories and other standardizations, tend to discourage such wholesome individual activities.

Of course, after talking of hobbies, I can not resist the temptation to tell you something of my own. Perhaps my most deeply rooted hobby is to understand the mechanism of simple and familiar natural phenomena. I will give only two illustrations, but these, I hope, will make you see how easy it is to find around us simple phenomena that are not well understood.

Every chemist knows that after he stirs a liquid in a beaker having a precipitate in the bottom, the precipitate collects near the center. Probably few of you know why this is so. It is not due to the slower velocity of rotation near the center, nor to the slower motion with respect to the glass. This is proved by the fact that if you put the beaker, with the precipitate in suspension in the liquid, upon a rotating table, the precipitate will collect in a ring as far from the center as possible, although the relative angular motion of the beaker and its contents are the same as before. A little study proves that the phenomena are due to unbalanced centrifugal forces. For example, when the liquid is stirred, so as to set it in rotation, centrifugal force produces a greater hydrostatic pressure near the walls of the beaker. But the liquid very close to the bottom surface of the beaker, because of friction, can not rotate so fast, and therefore the centrifugal force is not so great and does not counteract the radial hydrostatic pressure difference existing in the upper layers. The liquid in contact with the glass bottom is thus forced inwards and carries the precipitate with it.

The phenomena connected with the formation and the disappearance of ice in a large lake, such as Lake George, have interested me for years. One clear night at the end of December, when the water of a large bay was at a uniform temperature of not over 0.2° C. and the air temperature was −22° C., ice which formed slowly at some places on the shore, melted in a couple of minutes when pushed out a few meters from the shore. There was no wind in the bay, but a slight breeze over the central part of the lake caused a very slow circulation of water in the bay with a velocity of perhaps 1 or 2 cm. per second.

In contrast with this consider the phenomena observed one clear afternoon of the following April. The body of the lake was still covered with ice which was about 20 cm. thick, but close to the shore there were places where the ice had melted back for a distance of 5 meters or more. Although the air temperature was +3° C. and the water 10 cm. below the surface was at +2.5°, ice crystals about 50 cm. long formed in these pools in less than half an hour. After considerable analysis I believe I can explain this apparent paradox by the stability in the stratification of the water in April caused by the denser underlying warm water which had been heated by the sun. With this stability which prevented vertical convection the surface water could freeze because of the radiation into the clear sky. But in December the water temperature was so uniform that the differences of density were not sufficient to prevent vertical circulation, and thus the surface could not cool to the freezing point.

It appears then that a pool of water at +1° C., exposed to cold air with a slight wind can be made to freeze more rapidly if the water is heated from the bottom. Sometime I want to try this as an experiment.

All hobbies, however, stimulate individual action, and many develop wholesome curiosity. The child should acquire them early, and our educational system should foster them.

Irving Langmuir

Research Laboratories,
General Electric Company,
Schenectady

JAMES CAMPBELL TODD

James Campbell Todd died at his home in Boulder, Colorado, the evening of January 6, 1928, following a long illness.

Born in Shreve, Ohio, March 17, 1874, he graduated from Wooster College in 1897, with a degree of bachelor of philosophy. He continued his studies in the University of Pennsylvania School of Medicine, from which he received the degree of M.D., in 1900.

While in Wooster College he held the position of assistant in biology during 1895–96. From 1900–01 he was resident physician in the Allegheny General Hospital, Pittsburgh. About this time his health failed, and he moved to Colorado, where he located in Denver.

He soon became identified in the field of medical education, first as assistant of pathology in the Denver and Gross College of Medicine during 1904–05, then as lecturer from 1905–08, later as associate professor from 1908–10, and assumed the professorship of the department in 1910.

On January 1, 1911, the University of Colorado School of Medicine absorbed the Denver and Gross College of Medicine, the two faculties were merged, and Dr. Todd became professor of pathology in the Boulder Division. He also acted as the secretary of this division until 1916. Since 1923 he has been premedical adviser in the university.

As the study of pathology broadened he felt that he was losing the contact in the fields of hematology and parasitology he desired. So in 1916 he became professor and the head of the department of clinical pathology which had just been created at his request. These positions he held at the time of his death.

During these years ill health became an increasing handicap, but in the face of these difficulties he showed a determination and persistency of purpose that won the admiration of both students and faculty. And his enthusiasm for his work was transmitted to all who had the pleasure to work with him. He was ever willing to aid, and considered the rôle of a teacher as his highest ambition.

Early in his teaching career he found that little or nothing had been compiled in clinical laboratory methods of value to the general practitioner. The collecting and testing of such laboratory procedures became his life work. He kept the viewpoint of the average medical man before him, and simplicity of technic as well as the accuracy of results claimed his closest attention.

His book "Clinical Diagnosis by Laboratory Methods" first appeared in 1908, and in the different editions he placed all his writings, with the exception of a few early articles. This book has become established over the world as an authority in its field, and it has with few exceptions enjoyed as widespread a distribution as any medical book published in English. He was sole author of the first five editions. The sixth edition, which came out in September, 1927, was written in collaboration with Dr. Arthur Hawley Sanford of the Mayo Clinic. His determination and perseverance may be realized by the fact that the work on all editions of his book was done while bedfast or in a rocking-chair.

In recognition of his ability in his field Dr. Todd was the recipient of many honors. Modest to the point of bashfulness, he would seldom speak of his own work except in a reticent manner. But his opinions on diagnostic methods always demanded respect, for they were given only after due consideration, and then in a decisive manner.

He became a fellow of the American College of Physicians in 1922, was a member of Sigma Xi, and was given honorary membership in Phi Beta Kappa by his Alma Mater in recognition of his ability and learning. He was a fellow of the American Association for the Advancement of Science, a fellow of the American Medical Association, of the American Society of Clinical Pathologists, and an honorary member of the Colorado Society of Clinical Pathologists.

Four years ago he was compelled to give up active teaching, but kept in close touch with the affairs of his department, the university and the world. He read much, not only in his particular field, but on general subjects. He will be missed in particular by his old students, and by faculty members of the university, who enjoyed his ability as a conversationalist, who admired him for his accomplishments, respected his ability and scholarship, and whose memory will be cherished as that of a man whom all could well emulate.

E. R. MUGRAGE

DENVER, COLORADO

SCIENTIFIC EVENTS

THE ARNOLD ARBORETUM

CONTRACTS for a new and larger greenhouse and nursery for the Arnold Arboretum, according to the *Harvard Alumni Bulletin,* have been signed, and work will proceed at once. The land opposite the Jamaica Plain entrance, outside the arboretum, at the corner of Center and Prince Streets, on which the greenhouse now stands, has been sold. The new site is on the South Street side of the arboretum, on the rising ground of the Bussey Institution, adjacent to the Bussey greenhouse range.

A new feature of the greenhouse will be a laboratory fully equipped for research in plant pathology and genetics. The greenhouse will be about fifty feet long, and will have, also, a workroom for potting, and pits for the growth of woody plants. The nursery, a few feet away, will cover about three acres of land.

Professor Oakes Ames, supervisor of the Arboretum and of the Harvard Botanical Museum, and chairman of the council of botanical collections of the university, made the following statement in regard to the plans for the arboretum:

> We want to make the arboretum a world center not only of systematic dendrology, but of dendrology as a whole. The proximity of the new greenhouse to the Bussey Institution will make possible a closer cooperation than has been possible heretofore. The Arnold Arboretum is the only one in the United States which is connected with a university and can draw upon the specialists in its faculty for scientific help.
>
> Already we have in view for these courses two men in the first rank in their fields, although no definite arrangements have been made to secure their services. If we succeed in getting the right man for the course in plant pathology this work will begin about July 1. Dr. East, at the Bussey Institution, will supervise the work on genetics. We shall also add to the staff another systematic botanist whose field will cover the woody plants of tropical America.
>
> The assembling of rare species and varieties of plants will be continued, of course, so that the arboretum may remain in the forefront of gardens of its type. It is expected that Dr. Joseph F. Rock, who has returned to China and is conducting explorations for the National Geographical Society, will again serve the arboretum, and will classify many of the plants which he sent us from Kansu and Tibet. This spring, Professor J. G. Jack and Alfred Rehder, of the arboretum staff, will collect new plants at the Harvard Botanical and Zoological Station at Soledad, Cuba.

The arboretum is looking eagerly toward Spanish Honduras, at present, as very little is known of its plant life because it is a difficult country for the white man to explore. It is hoped to send an expedition there in the near future, as anything found there would be exceedingly valuable from a botanical point of view.

In cooperation with the University of California an expedition will be sent this year to New Guinea. It is also proposed to send a French botanist to explore the Island of Madagascar, where there is a very interesting flora, very few specimens of which have been brought to the United States.

J. E. Palmer, of the arboretum staff, will probably go to the southern part of Texas, near the Mexican border, to add to his findings from the botanically little-known Davis Mountains.

The arboretum, although under the supervision of Harvard University, has always had to raise its own budget. During Professor Sargent's lifetime he was able through his own efforts to secure sufficient funds to meet current expenses. Since his death, the Charles Sprague Sargent Memorial Committee has been trying to raise a million dollar endowment fund to carry on the work as he outlined it. About $765,000 has been contributed to date and $235,000 is needed. Contributions, of whatever size, should be sent to the Treasurer of Harvard University, to Henry S. Hunnewell, the Cedars, Wellesley, Mass., or to William C. Endicott, 71 Ames Building, Boston.

GIFTS TO THE COLLEGE OF PHYSICIANS AND SURGEONS BY THE ALUMNI ASSOCIATION[1]

To serve as a nucleus for a fund to establish an alumni professorship of pathology in memory of Francis Delafield, P. & S., instructor in pathology and the practice of medicine at the College of Physicians and Surgeons from 1876 until his retirement in 1901, members of the Association of Alumni of the College of Physicians and Surgeons have voted to turn over to Columbia University $127,822.70 belonging to various funds of the association.

This action took place at the annual meeting of the association on January 30 at the Faculty Club. Dr. Benjamin P. Watson, professor of gynecology and obstetrics, delivered a short address comparing medical education and practices in this country with those in England.

The money for the Francis Delafield professorship is to be held in trust until by its income and subsequent gifts it reaches $200,000, the amount necessary to endow a professorship. The sum represents the principal and unexpended income of four funds—the Alumni Fellowship Fund, the Alumni Publication Fund, the Cartwright Prize Fund and the Alumni Prize Fund. In the case of the prize funds, it has been impossible for several years to award the prizes under the conditions of the original gifts because of provisions of recent postal laws which specify that if a prize is offered, a prize must be given, whether contributions merit the giving of a prize or not.

The members also voted to turn over to the university $17,601.13, representing principal and unexpended income of the Cartwright lectureship fund, to be held in trust by the university, the income to pay for lectures on medical subjects at the medical school by prominent persons nominated from time to time by the school faculty.

Dr. Francis Huber, '77 P. & S., announced that $3,000 of the Huber Building Fund was being expended in furnishing an alumni room at the new medical center. Some money will be left in the fund to meet repairs and items of additional furnishing later on.

The executive committee of the association promised the sum of $1,000, $836 of which has been raised, to renovate portraits belonging to the school before they are moved up to the new medical center.

Before transferring the Cartwright lecture fund to the university, the sum of $1,500 was set aside to pay the expenses of bringing an internationally prominent medical man to deliver an address at the opening of the medical center.

[1] From the *Columbia Alumni News.*

RADIO BROADCASTS OF TWICE-DAILY WEATHER REPORTS

FOR several months past the U. S. Weather Bureau, with the cooperation of the Navy Department, has broadcast the morning weather reports from more than 200 stations in the United States and Canada. Beginning on February 1, the complete reports, both morning and evening, will be broadcast at 8:15 A. M. and 8:15 P. M. Eastern Standard time, in cooperation with the Office of Communications of the Navy Department by distant control connection with the Naval radio station (NAA) at Arlington, Va.

The reports are expressed in the regular Weather Bureau Code which may be translated at sight after a very short study of the key to the system. These broadcasts give the widest possible distribution of the twice-daily weather reports from all parts of the country for the use of both the army and the navy, commercial and government aviation fields, business organizations and individuals who may have need of the information at an earlier hour than has been possible heretofore to release and distribute it.

Two other broadcasts are made at 11 A. M. and 11 P. M. for the benefit of European weather services. The weather reports in these broadcasts are expressed in the International Numeral Code. Information relative to that code may be obtained on application to the Weather Bureau at Washington, D. C.—A. J. H.

DINNER IN HONOR OF DR. L. O. HOWARD

THE dinner held by the entomologists at the time of the annual meetings of the scientific societies affiliated with the American Association for the Advancement of Science, at Nashville, Tenn., during the Christmas holidays was observed as a testimonial to Dr. L. O. Howard, who recently retired as chief of the Bureau of Entomology, of the United States Department of Agriculture. Dr. H. A. Morgan, president of the University of Tennessee, who for many years was one of the leaders in entomology in the south, presided on this occasion and prominent entomologists throughout the United States and Canada paid tribute to the achievements of Dr. Howard which covered a period of nearly 50 years, during which time he has guided the entomological activities of the department, and has built up and stimulated a high degree of cooperation and good-will among the leading entomologists of the world.

Over 240 entomologists attended this dinner, representing all sections of the United States and Canada, as well as foreign countries, to express their respect and appreciation of Dr. Howard and his achievements.

A warm tribute was paid to Dr. Howard by Dr. C. L. Marlatt, the new chief of the bureau, who has been his associate for nearly forty years, in which he pointed out that Dr. Howard would continue his active research work with the bureau.

SCIENTIFIC NOTES AND NEWS

THE Geological Society of Stockholm has elected the following to corresponding membership: Professor Reginald Daly, Cambridge, Mass.; Professor Charles Schuchert, New Haven; Dr. E. O. Ulrich, Washington; Dr. F. A. Bather, London, and Professor P. Niggli, Zurich.

DR. L. H. BAILEY, of Ithaca, has been awarded the Veitch memorial gold medal by the Royal Horticultural Society of England "for scientific work on behalf of horticulture."

DR. HENRY FAIRFIELD OSBORN, president of the American Museum of Natural History, has been made a "corresponding academic" of the Italian Institute of Human Paleontology.

DR. TREAT B. JOHNSON, professor of organic chemistry at Yale University, has been appointed Sterling professor of chemistry in the university.

EDWARD BAUSCH, president of the Bausch and Lomb Optical Company, has been elected an honorary member of the American Microscopical Society "in recognition of more than fifty years of active interest in microscopy."

THE American Institute of Mining and Metallurgical Engineers has made the first award of the Hunt prize for the best paper on ferrous metallurgy by a member not more than 40 years of age to Charles H. Herty, Jr., of the United States Bureau of Mines, and the Johnson award for "the encouragement of research in ferrous metallurgy" to P. H. Royster, of the same bureau.

SIR GOWLAND HOPKINS, professor of biochemistry in the University of Cambridge, was recently presented with the Society of Apothecaries medal at a dinner.

ACCORDING to the *Bulletin* of the American Mathematical Society, the Lobachefsky prize of the Physico-Mathematical Society of Kazan has been awarded to Professor Hermann Weyl, of the Zurich Technical School, for his work as a whole and in particular for his contributions to the problems of space from the point of view of the theory of groups and for his researches on the representation of continuous groups. Earlier awards of this prize were to Lie in 1897, Killing in 1900 and Hilbert in 1903.

DR. RICHARD WETTSTEIN, vice-president of the Vienna Academy of Sciences and professor of systematic botany in the University of Vienna, has been elected an honorary member of the Russian Academy of Sciences.

PROFESSOR MANILOWSKI, who was recently appointed to the chair of anthropology in the University of London, was the chief guest at a luncheon given at the Lyceum Club on January 28 by the Polish Circle.

DR. VICTOR GOLDSCHMIDT, professor of mineralogy at the University of Heidelberg, celebrated his seventy-fifth birthday on February 10.

SIR JAMES WALKER will retire from the chair of chemistry at the University of Edinburgh at the end of the current academical year.

DR. J. PAUL GOODE, first professor of geography at the University of Chicago, will become professor-emeritus at the close of the present academic year. Professor Goode has been connected with the university since 1901.

THE seventieth birthday of Dean William Kuhns Hill, head of the department of chemistry of Carthage College, was recognized by a celebration consisting of a banquet, the presentation of a handsome chest for letters and a fireside chair presented by friends. The board of trustees have granted Dean Hill a sabbatical recess of one semester.

Drs. William J. Mayo and Alexis Carrel were guests of honor at a dinner at the Maryland Club on January 16, previous to their addressing the Johns Hopkins University School of Medicine on "The Splenomegalias" and the activities of tissue cells, respectively.

Dr. John Sundwall, professor of hygiene, public health and physical education at the University of Michigan, was elected president of the Michigan Public Health Association at its seventh annual meeting in Lansing on January 13.

Dr. Arthur P. Kelley, assistant professor of botany at Rutgers University, has joined the staff of the Allegheny Forest Experiment Station, as associate ecologist, with headquarters at the University of Pennsylvania.

Emanuel Fritz, associate professor of forestry at the University of California, has been appointed to the field staff of the West Coast Lumber Bureau, as technical authority.

Dr. T. Dwight Sloan, formerly professor of clinical medicine at the University of Nanking in China, has been appointed to succeed Colonel Louis G. Trimble as superintendent of the New York Post-Graduate Medical School and Hospital.

Alfred M. Bailey has been appointed director of the Museum of the Chicago Academy of Sciences. Mr. Bailey has been curator of birds and mammals in the Louisiana State Museum and in the Colorado Museum of Natural History.

Dr. E. Kidson, of the Central Weather Bureau, Melbourne, Australia, has been appointed to take charge of the Meteorological Bureau of New Zealand.

On invitation of Governor H. M. Towner, of Porto Rico, President Livingston Farrand, of Cornell University, accompanied by the dean of the New York State College of Agriculture, Albert R. Mann, and Dr. Lewis Knudson, professor of plant physiology, will sail for San Juan on March 1 to make a survey of agricultural conditions on the island, with particular reference to the problems of tropical agriculture and the opportunity for intensive scientific research in that field. President Farrand and Dean Mann while on the island will represent Cornell University at the twenty-fifth anniversary celebration of the University of Porto Rico.

Neil M. Judd, curator of American archeology, United States National Museum, returned to Washington on December 6, after six months' field work for the National Geographic Society at Pueblo Bonito, a prehistoric Indian village in northwestern New Mexico. The past summer marked the seventh and concluding season of the society's explorations at this most remarkable of all the pre-Hispanic pueblos of the southwest. Mr. Judd is now engaged upon preparation of his final reports to be published by the society.

Dr. George D. Birkhoff, professor of mathematics at Harvard University, is en route to Japan where he is to conduct some research work in pursuance of the mathematical principles of art.

Dr. Reuben L. Kahn, immunologist of the bureau of laboratories, Michigan Department of Health, has been invited by the health committee of the League of Nations to attend a serologic conference extending from May until July at Copenhagen, Denmark.

The Lane medical lectures, which are to be given at Stanford University by Dr. F. d'Herelle, directeur du Service Bacteriologique du Conseil Sanitaire, Maritime et Quarantinaire of Alexandria, Egypt, and discoverer of the bacteriophage phenomenon, have been tentatively fixed for the week commencing October 22, 1928. The subjects of the lectures will be as follows: "Bacteriophagy," "Bacterial Mutations," "The Nature of the Bacteriophage," "Infectious Diseases" and "The Phenomenon of Recovery." In addition Dr. d'Herelle will give a general lecture at Stanford University on "Logic in Biological Researches."

Dr. George Barger, professor of chemistry in its relations to medicine at the University of Edinburgh, whose appointment as non-resident lecturer in chemistry at Cornell University for the second term of the present university year was recently announced, will give lectures on the following subjects: The chemistry of hormones, the chemistry of vitamins, synthetic drugs, chemotherapy, the theory of the action of certain substances as depending on residual valency, illustrated by the analogy of the blue of adsorption compounds of iodine, the action of micro-organisms on carbohydrates and proteins, chemistry of sugars, proteins and purine derivatives and alkaloids.

Under the auspices of the H. K. Cushing laboratory of experimental medicine at Western Reserve University, Dr. Hugo Fricke, of Copenhagen, will give a series of fifteen lectures in biophysics at the medical school.

Dr. Sigmund Fraenkel, professor of medical chemistry at the University of Vienna, addressed the University of Wisconsin Medical Society on January 12 on "Chemistry of the Vitamins."

Dr. Bird T. Baldwin, director of the Iowa Child Welfare Research Station, will address a series of meetings in the United States and Canada during the last part of February on the subject of child development.

DR. W. F. G. SWANN, director of the Bartol research foundation of the Franklin Institute, lectured on "Recent Theories of the Atom" before the American Philosophical Society on February 3.

DR. HARRISON E. HOWE, editor of *Industrial and Engineering Chemistry,* has returned from Florida, where he was invited to speak before a number of open forums on the subject of "The New Competition."

THE centenary of the birth of Professor Eugène Koeberlé, the inventor of haemostatic forceps, has recently been celebrated at Strasbourg.

DR. CLIFFORD H. FARR, associate professor of botany in Washington University, St. Louis, died suddenly of pneumonia on February 10, aged thirty-nine years.

DR. KARL KONRAD KOESSLER, associate professor of medicine at the Rush Medical School and member of the Sprague Memorial Institute, died on February 14 at the age of forty-seven years.

DR. G. REESE SATTERLEE, specialist in gastro-intestinal diseases of the Fordham Hospital, New York, died on February 9 at the age of fifty-four years.

WADE TOOLE, professor of animal husbandry at the Ontario Agricultural College, died on January 12.

RICHARD KEARTON, well-known British naturalist, died on February 9 at the age of sixty-five years.

PROFESSOR R. W. GENESE, professor of mathematics in the University College of Wales, Aberystwyth, died on January 21, aged seventy-nine years.

GERMAN exchanges announce the death of the following scientific men: Dr. Valentin Haecker, professor of zoology and comparative anatomy at Halle; Dr. Antonin Prandtl, professor of psychology at Würzburg; Dr. Ludwig Milch, professor of mineralogy at Breslau; Dr. Richard Pribram, professor of physical chemistry at Vienna; Dr. Eilhard Wiedemann, professor of physics at Erlangen; Professor Hans Leo, formerly director of the Bonn Pharmacological Institute, and Dr. Joseph Thomayer, professor of neurology at Prague.

APPOINTMENTS to Ramsay fellowships in chemical science for this session have been made for the present session as follows, the institution selected by the fellow for his research being given: *British Fellowships:* Dr. R. F. Hunter, Imperial College of Science and Technology, London; Mr. A. M. Taylor, University of Cambridge; *Glasgow fellowship:* Mr. James D. Fulton, University of Manchester; *Canadian fellowship:* Dr. W. H. Barnes, Royal Institution, London; *Danish fellowship:* Miss Augusta M. Unmack, University of Oxford; *French fellowship:* M. Robert le Guyon, University College, London; *Italian fellowship:* Dr. Gastone Guzzoni, Royal School of Mines, London; *Japanese fellowship:* Dr. Yohei Yamaguchi, University College, London; *Spanish fellowship:* Senor Fernando Calvet, University of Oxford; *Swedish fellowship:* Mr. H. Liander, University College, London. The total value of the annual amount of the fellowships that is awarded is approximately £4,000, of which about £3,000 is provided by grants from dominion and foreign sources.

A SERIES of illustrated lectures on important developments and discoveries in various fields of engineering will be given by members of the staff of the Harvard Engineering School during the second half-year. These lectures will be open to the public, and will be given in 110 Pierce Hall on Thursday afternoons, at 4:30 o'clock, as follows: February 23.—"The Telephone and how it Works." Professor A. E. Kennelly, professor of electrical engineering. March 1.—"The Rusting of Iron and its Prevention." Professor Albert Sauveur, Gordon McKay professor of metallurgy and metallography. March 8.—"Steam Locomotives." Professor H. N. Davis, professor of mechanical engineering. March 15.—"The Purification of Municipal Water Supplies, with special reference to Cambridge." Professor M. C. Whipple, assistant professor of sanitary chemistry and sanitary inspector. March 22.—"Gasoline." Professor J. B. Conant, professor of chemistry. March 29.—"Electric and Gas Welding—One of the Most Useful Tools in Modern Industry." Professor C. A. Adams, Abbott and James Lawrence professor of engineering.

THE next International Mathematical Congress will be held at Bologna from September 3 to 10. *Nature* notes that, since the war, previous congresses have been held at Strasbourg in 1920 and Toronto in 1924, but the Bologna meeting will be the first since the war that will be strictly international in character, its two predecessors having been restricted as to membership to subjects of allied or neutral nations. The Italian prime minister takes great interest in the congress and has accepted the office of honorary president. Arrangements are actively proceeding for the various sections of pure mathematics and applications of mathematics to economics and to scientific and technical problems. In addition, excursions are being proposed for visiting the art treasures of Florence and Ravenna and some of the principal hydro-electric plants of Italy. Professor Pasquale Sfameni, rector of the University of Bologna, is organizing president, Professor S. Pincherle is president of the executive committee and the general secretary is Professor Ettore Bortolotti, Via Zamboni 33, Bologna.

The ninetieth meeting of the German Society of Naturalists and Physicians will be held at Hamburg from September 16 to 28. Special emphasis will be given in the general meetings and in the sections to the relationships of German science and medicine to maritime studies and to overseas countries.

According to *Nature,* the twentieth annual general meeting of the Institute of Metals will be held in London on March 7 and 8, under the presidency of Dr. W. Rosenhain, superintendent of the department of metallurgy and metallurgical chemistry in the National Physical Laboratory. The papers to be read and discussed include contributions from metallurgists in Germany, Japan and the United States, as well as Great Britain. The autumn meeting will be held at Liverpool from September 4 to 7.

The twenty-second Dutch Congress of Natural Science and Medicine will be held at Rotterdam from April 2 to 4, 1929, under the presidency of Professor P. E. Verkade, of Rotterdam.

The committee on scientific research of the American Medical Association invites applications for grants in aid of research on problems bearing on clinical medicine. Inquiries may be addressed to the committee at 535 North Dearborn Street, Chicago, Ill.

The council of New York University has accepted a $3,000 annual fellowship from Sherman M. Fairchild, president of the Fairchild Aviation Company, for research in air-cooled aircraft engines by a graduate of the Guggenheim School of Aviation.

The new $1,000,000 Chandler laboratories of Columbia University were formally opened on February 16, when members of the society of the Sigma Xi inspected them. The laboratories were built with an anonymous gift of $1,000,000 made to the university in honor of the late Professor Charles F. Chandler, who was head of the university's department of chemistry.

Max Epstein, who established the Max Epstein clinic in the University of Chicago, has given the university $100,000 to be subscribed to the building fund of the Chicago Lying-in Hospital. Mr. Epstein's contribution is to be used to establish in the Lying-in Hospital building, to be erected on the medical quadrangles, an out-patient department which shall be operated as part of the Max Epstein Clinic.

Work will start in the spring on an addition to the University of Minnesota Hospital to cost $890,000.

According to press reports, Albert Fuchs, Chicago millionaire, whose wife, Fanny Richter Fuchs, pianist, recently died of cancer, has announced an offer of all his wealth for cancer research. He is said to have sold his eastern holdings recently for $2,000,000.

Vanderbilt University announces the gift of $50,000 from Mr. Bernard Flexner, of New York City, for the establishment of a lectureship for the purpose of perpetuating the association of his brother, Mr. Abraham Flexner, in the recent reorganization of the school of medicine. The income from this donation will make it possible to bring leading scientific men to Vanderbilt to lecture on subjects in the field of medicine and possibly allied sciences. It is to be designated as the "Abraham Flexner Lectureship," which will serve to further emphasize the interest of the university in scientific work. By special provision of Mr. Flexner in making the gift, the first series of lectures will be given during the session of 1928–29.

According to the *Journal* of the American Medical Association, the board of trustees of St. Margaret Memorial Hospital, Pittsburgh, has received funds to establish a laboratory for clinical and biological research to be known as the John C. Oliver Memorial Research Foundation. The donor is Mrs. John C. Oliver, of Sewickley. The gift will provide generously for the equipment and maintenance of such a department in the hospital. A full-time biochemist will be in charge under the direction of a committee from the staff comprising Drs. Paul Titus, Ernest W. Willetts and Charles J. Bowen. The new department will not take part in routine laboratory work of the hospital, but will be available to the entire medical staff for research on any general medical problem.

The contract has been let for the new $500,000 dairy building at the Iowa Experiment Station. An insectary, especially for the study of the European corn borer, was also authorized by the legislature, and a section of the new horse barn and machinery shed has been completed. The old brick horse barn will be converted into a laboratory for the department of landscape architecture, while the old dairy building will afford much-needed additional room for other departments in the agricultural division.

The American Society of Mechanical Engineers has presented its gallery of forty-five portraits of noted engineers to Cooper Union. The gallery contains paintings of past presidents of the engineers' society. Among those represented are Charles M. Schwab, Ambrose Swasey, George Westinghouse and Admiral George F. Melville.

The French Academy of Sciences has awarded the Le Comte donation of 50,000 francs (triannual) to Dr. Alexander Yersin, director of the Pasteur Institute, Annam.

Nature states that on March 20 the king will open the eastern block of the new buildings of the Science Museum at South Kensington. First formed in 1856, the collections have occupied various buildings, but now for the first time they are shown in one designed for this purpose, though about a quarter of the collections still remain in buildings which were originally constructed for the exhibition of 1862.

A PRIZE of about $250 is offered by the British *Journal of Anesthesia* for the best research in anesthesia made in Great Britain during the coming year. This will be known as the Sidney Rawson Wilson prize, in memory of the late Dr. Wilson.

THE University of Edinburgh has received intimation of a bequest by the late James Sanderson, Galashiels of five shares of the residue of his estate, to be applied for the advancement or promotion in the university of technical and scientific study and research in the chemistry and engineering branches of the faculty of science. The amount of the bequest is estimated at about £35,000. The university has accepted the offer of an endowment contributed by former students and others associated with the work of emeritus Professor Robert Wallace, for the foundation of a university prize, to be known as the "Wallace Prize," to be awarded to the best degree student of the third year in agriculture.

ACCORDING to the report of the Royal Magnetical and Meteorological Observatory at Batavia for 1926, recorded in *Terrestrial Magnetism*, the electrification of the Batavia-Buitenzorg railway has made it necessary to move the recording magnetographs at Buitenzorg to the Island of Kuiper in the Bay of Batavia. The plans for the new building have been completed and construction was to begin shortly.

UNIVERSITY AND EDUCATIONAL NOTES

OF an allotment of $200,000 to the school of agriculture, Pennsylvania State College, for new buildings, $150,000 is to be used for the first unit of a biology building, primarily for botany. The remaining $50,000 is to be divided between a new sheep barn, an addition to the dairy barn milk room, a livestock hospital and the first unit of a new poultry plant.

COLUMBIA UNIVERSITY has announced twenty-eight gifts, aggregating $25,950, including one of about $10,000 from Dr. L. M. Waugh for the purpose of financing a research expedition to Labrador.

THE new Warner laboratory of mechanics and hydraulics at the Case School of Applied Science has been completed.

THE Dorr Memorial Research Laboratory of Temple University was dedicated on January 31. This laboratory was made possible through a $50,000 fund bequeathed by the late Dr. Henry Isaiah Dorr.

T. R. FERENS has given a further sum of £22,500 to the newly established University College at Hull. This brings his gifts to the college to about £300,000. Mr. Ferens has asked that £20,000 of his latest benefaction should be set aside for endowing a chair. The foundation stone of the new buildings will be laid on April 28.

DR. CHARLES K. EDMUNDS, formerly president of Canton Christian College, now Lingnan University, and later provost of the Johns Hopkins University, has accepted the presidency of Pomona College. He will assume office about May 1.

DR. MADISON BENTLEY, of the University of Illinois, has been appointed Sage professor of psychology at Cornell University to occupy the chair held for nearly thirty-five years by the late Edward Bradford Titchener.

DR. EDWARD U. CONDON, recently an International research fellow in mathematical physics at Göttingen and Munich and at present a special lecturer in Columbia University, has been appointed assistant professor in physics at Princeton University.

DR. P. W. WHITING, for the past year research investigator under the National Research Council stationed at the Bussey Institution, Harvard University, has been appointed assistant professor of zoology at the University of Pittsburgh.

ALBERT H. GILBERT, assistant professor of botany at the University of Vermont and associate plant pathologist for the Vermont Experiment Station, has been appointed professor of plant pathology and head of that department at Macdonald College, the Agricultural College of McGill University.

A. C. HARDY has been appointed the first professor of zoology at University College, Hull, England. Mr. Hardy acted as zoologist to the recent expedition to the Antarctic in the *Discovery*.

DR. EMIL RITTER VON SKRAMLIK, of Freiburg, has been appointed professor of physiology at Graz.

DISCUSSION AND CORRESPONDENCE

THE ICHNOLOGY OF TEXAS

IT it is almost one hundred years since the Reverend Dr. Duncan initiated the subject of ichnology by the description in the *Transactions of the Royal Society of Edinburgh* of some genuine tracks in the New Red Sandstone of Scotland. During the century that has passed there have been many contributions to the subject, and the last two years have been especially fruitful of studies, both in America and in Europe. Interest in these fascinating objects does not wane, but rather seems to be on the increase, in spite of the opinion of paleontologists that the study of tracks "leads nowhere," and "are so blind." To a true paleophilist fossil footprints are notes from the life of the animals of the past and give us some clue, not otherwise obtainable, of their daily life. The evidence is slight, it is true, but none the less the study of footprints aids us in our understanding of paleobiology, which we could not otherwise have.

Feeling thus as I do about the study of footprints, it was a source of delight to find here on the Pacific Coast other paleophilists who felt the same about the matter, and they possessed a collection of fossil footprints from the Red Beds of Texas, which I suggested would be well worth studying. The collection was then placed at my disposal. The tracks all represent small animals of types which are unknown from skeletal material. Williston saw some of the tracks in 1909 and suggested they might represent salamanders. During the twenty years which have elapsed since Williston published his short note, small collections of these objects have accumulated in several museums, and the time seems propitious to gain an insight into the small animals of the famed Texas Red Beds, by a study and description of this assemblage of new materials. The several hundred tracks represent a variety of animals, all of which are new to science.

We shall accept it as a well established matter that the usual rules of taxonomy apply to ichnological objects. This is a commonly accepted opinion of paleontologists and needs no defense. There are several new species, of different genera, represented in the present assemblage which it is planned to define as well as may be and place the matter where it can be at the disposal of other workers. The majority of the tracks measure under 15 mm. in length, the imprints looking amazingly like the foot-structure of the Microsauria whose anatomy I so delighted to study ten years and more ago. In addition to the vertebrate impressions, and making the study more fascinating still, are the trails of invertebrates and weather indications.

It has been more than a century since Pliny Moody pointed out to his friends the footprints of *Noah's Raven* on the red slab which formed a doorstep to his home in Massachusetts, and it is my purpose to regard this study of the Ichnology of Texas as a centennial celebration of man's study of the trails of his predecessors. It is my hope to see and study all materials of this nature and I hope that those who read this note and know of footprint assemblages from Texas will be so courteous as to let me know.

Roy L. Moodie

1021 Eleventh Street,
Santa Monica, California

DISCOVERY OF FOSSIL TRACKS ON THE NORTH RIM OF THE GRAND CANYON

Fossil tracks of quadrupedal animals were first discovered in the rocks of the Grand Canyon of the Colorado in 1915, but the abundance of their occurrence and their great variety of kind has only recently been made known.[1] During the past three years investigations carried on by the senior author show the presence of no less than 28 genera and 36 species of fossil ichnites. These represent three distinct faunas that named in descending order occur in the Coconino (Permian), Hermit (Permian) and Supai (Pennsylvanian?) formations. All of the specimens on which the above-mentioned determinations are based were obtained entirely from the south side of the canyon, and it is, therefore, of interest to find that fossil footprints also occur on the north side. Mr. Sturdevant, with the assistance of Mr. Charles Nash, made a special search for tracks on the north rim and on December 9, 1927, and was rewarded by finding well-preserved footprints in both the Coconino and Supai formations.

When collections have been made, it will be a matter of added interest to learn whether the tracks occur in the same horizons and also whether the same genera and species are to be found on both sides of the canyon, which are separated by a distance in an air line of fourteen or more miles.

Charles W. Gilmore,
U. S. National Museum
Glenn E. Sturdevant,
Grand Canyon National Park

A CORM ROT OF GLADIOLUS CAUSED BY A PENICILLIUM

The diseased corms have reddish brown lesions, firm but not hard, sunken, usually irregular in size and shape and without definite margins. The dark brown, moderately porous rot invades the corm tissues rather rapidly at temperatures between 12 and 23° C., eventually destroying the corm. At temperatures above 20° C. there is but scanty development of the blue-green conidia. Numerous sclerotia appear both on the surface and in the interior of the attacked corms.

The pathogenicity of the fungus has been proved by inoculation experiments and the connection of the sclerotia with the Penicillium has been definitely established.

[1] Gilmore, C. W., *Smith. Miscel. Coll.*, Vol. 77, No. 9 1926, pp. 1–41, 12 plates; *Smith. Miscel. Coll.*, Vol. 80, No. 3, 1927, pp. 1–78, 21 plates; *Smith. Miscel. Coll.*, Vol. 8, No. 8, 1928, pp. 1–16, 5 plates.

Both growing and stored corms become infected through even slight wounds but the fungus seems unable to penetrate the uninjured epidermis of corms.

Technical Description: Penicillium gladioli n. sp.

When grown at 20–24° C. on gladiolus corms or on favorable media such as Czapek's solution agar, or potato dextrose agar, the conidiophores are 50 μ to 2 mm. long by 2 to 3.6 μ in diameter; penicillus consisting of the main axis of the conidiophore with or without one or two branches, bearing few metulae 10–12 μ long and verticils of few sterigmata 12 to 14 by 1.5 to 2 μ with tapering rather than acute points, and conidia elliptical-fusiform, smooth, hyaline, 2.8 to 3.6 by 2.5 to 3 μ, adhering in long chains. When grown at 10 to 16° C. the conidiophores tend to be longer and coarser, with walls pitted or roughened, often forming conspicuous tufts, fascicles or complex branching coremia.

The sclerotia are 140 to 540 μ in diameter; cream to light pinkish tan, in age becoming pale brown or tan; smooth and composed of thick-walled cells 8 to 12 μ in diameter; retaining their vitality for several months.

On Czapek's agar the reverse color of the fungus growth is light pinkish cinnamon; drops of pale orange yellow fluid are more or less conspicuous on the mycelium; odor none.

The fungus described above has been identified from corms grown in such widely separated regions as Holland, New Mexico, Canada, Kansas and New York.

LUCIA MCCULLOCH
CHARLES THOM
U. S. DEPARTMENT OF AGRICULTURE,
WASHINGTON, D. C.

UNDULANT FEVER IN AMERICA

IN 1906 Craig[1] reported the first case of Malta (Undulant) fever originating in the United States. At the close of his paper he states: "(1) The probability of much wider distribution of Malta fever, even in temperate climates, than is generally supposed, and therefore the great importance of applying the serum test in all undetermined cases of fever in all regions. (2) That there are no pathognomonic symptoms of Malta fever. All the symptoms presented may occur in many other infections, and the cases are very few in which a diagnosis can be made without the aid of the serum reaction." The increasing number of cases reported since that time shows that Craig's prediction was correct.

The observation that the causal organism of Malta fever (*Alcaligenes melitensis*) and contagious abortion (*Alcaligenes abortus*) in cattle are closely related in their cultural, biochemic, serologic and pathogenic characteristics was reported by Miss Evans[2] and has been confirmed by numerous investigators. In addition to goats and cattle, hogs and horses are known to harbor the microorganisms.[3]

Of 35 strains studied by Miss Evans[3] 33 were of the abortus or melitensis A varieties. One strain which did not conform to the two common varieties is serologically closely related to paramelitensis of Négre and Raynoud.[4] These authors designated as paramelitensis in their morphologic, cultural and biochemic features, but failed to agglutinate or agglutinated slightly in melitensis serum. Absorption of agglutinins by paramelitensis from melitensis serum was only partial.

The writer has recently isolated a microorganism from the blood of a patient ill with a wave-like type of fever of long duration; with swelling and painful joints and sweats. Blood examination showed secondary anaemia, leucopenia and a marked increase in the percentage of the lymphocytes.

This microorganism was culturally, morphologically and biochemically melitensis, but it agglutinated in melitensis serum in the lower dilutions only, and it did not absorb very much of the agglutinins from the serum. Spontaneous agglutination in salt solution was marked. Perhaps this variety of melitensis is more widely spread than was formerly believed.

FREDERICK W. SHAW
MEDICAL COLLEGE OF VIRGINIA,
RICHMOND

[1] Craig, Chas. F., *Internat. Clinics,* 15 ser., 4, 115, 1906.

[2] Evans, Alice C., *Jour. Inf. Dis.*, 22, 580, 1918.

[3] Evans, Alice C., *Hygienic Lab. Bull.* no. 143, 1925.

[4] Négre, L. and Raynaud, M., *Compt. rend. Soc. de biol.* Paris, 72, 791, 1912.

ARE SALT SOLUTIONS MUSICAL?

TESTS in our laboratory with magnesium sulphate, salt, ammonium chloride and sugar convinced us that the change in pitch described by Dr. C. D. Spivak (SCIENCE, October 21, 1927) is due almost entirely to a change in volume of the solution with a consequent change in the length of the resonant column in our closed tube (air column over liquid in tumbler, beaker or graduate). Thus when magnesium sulphate is added to water the first increase in volume is equal to that of the dry magnesium sulphate; but as solution progresses, the volume of solution plus solid diminishes with a corresponding change in pitch. Solids on the bottom of the container produce a deadening of sound. The addition of sand deadened the sound and caused a change in pitch equal to that caused by the addition of an equal volume of water.

I wonder if Dr. Spivak has taken these points into

consideration? His finding that some salts are non-musical can be explained in this manner. If the length of the resonant column is long, the addition of salt or solid to the liquid below will cause only a relatively small change in the length of the resonant column. If, on the other hand, it is short to begin with, and has its length decreased by one half, a change of one octave will occur.

O. C. Magistad

University of Arizona

BANANA STOWAWAYS

Some time ago a couple of strange "mice" with prehensile tails, were brought to the laboratory from a neighboring grocery store. They proved to be Marsupials from some one of the Central American States, and belong to the genus Marmosa sp. A visit to the store resulted in the discovery of three more of this marsupial family making five in the single bunch of bananas. They were fed on grasshoppers and bananas and lived until the cold weather came on, when proper food could be secured no longer.

Many animals are imported in banana bunches and many insects, snakes and rats have been collected in the fruit commission houses, but this is the first time in the writer's knowledge that Marsupials of this genus have been included in the list of stowaways.

L. A. Adams

University of Illinois

ON THE VELOCITY OF SOUND

In an article entitled as above and published on page 381 of Science for October 21, 1927, an error was made in the value of a constant in the last line of the article. This line should read

$$V = 331.4 \left(1 - \frac{4.45 \times 10^{-3}}{d\,n^{.53}}\right) \frac{\text{meters}}{\text{sec}}$$

P. I. Wold

Geo. R. Stibitz

Union College

SCIENTIFIC BOOKS

Navigator. The Story of Nathaniel Bowditch. By Alfred Stanford. New York: William Morrow & Co. pp. 308. $2.50.

It is only an occasional book in the field of general literature that threads its story about the life of a scientific man. When such a contribution comes from the press it is a pleasing diversion from the technical aspects of one's subject and even from the more conventional types of scientific biography. Such a book is "Navigator" by Alfred Stanford, a recent Amherst graduate.

To one who is interested in things of the sea and the nautical aspects of a brilliant career this novelized sketch of the earlier days of Nathaniel Bowditch, of Salem, will prove a pleasing book.

It is more than a narrative of events in the life of a singular man. It is a book that wrests from the obscurity of eighteenth century science, a reticent but extraordinary personality.

To all who "go down to the sea" in ships, the name Bowditch is tantamount to Hoyle and "The American Practical Navigator" originally by Nathanial Bowditch is the recognized American epitome on navigation which has for so long been printed and reprinted by the Hydrographic Office that the number of its editions is now almost legion. If the aim of Mr. Stanford's book had been to show how and why this celebrated epitome of navigation came to be written, he could not have more strikingly portrayed his character, but his aim has been more than this. It is obvious that the author has solicited a wider circle of readers than mathematicians and astronomers by making human his unique character and detailing his varied experiences rather than his mathematical contributions.

Those who knew Bowditch more seriously through the authentic memoirs or the traditions of Salem's nobility, may find not altogether pleasing the intimacies of imagined conversations or descriptions of conjectured conduct, yet it is surprising and indeed gratifying, to find how consistent with fact is the main artery of events in this kaleidoscopic picture.

So far as the problems of the eighteenth century are concerned, Stanford has shown himself well informed. A scientific mind cringes a bit at the indiscriminate use of "straight line" for a "great circle" course to shorten sailing distances and the spelling of Laplace's celebrated work as "Mechanique Céleste." One might moreover gain the impression that a ship's position could be determined from lunar observations with a far greater degree of accuracy than was ever achieved in practice.

On the other hand, one should not minimize Bowditch's notable contribution to "lunars" in a day when chronometers were scarce and often wanting entirely in a ship's navigating equipment. While the author may have played up (or down) to romance with all allowable license in a book purportingly founded on fact, he has not obscured the Salem lad's love of figures as the *motif* of his career, nor has he failed to make mention of the high honors gained by his mathematical and astronomical attainments.

The final chapter is indeed a dramatic ending, and the more captivating for the knowledge that it is substantially according to fact. Rumor states that Captain Bowditch gained one glimpse of shore or of a familiar coastal light that piloted his landfall on the stormy return of the *Putnam* to Salem. Like Lindbergh's flight to Paris, aside from a piece of good navigating ability, it was probably a piece of good luck as well, that made possible the spectacular arrival. One might gain the impression that Bowditch's happy landfall was made possible by the accuracy of his newly developed "lunars," which, of course, is much overdoing it. Such a criticism is perhaps trivial for a book of much dramatic value, of distinctly human interest in things scientific, and perhaps on the whole as delightfully written as any fictional biography of the day. One can but wish equally competent authors would explore the fruitful and relatively untouched field of science for recreating in the literature of the day great personages of the past.

H. T. STETSON
HARVARD ASTRONOMICAL LABORATORY

REPORTS

AMERICAN SCHOOL OF PREHISTORIC RESEARCH

IN certain respects the work accomplished by the American School of Prehistoric Research in 1927 marks a departure from preceding years. In addition to the regular program there were four prospecting parties in the field. Moreover, during the term, the group of students was successfully turned over twice to former students of the school.

RECONNAISSANCE

Southern France.—The prospecting trip by the director and Mrs. MacCurdy was in southern France: the cavern of Aldène at Fauzan near Olonzac (Hérault); the Grottes des Fées on the Pic d'Ambouls near Nant (Aveyron); and the much discussed site known as Glozel near Vichy (Allier). Aldène is one more of the many caverns in southern France on the walls of which Paleolithic man left examples of his art; these were discovered in February, 1927. It has also yielded remains of Neolithic man including fine examples of pottery. The Grottes des Fées near Nant may also have been the abode of man in both Paleolithic and Neolithic times, but as yet only Neolithic remains have been discovered. As for Glozel, the prehistoric problems it has forced upon the attention during the past three years are now up for solution before an International Committee.[1]

Rumania.—One of our students, Dr. V. J. Fewkes, of the University of Pennsylvania, spent a part of June exploring a group of caves in the vicinity of Steierdorf, Rumania.

Austria.—Under the auspices of the school, a party in charge of Dr. Kurt Ehrenberg, of the University of Vienna, explored the newly discovered *Schreiberwand* cavern on the Dachstein mountain near Salzburg.

Greece.—After the close of the summer term, two of the students spent a month in Greece with a view to the checking up of prehistoric collections and sites.

SEVENTH SUMMER TERM

The seventh summer term of the school opened in London on June 27 and closed in Cologne on September 15. The special fields covered were southern England; a section of the Somme valley in the region of Amiens; Paris and St. Germain; Brittany; the region of Civray (Vienne), where the members of the school dug for a week as the guests of Mr. James T. Russell, Jr., a former student of the school; Charente; Dordogne with a season of digging at Castel-Merle near St. Léon-sur-Vézère and local excursions to important prehistoric sites and museums; an excursion to the caverns of Ariège and Haute-Garonne on the invitation of Count Begouen; Altamira, northern Spain; Neuchâtel, Zurich, St. Gallen, and Bâle, Switzerland. Attendance at the annual meeting of the German Anthropological Association marked the close of the term.

SUMMARY

Of the eleven students taking part, about half were unable to remain for the entire term; these were permitted to join for short periods. In addition to the student body, permission was granted thirty-four other persons interested in our work to take part in our program—especially in Brittany and the Dordogne.

Of the fifty conferences given, twenty were by the director and thirty by twenty-eight specialists. To the latter, the director desires to express his deep sense of appreciation. Sixty-three important prehistoric sites and thirty-five museums and special collections were examined. As a result of the twenty-five days of digging, collections were sent to seven contributing institutions. At the end of the season five students remained in the Old World for further study and field work.

PROSPECTS AND NEEDS

The school has demonstrated its ability to give a limited number of students intensive training in prehistoric archeology during the summers. It should be able to follow up these short periods of intensive training by taking the initiative in the location and development of new projects either alone or in cooperation with other existing institutions. During the

[1] This committee has since reported against the authenticity of the Glozel specimens.

past summer, invitations have come to us from members of Oxford University and the British School in Jerusalem to cooperate with them jointly in prehistoric exploring expeditions both in Iraq and in Palestine. Such a program renders highly desirable not only permanent headquarters for the school but also adequate endowment and if need be special funds for special projects.

With a permanent base, preferably at home, serving as a laboratory and repository for apparatus, books and specimens, branch bases could be established, or existing ones made use of, on the other side as the occasion demanded. With adequate endowment, professorships and lectureships might be maintained, at least one of which should be for distinguished foreign specialists. We already have the promise from an able foreign prehistorian and ethnologist that he will come to America and offer gratis a course of lectures as soon as such a center shall have been established. Surely we can not afford to be so lacking in appreciation of such a generous offer as to fail to take advantage of it.

BULLETINS

During the year two bulletins have been published by the school: Bulletin 2 containing the minutes of the first meeting of incorporators and trustees, the certificate of incorporation, and the by-laws of the school; and Bulletin 3 containing the report of the director on the work of the sixth season (22 pp. and 26 figures).

GEORGE GRANT MACCURDY

YALE UNIVERSITY

SPECIAL ARTICLES

ON THE DISTRIBUTION OF CRITICAL TEMPERATURES FOR SPAWNING AND FOR CILIARY ACTIVITY IN BIVALVE MOLLUSCS*

I

ORTON[1] classifies marine animals into three groups: (a) those which breed at a definite temperature, which is a constant for the species throughout its range; (b) those which breed at a particular temperature change, which may be at either the maximum or the minimum for the locality; (c) those which breed the year round.

Observations of the spawning temperatures of lamellibranch molluscs show that they fall within the first of these groups. Data gathered from the literature and collected by myself during some ten years of study of the marine lamellibranch larvae of our coastal waters show that of those bivalve molluscs which have been investigated each has its critical temperature for spawning. No species other than the American oyster has been studied extensively enough to determine the duration of the latent period after the critical temperature is reached before spawning begins. Since spawning occurs on a rising temperature in all forms thus far studied, it follows that the actual "trigger" temperature for these species is probably slightly below that of the water in which the first larvae are found.

The following species with their spawning temperatures represent those molluscs the larvae of which I have found, together with spawning temperatures gathered from the literature.

4– 5° C.	An as yet unidentified larva which appears in Barnegat Bay early in March.
10–12° C.	*Mytilus edulis, Mya arenaria, Astarte, Venericardium, Nucula.*
15–16° C.	*Ostrea edulis* (Orton[1]), *Ostrea lurida, Pecten irradians* (61.5° F. Belding[2a]), *Teredo navalis.*
20° C.	*Ostrea virginica* (J. Nelson[3], Townsend[4], Moore[5], Stafford[6], T. Nelson[7b], Churchill[8], Prytherch[9]).
24–25° C.	*Venus mercenaria* (76° F. Belding[2b]; 25° C., my finding). *Mytilus recurvus.*

One is impressed by the fact that these spawning temperatures fall into groups which differ by approximately 5° C. Setchell[10] studying the temperature limits for growth and fructification of marine algae, marine spermatophytes, and land plants has been led to assign as critical temperatures for the initiation of these processes: 5°, 10°, 15°, 20°, and 25° C. Crozier[11] has brought together a large amount of data on the temperature characteristics of vital processes of the most diverse sorts, and from these and other

* Publication No. 11, N. J. Oyster Investigation Laboratory.

1 Mar. Biol. Assoc. XII, 339, 1920.

2 Report upon the Scallop Fishery of Mass., 1910; (b) Report upon the Quaghog and Oyster Fisheries of Mass., Boston, 1912.

3 Report N. J. Exp. Sta. for 1890, 314; Contr. to Canad. Biol. for 1915–16, 53.

4 Report U. S. F. C. for 1889–91, 343.

5 Doc. 610, U. S. F. C., 1907.

6 The Canadian Oyster, Ottawa, 1913.

7 (a) Report N. J. Expt. Sta. for 1920, 317; (b) Bulletin 351, N. J. Exp. Sta., New Brunswick, 1921; (c) *Proc. Soc. Exp. Biol. and Med.* XXI, 90, 1923; (d) SCIENCE, LXIV, 72, 1926.

8 App. VIII, Report U. S. F. C. for 1919.

9 App. XI, Report U. S. F. C. for 1923.

10 *Am. J. Bot.* XII, 178, 1925.

11 *J. Gen. Physiol.* IX, 525, 1926.

data he determines the critical points to occur most frequently in the neighborhood of 4.5°, 9°, 15°, 20°, 25°, 27° and 30° C. As he points out, the agreement of these figures with those of Setchell can hardly be accidental. It may be assumed, therefore, that the temperatures for spawning of the lamellibranchs here listed fall where they do by reason of similar fundamental processes which control vital phenomena in the plants and animals considered by Setchell and by Crozier.

II

Although spawning has been the most extensively studied in relation to temperature of all vital processes in bivalve molluscs, observations of ciliary activity made thus far on lamellibranchs reveal a similar distribution of critical temperatures. Gray[12] showed in *Mytilus edulis* a progressive increase in speed of the cilia, with normal amplitude of beat, from 0° to 32.5° C. One may take 0° C. therefore as the critical temperature for the initiation of ciliary activity in this form.

In *Ostrea virginica* I have shown (Nelson, T. C., a, c, d.) that the critical temperature for ciliary activity and for shell opening of animals taken during cold weather is close to 5.6° C. Below this temperature ciliary activity is practically in abeyance. Galtsoff[13] finds that the cilia of the oyster come to a standstill at 5° C. This critical temperature of 5° for ciliary activity is accompanied by a spawning temperature of 20° C. Roughley,[14] working with the Australian oyster, *O. cucullata,* has shown that this form fails to open in water of a temperature lower than 10° C., whereas above this point the molluscs are active. This observer also notes that pulsations of the heart become slow and weak at 10° C. while above this temperature the beats are vigorous and more rapid. The spawning temperature for this species is not known, but from the restricted distribution of *O. cucullata* and from the observation of Roughley that in some seasons it does not spawn at all in the northern part of its range, it is probable that its spawning temperature will be found to be either 20° or 25° C.

Of interest in this connection is the observation of Takatsuki[15] that the pulsation of the heart of *Ostraea circumpicta* is abolished at 0° C. but begins at 5°–7° C. It is hoped that future work at the Asamushi Station will establish the critical temperatures for spawning and for ciliary activity in this little known species of oyster.

[12] *Proc. Roy. Soc.* 95, 6, 1923.

[13] SCIENCE, LXIII, 233, 1926.

[14] *Proc. Linn. Soc. N. S. W.*, LI, 446, 1926.

[15] *Scientific Report,* Tokhoku University, 4th Ser., II, 3, 1927.

The bearing of critical temperatures upon the distribution of these lamellibranchs is of prime importance, but can not be discussed here further than to mention the following facts. *Ostrea virginica,* the most valuable mollusc in the world, is barred from most of the otherwise favorable coast lines of the earth since the waters there rarely attain a temperature of 20° C. for a sufficient period to permit spawning. The inferior species *O. lurida* and *O. edulis* may thrive there since much of the coastline of the northern hemisphere rises to 15° C., or slightly above, for the time necessary to permit these species to spawn. *Teredo navalis* with the same spawning temperature has been carried into most of the ports of the world. *Mytilus edulis* with its still lower spawning temperature is the most widely distributed marine lamellibranch in the northern hemisphere. *Venus mercenaria,* the hard clam, on the contrary, is found only in a relatively few sheltered areas where subtropical spawning temperatures of 25° C. are attained at some time during the summer.

Many more observations of other species of pelecypods in widely different environments are needed to determine whether the critical temperatures shown above are characteristic for this group of animals as a whole. This preliminary paper is presented with the suggestion that study of the spawning temperatures of groups of aquatic species in the light of our newer knowledge of critical temperatures will prove a valuable method of attack upon problems concerning the distribution and behavior of such organisms.

THURLOW C. NELSON
RUTGERS UNIVERSITY

STARVATION KETOSIS OF THE PRIMATES

IN the course of experimental work on monkeys afflicted with "cage paralyses" the writer found that they excrete relatively large quantities of acetone bodies when starved, and, by analyzing the data in accordance with the ketogenic-antiketogenic conceptions of Shaffer,[1] the excretion (with the exception of the lemur) could be considered comparable in every way to that of man.

The following animals were used:

Black ape, *Cynopithecus niger* (Desmarest) (Celebes), male and female;

Bonnet Macaque, *Pithecus sinicus* (Linn.) (India), male and female;

Brown capuchin, *Cebus capucinus* (Linn.) (South America), male.

A mandrill, Papio sphinx (Linn.) (West Africa), male, on starving was found to excrete only traces of

[1] Shaffer, P. A., The Harvey Lectures (Series XVIII), Lippincott, 1924.

acetone bodies. The nitrogen excretion during starvation, however, was extraordinarily high. The animal weighed 5 Kg. and normally excreted 1.3–2 g. of nitrogen per day. After the withdrawal of food the nitrogen excretion rose to 4.5–5.3 grams per 24 hours on the three days of starvation.

A lemur *Lemur macaco* (Linn.) during two starvation periods of four days each excreted only faint traces of acetone bodies and the nitrogen excretion increased only slightly.

The animals were placed in metabolism cages and urine collections were made (without catheterization) at frequent intervals. The animals were very quiet, and would move away only when touched or frightened; however, they readily ate food when offered. They appeared to be in good condition—not noticeably emaciated. The urine contained much acetoacetic and β-hydroxybutyric acids after 24 hours starvation, and the excretion of these acids reached its maximum after 48 hours. The ketosis was promptly abolished on feeding glucose or carbohydrate-rich foods.

It will be noted that the starvation ketosis was equally severe in both the new and old world monkeys, and since it was found in monkeys of differing genus and living in widely separated regions, this behavior is believed to hold true for the anthropoidea in general. It is particularly interesting that a marked starvation ketosis has been observed only in the case of man and the anthropoidea. Thus a survey of the literature shows that the following do not develop a marked ketosis: dairy cow, steer, goat, pig, cat, dog, rabbit, guinea pig, rat.

There appears to be a real difference in the fat metabolism of man and the monkey on the one hand and the other animals enumerated above. It can not be explained by dietary habits, since it has been found to be slight in both carnivora and herbivora; nor can one accept the theory advanced by some that the absence of a starvation ketosis is due to adaptation. According to the popular theory fat metabolism proceeds in steps by β-oxidation, resulting finally in one of the acetone bodies, probably acetoacetic acid. The difficulty lies in the disposal of the latter. It is more logical to assume that organisms in general possess the means of *completely* metabolizing fats which are natural and necessary components of the cell. Putrefactive bacteria for example readily metabolize acetoacetic acid (Neuberg). The cat[2] and the dog[3] have a high tolerance and readily dispose of intravenously administered acetoacetic acid. The high tolerance and absence of a marked starvation ketosis is perhaps due to the presence of a "ketolytic" enzyme or catalyst which enables the cell to dispose of the acetoacetic acid formed from fat, etc. Entire loss or disfunction of this cell catalyst results in a ketosis. In the course of evolutionary development of the primates the "ketolytic" cell catalyst appears to have been lost. The acetone bodies do not normally appear in man because of a peculiar adaptation in which it appears that "the fats burn in the fire of the carbohydrates." Lacking metabolizable carbohydrate (as in starvation, phlorhizin diabetes, diabetes mellitus) the primates can not burn acetone bodies because of the absence of the ketolytic ferment. Because of the ease with which the lower animals dispose of acetone bodies they do not need to burn acetone bodies "in the fire of the carbohydrates," and metabolizing carbohydrate therefore probably is not antiketogenic, as in the case of the primates, because the necessary enzymes are not present. The slight starvation ketosis observed in the case of the lower animals, therefore, is not to be considered due to a lack of metabolizable carbohydrate, but is due rather to an altered condition of the cell which results from the low carbohydrate content. Restoration of the carbohydrate content of the cell to normal allows the cell to more efficiently burn the fats and hence leads to disappearance of the slight ketosis.

It is interesting in this connection to note several instances of severe ketoses, without apparent loss of carbohydrate tolerance, observed in cows. Sjollema and Van der Zande[4] report an "acetonaemia," etiology unknown, in milch cows following parturition. Although the animals received food, glucose was absent from the urine and the blood sugar was normal. A similar condition seems to occur in cattle poisoned by white snake root *Eupatorium urticaefolium*. From the meager data at hand, it appears that the carbohydrate metabolism in this condition also is not markedly disturbed. If a further study should confirm these observations, one may hazard the guess that the ketosis is due to blocking or a disfunction of the ketolytic ferment or hormone. A ketosis, in spite of a normal carbohydrate metabolism would confirm the view advanced above that glucose in these animals is not antiketogenic.

THEODORE E. FRIEDEMANN
DEPARTMENT OF BIOLOGICAL CHEMISTRY,
WASHINGTON UNIVERSITY

[2] Burn, J. H., *J. Physiol.* (1925), *60*, 16.

[3] Wilder, R. M., *J. Biol. Chem.*, *31*, 59 (1917); Friedemann, T. E., Somogyi, M., and Webb, P. K., *J. Biol. Chem.* (Proc.), *67*, 44 (1926).

[4] Sjollema, B., and van der Zande, J. E., *J. Metab. Res.*, *4*, 523 (1923).

SCIENCE

VOL. LXVII MARCH 2, 1928 No. 1731

CONTENTS

Physics and Politics: PROFESSOR WILLIAM BENNETT MUNRO 223
A Layman's View of History: PROFESSOR HENRY OSBORN TAYLOR 227
Samuel Garman: DR. DAVID STARR JORDAN and DR. THOMAS BARBOUR 232
Scientific Events:
The National Research Council of Italy; The Faraday Memorial Fund; The World Engineering Congress; The St. Louis Meeting of the American Chemical Society 233
Scientific Notes and News 236
University and Educational Notes 240
Discussion and Correspondence:
Notable Books on the History of Mathematics of the Greeks: PROFESSOR LOUIS C. KARPINSKI. *On Molecular Diameters in Gas Reactions:* PROFESSOR R. C. TOLMAN, D. M. YOST and R. G. DICKINSON. *Record of the Fresh Water Jelly-Fish:* C. M. BREDER, JR. *Transmission of an Acquired Character in Flax:* B. B. ROBINSON. *The Beginning of Winter:* DR. C. N. FENNER 241
Quotations:
One Tooth gone Wrong 243
Scientific Books:
Spearman's Abilities of Man: PROFESSOR EDWIN B. WILSON 244
Special Articles:
Telescopic Observation of Cathode and Anode Points: DR. CARL BARUS. *Factor H in the Nutrition of Trout:* DR. C. M. MCCAY, F. C. BING and W. E. DILLEY 248
Science News x

SCIENCE: A Weekly Journal devoted to the Advancement of Science, edited by J. McKeen Cattell and published every Friday by

THE SCIENCE PRESS

New York City: Grand Central Terminal.

Lancaster, Pa. Garrison, N. Y.

Annual Subscription, $6.00. Single Copies, 15 Cts.

SCIENCE is the official organ of the American Association for the Advancement of Science. Information regarding membership in the Association may be secured from the office of the permanent secretary, in the Smithsonian Institution Building, Washington, D. C.

Entered as second-class matter July 18, 1923, at the Post Office at Lancaster, Pa., under the Act of March 8, 1879.

PHYSICS AND POLITICS[1]

AN OLD ANALOGY REVISED

IT is just fifty-five years since Walter Bagehot wrote his "Physics and Politics," a very suggestive book in its day. He began the first chapter of this book with a reference to "the sudden acquisition of much physical knowledge" which had marked the second half of the nineteenth century, and declared it his purpose to show the bearing of these new ideas upon the political conceptions of mankind. That purpose he fulfilled with much ingenuity, pointing out the various lines along which the advance in natural science seemed to suggest modifications in the old theories of the state and government.

This was only a half-century ago; yet the new physics of Bagehot's day has already grown old. Its basic concepts have been turned inside out and upside down. Its laws relating to the indestructibility of mass and the conservation of energy have been radically amended. Even a generation ago the atom was held to be the ultimate and indivisible unit in the composition of the universe. It was the basis upon which the scientists of the nineteenth century built up an inclusive set of laws and principles relating to the structure of all creation.

To-day, all this is changed. The world is still composed of atoms; but we have discovered that they are not the last word in matter. On the contrary, they are themselves incessantly in process of division into still smaller, highly-energized particles known as electrons. These diminutive units of disembodied electricity, as they may be called, are continually in flight, yet they form part of every atom in the universe. It is quite possible, and even probable, that these electrons are engaged in the business of transforming matter into energy, and energy into matter. If this be so, there is nothing solid in the old sense, nothing static, nothing that is not continually in process of change.

Nor is this all. In Bagehot's day the science of physics was mainly concerned with visible and large-scale phenomena, with such mechanics of nature as were observable to the naked eye. To-day the physicist has shifted most of his attention to the study of

1 Presidential address delivered at the twenty-fourth annual meeting of the American Political Science Association, Washington, D. C., December 29, 1927.

small-scale and invisible things. The gross appearances no longer mean much to him. The general acceptance of the quantum theory has wrought a revolution in all the exact sciences. Even the chief corner-stone of the old physics, the law of gravitation, has been jolted out of place. Bagehot wrote in an age when scientists looked upon gravity as a force; to-day we are assured that it is merely one of the properties of space. And space itself is a concern of relativity, hence there is no such thing as absolute position or absolute movement. All things in the physical universe are relative to all things else.

It has been said that no metaphysical implications are necessarily involved in the quantum theory or in the doctrine of relativity, but it is difficult to believe that this can be the case. A revolution so amazing in our ideas concerning the structure of the universe must inevitably carry its echoes into all fields of human knowledge. New truths can not be quarantined. No branch of knowledge advances by itself. In its program it draws others along. By no jugglery of words can we keep mind and matter and motion in water-tight compartments, hence it is inconceivable that a greatly changed point of view, or a series of far-reaching discoveries in any one science can be wholly without influence upon the others, even upon those which are not closely allied. Science begins by altering the day's routine and ends by transferring our orientation towards the social cosmos.

The acceptance of the doctrine of evolution (to take an illustration from the past) did not confine its effects to biology, or even to the natural sciences as a whole. It compelled a general recasting of the older ideas concerning the origin of the state and of government; it threw political science into a new dependence upon history, and led Sir James Seeley to declare in one of his famous epigrams that history without political science could have no fruition. It impelled the student of politics to look upon public institutions as part of the whole evolving order of things, like the protoplasmic cell and the living organism.

And so the "sudden acquisition of much physical knowledge" which has marked the first quarter of the twentieth century would seem to suggest the timeliness of examining once again the old foundations of political sciences upon which we have built up our theories concerning the citizen's relation to his government. Natural science has moved a long way, not only from the teachings of Galileo and Newton, but even from those of Helmholtz and Kelvin; yet political science is still dallying fondly with the abstract formalism of Locke and Montesquieu, Austin, Blackstone and Bentham. It is still concerning itself with theories of absolute rights and duties, with old axioms about sovereignty and the general will, the sanction of law, the rule of public opinion, and the mass behaviorism of free and equal men and women who are assumed to be the ultimate atoms of sovereignty in the commonwealth.

It is still in bondage to eighteenth-century deification of the abstract individual man. Both the science and the art of government still rest upon what may be called the atomic theory of politics—upon the postulate that all able-bodied citizens are of equal weight, volume, and value; endowed with various absolute and unalienable rights; vested with equally absolute duties; and clothed with the attribute of an indivisible sovereignty. Under the influence of ideas which were borrowed from the old natural philosophy we continue to assume that the science of government can be a science only if it is based upon a series of fixed uniformities. Our vernacular and our thinking are still heavily saturated with the idea that there are laws and principles of human liberty to which all government must conform. And these principles we have embodied in a series of impostor axioms which stultify the free thought of the people and form the greatest of all obstacles to the orderly progress of social control.

So long as the social order was simple, without the unending complexities that have been infused into it during the past half century, these older formulas were not beyond the power of rational minds to accept—just as the old concepts of natural science were able to pass muster in the days when laboratory experiments were simple and few. But although we have now passed into an age when the vast laboratory of world politics is conducting experiments of every kind with unmeasurable rapidity, we continue the attempt to explain *our* electrodynamics in terms of mechanics—an attempt which the physicists abandoned a generation ago.

II

The American philosophy of government has exalted the individual citizen beyond all reason. It treats him as the incarnation of the Unknown Soldier. This is partly the result of our legacy from Puritanism, and in part the outcome of a pioneer insistence upon free scope for individualism. Hence it is the national habit to think of social control and individual freedom in terms of hostility to each other, whereas it is only through the one that the other can be realized. For even as every molecule of physical matter is conditioned and directed by those with which it interacts, so the individual citizen is similarly motivated and controlled by the influence of those with whom he associates. These influences, moreover, are not radiated upon him most strongly by society as a whole; they come from within his own orbit of life. They come directly from the immediate environment—his race, his religion, his political party, his labor union, his club, his newspaper and all the rest. He is the creature of his group-application. These influences are so penetrating, indeed, that for most of our citizenship the dogma of individual freedom is hardly more than a myth. Hence the first problem of political science is not that of adjusting social control to the interests of the individual citizen, but of securing and maintaining a fair balance between the various groups to which the individuals belong.

In other words it is time for political science to step up into line with the new physics by turning some of its attention to the sub-atomic possibilities. We should seek to discover the true reasons for that vast differentiation between good, bad and indifferent citizenship, which is perhaps the most obvious of all the phenomena of politics. We should enquire diligently into the nature and scope of the forces which make each civic atom what he is. And we should discard our allegiance to the absolute, for nothing would seem to be more truly self-evident than the proposition that all civic rights and duties, all forms and methods of government, indeed all principles of political science, are relative to one another, as well as to time and place and circumstance. They can not be stated compressed into rigid formulas.

III

Both in the physical world and in the body politic the atoms have this in common, that they are neither ultimate nor indivisible. The individual citizen, when you pull him apart, is a nucleus of heredity. He is the creature of a habit-system. But the whole training imposed upon us by civilization is based upon the assumption that human beings can be constrained or induced to modify their natural responses. More particularly they respond to the stimulus of ideas, the electrons of the social universe, and indeed our entire process of civic education—in the schools and colleges, by the press and at the forum—consists in bombarding the human nucleus with ideas. Some get attached, but the vast majority do not. The social atmosphere, like the physical universe, is filled with these invisible units of energy, moving at all rates of speed and penetrating power, gaining lodgment here and there, or departing from some human atom where they have been week-end guests. In the last analysis the weight of the individual citizen in the body politic is dependent upon the degree of his receptivity to these rays of intellectual illumination; it is proportioned to the number and quality of the ideas that he assimilates and retains. It is this variableness of response to the stimulus of ideas that largely accounts for the diversity among citizens in relation to their government.

Hence we have the hydrogen citizen. In his journey through the seven ages of man he manages to capture only one electron. His primal instincts have become modified by some single controlling obsession. Militant reformers, in any field, are drawn for the most part from among men and women who belong in this category. The same is true of the diehards at the other extreme, the reactionaries and the partisans of the hundred per cent. variety. They are what the physicist would call "stripped atoms." Neither of these elements ever contributes much to the orderly progress of government as an art or as a science. To continue the metaphor, it is the precious metals of mankind, not the light gases, that give both stability and movement to the social order. Even as the physical world is a composite of matter and energy, which are no longer regarded as separable, so the world of political opinion is to be looked upon as a composite of numbers and intensity, a product arising from the continuous redistribution of both. To the extent that energy is a substitute for mass, so the intelligence and the intensity with which convictions are held by a minority may offset a considerable deficiency in numerical strength.

Therein lies the flaw in such expressions as "the will of the majority" which suggests a purely quantitative measurement. The means by which a majority comes to be a majority is a matter of far greater importance than the mere existence of a majority as such. The actions and attitudes of the individual in politics become what they are by reason of the influences to which he is exposed, and more particularly the immediate influences, for the effectiveness with which a political idea or ideal can be transmitted is in part dependent upon the proximity of its source. The physicist is not content to know that the electron flies. He insists on knowing whence it cometh, whither it goeth, and to what purpose. The world is ruled by ideas which possess the power of penetration and lodgment. The electorate is merely the channel through which they become operative. Government is not, fundamentally, either an affair of laws or of men, but of imponderables behind both of them. To these imponderables, which constitute the invisible government, we have given far too little of our attention; yet we must do it if political science is to maintain an intimate contact with the realities.

IV

How, then, can the sub-atomic forces which make for the improvement of citizenship be singled out, strengthened and made more effective to the desired end? At present we have only a hazy notion of what they are and only in a crude way do we know how they operate. All around us gigantic campaigns of civic education are being carried on, by organizations of every kind, every bit of it inspired by the hope of improving the attitude of the citizen towards his government, and especially his sense of civic duty. A large part of this effort is based upon the naïve assumption that if you only exhort people with sufficient earnestness they can be induced to accept irrational ideas embalmed in the rhetoric of patriotism. No part of this nation-wide campaign for the promotion of better citizenship utilizes a technique that has ever been examined by scientific methods to discover whether it is at all adapted to the end in view. To a considerable extent the money that is being spent upon these so-called campaigns of civic education represents pure futility and waste. The ardent efforts of well-meaning men and women are frustrated by their sheer irrelevance to the end desired. Perhaps the most striking illustration of this has been afforded in recent years by expensive campaigns for improving the quality of our elective officials by the simple device of bawling at the voter to come out and vote. It is small wonder that these campaigns are accomplishing nothing, for they rest upon formulas concerning civic duty which are not merely unscientific but ridiculous.

Political science, to become a science, should first of all obtain a decree of divorce from the philosophers, the lawyers and the psychologists with whom it has long been in the status of a polygamous companionate marriage to the detriment of its own quest for truth. The philosopher, when he can not account for a phenomenon in any other way, ascribes it to some occult quality in the moral nature of man. The psychologist, in a like quandary, seeks the explanation by going through his inventory of standardized human traits, although it ought to be clear that political behaviorism can not be even described, much less accounted for, by the study of the individual in isolation. An increase in one knowledge of human behavior results at once in a modification of human behavior, hence it is rather optimistic to hope that social psychology will ever point us the way of explaining, much less controlling the actions of men in the body politic. The laws of science are not statistics which nature obeys, and the laws of political science, if ever such laws are formed, will not be rules which human nature obeys. They will be merely definitions which explain how men in groups respond to the stimulus of ideas. It is by the methods of science, not psychology, that we can hope to discover such laws. The essentials of the scientific method are accurate observation, careful experiment, and cautious inference. The earmarks of social psychology, thus far, have been crude generalizations and fantastic claims. Still it is only fair to say, on behalf of psychology, that it has taken the first step on the way to become a real science; it has already succeeded in providing itself with a technical jargon which is incomprehensible to the ordinary man. It has managed to translate many self-evident commonplaces into foggy language.

V

Government, as Emerson once said, is "the greatest science and service of mankind." Yet the science of government has been probably the least successful of all the sciences in building up a set of principles upon which any body of men can agree. Far from having the certitude and authority of physics or chemistry, it has not yet caught up with meteorology, which some people look upon as the least exact of all the natural sciences. As a result of this backwardness in what may be called the pure science of politics there has been almost no applied science of government worthy of the name. Government as an art has been so little perfected that as respects most of the serious problems encountered by the public authorities there has been no alternative but to rely on the promptings of political intuition.

The results are plainly visible in the great and ever-widening gap which separates government and technology. By the application of science to industry, transportation, communication and construction we have made unexampled progress during the past fifty years. But whether the world has made any progress at all during this half century, in the art of governing its people is a question that many of those best qualified to speak would answer in the negative. Our rulership over nature has become more commanding year by year; but man's rulership of man has made no such advance. The wheels of government have multiplied, and they are revolving at an increased speed; yet the electorate's control of them is certainly not firmer than it used to be. Surely there is an element of danger in a situation where our progress runs so fast in all the applied sciences except the one that ought to be the greatest. For although science may be the basis of civilization, government is the retaining wall that holds the entire structure in place. Science is producing wealth but there can be no such thing as wealth save under the protection of government.

Every new application of science to industry makes life more complex, and hence government more difficult, for the difficulties of efficient government in a democracy increase as the square of the newly-created human relations. That is why the big industrial city is so much harder to govern than is the rural area of equal population. The leaning tower of Pisa is deemed to be one of the greatest wonders of the world, yet it is an infinitely less complicated affair than an urban metropolis like Chicago in which one can find at this very moment, side by side, much of the best industrial technique and some of the worst municipal government on earth.

To be safe, our progress in the art of government ought to go faster than the advance of applied science, but unhappily it is doing nothing of the kind. It is steadily dropping behind. If the fathers of the Republic were to return to life, after their long sleep of a century, they would be equally appalled by the stupendous progress of the American people in all material things and by the relative lack of it in the art of government. Would they perceive any marked improvement in the way the laws are made, or the revenues raised, or the taxes spent? Would they note a conspicuous betterment in the caliber of the men elected to public office? Would they find our current political discussions above, or below, the plane represented by the letters in *The Federalist*? To ask these questions is to answer them.

Our immediate goal, therefore, should be to release political science from the old metaphysical and juristic concepts upon which it has traditionally been based; likewise to keep it clear of the sociologists and social psychologists who, if they could have their way, would only get us deeper into the morass of meaningless terminology. It is to the natural sciences that we may most profitably turn, in this hour of transition, for suggestions as to the reconstruction of our postulate and methods.

Political science should borrow from the new physics a determination to get rid of intellectual insincerities concerning the nature of sovereignty, the general will, natural rights and the freedom of the individual, the consent of the governed, majority rule, home rule, the rule of public opinion, state rights, laissez-faire, checks and balances, the equality of men and nations, and a government of laws. In place of these formulas it should seek to find concepts that will stand the test of actual operations, and upon them it should begin to rebuild itself by an intimate observation of the actualities.

By analogy from the new physics, moreover, it may well turn part of its attention from the large-scale and visible mechanism of politics to the invisible and hitherto much-neglected forces by which the individual citizen is fundamentally actuated and controlled. Three-quarters of a century ago the new biology suggested to us the abandonment of old ideas concerning the spontaneous creation of government; to-day the new physics may well suggest the discarding of our atomic theory of ultimate, equal and sovereign citizens in a free state. It is doubtless true that the natural scientist, as such, can never guide us to the true purposes and policies which should direct human action in matters of government; but it is equally true that only by paralleling his objectivity of attitude and his process of operational study can the political scientist ever hope to reach that goal.

WILLIAM BENNETT MUNRO

A LAYMAN'S VIEW OF HISTORY[1]

SOME time ago I received a pleasant letter from an honored officer of our Association. Among other things he said that his friends and colleagues would be glad to have one more book from me telling how it was that I came to write history. He added friendly words as to the interest of professional teachers of history in the thoughts of laymen like myself. So I am moved to give you a layman's view of history.

The muster-roll of laymen who have written histories is not a mean one. The old world offers us Herodotus, Thucydides, Xenophon, Polybius, Tacitus, no one of whom held a chair at any university. In modern times, in England, we pass from Gibbon down to Grote, and, in our own country, from Parkman to Rhodes. For myself, hovering, as I faintly hope, somewhere on the fringe of this rather Olympian company, I will endeavor to answer in a few words the query in the very friendly letter.

When I was a young man I became bent on devoting my mind and energies to the best things I could find. Not having original and creative gifts, I set myself to the study of what other men had deemed best, and had striven to attain in thought and work and conduct. I had ardently studied law, had practiced a very little, and had written a book on *Private Corporations*. But the law seemed too narrow—very far from covering the whole human field; and I turned to look beyond it. Being inclined toward the humanities rather than the sciences, I soon saw that I at least should find the most humanly interesting elements in the aim and the endeavor—the forming an ideal, and the struggle through the man's years, or perhaps through the longer life of a people, to accomplish it. The accomplishment itself, if indeed it is severable from the endeavor, might be beyond the strength either of individual or of race. Achievement lies on the knees of the gods. The true human story is a story of endeavor—the endeavor for the end conceived.

So I began with the ancient world, which is the pit

[1] Presidential address delivered before the American Historical Association at Washington, December 28, 1927.

whence we have been digged. And I devoted the ten years that were my supreme education to writing *Ancient Ideals*. That brought my notion of the story down to the time of Christianity. I gave all my time to the book, working eight hours a day, and traveling to see some of the things and countries I was studying. I had very little money, but I used it, and at last sweated blood to pay for the publication of my work.

Then, with the advantage of this discipline of knowledge, I devoted four years to *The Classical Heritage of the Middle Ages*. During two of them, I held a lectureship at Columbia, but gave it up as interfering with my real work. Profiting by this further time of studying and training, I next put ten enthusiastic years on *The Mediaeval Mind*, and, after that, six or seven years on *Thought and Expression in the Sixteenth Century*. There have been two or three smaller books, *Freedom of the Mind in History*, taking three years; and one that is now in the press bringing me to the present time.

Curiously enough I find that through all these books, if I have not been implicitly saying the same thing, I have, without intending it, been speaking with the voice of my first conviction as to the central human interest of the endeavor and the aim. Forty years, and all my mind and energy, have been put upon these books, which I mention to show the time they have taken. Such as they are, I could not have written them had my time been taken by teaching or academic administration. So much for this layman, now for his view of history.

Our ideas to-day of things about us are neither particular nor static. Rather we conceive a ceaseless movement to pervade the world; and we imagine that a like unbroken movement has brought all things to the present state of heterogeneous correlation as parts of a prodigiously variegated whole. Apparently it is one and the same universal movement that extends throughout our present world and reaches back through time. Within its sweep, past and present become a continuum, and our contemporary happenings are drawn into some real or conceptual unity. We recognize one vibrant current constituting an energizing and effective process. Each event is harnessed to the other, and the present emerges from the past. All seems an organic and possibly intelligent becoming. Perhaps this becoming is manifested most concretely in plants and animals. They *are* their past: phylogenetically as the present form of a somehow evolving species, and ontogenetically, since each living individual carries its line of ancestry to be handed on. These notions are not wholly new, yet they work in us to-day with new meaning.

If we turn from this universal process to our experience or knowledge of its phenomena, we find a like absence of barriers and separation. Fences are down between the fields of knowledge, which have become one vast *un*enclosure. Save for convenience of designation and prosecution, the sciences are no longer distinct and separate, but phases of each other, while philosophy would enfold them all in its consideration. Not unallied with them are philology, archeology, all scholarship if you will. Indeed, knowledge would conceivably become one, were there a mind genial enough to grasp it in its entirety.

Every element of our knowledge of the present world of man and nature is necessarily connected with our knowledge of that past through which man and the world he lives in have come to be what they are. We need make no distinction between our knowledge of living animals and contemporary human institutions and our knowledge of their antecedent stages. Every political or legal institution has come into existence gradually, or has arisen by notable mutation. The laws regulating corporations are of divers origin, yet there is continuity between the present body of corporation law and its multifarious past; and there need be no division in our knowledge of the past and present of this legal Briareus.

The continuity, or even oneness, between past and present is evident in the forms or provinces of knowledge. The science of physiology, for example, is a gradual and beautiful growth; its present state implies and includes its past, just as the animal organs, whose functions it treats of, contain their past genetically. Physics, so called, is also an emergence from its past, but more apparently by the way of mutation. Its fundamental conceptions appear to have suffered reversal. Yet if the old solidities of matter have been replaced by nimble units of electric energy, still the group of principles applying to the action of tangible bodies are as valid as they have ever been, and carry over the bulk of the science in its continuity. A more concrete illustration of mutation accompanying continuity is the manner in which relativity has, for a time at least, been grafted upon Newtonian gravitation.

And philosophy, that elastic method of ultimate consideration, of thinking any and all problems of the mind out to their final conclusions or despairs—this method or tissue of ultimate thinking assuredly becomes its whole self only in the oneness of its present with its past.

Yet changes come, and each age has its intellectual tendencies. Scientific or philosophic conceptions of the world are, of course, part of the thinking, even the temper, of a period. In modern physics the concepts of relativity and the substitution of electricity and motion for stolid matter are expressions of the spirit, the dynamic restlessness, of our times. So is our science of psychology, not to mention psychoanalysis specifically. A future age, with another temperament and mentality, may not be satisfied with them.

Knowledge is experience. But not all experience is knowledge, since experience may come in the guise of feeling or intuition. Such experience is direct, and is not apprehended through cognition and statement. Indeed much of our experience is rather untranslatable into knowledge or rational statement. Experience of the past, however, commonly takes the form of knowledge, or of doubt or conscious ignorance—the two latter being a mode of cognition or failure to know. Yet contemplation of a past event may stir our feeling and, as it were, arouse an intuitive sense of its import. To that extent our experience of the past might not take the form of knowledge.

In philosophy, realists and idealists still dispute as to the relation of all forms of experience to the assumed external world—the world past and present, I would add. Whatever be this relation, the point I wish to make is that our knowledge of the past and our knowledge of the present bear a like relation to the data or objects of their respective worlds. Knowledge of the past is the same sort of absorption or mirror of events as knowledge of the present. And if in any way knowledge of the present world should be held to reach practical identity with the assumed objective data, so one might hold as to knowledge of the past.

Again, as each man's knowledge, or other experience, of the present differs from that of his fellows, so will his knowledge of the past. This is strikingly true of historians living in different ages. Each age, with its own interests and view of life, will find in the past a different range of facts and interests. To different succeeding ages the past will appear, and even *be,* different.

As touching the intellectual identity in us of past and present, we should distinguish between evident forms of knowledge, like the sciences, and the material, for example, of past politics and war. The scholar may identify his knowledge of philosophy with philosophy's past as well as present, but will pause before identifying the Battle of Waterloo with his knowledge of it. In this respect, I should group religion and the fine arts of expression with philosophy and the sciences. For they also are an intrinsic part of the growth of the human spirit, of its feeling, its intuition; part, indeed, of the whole nature of man. To be sure, the whole nature of man, including reason, may exercise itself in battles. But in them there is more physical fact and violence than in the growth of poetry and painting, or the sweeter modes of religion.

With such rather crude distinctions in mind, I introduce the word "history." As applied to modes of human growth—science, philosophy, religion, and art—I regard their history as identical with the stages of their past, which is projecting itself into the present. This is one of the two current meanings of the term. For "history" is taken sometimes as descriptive narrative and sometimes as the subject-matter itself in its evolving course and processes. Both senses of the word exist, whatever be the topic. Thus the "history" of the earth may be either the narrative called geology, or may be the very changes which geology is attempting to describe. And a "history" of mankind may be the narrative, or, on the other hand, the very actual series of poignant human facts which follow on throughout the ages. In this sense the history of mankind would be mankind itself coming gradually to its present state; or the history of institutions would be the institutions themselves in the course of their growth; and, of course, the history of art or science would be art or science in its checkered course.

Clearly enough, if history, taken as narrative, is to be a thing of life and truth it must embody the verity, or veritable history, of the past; that is, must keep itself vitally one with the unfolding subject-matter which it is presenting. And it should absorb and re-express the elements of power moving the drama of mankind.

But a narrative composition is itself an event. It is part of the substance of its age, part of the intellectual conditions (which are actualities) of the time of its composition. The mind of Thucydides and the history which he wrote were elements of the period of the Peloponnesian War. So the sardonic Roman temper of Tacitus and the histories he composed were part of his epoch. Obviously contemporary documents and state papers are part of the event which they record. But Gibbon's *Decline and Fall* was one of the events of the eighteenth century, and part of the linkage between that century's consciousness of itself and understanding of the past. We may speak in the same way of Mommsen's very Prussian *History of Rome.*

More brilliant examples of things which are events and also narratives are the works of imaginative literature and the figurative arts. They too are records and also profoundly part of the substance of events. The *Iliad* or the *Divina Commedia* is a concrete manifestation, a supreme expression, of the qualities of an epoch. On the other hand, if these poems are not what are called historical narratives, they are records and masses of evidence. So the Parthenon, or Chartres Cathedral, is a document, a piece of evidence, even a vehicle of narrative. But each of these temples is also a concrete and monumental embodiment of the skill, the resources and capacities, and the intellectual and spiritual qualities of an epoch.

So the works of Plato and Aquinas are demonstrative evidence of the Greek and medieval minds. They are also part of the substance of their respective epochs just as truly as the Battle of Plataea or the Babylonian captivity of the Holy See.

For the purpose of this address, I am taking "history" in the more vital sense of the very life and actuality of the past, out of which the present has arisen. And the two points which I have endeavored to bring out are, first, the oneness between the present and the past, and, secondly, the view of "history" as this very living past and present which, as narrative, it seeks to bring to a descriptive statement.

There is a further point of view which seems proper for us. We are historians and scholars and I would say humanists, rather than physicists, mathematicians, or biologists. Whatever may be the view of our brethren the scientists, man is for us historians the centre of the world. We regard the sciences humanistically, as manifestations of the human mind and a phase of its growth. We are not investigators of the substantial data of the sciences, nor judges of their hypothetical accuracy or possible falsity as descriptions of the world. We are concerned with science as one of the modes of advance of human thought. And we bear in mind that physical science, and each branch of it, is a unity and a whole, made of its present and its past; so that the history of any science is verily that science itself in its entirety and continuous course from its beginning to what it is now and hereafter shall come to be.

We take similar interest in philosophy, that method and mass of ultimate consideration of fact or verity. We would regard it in its totality, which is its unity, and consists in an age-long and necessary mode of thought.

Many of us believe that religion is from God; but for us as historians it is another mode of the flowering of the human spirit, yet rather in the way of intuition and immediate conviction than by the gray path of reason. For us the past and present of religion, in all its manifestations, is one, even as philosophy is one. And we would make and keep our history of religion a true expression of its manifold growth and being.

In the same way we would work as historians of those glories of the mind which come to us in the forms of poetry and imaginative prose, and in the forms of the visual arts. And similarly would we view all human institutions, social, political, and belligerent—for man is a warring animal. We consider them in their time-unity, and, in studying them, should hold their past as one with their latest manifestations. So we weave into their growing web the salient events —battles, dynastic changes, executions, famines, and noisy revolutions, through which they have wound their course.

If we seek a further and universal unification of our conceptions of these manifold courses of human growth, perhaps we shall find it in a conception of humanity, of human life, one in its fruitful past and pregnant present. Human life may well be held a universal and dynamic unity in its manifestations, past, present, and to come; though for our intellectual and classificatory convenience we divide it into branches.

And now, if our considerations are valid, it becomes clear in what spirit and with what thoughts in mind we should write and teach history. We should strive to maintain this twofold unity, that of the time-dimension of past and present, and the pervasive unity of human life through its divers manifestations in religion, philosophy, science, institutions, and conduct. We should teach and write history as the veritable mirror, the *alter ego,* of this vibrant whole and unity of human growth. No one can compass this universal story. But each of us may set forth what he has to teach so that all the facts shall be constituent, and each fact shall appear in its topical relationship and exhibit its causal bearing. The story, and every part of it, is a linked emergent growth; and the facts which possess the broadest rational and connective value will best show its succeeding stages. Through the choice of such cardinal and potent facts, perhaps we may be able to present our topic in its furthest truth—as a chord in the symphony of man.

An awful time-honored figure looms before us, demanding to be dealt with. Its name is "historical fact." Since our history, taught or written, is to be truthful, the very *alter ego* of the course of events, one must take pains to be accurate. There is no telling when some small accuracy may prove a luminous link in the causal sequence. But usually accuracy relates to details and circumstances rather than to the larger features of the story. How can one be accurate about the Battle of Salamis or the assassination of Julius Caesar?—even though one were a contemporary with access to the newspapers of the following day. One will look to them for obvious details, which buzz about the fact. As for the event in its more essential nature, the historian will have to construct it out of his best knowledge and intelligence. Using our points of data, we form a conclusion as to how the event must have taken place, or probably took place. This is what every historian does of necessity. When he has determined the details, he has the more arduous task of their joinder and interpretation. Insight and judgment apply to this process, rather than accuracy. The result must be largely a matter of wise inference.

There are still two further considerations touching the conception of "historical fact." One is the human equation, and the other the multiple significance of every so-called fact.

Mark well the disturbing function of the human equation. Not merely is the fact's interpretation affected, in ways dependent on the interpreter's intelligence and bent of interest. But, beyond this, a molding and creative manifold of understanding enters and makes part of the fact itself. Caesar's death had different significance for each one of those Roman notables whose swords met in his body. It was differently intended, and also bore different results, according to the temperament, motives, and situation of each. Indeed it was for each a different fact. No fact can be in and of itself alone. Every fact comes to pass in its relationships and bearings, as well as in itself—if indeed there be any clearly marked and delimited *itself*. The causes of Caesar's death had worked up to it through the whole antecedent history of Rome—of mankind, if you will. More immediately it was brought about by the tempers and motives of the conspirators. Neither its causes, its manifold significance, nor its effects could be the same for an ethical intellectual like Brutus and for the sweaty mob about to take the air in Caesar's gardens beyond the Tiber.

Not only a striking event like Caesar's death, but every incident in life is exhaustless in its bearings; and since its substance extends to its relationships and effects, a multiplicity of actuality as well as meaning is very part of it.

But, furthermore, the understanding of a fact by contemporaries is part of its bearing and effect, and so part of the fact itself. This would, of course, apply to divergent understandings of it. Accounts that differ may be equally justifiable and equally true. Each one may set forth a different phase. Divergent histories, contemporary or future, may be each a receptacle and true expression of some actuality. But such histories are also part of the bearing and result of the fact, and so a part of it. And this is the ground of the justifiability, and indeed of the transcendent unity, of history as narrative and as one and the same with the course of the events described. As the events form an organic continuum, so should the expression be.

There is still a last complexity—perplexity it may seem. The very notion of fact, and what the real fact is, has varied marvellously among men; and this too, with no conscious weighing of the metaphysics of the matter. The phenomena, for example, of what we call the physical or natural world have been very differently viewed. Ordinary people accept them for what they appear. But the old Greek philosophers sought to find beneath them a profounder and causally explanatory fact. Such was the water of Thales, the atoms of Democritus, or the substance of Aristotle, or, if you will, the Ideas of Plato. None of these was either visible or tangible. Each was rather an explanation, an hypothesis, an assumed fact thrust forward, or thrust under, to explain things as they appeared. The nuclei and electrons of our modernized atoms may be a fact of this character. The ether at all events is such an explanatory fact, or hypothesis; and comes and goes at the call of physical theory.

Again, physical facts may be accepted symbolically; regarded as symbols of the verity which they carry, or which indeed they *are*, to the rightly instructed mind. The Church Fathers of the fourth and fifth centuries were prone to regard the facts of nature as symbols of the spiritual verity which it was their function to shadow forth. And, for some philosophers of the Middle Ages, the natural world, both in its creation and as presented before their eyes, was a divinely ordered allegory. Its actual reality, which appearances merely shadowed forth, lay in its spiritual and saving import.

As for so-called historical events, the Church Fathers, and after them the medieval theologians, admitted rather grudgingly the literal truth of the Old Testament narratives. That was but "the letter that killeth." The profounder verity, the deeper fact, was the salvation prefigured in them. It was their saving prefigurative meaning, which held "the spirit that maketh to live."

Some of us moderns, our Wordsworth for example, would still tend to find the deeper reality in the lesson, the teaching, the spiritual import of Nature. And in philosophy our extreme idealists, from Bishop Berkeley on, can find no reality beyond our thought.

Many of us to-day who are neither given over to allegory nor idealists of Berkeley's type still hesitate before our choice of fact or truth. We are haunted by the faith that the surest and most veritable fact is that which our whole human nature, passionate, spiritual and intellectual, might somehow conspire to substantiate. Fact may not be just as we see it, or scientifically observe it. And perhaps fact is not just as reason argues it. Assuredly it is not what impulse and emotional conviction would declare; our intuitions will not suffice. We crave the concurrent verdict—if we could only get it—of all the faculties of our cognitive and assertive selves.

Thus I have tried to set before you a layman's view, in which history shall not be mere narrative, nor merely the series of events forming the past; but shall incorporate and be the onward-striding thought, the interwoven tissue of event itself, the element of continuity without which nothing is or can ever have been. Every object in nature, every bit of science, every philosophic theory, every phase and kind of religion, and every constructive or destructive act of life, possesses the constituent of being and becoming which is time. And the history of politics, of science, of philosophy, of art, or of religion, is politics, science, philosophy, art or religion in its genesis, its emergent growth, its present, or even future, culmination and decay, through which its elements pass into other phases of the cosmic process.

Henry Osborn Taylor

SAMUEL GARMAN—1843–1927

Samuel Garman or Samuel W. Garmann, as he styled himself during his early life, was born on June 5, 1843, in Indiana County, Pennsylvania, and died on September 30, 1927, at Plymouth, Massachusetts.

Although he was for a while a student in the Lawrence Scientific School, he did not graduate but received an honorary degree of B.S. from Harvard University in 1898 and an A.M. in 1899. Garman told the junior author that as a young man he took part in surveying the routes for the Union Pacific Railroad and that having left home very early, he fought Indians and shot meat for the working crews while hardly more than a boy. This was a strange beginning for one who became almost completely a recluse.

In 1870 he became, for a year, the principal of the Mississippi Normal School and in 1871 taught natural science, again for one year, at the Ferry Hall Seminary in Illinois. Always keenly interested in natural history, he went to California, met Professor Agassiz at San Francisco when the *Hasslar* docked there after her voyage through the Straits of Magellan and Agassiz, immediately appreciating Garman's potential usefulness, hurried him on to Cambridge at once where he became one of his favorite pupils.

The senior writer's first acquaintance with Garman dates from the inception of the Anderson School at Penikese. Here Garman was one of the little group who, with Professor Agassiz, laid the floor of the barn with their own hands, on that memorable Sunday before the day on which the first modern marine biological laboratory ever opened its doors to students. Garman kept the books of the school and helped in practical as well as in scientific matters. Then, and later when he returned from the west after fossil hunts in the Bad Lands, he appeared in a broad hat and a flaming red necktie. But even as a young man he possessed a most firm dislike for personal publicity. He saw in the West the rivalry of Cope and Marsh to secure each other's specimens and to forestall each other's descriptions of their discoveries. Moreover, the somewhat unkindly attitude which they maintained towards each other's work evidently impressed him very deeply, for all his life long he maintained a singular reticence and it was only after years of intimate friendship that he would discuss any scientific work which he had in hand. Indeed he habitually put away his manuscript and the specimens which he was dissecting when a visitor rang the bell to his room. This was not by any means all from a fear that others might anticipate his results, although he did at times have this fear, as was so commonly the case with the zoologists of a few decades ago, but rather because he disliked discussing any of his work until his studies were completed. Those who came to know Garman early in their career, and the junior author was one who worked at his side almost daily for many years, appreciated that gradually he became more warm and kindly in his companionship, while his thorough and most accurate methods of work and his methods of training were always of the very best.

Johannus Müller was his guiding genius and of American workers he had vastly more intellectual respect for Jeffries Wyman than for most of his immediate predecessors. His affection for Louis Agassiz and his lifelong friendship for Alexander Agassiz amounted almost to hero worship and betokened a fine spirit of loyalty.

For many years his biography was not to be found in "Who's Who" nor even in "American Men of Science," although in his field of science he was easily one of the world leaders. The senior writer remembers a gathering on Penikese Island in 1874, six months after the death of Agassiz. Each one then present expressed in his own way his indebtedness to the great teacher. Finest of all were the words of Garman, depicting "the best friend that ever student had."

Garman, in 1874, accompanied Alexander Agassiz on his survey of Lake Titicaca and occasionally when in an unusually expansive and reminiscent mood he could be persuaded to tell how once while perched on a high Andean precipice catching frogs, he shot, with his suspender button, a gigantic condor which regularly swung past him on outstretched wings finally to fall a prey to his ingenuity. The details varied a little from time to time and while always told with the utmost seriousness there was nevertheless an unmistakable twinkle in his eye.

Garman also served for a while as Alexander Agassiz's assistant on *The Blake* and this gave him the opportunity to visit most of the Antilles and to make the collection of reptiles which he described on his return.

Once established in the Museum of Comparative Zoology, Garman seldom left Cambridge, but settled down to a life of persistent work on certain groups of fishes, a quiet career of graying age, one day much the same as another for over half a century. So seldom did he go upstairs to the museum library or exhibition halls that few students even knew him by sight, for he entered early and left late from his own little grilled door in the basement. Upwards of fifty papers on fishes, most of them of special value, and including new facts and new material are listed in Dean's "Bibliography of Fishes" from 1875 to 1913. Of these the most important is the one latest in date, "The Plagiostomia (Sharks, Skates and Rays)." In this are given detailed descriptions of the known species, with 77 excellent plates depicting nearly all of them. Of great value also is his report on the fishes of the deep seas collected by *The Albatross* under direction of Alexander Agassiz along the west coasts of tropical America. This is one of the most useful contributions to our knowledge of the fauna of the deep seas. Other papers of importance are the Selachians (sharks) of the voyage of *The Blake,* the accounts of *Chlamydoselachus* the frill-shark, regarded as the "oldest living type of vertebrates," which view is perhaps questionable; "The Discoboli," the "Cyprinodonts" and the "Chimaeroids," besides detailed anatomical studies and accounts of new species.

Garman was a man of medium size, latterly rather bent over and spare. He loved his garden and working there and with his bees kept himself in excellent physical condition until but a few years before his death. His library of fishes is one of the very largest ever gathered in private hands and by his generosity is now in the possession of the museum which he dearly loved and of whose staff he was one of the most distinguished members.

DAVID STARR JORDAN,
THOMAS BARBOUR

SCIENTIFIC EVENTS

THE NATIONAL RESEARCH COUNCIL OF ITALY[1]

HIS EXCELLENCY, PREMIER MUSSOLINI, the head of the government, on the first of the year, directed to the Honorable Guglielmo Marconi, president of the National Research Council, the following message, in which are fixed some of the fundamental objectives which should control the activities of the Council:

Mr. President:

The necessity of a coordination and regulation of scientific research, so intimately related at the moment to the technical and economic progress of the country, induces me to organize an instrumentality well equipped for this high national purpose. The interesting ("geniale") invention almost always originates in the brain of an isolated individual, but only the persistent work of patient investigators, with large and well adapted means, can efficiently develop and utilize it. A country like our own, poor in raw materials and dense in population, finds it absolutely necessary to have a thorough-going organization in order to be able to solve promptly difficult problems so as to avoid waste of energy, of money and of time.

To the National Research Council I have confided this duty, so full of responsibility. In its difficult task it can count upon my hearty support and to this end I intend to fix several fundamental objectives which should inspire its action and that of all of the bodies which will collaborate with it.

First. It is necessary to systematize in Italy research laboratories and well-equipped and live museums, in which the progress of science, of technology and of industry are rendered evident. A country does not spend in vain for such a progressive activity.

Second. The Research Council must have a care that Italian representatives in foreign parts, in the meetings so frequently held of technologists and scientists, should worthily represent our country and are dignified and well educated. I intend that these, my instructions, shall be respected in the most rigid manner. No official Italian delegation should go abroad to represent our country in the field of science or technology unless nominated by me on the recommendation of the Research Council. I beg that my colleagues in the government will assist in every way the directors of the council in discharging this not easy duty.

Third. The scientific and technical congresses which are held in Italy also, whether they are national or international, require to be regulated. These meetings will be authorized by me on the recommendation of the directors. No Italian delegate has the right to propose meetings in Italy of international scientific congresses without my specific authorization.

Fourth. I have intrusted the National Research Council with the not easy task of attending to the compilation of the Italian technical-scientific bibliography. The utility of this work is evident; it facilitates our scientific and technical progress which is essential to our economic welfare, and it is necessary for valorizing and recording in Italy the hard work done by our scientists also in comparison with other countries. It is necessary that everybody lends his cooperation with enthusiasm in this work of national interest, and everybody must answer with a ready response the questions asked by the National Council. It is my intention that all state, and public organizations in general, should support this truly Fascist undertaking.

Fifth. Very often government technical bureaus need

[1] From *La Tribuna,* of Rome, January 7, 1928. Translated and submitted to SCIENCE by Dr. John W. Lieb.

information and data about technical and scientific results accomplished in certain fields. The Research Council must see to it that the desired information is forwarded to the interested parties with promptness and accuracy. In this way, a service will be gradually unified, instead of having it, as it is now, divided amongst the various ministries with its great cost and waste of energy and which, on the whole, can be greatly reduced.

Mr. President, I am sure that the National Research Council will fully perform the task I am intrusting to it, and in that confidence I am sending my very best wishes to you and to the directors of the council.

January 1, 1928, VI.

Mussolini

This message of the chief of the government constitutes an event of outstanding importance for the scientific and technical development of the country and, from several points of view, can rank with the speech of Pesaro, which marked the beginning of the economic rehabilitation of Italy.

The head of the government, after having reestablished the authority of the state, reorganized the finances and stabilized the currency, is now taking up again genially with this message the policy of expansion and affirmation of our people in all fields of intellectual activity and he desires that Italy reconquer again the function of predominance in scientific research which had its birth and flourished in our midst.

The organ of this revival will be the National Research Council, which the lofty mind of the Duce has desired to be presided over by the most genial investigator which Italy to-day possesses, Guglielmo Marconi, and by a directorate on which serve men distinguished for ability and culture: His Excellency Giannini, minister plenipotentiary; the Honorable G. A. Blanc, Professor Parravana, General Vacchelli, His Excellency Bonaldo Stringer, manager, and Professor Magrini, secretary general.

A National Research Council has been in existence since 1921, but on account of its peculiar organization it has not been able to obtain all the expected good results.

The national government, fully aware of the great benefits which such an institution could render to the nation, decided to promptly reorganize it and better define its juridical status and it has accordingly made it a permanent consultative and informative organ of the head of the government, and of the ministry of public instruction, for everything concerning the development and progress of scientific activity at home and abroad.

At the same time, in order to obtain the necessary information, he has given to the council the freedom of approach to the institutions, laboratories and establishments where scientific research is carried on.

The constitution of the National Research Council is as follows: A board of directors and ten national committees, one for each of the principal branches of science.

At the head of each committee there is an executive board consisting of a president, a secretary and three members. Each national committee has a number of members varying according to the development attained by the scientific branch it represents.

In addition, the National Board of Directors may propose from time to time to the head of the government the appointment of special national commissions for the study of specific problems which have a practical importance in the life of the nation.

The organization of several of these commissions has already been determined upon, and two of them, that for food and that for national fertilizers, will very soon initiate their work.

The head of the government in his important message, when referring to the tasks assigned to the National Research Council, speaks of the institution of well-equipped research laboratories.

The Duce thus stresses, interestingly, one of the most important items of the activities of the organization and points out with accuracy one of our deficiencies which must be removed.

Italy, among the nations of great cultural development, is the only one which has not as yet any institution for pure scientific research, and all technical progress is intrusted to university laboratories, which, on account of their predominantly didactic functions, can not take care of the development of science with the necessary energy.

It is, therefore, indispensable to equip some great institution so that it may completely satisfy through books and magazines, apparatus and instruments, all of the exigencies of the investigators and thus place the country in a position to contribute, equally with other nations, to the technical progress of the world, and meanwhile this order of the Duce will be executed at once.

The importance of the other functions which the National Research Council is called upon to perform is self-evident but we wish especially to refer to the compilation of the technical and scientific bibliography and its diffusion abroad in every center of study in order that the patient and often valuable (geniale) work of Italian scientists may no longer be ignored by anybody.

THE FARADAY MEMORIAL FUND

William F. Castle, mayor of Southwark, writes as follows with regard to the Faraday memorial fund:

Michael Faraday was born in Southwark, the son of a

blacksmith whose forge stood not far from London Bridge and close to the present Southwark Town Hall and Central Reference Library.

To commemorate this great and unselfish pioneer worker, the council of his native borough purpose to form and maintain in connection with the Central Reference Library, a Faraday Memorial Library, to include a complete collection of portraits and biographies of Faraday and works containing contemporary references to him and his work; books showing the position of the physical sciences when Faraday began to work in them, and the best up-to-date works on those sciences and their latest developments.

For this purpose a Faraday memorial fund has been inaugurated, the annual income from which will be devoted to the acquisition of the best authoritative books as published year by year, and so keep the Memorial Library always abreast of developments in, and practical applications of, the sciences, especially electricity, for which Faraday did so much. In this way the memorial will have permanent vitality, perennial freshness, and ever-increasing usefulness, and like the benefits of Faraday's discoveries will be available for all who will to make use of it.

Some readers of SCIENCE may like to be associated with the Southwark Borough Council in this tribute to him. As mayor of this historic borough by the Thames-side, in whose annals are brilliant names of special interest to America—John Harvard, who, like Faraday, was born here, for example—I shall be happy to welcome tokens of America's interest, either in the form of contributions or of enquiries, addressed to me at the Town Hall, Southwark, London, S. E. 17.

THE WORLD ENGINEERING CONGRESS

A WORLD Engineering Congress is to be held in Tokio, October, 1929. The Congress proposes to discuss various engineering subjects in anticipation eventually of initiating and promoting international cooperation in the study of engineering sciences and problems in all its branches and to cultivate a feeling of brotherhood among the engineers of the world. Herbert Hoover, secretary of commerce, is honorary chairman of the American committee which is sponsoring the congress.

Seventy-eight prominent engineers in the United States have accepted appointments by Secretary Hoover, as members of the congress, including Thomas A. Edison, John Hays Hammond, Samuel Insull, William B. Mayo, of the Ford Motor Company; Charles M. Schwab, Samuel M. Vauclain, president of the Baldwin Locomotive Works; Daniel Willard, president of the Baltimore & Ohio Railroad; Orville Wright, Gen. William Barclay Parsons, James H. McGraw, of the McGraw-Hill Publishing Company; H. H. Westinghouse, of the Westinghouse Air Brake Company; Alfred P. Sloan, Jr., president of the General Motors Corporation; Michael I. Pupin, of Columbia University, and the following members of the General Electric Co.: E. W. Rice, Jr., honorary chairman of the board; Gerard Swope, president; C. C. Chesney, vice-president, and Professor Elihu Thomson, director of the Thomson Research Laboratory of the company.

Departments of various governments, universities, institutes and associations will take part in the sessions, which will cover a period of two weeks. Maurice Howland, secretary of the American committee, made the following statement:

> Some of the world's most pressing problems relative to public works, communication, transportation, power, chemicals, textiles and aeronautical and automotive engineering will come before the congress. At the outset, activity in these fields will be taken up under general groupings such as education, administration, statistics and standardization. The session will go on to specific problems under the heads of structural work, shipbuilding, mining and metallurgy, fuel, heating and ventilation, illumination, drainage, refrigeration, and the use of telephone and telegraph. Almost every activity of daily life as touched by modern science and invention will be reflected in the deliberations of the congress.

THE ST. LOUIS MEETING OF THE AMERICAN CHEMICAL SOCIETY

THE seventy-fifth meeting of the American Chemical Society will be held in St. Louis from April 16 to 19. Dr. William J. Mayo, of the Mayo Clinic, will address a public meeting on the evening of April 17 on "The Advancement of Learning in Medicine through Biochemistry."

Preliminary plans have been announced for the scientific sessions. All except the colloid, fertilizer and leather and gelatin chemistry divisions will meet.

The agricultural and food chemistry division, in addition to holding a meeting for the presentation of miscellaneous papers, will hold a symposium on insecticides and fungicides under the leadership of R. C. Roark.

The division of biological chemistry expects twenty to thirty papers on the biochemistry of soils, nutrition, vitamins, ultra-violet irradiations, endocrinology and the relation of chemistry to health and disease.

The cellulose chemistry division will hold two half-day sessions.

The division of chemical education will hold four half-day sessions at St. Louis. Two of these sessions have been allotted to a symposium on "Analytical Chemistry," in which several prominent chemists have already agreed to take part. One of these sessions will be held at the time of the general divisional meetings on Tuesday afternoon, April 17. The topics for this particular session are: "Objectives and Content of the Introductory Course in Qualitative Analysis"; "Objectives and Content of the Introductory Course of the Quantitative Analysis"; "Advanced and Graduate Work in Analytical Chemistry."

The history of chemistry division will hold one half-day session. The division expects to hold an exhibit of autograph letters, documents, medals, etc., relating to the French chemists of the French revolutionary period. Papers by H. M. Elsey, Orville E. May, Lyman C. Newell and Tenney L. Davis have been promised.

The division of industrial and engineering chemistry is planning to have round-table discussions on the following topics: "Lubrication," led by R. E. Wilson; "Filtration," led by D. R. Sperry, and "Equipment Construction," led by W. T. Read. The petroleum division will join in the discussion on "Lubrication."

In addition to a joint symposium with the division of physical and inorganic chemistry on "Atomic Structure and Valence," the division of organic chemistry will hold three half-day sessions.

The paint and varnish division will hold a symposium on "Settling of Pigments," with P. R. Croll as chairman. A number of other papers have been promised.

The petroleum division will hold three half-day sessions in addition to the joint round-table discussion on "Lubrication" with the industrial and engineering chemistry division. The division plans to visit one of the refineries in the neighborhood of St. Louis.

The division of physical and inorganic chemistry plans to devote a whole day to the joint symposium on "Atomic Structure and Valence." The purpose of this symposium is to try to bring physicists and chemists together in an effort to arrive at some common basis of understanding. The following speakers have promised to participate: K. K. Darrow, G. E. M. Jauncey, S. C. Lind, H. S. Fry, W. H. Rodebush, W. A. Noyes, W. D. Harkins, Herman Schlundt and W. H. Carothers.

The rubber chemistry division will hold three half-day sessions. It will also hold its regular banquet. The division of sugar chemistry will hold three half-day sessions.

At the meeting of the division of water, sewage and sanitation a group of papers will be presented on the treatment of water for railroad use, with special reference to softening; another group will have to do with recent advances in the softening of municipal water supplies; and the softening of water in the home will be discussed briefly. Some phases of the utilization of Colorado River water will be discussed in the light of new data on the dissolved mineral matter and the silt carried by the river.

The addresses of the secretaries of the divisions which will hold meetings are as follows:

Agricultural and Food Chemistry: C. S. Brinton, Food Inspection Laboratory, U. S. Appraiser's Stores, Philadelphia, Pa.

Biological Chemistry: M. X. Sullivan, Laboratory of Hygiene, Treasury Department, Washington, D. C.

Cellulose Chemistry: E. C. Sherrard, Forest Products Laboratory, Madison, Wis.

Chemical Education: R. A. Baker, Bowne Hall, Syracuse University.

Dye Chemistry: H. T. Herrick, Color and Farm Waste Division, Bureau of Chemistry and Soils, Washington, D. C.

Gas and Fuel Chemistry: O. O. Malleis, 5557 Woodmont St., Pittsburgh, Pa.

History of Chemistry: Tenney L. Davis, Massachusetts Institute of Technology.

Industrial and Engineering Chemistry: E. M. Billings, 343 State St., Rochester, N. Y.

Medicinal Products Chemistry: A. E. Osterberg, Mayo Clinic, Rochester, Minn.

Organic Chemistry: Frank C. Whitmore, National Research Council, Washington, D. C.

Paint and Varnish Chemistry: E. W. Boughton, New Jersey Zinc Co., 160 Front St., New York.

Petroleum Chemistry: Carl L. Johnson, The Manhattan Oil Co., Kansas City.

Physical and Inorganic Chemistry: Ward V. Evans, Northwestern University.

Rubber Chemistry: H. E. Simmons, Bierce Library, Municipal University, Akron, Ohio.

Sugar Chemistry: F. W. Zerban, New York Sugar Trade Laboratory, 80 South St., New York.

Water, Sewage and Sanitation Chemistry: W. D. Collins, U. S. Geological Survey, Washington, D. C.

SCIENTIFIC NOTES AND NEWS

PROFESSOR JAMES KENDALL, dean of the New York University Graduate School and formerly professor of chemistry in Columbia University, has accepted the chair of chemistry at the University of Edinburgh. Dr. Kendall will succeed his old teacher, Professor Sir James Walker, of Edinburgh, who retires at the end of the present academic year.

COLONEL WILLIAM B. GREELEY, since 1920 chief of the U. S. Forest Service, will resign on May 1, to accept a position with the West Coast Lumber Manufacturers' Association. Major R. Y. Stuart, now assistant forester in the forest service in charge of public relations, has been appointed to succeed Colonel Greeley.

THE British Iron and Steel Institute will award the Bessemer gold medal to Charles M. Schwab, chairman of the board of the Bethlehem Steel Corporation and president of the American Iron and Steel Institute. The presentation will take place at a meeting of the institute on May 3 and 4.

DR. MARCUS BENJAMIN, editor of the publications of the U. S. National Museum, has recently received the promotion from "Cavaliere" to "Officer" of the Order of the Crown of Italy.

THE grand cross, the highest rank of the Legion of Honor, has been conferred on Dr. Albert Calmette, of the Pasteur Institute, who has developed a preventive vaccine treatment for tuberculosis. His collaborator, Dr. C. Guerin, has been accorded the rank of officer.

DR. A. W. HILL, director of the Royal Botanic Gardens, Kew, who is on a visit, made possible by a grant to Kew from the Empire Marketing Board, to the botanical, agricultural and forestry institutions of Australia, New Zealand and Java, has been given the degree of D.Sc. by the University of Adelaide.

ACCORDING to the *British Medical Journal* the prize of the Marchiafava Foundation of the value of 8,000 lire for the best work on morbid anatomy and experimental pathology has been awarded to Professor Soli, who holds the chair of morbid anatomy at Palermo, for his investigations on arterio-sclerosis produced by *Spiroptera sanguinolenta,* and Professor Brancati, of the Surgical Clinic of Rome, for his investigations on internal tar cancer.

AT a meeting of the British Institution of Electrical Engineers held on February 2 a portrait in oils of Mr. Ll. B. Atkinson, past-president of the institution, was formally presented to the institution by the Cable Makers' Association. The portrait was painted by Mr. G. Harcourt.

DR. GUSTAV GIEMSA, director of the chemical section of the Hamburg Institute for Tropical Diseases and the inventor of a well-known stain, recently celebrated his sixtieth birthday.

PROFESSOR MINKOWSKI, who retired last year from the directorship of the medical clinic at Breslau, celebrated his seventieth birthday on January 13.

MORE than one hundred of his present and former associates and friends gathered at the Cosmos Club on the evening of February 3, 1928, to do honor to F. P. Veitch, who directs the research work on leather, paper, fabrics and naval stores of the Bureau of Chemistry and Soils. The celebration was to commemorate his twenty-five years of service in the Bureau of Chemistry. It took the form of a dinner, at which W. W. Skinner presided as toastmaster.

PROFESSOR SAMUEL C. LIND, director of the school of chemistry of the University of Minnesota, has been elected a member of the International Radium Standards Commission, to succeed the late Professor Boltwood, of Yale University.

DR. R. E. ROSE has been appointed a member of the advisory committee of the cancer research fund of the University of Pennsylvania.

STANLEY F. MORSE, consulting agricultural engineer, of South Carolina and New York, has been appointed chairman of the newly-organized division of consulting agricultural engineers of the American Society of Agricultural Engineers. The purpose of this division is to bring together in one organization the most competent men in the profession. The qualifications of applicants will be examined and only those of proper training, experience and reliability will be admitted to membership.

GEORGE A. STETSON has resigned as associate professor of heat-power engineering at New York University to become associate editor for the American Society of Mechanical Engineers.

PROFESSOR S. C. LANGDON has dropped his teaching work at Northwestern University to take charge of chemical research for the Curtis Lighting, Inc., of Chicago. He will continue to direct some of his researches at the university.

FACULTY members from foreign countries who will give summer quarter courses at the University of Chicago include P. W. Bryan, lecturer on geography at the University College, Leicester, England, and John Robert Charles Evans, geology, Brandon College, Manitoba, Canada.

L. C. COLEMAN, who was granted two years' leave of absence by the department of agriculture in Mysore, India, and has been, during that time, professor of plant pathology at Toronto University, has returned to India to again become director of agriculture in Mysore at Bangalore.

A. R. TRIST, research forester of Australia, has been sent to the United States by the Australian government for a stay of two years to study the organization of the forest experiment stations and the methods involved in forest research in the United States.

SIR WILLIAM B. HARDY, of Cambridge, England, will be the guest of honor at the sixth National Colloid Symposium, to be held under the auspices of the American Chemical Society in Toronto from June 14 to 16.

DR. JULIUS BAUER, professor of medicine at the University of Vienna and physician in chief to the Polyclinic, will deliver several lectures and also the convocation oration before the American College of

Physicians at the meeting in New Orleans, from March 5 to 9.

DR. WILLIAM CROCKER, director of the Boyce Thompson Institute for Plant Research, will address on March 15 the Columbia University chapter of the Society of Sigma Xi, on "Research on Plants as exemplified by the Work of the Boyce Thompson Institute."

DR. GERALD WENDT, director of the new Battelle Memorial Institute at Columbus, Ohio, will make a lecture tour of the West during the months of February and March. He will deliver three different lectures at a number of colleges and universities, including a popular lecture on "What is the World made of?" and two lectures of special interest to scientists, especially chemists, on the "Creative Artist in Research" and "American Chemical Research in 1928." This is the first of a series of lectures being planned for the institutions in the far west and is being arranged by Dr. J. L. St. John, head of the department of biochemistry in the State College of Washington.

DR. C. M. A. STINE, chemical director of the E. I. du Pont de Nemours Company, on a recent trip to the Pacific Coast, gave talks before various organizations. On January 13 he addressed the Society of Sigma Xi at the University of Washington on "High Pressure in Manufacturing."

DR. HENRY LAURENS, professor of physiology at Tulane University Medical School, recently gave lectures on "The Physiological Action of Radiant Energy," before chapters of the Society of Sigma Xi at the University of Missouri and the University of Kansas.

DR. ARTHUR H. COMPTON, professor of physics in the University of Chicago, lectured before the West Virginia Chapter of the Society of the Sigma Xi and the West Virginia Scientific Society on February 23. His subject was "What Things are made of."

DR. ULRIC DAHLGREN, professor of biology at Princeton University, read a paper on March 2 before the American Philosophical Society on "Equilibrium and Hearing."

ON February 11 Professor R. A. Gortner, chief of the division of agricultural biochemistry, University of Minnesota, delivered an address to the Royal Canadian Institute on the subject "Colloid Chemistry and Living Processes."

Industrial and Engineering Chemistry notes that the year 1928 marks the hundredth anniversary of Wöhler's preparation of urea from ammonium cyanate. That discovery marked the beginning of synthetic chemistry and the beginnng of the end of the older vitalistic ideas of organic chemistry. It is planned to celebrate the centenary by a special program at the Boston meeting (Swampscott) of the American Chemical Society in September, 1928.

THE centenary of the birth of Dr. Maximovitch, who was a distinguished Russian botanist, was recently celebrated by ceremonies in the town of Sapporo on the isle of Hocksido, Japan. The occasion was presided over by Professor Kingo-Miyabe, of the Institute of Natural Sciences.

A MEMORIAL plaque was recently unveiled in the medical clinic of Münster in honor of F. W. A. Sertürner, the discoverer of morphine, who was born at Neuhaus, near Padeborn, in 1783.

WILLIAM CORLESS MILLS, curator of the department of archeology in the Ohio State Museum, died on January 17, aged sixty-eight years.

JOHN ROWLEY, curator of mammals for the California Academy of Sciences, died in January, aged sixty-one years.

BRADSHAW HALL SWALES, of Detroit, honorary assistant curator of birds in the U. S. National Museum, died on January 23, at the age of fifty-two years.

WILLET MARTIN HAYES, formerly professor of agriculture at the University of Minnesota and later assistant secretary of the U. S. Department of Agriculture, died on January 15, aged sixty-nine years.

DR. EDWARD S. BURGESS, formerly professor of natural science at Hunter College, New York City, died on February 23, aged seventy-three years.

PROFESSOR JOSÉ RODRIGUEZ CARRACIDO, for many years rector of the University of Madrid, who worked chiefly on the action of alkaloids upon organisms and was the author of several text-books on biochemistry, has died, aged seventy-two years.

THE officers of the Louisiana Academy of Sciences met at Alexandria on January 28 at the Louisiana College. Those present were: I. Maizlish, H. L. Smith, Geo. Williamson, Jno. A. Hardin, F. M. Witherspoon, Leo J. Lassalle, Paul M. Horton, S. T. Sanders, H. V. Howe, A. C. Maddox, H. G. Shaw, F. G. Fournet, C. Cottingham, J. E. Guardia, O. B. Owens and A. L. Ducournau. Plans for the first annual meeting, which is to be held on May 5, were discussed as well as some of the future plans of the academy.

THE Ohio Academy of Science will hold its thirty-eighth annual meeting at the University of Cincinnati on April 6 and 7, under the presidency of Dr. Harris

M. Benedict, of the University of Cincinnati. Among the prominent outside speakers will be Dr. W. T. Bovie, of the Medical School, Northwestern University, and Dr. W. W. Lepeschkin, now at the University of Illinois, botanical department. The former will speak on the "Relation of Physics to Biology" and the latter on "Physico-Chemical Causes of Death." President Schneider, of the University of Cincinnati, will also speak. The Indiana and Kentucky Academies of Science have been invited to attend and participate.

THE executive committee of the American Society of Zoologists has voted to hold the 1928 meeting in New York from December 27 to 29, inclusive.

A CONFERENCE was held at the U. S. Bureau of Standards on March 2, to discuss the research work on electroplating that is completed or in progress, and to make recommendations regarding future studies, both by the bureau staff and by research associates of the American Electroplaters' Society.

THE American Society for the Control of Cancer will hold its annual meeting on March 3 in New York. In the morning, Dr. Francis Carter Wood will demonstrate modern cancer research at the Crocker Laboratory; Henry F. Vaughan, D.P.H., health commissioner of Detroit, will speak at a luncheon at the Biltmore Hotel on "Functions of Health Departments in the Control of Cancer," and Dr. Jonathan M. Wainwright, Scranton, Pa., on "What the Medical Profession should do about Cancer." Short discussions of cancer control in its practical aspects and a short business meeting will take up the afternoon.

THE date of the Third Annual Meeting of the Eastern Section at the University of Virginia (Charlottesville, Va.) has been arranged. The first session will convene on the afternoon of Monday, April 30. Sessions for the presentation of papers, etc., will occupy the afternoon of Monday, the morning of Tuesday and that of Wednesday, and, possibly, Wednesday afternoon also. Tuesday afternoon, May 1, will be devoted to excursions which are being arranged through the local committee. The chairman of the local committee is the president of the Virginia chapter of Sigma Xi, Professor Wilbur A. Nelson, University of Virginia, Charlottesville, Va.

AT a banquet in the Hotel Somerset on February 18 the centenary of the *Boston Medical and Surgical Journal* was commemorated. The first issue appeared February 19, 1828. With its next issue, the periodical will change its name to the *New England Journal of Medicine,* including also the states of Vermont and New Hampshire in its representations.

DR. HERBERT E. IVES, who was recently awarded the John Scott medal and premium, for his contributions to electrical telephotography and television, has donated the amount of the premium ($1,000) to the Optical Society of America, to found and endow a medal. This medal, to be awarded every two years, for distinguished work in optics, is to be named "The Frederic Ives Medal," in honor of the donor's father.

A JOINT resolution to provide $10,000 for expenses of an American delegation to the Eighth International Dairy Congress, in London during June and July, was passed by the House on January 26. Under terms of the resolution, the President will accept the invitation of the British government and appoint ten delegates to represent the United States.

THE U. S. Senate passed on February 6 the bill introduced by Senator McNary, of Oregon, authorizing an appropriation of $40,000,000 to be expended over a period of eight years to aid the various states in the purchase of denuded lands for reforestation purposes where reforestation is needed to protect the navigation of streams.

DESIGNATION of the American Green Cross as a national body for education and research work in connection with the protection of forests, flood control and allied problems, is provided for in a bill (H. R. Res. 196) just introduced in the House by Representative Evans, of Glendale, Calif. The bill authorizes appropriation of $120,000 to be placed at the disposal of the American Green Cross for the continuance and development of its organization. The bill was referred to the committee on education.

THE Iowa Lakeside Laboratory, situated on West Okoboji Lake in northwestern Iowa and operated in connection with the graduate college of the State University of Iowa, will be open to investigators during the season of 1928 from June 11 to August 17. No formal courses are offered, but research students in any field who find the conditions favorable for their work may be admitted to the laboratory. Supervision of research in experimental embryology and comparative physiology will be by Professor Emil Witschi and Otto M. Helff, of the department of zoology of the university, and in mycology by Professor G. W. Martin, of the department of botany. Professor Martin has been appointed director of the laboratory.

THE botanical specimens of the late Ellsworth Bethel, of Denver, have been given by the trustees of the State Historical Society to the Colorado Agricultural College and the University of Colorado. The Bethel collection proper consisting of some 10,000 mounted specimens and a much larger number of unmounted Colorado plants was received by the botanical department of the agricultural college. The collection is a valuable one as representative of the region.

The sum of $10,000 has recently been granted to the American Philosophical Association by the Carnegie Corporation of New York City for the preparation of a series of *Source Books in the History of the Sciences*. They will be under the general editorship of Professor Gregory D. Walcott, of Hamline University, St. Paul, Minn. The volumes will present the most important contributions of the most eminent scientists from the Renaissance to the present. Seven different fields of science are being covered by special committees under the supervision of the following: Frederick Barry, professor of chemistry, Columbia University; Joseph S. Ames, professor of physics, the Johns Hopkins University; Harlow Shapley, professor of astronomy, Harvard University; Alfred M. Tozzer, professor of anthropology, Harvard University; David Eugene Smith, professor of mathematics, Columbia University; Edwin G. Conklin, professor of zoology, Princeton University; R. T. Chamberlin, professor of geology, University of Chicago. The first volume, on astronomy, will be ready for publication within the next few months.

The Smithsonian Institution has engaged to prepare a series of twelve books to be known as the Smithsonian scientific series, under the general editorship of the acting secretary. It is the purpose of the series to give pictures of the activities of the whole institution and its branches. The publication is not intended for the specialist nor in any sense is it a collection of monographs, but is rather intended to present those features of the greatest interest to the average intelligent reader with no special training along technical lines. It is expected that the individual books of the series will come out at various intervals during the next two years.

At the recent meeting of the board of managers of the Wistar Institute of Anatomy and Biology, Philadelphia, the titles of professor and assistant professor were discontinued and a new series of titles designating members of the scientific staff were adopted. As the chief function of the institute is the promotion of research in biology the following titles were adopted as being most appropriate: Member, associate member, associate, and fellow. At the same meeting Dr. Helen Dean King was elected a member of the institute.

Errata. In the article by Dr. G. De Geer on the "Geochronology as based on Solar Radiation" (Science, 1927, LXVI, p. 458), in line 14 of the second column for "this" read "the," in line 22 of the fourth column omit the words "already made" and in line 37 of the fifth column for "non" read "now."

UNIVERSITY AND EDUCATIONAL NOTES

The income from a bequest of $100,000 from the late Thomas U. Coe, of Bangor, which has recently become available at the University of Maine, is to be used as a foundation for research. Projects bearing on the developing of the state are to be submitted by the faculty for approval under this fund.

The chemistry building of the South Dakota State College, Brookings, S. Dak., was totally destroyed by fire on February 4, 1928. All records and material are a total loss.

Sir Arthur Shipley, late master of Christ's College, left £5,500 to Christ's College for the endowment of a fellowship, along with various other bequests, including some relics of Darwin.

The Rio de Janeiro correspondent of the *Journal* of the American Medical Association writes that the president of the Minas Geraes has signed the law creating a state university. This will include at first four colleges, namely, law, engineering, medicine and odontology and pharmacy. The medical school will have an annual endowment of 600,000 milreis (about $72,000).

Dr. C. W. Hungerford, professor of plant pathology in the agricultural college of the University of Idaho, has been appointed assistant dean of the college of agriculture and vice-director of the Idaho Agricultural Experiment Station.

At the University of California, Dr. Chauncey D. Leake, associate professor at the University of Wisconsin, has been appointed professor of pharmacology, and Dr. Alfred C. Reed has been appointed professor of tropical medicine in the George Williams Hooper Foundation for Medical Research.

Dr. Laurence Selling, Portland, has been appointed clinical professor of medicine and head of the department of medicine of the University of Oregon Medical School.

Dr. Willis Dew Gatch has been appointed head of the department of surgery, including gynecology and orthopedic surgery, in the Indiana University School of Medicine, succeeding the late Dr. John H. Oliver.

Wilson F. Brown, instructor in chemical engineering at the Ohio State University, has been appointed to an associate professorship at the Kansas Agricultural College, to take charge of the work in industrial chemistry and chemical engineering.

Dr. Gustav Hertz, professor of experimental physics in the University of Halle, has been appointed to succeed Professor Kurlbaum as professor of physics at the Technische Hochschule, Berlin.

DR. F. HUND, of Göttingen, has been called to an associate professorship of theoretical physics at the University of Rostock.

DISCUSSION AND CORRESPONDENCE

THREE NOTABLE BOOKS ON THE HISTORY OF MATHEMATICS OF THE GREEKS

THE Belgian engineer, Paul Ver Eecke, inspector general of labor, has made three notable contributions to enrich our knowledge of Greek mathematical science. While the works of Archimedes, Apollonius and Diophantos have long been available to English students through the learned labor of Sir Thomas L. Health, there have not been available modern editions in French. The Belgian scholar performs this service for French readers. The titles of these works are as follows:

Les Oeuvres Complètes d'Archimède, (Paris-Brussels, 1921; LX, 554 pp. with 253 diagrams). Price 20 belgas.

Les Coniques d'Apollonius de Perge, (Bruges, Desclée de Brouwer & Co., 1923; LII, 645 pp.). Price 20 belgas.

Diophante d'Alexandrie. Les six livres arithmétiques et le livre des nombres polygones. Oeuvres traduites pour la première fois du Grec en français. Avec une introduction et des notes. (Bruges, 1926; LXXXXII, 300 pp.). Price 15 belgas.

These volumes are all fine specimens of the printer's art, an ornament to any library. A further volume is in preparation on the Spherics of Theodosius of Tripoli.

In all three volumes Mr. Ver Eecke demonstrates his familiarity with the field of Greek mathematics. The notes given constitute a source of information to which historians of science must have recourse in the many problems connected with these authors.

Particular attention has been paid by the author to the importance of the works of Archimedes, Apollonius and Diophantos in the development of European mathematics during the seventeenth and eighteenth centuries. It is highly desirable to stress this point since through these classical works the ancient mathematics became the source of inspiration for the modern mathematics. The birth of the analytical geometry and of the calculus connects thus directly with the mathematics of Greece.

It is the hope of the publishers that a number of American libraries will subscribe to the series. The price per volume is under three dollars and is much less than works of this character published elsewhere in Europe or in America. The publication performs a real service to scholarship, and must have constituted a serious financial problem at the present time for the publishers. The two later volumes have been issued with the support of the Fondation Universitaire de Belgique.

LOUIS C. KARPINSKI

UNIVERSITY OF MICHIGAN

ON MOLECULAR DIAMETERS IN GAS REACTIONS

IN a recent note published in this journal,[1] Dr. Bernard Lewis has called attention to a numerical error in our paper entitled "On Chemical Activation by Collisions."[2] We are of course very sorry that this error occurred and desire to thank Dr. Lewis for calling attention to it.

However, on the basis of the revised figures our friendly criticisms of the Fowler and Rideal[3] theory of chemical activation by collisions, using ordinary kinetic theory diameters for unactivated molecules, are not greatly altered.

It would still be necessary on the basis of the revised figures to assume that the *deactivational* diameter for N_2O_5 is considerably more than 60 times as great as the *activational* diameter, if the rate of activation is to be great enough to maintain the reaction first order down to a pressure of 0.05 mm. And this assumption is attended by the difficulties which we pointed out in the next to the last paragraph of our article, namely, that in a deactivational collision molecules which come within the large distance given by the deactivational diameter will mysteriously be drawn together to the much smaller distance corresponding to an ordinary kinetic theory collision and will then fly apart in deactivated states.

On the other hand, it no longer appears that the deactivational diameters would have to be so great that the effective volume of an activated molecule would be large enough to contain many ordinary molecules at 0.05 mm. pressure. Allowing, however, a reasonable excess in the rate of activation over that of reaction, we still find that the effective volume of the activated molecules is large enough to contain several other molecules and this is a notion which gives rise to considerable difficulty.

Finally, we may call attention again to a consideration which bears no relation to diameters, namely, that it certainly would be very surprising if the collision of chemically unactivated molecules having sufficient energy to activate one of them, should practically always result in the transfer of nearly all of the energy to one of the molecules.

RICHARD C. TOLMAN,
DON M. YOST,
ROSCOE G. DICKINSON

PASADENA, CALIFORNIA

[1] SCIENCE, 66, 331 (1927).
[2] *Proc. Nat. Acad.*, 13, 188 (1927).
[3] *Proc. Roy. Soc.*, 113, 571 (1927).

ANOTHER RECORD OF THE FRESH-WATER JELLY-FISH

DR. SCHMITT'S recent notice[1] in SCIENCE prompts the recording of the following data. On November 30, 1927, a small "balanced" glass tank in the laboratory of the New York Aquarium was noted to contain a number of medusæ. These were referred to the *Microhydra* stage of *Craspedacusta sowerbii* (Lankester). The conditions under which they appeared were as follows. The aquarium measured 20″ by 12″ by 12″ and was exposed to a strong northwestern light. The temperature of the water ranged from 20° to 28° C. It contained a dense growth of various kinds of aquatic plants, which for the most part were being choked off by a thick mat of algæ that, however, did not grow on the glass. There were living in it about ten young Pœciliidæ of undetermined species from San Domingo (probably *Heterandria versicolor* Günther). Most of the plants came from Wilmington, North Carolina, about a month earlier and it is supposed that they are responsible for the introduction of the organism, for the other plants had been living in the aquarium for at least a year. It is thought unlikely that the medusæ were brought from San Domingo with the fishes or that they were introduced with the tap-water used for this aquarium.

The medusæ increased in number up to about December 1, and from then on to the present date, December 22, have gradually fallen off, so that they number probably less than a dozen, whereas at their highest concentration there were at least four or five to the cubic inch. At all times they could be seen either pulsating their way upward or slowly descending in an inverted position.

Dr. Ruth Howland, of Washington Square College, has had one of her students, Mr. S. J. Gancher, studying their development and he has succeeded in finding a number of the hydroids. To date none has been seen to bud off medusæ, nor have the medusæ been seen to develop into mature *Craspedacusta*.

By transferring some of the plants into another tank a new colony was established, although it did not thrive very well and at this date none could be found.

C. M. BREDER, JR.

NEW YORK AQUARIUM

[1] "Additional records of the occurrence of the fresh-water jelly-fish." Schmitt, Waldo L., SCIENCE, Vol. LXVII, 1927, p. 591.

CONCERNING THE TRANSMISSION OF AN ACQUIRED CHARACTER IN FLAX

IN SCIENCE of September 30, 1927, Dean Henry L. Bolley suggested that the resistance of a plant to flax wilt is an indication of the transmission of an acquired character. The general conclusion drawn in his article does not seem to be warranted by the facts presented, especially since the inheritance of acquired characters has been so often disproved. The writer agrees with Dean Bolley in that a wilt resistant flax may be rapidly obtained and it can then transmit its resistance in succeeding generations. The point of criticism is that the wilt resistant characteristic is in all probability present in the beginning and is not observed so strikingly at first, due to the large percentage of susceptible plants that succumb to the disease. With the susceptible plants dead and no longer producing seed, the seed obtained from the wilt resistant plants, when sown another year, show a higher percentage of survival than the original planting. Thus, after a few years, a highly resistant strain of flax might be obtained due to the plants of different degrees of susceptibility dying off or merely a "survival of the fittest." While the above happens in many mixtures of flax it might also occur in the so-called pure line, the term pure line in these cases being relative and not absolute. A variety of flax may be called a pure line for certain characters because these characters have been studied and are known to be pure. However, if the wilt resistance is not one of the characters included in the previous study it may not be a pure line for wilt resistance. This is indicated by the results obtained in Michigan with selections that originated from a relatively pure line. When grown upon wilt-free soil these selections were not different from the parent in yields of seed, deseeded straw and fiber. The statistical odds determined by Students Method for six selections, for these three characters are 1:1. But when grown on wilt sick soil, the significant differences in performance of different strains indicate a rather wide variation in resistance to flax wilt. One selection, showing no difference under wilt-free conditions gave odds of 9:1 for germination (emergence of seedlings) and 500:1 for per cent. of normal plants to seeds sown. Another selection gave odds of 93:1 for germination in wilt sick soil and only 8:1 for per cent. of normal plants to seed sown. The seeds in these tests were of Russian origin and, so far as is known, had been grown upon non-wilt sick soil. The possibility of variation due to crossing must be considered. In Michigan, where the flax was grown, tests have shown from zero to three per cent. natural crossing, depending on the spacing and seasonal conditions. It seems probable that the variation in wilt resistance may be due to unselected factors in an otherwise pure line or possibly to natural crossing rather than a gradual change in a hereditary gene.

B. B. ROBINSON

FIBER INVESTIGATIONS,
U. S. DEPARTMENT OF AGRICULTURE

THE BEGINNING OF WINTER

IN the discussions relating to the beginning of winter that have appeared from time to time in SCIENCE, one phase of the question seems to have received hardly sufficient attention.

If we look up what the Century and Standard Dictionaries have to say about winter or the seasons, we find that historically and, apparently until recent times, popularly, the general conception of winter was that it covered the three coldest months of the year. The idea involved was simply our experience of average meteorological or climatic conditions. In most parts of the north temperate zone the interval from the first of December to the end of February was regarded as representing this period, and modern meteorological data seem to indicate that this does represent a satisfactorily close approximation. The exact beginning of the coldest period doubtless varies somewhat in different regions. In the District of Columbia it falls on the seventh of December;[1] in Minneapolis apparently about the third of December.[2]

More recently there has been manifest a growing tendency, especially in the United States, to change this conception and to assert that winter should be regarded as beginning with the winter solstice and ending with the vernal equinox. As nearly as I can ascertain, this is due to a certain number of astronomers, with the enthusiastic support of a multitude of newspaper scientists. The favorite expression of the latter group is that "astronomically considered, winter begins at the winter solstice." Of course, "astronomically considered," winter does nothing of the kind. If it is possible to consider astronomically an event which is not astronomical in nature, it is the middle of winter that, in the northern hemisphere, should be regarded as coinciding with the solstice, for it is at the solstice that the sun appears farthest to the south, the day is shortest, and the heat received per second on unit area of horizontal surface is a minimum. As a matter of fact, however, there is a lag in the seasons such that the coming of winter is considerably delayed, though not to the degree that would cause its beginning to coincide, even approximately, with the solstice. As far as winter is concerned, the solstice is the solstice, and nothing more.

In spite of ancient usage, it might be desirable to modify the conception of the term winter, if any good reason could be advanced for making the change, but all the argument seems to point in the contrary direction. To nearly every one, scientific men and laymen alike, the coldest quarter of the year, the hottest quarter, and the quarters of intermediate temperature are of direct personal interest and importance. They govern many of our daily habits, plans and activities. To very few people except astronomers are the solstices and the equinoxes of more than general interest. Educated people are supposed to have a fair idea of their significance and time of occurrence, but to enforce this knowledge by erecting them as monuments by which to date the seasons hardly seems wise. It is not the way to teach science or respect for science. In fact, it seems to be generating a distinctly wrong impression. Many people seem to have acquired the idea that something occurs at the solstice which, according to the laws of nature, definitely fixes this as the beginning of winter. They do not realize that to declare that winter begins at the solstice is as arbitrary as it would be to declare that it begins on the nineteenth or the twelfth or the twenty-fifth of December.

There is evident at times an unfortunate tendency on the part of one or another group of scientific workers to take a word of general usage and give it a special meaning which adapts it better to their particular purposes, and then to insist that this should be accepted as the essential meaning. If astronomers find it useful to have a name for the period from the winter solstice to the vernal equinox, it would be desirable, in order to lessen the misapprehension and confusion that are resulting, to choose another term than winter. Failing this, they should be especially careful to point out to inquirers that their use of the word is in a special sense, which does not affect and is not intended to supersede the old-established meaning.

C. N. FENNER

GEOPHYSICAL LABORATORY,
WASHINGTON, D. C.

[1] W. P. White: SCIENCE 62, 286.

[2] C. H. Briggs: SCIENCE 65, 424.

QUOTATIONS

ONE TOOTH GONE WRONG

THIS week's excitement about the "million dollar tooth" from Nebraska is a trifle belated. It is now two months since Dr. William K. Gregory, one of the original examiners of this famous tooth, decided that it had belonged neither to an ape nor a man and published this conclusion in SCIENCE. No evolutionist slept less well for this explosion of the tooth's significance. To correct conclusions that turn out to be false is a continual duty of scientific men, and even false assumptions not infrequently result in progress by uncovering facts or engendering ideas previously unknown. It is to be noted, too, that the scientists who now reject the man-like origin of the Nebraska tooth are the same who originally accepted it. They are merely correcting a mistaken theory which they previously proposed, something which all scientific men do almost daily and as a matter of course.

To imply that the theory of evolution is in the least endangered by this discovery of a mistake about a single fossil is as though a bridge builder abandoned his bridge and helped to destroy it because a single girder, not yet built into the structure, was found defective on the testing floor. Certainly no evolutionist believes that the theory is impaired. Had the tooth proved really to belong to some man-like or ape-like creature, that might have meant something about the history of the New World monkeys. It would neither have strengthened nor weakened materially the idea that evolution is a fact.

To have the public interested in science is a great advantage to both parties, but not entirely free from danger. Scientific research going on in a show window might mislead watchers who tarry too short a time to understand what it is all about. When first found the Nebraska tooth was heralded popularly beyond its real importance. Doubtless its fall will be too widely hailed now as another "mistake" of the scientists. In truth it is but a trivial incident in the slow rise of the edifice of science. The theory of evolution is far too hardy a creation to be ruined by losing one tooth.—*New York Herald-Tribune.*

SCIENTIFIC BOOKS

The Abilities of Man, their Nature and Measurement. By C. SPEARMAN. New York, The Macmillan Co., 1927. vi + 415 + xxxii pp.

THE Grote professor of philosophy of mind at the University of London has written an important book. It could not be otherwise when the book represents the cumulation of intellectual endeavor for a period of a quarter century by such as he. It may well be that he does not know exactly what his theories and facts signify; it is certain that I do not. The work has been supported during its progress by the collaboration of a multitude of Spearman's pupils and by others, it has drawn widely upon the investigations of other schools, it has also had constant opposition and the book has been severely criticized in a review in *Nature* (August 6, 1927, p. 180) which has led to an interchange of views between author and reviewer (*Nature,* November 12, 1927, p. 690). Into this difference I will not enter except to say that whether the book is mathematically complete or not does not interest me; this is unimportant. Science advances not so much by the completeness or elegance of its mathematics as by the significance of its facts. You can not upset the findings of the "Origin of Species" either by the contraposition of your religious convictions or by observing that Darwin's statistical technique was not up to standard. Science goes forward upon "evidence beyond reasonable doubt"; to that evidence incomplete mathematics may contribute valuable elements.

Spearman's chief thesis is that when a group of persons x, y, z, . . . are given a test *a,* say of arithmetic or spelling or literary interpretation, the marks m_{ax}, m_{ay}, m_{az}, . . . which they score represent in part their respective general intelligences g_x, g_y, g_z, . . . and in part their special abilities in the subject, s_{ax}, s_{ay}, s_{az}, . . . This would seem incontrovertible provided we mean by ability in the subject, ability to get scores in the test. The necessity for this proviso may be illustrated as follows. I have some general intelligence; I have some mathematical ability; yet if an examiner should set me a mathematical test in Yiddish, which might be "easy meat" for a lot of candidates for admission to our colleges, I should miserably fail. It may further be remarked that the scores m_{ax}, m_{ay}, . . . may depend on the manner of scoring used by the examiner or his clerk. For example, if the test be of the simple sort where a large number of questions are answered yes or no, one method of scoring is to count the number of right answers, R_x, R_y, . . .; another method is to take the difference between the numbers right and wrong $(R-W)_x$, $(R-W)_y$, ... If all the N questions are answered, the scores are equivalent since $W = N - R$ and the series of scores R_x, R_y, . . . and $2R_x - N$, $2R_y - N$, . . . are in the same order, will give the same correlations with other tests, etc. But if some of the questions are unanswered (U), the second series becomes $2R_x - U_x - N$, $2R_y - U_y - N$, . . . which need not be equivalent to R_x, R_y, ... How are we to compare the answers of two persons to 50 questions if one answers 40 all correctly and the other answers all 50 with 45 right and 5 wrong?

The next thesis is that when a battery of tests *a, b,* . . . are sufficiently different, so that the scores may be assumed to have in common only the general intelligence we may write for the nk marks of the n individual x, y, z, . . . on the k tests *a, b,* . . .

$$m_{ax} = c_a g_x + s'_{ax} \qquad m_{bx} = c_b g_x + s'_{bx}$$
$$m_{ay} = c_a g_y + s'_{ay} \qquad m_{by} = c_b g_x + s'_{by} \qquad (1)$$

in such a manner that the general intelligence g and the special abilities s′, are uncorrelated, *i.e.,*

$$\Sigma g_x s'_{ax} = O, \qquad \Sigma g_x s'_{bx} = O, \ldots \qquad (2)$$
$$\Sigma s'_{ax} s'_{bx} = O, \qquad \Sigma s'_{ax} s'_{cx} = O, \ldots \qquad (3)$$

when the summation runs over the individuals x, y, z, ... This leads to some correlation algebra to prove both that such a resolution of the marks is possible and that it is unique. I have read the proofs with care (including the references to the literature, not all of which has been reproduced in the book) and have found no errors in the mathematics. Yet I am not entirely happy, satisfied. I should like to have found at least one example worked out in detail—one set of nk scores for n individuals on k tests worked through to the determination of the n values g_x, g_y, . . . of the general intelligences of those individuals and of the nk values s'_{ax}, s'_{ay}, . . .; s'_{bx}, s'_{by}, . . .; . . . of their special abilities on each of the tests. Theorems which prove the existence of some possibility do not satisfy the practical applied mathematician—we do not so much want to know that there is a solution to the problem as to know what the solution is! I will work an example below.

What solution does the author offer us? (First he adopts scales which reduce the scores on each test so that they have the same dispersion about their means, we may take it as unity, which is also the dispersion of g.) If r_{ag} be the correlation coefficient between g and the test a, he shows that the solution is

$$g_x = r_{ag} m_{ax}$$

with a probable error of $.6745\ (1 - r^2_{ag})^{1/2}$. Note that the answer is a regression equation. We do not know the individual values g_x, g_y, . . .; we could write

$$g_x = r_{ag} m_{ax} + e_{ax}$$
$$g_y = r_{ag} m_{ay} + e_{ay}$$

where $e^2_{ax} + e^2_{ay} + \ldots = n(1 - r^2_{ag})$. If the author desires to prove that testing does not determine the general intelligence of the persons tested he has succeeded. Why did he pick on test *a* to determine g? Evidently one could equally well write

$$g_x = r_{bg} m_{bx}, \text{ etc.}$$

with a probable error $.6745\ (1 - r^2_{bg})^{1/2}$, etc. Practically we might choose that test as *a* which has the highest correlation with g. Better, he shows how to weight the different tests so as to get a combined score *t* which best determines g. In the example this best score gives $r_{tg} = .75$ so that the probable error in g_x is $.6745 \times .6614 = .446$. When we recall that the scale of g is such that the standard deviation of g is unity or that one half of the n values of g lie between $-.67$ and $+.67$, two thirds of them between -1.0 and $+1.0$, we can appreciate the significance of a probable error of .45. The solution for the special ability is likewise

$$s_{ax} = (1 - r^2_{ag})^{1/2} m_{ax}$$

with the probable error $.6745\ r_{ag}$. The better the test *a* estimates g the worse it estimates the special ability. Spearman's comment is: "We are faced by the fact that the current measurements of specific abilities—upon which have come to hang the weal or woe of countless individuals in industry and otherwise—are little more than the blind leading the blind." Rather pessimistic I call it, possibly unjustifiably so in view of such success as persons like O'Connor (West Lynn Works, General Electric Company) have in their placement work.

Spearman gives a long discussion of the attempts that have been made to define general intelligence. He does not define it, he computes it, and at that only by a regression equation, he does not measure it any more than he would weigh a person by computing his weight from his height through a regression equation of weight on height. He sets forth a hypothesis that the general intelligence is energy, the special abilities are engines, with apparently the will as engineer. This is allegory. If intelligence were energy it should be measured in ergs—but again he calls it a force (p. 414), so perhaps he thinks of measuring it in dynes. Or perchance the whole is mere logomachy. It would be interesting to enquire which of the technical physical terms is most like g, the general intelligence. Perhaps it might be efficiency! It would also be interesting to know just what he or Maxwell Garnett (a competent applied mathematician) means by the word unique in the proof that the resolution into g's and s's is unique. He can hardly mean that the regression equation $g_x : \sigma_g = r_{ag} m_{ax} : \sigma_a$ is unique since there is one such for each test and they give different results. If he means that given the nk grades m_{ax}, m_{bx}, . . ., m_{ay} . . . we can determine the actual values of g_x, g_y, . . ., why are we given the regression?

Example (preamble). If we can assign the k quantities c_a, c_b, . . . and the n values g_x, g_y, . . . equations (1) will determine the nk special abilities s′ from the nk grades m. Equations (2) if the n values g_x, g_y, . . . are known will determine the k values c_a, c_b, . . . as $c_a = \sigma_a r_{ag}/\sigma_g$. To have the intelligence g on a uniform scale we shall assume $\sigma_g = 1$ which gives one quadratic equation between the n values g_x, g_y, . . .

$$g^2_x + g^2_y + g^2_z + \ldots + g^2_n = n \qquad (4)$$

We must find the k coefficients r_{ag}. Equations (3) when expressed in terms of the m's and g's give the equations

$$r_{ag} r_{bg} = r_{ab}, \qquad r_{ag} r_{cg} = r_{ac} \qquad (3)$$

and if there be three or more tests enable us to solve for r_{ag}, etc., as

$$r_{ag} = \sqrt{\frac{r_{ab} r_{ac}}{r_{bc}}}, \text{ etc.} \qquad (5)$$

This requires that the values r_{ag} should be fractional or (if all the correlations r_{ab}, r_{ac}, r_{bc}, . . . between tests be positive, as is usually the case) that

$$r_{bc} \gtreqless r_{ab} r_{ac} \qquad (6)$$

or that the partial coefficients $r_{bc.a}$ shall all be positive, and, if there are more than three tests, that the so-called tetrad relations vanish, *i.e.*,

$$r_{ac} r_{bd} - r_{ad} r_{bc} = 0. \qquad (7)$$

These relations (6) and (7) are verified within the experimental error with respect to a large variety of intelligence tests. There is the equation

$$g_x + g_y + g_z \ . \ . \ . + g_n = 0 \qquad (8)$$

introduced to simplify the analysis and refer all g's to their mean. If the m's are also thus expressed, as is most convenient, the s's will be relative to their means. The k equations (5) are linear in the g's, *viz.*,

$$m_{ax} g_x + . \ . \ . + m_{an} g_n = n \ r_{ag} \sigma_a \qquad (5')$$

We have, therefore, in (5′), (8) and (4) the number k+1 of linear equations and one quadratic equation in the n quantities g. It would seem as though the n values g could be found with n−k−2 degrees of freedom, *i.e.*, that, as n is generally much larger than k+2, the solution should be indeterminate rather than unique.

Example (*solution*). Try a case. Let the marks of 6 students on 3 tests be (the first columns give the actual marks, the second columns give the differences from the means)

	a		b		c	
1	10	5	8	3	1	2
2	8	3	5	0	9	4
3	6	1	9	4	4	−1
4	4	−1	7	2	8	3
5	2	−3	0	−5	1	−4
6	0	−5	1	−4	1	−4
$6\sigma^2$		70		70		62

$$r_{bc} = .66, \quad r_{ac} = .73 \quad r_{ab} = .74$$

The equations to be solved are

$$5g_1 + 3g_2 + g_3 - g_4 - 3g_5 - 5g_6 = 18.5$$
$$3g_1 + 0g_2 + 4g_3 + 2g_4 - 5g_5 - 4g_6 = 16.7$$
$$2g_1 + 4g_2 - g_3 + 3g_4 - 4g_5 - 4g_6 = 16.3$$
$$g_1 + g_2 + g_3 + g_4 + g_5 + g_6 = 0$$
$$g^2_1 + g^2_2 + g^2_3 + g^2_4 + g^2_5 + g^2_6 = 6$$

The result of solving the first four for g_1, g_2, g_5, g_6 in terms of g_3 and g_4 and substituting in the last is

$$g_3 = .49 - .7g_4 \pm .89_4 \sqrt{(-g^2_4 + .40g_4 + .069)}$$

The radical is positive only if g_4 lies between −.14 and +.52 and any value of g_4 between these limits is possible. For the two limits the solutions for the g's are

				diff.
$g_1 =$	.91	$g_1 =$	1.43	−.5
$g_2 =$	1.21	$g_2 =$	.42	+.8
$g_3 =$	.59	$g_3 =$	.12	+.5
$g_4 =$	−.14	$g_4 =$	.52	−.7
$g_5 =$	−1.47	$g_5 =$	−.80	−.7
$g_6 =$	−1.10	$g_6 =$	−1.69	+.6

Notice that the ranges of possible intelligence for the six are different; we have a better line on 1 and 3 than on 6 and know least about 2.

Let us next compute the special abilities so standardized that their standard deviations are unity. The equations given by Spearman are like

$$m_{a1}/\sigma_a = r_{ag} g_1 + \sqrt{1 - r^2_{ag}} \ s_{a1}$$
$$m_{a1}/3.4 = .905 \ g_1 + .42 \ s_{a1}$$
$$s_{a1} = .7 \ m_{a1} - 2.1 \ g_1$$

On the basis of the extreme alternative solutions given above we have

				diff.
$s_{a1} =$	1.6	$s_{a1} =$	.4	+1.2
$s_{a2} =$	−.4	$s_{a2} =$	1.2	−1.6
$s_{a3} =$	−.5	$s_{a3} =$	.5	−1.0
$s_{a4} =$	−.4	$s_{a4} =$	−1.8	+1.4
$s_{a5} =$	+1.0	$s_{a5} =$	−.4	+1.4
$s_{a6} =$	−1.2	$s_{a6} =$	+.1	−1.3

Similarly we could compute for tests *b* and *c* the limits of specific ability. (The calculations given above have been carried to so few places that a positive check can not be expected, either for the zero mean or the unit standard deviation.) What we have shown is that the complete solution can be obtained but is indeterminate. We have had no need of any harder mathematics than the solution of a set of k+1 linear equations and 1 quadratic equation. We do not need the generalized Bravais distribution (as used by Garnett) and in view of Yule's wise comments on mental measurements (*Brit. J. Psych.*, vol. 12, p. 100.) to all of which I hereby subscribe, it would seem quite superfluous to introduce this higher mathematics, involving a probability theory which probably does not apply anyhow, to make determinate (if it does) that which without it seems indeterminate.

Do g_x, g_y, . . . whether determined or undeterminable represent the intelligence of x, y, . . .? The author advances a deal of argument and of statistics to show that they do. This is for psychologists, not for me, to assess. I believe he does not adequately emphasize the fact that they represent the intelligence only relative to the set-up of the tests. That this is so is evident from general considerations of the transformation theory of correlation algebra; but as even the term "transformation theory of correlation algebra" seemed unknown and unintelligible to a large group of persons professionally interested in statistics and in education when I recently mentioned it to them, I take the space, in a review already too long, to expound the obvious. 1°, If we have nk marks of n individuals x, y, z, . . . on k tests *a, b, c,* . . . we may combine these marks into new sets of scores, call them *a′, b′, c′,* . . . , in a linear fashion as

$$m'_{ax} = c_{11}\, m_{ax} + c_{12} m_{bx} + \dots$$
$$m'_{ag} = c_{11}\, m_{ay} + c_{12} m_{by} + \dots$$

$$m'_{bx} = c_{21}\, m_{ax} + c_{22} m_{by} + \dots$$

$$m'_{cx} = c_{31}\, m_{ax} + c_{32} m_{by} + \dots$$

with k^2 constants c_{ij}. These new scores m′ contain all the information of the old scores because they can be solved for the old scores m, but the information is differently assembled. It may be that these scores do not measure any particular ability such as spelling or literary interpretation or mathematical judgment, but they do represent scores involving certain weighted combinations of such abilities and with my limited knowledge of intelligence testing seem to represent some sorts of ability. 2°, Irrespective of whether the tetrad relations (7) are fulfilled, we can choose the constants c_{ij} in infinitely many ways so that the new scores are all uncorrelated, *i.e.,* $r'_{ab} = r'_{ac} = r'_{bc} = \dots = 0$. In this case the tetrad equations for the new correlation coefficients must vanish. Now if $g_x, g_y, \dots$ be the general intelligence of the persons tested the equations (3′) can no longer be solved as in (5) for $r'_{ag}, r'_{bg}, \dots$ because (5) become indeterminate; but inspection of the equations

$$r'_{ag}\, r'_{ag} = r_{ab} = 0$$
$$r'_{ag}\, r'_{cg} = r_{ac} = 0$$

shows that all of the correlations of g to the new scores must vanish except at most one. Which one? As the equations defining *a′, b′, c′,* . . . are largely arbitrary, the symmetrical and natural conclusion would be that none of them are correlated with g. Or we might so form one of them say *a′* as to agree that it represents the intelligence g with $r'_{ag} = 1$ and the others represent special abilities independent of g. Next, 3°, to be more specific we may take as one simple definition of *a′, b′, c′,* . . .

$$m'_{ax} = m_{ax}$$
$$m'_{bx} = m_{bx} - \sigma_b r_{ab} m_{ax}/\sigma_a$$
$$m'_{cx} = m_{cx} + \beta m_{bx} + \alpha m_a$$

and determine β, α, so that $r'_{ac} = 0$, $r'_{bc} = 0$, and so on. Now as we know r_{ag} by (5) as other than 0, it follows that $r'_{ag} = r_{ag} \neq 0$ and that the remaining values r'_{bg}, r'_{cg}, . . . all vanish. But from the definition of *b′*

$$0 = \sigma'_b\, r'_{bg} = \sigma_b (r_{bg} - r_{ab} r_{ag})$$
or
$$r_{bg} - r_{ab} r_{ag} = 0$$

This last equation is, however, impossible since we know that $r_{ag} r_{bg} = r_{ab}$. Hence, 4°, any set of values $g_x, g_y, \dots$ for the general intelligence of x, y, . . . which will go with the set-up of tests *a, b, c,* . . . can not possibly go with the set-up *a′, b′, c′,* . . . but must be replaced by new values $g'_x, g'_y, \dots$ approximate to that set-up. Yet the information we had in the nk scores of x, y, . . . on *a, b,* . . . is all contained in the nk scores assigned to x, y, . . . on *a′, b′,* . . .; the persons x, y, . . . are the same but their intelligences have changed—the old values whether indeterminate or unique will no longer do. What does this leave of the concept of the intelligence of an individual x as measured by g_x? Apparently only that it is relative to the set-up, which is the obvious proposition that I set out to prove.

The intelligence tester may object that the scores on *a′, b′* . . . mean nothing, are mere artificialities, whereas those on *a, b,* . . . are real things and mean something. I would not deny the objection. Although hypothetical unrealities may illuminate the significance of realities, it is the realities that make science. All I was trying to do was to supplement Spearman's discussion of the universality of g with a little contribution on the relativity of g—as might be expected of an erstwhile physicist! It seems to be an undeniable statistical fact that batteries of intelligence tests as given and as scored tend to be what has been termed hierarchical in that they tend to satisfy the tetrad relations (7). This fact means something, it needs to be explained, Spearman has offered an explanation. Possibly the explanation should have laid more emphasis on the tests and less on the general intelligence —I do not know—but in Spearman's system we have a method of examining our data, of discussing its implications, of organizing it into a philosophical system, just as we have in Einstein's, and at least for the immediate future the system propounded in "The Abilities of Man" can not be ignored by those working in its field. That is why I said that the Grote professor of philosophy of mind at the University of London has written an important book. Moreover, it is clearly, spiritedly. suggestively, in places even provocatively, written; intelligible and entertaining even to the general reader. The mathematics has been put out of the way in a highly compressed appendix. I have chosen to take the risk of misrepresenting the character of the book by writing a very lop-sided review with its emphasis chiefly on the appendix because I know that this has offered difficulties to some very intelligent readers, because it appears logically fundamental to the whole system, and because some of its important logical implications seem not to have been expressed by the author in the main text.

Edwin B. Wilson
Harvard School of Public Health

SPECIAL ARTICLES

TELESCOPIC OBSERVATION OF CATHODE AND ANODE POINTS

1. *Bright and dark sparks.* While the behavior of the anode in case of a mucronate electrode has been summarized,[1] further consideration of the cathode point is desirable. In this case the needle is to be critically set, so that the convection current is just about to pass into the spark condition. The set may often be made more sensitive, by waiting for some time until a convection current incidentally strikes and this may often be hastened by drawing sparks out of the cathode with a metal bridging the spark gap.

Since the U-tube interferometer is rather cumbersome for general observation, it may often be replaced by a suitable ear trumpet listening for the frequency of the crackle of sparks; or still better by a short range telescope (objective 6 or 8 inches off) refocussed on the cathode point. Whenever the convection current passes, a bright oval cathode glow is seen in the telescope like the nucleus of a comet, while in the dark even the convection current itself may be seen looking much like a cometary tail. As soon as any spark transfer takes place, this oval glow is extinguished.

The spark successions which follow the extinction of the cathode glow are not, however, of the same kind. There are two distinct types, bright and dark.

[1] *Proceedings National Academy of Sciences,* February, 1928.

The first consists of diffuse bright purple spark filaments, passing with marked crackling between many favorable points of the electrode plates, the needle point being ignored. Being relatively luminous, they are the most desirable, but they often refuse to appear or are not sustained.

The second type which I shall have to call by a misnomer dark sparks, show no spark lines at all, but consist of a faint violet surface glow at the edges of the anode plate. The cathode glow is none the less extinguished. They are apt to be the more usual (and undesirable) occurrence, particularly after long observation. There is no appreciable crackling heard in the ear trumpet. I have therefore (without certain evidence) regarded the bright sparks, since they nearly always appear when the cathode is earthed, as resulting from a promiscuous issue of positive electrons from preferred parts of anode plate (since it here has no needle point), whereas the so-called dark sparks may be the corresponding convection discharge of positive ions from such parts of the anode plate.

2. *Negatively charged body.* The most available instrument for extinguishing the cathode glow is the charged hard rubber rod. If this is highly charged and the critical set sensitive, the rod may be passed normally along the arc of a vertical circle even 50 cm in radius around the spark gap, from right to left, always keeping the glow dark (Fig. 1). As soon as the rod passes outside of the circle by a few centimeters, the glow at once relights. This may be repeated indefinitely. A brass ball, 8–10 cm in diameter on an insulated handle and charged at the cathode of the machine is also convenient, though it acts from a smaller radius (15 cm) from the spark gap. A proof plane is still weaker. Now if the negative rod at a radius of 50 cm (say) evokes a shower of bright sparks persistently, then it usually happens that at a smaller radius of say 20 cm these bright sparks disappear, to reappear at the radius of 50 cm again. This was at first a very puzzling observation; but as the cathode glow is kept extinguished, it is a passage of the bright type of spark into the dark equivalent

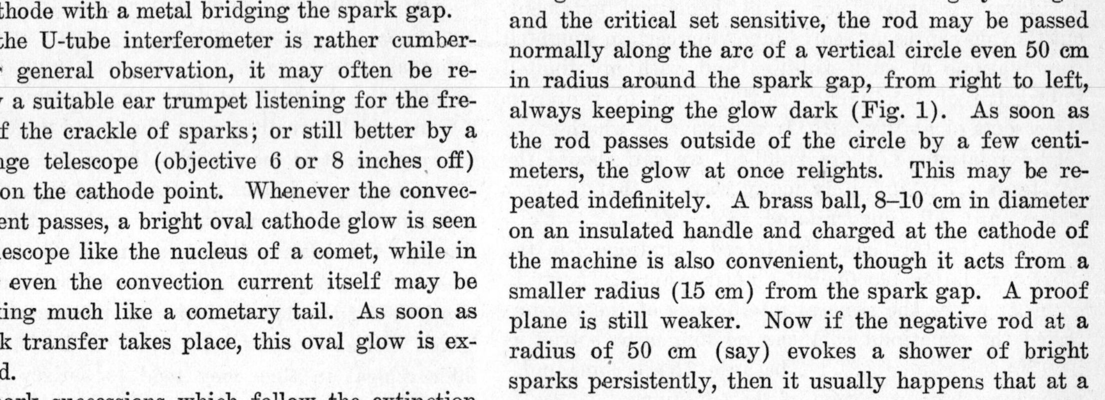

Fig. 1

just described. Since it requires a greater protrusion, y, of positive needle ($y > .3$ cm) to evoke the anode convection current than the anode spark succession ($y = .10$ to .14 cm for darts, $y > .14$ cm for cones), the above inference for bright and dark sparks is not unreasonable. The impression is often made as if the negative glow were transferred to the edge of the positive plate and became a positive surface glow.

Finally, since the negative body acts to extinguish the cathode glow from a definite radius, one may argue, as I have heretofore, that it imposes an effective negative increment of potential throughout the field of the spark gap.

3. *Telescopic anode reactions.* To obtain darts (snapping white linear sparks) from the cathode point in the absence of the anode needle has not been possible. They appear at the anode point (cathode point absent) as an integration of the earlier diffuse spark filaments for the narrow ranges of protrusion y, given, unless there is special stimulation (earthing the cathode, for instance) when darts appear sooner. The positive convection current does not appear until $y = .3$ cm or later, when a mere point of light tips the anode in the dark spark gap. Between these limits the dart degenerates into a purplish diffuse cone with its apex at the anode needle (see fig. 2). In the telescope the divergence is filamentary and scattering. As y ($< .3$ cm) increases, the cone grows narrower and weaker, and in the ear trumpet the crackling runs up into high frequencies. The spark gap is now in a good form for experiment. If, for instance, the negative rod[2] is put in the symmetrical position (1), figure 2, the straight symmetrical axis a of the cone changes to an axis b concave towards the rod, and more so as the rod is nearer. This proves adequately that the emitted rays, a, are positive ions and the method may be useful for measurement. Again let y be further increased until the luminous cone just vanishes and the dark convection current appears. Then it will be found that the negative rod at (2) on the anode side restores the cone a and keeps it; whereas the negative rod at (3) on the cathode side quenches the cone. The test may be repeated indefinitely. The negative rod at (2) or (3) is thus equivalent to a decrement or increment, respectively, of the protrusion y.

CARL BARUS

BROWN UNIVERSITY

[2] The magnetic field arising from a metal conductor is not convenient. The anode is much more capricious than the cathode. The convection current may strike too soon, or too late, or again not at all. The above data are good averages for the given machine and spark gap. Some control is possible, however, by the methods of § 3. The axial flexure of fig. 2 can not be obtained with the negative convection current.

FACTOR H IN THE NUTRITION OF TROUT

SINCE the time of Magendie, investigators have tried to develop purified rations which would meet all the requirements of the animal body for growth and reproduction. The greatest success in these attempts has undoubtedly been attained with the rat. That even the rat fails to show an optimum growth upon a simplified ration containing all the known elements, is evident from many experiments and especially from the recent reports of Osborne and Mendel,[1] and Palmer and Kennedy.[2]

The fact that many of the discoveries in nutrition that have been made in rearing rats have found ready applications in feeding the higher animals has led to the subtle assumption that the nutritional requirements of all species of animal life are the same. The reflection of such natural philosophy is seen in the wide-spread use of cod liver oil, yeast and other vitamin supplements in the hatcheries of the United States that are engaged in rearing trout. Although Laufberger[3] has stated that fish require vitamins in their food, his work fails to furnish convincing evidence that these are related to any of the known accessory substances required by the higher animals.

In order to furnish a more rational basis for feeding trout we have conducted a series of experiments upon their growth curves when they are fed diets of widely different compositions. These experiments have been performed at the Burlington hatchery in the state of Connecticut. This hatchery is unusually well equipped for such experiments, since it has a constant supply of pure spring water which exhibits very slight temperature variations. Each experimental group of trout contained fifty fingerlings which were confined in separate troughs with individual water supplies and outlets. The efficacy of a given diet was judged by the average growth rate and by the mortality rate.

In our first series of ten experiments we employed nine purified rations made up of casein, boiled starch, salt mixture, cod liver oil and yeast. In four of these the protein was incorporated at various levels from ten to seventy-five per cent. In two, lard was included at twenty-two and fifty-seven per cent. levels varying the other factors to secure adequate salt and protein intake. From one, cod liver oil was omitted; in another yeast was lacking and still another contained no salt mixture. For purposes of comparison a diet of dried skimmed milk was employed. For seven weeks all the fingerlings, except those upon the

[1] Osborne, T. B., and Mendel, L. B., *J. Biol. Chem.*, 1926, LXIX, 661.

[2] Palmer, L. S., and Kennedy, C., *J. Biol. Chem.*, 1927, LXXV, 619.

[3] Laufberger, V., *Physiol. Abstracts*, 1926, XI, 221.

ten per cent. protein diet, grew normally practically doubling their weight. Those upon the lowest protein level refused to grow but ate their ration readily and remained active.

At the end of seven weeks all groups commenced to die except those upon the low protein diet and those upon the dried skimmed milk. The latter continued to grow until at the end of sixteen weeks they averaged five times their initial weight. At this time they ceased to grow and began to die. The entire fifty had died at the end of the twentieth week.

At the end of the fourteenth week those upon the low protein diet began to die. This continued at a regular rate until the twentieth week when only seventeen remained alive. They were now divided into two groups. One of these received raw liver and the other remained upon the purified ration with the low protein level. Those fed raw liver immediately assumed an optimum growth rate and in nine weeks tripled their weight. Those kept upon the low protein diet did not grow and all died in the course of the next five weeks.

From these experiments we must conclude that raw meat contains some factors which is neither vitamin A, B or D and which is an unrecognized dietary factor essential for the growth of trout. Dried skimmed milk contains a small amount of this factor but not enough to permit continued growth for long periods, Furthermore trout require a diet containing more than ten per cent. protein for normal growth. In case they are stunted by a protein deficiency the power or resuming growth is not lost even at the end of five months. In the course of these experiments it was observed that trout which are stunted by protein deficiency do not develop the spots commonly observed upon this species of eastern brook trout while those that are allowed to grow develop these spots quite normally. The development of these is a function of growth and not of age.

In a second series of experiments twenty different rations were employed. One of these was a purified feedstuff of casein, starch, salt mixture, cod liver oil and yeast modeled after those previously used and commonly employed in work upon rats. This was accompanied by a ration of the same composition except that it contained orange juice. The trout showed a reaction that duplicated our previous experience. They displayed a slight initial growth followed by failure. Hence we must conclude that the unknown factor H which is found in raw meat is not vitamin C.

In this second group of experiments attempts were made to determine if this factor were sensitive to heat like that described by Dr. Wulzen[4] in her studies upon planaria. Comparative studies were made between raw liver and that which had been cooked and dried for other experiments upon blood regeneration, by the senior author.[5] Dried liver gave no response while fresh liver gave the usual excellent growth. From this, one must conclude that the factor in liver responsible for growth in trout is destroyed by heat. Furthermore it is an entirely different factor than that responsible for blood formation since the same cooked, dried liver produces excellent blood regeneration in rats, but fails to promote growth in trout. We have studied two commercial dried meats and find both of them entirely lacking in this growth stimulating power.

Two other diets which have been studied may be worthy of record. We have fed trout Sherman's stock ration for rats which consists of whole wheat, dried whole milk, calcium carbonate and sodium chloride. Trout consume this ration readily, but do not grow. From this we may infer that factor H is not related to vitamin E.

In order to determine whether the growth secured upon dried skimmed milk was the result of its composition or some extra factor which it contained, we prepared a synthetic product of casein, lactose and salt mixture and fed this supplemented with cod liver oil and yeast. Only slight growth resulted from this ration and the trout began to die at the end of the fifth week. This experiment is being repeated with part of the protein furnished by lactalbumin. We must conclude that natural dried skimmed milk contains factor H and "synthetic milk" lacks it.

Both the yeast and the cod liver oil employed in these experiments were products of tested potency.

The discovery of factor H to which we have called attention must be credited to those pioneers in the rearing and propagation of fish who long before our generation found that trout required raw meat for proper growth and would fail upon the dried products.

This work has been made possible through the Connecticut Board of Fisheries and Game and their representatives Mr. Titcomb and Mr. Cobb. We also wish to thank Professor L. B. Mendel, of Yale, and L. A. Maynard, of Cornell, for useful suggestions in the course of these experiments.

The complete data with growth curves will appear in the *Transactions* of the American Fisheries Society for 1927.

C. M. McCay
F. C. Bing
W. E. Dilley

Cornell University

[4] Wulzen, R., Science, 1927, LXV, 331.

[5] McCay, C. M., *Am. J. Physiol.*, 1928, LXXIV, 16.

SCIENCE

VOL. LXVII MARCH 9, 1928 No. 1732

CONTENTS

Wings for the Spirit: PROFESSOR HOWARD T. KARSNER ... 251
Commemoration of the Death of Newton: DR. FREDERICK E. BRASCH ... 255
Frank W. Very: J. GORDON OGDEN ... 262
Scientific Events:
The Expedition to Combat Sleeping Sickness in French Africa; Casting of a Large Disk of Optical Glass by the U. S. Bureau of Standards; Experiment Station of the Georgia State College; Award of the Charles Reid Barnes Life Membership in the American Society of Plant Physiologists ... 263
Scientific Notes and News ... 265
University and Educational Notes ... 269
Discussion and Correspondence:
Tree Frogs and Pitcher Plants: PROFESSOR E. A. ANDREWS. *The Occurrence of Conjugation in Paramecium Calkinsi:* DR. D. H. WENRICH and C. C. WANG. *Centrifuging Filterable Viruses:* H. H. MCKINNEY. *Colorimetric Methods in Biology:* DR. F. B. SUMNER. *Specialization and Cooperation in Research:* B. A. BEHREND. *A Function of Regional Scientific Societies:* THOS. LARGE. *Children who Run on all Fours:* ALEŠ HRDLIČKA ... 269
Scientific Books:
Moir on the Antiquity of Man: DR. H. F. OSBORN 273
Scientific Apparatus and Laboratory Methods:
A Photographic Plate that Penetrates Desert Haze: DR. ELIOT BLACKWELDER. *Modified Water Regulator:* DR. TAGE SKOGSBERG ... 275
Special Articles:
Devonian Plant Localities of New York: CHESTER A. ARNOLD. *Effect of Ultra-violet Light upon Digitalis Purpurea:* ADELIA MCCREA ... 276
Science News ... x

SCIENCE: A Weekly Journal devoted to the Advancement of Science, edited by J. McKeen Cattell and published every Friday by

THE SCIENCE PRESS

New York City: Grand Central Terminal.

Lancaster, Pa. Garrison, N. Y.

Annual Subscription, $6.00. Single Copies, 15 Cts.

SCIENCE is the official organ of the American Association for the Advancement of Science. Information regarding membership in the Association may be secured from the office of the permanent secretary, in the Smithsonian Institution Building, Washington, D. C.

Entered as second-class matter July 18, 1923, at the Post Office at Lancaster, Pa., under the Act of March 8, 1879.

WINGS FOR THE SPIRIT[1]

The dedication to-day of facilities for the prosecution of laboratory and research work of the Mount Sinai Hospital has far greater significance than the addition of a unit to the institution. The achievements of this great hospital are well known to its patients and to their friends. The medical profession is familiar with the professional skill of your staff of physicians and nurses and the high efficiency of your administrators. Adequately supporting these, stands a Board of Trustees, noted for philanthropy, loyal to and sympathetic with the ideals of a modern hospital. The example you have so generously set will serve as a stimulus to other hospitals not as yet so fully equipped. The new facilities mean an increased effectiveness in the care of patients. The influence of your staff, improving their work with the facilities now offered, will be felt by the entire profession. The nation will more and more perceptibly become awakened to the conception that hospitals must move forward with the newer knowledge available to medical science. Contributions to prevention, diagnosis and cure of disease, inspired by the conveniences now offered in these walls, will be of lasting benefit to generations yet unborn. In discussing with you the achievement which your generosity has brought to fruition, I hope to make clear to you some of the matters, spiritual and material, which you may expect to result from your benefaction.

The fact that the practice of medicine in a well-conducted hospital requires a laboratory for aid in diagnosis and treatment is not generally realized by those who have the responsibility for providing funds. It is but too well known that numerous hospitals are designed without adequate laboratory space and equipment; and, even in those so provided, it is not uncommon to find insufficient appropriation for personnel and maintenance. For our own benefit, and perhaps for a more far reaching purpose, it may be well to support the implication which opens this paragraph. The primary objective of the laboratory is to aid in diagnosis, which is fundamental to proper treatment. The laboratory may even take its part in the treatment, through consultation with surgeons and by the preparation of such things as vac-

[1] Address at the dedication of the Laboratory of Pathology, Mount Sinai Hospital, Cleveland, Ohio, November 8, 1927.

cines and serums. The laboratory is also, in a sense, the guardian of the health of the hospital. Its workers detect the presence of infectious diseases in patients and hospital personnel and may guide the authorities in preventing the development of an epidemic. The efficacy of sterilization of materials used in the surgery may be determined, and services may be equally useful in other similar matters.

The work includes diagnosis of tumors and other surgical diseases, the selection of donors for blood transfusion, the identification of bacteria and other parasites, as for example of tuberculosis meningitis, pneumonia and malaria, the chemical examination of the blood in order to aid in distinguishing between several otherwise confusing diseases, the performance of such tests as the Widal test for typhoid fever and the Wassermann test for syphilis, and numerous other procedures. Without an accurate diagnosis, treatment is entirely empirical, may be worthless and might be dangerous. The laboratory, then, is concerned largely with aid in the diagnosis of disease. It is to be noted that the laboratory rarely makes the diagnosis, for there are few diseases in which the laboratory has a test which is absolutely and finally conclusive.

A matter deserving the frankest discussion is the autopsy. The Jew is considered to be the most reluctant to permit autopsy of all those who constitute Occidental civilization. Much attention has been given the religious aspects of this question. It is said that the rabbis of the Talmud consented to the autopsy if it honored the dead or if it gave information of immediate value to someone suffering with the same disease as the deceased. The autopsy was to be forbidden if it desecrated the dead or if the benefit were to be of only general rather than immediately applicable value. The far reaching significance of science of all kinds was not appreciated at that time. Men know now what science has done for them and the prospects it has in store. The autopsy is the basis of much that we have learned about disease and will continue to contribute to our progress. Religion is not static but shows evolution. Modern opinion in the church is generally to the effect that the value of the autopsy to the relatives, to the community and to medicine outweighs regulations that were made at other times and under other circumstances. Rabbi J. B. Levinthal, of Philadelphia, is quoted as saying that the postmortem examination is not forbidden by the Jewish Rabbinical Law, and further, that "where a postmortem examination may result in the discovery of the origin or cause of some serious disease, it is my firm conviction that thus to serve humanity is sanctifying, rather than desecrating, the dead." Any autopsy may serve this purpose and no one can say in advance what the results will be. Hospital administrators and officers are generally of the opinion that "the history of a hospital fatality is not complete unless the (autopsy) report of the pathologist is included," and what applies to hospital patients applies equally to those who may die at home. We must demand of our pathologists that the dead body be regarded as the material remains of a loved soul and that they treat it accordingly. Only with rare exception is such a caution necessary. In spite of all sentiment and even superstition, the autopsy may well be regarded as an honor to the dead and is certainly a service to mankind. "When a patient dies a great debt is owed humanity in order that the patient shall not have died in vain."

The time is not so long past when the physician considered it beneath his dignity to touch the patient and employed a barber to perform the surgical operations. Physical diagnosis, including palpation, percussion and auscultation, is little more than a century old. We have then only recently emerged into a period, where, in addition to taking a history and making an inspection, the physician actually handles his patient to discover what is wrong. Once having taken the step, the physician was whole hearted about it, and in the middle of the last century the physician was tasting certain body fluids to detect diabetes and the pathologist tasting cerebro-spinal fluid in order to give an accurate description. Now the physician uses a thermometer to determine temperature instead of feeling for it, he uses a sphygmomanometer to determine blood and pulse pressure instead of depending upon his sense of touch, he uses an electrocardiograph to study cardiac irregularity instead of guessing at the cause, he examines materials by chemical tests instead of by taste, and in a wide variety of ways has improved his methods. He has not only enlarged his field of examination but continuously has developed increasing technical precision. In brief, he uses every means available to determine the nature of his patient's disease.

The young men now in our medical schools, the physicians of the future, are trained in the methods of the clinic and the laboratory and learn to evaluate the results of each. They wish to know what causes the disease, to eliminate it if possible, what organ or organs exhibit disease and how the functions are disturbed, to correct them if possible. The problem has become so intricate that no one man can master all its ramifications. Hence, specialties have developed and a group of men has grown up who have a particular interest in the laboratory side of medicine. These men are of a special mould, foregoing the glamour of practice and its rewards, because of a peculiar interest in the scientific aspects of laboratory work. They must have training and a proper equipment for work. The fact that in the past good work has been done and important discoveries made under adverse physical conditions should not divert us from the provision of better things. The world moves and the high speed of civilized life in general is reflected in the laboratory. If the commercial plant has labor saving devices, so should the laboratory. If the factory has special provision for light and ventilation, so should the laboratory. If the shop has precise instruments, so should the laboratory. The pathologist deals with affairs immediately concerned with human life and suffering. His is no eight-hour day. The import of his work is beyond question and he should be provided with equipment so that it may be conducted with convenience, speed and precision.

These notations have dealt with material conceptions, but only as the basis for the soaring of the spirit. This spirit is the series of motives which actuate medicine. First there comes to mind the spirit of service. This is the great humanitarian spirit of the votaries of medicine, but is shared in greater or less part by all professional and business activities engaged productively for the welfare of man. Ancillary is the spirit of sacrifice which in its highest form is vicarious. Typified in its extreme on the Cross of Calvary, it is found on the battlefield, in industry, in business and the professions. Medicine points with pride and humility to its list of heroes who have given their health and lives for the promotion of knowledge. Then there is the spirit of truth, truth for its own sake, truth without reward other than the supreme joy which its discovery gives. All problems put before us are no more than amplifications of the question, what is the truth?

The spirit of service and of vicarious sacrifice is inherent in the forward urge of mankind. It transcends the flesh. So also is the nature of the spirit of truth. The truth itself, however, requires constant search. Blessed are those who can provide wings for the search and even more so are those who can don them creditably. It is your privilege to provide the wings here, building, equipment, personnel, funds, and it is for us to show you the way of the flight.

Truth as we find it is not absolute, and may not be the same to-morrow as it was yesterday or is to-day. Truth is revealed by the demonstration of facts, which represent observations dependent upon methods. Human imagination and ingenuity evolve new and improved methods and, as circumstances alter, truth may alter with them. In the fifth century before Christ, Protagoras said, "Man is the measure of all things" and taught "that there is no absolute truth, that we know things only as they appear to us through the senses." Thus rational thinking through the ages has drawn attention to philosophical relativity, and we must face the fact whether dealing in pure reason or in material science.

This discussion is preparatory to a consideration of the truth as revealed in the laboratory. Without such a background misconceptions may arise in thinking our wings to be more sturdy than they are. When we say that the laboratory deals with facts, we mean that by methods of delicacy and precision which meet the rules of scientific procedure, a conclusion can be reached that, within the limitations of the methods available, the truth has been demonstrated. A truism of science is to the effect that it is wasteful to deal in the fourth decimal when the third decimal will provide the necessary information. The third decimal is not necessarily exact in such an instance, but for scientific purposes it represents the truth. When the laboratory furnishes a report, it must be regarded as exact within the factors of error inherent in human nature and in the methods of study available. Increasing precision of instruments and methods tends to obviate the fallibility of our unaided senses. Quoting a recent article of Peabody, "the popular conception of a scientist as a man who works in a laboratory and uses instruments of precision is as inaccurate as it is superficial, for a scientist is known not by his technical processes but by his intellectual processes; and the essence of the scientific method of thought is that it proceeds in an orderly manner toward the establishment of a truth."

As concerns the patient, the truth of a given situation may be provided by the laboratory, but the truth of the whole picture is made up of the results of laboratory and clinic correlated by orderly processes of thought. The methods of the laboratory are those of a high degree of exactitude and the material is in such form as to permit of direct study. This and this only gives the laboratory a distinct advantage over the clinic, and it is for this reason that the modern clinician asks the aid of his laboratory colleague. Many clinical examinations are of necessity by indirect methods, and the further information yielded by laboratory tests is often of inestimable value to the welfare of the patient. A noted hospital administrator, not a pathologist, Bluestone, has said that "broadly speaking no hospital is larger than its pathological laboratory," and that "the progressiveness of a hospital is in direct ratio to the laboratory spirit which it maintains." Permit me to point out that the maintenance of this spirit, springing primarily in the professional staff, must, in order to be effective, have not merely the assent of administration and trustees, but their cordial and enthusiastic sympathy and support.

You have provided not only a laboratory, but also

a center for research in the medical sciences. The activities of skilled physicians differ according to training, aptitude and opportunity. He who is a practitioner applies the knowledge of the day to the care of the patients of the present. He who teaches trains a group of students for the care of patients of the near future. He who investigates disease deals not merely in matters of the present, but rather of the future near and remote. Examples of how discoveries may reach far into the future are numerous, but a few will suffice. The discovery of the circulation of the blood by William Harvey has enlightened the world for centuries. The discovery of immune processes by Louis Pasteur has been of inestimable value long after his death and will be so permanently. The discovery of the insect transmission of disease brought forth amazing fruit within the lifetime of its discoverer. The discoverers of insulin are still young men.

Pasteur said that "in the fields of observation, chance favors only the mind that is prepared," a statement that might serve to clarify for you some of the features of investigative work that may have been puzzling. In the first place great discoveries often seem to come out of a clear sky, but this is not literally true. The investigations have been conducted by trained persons with the "prepared mind." Behind them is a background of experience personal to them and to others as recorded in the literature. The prepared mind is prepared partly by a reasonable familiarity with the work of others through conference, attendance on scientific meetings and access to the literature, and principally by experience in the methods of science and productive original work. When the "readiness is all," an isolated observation may open a field of vision for one who is prepared and may mean nothing for one who is not. An amazing example of this is given by the great physiologist Claude Bernard in his book, recently translated, "An Introduction to the Study of Experimental Medicine." The urine of well fed rabbits is usually cloudy and alkaline. Bernard, by chance, noticed that the urine of rabbits which had just been purchased for his laboratory was clear and acid, and found that they had not been fed for several days. By a series of experiments and further observations, this occurrence became the background for the discovery of pancreatic digestion, not only of singular novelty and significance to physiology but applied daily in the clinics of to-day. Kanavel wisely says "great knowledge acquired from reading and not from actual experimentation engenders a benumbing subservience to the written word." The worker has ever an opportunity to which the reader has no access. Nevertheless, the worker is in a superior position to profit by observations if he knows what has gone before.

In the history of science, it would seem that the world must be prepared for discoveries before their exploitation is possible. The receptiveness for new announcements seems to depend upon general world progress, contributed to in various domains of art and science, to the observation of facts that in themselves seem to be of little significance and to discoveries of outstanding importance. The use of the term exploitation is with all scientific reserve, but its importance to the common welfare should not be underestimated. The fact that the work of Mendel, which underlies the modern work on genetics and heredity, had to be rediscovered, was largely due to the fact that at the time it was not exploited. In your provision for research in this fine building, you have not completed the task until you make provision for the suitable publication of the results, and the workers in the laboratory have not fulfilled their trust until reports have been made in channels of publication where they will be most useful.

These implications are preliminary to a brief discussion of the costs of scientific research. All financial investments have an element of uncertainty. The most secure usually have the smallest rate of return. Generally speaking, this applies to research. There is this important difference, however, in that the research investments of apparently small return may, by accumulation or by chance observation, form the basis for a research investment of large return. A study, which from its inception is certain to give a useful result, positive or negative, may furnish what might be called one of the fragments of a puzzle picture. When a sufficient number of fragments is accumulated, a creative imagination, piecing them together, may see the way to providing the final fragment which will clarify the composite whole. The most recent example is the discovery of insulin. Studies of the changes of sugars within the body have been conducted for many years and formed small fragments of the complete picture. A large fragment was provided by von Mering and Minkowski in the discovery of the relation of the pancreas to the metabolism of sugar. Another larger fragment was contributed by Opie in relating changes in the human pancreas to diabetes. The vision and work of Macleod, Banting, Best and Collip, based on this background, furnished the final and immediately practical fragment which made the picture whole. Further studies along this line are directed toward filling in certain details of importance and rendering the practical features more satisfactory.

As with investments, the speculative factor must be considered. No wise investor indulges his gambling instinct in projects which examination shows are without the slightest guarantee of return. So the scientific investigator should not consume time and energy in studies which to the experienced student are without promise. There are, however, speculative investments where the promise of large return is as great as the promise of a total loss. The investigator frequently finds himself facing a position of this sort. It is for him to say whether or not he will chance his time and energy on the study and if he decide affirmatively, those who give him financial support should back him without stint, for he has more to lose than mere money and what he gains is for the benefit of mankind.

You repeatedly entrust your health and lives to the judgment of the physicians and surgeons of this fine hospital. There should be no hesitation in entrusting the funds which you give to it, in expanding amounts, to the judgment of those who give their lives and energy to the research work within its walls. A great philosopher, René Descartes, said many years ago that "if ever the human race is raised to its highest practical level, intellectually, morally and physically, the science of medicine will perform that service."

The designer of the aeroplane gives little to humanity if his machine is to remain without fuel and there would be no practical benefit without the adventurous spirit which through pioneering in unexplored fields leads on to progress and to newer and broader visions. The plane is built, the laboratory completed. All honor to the designers and builders. The fuel is not merely the material means of operation, but it must volatilize as faith in the pilot and his crew, faith in their productive capacity, faith in their guiding genius. The pilot has many mechanisms to oversee. These should be as nearly perfect as the mind and hand of man can devise, so that the spirit shall not be hampered. The pilot is the directing intellect of the flight. Give freedom to his imagination and energy. The time will come when his wings are no longer rigid and he can fly freely in the skies of truth toward his ultimate objective, the welfare of man.

My congratulations to the trustees, the director and the staff of Mount Sinai Hospital. May they live long and may their work prosper.

HOWARD T. KARSNER
WESTERN RESERVE UNIVERSITY

COMMEMORATION OF THE BI-CENTENARY OF THE DEATH OF NEWTON[1]

THE fourth annual meeting of The History of Science Society was held in pursuance of an act of its council of last year, to commemorate the bi-centenary of the death of Sir Isaac Newton. In view of this unusual occasion, and of the manifold interests Newton had, it was therefore considered expedient to ask those societies most interested to cooperate by appointing representatives on the committee preparing the program. The following names are those who served:

COMMITTEE ON PROGRAM

Dr. R. C. Archibald, Brown University Dr. E. W. Brown, Yale University Dr. Florian Cajori, University of California	The American Mathematical Society and The Mathematical Association of America
Dr. A. O. Leuschner, University of California Dr. Frederick H. Seares, Mount Wilson Observatory	The American Astronomical Society
Dr. Leigh Page, Yale University	The American Physical Society
Dr. David Eugene Smith, Columbia University, Chairman Dr. Henry Crew, Northwestern University	The History of Science Society
Mr. Frederick E. Brasch, Library of Congress	Secretary to the Committee

The meeting was called to order by the president of The History of Science Society, Dr. David Eugene Smith, at 10 o'clock A. M., Friday, November 25, 1927, in the Educational Hall of the American Museum of Natural History, New York City.

The two days' program consisted entirely of papers on various phases of Sir Isaac Newton's contributions to astronomy, mathematics, physics, chemistry, religion, problems of the mint, and the development of science since his day, also some indication of Newton's influence on the early science in the American Colonies from 1687 to 1779. Two papers were devoted to each subject and these were given by scholars of distinction—from both the United States and Canada. Twelve papers reviewing Newton's work from the present historical standpoint made what is probably one of the most notable of single contributions to scientific literature. These addresses are to be published (by the History of Science Society) in a memorial volume.

The object of this American commemoration was twofold, first to honor the great name of Newton, and

[1] Report of the meeting and exhibition under the auspices of the History of Science Society, held at the American Museum of Natural History, New York, November 25 and 26, 1927.

second to acquaint the younger generation of students, as well as the public at large, with the contributions made in the various fields of knowledge in which Newton labored. From the standpoint of interest and attendance, the meeting was successful.

Old England may justly feel proud of the recognition America (United States) has accorded her greatest philosopher. Similar celebrations have taken place. Particularly we note the program given in Grantham, Newton's birthplace, on Saturday, March 20, 1927, the exact date of the bi-centenary of his death, which was attended by many of the greatest scholars of the British Empire, as well as by representatives from abroad. Both commemorations will go down in history and furnish most interesting recapitulations of Newton's influence in the history of science and civilization.

Following the abstracts of papers presented, a brief account of the exhibition is given. Dr. David Eugene Smith, chairman of the first morning's program, gave the introductory address. He spoke of the occasion of the Commemoration and of the life of Sir Isaac Newton. He said in part:

We come here to-day for two major purposes: First, to pay our respects to the memory of a man who is rated by the world as one of its greatest geniuses; and second, to weigh once more, by modern criticism if not by scales of precision, the world's claim that its judgment is just.

Of the esteem in which Newton's work has been held for two centuries there is no question. Few men have ever fared so well. The justness of that esteem has, however, been seriously questioned by various scholars of reputation. There have been assertions that his word was not "as good as his bond"; that his influence upon British mathematics was not salutary; that he abandoned the altar of science for the fleshpots of Egypt; that the foundations of his greatest mathematical theory were weak and the theory was unstable; and that he stands as a fetich for the unthinking worship of the Anglo-Saxon. Nor have there been lacking expressions to the effect that, had he been the great genius that England asserts, his countrymen would long since have given to the public a definitive edition of his complete works, his correspondence, and his papers. Such editions are a common tribute paid by nations or societies to the memory of their great men. Why should England have published the monumental editions of Cayley's and Sylvester's works and yet have so neglected Newton and have allowed the Portsmouth papers to lie practically in oblivion? Was there not back of all the praise, a feeling that the nation had risen to his defense in an inglorious dispute, but that at heart it doubted his greatness?

These questions have not been raised merely by men of no intellectual capacity who seek a place in the limelight by decrying the work of others; by those who, as a French philosopher has put it, rail at greatness because they can not achieve it. They come from honest-minded men who really wish to know what it was that Newton accomplished to make him worthy of the acclaim that has been accorded him; who ask for an answer, without excess of praise, to the justifiable question, "What were Newton's real contributions to world knowledge?" To give and to receive this answer is one of the purposes of our meeting. The answer, however, can not be given with authority by any one man or by any small group of workers in a single field; it can come only from several men, representing the various major fields in which Newton showed an interest. It is with this thought in mind that representatives from different learned societies have been requested to place before other scholars a series of succinct but authoritative statements of his achievements.

When we review his life, his idiosyncrasies, his periods of contrast, and his doubts and ambitions and desire for place, may we not take some pleasure in thinking of him as a man—a man like most other men save in one particular—he had genius—a greater touch of divinity than comes to the rest of us?

The questions to be answered by the speakers will relate chiefly to Newton as a scholar, and upon the answers will depend our judgment of the justice of the praise that has been given him. One thing will not fail to stand out clearly, however, that few men have ever lived who explored so successfully as wide a range of human activities, and few who could so justly have used the well-known phrase,

Homo sum, et nihil humani a me alienum puto.

The second address was by Dr. Dayton C. Miller, of the Case School of Applied Science, who spoke on "Newton and Optics."

This convocation is held to commemorate the bicentenary of the death of Sir Isaac Newton which occurred in London on March 20, 1727. We are not now just discovering Newton's greatness; in his own life time he was regarded as the greatest man in intellectual achievement which the world had known; the greatest possible posthumous honors were done him. . . . Voltaire, a contemporary, said of Newton: "If all the geniuses of the universe were assembled, he should lead the band." The appreciation of his greatness has continually increased during the two centuries that have elapsed since his death. . . .

In the year 1668, Newton made the first reflecting telescope, but he had not yet discovered the nature of the spectrum, for in 1669 he helped Dr. Barrow in the publication of Barrow's lectures on optics, in which an erroneous theory of color is set forth. . . .

In the autumn of 1671, Newton made a second reflecting telescope and the fame of his researches, especially in optics, began to spread. He was proposed as a candidate for admission to the Royal Society in December, 1671, and was asked to send the reflecting telescope to the society for inspection. The instrument was sent to London, and was exhibited before the Society on January 11, 1672, at which time a description of the telescope was read, and Newton was elected a fellow of the society. This telescope has ever since remained with the society as one of its most cherished possessions. Newton was very much pleased with the honor of election to the Royal Society, and his acknowledgment to the secretary, sent one week later, says:

I desire that in your next letter you will inform me for what time the society continue their weekly meetings; because, if they continue them for any time, I am purposing them to be considered of and examined on account of a philosophical discovery, which induced me to the making of the said telescope, and which I doubt not but will prove much more grateful than the communication of that instrument, being in my judgment the oddest if not the most considerable detection which hath hitherto been made into the operations of nature.

This promise was fulfilled by a communication which was read just one month later and the "considerable detection into the operations of nature" proved to be the complete explanation of the nature of the solar spectrum, and the true theory of color. . . .

Nothing more was done in the domain of optics, until, in 1704, Newton published the first edition of his book called "Optics; or a Treatise of the Reflections, Refractions, Inflections and Colours of Light." There were slight additions made in the second edition which appeared in 1718. For our present purpose, it seems desirable to give a description of the contents of this book, which covers all of Newton's work in optics, and to make a kind of inventory of the optical developments due directly to his work, as interpreted in the light of the third century following their origin. . . .

Rays of Light, by impinging on any refracting or reflecting Surface, excite vibrations in the refracting or reflecting Medium or Substance, and by exciting them agitate the solid parts of the refracting or reflecting Body, and by agitating them cause the Body to grow warm or hot; that the vibrations thus excited are propagated in the refracting or reflecting Medium or Substance, much after the manner that vibrations are propagated in the Air for causing Sound, and move faster than the Rays so as to overtake them; and that when any Ray is in that part of the vibration which conspires with its Motion, it easily breaks through a refracting Surface, but when it is in the contrary part of the vibration which impedes its motion, it is easily reflected; and, by consequence, that every Ray is successively disposed to be easily reflected, or easily transmitted, by every vibration which overtakes it. But whether this Hypothesis be true or false I do not here consider.

The returns of the disposition of any Ray to be reflected I will call its Fits of easy Reflexion, and those of its disposition to be transmitted its Fits of easy Transmission, and the space it passes between every return and the next return, the Internal of its Fits. (p. 256.) . . .

It has been very generally stated that Newton adopted and developed the corpuscular theory of light, in which light consists of small particles and nothing else. This interpretation was really thrust upon him by his successors, for he was always exceedingly careful not to commit himself to any specific theory of the structure of light. Thirty years before his treatise appeared, when he was actively engaged in the optical researches, and was sending reports to the Royal Society, he wrote to Hooke, saying: "Were I to propound an hypothesis it should be this, that light is something capable of exciting vibrations in the ether." Again he says: "The hypothesis of light being a body, had I propounded it, had a much greater affinity with the objector's own hypothesis (Hooke's Undulatory Theory) than he is aware of, the vibrations of the ether being as useful and necessary in this as in his." . . .

The science of light to-day is indebted to Newton not alone for his discoveries in optics, but in a greater degree to his general influence upon the methods of philosophic thought. The discovery of universal gravitation is the discovery of the law of universal order, which is the basis and essential character of all science. The example of such profound and comprehensive philosophizing has been one of Newton's contributions to optics as well as to other sciences.

And now, two hundred years after the death of Newton, we in behalf of the science of optics, wish to join the great chorus of all the sciences in doing reverence to him, not for what he was, but for what he has been for these centuries, and for what he is now. We repeat the inscription on the Westminster Tablet which was erected in 1731:

LET MEN REJOICE
THAT SO GREAT A GLORY OF THE HUMAN RACE
HAS APPEARED

The third address was on Newton's Philosophy of Gravitation with special reference to Modern Relativity Ideas, by Dr. G. D. Birkhoff, of Harvard University.

Up to the time of the ancient Greeks, scientifically-minded men had accumulated comparatively few experimental facts. For the description of these facts ordinary geometrical space and measurable time, which seemed self-evident, were available. Copernicus took the space attached to the sun to be at rest. On this basis Kepler deduced his three laws of planetary motion and was led to correct ideas about the forces of gravitation. Newton's greatest achievement lay in overcoming many mathematical difficulties and establishing the laws of gravitation and of motion known by his name. It was stated that Newton's scientific procedure was according to the best general principles. The reason for the recent progress to the relativistic theory of gravitation was found in the accumulation of evidence that the physical universe is basically electro-magnetic, rather than dynamical. Nevertheless the Newtonian dynamical theory of space, time and gravitation will always stand, as the first and simplest approximation to the facts.

The final paper on the morning program was by Dr. W. W. Campbell, president of the University of California, upon "Newton's Influence upon the Development of Astrophysics."

Astrophysics is concerned with what the stars, comets, nebulae and other celestial bodies really are, and why they are as they are. Spectrum analysis, the most remarkable, the most fruitful system of analysis in existence, rests upon Sir Isaac Newton's discovery that white light—sunlight, starlight—contains light of all known pure colors—really an infinite variety of colors. When starlight is passed through a telescope and a spectrograph attached thereto, the light records a message on the photographic plate—the star's spectrum—which describes precisely the conditions prevailing in that star. The finding of spectroscopic Rosetta stones, by Kirchhoff in 1859, and by his many successors in our physical laboratories, is enabling us to read the messages which many thousands of stars have sent to us and written down for us. These messages tell us what chemical elements and compounds, in the form of vapors and gases, are present in the outer strata of the stars, in comets, in the many kinds of nebulae. They tell us that our chemical elements are widely—perhaps universally—distributed throughout the universe. They tell us whether a given star is approaching us or receding from us and with what speed; that a certain star is a giant or a dwarf star and how far away it is; and a seemingly endless procession of facts relating to the conditions existing in the stars and other heavenly bodies.

The law of gravitation, discovered by Newton, is enabling us to learn much concerning conditions in the interiors of the stars, the comets and other objects.

Sir Isaac, with his own hands, constructed and used the first reflecting telescope, the forerunner of the giant reflecting telescopes of to-day.

Newton developed a preference for the corpuscular theory of light, as opposed to the undulatory or wave theory. To this end he may have been influenced by the difficulty of understanding why light radiations escaped paying toll for their transmission through space by wave motion. In the last year or two many physicists—notably de Broglie, Schroedinger and others—appear to be advocating a combination of the corpuscular and undulatory theories of light, as Newton himself very definitely did. Astrophysicists will be tremendously interested to learn the real nature of light, so that they may apply its principles to the solution of many of their most difficult problems, such as those of stellar evolution.

Sir Isaac Newton was uniquely the great pioneer in astrophysics.

Dr. E. W. Brown, of Yale University, presided at the afternoon program and introduced Dr. M. I. Pupin, of Columbia University, as the first speaker, whose remarks were upon "Newton's Dynamics."

The bi-centennial commemoration of Newton's death turns our thoughts to his great achievements, and the greatest of them is his science of dynamics. This achievement is the crown of the scientific endeavors of the two centuries which preceded Newton.

The most precious part of the Copernicus, Brahe and Kepler triumph was the great dynamical problem which was suggested, and which can be stated in the form of the question: Why do the planets move in accordance with Kepler's laws? This question was a hopeless puzzle to the science of the sixteenth century.

The problems of pendulum motions and of the motions of projectiles yielded to Galileo, but his dynamical science could not answer the question: Why do the planets move in accordance with Kepler's laws? Neither could the dynamical science of Galileo's successors who preceded Newton answer it.

The momentum concept was created by Newton, and it is the most fundamental concept in his dynamics. His second law of motion expresses this fundamental character of the momentum concept by making its time rate of variation equal to the moving force. This measure of the acting and reacting forces not only conformed with the results of Galileo's experiments but, moreover, it shed new light upon them which was not visible to Galileo nor to any of Newton's predecessors. It also agreed with all impact experiments, particularly with their revelation that during the impact of elastic bodies no momentum is lost.

The analysis of these impact experiments in the light of the second law was very helpful in the formulation of the third law, the law of equality of actions and reactions. Newton's third law employs a terminology the importance of which can not be overstated.

Astronomical evidence supported Newton's answer and this assured the world that a new science, the science of dynamics, was born, and that Newton, inspired by Galileo, was its father. To this new science Newton added his great invention of a new mathematical art, the art of the differential and integral calculus.

Dr. Paul R. Heyl, of the U. S. Bureau of Standards, spoke on "Newton as an Experimental Philosopher."

Newton from his earliest years took delight in constructing mechanical devices, and his innate skill of hand served him well in later years.

Newton is sometimes called "the king of thought" but he was far from being merely a speculative philosopher. His reasoned conclusions were carefully tested by experiment wherever possible.

Newton turned his acquired skill in the making of lenses to what was then the new art of grinding and polishing reflectors for telescopes. So skilful did he become in the construction of such reflectors that the best London opticians could not equal those of his production.

Newton's skill with his hands was in part innate, but we must recognize that his superiority over the professional opticians of his time was doubtless due to the same cause that contributed to the excellence of the work of a certain painter, who when asked the secret of how he mixed his colors replied: "With brains, sir!" Newton's knowledge of geometry guided his technique, and furnished suggestions which could not have been expected to occur to the mind of the artisan of those days.

In his "Principia" as well as in the "Opticks" there is to be found evidence of Newton's skill of hand and experimental ingenuity.

Even the members of the Royal Society, a body of men selected for their excellence in scientific knowledge and attainments and, as the minutes of their meetings show, assiduous experimenters, bore witness to Newton's experimental skill. And yet I think that Newton would have been rather surprised had he heard himself described as an "experimental" philosopher, and would have considered the expression tautological. The scientific specialization of our time was unknown to him. The term philosopher meant then what its etymology signifies—a lover of wisdom, and wisdom (it was beginning to be recognized) was to be found by questioning nature by experiment.

The next paper related to the historical "Developments Following from Newton's Work," in which Professor E. W. Brown traced briefly the work of two centuries in following out the consequences of Newton's laws as applied to the moon and planets. To predict the future position of a heavenly body we must know how it has moved in the past. Some 100,000 observations of the sun and moon alone have been utilized, and besides these many hundreds of thousands of observations of stars have been made to regulate the clock which is of equal importance with the telescope to secure the necessary information. These masses of observations are all bound together into one whole by Newton's laws of motion and of gravitation. The development of the consequences of the laws must be done by mathematical methods and some of the ablest mathematicians have devoted large portions of their lives to the work.

But the laws are not only applicable to the motions of the heavenly bodies, but also to all our terrestrial machinery. The structure of a skyscraper, the safety of a railway bridge, the motion of a motor car, the flight of an airplane, the navigation of a ship across the ocean, the measure of time itself, depend fundamentally on Newton's laws. Many failures of our mechanical devices, especially of those which move at high speed, may be traced to lack of knowledge or lack of care in applying those laws.

The essential characteristic of Newton's laws is their power to predict with certainty. It is a remarkable feat to be able to foretell successfully within a second of time a century hence the moment when the moon or a planet will be observed due south. In the ordinary routine of the astronomer it is regularly done, even more accurately, five years ahead, and the leeway necessary when the interval is extended is known. We have now arrived at the place where we have been able to measure the deviations from the laws themselves as well as the deviation from correct running of our time keeper, the earth, in its daily motion round its axis, but this would not have been possible without the most careful working out of the consequences of the laws. Much remains to be done in applying them to stellar systems, especially globular clusters and spiral nebulae.

The paper from Dr. Florian Cajori, of the University of California, was read by Dr. Lao G. Simons, of Hunter College, who spoke in part upon "Newton's Twenty Years' Delay in announcing the Law of Gravitation."

It is well known that Newton in 1665 or 1666 first tested the law of universal gravitation, but that he did not announce the law until 1686. Before the year 1887, it was universally accepted that Newton's delay of about twenty years in announcing this great law was due to his having used in 1665 or 1666 too small a value for the size of the earth, so that in applying his gravitational hypothesis to the earth's attraction for the moon, he obtained a theoretical result for the distance a body falls from rest on the surface of the earth in one second which did not agree with the experiment, and that he could not get the two results to agree until the Frenchman, J. Picard, supplied a more accurate geodetic determination for the size of the earth.

At the two hundredth anniversary of the publication of Newton's "Principia," in 1887, the astronomer, J. C. Adams, and the mathematician, J. W. L. Glaisher, advanced another explanation of the twenty years' delay. They stated that in 1666 fairly accurate values of the earth's radius were known and that the real cause of the delay was the question how a sphere attracts an outside particle. This question Newton did not clear up until sometime in 1685, and not until then did he consider valid his proof of the law of gravitation, as applied to the earth and moon.

It is the purpose of this paper to make a searching study of what was really known in England respecting the size of the earth, before Picard made his measurements, and to subject the entire question of Newton's delay to a critical examination.

The paper was divided into five parts, which were as follows: British views of the size of the earth before 1671; Newton's gravitational calculation of 1665 or 1666; Newton's apparent indifference during 1666–1685 to earth measurements; an essential step in proving the law of gravitation, and conclusion.

The first paper for the second morning program was by Dr. L. C. Newell, of Boston University, who also presided at this session, and spoke on "Newton's Work in Alchemy and Chemistry."

Throughout his career as an experimenter in alchemy, Newton was a philosopher searching for a clue to some great generalization concerning the nature and properties of matter.

Although he conducted many chemical and alchemical experiments continuously for about thirty-five years, from 1661 to 1696, in his laboratory beside the great gate of Trinity College in Cambridge, his chief purpose does not seem to have been transmutation of base metals into fine gold, but rather a diligent search for a great principle, which would transform disconnected chemical phenomena into a philosophic system. He was not an alchemist in the usual meaning of the term, with its unethical implications.

Newton's early interest in chemistry is indicated by items in a note-book which has been assigned to his preadolescent years, Professor Newell went on to say. Among the "strictly chemical" items, which the boy had written down, were directions "for making allum water," "How to make lime water," "How to melt mettle quickly yea in a shel," and a prophecy of what chemists of the future were to strive for seriously, "a color for faces."

Newton experimented assiduously in chemistry and alchemy in the many years he spent at Trinity College, Cambridge, as a student, fellow and professor.

Commenting upon Newton's idea of atoms, as set forth in his work on "Opticks," Professor Newell stated that Newton was not far from certain aspects of our modern views on the constitution of matter. Indeed, if this statement of atoms, and if many of the queries propounded in the "Opticks," were stripped of their trappings and rewritten in modern terms, I think we would be compelled to appraise Newton's views as closely approximating modern interpretations of the constitution and behavior of matter.

Dr. George S. Brett, of the department of philosophy, Toronto University, presented a paper on "Newton's Place in the History of Religious Thought."

Newton's relation to the history of religious thought is defined partly by the actual work which he did on passages and books of the Bible, partly by the general influence which he exerted on the thought of the eighteenth century. In this paper reference is made to the specifically theological writings, but more attention is paid to the effects which his ideas of law and order produced upon writers who were concerned to follow his example in reconciling science with religion. The mechanistic philosophy of the eighteenth century was largely due to the attempt of the Newtonians to restate the principles of religion in a way that reconciled them with the idea of a universal reign of law. This idea of law as opposed to the purely sentimental or pietistic view of religion is taken to be the most permanent effect of Newton's work and is held to be the aspect of the subject which most clearly persists to the present time. Though this influence is indirect and is due to the application of Newton's ideas rather than to his own statements, it is the most important aspect of his relation to the progress of thought on religious questions.

George E. Roberts, vice-president of The National City Bank of New York, and formerly director of the United States Mints in Washington, D. C., spoke upon "Newton in the Mint."

Newton's appointment in the mint was eminently fitting in every respect, but not without a political bearing. He had represented the University of Cambridge in the Parliament which established William and Mary on the throne, and Macaulay says that he was the glory of the Whig party. The immediate occasion, however, was the problem which confronted the government in dealing with the coins in circulation, which had been clipped and debased until the currency situation was intolerable. Macaulay's account of the government's inability to make new coins circulate while this old money was in circulation at the same legal tender value is the classic illustration of Gresham's law that "bad money will drive out good money."

Newton was invited to accept the position of warden of the mint in 1696. It was not the highest office in the institution, but he was made master of the mint three years later, and held that place until his death in 1727. He discharged his official duties with fidelity and energy, particularly during the great recoinage which lasted three years.

The recoinage, however, did not end the monetary problems. When the old silver coins were completely replaced it was found that the new coins were being exported because they were undervalued in comparison with the gold coins, and thus the government was confronted with the problem which vexed the world for the next two hundred years, to-wit, how to make the two metals circulate concurrently upon equal terms under free coinage for both. The government addressed a letter to Newton asking his advice. He replied that silver was sent out of the country because it was more highly valued in proportion to gold elsewhere, and suggested that the gold coins might be reduced in weight, but intimated that it was hardly worth while because the relative values probably would change again shortly. His letter was a model of clarity as far as it went, but became a subject of a controversy between the partisans of bimetalism and the gold standard which lasted until practically the entire world had adopted the gold standard. Both sides sought to use the authority of his great name, but he proposed nothing more than a tentative adjustment of values, for which there were precedents. Evidently he fully comprehended the economic laws governing the fluctuations of the two metals, but he did not discuss the fundamental difficulty involved in trying to maintain two standards of value at the same time, or say anything about the theory of alternative standards.

The last paper, relating to "John Winthrop (1714–1779), America's First Astronomer and the First Disciple of Sir Isaac Newton in the Colonies," was by Frederick E. Brasch, of the Library of Congress, Washington, D. C.

The history of science in the American colonies centered itself in the work of John Winthrop, Hollis professor of mathematics and natural philosophy at Harvard College from 1738 to 1779. Winthrop graduated from the famous Boston Latin School and entered Harvard College where he became the leading scholar of his class. He was appointed to the professorship at the early age of twenty-four years and almost immediately assumed the honor position as a scholar of great ability. His principal work was, however, in the field of astronomy and he made such notable observations upon sun-spots, transits of Mercury and Venus, that he was honored by election as fellow to the Royal Society of London. With the cooperation of the college authorities and the colonial governor he was able to embark upon the first astronomical expedition that this country has ever undertaken, which was in 1761. Winthrop's mathematical ability led him to the more advanced studies which were now to be found in the works of the great Newton, and he soon secured for himself a copy of the "Principia Mathematica," third edition, 1726. This was the second copy known to be in the colonies. Yale College secured the first, namely, the second edition of 1713. The work resulting from Winthrop's studies of the "Principia" now revealed the true character of our scholar, for he was the first to introduce the subject of fluxion (calculus) in the colleges about 1751, also the first to establish a laboratory of physics for experimental purposes in 1746. All Winthrop's subsequent work in astronomy was based upon the "Principia." He was somewhat of a seismologist, as well as having advanced the science of meteorology by his long series of recorded observations, also of the northern lights. During Winthrop's long period at Harvard College he was offered twice the presidency, but refused due to not too good health. He was honored, however, as no man of his time, as a scholar and scientist as well as an ardent patriot, for he espoused the cause of Washington, Adams and others, whose friendship and counsel was always sought. Winthrop was the first scholar to receive the honorary degree of LL.D. of Harvard College, which he also received from the University of Edinburgh. His contemporaries at home and in England recognized Winthrop as the first Newtonian scholar in the colonies. His equals may have been Halley, Bradley and one other in England. Winthrop died at the age of sixty-five years in 1779, and lies buried in the King's Chapel churchyard in Boston, along with his ancestors, the first governor of Massachusetts and the first governor of Connecticut.

The great exhibition of books, portrait prints, letters, autographed documents and medallic illustrations of Sir Isaac Newton, and of his mathematical contemporaries, which supplemented the addresses, were all arranged in suitable cases in three sides of the hall in which the audience gathered. This most imposing collection probably will never be duplicated at any one time and in itself constituted one of the richest contributions to that phase of the history of science which goes to make this subject interesting and fascinating. The labor and excellent arrangement of these beautiful memorials was carried out under the personal direction of Dr. David Eugene Smith. From Dr. Smith's private collection came 125 of the most exquisite and beautiful portrait prints of Newton, of various ages and painters; also 25 medals of about that many engravers and also the largest assortment of letters and autographed documents. Dr. Smith loaned also over 40 various editions of Newton's "Principia," "Opticks," "Fluxions," "Universal Arithmetics," as well as essays on Newton's life and work.

Besides the Newton material from this same private collection came portraits and autographed letters of Halley, Barrows, Cotes, Wren, Wallis, Huyghens, Cassini, all friends and coworkers of Newton. There were also exhibited portraits of Flamsted, Leibnitz, Descartes, Bernoullis, Wolf, Gauss, LaPlace, Gassendi, Pascal, Kepler, Galileo and Copernicus. Most interesting probably was a collection of letters from Leibnitz to Newton with notes in Newton's handwriting. This copy of bound letters was from Newton's private library. Another collection of letters to Newton came from four generations of astronomers royal of France, the Cassini family, to whom Newton was indebted for his data on the size of the earth. From the Babson Institute, Wellesley, came also a magnificent collection of 36 items representing the various editions of Newton's work, the most interesting and valuable being a copy of the first edition of the "Principia Mathematica," 1687, and the reissue of the same book. The first item contained notes and corrections in Newton's own handwriting. Copies of the 1713 edition of "Principia," edited by Cotes, with an enlarged chapter on the "Lunar Theory and of Comets," and the 1726 edition edited by Pemberton, the last published during Newton's lifetime. There was also a copy of Newton's "Opticks," 2nd edition, with notes in his handwriting. All these contained Newton's book-plate and autograph, showing they were from his private library. Besides a collection of portrait prints of Newton, a cast of the sun-dial as well as of his inscription cut on the window sill of the Grantham grammar school made by the boy Newton.

From Mr. George A. Plimpton's (New York) great collection of rare arithmetics came 12 items of Newtonian collected works, as well as single volumes. One item was Newton's copy of a journal with his signature and numerous notes.

Through the courtesy of Dr. A. Koegh, librarian of Yale University, were loaned two books by Newton which have more than passing interest. A copy of the "Principia," 1713 edition, and of the "Opticks," 1706 edition, were presented to the colonial college in New Haven in 1714 by Sir Isaac himself.

Through the courtesy of Dr. L. C. Newell, of Boston University, Dr. S. Brodetsky, Leeds University and Grantham Public Library, came an interesting collection of prints, pamphlets and newspapers giving an elaborate account of the Newton birthplace, of his boyhood and of the bicentenary celebration at Grantham on March 20, 1927.

Six interesting photostat copies of various leaves of a precious commonplace note-book of Newton when a boy of seventeen years were exhibited. The original note-book is in the Pierpont Morgan Library, New York.

Mr. James Stokley, of Science Service, exhibited a copy of Riccioli's Almagestum Novum which came from Newton's library with his annotations, and Dr. Florian Cajori, University of California, exhibited single special items bearing upon Newton's religious writings.

Following are the members of the committee on arrangements: Dr. Lao G. Simons, *Chairman,* Hunter College; Dr. Vera Sanford, The Lincoln School; Miss Frances M. Clark, Teachers College; Miss Helen Walker, Teachers College; Dr. Lester S. Hill, Hunter College, and Mr. John A. Swenson, Wadleigh High School.

Frederick E. Brasch,
Secretary

Library of Congress,
Washington, D. C.

FRANK W. VERY

Supplementing the excellent article by H. H. Clayton, in a recent number of Science, concerning the passing of Professor Frank W. Very, may I be permitted the privilege of adding the sincere tribute of one of his former pupils?

From 1885 until 1895 it was the great privilege of the writer to be associated with Professor Very in the class room and in the field. Every Saturday afternoon, it was Professor Very's delight, in company with a number of young people, to go forth seeking the hidden treasures of field and forest, mine and hill-side, railroad cuttings, and ancient river beds and terraces. With scientific nicety he followed the wonderful trail made by old Mother Nature, and even the most arrant tyro among us was inspired by the keenness of our leader's perception, and the wonderful deductions made by him in the simplest language. We collected fossils, water-worn stones, cocoons, flowers, mosses, lichens, ferns, insects—in fact everything of scientific interest we happened to come across.

And then in the evening we assembled around his study table, either in the Allegheny Observatory, or in his own home, and went over the treasures of the day.

First of all, we were made to draw with scrupulous care the various objects, in order that we might see what was really there. Then there was a great hunting through the library for articles and descriptions. Professor Very superintended this research and illumined what we found with the light of his almost omniscient knowledge. It has never been my privilege to know a man more learned than he in so many different departments of science.

The writer is sure that throughout this broad land, there are thousands who have come under the gracious, kindly influence of Professor Very, and who will endorse these words of tribute to a great teacher.

J. GORDON OGDEN

FIFTH AVENUE HIGH SCHOOL,
PITTSBURGH, PENNSYLVANIA

SCIENTIFIC EVENTS

EXPEDITION TO COMBAT SLEEPING SICKNESS IN FRENCH AFRICA

THE organization of a government expedition to fight sleeping sickness in French equatorial Africa is reported by the New York *Herald*. Thirty-three French physicians and scientific men, under the auspices of the Pasteur Institute, will devote five years to combatting the disease and attempting to rid the colonies of the fatal tsetse fly.

Accompanying the decree authorizing the expedition was a letter from Leon Perrier, minister of colonies, to President Doumergue, stating that the present conditions in Africa made necessary special efforts to stamp out sleeping sickness above all other diseases.

The minister said sanitary conditions had become worse, due to the concentration of native labor in connection with railroad building. He suggested that, owing to the hazardous nature of the task and the length of service necessary, special awards be offered to those who volunteer. This was provided in the decree issued by the president. M. Perrier said he had suggested the expedition after consultation with the Pasteur Institute and that the director of the institute's branch at Brazaville had named a technical adviser for the expedition. Enlistment in the expedition is open to both army and civilian scientific men.

The decree signed by President Doumergue fixes the size of the party at ten physicians, ten hygienists, one veterinarian and twelve hospital attendants, all Europeans, and 105 natives. While the salaries are not unusually high—28,000 francs a year for the physicians and 18,000 and 13,000 for the other classes—they are offered many immunities from taxation and allowances for their families.

In addition they will be given a bonus of 10,000 francs after two years' service, 30,000 after four years and 60,000 if they enlist for an additional two years' service. The last clause implies that the government intends to keep the expedition in operation longer than the original five years mentioned in the decree.

The volunteers must pass three months in study at the Pasteur Institute in Paris or at the branch at Brazaville. They must enlist for two years' continuous service, followed by a vacation of six months, and then for another two years without interruption.

CASTING OF A LARGE DISK OF OPTICAL GLASS BY THE U. S. BUREAU OF STANDARDS

THE *Technical Bulletin* of the U. S. Bureau of Standards gives an account of the casting of a large disk of optical glass for Ohio Wesleyan University. On January 21 the mold containing the disk of optical glass, cast on May 7, 1927, was opened and the glass found to be very good. It appears to be quite uniform throughout, and although it contains some seeds and striae, they will not affect its value as a telescope mirror.

The cover was removed in the presence of several distinguished scientists, including Dr. S. W. Stratton, president of Massachusetts Institute of Technology; W. R. Warner, of the firm of Warner and Swasey, telescope makers, and Dr. George K. Burgess, director of the Bureau of Standards.

The disk, which is about 70 inches in diameter, 11 inches thick and weighs 3,500 pounds, will be used as a great concave mirror for the new reflecting telescope of the Perkins Observatory at Ohio Wesleyan University, Delaware, Ohio.

The money with which to establish this observatory was left to the university by Professor Hiram Mills Perkins, of Ohio Wesleyan, who during 50 years of hard work through most rigid economy and sound investment had been able to amass a small fortune, nearly a quarter of a million dollars. It was his desire to establish an observatory of the first rank at the university and that the entire equipment be of American manufacture. The mounting of the telescope was constructed by the American telescope makers, Warner and Swasey, of Cleveland, Ohio, but difficulty was experienced in getting any bids on the mirror from American glass manufacturers. In particular, no one was willing to state, even approximately, when the disk could be completed. Finally, the director of the observatory, Dr. Clifford C. Crump, called upon the Department of Commerce for assistance. Although the Bureau of Standards has been making optical glass since 1914, no task approaching the magnitude of the present one had ever been attempted.

After four unsuccessful attempts to obtain a disk of the size required a unique method was developed by the bureau's glass section. Cullet (broken glass of the same composition as the glass to be made) to the amount of 1,000 pounds and 4,600 pounds of sand and chemicals were melted in a single large pot in a gas-fired furnace.

The temperature of the glass when poured on May 7, 1927, was about 1,350° C. For one week the temperature was slowly lowered until it reached 600° C. The glass was held at this point for about four days to allow the temperature of the glass and furnace to become uniform throughout. At 600° C. this particular kind of glass (borosilicate crown) is quite rigid and yet sufficiently viscous to yield to cooling stresses without danger of cracking.

Beginning on May 18 the glass was allowed to cool slowly at an average rate of 2½° C. per day till 460° C. was reached. It was then annealed at this temperature for six weeks, during which time no variation greater than 1° C. was permitted. Final cooling was started on August 30, and room temperature was attained on January 16.

EXPERIMENT STATION OF THE GEORGIA STATE COLLEGE OF AGRICULTURE

THROUGH its president, Dr. Andrew M. Soule, the Georgia State College of Agriculture announces the establishment of an Experiment Station within the institution, this station to be supported *in toto* from the funds of the institution. For several years problems in farm management, fertilization of agronomical crops and fruit plants as well as ecological studies of the horticultural plants have been conducted. As soon after the first of January, 1928, as feasible, full-time research members of the staff will be appointed in the divisions of agricultural chemistry, agricultural engineering, animal husbandry, horticulture, poultry, marketing and home economics.

The experiment station will be in the hands of a committee of which President Andrew M. Soule is chairman. The responsibility for coordinating and general supervision of the experimental work will rest on the secretary of the research committee who has been designated for this position by the board of trustees.

The formation of the experiment station within the Georgia State College of Agriculture will be completed during the year of 1928. There will be ten full-time research members on its staff, and with these will be associated three Purnell workers already at the college in cooperation with the Georgia State Experiment Station.

It is with a great deal of pleasure that the announcement of this experiment station is made, for we feel that the agriculture of Georgia is certain to reap large benefits and profits from the work of these men who will be in a position to put their whole time on solving the problems of Georgia's farms and homes.

T. H. MCHATTON,
Secretary of Research

AWARD OF THE CHARLES REID BARNES LIFE MEMBERSHIP IN THE AMERICAN SOCIETY OF PLANT PHYSIOLOGISTS

AT the recent Nashville meeting, the second award of the Charles Reid Barnes honorary life membership in the American Society of Plant Physiologists was made to Professor Francis E. Lloyd, MacDonald professor of botany in McGill University, Montreal. This form of honorary life membership was inaugurated at the Kansas City meeting, in 1925, in memory of Charles Reid Barnes, who died at Chicago on February 24, 1910, in the midst of an active life. All who worked with Barnes at the University of Wisconsin or at the University of Chicago remember him as an exceptionally inspiring teacher, a man of untiring industry and wonderful ability. Through his publications and especially through his editorial work on the staff of the *Botanical Gazette* from 1882 to the time of his death, as well as through the work of those who received their training in his laboratories, Barnes left a permanent and indelible imprint of his remarkably clear and precise thought upon the whole science of plant physiology.

A Charles Reid Barnes honorary life membership is awarded each year, at the annual meeting of the American Society of Plant Physiologists. The first award was made at the Philadelphia meeting last year, to Burton E. Livingston, professor of plant physiology of the Johns Hopkins University and permanent secretary of the American Association for the Advancement of Science.

Professor Lloyd, who now becomes the second Charles Reid Barnes life member of the American Society of Plant Physiologists, was born in Manchester, England. He attended Lafayette College and Princeton University, receiving the degrees of A.B. and A.M. at Princeton in 1891 and 1895, respectively. He was a student at Munich in 1898, and at Bonn in 1901. He was instructor in biology at Williams College, 1891–92; professor of biology and geology 1892–95, and of biology 1895–97, at Pacific University, Oregon; adjunct professor of biology in Teachers College, Columbia University, 1897–1906. In 1907 he was connected for a brief period with Harvard University. He was a staff member of the Desert Laboratory, 1906; cytologist of the Arizona Agricultural Experiment Station, 1907; director of the department of investigation of the Continental-Mexican Rubber Co., 1907–08, and professor of botany in the Alabama Polytechnic Institute, 1908–12. Since 1912 he has held the MacDonald professorship of botany at McGill University. He has been a member of a number of scientific expeditions to Mexico, Puget Sound and Alaska, Dominica, Java and Sumatra.

For several years he was editor of *Plant World,* is now an associate editor of the *American Review of Tropical Agriculture,* and a member of the editorial board of *Plant Physiology,* the journal of the American Society of Plant Physiologists. Professor Lloyd has published many contributions in the field of botany, including the comparative embryology of the *Rubiaceae,* the morphology and physiology of the Mexican rubber plant guayule, the physiology of stomata, transpiration, tannin metabolism, fluorescent pigments, colloidal phenomena and the physiology of plant growth. His recent work, employing motion pictures to record the activity of conjugating cells of *Spirogyra* and the habits of *Vampyrella,* on which he has reported at recent meetings of the American Society of Plant Physiologists, has attracted much attention, and has thrown much light on the difficult field of protoplasmic physiology.

Professor Lloyd is a member of many scientific societies in this country and abroad, and is recognized as one of the most able and inspiring teachers and as one of the most distinguished investigators in American plant physiology. The American Society of Plant Physiologists expresses its appreciation of his important contributions in awarding to Professor Lloyd the second Charles Reid Barnes life membership in the society.

The Committee on the award of the first Charles Reid Barnes Life Membership of the American Society of plant Physiologists: Lee M. Hutchins, Walter F. Loehwing, Walter E. Loomis, James S. McHargue, Frank M. Andrews, chairman.

SCIENTIFIC NOTES AND NEWS

THE president and council of the Royal Society decided at their meeting on February 16 to recommend for election into the society the following fifteen candidates: Dr. Gleb V. Anrep, Professor Harry Bateman, Professor Carl Hamilton Browning, Mr. Stanley Smith Cook, Mr. William David Dye, Professor Clinton Coleridge Farr, Professor Major Greenwood, Dr. John William Heslop Harrison, Professor Walter Norman Haworth, Dr. David Keilin, Dr. Finlay Lorimer Kitchin, Dr. Francis Sowerby Macaulay, Professor Samuel Barnett Schryver, Professor Walter Stiles and Professor Robert Whytlaw-Gray.

IN connection with the tercentenary celebration by the College of Physicians of London of the publication of William Harvey's book, "De Motu Cordis," the Earl of Balfour, Sir Ernest Rutherford, Professors Ivan Petrovitch Pavlov and Karl Friedrich Wenckebach are to be made honorary fellows of the college.

DR. HENRY LE CHATELIER, honorary president of the French Society of Industrial Chemistry, has been made an honorary member of the American Society of Mechanical Engineers. The presentation was made on February 28 by Charles M. Schwab at a luncheon at the American Embassy in France.

DR. MICHAEL I. PUPIN, professor of electro-mechanics at Columbia University, was recently given the Washington award by the Western Society of Engineers at Chicago in recognition of his work on long-distance telephony and the radio.

PROFESSOR MAYNARD M. METCALF, of the department of biology of the Johns Hopkins University, has been elected a foreign member of the Société de Biogéographie de Paris.

DR. J. C. TH. UPHOF, professor of botany and head of the department of biology at Rollins College, Winter Park, Fla., has been elected a member of the Deutsche Botanische Gesellschaft.

DR. E. E. SLOSSON, director of Science Service, had conferred upon him the honorary degree of doctor of science at the founders' day exercises at Rollins College on February 20.

ON the occasion of the Washington Birthday celebration at the University of Pennsylvania, the honorary degree of fine arts was conferred upon Dr. R. Tait McKenzie, director of physical education at the university.

AT their annual meeting held on February 8, Dr. Charles Greeley Abbot, secretary of the Smithsonian Institution, was elected director of the Research Corporation of New York, to succeed the late Dr. Walcott.

JULIAN C. SMITH, vice-president and general manager of the Shawinigan Water and Power Company, Montreal, was installed as president of the Engineering Institute of Canada for 1928 at the institute's recent annual convention.

DR. LINSLEY R. WILLIAMS, former deputy commissioner of the State Department of Health, has been elected president of the New York Tuberculosis and Health Association to succeed Dr. James Alexander Miller, who retires after nine years' service.

The Sigma Xi Alumni Association of the University of Pittsburgh has elected the following officers for the year 1928: *President,* Dr. Oswald H. Blackwood (physics); *vice-president,* Dr. L. P. Sieg (physics); *secretary,* Dr. Alfred E. Emerson (zoology). The active membership of this association consists of 85 Sigma Xi alumni on the staff of the University of Pittsburgh.

The following officers and new members of the council of the Royal Astronomical Society have been elected: *President,* Rev. T. E. R. Phillips; *vice-presidents,* Professor A. S. Eddington, Professor Alfred Fowler, Dr. J. W. L. Glaisher, Lieut.-Col. F. J. M. Stratton; *treasurer,* Dr. E. B. Knobel; *secretaries,* Dr. John Jackson, Dr. H. Knox-Shaw; *foreign-secretary,* Professor H. H. Turner; *new members of council,* Professor S. Chapman, Sir Frank Dyson, Mr. W. M. H. Greaves, Dr. Gerald Merton, Professor E. A. Milne.

At the anniversary meeting of the Royal Anthropological Institute, held on January 24, Professor J. L. Myres was elected president in succession to Mr. H. J. E. Peake, whose term of office has expired. The vacancy for a vice-president was filled by the election of Professor H. J. E. Fleure, and Mr. G. D. Hornblower was elected honorary treasurer in succession to Dr. F. C. Shrubsall.

Perkins Coville, for the past five years instructor in forestry at Iowa State College, has been appointed assistant silviculturist, a new position in the U. S. Forestry Service. He will assume his new duties on July 1, in Washington.

Dr. Bernard O. Dodge, of the U. S. Department of Agriculture, has been appointed plant pathologist at the New York Botanical Gardens.

Ralph A. Morgan has resigned from the development branch of the Western Electric Company, to take charge of the research and development work for Black, Swalls and Bryson and their subsidiary corporation, the Cleaners' Equipment Corporation.

Dr. George N. Walcott, formerly entomologist at the Insular Experiment Station, Porto Rico, and more recently with Service Technique, Haiti, has accepted a position with the sugar-cane and cotton experiment station in Peru. He is sailing from New York on April 12.

At the Missouri Agricultural Experiment Station, Dr. Hans Jenny, of the Agricultural Chemical Experiment Station of Zurich, Switzerland, has been given an appointment in the department of soils, substituting for Dr. Richard Bradfield, who is spending a year's leave of absence at Kaiser Wilhelm Institute in Berlin.

Dr. Cornelis Lely, president and honorary member of the Netherlands Royal Institute of Engineers, was the guest of honor at a luncheon given at the Engineers' Club on March 6, under the auspices of the American Society of Civil Engineers, the American Institute of Mining and Metallurgical Engineers, the American Society of Mechanical Engineers and the American Institute of Electrical Engineers. Dr. John R. Freeman presided.

Walter Granger, paleontologist, and Leslie E. Spock, geologist, with their associates, James B. Shackleford and Albert Thomson, sailed from San Francisco on March 2 to join the Central Asiatic Expedition of the American Museum of Natural History. In Peking they will meet Dr. Roy Chapman Andrews, the leader, now getting together a camel caravan, with which it is planned to start for the desert of Mongolia by mid-April.

Professor R. A. Cooley, professor of zoology at Montana Agricultural College, will leave on April 1 for a year's leave of absence. He will spend part of the time in the interior of Africa with the Chicago zoological expedition and will study tick parasites.

Dr. Henry C. Sherman, Mitchill professor of chemistry at Columbia University, has been granted a leave of absence for the spring session.

Professor F. E. Wood, of the department of mathematics at Northwestern University, is spending the year in research in Bologna and Rome.

Dr. Albrecht Penck, professor of geography in the University of Berlin, has accepted invitations to lecture at the University of Chicago during June and at the University of California during July.

Dr. George R. Minot, professor of medicine at the Harvard Medical School, will deliver the fifth Harvey Society lecture at the New York Academy of Medicine on Friday evening, March 16. His subject will be "The Treatment of Pernicious (Addison's) Anemia."

Dr. Frank C. Mann, of the Mayo Clinic, delivered the fourth L. L. McArthur lecture of the Billings Foundation before the Chicago Institute of Medicine on February 24 on "Experimental Peptic Ulcer."

Professor Arthur H. Compton, of the University of Chicago, was the guest of honor at the annual banquet of the Iowa chapter of Sigma Xi on February 29 and gave an illustrated public address under the auspices of the society on the subject "What Things are Made of."

Dr. Irving S. Cutter, of Northwestern University Medical School, will give a Mayo Foundation lecture at the Mayo Clinic on April 6 on "Some Sidelights on the Etiology of Puerperal Fever." This lecture is one of a series on medical history.

DR. CHESTER DARROW, of the Institute for Juvenile Research, Chicago, delivered an illustrated public lecture at Colgate University on February 28 on "Recent Developments in the Use of the Galvanometer in Psychology."

ON February 18, Dr. L. R. Jones, professor of plant pathology at the University of Wisconsin, delivered an address to the Royal Canadian Institute on the subject "The 'Survival of the Fittest' in the Field of Plant Pathology."

THE council of the Royal Medico-Psychological Association has decided to commemorate the life work of the late Sir Frederick Mott by publishing a memorial book, and for this purpose has appointed a committee consisting of Drs. C. Hubert Bond, F. L. Golla, Douglas McRae, Thomas Beaton and J. R. Lord.

DR. HARRIS HAWTHORNE WILDER, since 1892 head of the department of biology at Smith College, died on February 27, aged sixty-four years.

DR. CHARLES F. DAWSON, formerly assistant chief of the U. S. Bureau of Animal Industry and professor of bacteriology at the University of Florida, died on February 28, aged sixty-seven years.

DR. R. S. HOLWAY, emeritus professor of physical geography at the University of California, died on December 2, aged seventy years.

DR. W. L. JOHANNSEN, professor of plant physiology in the University of Copenhagen, died on November 11.

THE United States Civil Service Commission announces open competitive examinations for associate agricultural engineer at a salary of $3,000 and assistant agricultural engineer at a salary of $2,400, applications for which must be on file with the commission not later than March 27. The examinations are to fill vacancies in the Bureau of Public Roads, Department of Agriculture, for duty in Washington, D. C., or in the field, and in positions requiring similar qualifications.

THE central petroleum committee of the National Research Council will meet in New York on March 17 to make recommendations to the American Petroleum Institute for research projects to be conducted during 1928–29 under the research fund contributed by Mr. John D. Rockefeller and the Universal Oil Products Company. Suggestions and proposals for research projects should be sent to the chairman of the committee, Professor Hugh S. Taylor, Princeton University, to reach him before March 15. Announcements on the research projects will be made before April 1.

FREE public lectures on medical topics will be given under the auspices of the Chicago Academy of Sciences and the North Side Branch of the Chicago Medical Society at the Chicago Academy of Sciences, at 3:30 P. M. on Sundays as follows: March 18, "Preventive Medicine," Dr. Nathan Smith Davis III; March 25, "Heart Disease in Childhood," Dr. Harold A. Bachmann; April 1, "Cults, Quacks and Cures," Dr. Morris Fishbein; April 15, "Tuberculosis," Dr. Ethan Allen Gray; April 22, "The Pre-School Child," Dr. Gustav L. Kaufmann; April 29, "The Prevention of Contagious Disease," Dr. Archibald L. Hoyne.

THE American Institute of Mining and Metallurgical Engineers, which recently held its annual meeting in New York, will convene in Boston next September. Electrical prospecting and the new geophysical methods now being used for the discovery of ore will be studied and discussed in technical sessions at this meeting.

PHI chapter of Tri Beta, honorary biology fraternity, was installed at Peru College, Nebraska, on February 13, by Dr. Wm. M. Goldsmith, of Southwestern College, Winfield, Kansas.

THE *British Medical Journal* states that the centenary celebration of the faculty of medicine at Cairo and an international congress of tropical medicine and hygiene will be held in association from December 15 to 22, 1928, in that town. In the provisional program which has just been issued, it is stated that various sectional meetings will be held and that special attention will be paid to ankylostomiasis and bilharziasis. In connection with this celebration a medical exhibition is being arranged, and it is possible that the foundation stone will be laid of a new building to replace the existing Kasr-el-Ani Hospital.

ACCORDING to the *Geological Magazine* the Geological Survey of Denmark will celebrate its fortieth anniversary in June, by a series of meetings and excursions to which foreign geologists are to be invited. Previous to the meeting in Copenhagen an excursion will be arranged to Bornholm, Denmark's outlying rocky island in the Baltic, which is replete with stratigraphical and all sorts of geological interest. Another party is to visit Moën and Zealand, where remarkable dislocations in the Senonian Chalk can be seen and studied. The conference will be devoted to lectures and discussions on the geology of Denmark, interspersed with inspections of the Copenhagen museums, with their collections of minerals, fossils and pre-historic remains. Afterwards, an eleven-day excursion will enable foreign geologists to visit and inspect a wide range of glacial phenomena in Zealand, Funen and Langeland, as well as on the mainland in Jutland.

IN view of the disastrous floods which have occurred in the United States during the past year and the fact that congress at its present session will discuss legislation relating to flood prevention, schools of engineering in the country will be interested in the visit of two distinguished men from Holland who will lecture on flood prevention as exemplified in the reclamation of land from the Zuider Zee. Dr. Cornelis Lely, the distinguished engineer of Holland who originated the plan of draining the Zuider Zee, is expected to visit the United States this winter, arriving the latter part of February. He expects to lecture in the colleges in the east during the month of March. Mr. Plate, president of the Shipping Association in Rotterdam, with many years of experience in engineering in Holland and the Dutch East Indies, will arrive in New York on February 15. He will lecture on the same subject *en route* to San Francisco and upon his return trip to Ann Arbor. The fact that these men will visit different parts of the country will make it possible for engineers to become familiar with the methods used in Holland with the reclamation of land from the Zuider Zee. The Institute of International Education, 2 West 45th Street, New York City, is arranging the itineraries of both of these lecturers.

AT the League of Nations assembly in September a report was presented on the work of the League's Committee on Intellectual Cooperation. The report, according to an account printed in *Nature*, directs special attention to the creation at the International Institute of Intellectual Cooperation of a coordination service of information offices attached to libraries, to the committee's proposals for coordination between the organs of bibliography for the various sciences, to the need of funds for the maintenance of the office for annual tables of constants and mathematical quantities, and to the steps taken in preparation for the Popular Arts Congress (to be held at Prague in 1928), for an international agreement with regard to casts, and for promoting the extension of the educational work of museums. It is also pointed out that additional funds are needed for the institute, grants to which are at present made only by the following countries: Austria, Czechoslovakia, France, Hungary, Italy, Monaco, Poland and Switzerland. The question how to protect and reward men of science and their discoveries by means of an international convention has been investigated during the past five years, and it is now thought that the matter is ripe for definite action. It is intended, therefore, to convene a committee of experts to prepare a draft convention. A separate report was submitted on the Italian proposal for the creation of an educational kinematographic institute. This proposal looks to the creation at Rome of an institute under the direction of the League of Nations, but to be carried on at the expense of the Italian government.

DR. WILLARD R. JILLSON, director and state geologist of the Kentucky Geological Survey, announces the completion of a unit set of thirty structural oil and gas and geological maps of eastern Kentucky. The maps are issued by the Kentucky Geological Survey at the scale of 1 inch to the mile, and taken as a unit constitute the largest area, structurally mapped on the same keybed—the Fire Clay coal—in the world. The district covers 10,500 square miles. This work initiated in 1918 has just been completed with the release of the Harlan County sheet.

A HISTORY of the world's development, told in chronological exhibits of the birds, mammals and terrain of each period, has been begun by Dr. Frank C. Baker, curator of the museum of the University of Illinois. Every general type of bird has been arranged in ordinal periods. The development of birds during each era, showing the types, nests, eggs, skeletons and reproductions or actual display of plumages, is illustrated. Partially completed now are exhibits of the Cambrian, Ordovician, Silurian, Devonian, Mississippian and Pennsylvanian periods.

THE Wilder medal, one of the highest awards made by the American Pomological Society, has been given to the Canadian Government Central Experimental Farm, Ottawa, for the Melba apple, which was originated at the Ottawa farm. This is the eighth time that the Wilder medal has been awarded to the Canadian Government Experimental Farm for notable varieties of apples.

DR. R. S. BASSLER, of the U. S. National Museum, writes that a pamphlet on the international rules of zoological nomenclature has been published by the Biological Society of Washington, copies of which can be had by addressing the secretary of that society, care of the U. S. Bureau of Entomology.

BEGINNING next September, a new department of agriculture will be inaugurated in Carthage College, Carthage, Illinois. A two years' course will be offered which will coordinate with the work offered at the University of Illinois.

THE Louisiana State University is adding to its summer curriculum a field course in zoology at some near seaside point, probably at the foot of Barataria Bay. The course is to be open to students who have had preliminary training and will be conducted with emphasis upon the local marine fauna. It is hoped that students from other southern schools and instructors interested in research upon local marine forms will join the undertaking.

A LARGE number of specimens of plants, birds, mammals and insects are included in the collections brought back by the Lee Garnett Day expedition to Mount Roraima, according to an announcement by the American Museum of Natural History. A total of 1,260 birds, some 350 mammals and many plants and insects were sent back by the party. The members of the expedition were G. H. H. Tate and T. D. Carter, of the museum's department of mammalogy, and Mr. Tate's brother, G. M. Tate, who joined them after traveling from Para, Brazil, up the Amazon and Negro Rivers to Manaos, thence by boat and canoe to the confluence of the Rivers Surumu and Cotinga. From there the journey was made in eleven days on foot.

PURCHASE of the plant collections of the late Dr. L. M. Umbach, of North Western College, Napierville, Ill., has added about 50,000 specimens to the University of Wisconsin herbarium. The acquisition practically doubles the collections of the university, and makes it one of the largest herbariums of middle west plants. Included in the addition are also collections from other parts of the country, from Europe, some from Asia and elsewhere.

IT is reported that the Rockefeller Foundation has given to the Stockholm High School 25,000 crowns for a building for a biochemical institute, with Professor Hans Von Euler as director. A like sum has been raised in Sweden.

THE Puget Sound Biological Station of the University of Washington, located at Friday Harbor, Washington, is erecting a fireproof store room 24 x 56 feet and a fireproof research laboratory, 31 x 73 feet. These are to be finished by June 1.

UNIVERSITY AND EDUCATIONAL NOTES

THE University of Chicago has received a gift of $250,000 from Mr. Julius Rosenwald to be used for graduate work and research in the departments of physics, mathematics and astronomy.

SIX friends of Wesleyan University have pledged a total of $600,000 to the centennial committee. The aims for the centennial year include a fund of $1,000,000 to raise the faculty salaries and to provide adequate pensions for retired faculty members.

DR. EDWARD HICKS HUME, former president of Yale-in-China, has been appointed to the newly created post of director of the Post-Graduate Medical School and Hospital at Yale University. Under the new organization, the dean of the medical school, the superintendent of the hospital and the principal of the school of nursing will all be responsible directly to Dr. Hume, who in turn will be responsible to the board of directors.

DR. GARY N. CALKINS, professor of protozoology in Columbia University, has been named executive officer of the department of zoology for three years.

HAROLD GOULDEN, formerly of the Squibb Laboratories, has been appointed an instructor in the department of biochemistry of the New Jersey College of Pharmacy.

ASSOCIATE PROFESSOR LAO G. SIMONS has been promoted to a full professorship and head of the department of mathematics at Hunter College.

A. J. WILSON, professor of analytical chemistry at North Carolina State College, has been appointed chairman of the department of chemistry for the remainder of the session, succeeding Frank E. Rice.

M. E. DELAFIELD, head of the department of public health and hygiene at University College, London, has been appointed to the university chair of chemistry as applied to hygiene tenable at the London School of Hygiene and Tropical Medicine.

DR. F. G. TRAYHORN has been appointed professor of chemistry at University College, Hull.

DR. SIGURD, of Freiburg, has succeeded Professor Trendelenburg in the chair of pharmacology at Berlin.

DISCUSSION AND CORRESPONDENCE

TREE FROGS AND PITCHER PLANTS

IT is well known that the regions where the southern pitcher plant (*Sarracenia flava*) abounds may also be the home of the carolina, or green tree frog (*Hyla cinerea*), but an association between them has not been noticed. However, the following observations seem to show that these frogs make use of the pitcher plant, though this may prove to be no general rule but only a local habit, possibly restricted to special conditions of weather.

In June and July, 1888, an examination of some of the pitcher plant leaves growing in abundance in the wet lands amidst pine groves close to Beaufort, North Carolina, showed that not a few of the leaves were inhabited by tree frogs. The leaves of this plant form beautiful yellow-green trumpets that stand straight up, in clusters, so high that one is naturally tempted to look down into their wide mouths to the water and insects that may be down in the narrowly pointed base. In this way it was noticed that now and then a leaf contained a tree frog. These frogs having exceptionally long legs and slender trunks seem especially well shaped to fit into any narrow cavity and as they sat holding to the side of the trumpet some distance down from its mouth where they yet had ample room, they presented very quaint and attractive pictures. The color of these frogs being a yellow-green with some golden spots, they harmonized excellently with the background illuminated by light in part transmitted through the walls of the leaf.

The frogs sat with their heads up toward the mouth of the pitcher or trumpet, and were advantageously placed to seize any insect that might come down into the cavity of the leaf. That this was a chance worth considering was perhaps indicated by the fact that in some cases small spiders had spun their webs across the opening of the leaves, thus being placed well to intercept the insects that might else have gone down to the frog.

In the latter part of June and the first of July as many as twelve frogs were found, on two days, a week or more apart, while looking into about six hundred leaves. That this occurrence of frogs in the leaves was not limited to the above cases was proved by a third examination made July 9, when just two hundred leaves were looked into as they came; one hundred in the locality previously visited and the other hundred in a new locality. In both cases the leaves examined were on plants growing along the edges of the woods where the frogs were probably more numerous than out in the open where the pitcher plants were more numerous. The first hundred leaves contained three frogs; the twenty-ninth leaf harbored two frogs and the thirty-sixth one. The second hundred contained five frogs; one in the fourth, in the fifty-sixth, fifty-eighth, sixty-sixth and eighty-seventh. Thus in these leaves skirting the woods some two to five per cent. contained frogs.

The season being then very dry the occurrence of the green-tree frog in the leaves of the pitcher plant may have been an unusual occurrence due to the frogs seeking protection from drying; on the other hand, this frog may have developed a special appreciation of the advantages of these retreats, both as affording food and as giving the comparative immunity from attacks of enemies that the protective resemblance of the frog to the leaf suggests.

E. A. ANDREWS

THE JOHNS HOPKINS UNIVERSITY

THE OCCURRENCE OF CONJUGATION IN PARAMECIUM CALKINSI

Paramecium calkinsi was described as a new species in 1921 by Woodruff[1] after he had carried pedigreed cultures of it for nearly a year and had made various tests to determine that the new species belonged to the genus Paramecium. Woodruff states that every effort was made to secure conjugation, but without success. He further states that during the life of his pedigree culture an intensive study of the nuclear conditions was made to detect endomixis if it occurred. There was no indication of endomixis, although there were rhythms in the rate of fission. So far as we are aware, neither Woodruff nor any other investigator has succeeded in inducing conjugation in *P. calkinsi* and we have seen no record of endomixis having been observed. One of us (Wenrich) has made repeated but unsuccessful efforts to induce conjugation in a strain of this species obtained from Professor Woodruff.

As a result of all these failures to observe conjugation or endomixis, the impression has been developing that these phenomena do not occur in this species. In view of the important theoretical implications of such an exceptional behavior on the part of a distinct species of Paramecium, it seems worth while to record here the fact that conjugation has been observed in cultures of *Paramecium calkinsi* secured originally at Woods Hole, Mass.

The original material was a sample of water taken from the pond on the east side of the Eel Pond at Woods Hole. The water in this pond is brackish, since at high tide sea water from the Eel Pond flows into it; at other times during the day, it drains into the Eel Pond. The material collected from the source pond on August 18, 1927, contained large numbers of *Paramecium calkinsi,* and some of it was distributed into syracuse watch glasses for more convenient culture and study. At the beginning of September, each of these cultures was placed into a vial and transported to Philadelphia. On September 5 each of these cultures was reestablished in a syracuse watch glass without change of media. On September 7 it was noticed that in culture number 5 many individuals had died, so a new culture, 5A, was made, by transferring about 200 individuals to another watch glass containing an infusion made by boiling together some timothy hay and wheat grains. The old culture was made over by taking out most of the fluid and replacing it with the infusion just mentioned. Within the next few days other cultures were replenished with the hay-wheat infusion. Examination on September 16 showed heavy populations in both cultures 5 and 5A and some dozens of pairs of conjugants. Conjugation has since been observed in five others of the

[1] "The Structure, Life History, and Intrageneric Relationships of Paramecium calkinsi," Sp. Nov. *Biol Bull.*, Vol. 41, pp. 171–180.

cultures brought from Woods Hole; and in the original culture, No. 5, a smaller or larger number of conjugating pairs were observed almost daily up to October 15, 1927.

The question presents itself as to the causes of the failure of Woodruff's strain to conjugate, in comparison with the apparent readiness to conjugate on the part of the Woods Hole strains. The differences may be attributed either (1) to the difference in the original habitat, (2) to different culture methods in the laboratory or (3) to inherent racial differences, or some combination of these. In regard to the first possibility, it will be remembered that Woodruff's strain came from a fresh-water source while the Woods Hole strains have come from brakish water. Experimental tests demonstrated that these brakish-water strains would live in an apparently normal condition in fresh water and in various strengths of sea water up to pure sea water, provided the changes to the higher strengths were made gradually. The brakish-water habitat may therefore be considered a normal one.

In regard to the second possibility, it may be pointed out here that we have subjected Woodruff's strain to the same cultural conditions that we used for the Woods Hole strains, but have not as yet been able to induce conjugation in this strain. The evidence at present available rather favors the third possibility—that of inherent racial differences.

Segregated strains are being established from exconjugants and it is hoped to make an intensive study of the conditions which will induce conjugation as well as to investigate thoroughly the cytological details of the process.

D. H. WENRICH,
C. C. WANG
ZOOLOGICAL LABORATORY,
UNIVERSITY OF PENNSYLVANIA

CENTRIFUGING FILTERABLE VIRUSES

I READ with interest the note by M. S. Marshall, entitled "Centrifuging Filterable Viruses," which appeared on page 219 in SCIENCE of September 2, 1927. There seems to be little doubt as to the accuracy of Marshall's computations, and it seems likely that his conclusions are correct for a pure virus in water. However, it should be pointed out that his conclusions do not hold for virus which is in the plant extract. The writer's studies show that the virus of tobacco mosaic can be concentrated by means of the supercentrifuge. These investigations were published in *The Journal of Agricultural Research,* vol. 35, pp. 13–38, July 1, 1927. It should be pointed out that the supercentrifuge has been used in this and in other laboratories for concentrating bacteria and other micro-organisms. See the article by C. Juday, in the *Transactions* of the Wisconsin Academy of Science, Arts and Letters, vol. 22, pp. 299–314. 1926.

The writer's studies indicate that physical and chemical treatments which cause coagulation and precipitation to take place in plant extracts, also cause or assist the virus to settle out of the extract. However, the relative advantages of the various treatments, and the exact relations between the virus particles and other particles which are precipitated out of the extracts, are not fully known. Some treatments are less desirable than others because they are toxic to the virus in varying degrees. Some treatments produce only very finely divided coagula which do not settle out on long standing. Frequently these are heavily charged with virus, and they can be removed almost completely by means of the supercentrifuge.

It should be emphasized that centrifuge methods are of unquestionable value in studies on the virus of tobacco mosaic, and thus far the writer has found the supercentrifuge to be one of the most useful pieces of apparatus in the laboratory.

H. H. MCKINNEY
CEREAL VIRUS DISEASE INVESTIGATIONS,
BUREAU OF PLANT INDUSTRY

COLORIMETRIC METHODS IN BIOLOGY

PAST discussions of colorimetry, in the pages of SCIENCE, and particularly the recent appeal by Irwin G. Priest for bibliographic references and reprints bearing on this subject, have emboldened me to call attention in your columns to a paper of my own, published during the past year. I refer to an article entitled "Linear and Colorimetric Measurements of Small Mammals," which appeared in *The Journal of Mammalogy,* vol. 8, no. 3, August, 1927, pp. 177–206.

I hope that this unseemly bit of self-advertising on my part will be condoned for the following reasons. The scope of the journal in which the paper was published would doubtless tend to conceal it from the view of many biologists who are not especially interested in the Mammalia. On the other hand, the methods therein described are doubtless applicable to a wide range of biological and even of inorganic objects.

The writer is far from wishing to pose as an expert on colorimetry, either practical or theoretical, but he has been dealing for many years with color differences in certain species of rodents, and has been obliged to treat these differences quantitatively. Since no recognized technique was available for the purpose, it was necessary to work this out through protracted experimentation. A type of instrument (the Ives Tint Photometer) was finally adopted, which was already in use for industrial purposes. Some further equipment was necessary, however, and the details of the procedure were not finally standardized until the lapse of several years. I have been fortunate enough to have had the advice of several persons who are far better informed in this field than I am.

These remarks are offered in the hope that they may be of service to some of those who wish to treat the colors of biological objects in a quantitative way. It is not claimed that the procedure adopted by me records absolute values, or ones which are accurate enough for the exacting requirements of physics. But it is, so far as I know, the only practicable method yet offered for measuring individual and racial differences of color and shade in the pelages of mammals, and it renders possible the treatment of these characters according to familiar biometric procedure.

F. B. SUMNER

SCRIPPS INSTITUTION
OF OCEANOGRAPHY

SPECIALIZATION AND COOPERATION IN SCIENTIFIC RESEARCH

PROFESSOR COMPTON'S interesting address delivered at Lehigh University and printed in SCIENCE of November 11, 1927, brings up pointedly the question as to whether the conception of mass production is to dominate the teaching of advanced physical science. Two remarkable statements on this subject have recently come, one from the Bishop of Ripon who pleaded for a ten-year holiday in research at the recent meeting of the British Association, and the other statement from Sir Ernest Rutherford, the president of the Royal Society, which was made at the opening of a new physics laboratory at the University of Bristol. "When I look back over the thirty years or more of my connection with research," says Sir Ernest, "I am conscious that I have always been looking for a breathing space when, for a few years, no advances of consequence would be made; when I should gain an opportunity for studying in more detail, at my leisure, the ground already won. Alas, that breathing space has never come, and I am sure will never come in my time."

A plea for limitation of the intensive methods of research which are at present advocated and practised in our universities is unpopular. But the intensive methods are bringing on very peculiar results. The quantity of "research" output has grown to be immense. It is not unlike the production of motor cars. The aim is not the very best, but something new and "salable." Anything that is good enough to hold its own is good enough to be produced as a piece of "research." An enormous amount of duplication has followed in the wake of this mass research. This is very noticeable in connection with the issue of electrical patents many of which are granted on devices which have been clearly described ten and twenty years previous to the date of the applications. Some very extraordinary examples might be cited in this connection besides the one referred to by Professor Compton.

The thesis work is growing more intricate and complex. In the majority of cases it must be difficult to secure proof of the accuracy of much of the work done. But it is new, or it appears new, and that suffices. Now, in the historical development of science we have the example of Darwin holding his manuscript of the Origin of Species for twenty years, checking and re-checking before publishing. It would not be difficult to name other examples though less noted. If this so-called research work were more carefully done, its rate of increase would slow down of its own accord. If scientific teaching was set into the proper historical relief, it would be more thoroughly done and there would be less of it. When we plead for the teaching of fundamentals it is this which we mean. It is not clear whether Professor Compton pleads for teaching the "easiest way" by following altogether the inclinations of the students. The kind of research work he refers to is a little like athletics and much of it can be done without a long systematic training but such training is the essence of science. If the test is to be utilitarian, science as we like to see it taught will depart. If the criterion is to be that taught and urged by such teachers as Huxley and Helmholtz, then it is the "truth" which is the standard. Constant care as to whether new work is worth publishing, whether previous workers have received the credit which their work deserves, whether experiments are accurately made, whether the theory is simplified to the point where it is something other than a cloud of symbols, such considerations would, of their very nature, slow down this high speed production and permit, to some extent, the realization of the hours of philosophic contemplation of the work already done for which Sir Ernest Rutherford makes his plea.

Mass production in science may prove to become as fatal as it is likely to become in industry, where it bids fair to be master instead of servant.

B. A. BEHREND

WELLESLEY HILLS, MASS.

A FUNCTION OF REGIONAL SCIENTIFIC SOCIETIES

ONE thing of prime importance to be stressed by regional groups of scientific workers which seems to have been entirely forgotten by the various secretaries of State Academies of Science as reported by Professor Segerblom, SCIENCE, October 16, is the incentive for young researchers which comes from being permitted to report their work in these meetings. The writer has distinctly in mind the attitude of the undergraduates toward a certain sophomore who had discovered the continuity of protoplasm between cells of a filamentous alga and had been permitted to report this before a State Academy of Science. The effect perhaps was as important on the sophomore as on his associates, for his name is now one of the starred list of botanists in American Men of Science. In itself the discovery may or may not have been important, but the effect was important on that student body. In this day of great stadia and unlimited honor to heroes of beef and bone, it should occur to scientists to devise some method of making scientific honors for undergraduates a thing worth the seeking. In those days of the Indiana Academy, when the influence of Jordan and Coulter was strong, democracy prevailed, and the student of science in the colleges of the state felt that to appear before the academy was almost as important as winning his degree. To the veteran it may be important to be reminded that the borders of the unknown are near at hand by bits contributed from unexpected sources. The best that can prevail for the promotion of research is that spirit which knows only the rank of ability.

Though not of the group of which the study was made, it may interest some to know that the models of the Indiana and the Wisconsin Academies were well in the minds of the organizers of The Northwest Scientific Association when that organization began four years ago. Here the senior or the young graduate meets on equal footing with the doctors and the deans of colleges, chancellor, president or professor, and fine fellowship prevails among all. The groups which were isolated and unknown to each other in the widely scattered colleges now meet and are getting well acquainted and learning to work together. The present membership is nearing three hundred. The program for December 28 and 29 announced seventy-four titles. Nine different sections are now under way and twenty-five sessions of breakfast, luncheon, dinner and general or section meetings convened.

Northwest Science, the official organ of Northwest Scientific Association, has now completed its first year and in a way represents the work accomplished by that organization. It has printed a history of the organization for three years of its existence, abstracts of papers presented at the meetings, some regional news, a few general papers and one issue devoted to the geology of the region on either side of the line between Idaho and Washington in the locality of Spokane.

THOS. LARGE

SPOKANE, WASHINGTON

CHILDREN WHO RUN ON ALL FOURS

IN the last two numbers of *The American Journal of Physical Anthropology* (Wistar Institute, Philadelphia), the undersigned publishes the account, with illustrations, of eleven children who before walking upright have spontaneously developed the habit of running effectively on all fours. This is a highly interesting phenomenon of nonpathologic nature, and he would be thankful for further reliable reports. The principal points on which information is desired are as follows: 1. Race and nationality; 2. Sex; 3. Health and robustness; 4. What child in numerical order; 5. Has the phenomenon been noticed in any other child of the same parents or among relatives; 6. At what age has the child begun to run on all fours and how long has it continued. To which should be added a description, as detailed as possible, of the performance itself, supplemented when this can be done by a photograph of the child in the act. The position of the hands (whether fully open or partly closed), and of the head, while running on all fours, as well as any other peculiarities of the child's behavior, are matters of interest.

ALEŠ HRDLIČKA

DIVISION OF PHYSICAL ANTHROPOLOGY,
U. S. NATIONAL MUSEUM

SCIENTIFIC BOOKS

The Antiquity of Man in East Anglia. By J. REID MOIR. Cambridge University Press, 1927.

THIS invaluable volume is not, like many of the contemporary works on the Old Stone Age, a restatement of current archeological knowledge or of current Continental research in archeology, but is an entirely fresh and convincing presentation of a series of wonderful discoveries in the newest field of prehistoric archeology which were made in the counties of Norfolk and Suffolk, a region collectively known as East Anglia.

The title chosen by the author does not fit the contents of this volume because he has assigned an age of only 500,000 years and the geologic epoch of merely Lower Pleistocene time to discoveries which in the reviewer's opinion belonged to a far more ancient period, namely, 1,250,000 years, and to a more ancient geologic epoch, namely, the close of Pliocene time. This is less surprising when we consider that English geologists for the most part still speak only of two glacial periods and, with the exception of Brooks, there is little serious attempt to connect these two ice invasions of British territory with a fourfold Ice Age of western Europe and of North America. The author, moreover, is under the very strong influence of Sir Ray Lankester, who insists that Upper Pliocene time in Great Britain corresponds to Lower Pleistocene time in other parts of Europe. Yet Lankester has rendered a courageous service to archeology in his strong support of Mr. Moir's contention for the artificial character, especially of the flints known as rostro-carinates, which are distinctive of what the reviewer would call the Upper Pliocene of Great Britain and thus far have not been found elsewhere, except as degenerate survivors in a subsequent archeological stage. These are the only two exceptions found by the present reviewer in this invaluable collection of most original observations in Norfolk and Suffolk, extending back to the year 1909 when the author made his first discovery and was attracted to this fascinating and absorbing subject. In previous writings, the present reviewer has also stoutly espoused the cause of Mr. Moir against much indifference and incredulity not only among English but among Continental archeologists, and has supported his successive discoveries as far ante-dating in geologic age those made in any other part of the world.

The author opens with the chapter entitled "The Pleasures of Flint Hunting." It is this pleasure or, more truly, this fascination guided by real genius that has led him to devote every spare moment of his time to thorough, repeated and well-rewarded research in localities which offered the best promise or prospect of revealing traces of prehistoric man. His outstanding discoveries are those of the Foxhall quarry and fireplace, which he suggests may be of the same age as the Piltdown skull, the rostro-carinate bed lying *beneath* the classic Red Crag of East Anglia and the giant Cromer flints on the foreshore of Norfolk in the most unpromising locality exposed only at low tide. In each case, he has been rewarded with most brilliant achievement and final recognition of the authenticity of his findings by such acute European archeologists as Breuil and Capitan. He is himself a master of the art of flint-making and has worked out many of the stages of early manufacture and adaptation, even of the long-disputed types of flints known as Eoliths. His firm opinion on this subject, as evidenced in the following quotations, is, therefore, entitled to a most serious consideration.

> The human origin of the Eolithic, Kentian, flint implement has been in dispute for a great number of years, but the weight of opinion is now in favor of the view that they were artificially flaked, especially as they are seen to conform to the criteria of man's work upon flints. The primitive appearance and profound antiquity of these specimens make them of the greatest interest to students of prehistoric man.
>
> Though, as has been shown above, there is very good reason to believe that the Eoliths of the Kent Plateau are of a very great antiquity, yet the gravel in which they are found is not covered by any other deposit such as would enable us to say, with certainty, that this gravel is of a particular geological age. It is fortunate, therefore, that examples of Eoliths, quite comparable with those discovered in Kent, have been found in Suffolk, in the detritus, or bone bed, below the Red Crag, thus showing that the very ancient people who made these implements inhabited East Anglia.
>
> * * * * * *
>
> The Eoliths are thus, evidently, of an extreme antiquity, and represent the most ancient works of man yet brought to light. In my opinion also these specimens show us the basic forms from which all later flint implements were derived, and I have been able to trace the manner in which the Eoliths developed into the later sub-Red Crag forms, and these, in their turn, to the still more advanced Palaeolithic specimens. It can not be too strongly urged that the evidence now to hand demonstrates the orderly development of flint implements from the very primitive Eoliths to the latest, symmetrical forms in use at the end of the Stone Age, and that this development, indicating as it must the slow, though sure, advance of man himself from a rudimentary pre-human state, provides further support, if such were needed, to Darwin's great theory of evolution.

In these passages, he not only commits himself to the theory of human origin of the Kentian Eoliths but goes still further back to those of Darmsden and Puy Courny. As to the latter, he says:

> . . . It is, therefore, of great interest to realize that at Puy Courny, in Central France, there is present a bed of gravel of Upper Miocene Age (the epoch immediately preceding the Pliocene) containing a large series of examples of cherty flint that assume very definite Eolithic forms. . . . There can not, fortunately, be any doubt as to the age of this deposit because in it have been found the remains of the following Upper Miocene animals, *Dinotherium giganteum, Mastodon longirostris, Rhinoceros Schleiermacheri,* and *Hipparion gracile.* The specimens in the Westlake collection impressed me strongly with their very primitive appearance, and I think it probable that they are comparable with the oldest series recovered by me from below the Red Crag of Suffolk. If this view is correct, then we can at last form some idea of the age of these earliest human implements, and realize that they must be referred to the end of the very remote Miocene epoch. . . . Henri Breuil, who has also seen this collection, regards the specimens it contains as of natural, rather than as of human, origin.

Altogether this is the most original and welcome contribution which has ever been made to Tertiary archeology as distinguished from Quaternary archeology which began with the great discoveries of the Chellean culture on the River Somme by M. Boucher de Perthes. Whether we accept Mr. Moir's interpretation of the Miocene Eoliths or not, we must give him first rank and accord to him the full priority of the discovery of indisputable flint work of man in Tertiary time. It is too early to draw all the theoretic conclusions regarding the antiquity and ancestry of man which may be deduced from these discoveries, but in the present reviewer's opinion, they vastly extend our conception of a truly human and pre-human type of Dawn Man rather than of an ape-man ancestry of our race.

H. F. O.

SCIENTIFIC APPARATUS AND LABORATORY METHODS

A PHOTOGRAPHIC PLATE THAT PENETRATES DESERT HAZE

GEOLOGISTS and others who have occasion to take photographs of distant mountains in the arid regions have often been afflicted by the presence of the blue haze that obscures the details of features more than a few miles away. This is presumably caused by the fine dust which the desert winds keep more or less continuously suspended in the atmosphere.

Ordinary photographic plates and films give but poor results under such conditions. The photograph generally shows much less of detail than the eye itself can see, and hence one is apt to be disappointed. By the use of ray filters or color screens, some improvement may be effected, but at best it falls far short of satisfaction.

By using panchromatic films and orange or red ray filters, very much better pictures can be obtained. Cut films or plates of this type are now rather generally used by the more experienced and painstaking photographers of mountain scenery. Unfortunately they are not yet available in the form of roll-films.

Further steps were taken some years ago by Messrs. Burns, Shane and Wright at the Lick Observatory (Mt. Hamilton, California), who, for the purpose of photographing distant landscapes, used plates treated with Krypto-cyanine, a dye which confers sensitivity to a narrow range of color near the red end of the spectrum. The plates have, of course, the usual sensitivity to blue and violet light, but, with the aid of a ray filter which excludes those colors, one may photograph a scene entirely by deep red light. In this way the blue rays, scattered by the dust particles, are eliminated, and a sharp clear picture may be obtained even at a distance of 25 miles and more. Even minor details stand out with a distinctiveness that is remarkable; and it is just such details that are generally the concern of the geologist.

With the addition of a suitable ray-filter (deep yellow or red) the red sensitive plates generally require, under normal conditions, an exposure of about one second, with stop f. 8 to 11.

It must be admitted that there are some objectionable features about the photographs thus obtained. The sky appears black; but if there are clouds present their whiteness relieves that appearance. Again, dry grass, and certain kinds of trees and shrubbery take on a whiteness that suggests a new fall of snow. However, these drawbacks may be considered of secondary importance, provided the chief need is for clear pictures through a hazy atmosphere. By means of these plates it is possible to obtain photographs that show details which the eye itself can not see at the time.

It was the sight of a remarkable photograph of the Sierra Nevada, taken by Mr. Wright from Mount Hamilton, that first drew the writer's attention to the red sensitive plates. The fact that Half Dome and other details of the Yosemite gorge could be clearly recognized although 115 miles away showed clearly that the ever-present blue haze had been definitely neutralized.

ELIOT BLACKWELDER
STANFORD UNIVERSITY,
CALIFORNIA

MODIFIED WATER REGULATOR FOR SMALL TANKS

IN the annual report of the department of oceanography of the University of Liverpool (London, 1925), H. C. Chadwick describes a new device for regulating the outflow of water from small aquaria. Since this device is quite practical and since its description is found in a publication (*Transactions* of the Liverpool Biological Society) of relatively small circulation in the United States, it may not be out of place to reprint Mr. Chadwick's original account in this journal.

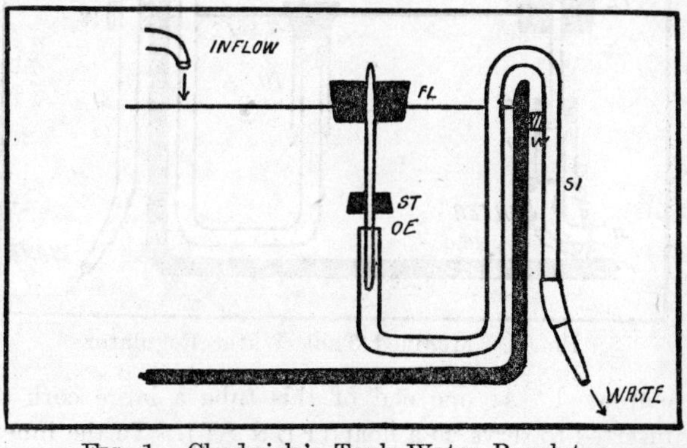

FIG. 1. Chadwick's Tank Water Regulator

The apparatus (Fig. 1) consists of a length of glass tubing 6 mm. in internal diameter, bent as shown in figure. The open end (OE) of the tube was ground on a fine carborundum stone, so as to be exactly at right-angles to the bore of the tube. FL is a good sound cork 1¼-inch in diameter and ¾-inch thick, rendered impervious to water by prolonged immersion in melted paraffin wax. Through a central hole is inserted a piece of glass tubing 4½ inches long and having both ends completely closed. It slides easily up and down in the vertical portion of the siphon SI. About an inch below the cork float, and sliding tightly on the tube so that its position may be varied, is a slice cut cleanly and exactly at right angles from a rubber cork (ST). To bring the apparatus into action it is immersed in the water of the tank (about 5 inches deep) and held in position by a wedge of cork (W) as shown in the figure. The water is drawn through the siphon (SI), and the longer end of the tubing carrying the cork float and the rubber stopper is dropped into the open end (OE), so that the stopper rests upon and closes it. Water is supplied to the tank, and as its surface level rises the rubber stopper is lifted from the aperture, thus allowing a rapid flow through the siphon. This slowly lowers the surface level until the stopper again rests upon the aperture and obstructs the flow. The waste aperture being only 2 mm. in diameter the siphon remains full until the stopper is again lifted. It has been found by experiments that the cork float should have ample buoyancy, so as to easily counteract the suction of the outgoing current.

The main shortcomings of this device are (1) that the glass rod to which the float and stopper are attached is entered into the siphon, thus impeding the free outflow of the water; and (2) that there is no way of preventing small organisms from being sucked into the siphon and thus lost.

These shortcomings, however, are readily removed in the following manner.

1. Instead of using a glass rod, a short glass tube (Fig. 2A, TU), somewhat wider than the siphon, is

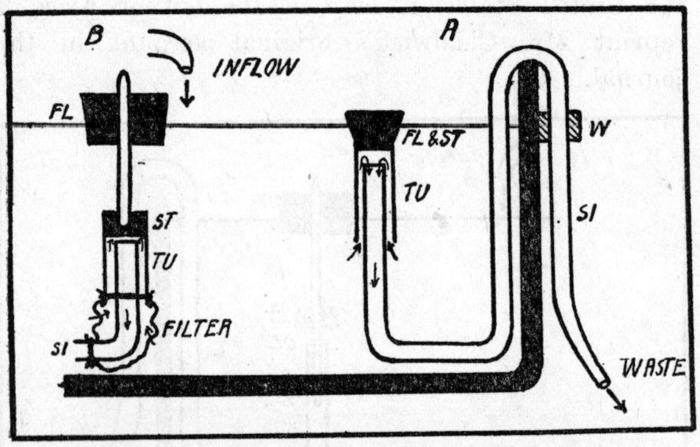

FIG. 2. Modified Tank Water Regulator

employed. At one end of this tube a large cork is inserted to serve as a float (FL & ST). To the inner end of this cork, a rubber gasket is attached in order to obtain a perfectly flat surface to close the open end of the siphon. The tube is now filled with water and placed over the inner end of the siphon in the manner shown in figure 2A.

2. The large float suggested by Chadwick is used in combination with the device described in the previous paragraph (Fig. 2B). However, the glass rod connecting the large float and the stopper should not be made to enter the siphon but should end inside the stopper. A tube of silk cloth (FILTER) should be tied to the lower end of the short glass tube (TU) and to the siphon, not tightly stretched, but in such a manner that the movements of the stopper are not obstructed.

The important points to be observed in making this apparatus are: 1. the tubing for the siphon should not be too wide gauged. 2. the open end of the siphon and the stopper should fit perfectly. 3. the float should be sufficiently large to overcome the suction in the siphon.

Finally, it may be added that instead of a one-sided wedge (W) to support the outer shank of the siphon, a pierced cork is more practical.

TAGE SKOGSBERG

HOPKINS MARINE STATION,
PACIFIC GROVE, CALIFORNIA

SPECIAL ARTICLES

SOME DEVONIAN PLANT LOCALITIES OF CENTRAL AND WESTERN NEW YORK

DURING the past few years a systematic investigation of possible plant localities in the Devonian outcrops of central New York has been in progress. As a result of these investigations plant material with preserved structure has been found in at least half a dozen localities, and there are good prospects of additional discoveries in localities yet to be investigated.

In 1924 Professor L. C. Petry[1] reported and briefly described a specimen from the Genundewa limestone on the west side of Canandaigua Lake at Cheshire, New York. This specimen showed mesarch primary wood strands at the margin of the pith, in contact with secondary wood in which the pits on the radial walls were segregated into groups of five to thirty-five each. These groups are arranged opposite each other in adjacent tracheids so that when the wood is viewed in radial section a characteristic cross banding is observed. To forms bearing these characters Zalessky[2] has assigned the generic name *Callixylon*.

[1] Petry, L. C., "On Fossil Plants showing Structure, from the Upper Devonian of New York." Paper read before the American Association for the Advancement of Science, Washington, D. C., 1924.

[2] Zalessky, M. D., "Etude sur l'anatomie du Dadoxylon Tchihatcheffi Goeppert sp." Mem. du Comité Geol. de Russe. Nouvelle Série 68: 29, 1911.

At Seneca Point, about five miles south of this locality, and in the Genundewa horizon, several more pieces of preserved wood have since been found. These specimens were enclosed mostly in nodular masses of grayish limestone and associated with the pteropod *Styliolina fissurella.* In the same locality, but in the Genesee shale immediately below, several excellent specimens have been found. Some of them represent complete woody cylinders but devoid of cortex and phloem, and range from one fourth inch to two inches in diameter. In some of these specimens the mesarch primary wood has been preserved and most of them show the grouped arrangement of the pits. These wood fragments were found in concretions of dark, dense limestone which are very abundant in the Genesee shale. However only a small per cent. of these concretions contain recognizable plant remains.

Directly across Canandaigua Lake from Seneca Point and in the Genundewa horizon more material was found. No preserved primary wood was found in these specimens, but in many cases the secondary wood was in good condition. The pits on the radial walls of the xylem cells are grouped in the same manner as described above.

On the west side of Cayuga Lake some well preserved plant material was found in a rock fall in the gorge just below the main falls of Taughannock Falls State Park. The secondary wood, which shows the grouped pitting, is in the best state of preservation of any material yet examined. The primary wood is in poorer condition. The exact horizon from which these materials came has not been determined, but the concretions within which they were enclosed closely resemble those of the Genesee shale. The Genundewa limestone is not recognizable above the Genesee shale in this locality.

During the autumn of 1926 several fragments of preserved wood were found in an outcrop of the Ithaca shale on the Cornell University campus. They consisted of both roots and stems, the largest being about three fourths of an inch in diameter. While the preservation in these specimens is rather poor, the nature of the primary wood and the pitting can be determined in some cases. A feature of interest in one of these specimens lies in the fact that the horizontal banding due to the grouping of the pits is not constant throughout the stem, but can be observed in only a few places. The majority of the tracheids show continuous pitting of the *Dadoxylon* type. These fragments did not occur in concretions as did the others but were in a bed of solid limestone of rather localized extent. Associated with the plant remains were numerous large brachiopods. This horizon is about five hundred feet above the Genundewa horizon where, or near where, most of the other material was found.

Mr. A. E. Alexander, a student at Cornell, has recently submitted a specimen from the Ludlowville shale, Spring Creek, Erie County, New York. In this specimen the wood structure has been preserved with marcasite. This material being perfectly opaque, the structure can not be studied in thin section. Consequently its exact nature has not been determined but the tracheids show two or three rows of alternately arranged hexagonal pits which are not grouped after the *Callixylon* fashion.

With the exception of the last the localities above described cover an east and west range of about fifty miles across central New York. The vertical range is about five hundred feet. They all belong to the lower part of the upper Devonian, and in every locality mentioned (except the last) *Callixylon* seems to be the predominating plant type. The locality in Erie County belongs to the middle Devonian.

The fragmentary nature of this material suggests that it was not deposited *in situ,* but represents pieces of drift wood which floated some distance before being buried and preserved. It is generally agreed that the Genesee shales, where some of the material was found, were deposited in a rather stagnant sea, and the material itself apparently represents dry land vegetation. No preserved cortex or phloem has been found in association with any of the material.

Some of the materials show faint suggestions of growth rings. In no case are they well marked and in many specimens there is no evidence of them at all. Where they do occur the cells we assume to be the summer wood have a slightly smaller radial diameter than the adjoining spring wood. In case of a stem which has been slightly crushed flattening of the cells seems to occur to a greater extent along the region of the ring.

CHESTER A. ARNOLD

CORNELL UNIVERSITY

EFFECT OF ULTRA-VIOLET LIGHT UPON DIGITALIS PURPUREA[1]

DURING the summer of 1927, an opportunity arose to test the influence of shorter rays of light upon a common medicinal plant, Digitalis purpurea or "Foxglove." In a five-section greenhouse, the center section was built of a special glass which transmits a considerable portion of the spectrum in the ultra-violet region.[2]

It was thus possible to develop the seedling plants

[1] Paper read before the Botanical Society of America, December 28, 1927.

[2] Acknowledgment is due The Vita Glass Corporation, of New York, for their cooperation in making this study.

under full exposure to these rays, while control plants in the same greenhouse were entirely out of range and received light only through ordinary, plain glass.

Seed was planted in the usual flats; and the experiment proper began when these seedlings were in the small, two-leaf stage. They were then arranged for study in two series as nearly identical as the eye could determine, each of which consisted of 160 plants.

Indoor Conditions

One series was placed under the special glass, the other under the plain glass. Henceforth, they were given identical care, keeping all other conditions uniform; soil, ventilation, moisture, and temperature as closely as possible. (A two or three degree higher temperature occurred at times under the plain glass, but at no time was it of any significance as plants were out of the greenhouse before this became high enough to be a factor).

For about six weeks, between late March and mid-May, plants were kept under close observation, and the advantage in growth was found to lie continually with those under the special glass. The second, third, and fourth pairs of leaves developed from two to four days earlier than the respective parts of the control plants. Treated plants were also somewhat larger and of darker green than the controls. Because these seedlings were to be used later in field work, no dry weight or ash determinations were made. Judgment was based upon careful consideration by four observers, including the gardener and the writer.

Seedlings used were of *D. purpurea,* and, so-called, *D. purpurea* var. *alba.* The former has typical purplish-red flowers; the latter, white flowers. The purple type, or "race," Group A-7, is somewhat sturdier than the white, Group C-23; but both give thrifty, typical plants.

Outdoor Disposal

To decrease the chances of accident, seedlings were hardened in cold frames only five days, after holding in greenhouse until danger from frost was over. They were then transferred to the open Demonstration Garden, May 24, 1927, and set out in four adjacent rows, placing plants one yard apart each way. At this time, all were good, vigorous seedlings; but those which had the benefit of ultra-violet light were unquestionably the better in appearance.

Michigan weather last summer was very dry, but, by very frequent cultivation to conserve moisture, all plants lived. Although, at the time of the first harvest, August 10, 1927, none of the plants were above normal in size, the treated ones were still the larger. The difference, however, was no longer so striking.

Physiological Test: First Cutting

Four samples were taken at this time, two from each group. To prepare a sample, the first twenty plants in a row were cut and the leaves well mixed. All samples were dried under uniform conditions. The crisp leaves were then crushed by hand and again thoroughly mixed before milling.

Tinctures were prepared by U. S. P. Method, and turned over with routine samples for physiological testing, which is done by the M. L. D. Frog-heart Method. Results obtained, shown in Table I, rather strikingly indicate that the stimulus received in seedling stage is carried over under field conditions.

Table I

First crop 8/10/27

Plants tested	Potency of Tincture: Exposed under special glass	Potency of Tincture: Exposed under ordinary glass	Increase of potency
Group A–7	500% of St'd.	400% of St'd.	25.00%
Group C–23	335% of St'd.	300% of St'd.	11.66%

Physiological Test: Second Cutting

To provide a check series, the cut plants were allowed to grow again until September 27, 1927, when a second test was made, extreme care being taken to repeat in every detail the previous procedure. For this cutting, plants were at least 50 per cent. larger than before, due to a very favorable fall season with continual fine weather and frequent warm showers. So far as the eye could detect, there was at this time no difference between the two series; the plants not treated had "caught up" to the treated ones in size and general appearance. It is, therefore, the more interesting to note, Table II, that the potency was again higher, in each group, in the drug exposed to the ultra-violet rays during development of seedling stages.

Table II

Second crop 9/27/27

Plants tested	Potency of Tincture: Exposed under special glass	Potency of Tincture: Exposed under ordinary glass	Increase of potency
Group A–7	400% of St'd.	300% of St'd.	33%
Group C–23	300% of St'd.	225% of St'd.	35%

These plants have all been mulched and, if they survive the winter, will be followed during their second-year stage. Meantime, it seems clear-cut that, so far as may be judged by one year's study, exposure to ultra-violet light is beneficial to both growth and potency of Digitalis purpurea.

Adelia McCrea

Parke, Davis and Company,
Detroit, Michigan

SCIENCE

VOL. LXVII MARCH 16, 1928 No. 1733

CONTENTS

American Association for the Advancement of Science:
Science and the Newspapers: PROFESSOR WM. E. RITTER 279
Malnutrition in Plants: PROFESSOR F. J. SIEVERS 286
Scientific Events:
Budget of the Bureau of Chemistry and the Bureau of the Biological Survey; The Giannini Foundation of the University of California; Presentation of the Charles P. Daly Gold Medal to Professor Alois Musil; National Research Fellowships in the Biological Sciences 288
Scientific Notes and News 290
University and Educational Notes 295
Discussion and Correspondence:
The Functional Nature of the Constant of Mass Action: DR. R. D. KLEEMAN. *Vegetative Propagation of the Apple by Seed:* DR. CHARLES F. SWINGLE. *Living Cells in Heart-Wood of Trees:* PROFESSOR J. H. FAULL. *A Prehistory Chart:* DR. E. A. HOOTON. *Philosophy or Irony, Which?* PROFESSOR M. M. GARVER. *The South African Station of the Harvard Observatory:* PROFESSOR HARLOW SHAPLEY. *Apparatus:* DR. WILMER SOUDER 295
Scientific Books:
Brooks' Climate through the Ages: DR. MALCOLM H. BISSELL 298
Scientific Apparatus and Laboratory Methods:
A Method for Cutting Glass Tubing: PROFESSOR I. P. TOLMACHOFF. *A Platinum Spoon for Isolating and Transferring Protozoa:* PERCY L. JOHNSON 299
Special Articles:
Statistics of Vocabulary: E. U. CONDON 300
Science News x

SCIENCE: A Weekly Journal devoted to the Advancement of Science, edited by J. McKeen Cattell and published every Friday by

THE SCIENCE PRESS

New York City: Grand Central Terminal.

Lancaster, Pa. Garrison, N. Y.

Annual Subscription, $6.00. Single Copies, 15 Cts.

SCIENCE is the official organ of the American Association for the Advancement of Science. Information regarding membership in the Association may be secured from the office of the permanent secretary, in the Smithsonian Institution Building, Washington, D. C.

Entered as second-class matter July 18, 1923, at the Post Office at Lancaster, Pa., under the Act of March 8, 1879.

SCIENCE AND THE NEWSPAPERS[1]

WHAT I bring this evening is a joint product. My partner-in-production is E. W. Scripps, the chief designer and builder of the Scripps-Howard newspaper enterprises. Of the great wealth gained by these enterprises Mr. Scripps saw fit to invest before his death a portion in such scientific ventures as the Scripps Institution of Oceanography at La Jolla, California, the Scripps Foundation for Research in Problems of Population at Miami University, Oxford, Ohio, and Science Service, Washington, D. C. The partnership lasted during the nineteen years of my incumbency of the directorship of the institution at La Jolla. Its purpose was to devote as many hours per week as possible to the personal discussion of all the problems humankind hath ever encountered or is likely ever to encounter—such having been the spiritual appetite of the senior partner.

THE NEWSPAPERS

By the popularization of science is understood in this address the promotion among people generally of that devotion to truth which is basic among the few people whose professional career is the pursuit of truth through scientific research. The scattering abroad of natural knowledge discovered by such research is regarded more in the capacity of that knowledge to promote devotion to truth than for any of the other uses to which such knowledge may be put.

To the making of our civilization many factors have contributed. Probably no two persons would agree on a list of the most important of these factors, or on a valuation of the different factors. But all would agree that among the foremost in influence are science and journalism. No phase of our life escapes the influence of both. From matches and beads to the ministry and birth-control nothing is out of reach of the penetrating gaze of science or the clatter and yell of the public press.

If evidence is wanted of the power of these factors, all that is necessary is to start something of major interest to the community. Launch a world war, or a world-wide health campaign, and note the instant and insistent appeal of the enterprise to both factors. Modern life depends vitally on both; yet its estimates

[1] Address at a general session, American Association for the Advancement of Science, Nashville, December 29, 1927.

of them, its attitudes toward them, are very different; and the estimate and attitude of each relative to the other is but a reflex of the generally prevailing estimate and attitude.

To the average member of the community and to many a newspaper man, pure science is as dry as dust and about as useful. True enough, now and then the researcher hits upon something, radium or "glands," that has a real kick in it. But this is accidental. Such lucky hits are not of the true nature of science. Indeed, the investigator is so blind to the business possibilities of the hits he occasionally makes that nothing of their real value is brought out until some practical chap—some good business man—comes along and converts them into dollars and cents.

Counterwise the typical investigator's conception of the average newspaper man, especially of the typical reporter, is that he is first and foremost "sensational." No matter how little or how much your typical scientist says in describing newspaper and newspaper men, that word, or some other containing the same meaning, must stand central in it.

On the whole, the newspaper press is sensational; some exceptions there surely are, but too few to affect the general situation. It is notorious that the occasional newspaper which is not sensational is apt to be a business failure. A daily newspaper that is not predominantly yellow is pretty sure to be predominantly red in its balance sheet.

"But," say the newspaper men who make their papers business successes by making them sensational, "the fact that people buy our papers is proof positive that we are furnishing them what they want; and surely we are not responsible for the people's tastes."

We find ourselves confronted at every turn by the problem of that in human nature which makes for emotionalism, for sensationalism. The aspect of the problem which we meet here is as to whether all mankind, save only the minute fraction known as scientists, are so constituted as to make them want what the sensational press gives them. Are scientists as a class wholly apart from the rest of mankind in this? By no means. As to matters outside their special interests and work scientists are obviously not fundamentally different from their fellow mortals. But even here they are not. The popular conception of science as something utterly unemotional—as flourishing only in the frigid zone of mental life—is all a myth. Effective inquiry into the hidden things of nature is no more possible without the energizing warmth of emotion than is creative effort in poetry or music. The real psycho-biological problem is as to the way reason and emotion are compounded in science as compared with the way they are compounded in art.

The special point to be made here concerns the particular effect the emotional responses of scientists have on the problem of making scientific knowledge comprehensible and accessible to the general public. No one who is familiar with the little class of scientific investigators needs to be told of the intensity, often the bitterness of the rivalry, that may exist there not only as to institutional and positional preferment but as to discoveries, conclusions and theories. The question of who of several rival experts in the same specialty are most competent—are the best authorities—is often very perplexing for those whose function it is to teach science to people at large, whether in classroom, on lecture platform, or through the printing press.

This is merely saying that scientific investigators like all normal members of modern civilized society are persons in whom rational life and emotional life have to get on together in some way, that way determining the measure of wisdom and usefulness of such persons to themselves and to the community. Hence it happens that the utterances by investigators themselves are in some instances distinctly tinged with yellow. Such instances are especially common where certain results suggest, though in a wholly tentative way, conditions and occurrences in the future which would greatly affect human life. In other words, scientists sometimes exercise altogether too little wisdom in their use of hypotheses touching matters of great human concern, departing in so far from allegiance to the true spirit and method of science.

Is it possible, then, for two such diverse agencies to find a ground on which to work together for the common good? Many scientists have not hesitated to answer "No, such a ground can not be found because it does not exist." And seemingly many newspaper men have held the same view.

On its face the history of journalism does not encourage hopefulness that it and science may find common ground on which to work. The only reference to science I find in one volume consulted is a brief narration of how the New York *Sun* increased its circulation by a yarn about the moon written by an educated reporter and boosted by Edgar Allan Poe. The hoax consisted of a lot of buncombe about an astronomical expedition to the Cape of Good Hope under the leadership of Sir John Herschel for investigation through a gigantic telescope of the moon and its vegetable and animal life. So well did the reporter and his booster do the job that the yellow and the white press and the scientists of the day are said to have swallowed the bait.

Science is the embodiment of rational life. Journalism is chiefly dependent on the emotional in life. The view is that these two lives are so antagonistic that it is folly to talk about bringing them onto a common ground. The kinship of journalism is held to be with art rather than with science. The newspaper is animated more by the spirit of *belles-lettres* than by that of exact, positive knowledge. A list of well-known names in the history of American journalism and another in American letters have many in common. Journalism in this country has been, as Dana, Watterson and others expressly regarded it, a form of literary art; and nobody seems to doubt that it is now an industry and a business.

No two men of the early period of our national history have actually lived through the whole of that history on into this very day more than Benjamin Franklin and Thomas Jefferson. Their continuous vital presence in the life of America is due to their having been men of learning—men of science in the broadest and best sense.

Both men were likewise giant figures in the journalism of their day. Franklin's newspaper, *The Pennsylvania Gazette,* and other journalistic and publishing enterprises (one of which was *Poor Richard's Almanac*) were his vocation for some forty years and the main source of his considerable wealth. During this period his fame as a scientific investigator was chiefly won; and his success in his vocation, his fame as a scientist and his reputation as a wise citizen were the basis and stepping-stone to his great but later career in diplomacy.

Jefferson's relation to science and to journalism was less direct and close and is much less known than Franklin's. He appears to have been the first to see clearly, as a professional statesman, the great significance of the newspaper as a factor in popular government, and of science and popular learning as factors in a democratic society.

Although he seems never to have had any connection either proprietary or editorial with any newspaper, yet he it was who could say "were it left to me to decide whether we should have a government without newspapers, or newspapers without a government, I should not hesitate a moment to prefer the latter. But I should mean that every man should receive those papers and be capable of reading them."

It was through the astonishing power Jefferson had of influencing other men to write for the papers that he made the press contribute so largely to the promotion of his social and political ideas.

As holders of public office it was inevitable that Franklin and Jefferson should have had to stand the lash of criticism, both fair and foul, through the press. It is consequently desirable to know what effect their experiences with this aspect of journalism had on their general views.

In an essay entitled "An Account of the Highest Court of Judicature in Pennsylvania, *viz.* the Court of the Press," Franklin gives us his views on the subject. As to the power of this court, he says, it "may judge, sentence, and condemn to infamy, not only private individuals, but public bodies, etc., with or without inquiry or hearing, at the court's discretion." Concerning the "natural support of this court," Franklin concludes that it "is founded in the depravity of such minds as have not been mended by religion, nor improved by good education." Then he goes on to ask what can be done about it.

Having convinced himself that no legislative control of the court's activities is possible that would not be "construed as an infringement of the sacred liberty of the press," he looks in other directions for the needed control. He thinks he has found an agency which will restore to the people a species of liberty of which they have been deprived by our laws. "I mean," he says, "the liberty of the cudgel."

"My proposal is to leave the liberty of the press untouched, to be exercised in its full extent, force, and vigor, but to permit the liberty of the cudgel to go with it, *pari passu.*"

Jefferson is not on record so explicitly as Franklin on the tendency of newspaper liberty to run riot. But he said enough to leave no doubt that he saw and felt this tendency. Not long after he became president, he spoke of newspapers as "a bear-garden scene into which I have made it a point to enter on no provocation." Printers, like the clery he said, "live by the zeal they can kindle, and the schisms they can create." Accordingly, they "can never leave us in a state of perfect rest and union of opinion."

As to what might be done about it, Jefferson's view was less heroic than Franklin's. He held that while Congress had no power to put the press in a strait-jacket, the individual states might do so to some extent. It does not appear, however, that he would have the states go farther than to punish slander. And he concludes: "However, the steady character of our countrymen is a rock to which we may safely moor; and notwithstanding the efforts of the papers to disseminate early discontents, I expect that a just, dispassionate and steady conduct will at length rally to a proper system the great body of our country."

A shallow dip into the history of American journalism is enough to convince one that for a long time the "bear-garden scene" of Jefferson's characterization held good and also that the "liberty of the cudgel" proposed by Franklin was a practical if not a legal reality.

The period of what might be called bellicose journalism may be roughly put as extending from the struggle between federalists and democrats during the beginning years of our present government to about 1850. Its peak may be regarded as having been reached with the use for advertising his paper (the New York *Herald*) James Gordon Bennett made of the cudgelings he got. Although Bennett appears to have come through all his personal encounters without permanent bodily injury, and to have profited greatly from them as publicity material, it may be inferred that to newspaper men generally this seemed rather too risky a form of advertising to justify its adoption on an extensive scale. For, on the whole, the "liberty of the cudgel" as a factor in journalism seems to have lost ground from about the end of Bennett's journalistic career.

It looks as though a close study of the subject would reveal Bennett's position to have had more significance than that of simply marking high-water in the physical bellicosity of journalism. He seems to have been one of the earliest discoverers that political journalism is bad. After an especially disappointing experience in this way shortly before starting the *Herald* in 1834 he declared himself through with politics. From about that time there seems to have gone on a slow but sure disentangling of journalism from party politics, and from alliance with any and all other special organizations and interests.

On the whole the freedom of the newspaper press has suffered more in America at least, from being tied up with special interests—political, business, religious, social or what-not—than from acts of government.

Our main contention is that although science is rooted more in man's life of reason than in his life of feeling, while journalism is rooted more in his life of feeling than in his life of reason, the devotion of both to truths peculiar to its own domain should constitute a ground on which the two may work together for the common good. The pursuit and dissemination of truth is as much the life of the newspaper press as it is of the research institution. Such a news-gathering agency as the Associated Press or the United Press *is* a research institution in a very real sense. A daily newspaper is essentially a collector from the community, and a narrator for the community, of information concerning the day-to-day happenings in the community. It is a sort of minute book of the community's daily life. Regardless of the extent to which news proper may be submerged in matters which have or seem to have no relation to news, after all, the news is the heart of the thing. Exactly what "news" is has been much debated. But whatever else it may be, it must include factual information chiefly about human life. Imagine any newspaper adopting a policy of making every news item as "sensational" as possible in utter disregard of the truth. How long would such a paper survive? Even if its plant escaped wreckage at the hands of an infuriated public, it could not escape financial wreckage.

The tendency to wholesale condemnation of the daily newspapers as "sensational" and "lying" ignores a great part of the most essential make-up of any given day's issue. The hundred-and-one notices of things that have happened and are scheduled to happen at home and abroad, in public affairs, in society, in school, in church, in sport, in business, in finance, in health, and so forth, concerning which there is no room for accusation of sensationalism, are forgotten when such condemnatory pronouncements are made. Except as legitimate interest is a form of sensation—of what is felt as contrasted with what is factually known—the basic substance of the newspaper is as true to life as is the basic substance of the most scientific treatise on human physiology or pathology, or on economics or sociology or politics.

Even as touching the most vital interests, that is to say, the most sensation-inducing interests, we find as emphatic expressions of allegiance to truth from journalism as from any calling whatever. Joseph Pulitzer's instructions to the editorial writers of the *Evening World* in connection with an election candidacy to the New York judiciary could hardly be surpassed in fidelity to truth.

> I want you to go into the Maynard case with an absolutely unprejudiced mind. We hold no briefs for or against him, as you know. I want you to get together all the documents in the case. I want you to take them home and study them as minutely as if you were preparing yourself for an examination. I want you to regard yourself as a judicial officer, oath-bound to justice, and when you shall have mastered the facts and the law in the case, I want you to set them forth in a four-column editorial that every reader of the *World* can easily understand.

Did a judge from the bench or scientist from the laboratory ever show more intelligent and determined effort in behalf of truth than that?

If the essence of journalism is the gathering and dissemination of truth in the form of news, and if the essence of science is the discovery and dissemination of truth concerning nature, then truth furnishes ample meeting ground for the two.

A single illustration of what this statement means, practically, must suffice. The extensive, though by no means universal support given to science by the newspaper in the Scopes' trial needs interpreting from two directions. Looked at journalistically it was a telling exhibition of that championship of freedom of speech and of the press for which journalism has always been famous. The attitude of many of the papers was primarily this: Regardless of whether the theory of evolution has been fully established or not, it is supported by a great number of incontestable facts and is believed by many persons specially qualified to speak on the subject. The rank and file of the community are therefore entitled to have it presented to them by all competent agencies of education, whether the school, the press, or any other. The right and freedom of the general public to learn is as vital as is the right and freedom of individuals to speak.

Then there was the genuine effort by many papers to get and publish data on the merits of the controversy. A considerable study by Science Service and by myself personally of the part the newspapers took in the affair suggests that scientists have not fully appraised the case as evidence of the possibilities there are of the usefulness journalism may have to science.

And unquestionably journalism has worked cooperatively with science in many other cases. This can not, however, blind us to the fact that in some situations newspaper practice is diametrically opposed to that of science. For instance, the apparent deliberateness with which some newspapers will publish almost anything about sex that is lascivious but almost nothing about it that is scientific, astonishes scientifically minded people and undoubtedly tends to moral havoc for great numbers of people.

At the same time it must be recognized that scientific research has as yet achieved little in the fields which involve human interest and welfare and hence emotion at its greatest intensity that is comparable in trustworthiness with what it has achieved in other fields. For instance biological investigation has enlarged knowledge enormously concerning those reproductive and sexual phenomena which are remote from immediate, personal human interest. Their manifestation in lower organisms, plant and animal, and their cellular aspects in higher organisms, have received wonderful illumination at the hands of investigators. Furthermore, medical science has penetrated deeply into certain of these phenomena. But such of them as implicate with greatest intensity the lives of men and women in their relations with one another are only now beginning to have the searchlights of rigid investigation turned upon them.

Hence there is ample justification for hesitancy on the part of teachers of the public whether in school or press to give adherence and general publicity to the fragmentary and tentative findings of science in these matters. All that can be properly desired is that just so far as the results of investigations become trustworthy as evidenced by being generally agreed upon by those devoting themselves to the special inquiries concerned, the essentials of the results shall be given adequate place in educational effort.

What is said about scientific knowledge of reproductive and sexual phenomena, and the general dissemination of such knowledge, would be essentially applicable to various other blocks of phenomena which involve mankind's interests and emotions almost if not quite equally closely. For instance, so much of economic science as deals with, or by rights should deal with, those phenomena which have given rise to the familiar dictum "self-preservation is the first law of life" seems to be almost as backward from the standpoint of scientific research as are the aspects referred to of reproduction and sex. And religious phenomena are in similar state.

Our study to this point has brought out that the problem of the relation between journalism and science is in large measure the problem of the relation between man's life of reason and his life of emotion. It is thus only an aspect of the problem by which humankind is confronted in every major concern of its existence.

SCIENCE

Early in this discussion the conviction was expressed that we now have enough scientific knowledge of the nature of man and of the world generally to justify the belief that truth as newspapers conceive and pursue it, and truth as science conceives and pursues it, is sufficiently the same to constitute a common ground on which journalism and science might work together for the common good.

Such a union of interests and efforts may be greatly facilitated by the broadened and deepened understanding of himself man is now gaining through the great advances of science.

Many sciences have contributed to this enhancement of man's self-understanding. But, as should be expected, the sciences of living nature, in which the sciences of man are of course included, have contributed most.

The advances in biology particularly are bringing about a transformation in our conception of the origin and nature of living beings. The theory of evolution is passing into a new and radically different phase from those it has before passed through. This phase will concern man as he actually lives from day to day much more particularly than have the phases through which the theory has been passing during the last half century and more. Once the character of the new phase catches the newspaper eye (more properly, I suppose, the newspaper "nose for news"), it is a safe guess that one of the most spacious and inviting common grounds for journalism and science will have been discovered.

What is this ground stated in language that might pass muster as journalistic science?

First, as to the name of the theory in its new phase: emergent evolution has already been applied to it so widely, especially since C. L. Morgan's book by that name, that this christening seems likely to stick. But it appears that the thing itself has been expounded by a number of biologists in quite different terminologies, the expounders not having been fully aware until recently that they were expounding essentially the same thing. Workers in widely separated subdivisions of the biological realm have come to essentially the same conclusion as to the general nature of the reinterpretation to which the phenomena of organic development must be subjected. H. S. Jennings has long championed the idea under the name "radical experimentalism"; and the small group, including C. M. Child and C. J. Herrick, have been whaling away at it for years under the name "the organismic conception." Under essentially this caption I have spoken in my own peculiar way for the idea rather extensively during more than a decade.

From the side of traditional philosophy the naturalism of John Dewey has much in common with the world view implied by emergent evolution; and the "evolutionary naturalism" of Roy Wood Sellars is perhaps as close to that view as it is practicable for a strictly philosophical treatment of a subject to approach a scientific treatment of the same subject. Furthermore, A. N. Whitehead's theory of "organic mechanism," coming from mathematical physics, is surely a close relative.

Three points concerning this new phase of the evolution theory may be presumed to interest everybody because recognizable as likely to bear upon everybody's personal well-being.

1. Living individuals of organic nature, including individual men and women, boys and girls, adolescents, young children and just-born babies, are going to loom much larger in biological science than they have heretofore. A period of scientific interest in individuals is impending. The scientific-poetic doctrine of nature's great care for the species and great carelessness for the individual is nearing the sunset of its long, somber day.

The idea of emergence traced to its physicochemical foundation finds a peculiar form of organized individual to be indispensable to the occurrence of phenomena which characterize bodies as being alive, or living. The conception of "living matter" as if it were something unindividuated or only secondarily individuated must be abandoned.

This coming of the individual organism more prominently into the field of scientific attention will shift the major theoretic interest for a time at least from *evolution* in the racial and species sense to *development* in the individual sense. We may anticipate that before long the present vogue in many aspects of modern life of the great place accorded the individual will be traced to its connection with this element in the revised theory of evolution. Under the caption "personality" the individual is gaining special prominence in education, in industry, in medicine and in social intercourse.

2. The second point of general human interest in regard to "emergent evolution" may be stated with reference to the doctrine of the fundamental independence and separableness of body and mind. Fix your attention on the individual as growing in the sense of *emerging* through its various stages, fertilized egg, early and late embryo, just-born infant, childhood, and the rest, and you fail to find a trace of evidence of such a thing as a body independent of a mind or a mind independent of a body. Could man's knowledge of himself have begun with a knowledge of the egg and various embryonic stages of his individual development, such a theory as that of the independence of his body and his mind would never have occurred to him.

Historically viewed all forms of the idea of mind as independent of body are genetically kindred to the numberless varieties of ghost ideas of primitive man. The theory of psychophysical parallelism can be traced to the dualism manifested in these terrific mental aberrations of our savage ancestors. This theory recognizes that man has a mind and also a body, but, it says, the phenomena which constitute mind and those which constitute body are so different that they can not have any causal relation with each other.

Viewed from the standpoint of common adult experience in broad daylight this is an astonishing theory. When it became linked with the theory of man's derivative origin revived by Darwin, the conclusion was almost inevitable that while the origin of man's body could be causally explained, the origin of his mind could not be so explained. It was first surmised, then dogmatically held, that since it is impossible to explain mind, its existence is only an illusion. Hence consciousness became an epiphenomenon, if it exists at all; ethical and esthetic feeling and action became by-products of mechanical processes; and religion became a trait of childhood to be outgrown by every normal individual, and, finally, by the whole race.

With the moral monstrosity of these speculations we are only secondarily concerned. It is their scientific monstrosity that concerns us. The most distinctive attributes of the human species as compared with all other species are those on the basis of which this species has produced agencies for human betterment and justice, science, art and religion. Yet here is a group of pre-scientific speculations espoused, elaborated and defended by science, that would deny the reality of these attributes, or reduce them to insignificance!

The theory of psychophysical parallelism, coupled with the mechanical theory of man's origin and fundamental nature, has infected man with the spiritual disease of misanthropy, cynicism and loss of self-respect. The contribution of the revised evolution theory to the cure of this affliction may be counted as one of the best fruits of the revision.

3. The last of the three points to be considered in connection with the new phase of the evolution theory concerns a probable shift of interest from the problems of when and how and where man originated to those of what he is, conceived as a *natural,* rather than in any part a *supernatural* being.

The conception of every individual organism as an emergent means that the degree of uniqueness, and the unifiedness which characterize the human organism, leaves no room for doubt of the objective reality of those attributes of man which make him a rational, a social, a moral, an esthetic and a religious animal, nor of the adequacy of the creative power of the natural order to produce man with all his physical and his spiritual attributes.

Man has arrived at a supremely critical stage in his millenniums of effort to make his positive knowledge of himself and of the world contribute in the highest measure to his own good. That stage is marked by the necessity of displacing the legendary, mythical and merely authoritarian knowledge which has constituted his theology by his verified and verifiable experiential knowledge of himself and the world, and of accomplishing this without impairing anything essential and valuable to the emotional aspect of his religion.

The chief lack of ability of both science and journalism (as of all other educational agencies) to face this tremendous situation is lack of preparedness to grapple rationally with three of man's attributes in which his emotional nature is most mightily involved. These attributes are his basic economic needs, his sexual impulsions, and his religious desires, hopes and fears.

Probably the most vital spot in this whole situation is the perception that religion is a response to the natural order; that it does not depend on a supernatural order or even a belief in such an order, as has been generally supposed. Man's belief in the supernatural seems to have resulted from his efforts toward a rational explanation of the peculiar form of his emotion here involved. The natural order to which this emotion is a response so vastly out-distances his factual knowledge and his scientific generalizations concerning it, that it is not surprising man should make hypotheses of the existence of bodies and powers quite outside of and above the natural order.

The contention that belief in the supernatural is a gigantic error into which man has been led in his effort to find a rational basis for the peculiar type of emotional response foundational to religion implies a change of attitude toward the natural order more deep and wide-reaching than any he has before had to undergo in his whole cultural history. It surpasses in human significance the change of attitude necessitated by the transition from the Ptolemaic to the Copernican astronomy because it implicates human life more directly.

Two considerations have impelled me to touch this ticklish subject. One is the composite nature of this production: My partner held, as a practical man, essentially the same views that I have sketched as a scientist. He would insist, were he with us, that once in the midst of such a treatment of our topic as that entered upon, we go through to the logical end, no matter how inadequately.

But the consideration that has pushed me hardest is the nature of the situation itself. That situation is, as previously indicated, before anything else, the problem of man's reaching a livable adjustment between his life of emotion and his life of reason.

If it is true that these conflicting aspects of man's nature are strictly natural phenomena and that the theory of evolution, especially in the phase now being entered, is the right approach to the great human problems involved, then it follows that the unified study and treatment of man in every aspect of his being is fundamental. We are faced with the necessity of bringing under one point of view for both research and practical treatment what are usually classed as "anthropology" and the "humanistic sciences," medicine, hygiene, human psychology and education ranging themselves within these two classes. Scientific research is already making considerable headway in some of the problems belonging to these intensely vital and hence equally emotion-manifesting domains of human life, and it is certain to push the efforts with more zeal and efficiency than ever in the future. But science must undergo a great renewal of self-illumination concerning its place in human life and its meaning for human welfare before it can achieve its greatest victories in such research.

A grave charge often made against science is that many of its devotees are disregardful of the sensibilities of persons who hold what the specialists know or believe to be erroneous ideas on points of vital human concern. In some instances this disregard has been heartless, even to brutality. The psychologist who could tell his class to "park their souls out of doors" when they came to his class room, had at some time somehow suffered a bad twist to his mental and moral make-up. When and how the twisting happened, it may be impossible to tell exactly. But an important factor in it may be confidently supposed to be failure to recognize one of the most important differences between the physical sciences and the sciences of man. The difference referred to inheres in the different relation held by the investigator to what is investigated. The physical sciences are motivated entirely in the gaining of knowledge of, and control over, the objects and processes investigated. The well-being of what is investigated is considered not at all by the investigator. He may exploit his experimental materials without let or hindrance so far as their rights are concerned.

Quite otherwise is it in the sciences of man. In all these, knowing and controlling the objects and processes investigated are and must be subordinate, speaking broadly, to the wellbeing of the objects studied. The surgeon at the operating table may be taken to typify the essential relation between investigator and investigated in the whole group of sciences of man. Technical knowledge of investigator and skill of operator are here dedicated wholly to the purpose for which they primarily exist, namely, human welfare in the form of restoration to health of individual human beings. Obviously not in all these sciences can the objects studied become the beneficiaries of knowledge in such immediate personal way as in the case of the patient needing operative treatment.

How, then, are the benefits to be extended? Undoubtedly in many different ways, but most importantly through the increased intelligence of the public concerning the knowledge gained by the researches.

But again, how is such extension of intelligence to be accomplished? To illustrate, what part should school education play in making people at large effectively acquainted with the established results of investigations into the relation between the human sexes? What part should the newspapers play? What part should be taken care of in the home?

The evidence of the intellectual decadence of New England, so startlingly emphasized by Dr. Cattell's just-published résumé of his study of the distribution of scientific men in the United States, is too obvious in its sinister bearing on the future of our country to be missed by anybody who becomes acquainted with the facts. Is this study to be followed up so as to learn what factors are responsible for the decay, whether it affects all aspects of New England's cultural life, whether the disease is likely to extend to the entire nation? Suppose science should get certain or highly probable answers to these questions, how is the truth to be so brought home to the general public as to make it effective in the national life?

Because of the nature and complexity of the situation, I am going to do no more than make a suggestion which, if carried out, might do much to promote the desired end so far as journalism and science are concerned.

I suggest that the special efforts made at this meeting of the American Association toward increasing the dissemination of science to the public be the beginning of efforts in this direction that shall go much farther than anything of the sort this country has ever seen.

I suggest that the symposium held yesterday on publicity for science be repeated, perhaps many times, either under the auspices of this association or some equally competent agency, but extended in scope so as to secure the joint discussion between the very foremost representatives of the sciences and of the newspapers of the almost numberless points at which they impinge on each other, sometimes in friendliness, but sometimes in hostility.

Do not the indications of growing desire by newspapers for scientific news and opinions justify the belief that the time is favorable for such a move? It seems to me the results of the study just reported by the Permanent Secretary of the American Association of the space given by newspapers to the scientific proceedings of recent meetings of the association may be interpreted in this way. This instance by no means stands alone on the side of journalism itself in affording like encouragement. Is it possible that journalism is more ready than science for such a move?

We are all patriotic Americans. As men of science we may claim more. We may claim that our patriotism embodies knowledge of, and devotion to, the best ideals and traditions of Americanism. A few critics of America, some foreign and some of our own number, are saying that American ideals as held by the founders of the Republic have gone by the board. I would like this partnership address, as I have called it, to be viewed as an attempt by one journalist, E. W. Scripps, and one scientist, myself, to join forces in support of the basic ideas of journalism, of science, and of Americanism that were held by those two master builders of our Nation, Benjamin Franklin and Thomas Jefferson.

WM. E. RITTER

SCIENCE SERVICE, WASHINGTON, D. C., AND
UNIVERSITY OF CALIFORNIA

MALNUTRITION IN PLANTS

NUTRITION problems are quite as common in plant as they are in animal life, and in both cases these problems become most evident where the living organism is forced to develop under unnatural environmental conditions. In plant life when plants are fed artificially, many disorders are common and recognized, and these disorders are most evident in plants when their culture is attempted under climatic and soil conditions to which they are not naturally adapted. The orchard industry as practiced in the more or less arid sections, both with and without irrigation, furnishes an outstanding illustration of this fact. In nature, orchard trees are best adapted to humid regions having a soil comparatively well supplied with organic matter and nitrogen, and where the precipitation is so distributed as to cause the plant food in the soil to become available through bacterial action in about the proper amount and proportion to meet the demands of the growing plant. When attempts are made to grow such trees in the arid regions where soils are primarily not abundantly supplied with organic matter and nitrogen and where moisture must be furnished either by irrigation or by conservation through clean cultivation, nature's influences are decidedly modified.

Among the apparent nutritional disorders of orchard trees in the arid regions the "disease" sometimes referred to as "roseatte," or "small leaf," or "die back," or "mottled leaf," or "multiple bud," is quite common. Its main symptom is that large numbers of small leaves develop in clusters in a more or less roseatted arrangement on the ends of twigs. Cultural indications are that soil nitrogen is a contributing factor to this abnormal condition. The influence of available nitrogen on the development of some of our annual plants is fairly well understood. For instance, large supplies of soluble nitrogen when present in the soil during the tillering stage of wheat will cause the plant to set many stools, when present after the jointing stage they result in luxuriant vegetative growth and during the fruitation stage their tendency is to produce a grain high in protein. While the influence of nitrogen in the development of a perennial plant like an orchard tree is not so easily traceable, and therefore, not so well understood, it is only reasonable to suppose that such influences may be quite as evident and prove quite as effective once it is learned how they may be detected. Using the "disease" referred to as an illustration of a case of malnutrition let us see what the conditions are under which it develops and the practices that have been effective in its control, so that a proper basis for a diagnosis may be established.

This roseatted condition develops under both irrigated and non-irrigated conditions in the more arid sections of the state of Washington where trees are grown under clean cultivation. When this "disease" which interfered so materially with the production of marketable fruit that it made the business unprofitable, was first experienced the more radical growers pulled up their orchards and resorted to the production of other crops from which the required returns could be derived. The more conservative orchardist left his trees but attempted to grow a crop between the rows. Alfalfa was known to be well adapted and it was introduced. This crop not only proved fairly profitable, but to the grower's surprise the orchard trees took on a deeper green foliage, made a more luxuriant leaf and wood growth and the roseatted condition rapidly disappeared. The natural effect of this beneficial influence on the trees was that not only alfalfa but other legumes were rapidly introduced in the growing orchards so that now there is little clean cultivation practiced where the irrigation water supply is adequate to make intercropping possible. The first reaction from such results might well lead to the conclusion that the beneficial effect of legumes in this relationship is traceable to their nitrogen fixing power and this is justifiable on the basis that most of the irrigated soils are, even in their virgin state, not over well supplied with nitrogen. Where intercropping with legumes was considered impracticable due to prejudice or to the lack of sufficient irrigation water, it was concluded, and reasonably so, that the same benefits could be derived if the trees were supplied with a readily available nitrogen fertilizer. In actual practice, however, this did not follow because it proved that the beneficial results produced by the legume could not always be duplicated in that way. Furthermore, roseatted trees were not always associated with nitrogen deficiency in the soil, because in a few cases trees growing in hog lots where there was every evidence of an adequate nitrogen supply also developed the "disease." Animal manures, on the other hand, when applied to roseatted orchards in liberal amounts were just as effective in overcoming this nutrition problem as were legumes.

Although these apparent inconsistencies may be difficult of complete explanation on the basis of actual controlled experimental work, it is reasonable to conclude that the form in which the nitrogen is applied and the time at which the application is made is a very important factor. In the orchard sections of the State of Washington it is not uncommon to have long periods of comparatively warm weather and considerable rainfall after the trees have reached their dormant state in the fall. This warm weather and the optimum soil moisture supply promote nitrifying bacterial activity with the result that in clean cultivated soils where there is no vegetative growth to utilize the nitrogen so made available, large amounts of nitrogen frequently accumulate in the autumn season. Where the succeeding winter precipitation is not sufficient to cause the accumulated nitrates to be leached into the drainage system, a condition that prevails in most irrigated sections, a comparatively large amount of available nitrogen will be present in the soil and ready to function as soon as the growing season begins in the spring. Such supplies of available soil nitrogen are not possible in the humid climates naturally adapted to tree growth and it is only reasonable to suppose that this abnormal food supply in the spring will produce abnormalities in tree development.

Liberal supplies of available soil nitrogen are conducive to excessive vegetative growth and in the case of trees nitrates, present in large amounts in the very early spring, may serve as a stimulant for the development of a large number of buds and leaves. When later in the season this supply of nitrates is exhausted as is likely to be the case with these soils, which are at best not abundantly supplied with total nitrogen, there is no corresponding twig growth and elongation. The result is that the leaves are left in a light green colored, partly developed state, grouped close together near the ends of branches. The use of a nitrogen fertilizer, instead of overcoming this condition, as was at one time supposed, may even aggravate it if the application is made at the wrong time of the year. Surely it would seem illogical under such conditions to make heavy applications of readily available nitrogen fertilizers in the late fall, winter or early spring.

In orchards where legumes are grown to supply the nitrogen, the situation is different. The conditions that are conducive to the bacterial activity essential for nitrogen fixation by legumes and for the decay of soil organic matter necessary to release nitrogen for plant use, are the same conditions that promote best tree growth. There should be little danger, therefore, of the accumulation of an abnormal supply of available nitrogen, under conditions where that element of plant food is supplied by legumes or by slow acting organic fertilizers. That this is borne out where legumes are grown has been shown and it is also known that the roseatted condition does not develop but can be overcome when animal manures are used to supply the nitrogen. The property of manure to supply regular and normal amounts of available nitrogen in the proportion that the growing plant demands them has caused this fertilizer to become known as being "fool proof." When plants are fed with artificially prepared fertilizers of high availability an attempt should be made to apply such fertilizers at the time and in the proportion that they are required if best results are to be obtained, and this is especially true where perennial plants are grown and when the quality of the product is a factor. If these relationships are once properly understood many malnutrition problems can be controlled and commercial fertilizers may be used to exert influences on yield and quality never before credited to or claimed for animal manures.

F. J. SIEVERS

STATE COLLEGE OF WASHINGTON,
PULLMAN

SCIENTIFIC EVENTS

BUDGET OF THE BUREAU OF CHEMISTRY AND THE BUREAU OF BIOLOGICAL SURVEY

THE budget of the U. S. Department of Agriculture for the fiscal year 1929 (see SCIENCE, LXVII, page 186), which has been transmitted to congress by the president, includes the following recommendations for the work of the Bureau of Chemistry and Soils and for the Bureau of the Biological Survey:

Bureau of Chemistry and Soils, $1,244,963, which includes increases of $15,000 for studying methods for diversifying products made from sugar-cane and originating new products; $10,000 for food research, including a study of the deterioration of foods due to micro-organisms, chemical agencies, etc.; $10,000 for a study of the commercial utilization of citrus fruits, pomegranates, avocados, pears, prunes and other fruits; $10,053 for experiments and demonstrations in proper methods of removing and curing hides and skins, and study of little-used native tanning material and of foreign tannin-bearing plants; $5,000 for fundamental investigation of the chemical properties and utilization of lignin; $3,000 for extension of studies on the composition and utilization of vegetable oils and fats; $10,000 for investigating the possibilities of utilizing sweet-potato culls for the production of starch and conversion products; $10,000 for the development of new insecticides and fungicides; $10,000 for enlargement of research work on the causes and methods of control of farm fires; $5,000 for inaugurating studies of new processes and equipment for the production of naval stores, in cooperation with producers and the Forest Service, as well as a study of the adaptability of naval stores for various uses; $5,000 for expanding the work necessary to properly coordinate the chemical investigation of soils with the classification and mapping of soil types; $6,060 for investigation of methods of producing nitrogen fertilizer; $5,000 for a study of the production of phosphoric acid in a more desirable form than acid phosphates, and for potash investigations; $6,000 for bringing up to date the soil-survey map drafting work; $9,485 for studying the causes and developing methods for remedying destructive soil erosion; $4,650 for further crop experiments with air-derived nitrogen and other concentrated fertilizers; $2,350 for soil fertility and fertilizer studies on sugar-cane soils in Louisiana, Florida and other southern states, and $3,360 for additional editorial assistance and other general administrative work.

Bureau of Biological Survey, $1,078,500, which includes

increases of $1,480 to provide for additional clerical assistance in the general administrative work of the bureau; $2,500 for laboratory and field work on the perfection of rodent and predatory animal poisons; $6,000 for extension of the campaign for the destruction of injurious rodents; $10,000 for predatory animal control operations; $3,500 for researches on the food habits of water-fowl; $8,000 for extending the study of food habits, diseases and parasites of game animals, fur-bearing and predatory animals; $5,000 for the employment of additional game wardens, and $14,000 for administrative expenses in connection with the acquisition of land for the upper Mississippi River wild-life and fish refuge. There is an apparent decrease of $3,000 in the item for maintenance of mammal and bird reservations, but, due to the release of $18,000 provided in 1928 for fencing on the Wind Cave Game Preserve in South Dakota, there is actually $15,000 additional available for other work, as follows: $600 for minor construction work on the Big Lake Bird Reservation, Arkansas; $3,000 for work incident to the disposal of surplus animals in big-game preserves; $7,230 for the construction of various buildings and shelters and for necessary implements at big-game preserves; $1,000 for water development work on the Wind Cave Game Preserve; $900 for fencing at Sully's Hill Game Preserve, North Dakota, and $2,270 for care and maintenance of lands donated to the government by the Izaak Walton League as an addition to the winter elk refuge in Wyoming. A decrease of $4,000 is made in the fund for the purchase of land for the upper Mississippi River wild-life and fish refuge, the balances from prior appropriations being sufficient, under present purchase limitations, to take care of payments under contractual obligations during the fiscal year 1929.

THE GIANNINI FOUNDATION OF THE UNIVERSITY OF CALIFORNIA

FORMAL tender of a gift of $1,500,000, to be devoted to the study of agricultural economics, has been made to the regents of the University of California by Bancitaly Corporation, "in tribute to A. P. Giannini, of San Francisco, and to be named after him." As already recorded in SCIENCE, one third of the gift is to be used for the construction of a building for the College of Agriculture, to house the works of the Giannini Foundation, and $1,000,000 to be used as an endowment for the foundation.

In making the announcement, President W. W. Campbell, of the University of California, said in part:

As a result of Mr. Giannini's feeling, expressed to me some months ago, that he wanted to do something for the agriculturists of the state, that it is the very opposite of his philosophy of life that a man be rich at the time of his death and that he wanted to do something through the University of California for the farmers of California, conferences have been held since that time getting these ideas clarified; and Mr. Giannini has decided to extend to the regents of the University of California a gift of a million and a half dollars to establish and support a foundation of agricultural economics. Of course I shall recommend that it be designated as the Giannini Foundation of Agricultural Economics, although neither Mr. Giannini nor any of his friends have made any such suggestion.

My recommendation that we complete the agricultural college group of buildings now consisting of Agricultural Hall and Hilgard Hall by the construction of a counterpart of Hilgard Hall, the three buildings to enclose the agricultural quadrangle on as many sides, part of the building to accommodate the activity in agricultural economics, met his approval. This will call for approximately half a million dollars.

The activities of the foundation are to be embraced by the great field of agricultural economics, and relate to such subjects as: (*a*) the economic consideration of increased production, which results from improved seed grains, improved nursery stock, improved livestock, improved methods of farming, all these brought about largely through researches conducted by colleges of agriculture, and from the use of improved farm machinery; (*b*) the economic consequences of overproduction and underproduction arising from unusually favorable seasons or unusually unfavorable seasons as to weather and other conditions in the nations producing the agricultural product concerned, such as grains, cotton, etc.; (*c*) relations between conditions existing in the farming industry and the general economic conditions prevailing in the nation and internationally; (*d*) the methods and problems of disposing of farm products in the markets of the world on terms or conditions giving the maximum degree of satisfaction to the growers; (*e*) the economic questions which concern the individual farmer and the members of his family, and affect their living conditions, and so on.

It may be assumed that the Giannini Foundation of Agricultural Economics will be privileged to produce results of enormous value to the agricultural industry in California, not only in the years and decades immediately ahead but as a continuing foundation in perpetuity.

The offer of the gift was accompanied by a check for $25,000; this is to be followed by another for $475,000 within two months, and the remaining $1,000,000 to be made available as it is needed.

PRESENTATION OF THE CHARLES P. DALY GOLD MEDAL TO PROFESSOR ALOIS MUSIL

ON the evening of February 21, at a meeting of the American Geographical Society of New York, the Charles P. Daly gold medal of the society was presented to Professor Alois Musil, of Charles University, Prague, in recognition of a lifetime devoted to explorations in northern Arabia and Mesopotamia and to historical researches relating to this part of the world. After the ceremony, Professor Musil delivered a lecture entitled "Desert Life in Northern Arabia." We have received from the American Geographical

Society the following account of Professor Musil's work:

Professor Musil is now recognized as the foremost living authority on the topography, history and folklore of the desert tracts lying between the settlements of Palestine and Syria on the west, the Tigris on the east, and the oases of Nejd on the south. Since 1896 he has spent many seasons in the field in the course of journeys on camel-back covering a total distance of no less than 13,000 miles. An extremely close observer, Professor Musil has recorded on his maps detailed topographic features and place-names over broad districts previously wholly unexplored. By comparing the results of his field work with the ancient documentary sources, he has been able to reconstruct the probable course of historical events that have hitherto proved enigmas to students of the Old Testament, and to Assyriologists, classicists and Arabicists. His most sensational discovery was made in 1898 on the edge of the desert east of the Dead Sea. Here he found the Kuseyr 'Amra, well-preserved ruins of a summer residence built by the Omayyad caliph Walid II in the eighth century of our era. The interior walls of this structure were decorated with paintings illustrating the adventures of the caliph in the hunting field and with portraits of the fallen rulers of the various countries which had been brought under Moslem subjection—among them one of Roderick, the last Visigothic king of Spain. From the geographical point of view Professor Musil's most striking work was the determination of the position of the main watershed of northern Arabia and the exploration of the fringes of the Nefud, or great sand waste that lies between Nejd and the Hamad steppes (sometimes called the Syrian desert). Professor Musil also traced the lower course of the River Tharthar, in the interior of Mesopotamia, to its outlet in an unexplored salt lake on the floor of a depression fifty meters below sea-level. Reports of this stream may have given rise to the classical legend of Tartarus, river of the underworld.

Professor Musil has made an extremely important contribution to our knowledge of Bedouin folklore. Accepted as a member of the Rwala tribe, on equal terms with their head chief, he was enabled to study the life of these nomads in its minutest details. He records, translates and explains several hundred of their songs in his volume, "The Manners and Customs of the Rwala Bedouins."

The results of Professor Musil's researches prior to 1908 were published in two great series by the Vienna Academy of Science: "Kusejr 'Amra" (in 2 volumes) and "Arabia Petraea" (in 4 volumes); the latter is accompanied by a map of Arabia Petraea on the scale of 1:500,000. His field work of 1908–1915 is described in a series of six volumes, the publication of which by the American Geographical Society has been made possible through the generosity of Charles R. Crane, Esq. Five of these six volumes are devoted to the narratives of the explorer's itineraries and to historical essays on the various regions visited. Three volumes are now in print ("The Northern Hegâz," 1926; "Arabia Deserta," 1927, and "The Middle Euphrates," 1927). Two more will be published in the course of 1928 ("Palmyrena" and "Northern Negd"), and the sixth volume of the series ("The Manners and Customs of the Rwala Bedouin") will also appear before the close of the present year. Forming an integral part of this series are three maps: The Northern Hegâz, 1:500,000; Northern Arabia, in four sheets, 1:1,000,000, and Southern Mesopotamia, 1:1,000,000.

NATIONAL RESEARCH FELLOWSHIPS IN THE BIOLOGICAL SCIENCES

THE Board of National Research Fellowships in the Biological Sciences met on February 10 and 11 and made the following awards for the year 1928–29:

Reappointments

Kenneth Cole—Biophysics
Robert Emerson—Botany
M. B. Linford—Botany
Louis W. Max—Psychology
G. G. Pincus—Zoology
Jack Schultz—Zoology
R. H. Wallace—Botany

New Appointments

F. M. Carpenter—Zoology
F. E. Clements—Anthropology
S. H. Emerson—Botany
Eileen W. Erlanson—Botany
Clay G. Huff—Zoology
C. F. Jacobsen—Psychology
D. A. Johansen—Botany
P. A. Readio—Zoology
D. C. Smith—Zoology
M. T. Sonneborn—Zoology
R. C. Tryon—Psychology

The second meeting of the board for further appointments for 1928–29 will be held the latter part of May, and applications for consideration at that time are requested by April 15. The necessary forms and information for making application may be secured from the Secretary, Board of National Research Fellowships in the Biological Sciences, National Research Council, Washington, D. C.

FRANK R. LILLIE, *Chairman,*
Board of National Research Fellowships in the Biological Sciences

SCIENTIFIC NOTES AND NEWS

IN recognition of his research work in the field of catalysis, the Nichols medal was formally awarded to Dr. Hugh Stott Taylor, David B. Jones research professor of chemistry at Princeton University, on March 9. The presentation of the medal followed a dinner at the Chemists' Club, given by the New York section of the American Electrochemical Society, the Society of Chemical Industry and the Société de Chimie Industrielle. After speeches by Dean James Kendall, of New York University, and Professor Wilder D. Bancroft, of Cornell University. Professor Arthur W. Thomas, of Columbia University, chairman of the jury of award, presented the medal to Professor Taylor, who then described his work on catalysis.

THE Messel Medal of the British Society of Chemical Industry has been awarded to Dr. R. A. Millikan, director of the Norman Bridge laboratory at the California Institute of Technology, in recognition of his achievement in measuring the electrostatic charge of the electron.

PROFESSOR W. H. WRIGHT, astronomer of the Lick Observatory, has been appointed George Darwin lecturer for 1928 of the Royal Astronomical Society. The lecture will be delivered in June, and will probably deal with the photography of the planets with different color filters.

DR. LAWRENCE J. HENDERSON, professor of biological chemistry at Harvard University, is giving the Silliman lectures for 1928 at Yale University on "Blood: A Study in General Physiology." The course will consist of six lectures, is given on Mondays, Wednesdays and Fridays, from March 12 to 23, inclusive.

DR. OYARTZUN, curator of the Anthropological Museum, Santiago, Chile, has been awarded the gold medal of the University of Würzburg.

DR. PAUL FLECHSIG, professor of psychiatry at the University of Leipzig, has been elected an honorary member of the Psycho-Neurological Academy of Leningrad.

THE rank of officer of the Legion of Honor has been conferred on Dr. Pierre Fredet, a well-known Paris surgeon and senior medical officer of the Paris, Lyons and Mediterranean Railway; Dr. Loeper, professor of therapeutics in the Paris faculty of medicine; Dr. Abadie, professor of nervous and mental diseases at Bordeaux, and Professor Léon Blum, of Strasbourg.

PROFESSOR CLEMENS PIRQUET, of Vienna, has been elected president of the International Union of Child Welfare in succession to the Duke of Atholl.

PROFESSOR WILLIAM H. WELCH, of the Johns Hopkins University, has been appointed a member of the Baltimore Revision Commission. The commission will consider the revision or amendment of the City Charter and the City Code.

DR. ELLIOTT C. CUTLER, of Cleveland, has been elected to succeed Dr. Montrose Burrows as chairman of the committee on the protection of medical research of the American Medical Association.

DR. RICHARD P. STRONG, professor of tropical medicine at the Harvard Medical School, was guest of honor at a dinner given by the Harvard Union on March 1, where he exhibited moving pictures taken last year in Africa on an expedition under the auspices of the Medical School of Harvard University.

STANLEY P. YOUNG, of Colorado, has been appointed head of the division of economic investigations of the U. S. Bureau of Biological Survey, in charge of the department's rodent and predatory-animal control operations. He succeeds Dr. A. K. Fisher.

DR. OLIVER BOWLES, formerly supervising engineer of the Non-metallic Minerals Experiment Station of the U. S. Bureau of Mines at New Brunswick, N. J., has been transferred to the economics branch of the bureau to be chief of a new structural materials section, having charge of economic studies in the major non-metallic minerals and their products.

WILLIAM L. HALTOM has been appointed curator of the Alabama Museum of Natural History, to succeed H. E. Wheeler, resigned.

PROFESSOR RICHARD R. FENSKA is spending his sabbatical year from the New York State College of Forestry as forester for the Massachusetts Forestry Association.

RAYMOND L. DITMARS, curator of reptiles at the New York Zoological Park, sailed for Honduras on March 6, where he will collect poisonous snakes for the production of serum.

GREGORY MASON, explorer and author, sailed from New Orleans on February 7, at the head of an expedition being sent out by the Museum of the American Indian, of New York, to search for evidences of Mayan civilization.

PROFESSOR J. E. HOFFMEISTER, of the University of Rochester, and Professor H. S. Ladd, of the University of Virginia, will sail early in April for the South Pacific to continue geological field work begun in 1926. Professor Hoffmeister is studying the geology and paleontology of certain islands in the Tonga Group, while Professor Ladd is carrying on similar work in Fiji. They will return about the middle of September. The work is being done under the auspices of the Bernice P. Bishop Museum of Honolulu.

DR. STANLEY COBB, Bullard professor of neuropathology at the Harvard Medical School, is on leave of absence for the second half of the current academic year and will go to Munich to work in neuropathology and psychiatry.

AFTER nine months' absence in Africa, L. W. Kephart and R. L. Piemeisel, plant explorers of the U. S. Department of Agriculture, have returned with more than 160 lots of seed of different grasses and forage plants and 400 specimens of other plant life. It is hoped that some additions to the pasture and meadow forage of the United States will result from this expedition.

Miss Mary Proctor, the astronomical author, arrived in New York on March 6 for an American lecture tour during which she hopes to raise money for the construction, probably in southern California, of the world's largest astronomical telescope.

Dr. Nils G. Hörner, of Uppsala, Sweden, Scandinavian-American fellow, has spent the fall and winter as a visitor in the department of geology at Harvard University. He has recently been appointed a fellow of the Liljewalch fund of Uppsala University, which will enable him to make a geological excursion in Western United States beginning about March 15.

The first lectures under the William Sydney Thayer and Susan Read Thayer lectureship in clinical medicine at the Johns Hopkins University School of Medicine will be delivered by Sir Humphry Rolleston, Regius professor of physic in the University of Cambridge, England, on March 20 and 21. The titles of the lectures are "Hereditary and Familial Diseases of the Blood Forming Organs" and "Diseases Peculiar to Certain Races."

Dr. George Barger, professor of medical chemistry at the University of Edinburgh and non-resident lecturer in chemistry at Cornell University during the present semester, will give three Dohme lectures at the Johns Hopkins University early in May.

The annual William Lowell Putnam memorial lecture will be delivered on March 21 by Professor Constantin Carathéodory, of the University of Munich, who will speak on "Selected Problems in the Calculus of Variations."

Professor Albert Einstein, of the University of Berlin, will deliver the inaugural lecture of a first course of international university extension lectures, to begin at Davos on March 18. The object of the institution is to enable students in delicate health to continue their studies in the Alps.

The thirteenth Guthrie lecture of the British Physical Society was given by Sir Joseph Thomson, F.R.S., on "Electrodeless Discharge through Gases," on March 9, at the Imperial College of Science and Technology.

The College of Physicians of Philadelphia will commemorate on March 22 the tercentenary of William Harvey's discovery of the circulation of the blood. Addresses will be delivered by Sir Humphry Rolleston, of Cambridge, England, and Professor J. J. R. Macleod, of Toronto. There will also be an exhibition of Harveyana.

On February 29 the central Pennsylvania section of the American Chemical Society celebrated the one hundredth anniversary of the birth of Dr. Evan Pugh, well-known agricultural chemist and the first president of the Pennsylvania State College. Dr. Erwin W. Runkle, college historian, gave the principal address entitled "Evan Pugh—Teacher, Scientist, President."

The bridge over the Arthur Kill between Elizabeth, N. J., and Howland Hook, S. I., will be named in honor of the late General George W. Goethals, under the terms of a resolution recently passed by the Port of New York Authority.

Dr. Samuel A. Matthews, professor and head of the department of physiology, therapeutics and pharmacology at Loyola University School of Medicine, Chicago, died on February 19.

Dr. M. G. Schlapp, professor of neuropathology at the New York Postgraduate Medical School, died on March 5, at the age of fifty-eight years.

Dr. Robert Abbe, associate in surgery at the College of Physicians and Surgeons, Columbia University, died on March 7, aged seventy-seven years.

Professor Ludwig Milch, director of the Institute of Mineralogy and Petrology at the University of Breslau, died on January 5, aged sixty years.

The United States Civil Service Commission announces open competitive examinations for the positions of associate aquatic biologist, and assistant aquatic biologist, at entrance salaries of $3,000 and $2,400 per annum, to be held not later than March 27, 1928. Two vacancies in the position of assistant aquatic biologist, for duty at Fairport, Iowa, and Ann Arbor, Mich., and vacancies occurring throughout the United States in these positions or in positions requiring similar qualifications, will be filled from these examinations, unless it is found in the interest of the service to fill any vacancy by reinstatement, transfer or promotion. The subjects to be considered are (1) education, training and experience, weight 70; (2) writings (publications or thesis, to be filed with application), weight 30. The ratings on the first subject will be based upon competitors' sworn statements in their applications and upon corroborative evidence.

The two hundred and twentieth meeting of the Washington Academy of Sciences was held in the auditorium of the National Museum on March 15. The program consisted of a moving picture entitled "Mechanics of the Brain," prepared by Professor Ivan P. Pavlov, director of the physiological laboratories in the Russian Academy of Sciences. The picture presented a series of experiments on children and animals chosen to illustrate the mechanism of their reactions to various external stimuli. Especial attention is paid to the development of "conditioned reflexes," which has been one of the principal subjects studied by Professor Pavlov and his collaborators. This film was exhibited through the courtesy of the American Society for Cultural Relations with Russia.

A SERIES of four addresses on the general subject "The Measurement of Mankind" is being delivered under the auspices of the Minnesota chapter of the Society of the Sigma Xi. These lectures are as follows: February 16, "The Measurement of Man in the Mass," Professor J. Arthur Harris; March 7, "Body Growth in Infancy and Childhood," Professor R. E. Scammon; March 28, "Normal and Abnormal Human Types," Professor C. M. Jackson, and April 18, "Mental Development in Relation to Physical Development and Types," Professor D. G. Paterson.

DR. JOSEPH EUGENE ROWE, professor and head of the department of mathematics and director of extension in the College of William and Mary, has been granted two sets of letters patent on the trinometer and associated instruments. The first of these consists of nine claims on the trinometer, which is an instrument that makes possible the mechanical solution of triangles and the finding of their areas by simple means. The second patent consists of improvements on the original instrument and extends it to the solution of quadrilaterals and other polygons.

THE polar ship *Morrissey,* with Captain R. A. Bartlett in command, sailed north on March 4 from Balboa, bound for the Aleutian Islands and Northern Siberia, by way of Seattle, to search for post-glacial mummies and explore little-known lands. The *Morrissey* arrived at Balboa from New York on February 29. The present expedition is headed by Dr. Frank Chapman and includes five others.

THE Field Museum of Natural History, in Chicago, has arranged an exhibition showing the results of five recent zoological expeditions. These are the Chicago *Daily News*-Field Museum Abyssinian expedition, the Marshall Field Brazilian expedition, the James Simpson Roosevelt Asiatic expedition, the John Borden-Field Museum Alaska Arctic expedition and the Conover-Everard African expedition.

AT a meeting of the directors of the Guggenheim Medal Fund at the offices of the Guggenheim Foundation for the Promotion of Aviation the following officers were elected: Elmer A. Sperry, *president;* Edward P. Warner, assistant secretary of the Navy in charge of aeronautics, *vice-president,* and Alfred D. Flinn, secretary of the United Engineering Societies, *secretary and treasurer.* The fund was established to award from time to time a gold medal to "that person who performs some notable achievement tending to the advancement of aeronautics." The rules require that the names of the recipients must be under consideration at least a year before the award is made.

A MARINE zoological laboratory and summer camp on the Isles of Shoals will be a project of the department of zoology of the University of New Hampshire this summer, according to Professor C. Lloyd Jackson, head of the department. Full credit at the camp may be received for either graduate or undergraduate work, since, in addition to research work, full courses will be offered in ecology, systematic zoology, comparative anatomy and embryology.

THE National Park Service has announced that the Yosemite School of Field Natural History will open on June 25 for its fourth season, as a summer school for the training of naturalists, nature guides and teachers of natural history. The Yosemite Museum is headquarters for the school. The work was originated by the California Fish and Game Commission and is also participated in by the Yosemite Natural History Association. There are seven members of the staff, including A. F. Hall, chief naturalist; C. P. Russell, park naturalist, and H. C. Bryant, director of the school and nature guide.

A GIFT of $5,000,000 has been made from the Laura Spelman Rockefeller Memorial to the Great Smoky Mountain National Park fund. The sum of $4,913,000 has already been raised by subscription and by appropriations of the North Carolina and Tennessee legislatures. The Rockefeller gift brings the total almost to $10,000,000, which, it is believed, is more than enough to purchase the land for the park. The park will lie partly in Tennessee and partly in North Carolina. It will be some 700 square miles in area and will take in almost all the Smoky Mountain territory.

THE State of Rio de Janeiro, Brazil, has announced the offer of a prize of approximately $1,200 to a scientific man, either Brazilian or foreign, who prior to December 31, 1928, determines in an accurate and scientific manner the etiology of sugar cane mosaic and an effective method of combatting it, and presents the best thesis on this subject, this thesis to be published for the use of the public. Further information can be had from Dr. Enrico Teixeira Leite, director, Instituto Fomento e Economia Agricola, Ministerio da Agriculture, Rio de Janeiro, Brazil.

ACCORDING to the *Journal* of the American Medical Association a bill, authorizing the maintenance of the Gorgas Memorial Laboratory on the Isthmus of Panama and providing that $50,000 annually be paid to the Gorgas Memorial Institute of Tropical and

Preventive Medicine, Inc., for the operation of the laboratory, has been approved by the committee on foreign affairs of the House of Representatives on condition that it be constructed within five years; that each of the Latin American governments be invited to contribute annually toward its maintenance, and that the United States be represented permanently on the board directing the administration of the laboratory, while the Latin American governments contributing have the privilege of being represented on the board.

Creation of the "Textile Alliance Foundation" to administer a fund of approximately $1,500,000, accumulated during the world war, for educational research in the development of the textile industry, would be provided in a bill introduced by Representative Merritt, of Stamford, Conn. The bill was referred to the house committee on interstate and foreign commerce.

The valuable collections of fungi collected by the late Curtis G. Lloyd, who died a year ago, will probably go to the Smithsonian Institution, because the trustees in Cincinnati are unable to properly care for it. The Central Trust Company has filed suit to end its trusteeship and obtain authorization to give the Lloyd collection to the institution.

Dr. Willard Rouse Jillson, state geologist of Kentucky, announces the passage through the legislature and approval by the governor of Kentucky of an emergency appropriation bill of $34,000. This sum is immediately available for all general administrative purposes of the Kentucky Geological Survey. The annual appropriation of the Kentucky Geological Survey is $90,000, to which sum this appropriation has been added this year.

Under the will of the late Dr. W. Gilman Thompson, a former president of the New York Botanical Garden, the garden is to receive the sum of $5,000.

Announcement is made that subscriptions to the Charles Sprague Sargent Fund for the endowment of the Arnold Arboretum now amount to $793,307, or nearly three fourths of the $1,000,000 goal.

The United States Shellac Importers' Association has founded a research fellowship in shellac, known as the Shellac Research Bureau, at the Brooklyn Polytechnic Institute. The work is to be done under the direction of J. C. Olsen and W. F. Whitmore.

Oxford University has authorized the expenditure from the government grant of a sum not exceeding £2,800 on an addition to the department of chemistry at the University Museum so as to provide an additional workshop on the ground floor and a research laboratory on the first floor.

Dr. R. M. Appert, who recently died at San Remo at the age of sixty-five years, has bequeathed the Pasteur Institute of Paris a sum of 2,000,000 francs.

Another addition to the University of Chicago's medical center on the Midway has been made public by President Max Mason, who announced that an arrangement had been made by which the Home for Destitute Crippled Children will transfer its main hospital to the south side, where new buildings providing one hundred beds will be in operation by the summer of 1929 as one of the series of university clinics. A part of the program is made possible through a gift to the home of $300,000 by Mrs. Elizabeth S. McElwee for the erection and equipment of one of the buildings. Another gift of $300,000, made by Mrs. Gertrude Dunn Hicks to the university last September for an orthopedic hospital, is to be used for the erection of the other division of the building to house the home.

A special clinic and laboratory has been opened by New York University at the new Sydenham Hospital. The clinic is designed to study exclusively cases of asthma, eczema, hives, hay fever and other allergic diseases of children from infancy up to puberty. It was made possible by the gift of $30,000 by a friend of the university. Adequate hospital and laboratory facilities have been arranged for an intensive study of these diseases. Dr. Bret Ratner, of the New York University and Bellevue Hospital Medical College staff, who will direct the work of the clinic, began his investigations several years ago in the physiology department of the late Professor Holmes C. Jackson when an initial gift of $15,000 for research in this field was given the university by the same donor. The experimental work involving tests on animals will continue to be done in the university laboratories. The clinic which will be open for patients immediately will be under Dr. Ratner and a special staff.

The medical school of Stanford University has received $500 from Mr. Edward M. Mills for free beds for children; $1,000 from Miss Helen E. Cowell for physiotherapy treatments for indigent deserving patients; $100 from a grateful patient to be used for surgical research; $610.69 from the estate of Mrs. Ann Whitney Sperry to be used for the benefit of Protestant and Catholic crippled or orphaned children of San Francisco; $2,500 from Mr. Roy N. Bishop, and $500 from Mr. George T. Cameron as contributions to the Wellington Gregg Fund for the study of nephritis. Pediatrics, which so far has been a division of the department of internal medicine, has been made a full department in the medical school.

A research institute for psychiatry, consisting of serological, genealogical, chemical, histological, anatomical and psychological departments, for which the funds have been provided by the Rockefeller Foundation, will be opened at Munich next May.

Nature states that it has been decided to found an institute at Prague for the scientific investigation of coal. It will have the support of the state and of the various coal undertakings in Czechoslovakia.

AN anonymous donor has presented to Cornell University five hundred acres of abandoned farm land in Newfield, which will be used for experiments and instruction in forestry and as an observation ground for botanists.

AN archeological expedition sponsored by Captain Marshall Field has gone to British Honduras to seek new facts concerning the ancient culture of the Mayas and to collect material illustrating their civilization for exhibition in the Field Museum of Natural History. The expedition has for its leader J. Eric Thompson, assistant curator of Mexican and South American archeology at the museum. Its center of operations will be Belize.

WITH all construction details completed and with a large stock of rabbits on hand, the rabbit experiment station maintained by the division of fur resources of the U. S. Bureau of Biological Survey in cooperation with the National Rabbit Federation and local rabbit breeders at Fontana, California, was formally opened on March 3. The chief of the biological survey, Paul G. Redington, represented the U. S. Department of Agriculture. The station will be under the directorship of D. Monroe Green, formerly of the Washington office of the U. S. Biological Survey, who went to Fontana several months ago to take charge of the erection of the station. Assisting Mr. Green will be John W. Meyer, formerly of the office of exhibits of the Department of Agriculture.

UNIVERSITY AND EDUCATIONAL NOTES

DR. HARVEY NATHANIEL DAVIS, professor of mechanical engineering at Harvard University, has been chosen president of the Stevens Institute of Technology at Hoboken, N. J. Dr. Davis takes office on September 1, succeeding the late Dr. Alexander C. Humphrey.

DR. EDWARD HICKS HUME, formerly president of the Colleges of Yale-in-China, has been appointed director of the New York Post-Graduate Medical School and Hospital, and not of the Yale Graduate School as was erroneously reported in the last issue of SCIENCE.

DR. HARRY CLARK, of the biophysics division of the Rockefeller Institute for Medical Research, has been appointed acting professor of physics for the summer session at Leland Stanford University.

DR. JOSEPH T. WEARN has been promoted to be associate professor of medicine at Harvard University.

DR. CHARLES HUNTER has been appointed professor of medicine at the University of Manitoba, to succeed Dr. Edward W. Montgomery, now minister of public welfare of Manitoba.

PROFESSOR J. H. DIBLE, professor of pathology in the University of London and honorary pathologist to the Royal Free Hospital, has been appointed to the chair of pathology in the Welsh National School of Medicine in succession to Professor E. H. Kettle.

THE first professorship of the geology of fuel (petroleum and coal) at a German technical school has been created at Freiberg in Saxony. The occupant is to be Dr. Otto Stutzer, who has also been elected director of the new fuel institute at the School of Mines.

PROFESSOR ROBERT KÖNIG, of the University of Münster, has been appointed professor of mathematics at the University of Jena.

DISCUSSION AND CORRESPONDENCE

THE FUNCTIONAL NATURE OF THE CONSTANT OF MASS ACTION

THE thermodynamical proof given by van't Hoff that the constant of mass action is a constant at constant temperature depends on the tacit assumption that molecules while getting transferred from one chamber to another in a certain isothermal process do not decompose. This is a difficulty in the process which has been recognized, but is usually ignored. Attempts have been made to overcome it by supposing that either, (a) the molecules are so rapidly transferred that they have not time to decompose, or (b) decomposition is prevented by a catalytic agent. But (a) does not give an isothermal process, and (b) would radically change the nature of the molecules. The writer has shown in a paper that will appear shortly in the *Philosophical Magazine,* that if all the thermodynamical conditions of equilibrium are satisfied, the constant of mass action can be shown to be a function of the volume of the interacting gas, the masses of the constituents, as well as of the temperature. It may of course be in most cases *approximately* independent of all variables except the temperature.

If this result is true, we should expect that thermodynamical differential equations exist which determine the functional nature of the constant of mass action. These the writer has obtained and will be given in a subsequent paper. They are evidence of the truth of the result obtained; additional evidence presents itself from many directions which can not be dealt with here.

From kinetic considerations we would also expect this result to hold. The number of molecules ae that are formed per second from molecules a and e in a gas is usually written $k_1C_aC_e$, where C_a and C_e denote the concentrations of the molecules a and e, respectively, and k_1 the chance of a molecule a encountering a molecule e in a second. But what happens during an encounter most likely depends on the state of the molecules, which would depend on previous encounters with other molecules, during which they get activated so to speak, or we should write $\varkappa_1k_1C_aC_e$ for the number of molecules formed, where $\varkappa_1$ may be called the activation constant, and is the fraction of the encounters at which the molecules were sufficiently activated to form new molecules. Similarly the number of molecules ae breaking up per second is usually written k_2C_{ae}, where C_{ae} denotes the concentration of the molecules ae, and k_2 the chance of a molecule breaking up during a second if left to itself. But this chance may depend on previous encounters with other molecules, or we should write $\varkappa_2k_2C_{ae}$ for the number breaking up per second, where $\varkappa_2$ denotes the activation constant. When equilibrium exists

$$\varkappa_2k_2C_{ae} = \varkappa_1k_1C_aC_e$$

and hence

$$K = \frac{\varkappa_2k_2}{\varkappa_1k_1}$$

The quantities k_1 and k_2 depend on the temperature only. Hence unless $\varkappa_2 = \varkappa_1$ the constant of mass action is a function of the volume of the interacting mixture and masses of the constituents, since $\varkappa_1$ and $\varkappa_2$ are functions of these quantities, besides of the temperature.

R. D. KLEEMAN

SCHENECTADY, N. Y.

VEGETATIVE PROPAGATION OF THE APPLE BY SEED

IN a recent article[1] dealing primarily with chromosome studies, Kobel, of the Swiss Versuchsanstalt für Obst-, Wein- und Gartenbau (Wädenswil), has reported several instances of apparent apogamy in the apple. Using the variety known there as Transparent de Croncels (but which may possibly be Yellow Transparent), several emasculated and bagged flowers have in different years set seeds, some of which have been cytologically examined at various stages of development, while others of these seeds have been grown to bearing trees. The writer of this note saw on the Wädenswil experimental grounds, the 4 seedlings which are now in bearing; their apparent identity with the seed-mother tree, together with the results of Dr. Kobel's cytological studies seem to warrant the conclusion that under certain conditions (not as yet defined), unfertilized ovules of this variety may set viable seeds, genetically constituting true vegetative reproduction. These results differ from the somewhat similar observations by Frost,[2] in that in Citrus the stimulus proceeding from fertilization seems necessary for the production of such "asexual" seeds, while in the apple they may arise entirely without fertilization.

As Kobel points out, the importance of such apogamic seeds as a means of obtaining uniform, clonal rootstocks, should be at once apparent. Although under the conditions of his experiments, Kobel was not able to get a high enough percentage of such "asexual" seeds to make them a factor in the production of uniform rootstocks, still his results point very strongly toward the desirability of carrying out extensive emasculation and bagging experiments with as many different varieties of apples and under as many different conditions as possible, with the expectation that the proper combination of varietal and environmental conditions will be found which will make such "vegetative propagation by seed" feasible.

CHARLES F. SWINGLE,
National Research Council Fellow in Botany.

THE UNIVERSITY
LEEDS, ENGLAND

[1] Zytologische Untersuchungen an Prunoideen u. Pomoideen. *Archiv Julius Klaus-Stiftung f. Vererb., Soz., u. Rassenhygiene.* 3(1): 1–84. 1927. Zürich.

[2] Polyembryony, heterozygosis and chimeras in Citrus. *Hilgardia.* 1(16): 365–402. 1926.

LIVING CELLS IN HEART-WOOD OF TREES

IN a special article entitled "Long-lived Cells of the Redwood," published in SCIENCE of November 11, 1927, D. T. MacDougal and G. M. Smith state that "We can not find any definite statement of living cells in heartwood," and conclude that the facts they present in connection with their study of redwood "seem to constitute the first announcement of living cells in heartwood."

They have evidently overlooked a paper by J. H. White, "On the Biology of Fomes applanatus (Pers.) Wallr." published in the *Transactions* of the Royal Canadian Institute, pages 133–174 of Vol. XII, 1919. Dr. White described the path of entrance of the fungus into the heartwood, and then the character of the changes induced. "A study of the living wood of trees attacked by *F. applanatus* shows, as I have already indicated, a feature not found in dead wood. I refer to a brownish discolored zone which marks the extreme limit of advance of the fungus," (p. 155). Within this band there were found deposits of wound gum, but more striking still "Tyloses constitute another remarkable feature of the brown zone." "I have found them in attacked sapwood and heartwood of several species in which search was made for them, including beech, sugar maple, and red oak." Convincing demonstration is especially easy in red oak.

These do not occur similarly in adjacent sound wood.

There had been such a prevalent opinion among pathologists that heart-rotting fungi are not truly parasitic, because of the commonly accepted assumption that the heartwood is dead, that White took pains to show that such views were erroneous. After discussing evidence to be drawn from the "wound gum," he continues, "Tyloses fortunately do not suffer such variant opinions; they can be produced only by living cells. Their occurrence, then, proves that the invaded tissues are living . . . The tyloses arise as the result of a stimulation primarily induced by the fungus." (p. 163.)

J. H. FAULL

DEPARTMENT OF BOTANY,
UNIVERSITY OF TORONTO

A PREHISTORY CHART

Professor A. E. Jenks, of the Department of Anthropology at the University of Minnesota, has designed a chart illustrative of the chronological sequences of archeological periods in prehistoric Europe and of typical artifacts of each period. The dimensions of this chart are three feet by four feet. The upper half is devoted to a chronological diagram of culture sequences in which the various glacial advances are represented by peaks and the interglacial periods by valleys. The associated cultures are distinguished by the varied colors of the different portions of this Pleistocene range. The several types of fossil man have their positions in the landscape indicated by guide posts.

The lower half of the chart shows drawings of characteristic implements of the successive periods, excellently delineated and clearly labelled. The selection of artifacts representative of the Paleolithic periods is very good. Limitations of space prevent an equally satisfactory display of objects characteristic of the Neolithic, Bronze, and Early Iron Ages. Nearly all of those represented on the chart come from the Scandinavian area. But the author has chosen carefully and well.

Teachers of history and of prehistoric archeology will find that Professor Jenks' chart is a valuable aid to themselves and to their students. Ten minutes' study of this chart will fix in the mind of the reader facts which ordinarily require for their absorption hours of concentration and much thumbing of leaves of text-books.

E. A. HOOTON

HARVARD UNIVERSITY

PHILOSOPHY OR IRONY, WHICH?

IN the current number of SCIENCE, January 13, I read Dr. Stetson's short, but appreciative, review of Professor Eddington's "Stars and Atoms" and noted what the reviewer says of the author's sense of humor. However, there is one sentence in particular in which the humor is so "dry" that the casual reader may be led to draw the erroneous conclusion that Professor Eddington endorses the views expressed in the first two paragraphs of Bertrand Russell's "What I Believe." These two paragraphs are sufficient to convince the reader that the author finds his *Ultima Thule* in the electron.

There is nothing in the context leading to the sentence referred to above—nothing but the absurdity of the conclusion itself—that would lead one to regard the sentence as ironical; but I take it, in reality, to be a "sly dig" at Russell and his school. After showing the possible complexities to be expected under conditions due to terrestrial temperatures compared with the simple structures found associated with the high stellar temperatures, Professor Eddington concludes, p. 84:

> Our earth is one of those chilly places and here the strangest complications can arise. Perhaps strangest of all, some of these complications can meet together and speculate on the significance of the whole scheme.

My reason for regarding the above excerpt as ironical may be best expressed in Professor Eddington's own words as given in "Science, Religion and Reality," p. 214.

> Is the motion of the editor's pencil to grammatically amend the split infinitive in this sentence simply the automatic response under physical laws of a complicated configuration of electrons to the external stimulus of this smear of ink on paper? Such an extravagant hypothesis might conceivably appeal to the crude materialist who supposes that the world of electrons is the fundamental reality.

Verbum sap.

M. M. GARVER

THE SOUTH AFRICAN STATION OF THE HARVARD OBSERVATORY

A NOTICE in SCIENCE, January 20, 1928, on the new South African station of the Harvard Observatory was taken indirectly from an unedited article in a student publication; it contains several mistakes and extravagant statements, three of which perhaps justify correction.

1. Mazel's Poort where the Harvard station is located is not a city; it is the water works station of the city of Bloemfontein. The new road and other assistance are being provided by Bloemfontein.

2. The Harvard Observatory is constructing one 60-inch telescope, not three, for the southern station.

3. Mr. W. F. H. Waterfield leaves Cambridge for

Bloemfontein in the near future to act as assistant to Dr. Paraskevopoulos, the superintendent of the southern station.

Harlow Shapley

APPARATUS

While we are polishing up our pronunciation of scientific terms why not smother the "rat" so frequently heard in ap pa "rā′" tus?

Wilmer Souder

SCIENTIFIC BOOKS

Climate through the ages: A study of the climatic factors and their variations. By C. E. P. Brooks. 439 pp., 39 figs. London: Ernest Benn.

There are two principal difficulties in the way of a satisfactory explanation of the great climatic changes of geologic time. In the first place, the problem is both meteorological and geological, and requires a command of both of these fields which is practically beyond the power of either the meteorologist or the geologist alone. Secondly, it necessarily rests upon a fragmentary and uncertain knowledge of past conditions, both of climate and physiography, which is often interpreted in very diverse ways by different students of the subject.

Both of these difficulties are illustrated in the latest excursion into the field by the distinguished British meteorologist, C. E. P. Brooks. Nevertheless, his book is one of the most valuable contributions to the problem that has yet appeared. Perhaps its most praiseworthy feature is its emphasis on the quantitative point of view, in contrast to the glittering generalities so prevalent in discussions of paleoclimatology. Even though this does in some cases result in an impression of mathematical exactness hardly warranted by the accuracy of the data involved, it certainly is a step in the right direction.

The book is divided into three parts, the first and longest being a discussion of "Climatic Factors and their Variation," the second dealing with geological climates and their causes, and the third with the climates of the historical past. Climates are broadly classified as "glacial" and "non-glacial," the distinction being based on the presence or absence of a polar ice-cap. It is clearly demonstrated that this factor is of paramount importance in determining the climate of a given period, and hence the classification into "glacial" and "non-glacial" climates is fully justified.

The discussion of the "critical temperature" which determines the expansion of a small winter-formed polar ice-cap into an ice sheet of continental dimensions is highly significant, and should be read by every student of climatic changes. It is shown that a very small fall of temperature—not more than 0.6° F.—may, under proper conditions, produce an ultimate lowering of winter temperature by about 45° F. The importance of this fact in the problem of Ice Ages is evident.

Wegener's hypothesis of continental drift is given considerable attention from a climatic point of view, the conclusion being that it is not necessary to explain even the low-latitude glaciation of Upper Carboniferous time, which Brooks accounts for by purely geographic factors. In spite of some very questionable assumptions, such as the figures for mean cloudiness and amount of solar radiation reflected from cloud surfaces, both of which are based on data applying to special cases, the argument is a strong one.

This dominance of geographic factors is the general theme of the book. While all climatic factors are recognized, and particular significance is given to volcanic dust and solar variations in special cases, the changing relations of land and sea, and the elevation of mountain ranges, with their resultant effects on winds and ocean currents, are shown as capable of bringing about even the major climatic fluctuations of geologic time. No resort to astronomic causes or to special hypotheses is necessary. In the case of historical changes of climate, which Brooks considers to be fully established, solar influences are given a prominent part.

The book is not without serious faults. It shows evidences of hasty and careless writing and insufficient proof-reading. The discussion on p. 75 is a hodgepodge of blunders, in which the direction of winds around a center of high pressure in the northern hemisphere and the direction of the Equatorial Current are both given incorrectly. The reason given on p. 182 for the vertical decrease of temperature gradient is also incorrect. No authority is quoted for the statements on pages 162 and 163 regarding the percentage of water in the Gulf Stream which reaches the Arctic Ocean and the melting of the ice floor in Spitzbergen about 3000 B. C. The figures on p. 166 and the diagram on p. 167 to which they refer are both wrong, leading to much confusion. On p. 210 "windward" is used where "leeward" is meant. Other mistakes and omissions occur all too frequently.

Geologists will take exception to many statements in the book. Some of these, like that on p. 128, where the area of the Pleistocene ice-sheets is given as 1,000,000 sq. miles greater than the present area, are inexcusable. It is far from true that "the accession of salt to the oceans is at present derived almost entirely from sedimentary rocks" (p. 93). Nor is there any adequate basis for asserting that deserts were extensively developed in southeastern United States during the Mesozoic (p. 273). The reference is presumably to the areas of Newark rocks, which do not extend south of North Carolina and do not represent true desert conditions. The more southerly of these areas indicate distinctly less arid climates than those farther north, and even contain appreciable quantities of coal, which Brooks interprets as a product of equatorial rain forests.

It is perhaps too much to expect a meteorologist to be fully qualified to deal with purely geological questions, but when he ventures into a field in which geology plays almost as important a part as meteorology, the active collaboration of a geologist of recognized standing would appear to be a highly desirable safeguard. It would at least prevent such violence to terminology as the indiscriminate use of the word "period" to describe any and all intervals of geologic time, from "Mesozoic period" to "Pliocene period."

Although marred by too frequent errors such as those mentioned, the book is nevertheless a remarkable and highly valuable work. A prodigious amount of labor has gone into its preparation. It is to be hoped that it will have a salutary effect on those who see in new and fantastic hypotheses the only solution to the problem of geologic climates.

MALCOLM H. BISSELL

CLARK UNIVERSITY

SCIENTIFIC APPARATUS AND LABORATORY METHODS

A METHOD FOR CUTTING GLASS TUBING

READING the note by Herman E. Seemann on a "Method for Cutting Glass Tubing," SCIENCE No. 1726, I have remembered a method used to the same effect at laboratories of the University of St. Petersburg, Russia.

By means of a fine triangular file a circular furrow used to be made around a tube and then a melted glass stick applied to the cut in such a way as to press melted glass into the furrow. Usually the tubing cracked immediately and very regularly following the direction of the cut. Rather seldom it was necessary to apply melted glass repeatedly. The method, so far I am able to remember now, never failed and gave everybody a complete satisfaction. Especially it was used to open heavy glass tubings containing some preparation for analysis, for example, minerals or rocks under great pressure heated for a number of hours with sulfuric acid in a closed tubing. Any other method of cutting, for example, the one offered by Hermann E. Seemann, might not be applied in this case.

A furrow might be rather shallow, about a half of a millimeter was found quite sufficient, but has to be made accurately without lateral incisions even short ones. The whole operation, including the making a furrow, used to take less than a half of an hour even in the case of heavy tubing of a large diameter.

I. P. TOLMACHOFF

CARNEGIE MUSEUM,
PITTSBURGH, PENNSYLVANIA

A PLATINUM SPOON FOR ISOLATING AND TRANSFERRING PROTOZOA

IT is often desirable in investigations on protozoa, especially in those concerning life-histories, to secure the animals free from other organisms and detritus. The use of the capillary pipette in isolating organisms is very satisfactory in most cases if the animals are sufficiently washed. The author has experienced considerable trouble in washing to eliminate all other organisms. In an attempt to obviate this difficulty he has found that if only a few specimens are required, the instrument described below (Fig. 1) has some advantages over the pipette.

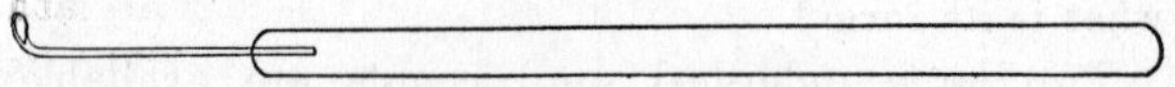

FIG. 1

The tip of an ordinary platinum bacteriological needle is flattened so as to form a circular disk about .2 mm. thick and .5 mm. to 1 mm. in diameter according to the needs. The surfaces and edges are then smoothed off so that the animal will not be injured. With a stylus or some other blunt instrument a depression is made in one of the flat surfaces of this disk forming a concavity, holding just enough water to cover the individual to be isolated.

The spoon is used as follows: A specimen desired for isolation is selected and if lying on the bottom of the dish, the instrument is lightly passed beneath it, then with a jerk it is brought to the surface by the currents produced; the spoon is now placed directly under the individual and gently raised through the surface film. In this way one can transfer active as well as sluggish animals, *e.g.,* didinia, paramecia, amoebae, etc. With a little practice specimens as small as 150 micra can be isolated under the low and high powers of the microscope.

The use of the instrument has the following advantages: It can be easily and thoroughly sterilized, a thing which is often desirable in protozoan studies; it is not fragile, an item of considerable importance as a labor saving device; and lastly, such minute quantities of fluid are transferred with the animals that the effect of it on the new solution becomes negligible after a few transfers and the possibility of contamination less.

PERCY L. JOHNSON

THE JOHNS HOPKINS UNIVERSITY

SPECIAL ARTICLES

STATISTICS OF VOCABULARY

WHILE studying some data on the relative frequency of use of different words in the English language, I noticed a rather interesting functional relationship which is here communicated. The note which follows, admittedly incomplete, is published in this form because the subject is one which I can not pursue and which may be of interest to those who are actively engaged in the study of language.

Suppose one takes a large representative sample of written English, counts the number of times each word appears and arranges the words in order of decreasing frequency of occurrence. The nth word in such a list will then occur with an observed frequency which is a function of n, call it f(n). This function is clearly a monotonicly decreasing function of n, from the way the data have been arranged. But what is its form?

Two large published word counts are available. One is that of L. P. Ayres, "A Measuring Scale for Ability in Spelling," Russell Sage Foundation, 1915, and the other is that of G. Dewey, "Relativ Frequency of English Speech Sounds," Harvard University Press, 1923. Each of these writers analyzed samples of 100,000 words of written English.

In the accompanying figure is plotted the logarithm of the observed frequency of the nth word against the

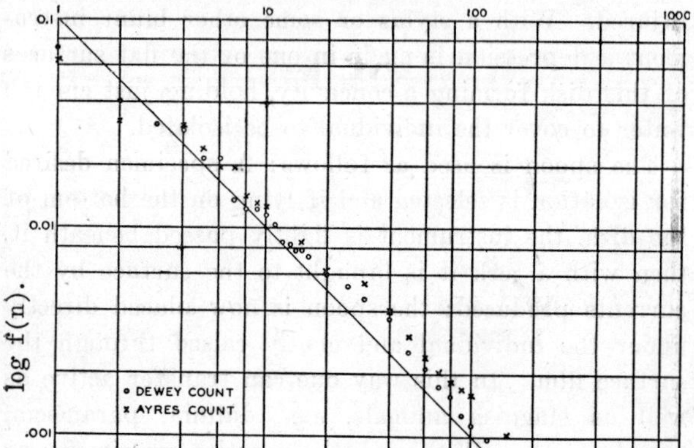

FIG. 1

logarithm of n. The circles are based on Dewey's count while the crosses are based on that of Ayres. The close approximation of the points to a straight line with unit negative slope is at once remarked. This suggests that there is something about the way in which man uses his language (Is the relation true for other languages?) which makes the frequency of occurrence of the nth word be given by a formula of the form,

$$f(n) = \frac{k}{n}.$$

On this form some comments will be made at the close of this letter. An interesting question concerns the value of the constant, k. Supposing the law to be valid over the entire range of the language, k must have such a value that the result of summation over all the different words in the sample will equal unity. That is, k is determined by the equation,

$$k \sum_{n=1}^{m} \frac{1}{n} = 1.$$

Since for large values of m (the number of different words in the sample) the summation can be replaced by $\lambda + \log_e m$, where $\lambda = 0.5772$, is Euler's constant and the logarithm is to the natural base, one has a ready means of computing the value of k from the total number of different words in the sample. Dewey found 10,161 different words in his sample, accordingly the value of k is 0.102.

A sort of check on the accuracy of this representation is given by assuming that the most infrequent word occurred just once and inferring from that fact and the value of k the total size of the sample. The value would clearly be 10,161 divided by k, or 99,500., which checks well with the actual size of sample counted, *i.e.*, 100,000.

On the figure the solid line has been drawn to represent the function with $k = 0.100$. It is seen to fit the data quite well, although there are systematic deviations.

Supposing the law to be substantially correct, the writer ventures to point out that it is perhaps a quantitative appearance in language of the Weber-Fechner law of psychology. In the language of the economist, it is a quantitative law of diminishing utility in vocabulary. The frequency of use of a word measures in some way its usefulness in transmitting ideas between individuals. Considering a vocabulary of n words it appears that the marginal increase in idea-transmitting power which can be accomplished by the addition of another word to the vocabulary is smaller the greater the value of n, according to the same law which governs the relation between the psychological increase in sensation accompanying an increase in the total intensity of the physical stimulus.

E. U. CONDON

BELL TELEPHONE LABORATORIES,
NEW YORK CITY

SCIENCE

VOL. LXVII MARCH 23, 1928 No. 1734

CONTENTS

George Sumner Huntington: PROFESSOR CHARLES F. W. MCCLURE 301

Ideals of the Engineer: GENERAL JOHN J. CARTY 307

Scientific Events:

Conference of Lake Erie Biologists; Meeting of the Electrochemical Society; Election of Fellows to the Royal Society of Edinburgh; New Chapters of the Society of Sigma Xi 309

Scientific Notes and News 311

University and Educational Notes 314

Discussion and Correspondence:

Oxidation-Reduction Reactions: PROFESSOR WILLIAM T. HALL. *Pseudo-Artifacts from the Pliocene of Nebraska:* N. C. NELSON. *The Life History of Varanus Niloticus:* RAYMOND B. COWLES. *Trinitasia—A New Molluscan Genus:* DR. CARLOTTA J. MAURY. *The Behavior of Mallard Ducks:* BIRGER R. HEADSTROM. *Wanted—A Word to Replace Believe:* DR. E. C. L. MILLER. *The Pronunciation of Research:* DR. NICHOLAS KOPELOFF 315

Scientific Books:

Hirmer's Handbuch der Paläobotanik: PROFESSOR EDWARD W. BERRY 319

Scientific Apparatus and Laboratory Methods:

A Constant Rate Aspirator: DR. CHAS. F. HOTTES and A. L. HAFENRICHTER. *A Simplified Plankton Bucket:* ARTHUR S. CAMPBELL 320

Special Articles:

Heating Hay in Flooded Regions: DR. LAWRENCE H. JAMES and DAVID J. PRICE. *Boron and the Growth of the Tomato Plant:* DR. EARL S. JOHNSTON and PROFESSOR W. H. DORE. *Triassic Fossils from Wyoming:* DR. E. B. BRANSON and DR. M. G. MEHL 322

Science News x

SCIENCE: A Weekly Journal devoted to the Advancement of Science, edited by J. McKeen Cattell and published every Friday by

THE SCIENCE PRESS

New York City: Grand Central Terminal.

Lancaster, Pa. Garrison, N. Y.

Annual Subscription, $6.00. Single Copies, 15 Cts.

SCIENCE is the official organ of the American Association for the Advancement of Science. Information regarding membership in the Association may be secured from the office of the permanent secretary, in the Smithsonian Institution Building, Washington, D. C.

GEORGE SUMNER HUNTINGTON, ANATOMIST[1]

TO-NIGHT there are gathered here the colleagues and friends of the late George Sumner Huntington to do honor to him whom all of us admire and respect for his works, to whom many of us are held by the strongest and closest bonds. Posterity knows a man through his accomplishments; his personality lives only in the memory of those with whom during his lifetime he was intimately associated. It would seem appropriate that in this company I should dwell more on the man, on his great and compelling personality, than was possible in the address that I recently delivered before the American Association of Anatomists.

My own acquaintance with Huntington dates back to 1890 when I was a student of his in the College of Physicians and Surgeons. It was not until the autumn of 1903, however, that I was brought into close working association with him. His associate, Dr. Churchill Carmalt, was then greatly interested in certain work going forward in my laboratory, and on one of his week-end trips to Princeton, he was accompanied by Huntington. It happened that at this time both Huntington and I were actively developing our respective collections in comparative anatomy; through our community of interest in these, there grew the close friendship and professional relationship that existed between us to the end of his life. Very soon we were deeply engaged in joint investigations on two problems of the vascular system. It is because Huntington and I worked so closely on these through a period of twenty odd years, collaborating in the publication of work carried on both together and independently, that I was so intimately acquainted with him professionally and personally, and so was asked to address you this evening on the subject of his life, character and accomplishments.

Rarely is there such a man as George Sumner Huntington. I wish I might draw a picture of him as I really knew him. He began life as a professional anatomist at the time when in this country anatomy was merely an adjunct to surgery; he died as one who had played a leading and dominant rôle in raising anatomy to the high status it now has in America—that of an independent science. We who were well acquainted with him realize that in any field of action he

[1] An address delivered before The New York Academy of Medicine, on January 20, 1928.

had chosen he would have become a leader. Marked physical and mental energy, indomitable perseverance, brilliant intellect, great power of concentration, unbounded enthusiasm—these are characteristics that we all know. Added to these were his charming, magnetic personality, his unfailing loyalty, his great capacity for deep and enduring friendship.

It is interesting to follow the early training and education of a man who, like Huntington, attains real eminence, and to observe the influence that environment may have played in forming his general character, and in moulding him for his chosen profession. While still an infant, Huntington was taken by his mother to Germany and remained there until he had completed his course in the German Gymnasium. He obtained his later education, both college and professional, in this country. The influence of the years in Germany, however, is most evident throughout his life. His thorough and methodical training in the Gymnasium accounts for the exactness and the attention to detail so characteristic of all his investigations. In Germany, too, he acquired his knowledge of the classics and his love for them—a love which he never lost even through the period of his most strenuous scientific career. In later years, when he had occasion to refer to Latin treatises on anatomy and medicine, he was able to read them with great facility. Although his research was of a most highly specialized character, the broad culture of the man was always apparent. Evidently during these early years abroad his mind was directed toward the subject that was to become his profession, for while there he began to collect books on anatomy. These anatomies, collected during his boyhood, with his name and the dates inscribed in them, still form a part of that great collection of books which he has left behind him.

On his return to this country in the autumn of 1877, Huntington was well prepared to enter Trinity College (Hartford) as a member of the class of 1881. Here, as in Germany, his general course continued to be broadly cultural; but the ever-increasing number of electives in chemistry, botany and zoology indicates that he had determined to adopt a scientific career. In his sophomore year he was awarded the Pascal-Fenelon prize for the best examination in Pascal's "Pensées"; in his senior year he received the chemical prize for an essay on explosives. He was graduated with the degree of Bachelor of Arts, *cum honore,* receiving honors in mental, moral and political philosophy, in chemistry and in the natural sciences.

The autumn after his graduation he entered the College of Physicians and Surgeons, then located at Twenty-third Street and Fourth Avenue, New York City. At his graduation from Trinity College, Huntington had ranked seventh in a class of nineteen. In 1884, at his graduation with the degree of M.D. from the College of Physicians and Surgeons, he ranked second in a class of one hundred and twenty-five. In a competitive examination, taken by the first ten men in the graduating class, he won the first prize of five hundred dollars. At the same time he won also a prize for the best clinical reports at the New York Hospital. At the time he had graduated from the College of Physicians and Surgeons, Huntington had given unmistakable indication of the extent of his great natural abilities and of the brilliance of his future career.

After graduation from the medical school, Huntington chose surgery as a profession and entered the Roosevelt Hospital as a member of the House Staff, where he remained until 1886, when he was made an assistant demonstrator of anatomy in the College of Physicians and Surgeons. Between 1886 and 1889, he continued as demonstrator in anatomy; and, for part of this time, assisted Dr. Henry B. Sands in his private practice. He acted also as visiting surgeon to the Bellevue Hospital, as junior assisting surgeon to the Roosevelt Hospital and as chief of clinic of the surgical department of the Vanderbilt Clinic.

In May, 1889, Huntington was appointed to a full-time professorship of anatomy in the College of Physicians and Surgeons. So far as I have been able to determine, no medical school in this country had ever before appointed a man whose full time was given to the teaching of anatomy and to the investigation of anatomical problems. It had been the custom to appoint to the chair of anatomy a man whose time was divided between the practice of surgery and the teaching of anatomy, but whose interest lay chiefly in surgery. As a result the teaching of anatomy had been wholly perfunctory, and no attempt had been made to interpret the structure of the human body in a scientific manner. In America anatomy had not at this time attained that development, that preeminence as a separate science, which already it held in Europe; it was too often presented as a mass of unrelated detail which medical students learned in the hope that at some future time the information might be of practical service. At the time Huntington was called to the chair of anatomy at the College of Physicians and Surgeons, anatomy was entirely subordinate to surgery.

During the three years that he served as demonstrator, Huntington must have been dissatisfied with the prevailing method of teaching anatomy; for in 1889, the year that he was made professor, he abandoned the system then in vogue in all American medical schools—that of giving didactic instruction by lecturing to large sections—and substituted teaching by demonstration of the actual objects to small sections of the class. This plan, inaugurated by Huntington, prevails at the present time throughout the country; he was the pioneer in effecting the change. It would have taken a man of no less ability and personal force than Huntington so quickly to revolutionize current methods of teaching. Soon, however, he was to exert a still greater influence by his recognition and application of the fact that anatomy is not an offshoot of surgery, but is a science by itself, and should be regarded and taught as such.

Having reorganized the method of teaching anatomy in the college, he soon recognized the inadequacy of the system in which the subject was presented to the students. Being a close student of evolution and having been deeply influenced by Darwin, Huxley, Owen and Gegenbaur, he now adopted morphology as a means of interpreting the structure of the human body. In doing this he was instrumental in influencing the whole of anatomical study in the medical schools in America; he gave importance to comparative anatomy, and so vitalized the whole subject. There had been other comparative anatomists in this country; Huntington was the first man in America, however, with the vision to see the importance of emphasizing the comparative method in the study of human anatomy, and to make clear the fact that the multitudinous detail which the structure of man offers can be interpreted from the standpoint of the morphology of the different organ systems, and in relation to the application of structure to function. The significance and importance of the structural peculiarities of man he accentuated and illustrated by comparison with the morphology of corresponding structures in the lower vertebrates. In his own words: "There is no region or part of the human body, which is not more readily and permanently comprehended through the comparison with the corresponding structures in the lower vertebrates." With the adoption of the laboratory method of teaching, Huntington radically changed the character and significance of his lectures. The old-fashioned recital of unrelated detail was replaced by a lecture on a much higher plane. Such, in brief, were the new methods of teaching and the general conceptions of anatomy which were initiated by Huntington in 1889, and were consistently followed by him during the thirty-five years that he was professor of anatomy in the College of Physicians and Surgeons.

I have emphasized the methods employed by Huntington in presenting to his students the subject of anatomy. At the time of his appointment as professor, he already had the practical acquaintance with the cadaver and the detailed knowledge of all its parts which were essential to the old-time teacher. When he made comparative anatomy the basis of his new course, however, he was confronted with the necessity of acquiring a first-hand, detailed knowledge of the structure of vertebrates in general; throughout our acquaintance he again and again emphasized his opinion that it is only through observation and practical experience, not through books, that an understanding of anatomy, both human and comparative, is to be gained. He at once began an intensive study of the comparative anatomy of vertebrates, and this work he carried over a period of thirty-five years. The number of vertebrates that he personally examined, dissected and prepared is almost unbelievable; to his associates it has always been a source of wonder how, in addition to attending to numerous other duties, he was able to do work so thorough and detailed on the many animals that came into his possession.

Huntington spent a lifetime in the study of comparative anatomy; in this field no one in America has ever equalled him either in practical experience or in the extent of information. With his experience and his profundity of knowledge, and with his great variety of preparations, Huntington was able to teach and illuminate the subject of human anatomy as before him no one had done in this country. As an inspired and inspiring teacher his name will long remain a tradition in the College of Physicians and Surgeons.

The development of his extensive human and comparative anatomical collection was a natural necessity of Huntington's method of teaching; and, as the collection gradually grew in size and importance, Huntington saw that in its future development he must adopt some definite plan leading to the establishment of what he hoped would be a permanent museum of comparative anatomy. Such a plan was formulated by him and was published in Science in 1901, under the title: "The Morphological Museum as an Educational Factor in the University System."

The Huntington collection now consists of nearly 6,000 mounted exhibits, practically all of which were prepared and mounted by Huntington himself. In addition to this there is in storage a large amount of material which is classified and catalogued, but remains still to be prepared. The collection is the most extensive and complete of its kind in this country and the technique displayed in the dissection and mounting of the exhibits is unexcelled by any in existence. It was Huntington's intention that in its complete state the collection should constitute a kind of general morphological reference library for the organs and organ systems of vertebrates; for, he says, "In this sense the museum fulfills its highest functions, stimulating and directly promoting investigation and rendering such investigations fruitful and effective by contributing the series necessary for comparison and reference."

The plan adopted by Dr. Huntington was very comprehensive; it serves to emphasize the thoroughness and attention to detail he invariably displayed in all matters in which he was professionally interested. The facilities for exhibiting the collection in accordance with his plan were notoriously inadequate in the College of Physicians and Surgeons, so that during his lifetime he was unable to organize it along the lines projected. This accounts for his unwillingness to open the collection to the general public, for which in the past he was sometimes unjustly criticized. He had hopes, however, that the foundation laid by him might be built upon by his successors, so that in time and under more favorable conditions, the museum would rank in prestige and in importance to the medical community, as does the Hunterian Museum of Comparative and Human Anatomy in the Royal College of Surgeons in London, now under the directorship of Sir Arthur Keith, the eminent British anatomist. This great Hunterian collection, illustrating both human and comparative anatomy, had its origin in much the same manner as did that of Huntington, and the greater part of the dissections were prepared by the founder, John Hunter. Following this tradition, the Federal Government of Australia has recently founded a National Museum which is to be a center for the advancement of comparative anatomy in its application to modern medical practice. This and the fact that the Hunterian Museum continues to be a growing and active institution, indicates the attitude of British anatomists toward the value of comparative anatomy as a means of elucidating man's structure.

It is to be hoped that the temporary reaction against morphology will not prevent the College of Physicians and Surgeons or some other institution of like standing from carrying out the plan formulated by Huntington and from making the Huntington Museum of Comparative Vertebrate Morphology, like the Hunterian Museum in London, a Mecca for American anatomists.

During the more recent years of his life, Dr. Huntington had observed the rôle played by experiment in influencing the methods of teaching anatomy and the investigation of its problems. It was always fixed firmly in his mind, however, that the experimental aspect of anatomy and of development can not precede the comparative aspect; otherwise, one would have to build and to elaborate theories based on materials he neither knew nor understood. Comparative morphology and experimental morphology are not opposing branches of science, but are complementary methods of attacking one and the same subject. A thorough knowledge of comparative anatomy and of comparative embryology he always maintained is a necessary prerequisite for the experimentalist.

Dr. Huntington has left forty-five publications which were written between 1892 and 1920. In addition to these there are several unfinished manuscripts; and there is one other, completed in 1923, but still unpublished, on the history of anatomy and medicine. These publications cover a wide range in the field of vertebrate morphology, and include investigations on the comparative anatomy and development of the digestive, genito-urinary, respiratory, nervous, muscular, lymphatic and cardio-vascular systems. Seven papers on the development of the vena cava posterior and of the lymphatic system were published jointly with me, between 1903 and 1920.

Between 1892 and 1903, when Huntington was especially interested in developing his teaching and in preparing his museum collections to be used in his course in anatomy, his papers were largely anatomical in character. After 1903, however, his interest was centered primarily on the embryology of the organ systems. His extensive collection of wax reconstructions gives evidence of the vast amount of work he accomplished in this direction.

His earlier investigations dealt largely with the morphology of the digestive system, and between 1892 and 1898 he published a number of papers on this topic. These earlier investigations on the digestive system finally led to the publication of an extensive comparative treatise on the subject, which appeared in 1903 under the title of "Anatomy of the Human Peritoneum and Abdominal Cavity." This book is profusely illustrated by 582 figures, the greater number of which are drawn or photographed from his own dissections. The book well represents Huntington's conception of the value of comparative anatomy and embryology "in elucidating the difficult and often complicated morphological problems encountered in the study of human adult anatomy."

Variations in anatomical configuration as observed especially in different mammals of the same species were always of great interest to Huntington. In this connection a series of five papers were published by him between 1895 and 1904, on variations of the muscular system in the lower primates and in man, with reference to their classification and morphological significance. In his Harvey lecture in 1907, on "The Genetic Interpretation and Surgical Significance of some Variations of the Genito-Urinary Tract," he described such variations of the genito-urinary tract in man as would probably be encountered by surgeons. Here he shows that all such variations can be interpreted by certain definite and recognized modifications possible in the embryonic ground plan of the genito-urinary tract of mammals.

Among his earlier publications was one appearing in 1898 on "The Eparterial Bronchial System of the Mammalia." It was written in refutation of a theory advanced by Aeby in explanation of the asymmetry which exists in mammals between the right and the left pulmonary arteries and the most proximal branches of the stem bronchi. This paper was the forerunner of a series of others published between 1916 and 1920 on the comparative anatomy and development of the mammalian respiratory organs.

In one of these papers published in 1917 on "The Morphological Basis for the Dominant Pulmonary Asymmetry in the Mammalia" he demonstrates by an embryological study the incorrectness of Aeby's view. He shows that the asymmetry which in the adult exists between the right and the left pulmonary arteries and the bronchial tree, has been brought about in the embryo by a rotation of the gut and the heart in opposite directions. As the result of this rotation the left pulmonary artery is shifted dorsad so that the most proximal branch of the left stem bronchus must necessarily grow out into the interval caudal to or below the left pulmonary artery.

At the time of his death Huntington had almost completed an extensive investigation on the morphology of the lungs of vertebrates, with special reference to mammals. This investigation, which extended over a long period, consists of a comparative study of the development of the lungs of vertebrates. For this he made nearly 500 wax corrosions of the lungs of mammals and of other vertebrates. A large portion of the manuscript, including the plates for figures, is ready for the press and it is to be hoped that funds will be forthcoming to insure its publication, even though the investigation is still uncompleted. Still another important series of investigations made by Huntington deals with the morphology of the salivary glands of mammals. In collaboration with Doctors Churchill Carmalt and Herman Von W. Schulte he published in 1913 a monograph on this subject. His personal contribution to the monograph deals with the development of the salivary glands in the lower primates and gives an interpretation of the primate alveolingual salivary area. This monograph is the most extensive and complete exposition of the subject in existence and must long remain a standard authority.

The above brief outline of some of Huntington's investigations gives a general idea of the character of his work and of the attitude held by him toward the investigation of anatomical problems.

It was in 1903, when his interests were becoming largely centered on embryological problems, that I became associated with Huntington as a collaborator and joined with him, as I have stated above, in making two extensive investigations. At the time of his first visit to Princeton, I was engaged in work on the development of the veins, and especially on the atypical conditions presented by the mammalian posterior vena cava. On account of the interest Huntington showed in my investigation it was suggested that we undertake a joint study. We decided that the development of the veins in the cat furnished material on which to establish an ontogenetic plan that would interpret these atypical conditions. On the basis of this investigation we have been able to classify under 17 main types the variant conditions of the vena cava posterior which in the adult cat are potential; also, we found that all caval variations thus far observed in man could be classed under these same types. This investigation led us directly to one still more important, on the development of the lymphatic system, which occupied us for over 15 years.

In the course of our work on the development of the veins, we observed that the formation of the jugular lymph sacs and thoracic ducts in the cat did not bear out a view advanced in 1902 by Florence Sabin regarding the development of lymphatics in the pig. Accordingly, postponing further work on the veins, we at once transferred our attention to the development of the lymphatic system; and our paper on the development of the veins in the cat did not appear in complete form until 1920.

An examination of any one of the current textbooks on embryology published prior to 1902 will show that up to that time no exact knowledge existed regarding the development of the lymphatic system. It was in 1902 that Florence Sabin advanced the view that the lymphatic system of the pig embryo begins as four blind ducts which in the neck and inguinal regions bud off from the endothelium of the veins and then grow continuously in a centrifugal direction, without discontinuity, throughout the body of the embryo to form the endothelium of the lymphatic system. In other words, she claimed that the endothelium of the lymphatics is invariably derived from the endothelium of the veins.

This view of Sabin's accorded with the angioblast theory of His, who maintained that all intraembryonic endothelium is derived from a unit vascular anlage situated, in the chick embryo, on the yolk sac, from which the endothelium grows continuously, without discontinuity, into and through the body of the embryo. In both these views the idea of the specificity of intraembryonic endothelium is especially involved, since both claim that it comes from a unit vascular anlage and is incapable of arising from any other source or in any other manner.

In 1906 Huntington and I read a joint paper before the American Association of Anatomists in which we maintained that the main lymphatic vessels of the embryonic cat do not develop from the endothelium of the veins, as claimed by Sabin, but develop *in loco,* independently of venous endothelium, from embryonic mesenchyme.

The appearance of this paper marked the beginning of an active controversy which lasted for about fifteen years. Following Sabin's first paper in 1902, nearly 100 others have appeared in substantiation of one or the other view and, with very few exceptions, they have all been written by American anatomists. The living embryo was studied and both the morphological and the experimental methods of investigation were employed.

In the heat of debate one is likely to lose sight of the broader aspects of a question. During the early years the problem was approached chiefly from the standpoint of a unit vascular anlage and of the specificity of lymphatic endothelium alone. Later on, however, as it became apparent that the lymphatic system is merely a part of the general vascular system the problem developed into the broader question of the genesis of endothelium in general, including that of the lymphatics, arteries and veins.

Without entering further into details, it can be stated that as a result of this long controversy, the morphological evidence favoring the local genesis of intraembryonic endothelium from mesenchyme has been completely confirmed by experiment and that the Angioblast Theory of His no longer holds. Furthermore, it is a matter of record that the principle of the local genesis of intraembryonic endothelium from mesenchyme is now generally accepted by anatomists, even by those who at one time most strenuously opposed this view.

Huntington's own personal contributions toward the solution of this problem will continue to be important as long as such pioneer work is of interest to anatomists. The great influence he exerted in stimulating his coworkers and in directing the endothelial problem toward its final solution will not soon be forgotten. He was instrumental in initiating two important experimental investigations by his own associates, McWhorter, Miller and Whipple, in the College of Physicians and Surgeons; these were outstanding contributions in our effort to establish the local genesis view.

The conclusions reached in the investigations which this controversy provoked will ever form a firm foundation on which future investigators may base their work dealing with the genesis of vascular tissues.

Huntington's unusual and striking personality was a dominant factor in his power as a teacher and contributed greatly to his professional success. His sense of humor and his gracious manner endeared him to all who came in contact with him. His innate fineness, his ready sympathy, his keen insight and his broad culture won him friends wherever he went. Every one who saw him was impressed with his vitality, with his indomitable strength—when he was roused in argument, with his alertness and pugnacity and power. Combined with these, he had a charm of virile manhood that is entirely indescribable to any one who did not know and feel it at first hand. All Huntington's activities were characterized by enormous vigor. When a young man, his daily exercise was taken with a professional wrestler. He was an incomparable woodsman and hunter. On his extensive camping trips in Canada, he went without guides, preferring to do all the hard work himself.

In his laboratory, he showed the same indomitable qualities. He loved his work, could never get enough of it. From the time he reached the college in the morning until he left for home at night, he worked incessantly. He was oblivious, insensitive to everything but the idea he was pursuing. In the height of our investigations, he would often in the evening call me over the long distance telephone to compare with me the results that the day's work had brought. It was a joy to collaborate with a man who never failed in eagerness and enthusiasm to share the results of his toil and mine.

At home his hospitality had the charm that characterized his every activity. When sometimes I would accompany him there after long hours of work, he showed no fatigue; his active mind would then often play over ideas that had been occupying us in the laboratory but it was from a new angle. He would comment on the broad aspects of our task, he would laugh over humorous incidents of the day, would sketch plans for the future. The evenings I spent with him by the fireside were among the most delightful of my life.

Although Huntington was that type of intensive individual investigator whose mind is strongly focussed on his own work, I know of no teacher who has been more solicitous for the success of his students, or who has done more to further their interests. He was always ready to discuss their problems and to aid them in their work. During the years that I collaborated with him he was surrounded by a brilliant group of young men; and between the years 1895 and 1919 thirty-nine investigations were published from his laboratory, not including those that he himself wrote. No one could be long with him without being fired by the enthusiasm that he had for his work. Some of the most prominent medical men in this country worked in his laboratory and owe to George Huntington much of the impulse and ambition that has brought them their professional success. It was always a great pleasure to me to accompany him here and abroad to meetings of the Anatomical Association, where he invariably played a leading rôle. He almost always took part in every discussion; and in debate no one could surpass him when he was discussing his own specialty or other subjects where he was convinced that his opinions were correct. His early experience as a surgeon made him a consultant peculiarly valuable to the medical profession at large; he was alert to the practical significance of his anatomical work, and was always ready to give advice to those who sought it. As an anatomist, as an investigator in fields far removed from surgery, he never lost sight of the fact that the training of surgeons was one of his chief aims. The combination of a professional anatomist of highest standing, with a surgeon of rare skill is unique; in these days of high specialization, it is not likely to occur soon again.

Those of us who were Huntington's intimate friends will always regard him as highly for what he was, as for what he accomplished. His charm of manner, his humor, his deep loyalty to friendships, his masterful energy, his whole dominant personality we shall not forget. He was a rare man, a remarkable friend.

CHARLES F. W. MCCLURE
PRINCETON UNIVERSITY

IDEALS OF THE ENGINEER[1]

IN receiving this great honor, I do so with feelings of deep gratitude and not without a sense of humility, for I realize that the brain of the individual has its limits as a storehouse, and that with knowledge continually increasing, any one mind can take in only a small portion of the rapidly accumulating body of engineering information. In these days, intellectual specialization is absolutely necessary, and whatever I have been able to accomplish is the result of specialization and the cooperation of many individuals.

In order to be of use to society, the ideas of the engineer in every department, in transportation, communication, and architecture, must first be embodied in physical form, and because of this he has achieved such a mastery over material things that he is regarded as preeminently the exponent of a material age. The great utility and economy resulting from his activities are so sensational as to conceal from view the ideals which form the basis of his creative work.

If seeking the truth and applying the truth to the affairs of man is a spiritual thing, then the engineer must be absolved from the charge of materialism. He is an advocate for truth. His works must be tried in the inexorable court of Nature, where no errors are committed and no exceptions granted. The work of the engineer is dedicated to the use of mankind, and the pecuniary compensation which he himself obtains is slight compared with the great benefits received by society. He finds inspiration and reward in achievement, and his real compensation is the good which others derive from what he has done.

Let us consider briefly the ideals of the engineer and the nature of his functions in the light of modern theories of evolution.

We are told that man has come from a lowly origin, and that during ages of time incalculably long he has advanced to his present position at the head of the animal kingdom. It has been supposed that in man himself this evolutionary process is still at work, and that, therefore, in the course of the ages he will evolve into a superlative type, and then perhaps all will go well.

Inasmuch as this evolutionary process in man himself is said to have taken vast periods of time, it is not unreasonable to expect that further ages must elapse before salvation by this form of evolution could be achieved.

Such a view does not afford much comfort nor does it provide any basis for a practical program to guide us. Even speaking in terms of the life of a nation, such a process is too slow. We must reckon with man as he now is. Our problems must be solved by working upon him and through him, and can not wait for the arrival of the hypothetical superman. Indeed, it is stated by an eminent authority that there are no indications that future man will be more perfect in body than the most perfect individuals of the present, or than the most perfect men and women in the days of Phidias and Praxiteles. There seems to be no general agreement as to whether this process in man himself has actually ceased; but I believe it is safe to say, in any event, that it is too slow in its operation to afford a solution of any of the problems that now confront us.

But this is not all that evolution has to offer. For, even if this one pathway should be closed to further great progress during our age, we are assured by that eminent authority, Professor Edwin Grant Conklin,[2] that there are two others which are open to us.

The first of these to be considered is one which is preeminently under the control of the engineer. Conklin tells us that the evolution of man, the individual, is no longer limited to his body or mind;

1 Address of John J. Carty upon receiving the John Fritz Gold Medal, February 15, 1928.

2 "The Direction of Human Evolution," Edwin Grant Conklin.

but by adding to his own powers the forces of nature, man has entered upon a new path of progress. The differentiations of various members of a colony of ants or bees, he tells us, are limited to their bodies and are fixed and irreversible. But in human society, differentiations are no longer confined to the bodies of individuals, but have become as it were extra-corporeal. And by his control over nature, man has taken into his evolution the whole of his environment. Although he is not as strong as the elephant, nor as deft as the spider, nor as swift as the antelope, nor as powerful in the water as the whale, nor in the air as the eagle; yet by his control of the forces of nature outside of his body, he can excel all animals in strength and delicacy of movement, and in speed and power, on land, in water, and in air.

The true object of engineering is not to create machines to which men will be bound by the chains of necessity, or mechanisms to which they will become slaves. The mission of the engineer is to obtain such a mastery in the application of the laws of nature that man will be liberated and that the forces of the universe will be employed in his service. According to Conklin, this new path of progress is in all respects the most important which has ever been discovered by organisms, and no one can foresee the end of this process of annexing to our own powers the illimitable forces of the universe.

Concerning the other pathway of evolution, he tells us that progress in intellectual evolution, no less than in physical, lies in the direction of increasing specialization and cooperation. But this progress, he says, is no longer taking place within the individual, but in the specialization and cooperation of many individuals. The intellectual evolution of the individual may have come to an end; but whether or not this is true, it is certain that the intellectual evolution of groups of individuals is only at the beginning. In social evolution—the evolution of human society—Conklin says a new path of progress has been found, the end of which no one can foresee.

Progress along this pathway, also, is vitally dependent upon the work of the engineer, for the perfection of all forms of communications and transportation is essential in order that this new super-organism, human society, shall achieve its destiny.

Emphasizing the importance of this, Trotter,[3] another distinguished writer on evolution, tells us that the capacity for free intercommunication between individuals of the species has meant so much in the evolution of man, and will certainly come in the future to mean so incalculably more, that it can not be regarded as anything less than a master element in the shaping of his destiny.

The use of the spoken word to convey ideas distinguishes man from all other created things. It is the function of the engineer to provide for the extension of the spoken word by means of electrical systems of intercommunication which will serve to connect the nervous system of each unit of society with all of the others thus providing an indispensable element in the structure of that inconceivably great and powerful organism which it is believed will be the ultimate outcome of the marvelous evolution which society is to undergo.

There is one element and only one, which stands in the way of the realization of this inspiring vision. That is man himself for he is the unit or cell out of which the new organism is to be evolved. In the individual animal organism, the units or cells are physically joined to each other; but in the social organism, the units are individuals, not physically joined but free to move about at will. The connection between these separate and mobile units is accomplished by communications, which convey information, ideas, and impulses from one mind to another. Whether these communications shall be employed in peaceful, constructive cooperation, or whether they shall be used to engender conflict and confusion, depends upon man himself.

Already, the applications of science to human affairs have far outrun the ability of man to use them wisely. The engineer has provided agencies of incalculable value in time of peace, but they are also endowed with prodigious powers of destruction which can be loosed in time of war. Unless we solve the problem encountered in man himself, the outlook is dark indeed, and it may even be questioned whether our civilization will endure.

Human behavior presents the most important and the most formidable problem of all the ages. Its solution can be achieved only by profound and prolonged researches, which shall bring to bear upon every phase of the subject all of the resources of science.

While, in such a consideration as this, it would be folly to ignore the claims of religion and philosophy, it would be a grave error to conclude that, in order to avoid disaster, we must restrict progress in the application of science to material things. On the contrary, we must accelerate progress in all the sciences, for the knowledge thus gained will be required in preparing the individual man to function as a sane and peaceful unit in the ultimate social organism.

Scientific research in our universities and elsewhere,

[3] "Instincts of the Herd in Peace and War," W. Trotter.

conducted solely for the increase of knowledge, should receive more adequate financial support, so that it may be prosecuted with ever-increasing vigor. If this is done, I believe that in the fulness of time, by further scientific discoveries, the physical development of man will be improved, that many diseases will be entirely eliminated, and that immunity to the others will be achieved, and that feeble-bodiedness and feeble-mindedness will disappear. Thus will be removed some of the greatest barriers to social progress.

In the great plan of evolution, the part assigned to the engineer calls for the highest exercise of his creative faculties, for he is to direct the evolution of man's extra-corporeal powers, providing him with more numerous and still more powerful additions to his feeble bodily equipment.

The ideals of the engineer will not be realized until man has achieved his destiny in that social organism which is foreshadowed "with its million-minded knowledge and power, to which no barrier will be insurmountable, no gulf impassable, and no task too great."

JOHN J. CARTY

AMERICAN TELEPHONE AND TELEGRAPH CO.

SCIENTIFIC EVENTS

CONFERENCE OF LAKE ERIE BIOLOGISTS

SINCE the initiation of active field investigations in Lake Erie by the U. S. Bureau of Fisheries in the summer of 1927, it has become evident that several investigators and research institutions are already interested in biological research in these waters and that others are either planning to undertake such studies or are in a favorable position to do so.

To stimulate interest in Lake Erie and to center attention upon fisheries conservation, the commissioner of fisheries called a conference of the various biologists working independently or as members of the staffs of research institutions and universities with the hope of effecting closer coordination of the work and to prevent duplication of effort. Dr. Francis H. Herrick, of Western Reserve University, offered the facilities for the meeting, and the conference, therefore, was held in Cleveland on February 6.

The New York Conservation Department was represented by Alexander McDonald, commissioner, and Dr. Emmeline Moore; Dr. R. H. Pegrum represented the Buffalo Society of Natural Sciences; N. R. Buller, Fisheries Commissioner of Pennsylvania, was present; Dr. R. C. Osburn, of Ohio State University; E. L. Wickliff, W. M. Tidd, and M. K. Young, of the Ohio Division of Fish and Game, and Dr. R. V. Bangham, of Wooster College, Wooster, Ohio, also were present. A number of the faculty of Western Reserve University attended, including Dr. Herrick and Dr. J. Paul Visscher. The Ohio State Department of Health was represented by Messrs. B. F. Hatch and Paul Mason; G. F. Simmons represented the Cleveland Museum of Natural History. Michigan was represented by C. L. Hubbs, curator of fishes of the State University, and the Province of Ontario by W. J. K. Harkness and J. L. Hart, of the University of Toronto. Besides Commissioner Henry O'Malley, who presided at the conference, the Bureau of Fisheries was represented by Lewis Radcliffe, Elmer Higgins, Dr. John Van Oosten, Stillman Wright and E. J. McClure. In addition to these official delegates a number of commercial fishermen and fish merchants evidenced their interest in the solution of fishery problems in Lake Erie by attending the conference and entering into the discussions.

After an address of welcome by Dr. Herrick, Mr. O'Malley took the chair and the following program was taken up:

1. Conservation in Lake Erie and the need for cooperative investigation, Henry O'Malley.
2. The condition of the Great Lakes fisheries, Lewis Radcliffe.
3. Review of the present state of knowledge concerning the biology of Lake Erie, Dr. R. C. Osburn.
4. Biological problems in Lake Erie, Dr. C. J. Fish (read by Dr. R. H. Pegrum).
5. Survey of research programs and research facilities:
   a. State of New York, Mr. McDonald and Dr. Moore.
   b. Buffalo Museum of Natural Sciences, Dr. Pegrum.
   c. State of Pennsylvania, N. R. Buller.
   d. State of Ohio, Dr. R. C. Osburn.
   e. Western Reserve University, Dr. J. Paul Visscher.
   f. University of Toronto, W. J. K. Harkness.
   g. University of Michigan, Carl L. Hubbs.
   h. U. S. Bureau of Fisheries, Dr. John Van Oosten.
   i. Other agencies:
      1. Cleveland Museum of Natural History, G. F. Simmons.
      2. Ohio State Board of Health, B. F. Hatch.

The fisheries situation in Lake Erie and the need for further investigations were discussed freely by various members of the conference. In surveying the research programs and research facilities of the various organizations it was apparent that the States of New York and Ohio are contemplating further investigations in Lake Erie on an extensive scale during the coming year. Included in the program of the State of New York is the employment of personnel from several cooperative institutions, such as Cornell University, Syracuse University, Rensselaer Polytechnic Institute and the Buffalo Museum of Natural Sciences. At the western end of the lake the Ohio Division of

Fish and Game is joining forces with the state university and the Franz Theodore Stone Laboratory in conducting studies there. In the central part of the lake the Fish and Game Department of Pennsylvania has promised cooperative action, together with the biologists of Western Reserve University. The province of Ontario is unable to cooperate actively because of the fact that biologists of the University of Toronto are already engaged in fishery problems in Lake Ontario; and while undertaking no active field work, the University of Michigan offers cooperation in problems concerning technical ichthyology. The bureau's staff of investigators, under the direction of Dr. John Van Oosten, is being built up, and by early summer seven workers will be engaged in investigations dealing directly with the fisheries.

At the close of the discussions, in which every one was given opportunity to express his views, it was determined that the Commissioner of Fisheries should appoint an executive committee to draft plans for coordinated research on Lake Erie, based on the individual plans submitted. Mr. O'Malley appointed Elmer Higgins chairman and Drs. R. C. Osburn and Emmeline Moore as members of this committee with instructions to draft the program and refer it back to the individual cooperative investigators for their approval and action. The committee was directed further to prepare a bibliography on equipment, with special reference to experimental fishing gear, and to make an effort to standardize collecting equipment among the investigators as far as possible. It is believed that material progress has been made in stimulating research on the problems of conservation and the rebuilding of a valuable but sadly depleted fishery in Lake Erie.

ELMER HIGGINS

U. S. BUREAU OF FISHERIES

MEETING OF THE AMERICAN ELECTRO-CHEMICAL SOCIETY

THE American Electrochemical Society will hold its annual meeting at Bridgeport, Conn., on April 26, 27 and 28. This district was chosen owing to the epoch-making developments in the electric manufacture of brass. The president of the society is Professor S. C. Lind, head of the department of chemistry of the University of Minnesota and the American representative of the International Radium Standards Commission. Professor Lind will show the members a number of gas reactions brought about by radium emanations.

On April 26, the society will convene at the new Hotel Stratfield, and will devote Friday morning to the discussion of electric heating, molting and electric furnace linings. Among those who will participate in this discussion are Mr. R. E. Talley, president and chief engineer of George J. Hagan Company, Pittsburgh; Mr. R. M. Keeney, industrial heating engineer of the Connecticut Light and Power Company; Mr. John L. Christie, metallurgist of the Bridgeport Brass Company; Dr. B. D. Saklatwalla, vice-president of the Vanadium Corporation of America, and others.

The Thursday morning session at the Hotel Stratfield will be devoted to a discussion of new batteries, and Dr. George W. Vinal, of the U. S. Bureau of Standards, will preside. Owing to the development of the radio industry, the battery business has increased by leaps and bounds. The Burgess Laboratories of Madison, Wisconsin, will present the results of their latest discoveries. The storage battery will be analyzed by experts in this field, and there will be reports on improved types of wet primary cells such as the Edison and Waterbury cells. Finally, there will be a demonstration of new rectifiers and eliminators. On Thursday afternoon the members will proceed upon a tour of inspection of the factories in Bridgeport and vicinity. On Thursday evening there will be a public lecture by Professor Bergen Davis, of Columbia University, who will demonstrate the use of the X-ray in the study of metals and compounds.

The local committee is headed by Mr. John L. Christie, metallurgist of the Bridgeport Brass Company. Mr. Christie has been working for many weeks in arranging for plant visits and social functions. Other members of his committee include the following: Messrs. F. M. Turner, Charles J. McElroy, W. G. Stratten, Raymond O'Connor, W. O. Mitscherling, Karl Pitschner, Walter M. Bradley, William Delage, George B. Hogaboom and J. C. Bradley. The main social event of the electrochemists' convention will be a dinner and dance on Friday evening.

The final session will be held Saturday morning, and will be devoted to the presentation of papers on electroplating of nickel, gold, silver, chromium and thallium. Professor E. M. Baker, of the University of Michigan, and expert for the G. C. Spring and Bumper Company, will preside over this session.

ELECTION OF FELLOWS TO THE ROYAL SOCIETY OF EDINBURGH

THE following candidates have been recommended by the council for election as Fellows of the Royal Society of Edinburgh:

Baker, Edwin Arthur, assistant at the Royal Observatory, Edinburgh; Barbour, George Brown, professor of geology, Yenching University, Peking, China; Brown, Hugh Wylie; Bruce, William Straton, parish minister of Banff; Clark, Alfred Joseph, professor of materia medica in the University of Edinburgh; Coutie, Alexander, assistant in the chemistry department, University of Edinburgh; Cumming, William Murdoch, senior lecturer on organic chemistry, Royal Technical College, Glasgow; Dawson, Warren Royal, fellow of the Royal Society of Medicine; Fenton, Edward Wyllie, lecturer in agricultural botany, Edinburgh and East of Scotland College of Agriculture; Forrest, James, lecturer in physics, University College, Dundee; Fraser, John, Regius professor of clinical surgery in the University of Edinburgh; Fraser, Kenneth, deputy county medical officer of health, Cumberland; Harding, William Gerald, Christ Church, Oxford; Hobson, Alfred Dennis, lecturer in zoology in the University of Edinburgh; Hodge, William Vallance Douglas, lecturer in mathematics in the University of Bristol; Hunter, Arthur, vice-president and chief actuary of the New York Life Insurance Company; Johnston-Saint, Percy Johnston, secretary, Wellcome Historical Medical Museum, London; Johnstone, Robert William, professor of midwifery and diseases of women in the University of Edinburgh; Jones, Tudor Jenkyn, lecturer in anatomy in the University of Liverpool; MacDonald, Thomas Logie, secretary of the West of Scotland branch of the British Astronomical Association; Mackie, Thomas Jones, professor of bacteriology in the University of Edinburgh; Matthai, George, professor of zoology, the Government College, Lahore, India; Nichols, James Edward, research assistant in genetics at the animal breeding research department, University of Edinburgh; O'Donoghue, Charles Henry, lecturer in zoology in the University of Edinburgh; Percival, George Hector, assistant physician, skin department, Royal Infirmary, Edinburgh; Pilcher, Robert Stuart, general manager and engineer, Edinburgh Corporation Tramways and Motors; Price, Charles Edward, formerly M.P. for Central Edinburgh; Roberts, Owen Fiennes Temple, lecturer in astronomy and meteorology in the University of Aberdeen; Senior-White, Ronald, malaria research officer, Central Malaria Bureau, Kasauli, India; Smith, Alick Drummond Buchanan, assistant animal breeding research department, University of Edinburgh; Watters, Alexander Marshall, rector of Hawick High School; Whittaker, John Macnaghten, senior scholar of Trinity College, Cambridge, and lecturer in mathematics in the University of Edinburgh; Williamson, John, lecturer in mathematics in the University of St. Andrews.

NEW CHAPTERS OF THE SOCIETY OF SIGMA XI

THE Arizona chapter of the Society of Sigma Xi was installed at the University of Arizona on the afternoon of February 22, Dr. W. F. Durand, of Stanford University, acting in the capacity of installing officer. In the evening a banquet was held, followed by the first Sigma Xi lecture, entitled "Science and Civilization," by Dr. Durand. The officers of the newly-installed chapter are: Dr. P. S. Burgess, *president;* Dr. G. T. Caldwell, *vice-president,* and Dr. H. B. Leonard, *secretary-treasurer.*

The college of medicine of the University of Illinois chapter of the Sigma Xi was installed on March 9 by the national president, Dr. F. R. Moulton, and Professor George Baitsell, of Yale University, head of the executive committee. There are twenty-eight charter members. Dr. D. J. Davis, dean of the college, was elected president, and Dr. William H. Welker, *secretary;* Dr. I. Pilot, *treasurer,* and Drs. William F. Petersen, H. A. McGuigan and Dr. V. E. Emmel *to membership in the executive committee.*

A chapter of the Society of the Sigma Xi was installed at the Kansas State Agricultural College on March 3. The chapter members, 58 in number, were all alumni members of Sigma Xi, representing 22 different institutions. The installing officer, Professor George A. Baitsell, of Yale University, gave the installation address on the subject "Coagulation in its relation to Tissue Formation."

There has recently been organized at Louisiana State University a Sigma Xi Club composed of nineteen members from the departments of botany, chemistry, geology, mathematics, physics, zoology and the experiment station. The purpose of the club is to further the advancement of research in the university and to give the university community the opportunity when possible to hear prominent speakers on scientific subjects.

SCIENTIFIC NOTES AND NEWS

PRESENTATION of the Bruce medal of the Astronomical Society of the Pacific to Dr. Walter S. Adams, director of the Mount Wilson Observatory, will be made on April 16 by Dr. W. W. Campbell. On this occasion Dr. Adams will give an address on "The Past Twenty Years of Physical Astronomy."

DR. HIDEYO NOGUCHI, of the Rockefeller Institute for Medical Research, has been elected a corresponding member of the Vienna Microbiological Society.

IN recognition of his distinguished service to the British government in the field of tropical medicine, the honor of knighthood has been conferred on Dr. Aldo Castellani, professor and director of the department of tropical medicine, Tulane University of Louisiana School of Medicine, and director of tropical medicine and physician in the Ross Tropical Institute and Hospital, London.

DR. ARISTIDES AGRAMONTE, of Havana, who was a member of the group of army officers—Reed, Carroll, Lazear and Agramonte—which was appointed by the United States to conduct the yellow fever investigation in Cuba, at a special meeting of the faculty, members of the American College of Physicians and students and citizens of New Orleans, was awarded the degree of doctor of laws by Tulane University.

THE Academy of Natural Sciences of Philadelphia announces that its committee on the Joseph Leidy

Memorial Award for 1928 has selected Dr. Henry Augustus Pilsbry, chief of the department of mollusca at the academy, as the recipient of the award. The report of the committee states that "the award is made in recognition of his researches on the phylogeny of the terrestrial mollusca, in which field he is universally regarded as a leading authority, and for his work on the classification of the Cirripedia which constitutes the most notable contribution to the subject in recent years." The award consists of a bronze medal and honorarium, given once in three years for outstanding work in the natural sciences. It was founded in 1923 and its first recipient, in 1925, was Dr. Herbert Spencer Jennings, of the Johns Hopkins University. The committee which made the 1928 award consisted of Dr. Witmer Stone, *chairman*, Dr. Edwin G. Conklin, Dr. William B. Scott, Dr. J. Percy Moore and James A. G. Rehn.

S. G. BLAYLOCK, general manager of the Consolidated Mining and Smelting Company of Canada, will be the recipient this year of the James Douglas medal, awarded annually by the American Institute of Mining Engineers for distinguished achievement in nonferrous metallurgy.

THE Thomas Hawksley gold medal of the British Institution of Mechanical Engineers has been awarded to H. L. Guy for his paper entitled "The Economic Value of Increased Steam Pressure," which was presented in November, 1926.

BOYLE medals have been awarded by the council of the Royal Dublin Society to Dr. W. R. G. Atkins (pure science) and to Professor W. E. Adeney (applied science) and were presented at a special scientific meeting of the society on February 15.

DR. JOHN H. MUSSER, professor of medicine at Tulane University, was elected president-elect of the American College of Physicians at the New Orleans meeting on March 8; Drs. Aldred S. Warthin, Ann Arbor, and Solon Marx White, Minneapolis, were reelected vice-presidents; Dr. Williams McKim Marriott was elected third vice-president, and Drs. Clement R. Jones, Pittsburgh, and George M. Piersol, Philadelphia, were reappointed treasurer and secretary-general, respectively.

DR. EDWARD L. KEYES, professor of clinical surgery at the Cornell University Medical College, has been elected president, and Dr. Donald R. Hooker, of Baltimore, secretary, of the American Social Hygiene Association for 1928. Dr. William H. Welch is honorary president.

PROFESSOR R. C. WALLACE, of the University of Manitoba, has been made chairman of the Manitoba hydro-electric commission.

DR. ANDREW M. SOULE, president of the State College of Agriculture, Athens, Ga., has been named president of the Southern Appalachian Power Conference.

RAPHAEL ZON, director of the Lake States Forest Station at St. Paul, has been transferred to Wisconsin and has been appointed non-resident professor in the university. He will direct forestry investigations under the supervision of the Wisconsin Conservation Commission, the United States Forest Service and the State College of Agriculture. The experiments will be conducted in different sections of the state.

DR. CLIFFORD L. DERICK, assistant resident physician at the Rockefeller Hospital, New York City, has been appointed physician to the Peter Bent Brigham Hospital, Boston, Massachusetts, to succeed Dr. Cyrus C. Sturgis, recently appointed professor of medicine at the University of Michigan.

DR. A. L. MELANDER, head of the department of biology in the College of the City of New York, has declined the post of state entomologist for New York.

COMMANDER JOHN C. THOMPSON, doctor at the Pearl Harbor Navy Yard; W. M. Giffard, amateur entomologist, and Bruce Cartwright, student of Hawaiian ethnology and history, have been appointed research associates on the staff of the Bernice P. Bishop Museum, Hawaii.

DR. H. E. BARNARD recently resigned the presidency of the American Institute of Baking, and has organized the firm of H. E. Barnard, Inc., in Indianapolis, for consultation on problems relating to food production.

DR. C. L. SHEAR, who spent the past winter collecting fungi in the Hawaiian Islands, is expected to arrive in Washington sometime during April. Dr. Neil E. Stevens, who accompanied Dr. Shear during much of his trip, devoted especial attention to the diseases of strawberries.

DR. H. A. GLEASON, of the New York Botanical Garden, sailed on March 22 for Europe, and will devote the ensuing six months to a continuation of his studies on the flora of British Guiana.

MAURICE H. BIGELOW, of Concord, Mass., who for the past three years has been head of the department of sciences in the American College of Salonica, Greece, plans to return in June, to engage in industrial chemistry and to give a course of lectures on "Industrial Openings in the Near East."

THE third course of two lectures under the Morris Herzstein lectureship on diseases of the Pacific Basin including tropical diseases will be given by Dr. Richard P. Strong, professor of tropical medicine of the Harvard Medical School, on May 2 and May 3, at the Stanford Medical School. The title of Dr. Strong's lectures will be "Recent Advances in Tropical Medicine."

THE first address under the Abner Wellborn Calhoun lectureship of the Medical Association of Georgia will be given on May 9, by Dr. George E. de Schweinitz, of Philadelphia, on "Headaches."

PROFESSOR LYMAN C. NEWELL, of Boston University, will deliver the address at the exercises commemorating the one hundred and seventy-fifth anniversary of the birth of Count Rumford which will be held on March 26 at Woburn, Mass., where Count Rumford was born. The title of the address is "Count Rumford—Scientist and Philanthropist."

DR. GEORGE BARGER, professor of chemistry, University of Edinburgh, lectured at the Medical School of Harvard University, on March 9, on "Thyroxine and the Thyroid Gland." On March 16 Dr. Barger gave a lecture on the same subject before the New York University chapter of the Sigma Xi.

DR. DEAN D. LEWIS, professor of surgery in the Johns Hopkins University, delivered the Hodgen lecture on March 20, before the St. Louis Medical Society on "Reconstruction Surgery."

V. K. LA MER, assistant professor of chemistry at Columbia University, lectured on "The Influence of Electric Properties on the Behavior of Solutions" before the Cleveland, Columbus, Cincinnati, Ann Arbor and East Lansing, Michigan, sections of the American Chemical Society from March 9 to 16. His lecture before the Indianapolis section on March 14 dealt with "Oxidation Potentials and their Biological Significance."

PROFESSOR CHANCEY JUDAY, of the University of Wisconsin, gave a public lecture at the University of Michigan on March 9 on "Recent Aspects of Limnology."

DR. C. J. DAVISSON, of the Bell Telephone Laboratories, Inc., addressed the Franklin Institute on March 21 on "Are Electrons Waves?"

DR. O. E. MEINZER, of the U. S. Geological Survey, recently delivered a lecture entitled "Well Water and Well Problems in Different Parts of the United States," before the Illinois Water-Well Drillers Association, in Urbana, and the Minnesota Well Drillers Association, in Minneapolis.

DR. ROBERT G. AITKEN, associate director of the Lick Observatory, addressed the Astronomical Society of the Pacific on March 19 on "Multiple Stars."

DR. OSCAR RIDDLE, of the Carnegie Station for Experimental Evolution, Cold Spring Harbor, N. Y., addressed a meeting of the section of biology of The New York Academy of Sciences on March 12 on "Studies on Thyroids and Gonads."

DR. W. F. G. SWANN, director of the Bartol Research Foundation of the Franklin Institute, lectured on "The Earth's Magnetic Charge" at the meeting of the American Institute of Electrical Engineers in New York on February 13, and also on "Recent Theories of the Atom" at the joint meeting of the Physical Society and Optical Society at Columbia University on February 24.

THE thirteenth Guthrie lecture before the British Physical Society on electrodeless discharge through gases was given by Sir Joseph Thomson on March 9 at the Imperial College of Science and Technology, South Kensington.

THE Romanes lecture at the University of Oxford for this year will be delivered by Dr. D. M. S. Watson, Jodrell professor of zoology and comparative anatomy in University College, London, on May 4. His subject will be "Paleontology and the Origin of Man."

As a tribute to the thoroughness and accuracy of the exploratory and geological investigations of the late Dr. G. M. Dawson, at one time a member and later director of the Geological Survey of Canada, a monument is to be erected by Mr. Fenley Hunter, of New York, on the bank of the Liard River in Yukon territory.

IT was announced on March 14 that the half-way mark had been passed in New York's quota of $500,000 toward the completion of the $2,000,000 Leonard Wood memorial for the eradication of leprosy.

DR. THOMAS BRUCE FREAS, professor of chemistry at Columbia University, died on March 15, aged fifty-nine years.

CHARLES WILSON EASLEY, professor of chemical engineering at Syracuse University, died on January 27, at the age of fifty-two years.

AUSTIN BRADSTREET FLETCHER, consulting engineer for the Bureau of Public Roads of the U. S. Department of Agriculture, died on March 8, at the age of fifty-six years.

SIR DAWSON WILLIAMS, who retired last January from the editorship of the *British Medical Journal* after thirty years of distinguished service in that office, died on February 27, aged seventy-three years.

A CORRESPONDENT writes that Professor Charles Walter Howard, who in September last returned to this country from China to head the department of zoology at Wheaton College, died on March 1 from injuries received when he was struck by an interurban trolley. Professor Howard was an entomologist of wide experience in this country, in Africa and in China. For the past eleven years he was connected with Lingnan University at Canton and since 1923 he was director of the Government Bureau for the Improvement of Sericulture in Kwongtung Province, a position which he held at the time of his death. He was fellow of the London Entomological Society and member of the Pan-African Trypanosomiasis Commission and was a member of the First International Congrèss of Entomology held in Brussels in 1909. He was to have served as chairman of the sericultural section of the Fifth International Congress of Entomology, meeting in August of this year in Ithaca.

THE annual meeting of the Kentucky Academy of Science will be held on May 12 at the University of Kentucky. The invited speaker will be Dr. E. C. Stakman, plant pathologist of the University of Minnesota, who will also represent the American Association for the Advancement of Science at the meeting. Dr. A. M. Peter, of Lexington, is secretary of the academy and the division secretaries are: Physical sciences, Professor C. S. Crouse, University of Kentucky; biological sciences, Professor E. N. Fergus, Experiment Station, Lexington; philosophy and psychology, Dr. M. A. Caldwell, University of Louisville.

A GROUP of scientific men at Princeton who are interested in "analysis situs" is organizing an informal conference on the subject immediately preceding the April meeting of the American Mathematical Society in New York City. At that meeting there will be held an extensive symposium on all phases of analysis situs, but it is believed that a conference such as planned will provide closer contact and a more thorough exchange of ideas than can take place at a general meeting of the society. The topic to be considered will be "The Ideal Organization of the Subject Matter of Analysis Situs as it Stands To-day." There is, however, no idea of holding to this subject should the discussion develop in some other direction. The formal meetings of the conference will take place on Wednesday and Thursday, April 4, 5, at 2:30, Room 312, Palmer Physical Laboratory. In addition to the members of the Princeton group (Alexander, Alexandroff, Hopf, Lefschetz and Veblen) the participation of Professors Chittenden, Kline and Morse has been assured.

AT the annual council meeting of The History of Science Society, held in New York at Teachers College, Columbia University, on February 25, officers for the year were elected as follows: *President,* Dr. Edgar F. Smith, University of Pennsylvania; *Vice-Presidents,* Dr. John C. Merriam, Carnegie Institution of Washington, and Dr. James Harvey Robinson, 173 Riverside Drive, New York; *Recording Secretary,* Dr. Harry Elmer Barnes, Smith College; *Corresponding Secretary* and *Treasurer,* Mr. Frederick E. Brasch, Library of Congress; *Editor of Isis,* Dr. George Sarton, Harvard University; Members of the Council to serve until 1930, Dr. J. McKeen Cattell, editor of SCIENCE; Dr. Florian Cajori, University of California; Dr. George S. Brett, Toronto University; Dr. Lao G. Simons, Hunter College, New York, N. Y., and Dr. C. A. Browne, U. S. Bureau of Chemistry.

THE Civil Service Commission announces an examination for the position of chief of the Bureau of Dairy Industry, Department of Agriculture. The examination will consist solely of the consideration of qualifications by a special examining board. The entrance salary for the position is $6,000. Applications must be on file with the commission in Washington not later than April 3.

UNIVERSITY AND EDUCATIONAL NOTES

THE Columbia University-Presbyterian Hospital Medical Center, which has been under construction for three years, was opened to public inspection for the first time on March 16. Six units were opened. They were the Presbyterian Hospital, the Sloane Hospital for Women, the Squier Urological Clinic, the Presbyterian Hospital School of Nursing Practice, the Harkness Pavilion and the Anna C. Maxwell Hall for Nurses. On March 19 the Presbyterian Hospital will begin to move to its new quarters. The College of Physicians and Surgeons, the School of Dental and Oral Surgery and the State Psychiatric Institute will move to the Center during the coming summer.

GIFTS amounting to $2,000,000 have been made to the $15,000,000 endowment fund for the six American colleges in the Near East since the nation-wide campaign for funds started on December 2. These gifts bring the total endowment up to $9,010,760, plus the $1,000,000 from the Rockefeller Foundation for Medical Work at the University of Beirut.

GROUND has been broken at the University of Washington for a new physics building to be built at a cost of $465,000. This will be the first unit of a science group at the university. The building, a four-story structure of Gothic design, will cover an area of 80 by 230 feet and will be from 50 to 60 feet in height. The building is expected to be ready for occupancy by November of this year.

ACCORDING to the *Journal* of the American Medical Association, Tokyo Imperial University has decided to establish a course in hormone chemistry in the medical department beginning in April. This is said to be the first course of its kind. The cost of maintaining the laboratory for the course has been donated by the Society for the Advancement of Pharmacology in an amount believed to be between 200,000 and 300,000 yen. Dr. Akira Ogata will be promoted to the rank of professor and placed in charge of the laboratory; he has been studying hormone chemistry in Europe for two years.

WILLIS A. SLATER, engineering physicist of the U. S. Bureau of Standards, has been elected research professor of engineering materials and director of the Fritz engineering laboratory in the department of civil engineering at Lehigh University.

DR. BENJAMIN ALLEN WOOTEN, professor of physics at Washington and Lee University, has been appointed head of the department of physics of the University of Alabama. Dr. Robert W. Dickey, professor of electrical engineering in the university, will replace Dr. Wooten as head of the physics department for the coming year.

DR. T. L. PATTERSON, professor of physiology at the Detroit College of Medicine and Surgery, has been appointed acting professor of physiology for the summer quarter of 1928 at Stanford University and will be located at the Hopkins Marine Station, Pacific Grove, California.

THE summer session of Cornell University, which will open on June 30, will have on its teaching staff thirty professors from colleges and universities in addition to regular members of the Cornell faculty. These include in geography and geology: Dr. Collier Cobb, of the University of North Carolina; Professor Harry Leighton, of the University of Pittsburgh; Dr. J. P. Rowe, of the University of Montana; Professor M. H. Stow, of Washington and Lee University. In physics: Dr. William F. G. Swann, of the Franklin Institute; Professor Robert E. Loving, of Richmond College; Carl A. Heeler, of Columbus, Ohio.

WILSON F. BROWN, instructor in chemical engineering at the Ohio State University, has been appointed to an associate professorship at the Kansas Agricultural College to take charge of the work in industrial chemistry and chemical engineering.

THE electors to the newly-established Rouse Ball professorship of mathematics at the University of Cambridge have elected John Edensor Littlewood, F.R.S., fellow of Trinity College and Cayley lecturer in mathematics, to the professorship.

DR. GEORG B. GRUBER, of Innsbruck, has been appointed professor of pathology at Göttingen.

DISCUSSION AND CORRESPONDENCE

OXIDATION-REDUCTION REACTIONS

IN a recent delightful address of Professor Albert P. Mathews[1] he states that it remained for the *physical chemist* to discover what was really at the bottom of oxidations, namely, that when an oxidation takes place one or more electrons are lost by the substance oxidized. This view does, indeed, prevail to-day but in the numerous recent papers which have been written to explain oxidation in the light of the electron theory, no one, apparently, has attempted to trace back this idea to its origin. The reason for this is probably that the original publication took place long before the electron theory had been enunciated and our present conception of oxidation-reduction reactions was not due at all to one who might be called a "physical chemist."

In the third edition of Douglass and Prescott's "Qualitative Analysis," published in 1880, special attention is called to the chapter on oxidation-reduction written by Otis Coe Johnson on the basis of the theory of *negative bonds.* This section appears as Part IV of the fourth edition published in 1883, and the section by Johnson is mentioned on the title page of this fourth edition as well as in the preface to the third edition. Later editions of this well-known book bear the name of Prescott and Johnson as authors. If one substitutes the word *electron* for what Johnson called a *negative bond,* it is clear that his theory is exactly the same as that which has been rediscovered by so many of the younger chemists during recent years. Inasmuch as it is not very far-fetched to call an electron a negative bond, it seems rather remarkable that Johnson in 1880 should have anticipated so closely the present electronic conception of oxidation.

Another statement occurs in Professor Mathews' address which illustrates how long an old theory will persist in literature. He writes "And when the electrical and electronic nature of valence was finally understood, *a few years ago,* it was seen that in every case of oxidation the oxidized substance lost a negative electron and thus gained a positive charge, in other words in every oxidation there is always a *flow of positive electricity, since the current is always supposed to be in the direction of movement of the positive, from the oxidizing to the oxidized body.*"

Such a statement is likely to lead to confusion. Since even the high-school pupil of to-day knows that the so-called "flow of electricity" is theoretically a flow of electrons, it is absolutely inconceivable that there should be such a thing as a flow of positive electricity. It is quite true that some fifty years or so

[1] "Some Applications of Physical Chemistry to Medicine," SCIENCE, 66, 606, 1927.

ago there was a single fluid theory which was practically the reverse of our present electron theory. In terms of this old theory, the positive electricity flowed in the positive to negative direction. According to a later theory, the positive electricity moved in one direction and the negative electricity in the other, but now this double fluid theory has been discarded and it is quite generally believed that only the negative electricity moves in the passage of an electric current through, or over, a wire and in oxidation-reduction reactions. To be sure, a positively-charged body is attracted to a negatively-charged one, and if the former is fixed in position, as the cathode when dipped in an electrolytic cell, then the positively-charged body will move, but in every case of a transfer of electricity it is the light electron that changes position and never the heavy proton. Consequently, in oxidation-reduction reactions there is a flow of negative charges from the reductant to the oxidant and never a flow of positive electricity from the oxidizing to the oxidized body.

Teachers who persist in indicating the direction of an electric current in terms of discredited theories help to bring confusion into the minds of their pupils.

William T. Hall

PSEUDO-ARTIFACTS FROM THE PLIOCENE OF NEBRASKA

In Science of May 20, 1927, there appears, on page 482, a genealogical diagram by Henry Fairfield Osborn, showing his recently modified conception of the origin of man and of his culture. Near the base of the family tree is indicated the geological position of the well-known Hesperopithecus tooth and of certain accompanying fossil bone fragments, thought to be implements. Indirect textual references to the latter are to be found in the same issue (Science News, page xiv) and also in Science of May 6 (Science News, page x).

In Science of December 16, Professor W. K. Gregory published a belated article setting forth his matured views regarding the famous tooth under the explanatory title, "Hesperopithecus apparently not an Ape nor a Man." It seems timely, therefore, that available observations on the associated bone "implements" should also be made known without further delay and I accordingly submit my findings as originally set down in August.

The occurrence of anthropoid remains in the Snake Creek beds at Aldine, Nebraska, being still under dispute, the existence in these Pliocene deposits of bone objects suggestive of a tool-making being becomes a subject calling for more than ordinary caution. Observation, unfortunately, is further limited by the fact that in the absence not only of human skeletal remains and of hearth-sites, but also of stone implements such as could have been used in the production of bone artifacts, the question of man's presence comes to depend entirely on the evidence furnished by the peculiar bone specimens themselves.

Having been requested for an opinion concerning these bones, it was at once assumed that the occasion demanded something decisive. The entire available collection—or rather selection—has therefore been subjected to systematic study. To check my own observations, the material was looked over independently by a laboratory assistant who had previously shown some aptness, *e.g.*, in detecting frauds among our old Indian collections. More precisely stated, this examination involved the scrutiny of nearly 3,000 specimens with a magnifying glass and by the aid of the best obtainable light. In short, all reasonable mechanical precautions have been observed. By way of further precaution I have also, as a matter of course, asked myself these questions: What now is it you are looking for? What precisely are the standards by which you are to measure these specimens? Expressed in other terms, what are the diagnostic characters indicating bone artifacts?

Without giving a complete inventory of primitive bone implements and ornaments, it may here suffice to say that implements divide into two major groups or classes, *viz.*, sharp-pointed and sharp-edged. The ornaments, or at any rate the objects less distinctly utilitarian, separate into tubular forms (cylindrical beads, flutes, etc.), and thin flat forms of varying outlines, rectilineal and curvilineal. And what distinctive features normally characterize each and all of these four outstanding classes of objects? First of all, a certain more or less easily recognizable shape or design. In the second place, implements are generally marked by evidences of wear, often resulting in a high degree of polish. Generally, too, they are marked by abrasions, if not actual perforations; and they almost invariably show certain unmistakable straight-line cuts and scratches running diagonally or transversely across the natural striations of the bone itself. Assuming, therefore, that the bone specimens to be examined were worked or utilized in a fresh state, and that at least some of the more deep-going evidences of artificial treatment have been preserved in the fossilized objects now available, we have remaining these criteria: shape, wear, polish, cutting marks, chopping marks, abrasions and perforations. These are perhaps not infallible proofs but they are all that we have. In matters of observation pertaining to objective facts no man is entitled to call up a standard for judgment out of his own inner consciousness.

By the light, then, of these deliberate precautions, the cursory examination of all the material and the repeated critical study of the several suspect pieces were undertaken. The result is, in brief, that I find no positive evidence either of intentional design or of artificial workmanship.

It is true there are several pointed forms resembling awls and also some tubular bone sections resembling beads, which, if found, say, in an Indian shell-heap would cause a careful archeologist to look at them several times before discarding them. But, after all, aside from their suggestive shape—simulating not finished articles but rather improvised forms often adapted from accidental bone fragments—they carry none of the real telltale marks above enumerated. When, therefore, it is alleged (Science News, May 10, p. xiv) that "eighteen of the [Nebraska] types of tools have been matched with counterparts found in the ruins of cliff-dwellers," two observations become imperative. One is, that with two exceptions—awls and tubular beads—the "eighteen counterparts" are not designed tools or ornaments but merely accidental fragments, a few of which have served temporary purposes. The other is that the "matching process" referred to involved on the discoverer's part the culling over of many thousands of fossil bone fragments. We have here, in other words, a close parallel to the selective procedure of which Europeans have made so much in the accumulation of eoliths. But, as in the case of eoliths, it is pertinent here to remark that given the proper raw materials and the right natural conditions for their manipulation, nature produces many things more or less suggestive of human handiwork, and the collector by taking pains can easily gather an array of imitations which considered by themselves are sometimes deceptively impressive.

It is true also that the Nebraska collection affords several bone specimens marked by worn U-shaped grooves of varying and rather large dimensions and of unexplainable origin. These grooves are, however, weathered irregularly, and taken by themselves are meaningless, being in no sense characteristic of true artifacts.

Lastly, there are two, perhaps three, bone fragments which carry decidedly suggestive markings. Two of these specimens are so striking that once more the writer would say that if they had been found in a refuse heap one might conceivably have retained them as showing certain accidental and purposeless indications of human activity. One of these pieces is a rib fragment with some shallow irregular cut-like markings on the inner face. No one can say that these are or are not artificial. They may, however, be nothing but tooth marks. The other piece is a tibia fragment, the sharp natural angle of which carries four slantingly transverse chop-like marks. These markings, though fairly deep, are not sufficiently clean cut to enable any one to say positively that they are artificial; and close to them, moreover, are several other fainter and more irregular markings which are certainly not artificial and which therefore weaken the original possibilities.

There remains the difficult question of accidental fracture. The success of the collector's matching process is really dependent on this feature. And it can not be denied that some of the longitudinal and diagonal breaks exhibited by the Nebraska specimens resemble the breaks to be observed in the animal bones so abundant in our shell-heaps and ruins everywhere and which can with reasonable certainty be attributed to human agency. Some of these fractures in the Nebraska finds are probably old and may have been produced while the bone was green or fresh. But who is prepared to tell us of the finer distinctions—if any—between fresh bone crushed by a carnivor and fresh bone crushed by a man between two stones? Certain other longitudinal fractures characteristic of the Nebraska bones, especially those carrying the split clear through the condyles, are distinctly unhumanlike performances; besides, they seem to me to have been made since the bones were fossilized. Belonging to this latter class are also many clear-cut transverse fractures, which certainly could not have been produced in fresh bone. Finally, the various facets on the fractured pieces often show different degrees of wear and polish, suggesting again that the breaking-up process has been prolonged and at least in part subsequent to fossilization. The more or less uniformly worn or semi-polished condition of certain of the specimens is a matter which may be left for others to explain, but it can scarcely be regarded as the work of man.

The inevitable conclusion is, therefore, in my judgment, that the presence of artifacts in the Snake Creek deposits is not established and can not be established by the collections examined to date.

N. C. Nelson

The American Museum of Natural History

THE LIFE HISTORY OF VARANUS NILOTICUS

A paper giving a detailed account of the entire life history of the Nile monitor, *Varanus niloticus,* is being prepared for publication, but a brief description of one of the most interesting chapters of its life will not be out of place at the present time.

The monitor is a large reptile which is fairly common in many parts of Africa, its range extending throughout the continent wherever proper conditions exist. Although it is one of the largest lizards within its range and is not rare even in the more settled districts, comparatively little is known concerning its more intimate activities. The few accounts dealing with the habits of the Nile monitor come from observers who have worked in the tropics rather than in the more temperate regions of South Africa, which probably explains the great difference between the following observations and those previously made by other observers. (For one account of the egg laying, see Roosevelt: "African Game Trails," pp. 411.)

Throughout the section of Natal, South Africa, where these observations were made, there are large numbers of hard clay nests made by one of the most common termites, *Eutermes trinervius*. These nests are cellular in structure, being perforated in all directions by numerous small intersecting passages. The outside of the nest is composed of the same material as that used within, clay, but becomes much harder and offers a good deal of resistance to penetration with a hoe or even a spade.

During the rains the outer covering of the nest becomes soaked with moisture and can be broken into very easily. At this season of the year the monitor digs its way to the center of the nest and lays from a dozen to thirty eggs, about the size of hens' eggs, covered with a tough, leathery integument. As soon as the parent is through laying she returns to her regular habitat, in some cases at least without having made any attempt to cover the eggs. The termites, which are always exceedingly active in a healthy colony, repair the break and in a few hours at most only the presence of a slightly damper area on the surface of the next remains as evidence of what has occurred.

At the end of ten months, which brings the date to the spring of the year, the eggs hatch out, and through their own efforts aided by the softening effect of the excess liquid contained in the old egg "shell," the young make a vertical tunnel and finally emerge from the top of the termite nest. As soon as they have left the nest they make for the nearest stream where they will be found hunting for food and basking on the banks or swimming and diving as readily as do the adults.

Raymond B. Cowles

University of California
at Los Angeles

TRINITASIA—A NEW MOLLUSCAN GENUS FROM SOUTH AMERICA

In 1925, I described and figured from the Miocene of Manzanilla, Trinidad, W. I., a shell of very striking form, as *Thyasira sancti-andreæ* (*Bulletin of American Paleontology,* No. 42, p. 166, pl. 30, figs. 2, 3, 1925). The hinge of all the Trinidad specimens was concealed, and they were only provisionally referred to the genus *Thyasira,* on the advice of Dr. W. H. Dall, our greatest conchologist, to whom they were submitted because of their puzzling generic position.

Subsequently I studied a series of shells and molds from northern South America, which graded in size from small individuals to those equalling the Trinidad type and exactly like it in form. Several of the smaller molds showed in reverse traces of strong cardinal hinge teeth. These were certainly not *Thyasira,* which is practically edentulous; and Dr. Dall pronounced them unlike anything he knew. Clearly they represented a new genus, but the larger members of the series did not show their hinge characters, and although they had the same form, one could not be certain that they possessed hinge teeth like the smaller specimens.

Lately, however, I had in hand a full-sized shell, equaling the Trinidad type, and by a happy accident, its very thin and delicate substance was abraded at the beak and marks of about three strong, rather long, cardinal teeth were clearly shown in reverse upon the internal filling. I hope later to figure the hinge structure.

For this interesting Miocene genus of Trinidad and northern South America, I propose the name *Trinitasia,* the genotype being the form described, in the citation above given, as *Thyasira sancti-andreæ* Maury, from the Miocene of Manzanilla, Department of St. Andrews, in southeastern Trinidad.

Carlotta J. Maury

Yonkers, N. Y.

THE BEHAVIOR OF MALLARD DUCKS

During the recent cold period a very interesting experience was afforded by a flock of about twenty-five Mallard ducks who make their home in a small stream known as Muddy River, in the Fenway section of Boston. With the fall in temperature, and the consequent freezing of the water, it seemed inevitable that the ducks would be driven from their swimming pool. Yet, from watching them, it became apparent that they were not to be driven from their home without a struggle. The ducks began to circle round and round in a radius of about 15 feet with a speed and determination that was amazing. Throughout the entire night, they plied about in their little pool, and though the bitter cold and fast-forming ice, which tried to hem them in, were sufficient to discourage the most courageous, the ducks were not to be denied, and daybreak found them still in possession. Yet, it was not until the sun was high in the sky that they felt it safe to leave their pool and rest on the edge of the ice.

These ducks serve as the center of attraction for the thousands that daily pass through the Fenway; and as one studies them there seems to be an air of triumph about them as if conscious of having successfully combated the first and most severe thrust of King Winter.

BIRGER R. HEADSTROM
MEDFORD HILLSIDE,
MASSACHUSETTS

WANTED—A WORD TO REPLACE "BELIEVE"

FOR some years the writer has avoided the use of the expression "I believe" feeling that it did not adequately express the scientific attitude of mind. Belief is a religious attitude of mind and implies something which the person considers precious and immutable, which he is ready to defend, and for which he is willing to sacrifice even his life. There is nothing in the scientific attitude of mind corresponding to this. Our hypotheses and assumptions and so-called facts are subject to change over night and no one sheds a tear.

Not only does the word "believe" fail to express the scientific attitude of mind, but it is particularly unfortunate to use it because of the effect produced on the non-scientific persons. One reason why the rabid fundamentalists fail to understand the scientist is that they have no adequate conception of our mental attitude in such matters. Their whole attitude of mind is one of belief and they naturally assume that our attitude is similar. They assume that we hold to the theory of evolution as they hold to the (theory of) atonement. Under these circumstances, for us to continue to use the word "believe" simply confirms them in their error.

However, when one attempts to eliminate the word from his vocabulary he finds that it is a very convenient word and one for which it is hard to find a substitute. It is widely used and well understood by the people in a rather loose sense. It is widely used because the corresponding attitude of mind is so universal; it is used in a loose sense because religion has so largely lost its meaning. We who have found the better way still continue to use the old words though we have been warned about putting new wine in old wine skins.

It certainly would be a great improvement if we could find an adequate substitute and even if we can not, it is desirable to eliminate the word from our vocabularies even at the cost of some circumlocutions. If any one can suggest a substitute please speak up.

E. C. L. MILLER
MEDICAL COLLEGE OF VIRGINIA,
RICHMOND, VA.

THE PRONUNCIATION OF RESEARCH

As pointed out by R. H. Smith, in the issue of January 20, 1928, the average scientist is likely to have certain foibles in pronunciation. Even more annoying to me than the mispronunciation of "data" is the mispronunciation of "research." There was a time when I used to pronounce this word correctly, with the accent on the last syllable, but overwhelming usage seems to place the accent on the first syllable.

NICHOLAS KOPELOFF
PSYCHIATRIC INSTITUTE,
WARD'S ISLAND, N. Y.

SCIENTIFIC BOOKS

Handbuch der Paläobotanik by MAX HIRMER, with Chapters by Julius Pia and Wilhelm Troll. vol. 1: *Thallophyta, Bryophyta, Pteridophyta.* 624 pp., 817 figs., R. Oldenbourg, Munich and Berlin, 1927.

THIS pretentious work has the usual merits and defects of such an undertaking. It starts off with a rather good 30 page discussion by Pia on methods of preservation. The Thallophyta are also treated by Pia, who probably knows more about the fossil forms than any other living student. This is gotten into 106 pages and is on the whole very well done, although some sections such as that on the Diatoms are too brief to be of much service.

The part on Bryophyta is by Troll and occupies but 9 pages. It is not at all notable and the author does not seem to be familiar with the literature, as many fossil forms are missing. For example no fossil mosses are recorded from North America.

The bulk of the volume, nearly 550 pages, is devoted to the Pteridophyta. As conceived by the author, the term Pteridophyta is quite as broad and comprehensive, and consequently as meaningless as the term Thallophyta. One might forgive the author for not having heard of several more or less valid proposals for segregating the diverse assemblage included under the term Pteridophyta if only his ears were not so keenly attuned to such, to the reviewer, ill advised proposals as the group Protoarticulatineae, suggested recently by a fellow countryman.

The Pteridophyta are segregated in 6 main stocks which unfortunately are given with the *ales* endings universally applied to groups of ordinal rank by botanists. These 6 stocks are Psilophytales, Lycopodiales, Psilotales, Articulatales, Cladoxylales and Filicales, the first four microphyllous and the last two megaphyllous (wrongly termed macrophyllous). The Psilophytales are thoroughly described and to it the following 5 families are referred: Rhyniaceae, Horneaceae, Pseudosporochnaceae, Psilophytaceae and Asteroxylaceae. One might well question the propriety of making the imperfectly known Pseudosporochus the type of an independent family.

The Lycopodiales are considered to include the following 6 families: Lycopodiaceae, Selaginellaceae, Isoetaceae, Lepidodendraceae, Sigillariaceae and Bothrodendraceae, and aside from certain questions of relative values, are fairly well done.

The Articulatales stock is divided into 5 groups which I suppose have the rank of orders. These with their contained families are: Protoarticulatineae with the families Calamophytaceae and Hyeniaceae, which is considered the most primitive group, although actually based upon 3 highly interesting but imperfectly known and possibly misinterpreted species: Pseudoborniineae with the single family Pseudoborniaceae, also imperfectly known: Sphenophyllineae with the family Sphenophyllaceae: Cheirostrobineae with the family Cheirostrobaceae: and Equisetineae divided into the three families Asterocalamitaceae, Calamitaceae and Equisetaceae.

The fifth main stock, the Cladoxylales, with the single family Cladoxylaceae, seems particularly unfortunate. The group is remarkable enough in its combination of characters and is evidently an isolated one, but no one certainly knows that it is a Pteridophyte. Paul Bertrand, who knows considerably more than the present author about these forms, thinks that they were seed plants. We know something of the habit of the middle Devonian *Cladoxylon scoparium* but its foliage is less deserving of the term megaphyllous than is that of Pseudobornia or Asterocalamites and the supposed association of *Sphenopteris refracta* Goeppert with Voelkelia is by no means established.

The Filicales are treated as Eusporangiatae, Protoleptosporangiatae, Leptosporangiatae, and those of uncertain systematic position. The first includes the Coenopteridineae with six families, and is well done to the extent to which the facts are available; the Ophioglossineae and the Marattiineae. The Protoleptosporangiatae comprise the single family Osmundaceae, and the Leptosporangiatae are divided into 12 families. The volume closes with brief and unimportant chapters on the general morphology of the Filicales and the comparative morphology of the Pteridophytes.

The book is well printed and profusely illustrated, a considerable number being original. It seems to me that the discussion of impressions of Lepidodendron and Sigillaria is well done. The somewhat difficult anatomy of the Coenopteridineae is made rather clear, and there is a full discussion of the diverse forms of Psaronius. The author evidently believes that Thomas has demonstrated that Sagenopteris is the foliage of a seed plant, since it receives no mention in the present volume.

Opinions will naturally differ regarding the success with which Hirmer has performed his self-assigned task. Many omissions could be pointed out, but such are inevitably present in a work of such scope. On the whole I believe that the book will serve a very useful purpose. Its chief defect, in addition to the lack of judgment in the classification adopted which has already been alluded to, is the failure to exhibit any acquaintance with the American literature. For example I find no Mesozoic Lycopodiums recorded from North America, nor any mention of Harder's work on fossil bacteria, or of the important Lepidophyte fructification Cantheliophorus, and I might easily mention a great many other instances. However, no one but a German author seems to have the industry to produce a work of this sort, and no one but a German publisher would undertake to print such a work, so that botanist, paleobotanist and geologist should alike be thankful and give it their blessing.

EDWARD W. BERRY

THE JOHNS HOPKINS UNIVERSITY

SCIENTIFIC APPARATUS AND LABORATORY METHODS

A CONSTANT RATE ASPIRATOR

IN a study of the factors affecting the rate of respiration in plants,[1] it became apparent that a constant rate of aspiration was one of the most desirable features. Several well-known types of aspirators were tried but in every instance it was found that the desired constancy could not be maintained. A new type of aspirator was developed which combines simplicity, unvarying rate, a wide range of force and portability. The features of this instrument are such that we believe it will prove of value to investigators in all branches of scientific research where a constant rate of aspiration is desired.

The device consists in an arrangement employing the well-known principle of Mariotte's bottle. Two bottles, the size of which depends upon the use to which the operator puts his instrument, are arranged so that one is supported in an inverted position directly over the other as in Figure 1. The inverted bottle is fitted with an intake tube A bent upon itself in the manner illustrated with the open end at x–x′. The reason for bending this tube will be shown later.

[1] Article to appear in a forthcoming issue of *The Botanical Gazette.*

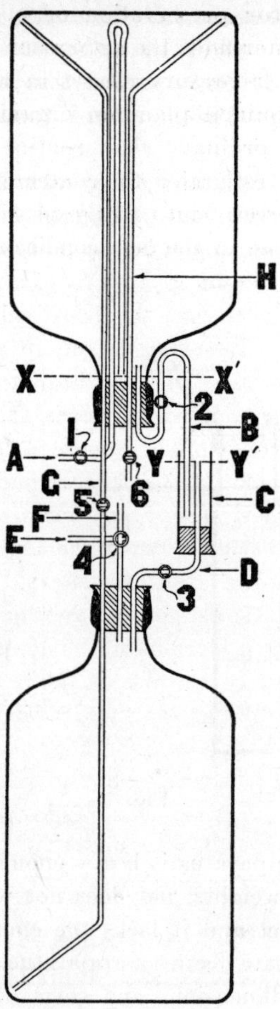

FIG. 1. A constant rate aspirator. Explanation in the text. The mechanical support for the bottles is not shown.

The outlet tube B is bent in the form of an S or a reverse curve with the intake end arranged so that it is well above the open end of A at x–x′ and with the second curve above the level of the intake end. The open end of B extends below the level of the liquid y–y′ in the automatic level device C. When the aspirator is in operation the flow of liquid from the inverted bottle through tube B, automatic level device C and discharge tube D into the lower bottle exerts a negative pressure in the inverted bottle. This negative pressure operates through intake tube A which is attached to the instrument in which a constant rate of aspiration is desired. The rate of flow of gas through intake tube A is determined by the distance between x–x′ and y–y′ minus the resistance offered in the instrument attached to A. When the latter is determined the rate of aspiration is adjusted by controlling the distance between x–x′ and y–y′.

The arrangement in Figure 1 facilitates the rapid refilling of the inverted bottle with the liquid that has been collected in the lower one while the instrument was in operation. This makes possible the reusing of the same liquid. Further, the gas collected in the inverted bottle can thus be analyzed by gasometric methods. Assuming the latter to be the case, air pressure is applied to E through three-way valve 4. Stopcocks 1, 2 and 3 in tubes A, B and D respectively, are closed. Stopcocks 5 and 6 in tubes G and H are opened. The air pressure in the lower bottle returns the liquid through tube G into the inverted bottle, the displaced gas being forced out through tube H. To this tube a gas meter and burette are attached. When all of the gas in the inverted bottle is displaced stopcocks 5 and 6 are closed and the three-way stopcock 4 is opened to F. The instrument is ready for operation when stopcocks 3, 2, and 1 are opened in the order named, tube F serving as an exhaust for the lower bottle.

When this aspirator is used for collecting the gas passing through the instrument attached to A it is essential that the construction of the former precludes the entrance of air. The greatest error from such a source is obtained when the volume of gas changes quickly in the inverted chamber with a lowering temperature. This tends to draw the liquid back through the reverse-curve tube B. To insure the sealing of this tube, constant level device C is made large enough to contain sufficient liquid to compensate volume changes due to temperature variations under the conditions of operation. The construction of the instrument also obviates the possibility of a loss of aspirated gas outward through B. This is obtained by having the level of the outlet of the tube A below the level of the intake of tube B and the second curve of B above its intake end. By this arrangement the aspiration ceases as soon as the level of the liquid in the inverted bottle reaches the intake of tube B. It is desirable not to allow the instrument to operate until the liquid reaches this level, especially if the temperature of the surrounding air is likely to increase.

If tube A is not constructed as shown it is almost impossible to keep the liquid from entering it when refilling the bottle. Should this happen the rate of aspiration is seriously affected. To prevent it, the tube is carried to the top of the bottle before being recurved.

This aspirator has been used successfully in the study of the respiration of plants both under laboratory and field conditions. It is constructed from 40 liter or 20 liter bottles when used in the laboratory and from 10 liter bottles when used in the field. Pyrex tubing with a 4 mm. inside bore is used throughout. A special liquid is employed when gasometric methods are used. It is known to absorb only slight traces of carbon dioxide and was obtained from Layng and Crum[2] of the chemistry department of the University of Illinois. It consists of a 35 per cent. aqueous solution of zinc sulphate to which 14 grams of concentrated sulphuric acid are added per liter of solution.

Chas. F. Hottes
A. L. Hafenrichter

A SIMPLIFIED PLANKTON BUCKET

Many users of the old fashioned naturalist's plankton net who may object to its crudeness or who have employed the commoner expedient of tying a glass bottle into a silk net, will appreciate a simple device which serves the same end much more efficiently. There are a number of elaborate plankton buckets described which serve various purposes but none of these are quite simple or inexpensive enough for the ordinary biological teacher or investigator who purposes only a qualitative collection for classroom demonstration or technical use.

The writer uses, both for class work and for his own investigations, conical fine silk nets of number twelve and twenty grade, and a plankton bucket of his own design. While not especially new in principle, the bucket is simpler and more inexpensive than any he has seen or used before. It may be constructed by almost any one. The bucket is made up of four parts: First, there is an inverted and truncated cone with a fairly long threaded tube attached to the truncated end, secondly, there is another cone exactly like the first one but without the tube, which fits closely over the other of the two cones. A threaded ring which screws on the tube of the first cone is the third part. The first cone is dropped *into* the net and its tube is arranged to project below, outside the net. The second cone is then fitted to the first from the *outside* of the net with the silk between the two. The two cones are now clamped together and held tightly by the threaded ring; they lock the device to the apex of the net. The fourth part of the apparatus is the bucket, a simple cylinder closed at one end and threaded at the other to fit the tube of the inner of the two cones. The cylinder is of uniform diameter and may or may not have a flange at its threaded end to give weight to the apparatus. The cylinder is screwed to the tube and the bucket is ready for use at once. All parts are constructed of brass.

The net arranged as above may be used exactly as other rigs, but one needs only to unscrew the cylinder to release the catch, and pour the collected plankton into a bottle for preservation or observation while alive. The writer finds the apparatus a very valuable adjunct to his laboratory classes in which a number of plant and animal plankton organisms lend much interest to the ordinary class routine. In collecting material for investigation the contents of the cylinder may be put directly into fixing reagents in the field and carried home in the best condition.

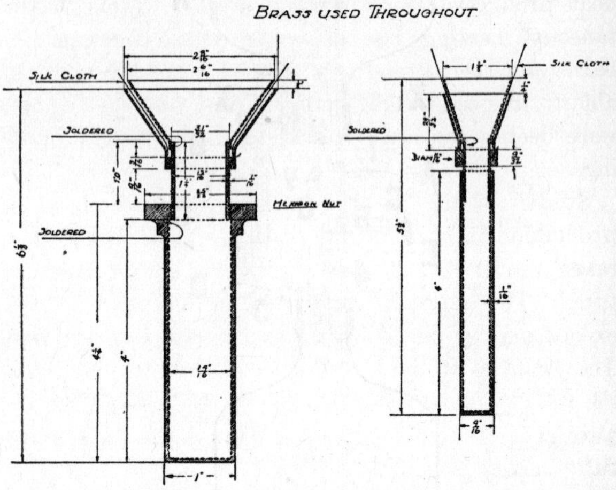

Fig. 1

The whole apparatus is heavy enough to sink easily without extra weights, but does not weigh enough to tear the wet net and it lacks the cumbersomeness of the more elaborate deep-sea apparatus. The diagrams illustrate the dimensions and form of two rigs used by the writer (Fig. 1). Others may be used of course to fit different nets and purposes.

Arthur S. Campbell
The San Bernardino Valley
Union Junior College,
California

SPECIAL ARTICLES

OBSERVATIONS ON HEATING HAY IN THE FLOODED REGIONS OF NORTHERN VERMONT

Many interesting reports of the devastations wrought by the recent floods in Vermont and Massachusetts have been written. Little mention has been made, however, of the effect of the floods upon the tons of feeding stuffs stored on the farms for winter use. The agricultural pursuits of the farmers in the valleys of the Vermont rivers have been confined largely to dairying, most of the flat valley land being used for hay production. In New England the length and severity of the winter season make it imperative that the farmer be well supplied with hay for his stock.

[2] Layng, T. E., and S. A. Crum, "On Examination of Methods of Gas Analysis." Unpublished paper, University of Illinois.

In order to store the hay properly, large barns with deep bays or open sections extending usually from the ground to the roof have been constructed. The recent floods, coming early in November, found practically every barn filled with good meadow hay. The flood waters entered many barns, covering as much as 17 feet of the hay piles. When the flood waters receded, masses of wet hay remained, in which intense heat production soon became evident. This "spontaneous" heating was so severe as to endanger the barns and their contents with fire. One fire attributable to this cause had been reported, and the farmers were deeply concerned for the safety of their buildings.

Studies of the problem of the "spontaneous" heat production in agricultural products have been undertaken in the United States Department of Agriculture.[1] The unusual conditions in Vermont offered exceptional opportunities for further investigation. The facilities of the University of Vermont, including the College of Agriculture and the Extension Service, were generously placed at our disposal and are gratefully acknowledged.

Studies were made of the conditions on 13 farms in Northern Vermont, in the valleys of the Winooski, Lamoille and Mississquoi Rivers. The wetting and heating of the hay at these places were said to be typical of those throughout the entire flooded area. In many cases actively steaming hay had been removed from the barns before our arrival, and many other lots were then being thrown out as rapidly as possible with the limited amount of help available. A brief résumé of the data gathered at the thirteen farms is given below. Eight of the farms are in the valley of the Winooski River, and five are in the valleys of the Lamoille and Mississquoi Rivers.

The floors supporting the hay in a few of the barns consisted only of boards resting directly upon the ground. In the majority of the barns visited, however, the hay was piled above the first-floor level, and the stock was housed in basement stalls beneath. The rising waters entirely covered the stalls and immersed as much as eight feet of the hay piles.

"Spontaneous" heat production had begun in the bottom wet layers of the hay, and the hot gases rising through the stacks led to the production of strong draughts or "flues." The moisture thus carried upward condensed in the cooler parts of the hay or in the air above, wetting the hay in the immediate area. So many of these draughts had existed in some piles as to soak the hay thoroughly. Similar draughts were observed in all heating piles of hay. Temperatures in typical "flues" ranged from 47° to 74° C.

When we arrived the period of most marked heating had passed, and the temperatures were then on the decline. Many piles of hay had shown such marked steaming as to prompt the farmers to remove them immediately to the open. A large number of the men students of the University of Vermont, at Burlington, cheerfully gave their full time and energies to the pitching of the hot hay out of the barns. While forking over the hot material, only one farmer had observed any evidence of charring.

One clear-cut case of "spontaneous" ignition of heating hay occurred on a farm near Middlesex, Vermont. This farm is in a narrow portion of the valley of the Winooski River where the flood waters rose exceptionally high. The barn held about 50 tons of meadow hay and a little alfalfa. The hay had been kept in a bay in the rear of the barn and rested upon boards laid flat on the ground. The contents of the bay at the time of the flood, as shown in the accompanying diagram, considered from the bottom to the top consisted of:

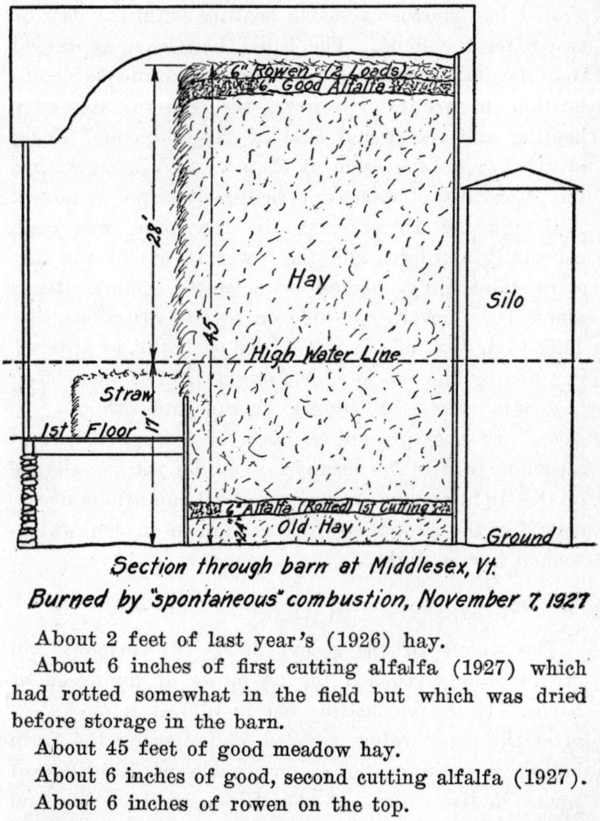

Section through barn at Middlesex, Vt.
Burned by "spontaneous" combustion, November 7, 1927

About 2 feet of last year's (1926) hay.

About 6 inches of first cutting alfalfa (1927) which had rotted somewhat in the field but which was dried before storage in the barn.

About 45 feet of good meadow hay.

About 6 inches of good, second cutting alfalfa (1927).

About 6 inches of rowen on the top.

There was also a small pile of old dry straw on the barn floor.

The flood waters covered 17 feet of the pile of hay and most of the straw. No heating of the hay had been noticed before the flood, but considerable steam-

[1] James, L. H. "Microbial Thermogenesis." I. SCIENCE, LXV, May 20, 1927, 504–6; II. *Jour. Bact.*, XV, February, 1928, 117–41.

ing was in evidence 24 hours after the waters had receded. The crest of the flood occurred early on Friday morning, November 4, and the barn burned between 4:00 and 5:00 P. M. on Monday, November 7, or about two days after the flood waters receded. On Sunday much heating had been noticed and on Monday a distinctly charred odor was noticed before the fire started. The barn burned to the ground and a silo, close to it, fell over and also was destroyed. It is interesting to note that owing to the contour of the land, the barn and hay stood in about 3 feet of water when the fire broke out.

A number of veteran farmers living close to the Canadian border were visited. Several claimed to have had marked success in stopping "spontaneous" heating of hay by the application of large quantities of salt.

It is unfortunate from the standpoint of the accumulation of scientific data that observations of the heating hay piles were not begun for about six days after the flood waters had receded. Discussions with county agents, agricultural men and farmers revealed that practically every lot of hay which had been wetted had shown excessive heating within a day or two after the flood. The belief had been expressed that the season was too cold for "spontaneous" combustion to occur. However, the general excessive heating and the actual case of "spontaneous" firing of the hay on the farm at Middlesex, Vt., show that the possibility of dangerous heating was not removed. Although the air entering the hay piles was cool, especially at night, and the lower layers of the hay were thoroughly soaked with water, temperatures above 70° C. were recorded on several occasions.

The question of the possibility of botulism appearing among the stock which might be fed the rotted hay was raised by county agents and others. No cases of such poisoning have been reported, and although it is by no means impossible yet the chance of the simultaneous occurrence of all conditions necessary for the growth of this organism in the water-soaked hay is slight.

Summary

The waters of the recent floods in Vermont and Massachusetts reached the haymows of hundreds of barns. Excessive heating set in almost immediately after the flood waters receded, endangering the farm buildings. Observations were made at 13 different farms in the valleys of the Winooski, Lamoille and Mississquoi Rivers. These observations are summarized in the following statements:

1. From half a foot to seventeen feet of the piles were under water.

2. In every pile of wet hay observed some "heating" had taken place, frequently to the point of being considered dangerous.

3. Heat was generated in the bottom layers of the piles and, escaping up through the hay, led to the production of draughts of hot gases or "flues" rising to the surface.

4. The large quantity of moisture carried with the hot gases from the lower layers was condensed on the upper, cooler hay, or in the air above. Many hay piles had been soaked throughout by the falling condensed moisture.

5. While the hot hay was being removed from the barns only one farmer had observed any charred materials.

6. The maximum temperature found (besides one case of fire) was 74° C., though temperatures above 70° were recorded in other places.

7. The most marked evidence of excessive heating was observed (by the farmers) on the second and third days after the recession of the flood waters.

8. One authentic case of "spontaneous" combustion of hay caused by the flood was reported. The outstanding features were:

a. The lower two feet of the pile consisted of old hay from the preceding season (1926).

b. Covering this lower 2-foot section of old hay was a 6-inch layer of first cutting alfalfa.

c. Two feet beneath the top surface of the 42-foot pile was another 6-inch layer of alfalfa (second cutting).

d. This hay pile which fired "spontaneously" was the only one containing even a small quantity of alfalfa.

The urgent need for extensive research upon the problem of the "spontaneous" heating of farm products was emphasized by the lack of scientific knowledge with which to meet the situation.

Lawrence H. James
David J. Price
U. S. Department of Agriculture

THE RELATION OF BORON TO THE GROWTH OF THE TOMATO PLANT

It is surprising to note the prevalence of the old idea that the number of elements essential for normal plant growth is limited to ten. To this list of "preferred" elements, to use the expression of Sommer and Lipman,[1] have been added manganese, zinc, boron and without a doubt several others will be annexed as methods and technic become more and more refined. There is little doubt that in the past, failure to obtain good plant growth in numerous water-culture experi-

[1] Sommer, A. L., and Lipman, C. B., "Evidence on the Indispensable Nature of Zinc and Boron for Higher Green Plants," Plant Physiology *1*: 231–249. 1926.

ments was due to a deficiency of some of the above-mentioned elements so long overlooked. An illustration with regard to boron will serve as an example.

In a series of experiments dealing with certain potassium relations of the tomato plant, it was found impossible to obtain anything that even approximated normal growth in water cultures without the addition of a small quantity of boron. This circumstance was especially interesting since no attempt had been made to purify the ordinary C. P. chemicals used in the solutions. These observations led to a series of experiments dealing with the relation of boron to the growth of the tomato plant. It is believed that some of the results obtained are interesting enough to warrant this brief preliminary paper. Both the appearance of the plants as well as actual measurements and analyses clearly showed boron to be absolutely essential.

Most of these experiments were carried out in the division of plant nutrition at the University of California, with the variety Santa Clara Canner. Some of the experiments have been repeated at the University of Maryland with this same variety and with Marglobe. Boron was supplied as boric acid in a concentration of 0.5 p. p. m. Plants grown in nutrient solution containing this concentration of boron grew normally and produced blossoms. Plants grown in the boron deficient solutions ceased to grow at the end of three or four weeks. In the Maryland experiments the first signs of injury were noticed after nine days. One of the early visible symptoms of boron deficiency is the blackened appearance at the growing point of the stem. New leaves and branches often start growing just below this dead portion and give to the plant a short bushy appearance. Often the leaves grow in length, but not in width. Chemical analysis in the case of the Berkeley experiments showed approximately twice as much total sugars in the leaves of the boron deficient plants as in those from normal plants grown in a similar manner, but in solutions containing boron. The leaves from the boron deficient plants also contain more starch than those from the normal plants. On the other hand, the quantity of total sugars in the stems of the boron deficient plants is only about two thirds of that in the stems of normal plants. The leaves of the boron deficient plants at College Park developed, after 13 days, a distinct purple color, probably anthocyan, which is frequently associated with an excess sugar accumulation. Another very striking characteristic of the boron deficient plants is the extreme brittleness of the leaf petioles. This brittleness is not that characteristic of turgid stems, which break with more or less snap, but it is one that may best be described as similar to the breaking of a piece of cheese.

Both the chemical analysis and later observations on an entirely different variety indicate a failure on the part of the boron deficient plants to remove sugar from their leaves. This seems to be related to a breaking down of the conducting tissues. Microscopic examinations of the petioles and stems made by Professor J. H. Priestley on a few of our plants seem to bear out this view. In the boron deficient plants the phloem was broken down and apparently gave a much more acid reaction than the corresponding regions of the normal plants.

These general conclusions are in agreement with the anatomical studies of Warington[2] on *Vicia Faba* (broad bean) grown in boron deficient solutions. She states, "The vascular bundles in particular are affected, the xylem often appearing unusually remote from the phloem or even broken up into small groups of elements . . . an unusual development of the cambium is chiefly responsible for this abnormal appearance." The phloem is described as becoming compressed or displaced and the xylem itself may degenerate. Frequently the lumen of the tracheides become completely blocked. These conditions of the broad bean seem to be very similar to those occurring in the tomato when grown in boron deficient solutions.

EARL S. JOHNSTON,
UNIVERSITY OF MARYLAND

W. H. DORE
UNIVERSITY OF CALIFORNIA

TRIASSIC VERTEBRATE FOSSILS FROM WYOMING

DURING the past summer the writers, with the able and enthusiastic assistance of Mr. N. H. Brown and his son, Newton, of Lander, Wyoming, added materially to the University of Missouri collections of vertebrate fossils from the Triassic of Wyoming. All the fossils came from the Popo Agie beds of the Chugwater formation, but from several scattered localities. Chief of these are the quarries on Bull Lake Creek and Sage Creek, Fremont County.

The collections include both reptilian and amphibian remains, the latter in much the greater abundance. Among the amphibian materials are two nearly perfect skulls similar in many respects to the specimen from Texas described by Case as *Buttneria perfecta*.[1] There is in addition a considerable part of four other skulls; at least two distinct types of clavicular girdles,

[2] Warington, Katherine, "The Changes induced in the Anatomical Structure of *Vicia Faba* by the Absence of Boron from the Nutrient Solution," *Ann. Bot. 40*: 27–42. 1926.

[1] E. C. Case, "New Reptiles and Stegocephalians from the Upper Triassic of western Texas," Carnegie Inst. Wash. Publication No. 321, pp. 13–25, 1922.

each represented by several specimens, some of which appear to be complete; several mandibles, and numerous limb bones and vertebrae. Lower jaws, limb bones and clavicles were found rather closely associated with two of the skulls.

The reptilian remains consist of several imperfect phytosaur skulls, isolated limb bones, vertebrae of several types, teeth not yet identified, and several footprints of such a nature that the stride can be determined. It is thought that the phytosaur material will clear up some of the doubtful points in two little known genera, *Palaeorhinus* Williston and *Angistorhinus* Mehl. In two of the quarries a large amount of bone remains to be excavated.

The study of this new material has progressed little beyond the point of raising again the entire question of Triassic correlations. It appears to the present writers, who have been in intimate contact with Triassic problems in one capacity or another for many years, that in correlations much stress has been placed on paleontological evidence of a very unsatisfactory nature, particularly in the use of the vertebrates. Attempts have been made to designate various horizons as Lower, Middle or Upper Triassic on the basis of "primitive" or "advanced" forms. One of the more recent of such attempts is that by Huene.[2] Here, as in an earlier and more elaborate correlation table,[3] a rather meager list of "primitive" forms, genera for the most part inadequately known and of very limited geographic range, serves to place much of the bone bearing western Triassic as equivalent to the European Muschelkalk or even lower.

In time these assumptions may prove to be well founded, but at present they seem little better than guesses without particular merit. The writers place little confidence in such long range correlations based on present vertebrate evidence and they are not entirely enthusiastic over future possibilities, the abundance of recent additions to the collections notwithstanding. In the first place, while there seems to be no great difficulty in determining primitive and advanced forms, except that the individual is often a peculiar combination of the old and the new, there is no assurance that one can differentiate between earlier and later forms by this means. On the other hand, there is evidence that during Triassic times primitive and highly specialized forms were often contemporaneous. *Acompsosaurus* Mehl, listed by Huene with the Middle Triassic forms from New Mexico and Arizona, was based on a pelvic girdle with peculiarly down-turned pubes, a character scarcely to be designated as primitive. In this particular, *Acompsosaurus* resembles Huene's phytosaur genus *Angistorhinopsis* except that in the former the down-turning is much more pronounced. *Angistorhinopsis* is found only in the uppermost Keuper.

The insecure foundations of present Triassic correlation are further evidenced by the difficulties encountered in placing the members of a single formation in a limited area. The Chugwater formation of central and southern Wyoming illustrates the point. The Jelm of southern Wyoming is commonly correlated with the Popo Agie beds of central Wyoming, apparently because both members contain vertebrate remains and because of the assumption that both are of the Upper Chugwater. So far as the writers know, dependable fossil evidence has not been found in the Jelm. During June of the past year Branson examined the Jelm with the view of obtaining identifiable fossils, but found only scraps. The Popo Agie beds are the source of the recognizable Triassic vertebrates throughout central Wyoming. As recently emphasized by Branson,[4] these beds do not form the upper part of the Chugwater of this region, but are near the middle. The Popo Agie and the Jelm are both near-shore or actual land phases of the Chugwater. The conditions recorded by these members undoubtedly existed over limited areas from time to time throughout the Chugwater, and are not evidence of contemporaneity.

The point the writers wish to emphasize is that vertebrate fossil evidence must be used with the greatest caution in Triassic correlations and that present vertebrate summaries do not lend themselves to such usage. It is the intention of the writers to publish a series of papers describing the Triassic vertebrate remains in the University of Missouri collections. At present they are preparing descriptions and summaries of the amphibians from the Triassic of Wyoming. Later, amphibian materials from New Mexico and Arizona will be included. It is hoped to present in a similar way the Triassic reptiles. As a start in this direction Mehl is preparing descriptions of the new or little known phytosaurs represented in the collections.

E. B. Branson
M. G. Mehl
The University of Missouri

2 F. R. von Huene, "Notes on the Age of the Continental Triassic Beds in North America with remarks on some Fossil Vertebrates," *Proc.* U. S. Nat. Mus., Vol. LXIX, pp. 1–10.

3 "Neue Beiträge zur Kenntnis der Parasuchier," *Jahrbuch der Preussischen Geologischen Landesanstalt*, Band XLII, Heft 1, pp. 59–160, 1921.

4 E. B. Branson, "Triassic-Jurassic 'Red Beds' of the Rocky Mountain Region," *Jour. Geol.*, Vol. XXXV, pp. 607–630, 1927.

SCIENCE

VOL. LXVII   MARCH 30, 1928   No. 1735

CONTENTS

Some Applications of Paleontology: PROFESSOR WILLIAM BERRYMAN SCOTT 327

The Contribution of Biology, Chemistry and Physics to the Newer Knowledge of Rickets: DR. ALFRED F. HESS 333

Acoustics of Auditoriums: PROFESSOR F. R. WATSON 335

Scientific Events:

The Population of the United States; Appropriations by the Commonwealth Fund; The Fourth Pacific Science Congress; Award of Fellowships by the Guggenheim Foundation 339

Scientific Notes and News 341

University and Educational Notes 344

Discussion and Correspondence:

Science and Secretaries: DR. BAILEY WILLIS. *Re Speciation without Climatic Change or Geographic Isolation:* J. T. NICHOLS. *Weight and Humidity:* PROFESSOR ARNOLD ROMBERG and L. W. BLAU. *Lepidoptera of New York:* PROFESSOR WM. T. M. FORBES. *The Eastland Horned "Toad":* WILLIS G. HEWATT. *The Brasso Fossiliferous Miocene of Trinidad:* DR. CARLOTTA J. MAURY 345

Scientific Books:

The Cephalaspidae: DR. ROY L. MOODIE 348

Scientific Apparatus and Laboratory Methods:

A Universal Muscle Lever: ALVAH R. MCLAUGHLIN. *Method for Growing Small-seeded Plants under Sterile Conditions:* A. B. BEAUMONT and G. J. LARSINOS 349

Special Articles:

The Overwintering in Massachusetts of Ixodiphagus Caucurtei: F. LARROUSSE, ARTHUR G. KING and S. B. WOLBACH. *An Efficiency Formula for Dairy Cows:* PROFESSOR W. L. GAINES 351

Science News x

SCIENCE: A Weekly Journal devoted to the Advancement of Science, edited by J. McKeen Cattell and published every Friday by

THE SCIENCE PRESS

New York City: Grand Central Terminal.

Lancaster, Pa.   Garrison, N. Y.

Annual Subscription, $6.00.   Single Copies, 15 Cts.

SCIENCE is the official organ of the American Association for the Advancement of Science. Information regarding membership in the Association may be secured from the office of the permanent secretary, in the Smithsonian Institution Building, Washington, D. C.

SOME APPLICATIONS OF PALEONTOLOGY[1]

PERHAPS the most remarkable feature in Dr. Joseph Leidy's mental make-up was the immense variety of his scientific interests and achievements. I would use the word *versatility* to describe him, were it not that that term usually implies a certain degree of superficiality, which was utterly foreign to Leidy's mind, for thoroughness and minute accuracy were characteristic of him.

Last year, the centenary of Dr. Leidy's birth was celebrated in the Academy of Natural Sciences in Philadelphia, at which each one of a number of speakers dealt with his own specialty and with Leidy's activity in that particular branch of science. I think that every one who attended that celebration was astonished to hear that fields which they had never associated with Leidy's name had been successfully cultivated by him. For instance, I imagine that very few people knew anything of Leidy's work in botany, or in geology, matters which lie outside of the range of work with which his name is usually associated, even by those to whom he was more than a name in America's honor-roll. Among all those strikingly varied fields which he cultivated so successfully, there is none, I think, which has so contributed to his fame throughout the world as that of paleontology, especially of the vertebrates. In this work Leidy was a pioneer. There had been some work done by such men as Wistar and Harlan in Philadelphia, Mitchill and DeKay in New York; but these men had dealt with such fossil remains as are found in the Eastern States, occurring near the surface of the ground and of very late geological date, including mastodons, horses and ground sloths. It was once thought, both in this country and in Europe, that North America contained no fossil vertebrates of any particular interest or importance, and that, in this respect, we should have to admit inferiority to South America and to the Old World. The first breach in this tradition was made by Leidy, when he began to receive through Dr. Hiram Prout, of St. Louis, fragmentary fossils brought in by the fur-traders from that marvellous and inexhaustible field of discovery, the White River Bad Lands of what was then Nebraska Territory.

[1] No. IV of the Leidy Memorial Lecture Series. Delivered at the University of Pennsylvania.

The White Earth River, to give its full title, is a muddy stream which flows into the Missouri, its course nearly parallel with that of the Cheyenne. Between these two rivers, and on both sides of them, especially south of White River, is the vast area of bad lands, 150,000 square miles or more in extent; and it was with the fossils collected from this region that Leidy's most important contributions to paleontology were made. This is not to overlook the value of his investigations among Eocene mammals and reptiles and Cretaceous reptiles of the Far West, but merely to emphasize the greater importance of his work on the White River fauna. Aside from the great number of short papers published in the *Proceedings* of the Philadelphia Academy of Natural Sciences, the two great monographs of 1853 and 1869 are his monuments, and they form the foundation upon which the great edifice of subsequent work has been erected.

Leidy himself did not collect from the Western fossil grounds; unless I am mistaken, his first visit to those regions was made in 1877, when I met him at Fort Bridger at the house of his friend Dr. Carter, who had sent many Eocene mammals to him. It must be emphasizeed that the art of collecting vertebrate fossils was quite undeveloped in the United States, and that the material sent to Leidy was nearly always made up of such bones as had been weathered out of the soft bad land rocks and were picked up, in a more or less fragmentary condition, so that only skulls and jaws and a few occasional limb bones were included. He had no skeletons to deal with, nor even a single well-preserved foot, only a few good skulls and a great quantity of fragments. Another reason why collections from the White River beds were so hastily and unskilfully made was that till quite late in the century the region was unsafe for white men. My first expedition to the White River bad lands was in 1882, and the U. S. Indian agent at the Pine Ridge Agency warned me that my enterprise was a dangerous one, and advised that my camps should be guarded day and night. So late as the winter of 1890-91, there were fierce battles with great loss of life between the Sioux tribe and the U. S. Army; since that time the region has been entirely safe for the collector.

One of Leidy's most serviceable friends was Dr. F. V. Hayden, long the director of the U. S. Geographical and Geological Survey of the Territories, who from 1856 till 1880 was constantly engaged in surveying and collecting in what were then the "Territories," and was thus able to send much valuable material to Leidy. Even such fossils as were assigned to the collections of the Smithsonian (there was no U. S. National Museum in those days) were first determined and described by Leidy. Hayden's collections were, in large degree, the basis of Leidy's splendid quarto monographs of 1853 and 1869. Hayden enjoyed among the Sioux the enviable reputation of being mad, and therefore his person was under divine protection and inviolable; this enabled him to go about freely, breaking rocks and picking up old bones, where other white men would not have dared to show themselves.

Before proceeding farther, it will be useful to stop for a moment and explain the oft-used phrase "bad lands." The term is a partial translation of the expression used by the French Canadian *voyageurs*, "mauvaises terres à traverser," bad lands to cross. Our abbreviated form of the term gives a false impression of utterly barren and useless grounds, whereas, in many regions, the flats and bottoms are covered with grass and form an excellent winter range for cattle. The term "bad lands" applies to the gullied and cut-up shapes of the valleys and hillsides, which are worn and gashed by the rain and melting snows. Wherever soft and easily weathered rocks are widely exposed in an arid or semi-arid climate, then bad land topography is developed, and many hundreds of thousands of square miles of these peculiar regions, often presenting views of the wildest and most unearthly scenery, extend through the Far West from Alberta to Mexico, and ranging in geological time from the Cretaceous to the Miocene. Very often, but not always, the bad lands are a paradise for the collector of fossils, because of the immense areas which are exposed to view, and if the beds, so worn and gashed, are richly fossiliferous, then great numbers of fine specimens are weathered out of the enclosing rock. Of course, if the beds were originally barren, weathering will not supply them with fossils.

What I especially wish to talk about this evening, the main subject to this lecture, is a consideration of the reasons why Dr. Leidy should have been interested in these things. Why should any one care about a lot of old bones, and why do the universities and museums spend vast sums to obtain them and prepare them for exhibition? Could anything seem more absurd than for the American Museum, in New York, to equip and maintain costly expeditions to India, to the Gobi Desert of Mongolia, to South America, merely to gather more or less petrified bones? Not only bones, but shells and tests, insects, corals and plant-impressions, are all fish for the paleontologist's net and to the uninitiated it must seem a singularly futile type of child's play. It was Darwin's great book, published in 1859, that gave a new impetus to the study of these things; before that time it was believed among geologists that the earth's history consisted of a succession of periods of calm and quiet rock-formation, interrupted at intervals by great cataclysms, which destroyed all the life of the earth.

When tranquillity was restored, a new creation was made to replace the old. This was the catastrophic theory of Cuvier, which, so far as the rocks were concerned, was gradually replaced by Sir Charles Lyell's theory of uniformity, according to which the earth's history was an uninterrupted sequence, but Lyell did not venture to suggest the evolutionary conception of plants and animals and their gradual development by natural agents.

From the beginning of the Nineteenth Century, geologists had made most careful studies of the fossil invertebrates, which were (and are still) an indispensable means in arranging the rocks of the earth's crust in chronological order. Fossil vertebrates, on the other hand, were of much less use for such purposes, because of their comparative scarcity, and therefore but few men took any interest in them. When new ones were found, they received names, were catalogued in their proper systematic order, put into glass cases, and ignored. According to the dominant theory of special creation, which taught that every species of animal and plant was unchangeable, save within very narrow limits, and owed its existence to a creative fiat, vertebrate paleontology could be little more than a descriptive catalogue of the animals which had successively appeared on the earth. Darwin's book, which immediately divided civilized mankind into two opposite and warring camps, completely changed the status of paleontology. Every one recognized that the fossils offered one of the best means of putting this newfangled theory of evolution to a crucial test. Since the fossils were the actual remains of the animals that once had lived on the earth, and since the rocks gave us their order of succession in time, then the fossils ought to make manifest whether they formed genetic series, connected by a real blood-relationship of ancestor and descendant, or whether they were due to separate acts of creation, related only ideally in a common creative plan. None of the biological sciences was so completely transformed and rejuvenated by Darwin's work as was the paleontology of the vertebrates, which thus received an entirely new content and significance, causing it to thrive and flourish mightily. I may remark here, incidentally, that some of the strongest and most convincing proofs of Darwin's views have been supplied by paleontology.

It is time for us to have done with this preliminary discussion and turn to a consideration of the topics announced in the title of this lecture, *viz.,* some of the applications of paleontology. Nature is one and indivisible, and the important discoveries made in one branch of science are sure to effect more or less radical changes in other branches. When M. and Mme. Curie announced the discovery of radium and the amazing phenomena of radio-activity, no one could have foreseen that these newly discovered phenomena were to affect profoundly the sciences of astronomy and geology. Such has been their effect, nevertheless. The discoveries of paleontology have modified biology, geology, geography, and even, strange to say, the seemingly remote science of astronomy.

The first and most obvious application of the modern paleontology, which was so fertilized and stimulated by Darwin's writings, was to explain the facts of zoology and botany; but another, and very much older, application was as a means of arranging the earth's history chronologically and correlating the histories of the various continents and seas into a single consistent and harmonious earth-history. This use of fossils does not depend upon any theory of the origin and succession of living forms. Familiarly and universally employed for sixty years under the prevailing belief in special creation, it still continues to be employed as widely now that all the world has accepted a belief in evolution. I refer to the use of fossils as a means of arranging the rocks in chronological order. This great and fundamental discovery was due to William Smith, an English engineer, though Cuvier and Brongniart made the same discovery in France almost at the same time.

Last summer I had the good fortune to be in Bath, and was invited to take part in the ceremony of unveiling a tablet to the memory of William Smith. This tablet was placed on the outer wall of a house in which Smith, in 1799, had dictated to a friend "the order of the strata." That was the beginning of historical geology. Smith had observed that the strata, or beds of water-laid rock, were arranged in a certain order, one over the other; further, he noted that each group of beds was characterized by a particular assemblage of fossils, such as occurred in no other beds, and that, from the succession of beds the succession of fossils might be made out. Having determined the succession of fossils, it was possible to apply it in new regions, and it was found to apply in other parts of England, in France and in Germany, and gradually its application became world-wide. It can be employed in America, Africa, Australia, or any other part of the earth's surface.

The principle is extremely simple, and is widely made use of in historical and archeological inquiries of all sorts. For example, the student of handwriting has learned from a careful study of *dated* manuscripts that the handwriting of the mediaeval copyists underwent changes in a certain definite order; having learned the order of change, it is possible to use that order to place *undated* documents from their handwriting alone. One needs but little experience to distinguish writing of the eighteenth century from that of the nineteenth or the seventeenth, and expert paleographers can determine the date of a document within a decade of its writing. Though simple and obvious, this principle has been persistently misunderstood, and from time to time it has been attacked. Even so great a man as Herbert Spencer could not see that it did not involve reasoning in a circle, and declared that it was unscientific. But such an inference is due to a failure to grasp the significance of the method.

The progress of life from the lower and simpler to the higher and more complex upon which Smith's system is founded is substantially the same everywhere. This is because the fossils which are employed for chronological purposes are chiefly those of marine animals; and as all parts of the sea are in communication with one another, the only barriers which prevent the universal spread of marine organisms are those due to temperature, so that the inhabitants of warm seas are very different from those of cold waters. In former ages of the earth, however, when a more uniform temperature prevailed and climatic zones were but faintly indicated, the inhabitants of the different oceans were much more nearly alike than they are now.

The paleontology which was rejuvenated, almost re-created, by Darwin proved to be an indispensable means of explaining the anomalous distribution of land animals and plants in the various continents. Before Darwin's day, much interest was taken in the geographical distribution of animals, but merely as so many statistical facts, for which no explanation could be found. As Darwin tells us in his autobiographical sketch, it was the facts of paleontology and of the geographical distribution of animals, which he observed in South America, that first led him to question the truth of the then almost universally accepted dogma of special creation. He felt assured that if the theory of evolution were to be accepted as true, it must be able to explain distribution. The present order of things on the earth, geographical, climatic, and biological, is, according to the evolutionary theory, the necessary outcome of an unimaginable series of changes throughout hundreds of millions of years; and, if that theory is to be accepted as true, it must be able to offer a reasonable explanation of this present order. If the geographical arrangement of animals in existing lands is not due to special creative fiat, but to natural causes, and is the inevitable result of the long sequence of past changes, then paleontology should be able to offer an explanation of the anomalies and paradoxes in that arrangement.

For example, the camel family is divided into two sub-families, the true camels of the Old World, native to Asia, and the llamas, guanacos, etc., of South America. This seems to be a very anomalous kind of distribution, to have the two parts of the same family separated as far as the size of the globe will permit; yet the history of the family, as recorded by the fossils, offers a simple explanation. The group originated in North America and for long ages was confined to that continent; at first, there was but a single series without distinction of sub-families, and this series shows in each successive division of geological time a continuous advance and development. Finally, the series gives off two branches; the true camels, which passed into Asia by way of the raised bottom of Bering Sea; the other, the llamas, into South America. For a time both sub-families were present together in North America, and were completely wiped out by the great Pleistocene extinctions. It is their extinction in North America which has brought about the wide separation of the surviving species.

This explanation is typical of a great many cases of what is called "discontinuous distribution;" whenever the history is known, it is found that the group in question once occupied the intervening area and then became extinct in that area. Not that all cases can be explained, by any means; in such cases the history of the animal group has not yet been recovered and deciphered, perhaps never can be. But it may be stated as a rule, without known exception, that whenever the history and development of a group has been made clear, its modern distribution is thereby explained. This could not be true were each species an immutable entity, separately created.

The present distribution of the tapirs exactly parallels that of the camels and llamas; they are found only in southern Asia and in Central and South America. Throughout nearly the whole of the Tertiary period, these curious creatures were distributed all around the northern hemisphere; in this country fossils of them have been collected from Los Angeles to Port Kennedy on the Schuylkill and southeast to Florida. Then, for some unknown reason, they disappeared from all lands save those in which they still occur. Like the camels, the tapirs probably originated in North America; at all events, they have been found here in rocks more ancient than in any other known region.

As a last illustration of the manner in which paleontology explains distribution, we may take the case of the Proboscidea (elephants and their close relatives, the mastodons). The mastodons are extinct, and the present occurrence of elephants would seem to require no particular explanation, for they are found only in the warmer parts of Asia and Africa, between which there is land connection now. In the epoch immediately preceding the present, Proboscidea were found in all the continents, perhaps even including

Australia; only elephants in the Old World, from Great Britain to South Africa and eastward to China and Siberia. In North America elephants and mastodons ranged together, but only the mastodons extended into South America. In the late Tertiary (Pliocene epoch) the facts were the same, except that the mastodons were also present in all lands of the Old World. In the middle Tertiary (Miocene) only mastodons were in existence, the true elephants having been subsequently derived from them. The mastodons appeared in North America and Europe almost simultaneously (in the geological sense of that word); but for a long time we were ignorant of their place of origin, for their appearance in the northern regions was entirely unheralded, and nothing was known in the earlier epochs which, by any stretch of the imagination, could be regarded as ancestral to these Miocene mastodons. By a process of elimination that region of origin could be narrowed to the warmer parts of Asia and Africa; and there the desired ancestors were at last found, first in the Oligocene and Eocene of Egypt, carrying the genealogy back to a much earlier time and more remote antecedents than in the northern lands.

Last year, I presented a paper before the American Philosophical Society on "The Isthmus of Panama as the Strategic Point in the Distribution of North and South American Life." In this paper I brought forward evidence to show that in the Cretaceous period the two western continents were joined by continuous land, while in the earlier half of the Tertiary period, they had been divided by a sea which occupied the site of Central America and the Isthmus. This separation brought about complete difference in the North and South American faunas; and the final re-elevation of the land accounted for the many animal groups which are now common to the two continents.

I do not mean to leave with you the impression that all the problems of animal distribution have been solved, for this is far from being the case. Many such problems still await the solution which may never be found. On the other hand, it is a highly significant fact that whenever the fossils enable us to reconstruct the history of a group of plants or animals its distribution, present and past, is thereby explained; and the cases of distribution which we cannot explain are those of which we do not know the history.

A third application of this science, to which Leidy devoted the most fertile years of his life, is that which enables us to follow the past climatic changes which have succeeded one another upon the earth. The climatic history of the earth is one of the most wonderful parts of its marvelous story and has wide astronomical bearings, as well as geological and geographical. That life has existed on the earth without interruption for a billion years or so is now a familiar fact and when it is remembered within what narrow limits of temperature terrestrial life is possible, the constancy of solar radiation throughout that unimaginable lapse of time is all but incredible. Thirty years ago Lord Kelvin's calculations of the age of the sun were very generally accepted and, according to these, the sun could not be more than 20,000,000 years old. The discoveries in the field of radio-activity have indefinitely extended the time involved in the history of the solar system.

While the climatic changes through which the earth has passed have never been so extreme as to exterminate all living things, they have, nevertheless, sufficed to bring about very remarkable results. Throughout much the greater part of the earth's recorded history, its climate has been so mild and nearly uniform that the temperature-zones, so familiar to-day, are scarcely or not at all indicated; and this fact led to the widespread belief among geologists that the glacial ages of the Pleistocene had been altogether exceptional, and due to some transitory cause from which the present amelioration was a slow recovery. Subsequently it was learned that there had been several glacial times recorded in the rocks, the oldest of which antedated the fossiliferous rocks; and there is now reason to believe that these times of refrigeration were rhythmically recurrent, at intervals of approximately 250,000,000 years. The evidence of former glaciations is mostly to be found in the rocks themselves; the fossils, which sometimes give corroborative testimony, are often unavailable, but for the less extreme fluctuations of climate paleontology gives the only evidence which can be trusted. All classes of organisms may give proofs of climatic changes, but the most useful are fossil plants.

The Mesozoic era and the earlier part of the succeeding Tertiary period had climates, not only free from other than local glaciation, but even much milder and more uniform than those of the present day. Greenland, for example, which now can support only dwarf willows and birches, 2 or 3 inches high, then had abundant forests of temperate zone type. Great palms were growing as far north as Idaho and Montana, and large crocodiles accompanied them. In the Jurassic period, the Antarctic continent, the most lifeless and desolate of all existing lands, had plants like those of England. The enormous reptiles which throughout the Mesozoic era inhabited all the continents and oceans, even in the far North, could not have endured the Arctic climate of the present. The gradual refrigeration of the climate, leading to the Glacial epoch, is likewise clearly recorded by the fossils, also the very curious fact that interglacial climates were milder than those of the present time. The term "interglacial" requires a word of explanation. After Agassiz's conception of a glacial time, when the northern parts of Europe and North America were, like modern Greenland, buried under great sheets of moving ice, had been almost universally accepted, evidence began to appear that the Glacial age had not been single, but multiple; and the proof which has accumulated in many lands has convinced nearly all students of the problem that Pleistocene glaciation consisted of at least four Glacial stages, separated by three Interglacial stages when the climate was warmer than at the present time. On the north shore of Lake Ontario, near Toronto, there is a series of bends, laid down in water, the interglacial nature of which is shown by the two glacier-made boulder beds, between which the sediments deposited in water are contained. The water-laid beds are in two series, of which the lower one has preserved many leaf-impressions, and these plainly indicate a climate considerably warmer than that of present-day Ontario. Other interglacial deposits on the shore of Hudson's Bay and in the Great Plains region contain fossils of plants and animals indicative of a relatively warm climate, milder than the climate of the same localities in recent times.

Similar facts have been observed in Europe, and in few places are the climatic indications more beautifully clear than at Mauer, where the famous jaw of the Heidelberg Man (*Homo heidelbergensis*) was discovered. This lower jaw was found in a sand-pit some forty feet below the surface of the ground; and in the same bed as the human remains, and evidently contemporary with them, were found the bones of many mammals, such as the southern elephant, hippopotamus, etc., which plainly suggest a climate warmer than that which now prevails in Central Europe. Not far above this bed are numerous bones which show the renewed refrigeration which was to lead to another glacial stage, as must be inferred from the bones of the boreal mammals which are there found. The southern animals have all disappeared from the region, and their place is taken by cold-country creatures, such as the mammoth, or woolly Siberian elephant, reindeer, and the like. The climatic inferences to be drawn from these two sets of animals are quite unmistakable, and it is interesting to note how closely the facts in Europe and North America correspond.

The whole process of reconstructing the earth's past history, the arrangement and changing connections of the great land-masses of the various seas, is dependent upon the study of fossils, which give a record of changes in their order of chronological succession. That is where geology has a great advantage over so exact a science as astronomy, for the exactitude of astronomy is confined to the present order of things; and in dealing with historical problems concerning the origin of stars and planetary systems, there is great vagueness and little certainty. For over a hundred years, the Nebular Hypothesis of the great French astronomer, La Place, was accepted by astronomers and geologists with practical unanimity, as explaining the origin and history of the solar system. Now that hypothesis has no standing with astronomers and among the geologists of England and America, the ancient hypothesis is completely abandoned, for it has been conclusively shown that La Place's conceptions are mechanically impossible. Nevertheless, many if not most of the German geologists still adhere to the scheme of La Place, chiefly because they are not convinced of the truth of the hypotheses which have been propounded to take the place of the discredited nebular theory. Astronomers have no such record of the past as the fossils offer to geologists and, in the lack of that record, they can not solve historical problems with confidence.

Needless to say, I hope, this statement is not meant to belittle the astounding achievements of astronomy, which include the highest attainments of the human intellect. Nor would any prudent man be so foolish as to attempt fixing any limit to the progress of astronomical discovery. What methods of investigating and determining the origin and development of the celestial bodies may hereafter be devised, no man can predict. At present, however, astronomy can not deal with these historical problems in an assured way.

To many minds the most interesting and important of the applications of paleontology is the testimony which the fossils give to the theory of Evolution. As we have seen, it was Darwin's book that rejuvenated the study of fossils and gave it an unheard of extension. It was immediately and generally recognized that the most crucial test of Darwin's theories would be, whether it was in harmony with the facts of the geological record, or in hopeless conflict with those facts. Even more exacting and severe was the test of future discovery. It has often happened in the history of science that a theory which satisfactorily explains and coordinates the facts known at the time it is first enunciated, is gradually undermined by the discovery of new facts, which do not harmonize with it, until the exceptions outweigh the rule and the theory collapses.

When Darwin published his great book, he showed in a famous chapter that the facts of paleontology agreed with his theory as well as could be expected in view of the admitted incompleteness and imperfection of the geological record. Since that date, the geologist has extended his exploring and collecting work to all lands that can be reached and studied. Wonderful series of fossils have been found in western North America, a work of collecting which had just begun in Darwin's day, when no one had any conception of the astonishing museum of long-vanished animal life which is entombed in the rocks of arid and semi-arid America. As we have already learned, one of Dr. Leidy's securest titles to fame is the great work which he did in revealing and reconstructing this record. Likewise, Africa, Asia, and even parts of Europe, have all yielded up treasures of fossils, of which Darwin had no inkling. He himself was one of the first to discover the richly fossiliferous beds of Patagonia, but he had not the smallest conception of what was to be found there sixty years and more after his explorations in South America.

There has thus been a veritable flood of new discoveries which put the evolutionary conception to the severest possible test. The result has been that that conception has been supported and strengthened in a wonderful way, and is far stronger and more universally accepted than it was sixty years ago. No competent person would maintain that all problems have been solved and all difficulties removed; far from it, but those difficulties are plainly due to lack of information. The record of the development of living things which is contained in the rocks is like a book from which many pages, even whole chapters, have been torn out. On the other hand, many chapters have been preserved, of which the fullness and precision make a perfectly unambiguous and most eloquent support of the theory. More than ever is it true, that by far the best, most probable and most convincing interpretation of the facts of paleontology is that offered by the theory of evolution.

This result is all the more striking when the state of the other sciences in 1859 is taken into consideration. Physics, chemistry, astronomy, and even mathematics, have been more or less completely reconstructed since that time. The principal theories which then dominated physics and chemistry have nearly all been abandoned in favor of newer interpretations. The advance of discovery has been fatal to the older conceptions. This is not true of the theory of evolution which, as stated above, is more thoroughly established and more universally accepted than ever before.

In 1876-7 Huxley delivered a series of lectures on evolution in New York; and the lecture entitled (I quote from memory) "The Demonstrative Evidence of Evolution" was devoted to the discoveries of American paleontology, and more particularly to the genealogy of the modern horses, as that had been worked out by Professor Marsh. Huxley himself had been the first to attempt a scheme of equine evolution; but, as he had access only to European material, he could make but an approximation to the later conceptions. When he saw Marsh's finely preserved fossils, arranged in chronological order, he was convinced that he had before him an actual and positive demonstration of the evolutionary theory. It wasn't that, perhaps, but it was evidence of so high a degree of probability as to be convincing. That Leidy, though a thorough-going evolutionist, has little to say concerning the interpretation of the fossils, which he discovered and described, seems at first sight surprising. But he was, in fact, laying the foundations of the theoretical structure. It was he who first showed the chronological stages and modifications in the history of many families, horses, camels, rhinoceroses, wolves, cats, etc.; and that he did not categorically draw the obvious conclusions was due to his belief that theoretical discussions should wait upon the acquisition of more complete material.

These are the more important of the applications of paleontology. Can it be a matter of surprise that Leidy, with his remarkably clear and broad outlook over the world of nature, should have felt that paleontology was the main work of his life?

WILLIAM BERRYMAN SCOTT
PRINCETON UNIVERSITY

THE CONTRIBUTION OF BIOLOGY, CHEMISTRY AND PHYSICS TO THE NEWER KNOWLEDGE OF RICKETS[1]

THE investigation of rickets is an outstanding example of the value of interweaving the basic sciences with clinical medicine and may well serve as a text to illustrate "the contributions of other sciences to medicine." It is an axiom that many disorders have been elucidated only with the aid of chemistry and animal experimentation, but the instances are few in which biology, inorganic and organic chemistry and various forms of physics have been resorted to so frequently and to such a degree. Although decreasing in incidence and severity, rickets still undoubtedly is the most common nutritional disorder of early childhood in the temperate zones. It has been the object of intermittent study ever since Glisson first described signs and symptoms of the "Englische Krankheit" in 1650. Our acquisition of knowledge concerning its various aspects may

[1] Presented as part of a symposium on "The contributions of other sciences to medicine" at the annual meeting of the American Association for the Advancement of Science, Nashville, Dec. 28, 1927.

be divided broadly into two periods, the one—which may be termed the clinical and pathologic era—comprises the long span between 1650 and 1918, and the other—that of "the newer rickets"—embraces less than a decade, from 1918 until to-day. The latter period, which is still in full fruition, is an indirect result—a by-product—of the discovery of the vitamins. Using this new concept as a fulcrum, and abandoning the old and fixed idea of producing rickets experimentally by limiting the intake of calcium, Mellanby successfully brought about this disorder in puppies by depriving them of a specific fat-soluble factor. It is true that he mistook what we now recognize as the fat-soluble vitamin for the antirachitic factor, but there can be no doubt but that he succeeded in inducing true rachitic lesions. Shortly thereafter investigators in this country—McCollum and his coworkers, as well as Sherman and Pappenheimer—produced typical histologic lesions in the rat by means of rations deficient in phosphorus.

The first factor which led to the era of "the newer rickets" emanated therefore from the biologic or physiologic laboratory and, as has been the case so often in connection with infectious as well as nutritional disorders, consisted of the ability to reproduce at will a disorder in an experimental animal. The second propelling influence following on the heels of the first, although having no connection with it, was the demonstration by Huldschinsky in 1918 of the importance of light, of the fact that ultra-violet radiations are a specific preventive or curative antirachitic agent. From this time until to-day, rickets—which for two and a half centuries had awakened but a fitful interest in the clinician—has been the object of intense investigation in many of the biologic, chemical and physical laboratories both in this country and abroad.

The earliest and simplest chemical studies were carried out in the clinic. Iverson and Lenstrup, of Copenhagen, as well as Howland and his coworkers in this country, showed the old conception to be erroneous which held that a deficiency of calcium is the essential disturbance in rickets, and proved that it is the phosphorus ion which dominates the metabolic picture. The inorganic phosphorus of the blood was found to be low. Indeed, due to the wide prevalence of rickets, it was shown later that there is what may be termed "a phosphate tide" in the blood of infants, an ebb during the winter months followed by a flood in the spring with the advent of sunshine. We shall find that the later chemical studies, those on the sterols, have been far more complex and have taxed to the utmost the resources and ingenuity of experienced organic chemists.

Up to this time chemistry and pathology had aided the clinician in the solution of his problems. As soon as it had been demonstrated that certain light waves are a specific curative agent, it was necessary to turn to physics for information. Naturally, the first point of attack was the segregation and definition of the specific radiations which were endowed with this remarkable therapeutic property. By means of filters of known penetrability it was soon found that ultra-violet radiations of greater length than about 320 μμ, or 3,200 engstrom units, were unable to protect animals from rickets which were fed a diet deficient either in phosphorus or in calcium. This observation proved to be of interest not only to clinicians but to the large number of workers who were actively engaged in studying various biological processes, for example, the growth of plants, or the factors involved in egg production and fertilization or the rôle of light in the cultivation of cells *in vitro*. *To-day rickets has become the established criterion for appraising the biologic action of ultra-violet waves in the region of 300 millimicrons.*

In 1924, less than four years ago, it was shown by me and almost simultaneously by Steenbock that the specific ultra-violet radiations exert their action not only on animals exposed to their influence, but also indirectly on various foodstuffs. As is well known, milk, flour, oils, cereals, etc., can be rendered antirachitic by this means—activation being restricted to the same band of ultra-violet light as in the case of animals. This newer knowledge, combining as it did physical and chemical aspects, led to renewed activity in these fields of endeavor. The first question was to attempt to discover the substance in the food which underwent this remarkable transformation. This study, although having made steady progress, is still incomplete and is being actively pursued in various laboratories both in this country and abroad. It was ascertained within a few months that it is the non-saponifiable fraction and not the fat in the foods which is essential to activation. At the end of 1924 both Steenbock and I were able to report that it is the cholesterol in the animal cell, or phytosterol, its counterpart in the vegetable cell, which undergoes specific alteration. Cholesterol purified by repeated crystallizations, which from the standpoint of rickets is inert, could be rendered highly antirachitic by subjection to ultra-violet irradiation for a minute or less. Its melting-point, specific rotation and chemical constitution had undergone no apparent change in the course of the procedure, and it seemed as if the new product were an isomer of cholesterol. During this period studies were being carried out concurrently in the physical laboratory. The problem of the activation of cholesterol lent itself readily to an investigation by means of absorption spectra. It was found that the well-known absorption bands of cholesterol were definitely altered as a result of irradiation, that the sterol becomes more permeable to certain definite wave-lengths of ultra-violet light. This work, into which we shall not enter in detail, was first undertaken in this country, and has more recently been refined and extended by Heilbron in Liverpool, and Pohl in Goettingen. Furthermore, by means of the use of monochromatic ultra-violet light, it was shown that the uppermost limit of the antirachitic field may be placed at 313 $\mu\mu$, and that even at this point its action is feeble. When we bear in mind that the shortest rays of the sun which reach the surface of the earth rarely are less than 300 mm. in length, it is evident how circumscribed is the area of specific solar radiations. *A difference of a few millimicrons or millionths of a millimeter determines whether or not waves are specific or ineffective.*

It was soon evident that only a very small fraction of the cholesterol becomes activated following irradiation, less than one per cent. This observation raised the question in the minds of several investigators, as to whether it is truly the cholesterol which is transformed or some associated sterol—a subject which during the past year has been studied by Windaus and myself, as well as by Rosenheim and his coworkers in London. It developed that another unsaturated sterol—a sterol with 3 unsaturated bonds—is mainly concerned in the elaboration of the antirachitic factor, namely ergosterol, which heretofore has been extracted from ergot and from yeast, but which is now being found more widely distributed in nature. It would lead too far afield to discuss the moot question of the activation of cholesterol and other sterols. In brief, it may be stated that it has not been shown definitely that cholesterol, as well as ergosterol, can not be activated. In this connection, the minuteness of the amount of irradiated ergosterol required to protect an animal should be emphasized; it has been found that *1/10,000 of a milligram or 1/10,000,000 of a gram daily is sufficient to confer protection.* When we bear in mind that this infinitesimal amount is given by mouth, it is difficult to conceive that the specific antirachitic factor exerts its curative action directly and bodily on the various epiphyses throughout the body.

Parallel with these investigations on ultra-violet radiations and the sterols, which engaged the attention of the physicist and of the chemist, the question was being considered as to how these newer ideas could be brought into consonance with the well-established fact of the specific antirachitic properties of cod-liver oil. At first the two phenomena seemed irreconcilable, but, as you know, it soon was demonstrated that the activity of cod-liver oil in rickets rests on the same basis as that of foods which have been subjected to irradiation—that both are dependent on the action of a specific sterol. In passing, it should be added, however, that it has not been shown that the therapeutic activity of cod-liver oil is confined to the effect of this sterol.

In my review of this subject, it has been necessary to treat the advances in the fields of biology, chemistry and physics as if they took place consecutively. As a matter of fact, they have progressed at one and the same time, new discoveries by the physicist being made at once the basis for some newer chemical investigation and both in turn leading perhaps to interesting developments in the provinces of experimental biology or clinical therapeutics. Some of these studies have been carried out in conjunction or close cooperation with the clinic, others have been made in laboratories devoted solely to investigations in pure science. In the light of recent studies of the vitamins and hormones, it would seem that, in general, this probably will be the method—if it can be called a method—of advancement in the future. It is questioned often whether newer technics and discoveries in medicine will be evolved by the clinician in ward and laboratory, or whether, as it becomes necessary to delve ever deeper into the realms of pure science, the clinician, in spite of his modern training, will not become dependent upon the discoveries of the physicist, the chemist and others occupied with the basic sciences.

No one can answer this question with any degree of certainty. It seems probable nevertheless that for some time to come the clinician—owing to his strategic position in the broad realm of medicine—will continue to make valuable and even basic contributions to our store of knowledge, and that the recent experience in the field of rickets will from time to time be repeated in other provinces of clinical medicine. It can, however, be safely predicted that in order to gain this newer knowledge we must once more call to our aid in varying degree biology, chemistry and physics.

ALFRED F. HESS

NEW YORK, N. Y.

ACOUSTICS OF AUDITORIUMS*

A CONSIDERATION of recent investigations led the writer logically and unexpectedly to the conclusion that good acoustics in an auditorium may be obtained by making it like the outdoor theater of the Greeks. Also, it is concluded that better acoustics appears likely if a study is made of the way in which speech and music are generated, with special consideration

* An address given March 1 at the Physics Colloquium, University of Illinois.

of the effect of the sound reflected from walls near the speaker or musician.

Very little was known scientifically about acoustics of auditoriums until W. C. Sabine, about 1900, began to publish the results of his work.[1] Aside from occasional minor faults or interference and resonance, Sabine concluded generally that the acoustics of a room depended mainly on the reverberation or decay of sound. He conducted an extensive and careful series of investigations which showed that the time taken for a standard sound to die out in a room depended on the loudness of the sound and on the volume of the room, and inversely on the absorption of the surfaces in the room. Most of the investigations since then have only amplified and extended Sabine's fundamental conclusions.

As a result of these efforts, auditoriums have been greatly improved in acoustical qualities, so much so that attempts have been made to specify "optimum" conditions,[2] with the hope of securing perfect acoustics. Auditoriums adjusted according to these conditions, while generally satisfactory, have not always given the expected perfect effects. In some cases, speakers and musicians have voiced objections without being able to state clearly what the trouble was.

In the meantime, within the past two or three years, several publications have appeared that yielded information from different viewpoints than those given originally by Sabine and that furnish possibilities of improving acoustic effects. That is, while Sabine investigated primarily the reverberation and decay of sound, these later studies deal more particularly with the growth of sound in a room.

For instance, Petzold[3] has shown that blurring (Verwischung) will be set up if two identical speech sounds reach an auditor with a time interval between them of .05 second or more. This would be the case if two speakers were separated about fifty-six feet and uttered the same words simultaneously. While it is practically impossible for two speakers to do this, the effect may be obtained by a single speaker who stands near a reflecting wall so that his acoustic image on the other side of the wall may be thought of as saying the same words as the speaker and at the same time. The image is really due to the reflected sound. For music, Petzold finds a shorter time limit between two sounds of .035 to .042 second, depending on the character of the music.

This conclusion of Petzold's indicates the importance of studying the reflecting surfaces near speakers and musicians to avoid blurring effects. Usually in auditoriums, the space about the performer has been decided by other requirements than acoustics. The large stage house of the modern theater gives little practical opportunity for suitable reflecting walls. In smaller auditoriums, it would be easier to design such reflectors, without the usual heavy absorbing curtains.

Such reflecting surfaces should preferably be plane, and situated not more than about twenty feet from the performer—a smaller distance would give better results—and inclined so as to reflect sound to the audience. Under these circumstances, the direct sound from the performer is reenforced without distortion by a number of images, all giving simultaneously the same sound.[4]

Not only are the auditors benefited by this arrangement, but the performer himself gets an immediate response to his effort that allows him to adjust his speech or music to get the best effect. Without this, the performer feels lost, and the resulting sound, particularly music, lacks perfection. Musicians state that they prefer to sing or play near a wall—and always with a resonant stage floor, without carpet—presumably because of the reassuring support given by such reflecting surfaces.

An experiment of this nature recently performed by the writer supports this view. A reflector, twelve by fourteen feet, was hung horizontally over a band stand, and, by means of ropes and pulleys, could be raised or lowered. When the reflector was lowered successively to positions twelve, ten, eight and seven feet above the players, the acoustic conditions were improved. The comments of the players were: "Plays easier," "Tones are more natural," "Gets better as the reflector gets lower," "Tones are smoother," etc. The resultant music in the hall for auditors was also better as the reflector was lowered.

Petzold[5] describes some uses of reflecting surfaces about orchestras and choruses. An orchestra pit, for instance, is a resonant enclosure that allows the music to be reenforced and blended beneficially before it goes out to the audience. "Sounding" boards are advantageous if they have sufficient size and if placed intelligently in accordance with acoustic principles.

Another investigator[6] obtains values of the resultant sound as it builds up and dies out at various points in an auditorium. By means of a condenser-transmitter, amplifying device and oscillograph, he obtained curves

[1] "Collected Papers on Acoustics," 1922.

[2] S. Lifshitz, *Physical Review*, 25, 391, 1925; 27, 618, 1926; F. R. Watson, *Architecture*, LV, 251, 1927.

[3] Ernst Petzold, "Elementare Raum Akustik," 1927, p. 8.

[4] F. R. Watson, "Acoustic Design of Churches," *Western Architect*, XXXVI, 178, 1927.

[5] *Loc. cit.*, Chap. 10.

[6] F. Trendelenburg, "Experimentalbeitrag zur Raumakustik," *Zts. für Tech. Physik*, No. 11, 1927.

of the resulting sound. In certain positions near the source of sound, where the reflected sound arrived some time after the direct sound, it was easy to understand the speaker. At considerable distances from the speaker the reflected sound was of more influence and the understanding of speech was difficult. He concluded that good speech understanding would be obtained only at points where the direct sound predominated.

In another connection, Petzold[7] calculated the value of the direct sound at a point 18.1 meters from the source in a room 30 x 20 x 12 meters in volume, and estimated also the added effect of the reflected sound. Neglecting interference phenomena, he assumes that the direct sound gives 10,000 "Vox" (where the Vox is the arbitrary unit of intensity of a sound produced by a special organ pipe used). To the direct sound, the beneficial reflections, that is, those that arrive quickly enough to avoid blurring the direct sound, add enough to give a total of 31,210 Vox. The resultant is then about three times as intense as the direct sound, but the loudness, as perceived by a listener, is less than this, being proportional to the logarithm of the intensity. The relative effects for auditors are the logarithms of 10,000 and 31,210, or 4 and 4.5, respectively; that is, the beneficial reflected sound contributes one half unit to the four units of the direct sound, or only one ninth of the total sound.

From these calculations, it would appear that the reflected sound could be omitted entirely without vital consequence—a conclusion that is quite contrary to the usual conception of auditorium acoustics, where the reflecting walls are supposed to be quite beneficial in increasing the loudness. Omitting the reflected sound would have the advantage of eliminating any possible blurring defects of reflection, as previously described. But this arrangement surprisingly suggests the open-air theater, such as was used by the Greeks, with no reflecting surfaces except the wall at the rear of the stage, and generally regarded as having very good acoustics.

A book[8] on outdoor theaters bears out this supposition about satisfactory acoustics. For example, we read, "Outdoor theaters differ considerably with regard to acoustic qualities, but in general it is surprisingly easy in any of them to hear what is said or sung on the stage." Regarding the Garden Terrace Theater at Yankton, South Dakota, the author writes, "The acoustic properties are a surprise to every one. At the extreme rear, 180 feet from the stage, an ordinary stage or platform voice is perfectly clear and satisfactory." In the Greek theater at the University of California, that holds an 8,000 audience, one can see and hear in every seat. Again, "The acoustic qualities of the theater (Isis Theater, Point Loma, California), like those of every other outdoor theater without exception, are spoken of as remarkable." And so on for other theaters.

An experiment by the writer furnishes a suggestive example. In an investigation on "Optimum Conditions for Music in Rooms,"[9] the fact was brought out that musicians preferred a reverberant space to play in, but that auditors found "dead" surroundings preferable for listening. What was done was first to adjust a room of approximately 6,500 cubic feet volume to give "optimum" reverberation by placing sound-absorbing material about the walls. A quartette of musicians (three violins and a cello) then played at one end of the room. They did not like the musical effects, nor were the auditors pleased. But when the absorbing material was transferred from the walls about the musicians to the end of the room occupied by the listeners, the musical effects for both playing and listening improved until, in the final stage, they were thought "perfect." This arrangement appears to imitate an outdoor theater. The "dead" conditions surrounding the listeners are repeated outdoors by the perfect absorption of the open sky, but there would be some reflection from the leaves of trees and plants.

An experiment by Sabine[10] was performed in which absorbing material was brought into a music studio until the musicians present thought the conditions were satisfactory. This was repeated in several other similar studios. Sabine then found in subsequent experiments that the average time of reverberation for rooms of this size was 1.08 seconds, thus indicating that an optimum reverberation exists for players, that is, for the generation of sound.

Lifshitz[11] conducted a similar experiment in a room of 265 cubic meters volume holding an audience of 120 persons. By varying the number of auditors he could conveniently change the absorption—due to clothing—and thus control the time of reverberation. Opinions were given concerning the acoustic effects, so that he arrived at an average optimum time of 1.11 seconds. Earlier experiments in a room of 126 cubic meters volume gave 1.03 seconds as the optimum. Averaging four values—Sabine, 1.08 sec., Watson ("Acoustics of Buildings," p. 51), 1.04 sec., Lifshitz, 1.11 and 1.03 sec.—he obtained 1.06 seconds as the

[7] *Loc. cit.*, p. 74.

[8] Frank A. Waugh, "Outdoor Theaters," 1917.

[9] SCIENCE, LXIV, 207, 1926.

[10] "Accuracy of Musical Taste," Proc. Amer. Acad. Arts and Sciences, XLII, June, 1906.

[11] "Mean Intensity of Sound in an Auditorium and Optimum Reverberation," *Phys. Rev.*, 27, 618, 1926.

optimum value for reverberation for rooms of this size. While these experiments allowed an optimum to be estimated for the reverberation or decay of sound, the writer is led to ask if the listening musicians in each case did not primarily pronounce an opinion on the generation of sound rather than the decay.

Experiments by Knudsen[12] show that speaking is better understood as an auditorium is made successively "deader" with sound-absorbing materials, thus imitating an outdoor theater. He found[13] for an open-air theater (Hollywood Bowl, Los Angeles) that a listener one hundred feet from the speaker could understand speech better than in the most satisfactory Los Angeles theater. Lifshitz (*loc. cit.*) found the same effect, but thought the speech lost its musical quality and became dry and lifeless.

The Eastman Theater, Rochester, New York, gives further information in this regard. Some apprehension was felt in designing the acoustics of this theater[14] whether or not music would be heard distinctly on the mezzanine balcony. The opening to this balcony, under the main balcony, was comparatively small and it seemed likely that only a small amount of sound would enter. Also, this space was furnished with a considerable amount of sound absorption in the upholstered seats and carpet. On completion of the theater, however, the reception of music on this floor was thought superior to other locations. Here again it appears advantageous to have conditions for listening quite dead acoustically.

From the investigations cited in this article, the writer is led to draw certain conclusions and to make suggestions for further experimental work. That is, the problem of the acoustics of auditoriums is twofold—first, a study of the generation of sound and its building-up processes, which are practically completed in one or two tenths of a second; and second, a study of the decay of sound. The latter feature has been studied extensively by Sabine and his followers, but further investigation of the growth of sound appears promising in securing important information.

The growth of sound and the decay of sound are not independent processes, because the absorption of the room affects both. What is desired apparently is to have the time of reverberation shortened sufficiently so that the successive sounds of speech and music will be given opportunity for suitable development without possibility of serious overlap and distortion.[15] Increasing the absorption allows a sound to rise more quickly to its maximum value, and also increases advantageously the rate of decay so that the field is cleared for the next sound.[16]

Further information on the relative adjustment of the growth and decay of the sound is given by the investigations of the "masking" of one tone by another. For instance, Wegel and Lane[17] showed that the masking of two tones was greatest for tones nearly alike. Also, they found that loud tones more easily masked tones of high frequency than those of low frequency. Knudsen[18] showed that noise had more effect than a pure tone on another tone. He states also, "For good hearing in an auditorium, the speech energy should be from 1,000 to 10,000 times the energy of any interfering noise." These investigations would indicate how much two sounds could overlap without serious distortion.

The various investigations discussed lead the writer to suggest the possibility of an "indoor-outdoor" theater; that is, an indoor theater that incorporates the good acoustics of an outdoor theater. An investigation should be made to improve, if possible, the stage conditions of the outdoor theater.[19] A stage with a wooden floor, a vertical rear wall, diverging side walls and a sloping ceiling gives promise of beneficially reenforcing speech and music and also of developing enough resonance so that the speaker can better judge the effect of his voice. The use of thin, resonant reflecting boards would yield some interesting effects. On the other hand, it would be instructive in an indoor theater, to have the auditorium quite dead—comparable with outdoors—but to try a stage similar to the one just described. Additional information is needed about the resultant speech effects at different points in a room; that is, a photograph of the vibrations set up by words and music of different kinds when sound-waves cross each other. Some attempts in these directions are being tried by the writer, but cooperation of others in this apparently important development appears desirable.

F. R. Watson

University of Illinois

12 V. O. Knudsen, *Physical Review*, 26, 287, 1925.

13 *The Architect and Engineer*, September, 1926.

14 Watson, "Acoustics of Buildings," p. 49.

15 Trendelenburg, *loc. cit.*; E. A. Eckhardt, "The Acoustics of Rooms," *Jour. Franklin Inst.*, 195, 799, 1923; E. Michel, "Horsamkeit Grosser Räume," p. 8.

16 Watson, "Acoustics of Buildings," p. 16.

17 "Auditory Masking of One Pure Tone by Another," *Phys. Rev.*, 23, 266, 1924.

18 "Interfering Effect of Tones and Noise Upon Speech Reception," *Phys. Rev.*, 26, 133, 1925.

19 R. Berger, "Die Schalltechnik," p. 61; Davis and Kaye, "The Acoustics of Buildings," chap. VII.

SCIENTIFIC EVENTS

THE POPULATION OF THE UNITED STATES

THE Department of Commerce announces an estimate of the population of the United States made by the Bureau of the Census. This gives a total estimated population of 120,013,000 on July 1, 1928, as compared with 105,710,620 on January 1, 1920. The total is arrived at by estimating the increase since 1920 upon the basis of the available data regarding births, deaths, immigration and emigration. The population of the several states is then estimated by distributing the total increase for the United States upon the basis of the increase by states from 1910 to 1920 or, where there has been a state census, from 1920 to 1925, except that where there was a decrease between 1910 and 1920 or between 1920 and 1925, the 1920 or 1925 census figure is retained, and no estimate is made:

	Census Jan. 1, '20	Estimated July 1, '28
United States	105,710,620	120,013,000*
Alabama	2,348,174	2,573,000
Arizona	334,162	474,000
Arkansas	1,752,204	1,944,000
California	3,426,861	4,556,000
Colorado	939,629	1,090,000
Connecticut	1,380,631	1,667,000
Delaware	223,003	244,000
District of Columbia	437,571	552,000
Florida	968,470	1,411,000
Georgia	2,895,832	3,203,000
Idaho	431,866	546,000
Illinois	6,483,280	7,396,000
Indiana	2,930,390	3,176,000
Iowa	2,401,021	2,428,000
Kansas	1,769,257	1,835,000
Kentucky	2,416,630	2,553,000
Louisiana	1,798,509	1,950,000
Maine	768,014	795,000
Maryland	1,449,661	1,616,000
Massachusetts	3,852,356	4,290,000
Michigan	3,668,412	4,591,000
Minnesota	2,387,125	2,722,000
Mississippi	1,790,618	1,790,618†
Missouri	3,404,055	3,523,000
Montana	548,889	548,889‡
Nebraska	1,296,372	1,408,000
Nevada	77,407	77,407†
New Hampshire	443,083	456,000
New Jersey	3,155,900	3,821,000
New Mexico	360,350	396,000
New York	10,385,227	11,550,000
North Carolina	2,539,123	2,938,000
North Dakota	646,872	641,192§
Ohio	5,759,394	6,826,000
Oklahoma	2,028,283	2,426,000
Oregon	786,389	902,000
Pennsylvania	8,720,017	9,854,000
Rhode Island	604,397	716,000
South Carolina	1,683,724	1,864,000
South Dakota	636,547	704,000
Tennessee	2,337,865	2,502,000
Texas	4,663,228	5,487,000
Utah	449,396	331,000
Vermont	352,428	352,428†
Virginia	2,309,187	2,575,000
Washington	1,356,621	1,587,000
West Virginia	1,463,701	1,724,000
Wisconsin	2,632,067	2,953,000
Wyoming	194,402	247,000

* Provisional estimate data regarding births, deaths, immigration and emigration from 1927 to 1928 not being available.

† Population, January 1, 1920; decrease 1910 to 1920.

‡ Population, January 1, 1920.

§ Population, State Census, 1925.

APPROPRIATIONS BY THE COMMONWEALTH FUND

THE board of directors of the Commonwealth Fund at their February meeting appropriated $358,438 for the fund's rural hospital program. During the last two years five awards have been made under this program for hospitals in Farmville, Va.; Glasgow, Ky.; Farmington, Me.; Beloit, Kans., and Wauseon, Ohio. In each case the Commonwealth Fund provides two thirds of the cost of construction and equipment, while the community pays the remainder of the cost and assumes the expense of operation.

At the same meeting $27,000 was appropriated for fellowships in psychiatry at the University of Colorado Medical School. Six such fellowships, each with a stipend of $4,500 for two years' study, will be offered to graduates of class A medical schools who intend to specialize in psychiatry. The University of Colorado, in affiliation with the Colorado Psychopathic Hospital, which was opened three years ago under the direction of Dr. Franklin Ebaugh, is regarded as offering unique opportunities for the training of psychiatrists in that part of the country.

Five three-year fellowships for psychiatrists at the Henry Phipps Psychiatric Clinic, under the direction of Dr. Adolph Meyer, the Johns Hopkins University, Baltimore, were also provided for with a grant of $45,000.

A grant of $4,750 for operating expenses was made to the New York City Committee on Mental Hygiene with a possibility of renewal for two subsequent years. This committee was organized in May, 1927, as one of the local branches of the New York State Committee on Mental Hygiene affiliated with the State Charities Aid Association. Dr. C. Floyd Haviland, superintendent of the Manhattan State Hospital, is chairman of the committee and Mrs. Sydney C. Borg, of the Jewish Board of Guardians, is vice-chairman. The committee will function as the mental hygiene section in the health division of the Welfare Council of New York City and it expects to develop a unified mental hygiene program for New York City.

Other appropriations made at the February meeting included $10,000 to the National Probation Association for the further development of its field service department; $15,000 to the Foreign Language Information Service; $3,800 for the cardiac clinic of the Johns Hopkins University Hospital, and $2,000 for scholarships at the Southern Pediatric Seminar. The latter grant renews one of the same amount made for the summer of 1927, under which 35 scholarships were awarded to physicians from six southern states to attend this seminar, which is held for two weeks each summer in Saluda, N. C., in order to enable general practitioners to gain further clinical information concerning methods of diagnosis, treatment and prevention of children's diseases.

At the preceding meeting of the board of directors of the Commonwealth Fund, held in December, the following appropriations were made. For the child health program of the Commonwealth Fund, $230,000; for projects in legal research to be conducted by the law schools of Chicago, Yale and Harvard Universities, $25,000; for surveys of rural health work, under the direction of the Committee on Administrative Practice of the American Public Health Association, $22,500; to the National Conference of Catholic Charities for a study of child-caring homes, $16,500; for a two-year study of encephalitis cases at the Pennsylvania Hospital, $10,000; for the general budget and the department of institutional care of the Child Welfare League of America, $10,000; for the cardiac work of the New York Tuberculosis and Health Association, $7,500.

THE FOURTH PACIFIC SCIENCE CONGRESS

Announcement has recently been made that the fourth Pacific Science Congress, sponsored by the Pacific Science Association, will be held under the auspices of the Netherlands Indies Pacific Research Committee in Batavia and Bandoeng, Java, from May 16 to 25, 1929.

The program for the congress will be organized in three divisions, including physical sciences, biological sciences and agricultural sciences, the latter group having been added to the major divisions recognized at earlier congresses because of the dominating economic and scientific interests of agriculture in the colonies of the Netherlands Indies. As in the previous congresses most of the sessions of the divisions will be given over to symposia upon selected problems.

Papers for these symposia are invited from American scientists upon any important scientific problems pertaining to the Pacific region in these three general fields. The plan for organizing the program for the congress contemplates requesting men who are competent to speak upon the scientific problems of the region to summarize groups of related papers offered and to present briefly at these symposia a coordinated review of these contributions, in order to relate each group of papers to its problem as a whole and preserve as large an opportunity as possible for discussion. Abstracts, in duplicate, of all papers offered for the program of the congress should be in the hands of the first general secretary of the congress, Dr. H. J. Lam, Botanical Gardens, Buitenzorg, Java, by January 1, 1929, and the complete papers, also in duplicate, should be forwarded to Dr. Lam as soon as practicable after that date, so as to permit adequate consideration of the papers in the preparation of the program.

For several days both before and after the period of the scientific meetings, excursions have been planned which will make it possible for visiting scientists to see many things in Java which are of particular scientific significance, as well as the scenic features of the island and its agricultural developments.

Vernon Kellogg

National Research Council

AWARD OF FELLOWSHIPS BY THE GUGGENHEIM FOUNDATION

Fellowships of an aggregate value of $173,000 have been awarded by the John Simon Guggenheim Memorial Foundation to seventy-five young American scholars, scientists and artists. The usual stipend, $2,500, for one year, will enable the beneficiaries to spend all or part of the coming year in study and research abroad.

The following is a list of awards in the field of science:

Dr. Willem Jacob Luyten, assistant professor of astronomy at Harvard University: to photograph the southern sky with the Bruce telescope of the Harvard Observatory at Mazelspoort, South Africa, with a view to comparing these plates with similar plates taken between 1896 and 1905 to obtain information concerning the numbers, velocities and intrinsic brightnesses of the stars in the neighborhood of the sun.

Dr. Otto Struve, assistant professor of astrophysics at the University of Chicago, a theoretical study of the distribution and physical properties of diffuse matter in interstellar space, with Professor A. S. Eddington, at Cambridge University.

Dr. Olive C. Hazlett, assistant professor of mathematics at the University of Illinois: to study the arithmetics of linear associative algebras together with their application and interpretation in other lines of mathematics, in Europe.

Dr. Perry Byerly, assistant professor of seismology in the University of California: to study mathematical geophysics in order to apply data already obtained in the study of the Montana and other American earthquakes to the problems of the nature and position of these discontinuities in the earth's structure which lie above the central core.

Dr. J. J. Hopfield, assistant professor of physics at the University of California: to study the Zeeman effect of the infra-red spectra of oxygen and nitrogen with reference to the classification of the extreme ultra-violet spectra of these elements, with Professor F. Paschen, at the Imperial Physico-Chemical Institute, Charlottenburg, Germany.

Dr. R. J. Kennedy, research associate in physics at the California Institute of Technology: to do research towards establishing a consistent theory of radiation, with Professor Sommerfeld at Munich and Schrödinger at Berlin.

Dr. Noel C. Little, professor of physics at Bowdoin College: to determine the thermo-magnetic properties of gaseous molecules by a new method of convective flow with a view to the study of their structure and special quantitization, with Professor W. Gerlach at Tubingen.

Dr. F. W. Loomis, associate professor of physics at New York University: to make a study of the new quantum mechanics, especially in relation to problems in band spectra, with Professor T. Frank at Göttingen and Professor Schrödinger at Berlin.

Dr. L. E. Reukema, assistant professor of electrical engineering at the University of California: to make a theoretical and experimental study of electric discharge of gases at high frequencies and of the breakdown of solid insulating materials under high electric stress, with Professor W. O. Schumann at Munich.

Dr. W. W. Watson, assistant professor of physics at the University of Chicago: to study molecular spectra under Professor Frank of Göttingen and Sommerfeld of Munich, with a view to learning more about the structure of molecules and the nature of chemical reactions.

Dr. Richard Bradfield, assistant professor of soils at the University of Missouri: to investigate some of the principles involved in the purification of colloids by electrodialysis (reappointment).

Dr. G. H. Coleman, assistant professor of chemistry at the State University of Iowa: to carry out an experimental study of a new method for the preparation of amines by the reaction of organomagnesium halides with chloramines and related compounds, with Professor Victor Grignard at the University of Lyons.

Dr. Earl C. Gilbert, associate professor of chemistry at the Oregon State College: to make an experimental study of some hitherto uninvestigated reaction of hydrazine from the standpoint of modern theories of solution, catalysis and electronic structure; principally with Professor J. N. Bronsted, of the Polytechnic Institute, Copenhagen.

Dr. Ralph E. Cleland, associate professor of botany at Goucher College: to make studies of the chromosome constitution and behavior in the evening primrose.

Dr. R. B. Harvey, associate professor of plant physiology and botany at the University of Minnesota: to investigate the effects of low temperature on plants, in Northern Russia.

Dr. Warren K. Stratman-Thomas, research pharmacologist of the University of Wisconsin: to determine by clinical trial the therapeutic value of certain new arsenical compounds in the chemotherapy of sleeping sickness, with Dr. Clement C. Chesterman, in the Belgian Congo.

Dr. Homer W. Smith, professor of physiology at the University of Virginia: to go to Naples, Cairo and Khartum to make physiological studies of rare species of lung fishes surviving in the waters of the Nile and Mediterranean.

Dr. Dwight E. Minnich, associate professor of zoology at the University of Minnesota: to make physiological studies on the chemical senses of insects, principally with Professor Karl V. Frisch, director of the Zoological Institute at the University of Munich.

Dr. Emmett R. Dunn, associate professor of zoology at Smith College: to carry out researches on Central American reptiles and amphibians, and on the salamanders of the family Ambystomidae, field work in Mexico and Costa Rica and study in European museums.

Dr. William V. Cone, instructor in surgery at the Columbia University College of Physicians and Surgeons: to study the reactions of the interstitial cells of the central nervous system, with Dr. Gordon Holmes at the National Hospital for the Paralyzed and Epileptic in London.

Dr. R. R. Dieterle, instructor in psychiatry at the University of Michigan: to study the spirochetosis of the central nervous system in the syphilitic diseases affecting the nervous tissues, with Professor F. Jahnel, in Munich.

Dr. John C. McKinley, associate professor of neuropathology at the University of Minnesota: to make quantitative studies on human muscle tonus at the University of Breslau, Germany.

SCIENTIFIC NOTES AND NEWS

SIR THOMAS HOLLAND, of the Imperial College of Science and Technology, has been nominated by the council to be president of the British Association for the Advancement of Science for the 1929 meeting, which is to be held in South Africa.

ON the occasion of the Harvey tercentenary meeting of the Philadelphia College of Physicians on March 22, Jefferson Medical College and the University of Pennsylvania conferred the honorary doctorate of laws upon Sir Humphry Davy Rolleston, physician-in-ordinary to King George of England, and the degree of doctor of science on Dr. J. J. R. Macleod, professor of physiology in the University of Toronto.

DR. ADOLPH ENGLER, professor of botany at the University of Berlin, has been elected an honorary member of the Russian Academy of Sciences.

M. BOUIN, professor of histology in the University of Strasbourg, and M. Bardier, professor of pathology in the University of Toulouse, have been elected corresponding members of the French Academy of Medicine.

DR. PAUL KOEBE, professor of mathematics in the University of Leipzig, has been awarded the international mathematics prize of the Swedish Academy of Sciences.

PROFESSOR W. H. HOFFMANN, of the Finlay Laboratory, Havana, has been elected a fellow of the Royal Society of Tropical Medicine and Hygiene, London.

SEBASTIAN L. DE FERRANTI, past-president of the Institution of Electrical Engineers of Great Britain, has been elected a fellow of University College, London.

THE February issue of the *Deutsche Zeitschrift für Chirurgie* is dedicated to Professor Alexander Fraenkel, director of the surgical division of the General Policlinic of Vienna, on the occasion of his seventieth birthday.

DR. L. A. ROGERS, director of the research laboratories of the U. S. Bureau of Dairy Industry, who, on July 1, completed twenty-five years of continuous service in the Department of Agriculture, was guest of honor at a dinner given at the Cosmos Club on the evening of March 3. The occasion was the formal presentation of the book entitled "Fundamentals of Dairy Research," written by Dr. Rogers's associates and dedicated to him in recognition of his leadership and his many outstanding scientific contributions and as an expression of the high regard in which he is held.

A WILLIAM SNOW MILLER lectureship has been established at the University of Wisconsin Medical School by the Phi Beta Pi fraternity in connection with the seventieth birthday of Dr. William Snow Miller, emeritus professor of anatomy at the university. Dr. T. Wingate Todd, of Western Reserve University, will discuss "The Medieval Physician" soon as the first of the series of lectures.

DR. CHARLES SHEARD, of Rochester, Minn., and Dr. Howard C. Doane, president of the Massachusetts Board of Registration in Optometry, have been selected as recipients of the first gold medals of the Distinguished Service Foundation of Optometry.

PROFESSOR C.-E. A. WINSLOW, Lauder professor of public health in the school of medicine at Yale University has been awarded the Ling medal by the Ling Foundation of Los Angeles, "in appreciation and recognition of Professor Winslow's active and unselfish work in behalf of the health progress of school children."

ON account of blindness, Professor Thomas E. McKinney, of the department of mathematics and astronomy at the University of South Dakota, will retire from service at the end of the present university year.

PROFESSOR CHARLES B. BREED, of the Massachusetts Institute of Technology, was elected president of the Boston Society of Civil Engineers at its eightieth annual meeting.

DR. L. H. ADAMS, of the Geophysical Laboratory of the Carnegie Institution, has been appointed secretary of the central petroleum committee of the National Research Council, which acts as adviser of the American Petroleum Institute in expending the funds for fundamental research on petroleum donated by Mr. John D. Rockefeller and the Universal Oil Products Company.

THE following officers were elected at the annual general meeting of the Geological Society of London, held on February 17: *President,* Professor J. W. Gregory; *vice-presidents,* Dr. F. A. Bather, Professor E. J. Garwood, Dr. E. Greenly and Mr. H. W. Monckton; *secretaries,* Mr. W. Campbell Smith and Dr. J. A. Douglas; *foreign secretary,* Sir Arthur Smith Woodward; *treasurer,* Mr. R. S. Herries.

M. MANGIN, director of the National Museum of Natural History, Paris, has been elected vice-president of the French Academy of Sciences to take the place of the late M. Henneguy.

THE Chicago Academy of Sciences has appointed Mr. Alfred M. Bailey as director. He was recently assistant on the Abyssinian expedition of the Field Museum, Chicago, and has been actively engaged in museum and field work during the past ten years.

WALLACE H. CAROTHERS has resigned his instructorship at Harvard University to accept a position with the E. I. du Pont de Nemours and Company, where he will engage in fundamental research in organic chemistry at the experimental station, Wilmington, Del.

PROFESSOR N. H. FURMAN, of Princeton University, has resumed his duties after a year's leave of absence, during which he visited university and research laboratories and chemical plants in England, France, Germany and Austria.

HUGH B. FREEMAN returned from Chile on March 10, where he has been director of the Mt. Montezuma solar radiation station of the Smithsonian Institution for the past three years. M. Keith Baughman sailed for Chile on March 15 to take up the duties of assistant to Mr. Zodtner, the present director of the Mt. Montezuma station. Mr. Baughman expects to remain in Chile three years.

DR. C. E. MYERS, professor of plant breeding at the Pennsylvania State College and Agricultural Experiment Station, will be on sabbatical leave from April 1 to August 1. During this time he will tour the South Atlantic, Gulf, Western and Northern States. He will visit a number of the agricultural experiment stations and educational institutions and also some of the leading trucking and seed-producing sections.

CHESTER WASHBURNE, geologist, of New York, returned from Venezuela in March, and has since departed for São Paulo, Brazil.

DR. CHRISTIAN POULSEN, curator of paleontology at the Mineralogical Museum, Copenhagen, has returned to Washington for three months' research work on the U. S. National Museum's early Paleozoic invertebrate fossils in connection with his studies on these same faunas from Greenland.

DR. KARL BÜHLER, of the University of Vienna, who was visiting professor of psychology at the Johns Hopkins University during the first semester, is lecturing at Harvard University during the second semester.

SIR HUMPHRY ROLLESTON, Regius professor of physics at the University of Cambridge, will be in residence at the Peter Bent Brigham Hospital, Boston, for the week beginning March 25, as the fourteenth physician-in-chief, *pro tempore,* in charge of the medical service of Dr. Henry A. Christian, Hersey professor of the theory and practice of physics at Harvard University and physician-in-chief of the Peter Bent Brigham Hospital.

PROFESSOR W. E. BRAGG, of the University of Leeds, gave a lecture at the Rockefeller Institute for Medical Research on March 19 on "The Scattering of X-rays by Atoms."

DR. E. J. LONDON, director of physiology in the University of Leningrad, will deliver the sixth Harvey Society lecture at the New York Academy of Medicine on Friday evening, April 13. His subject will be "Experimental Fistulae of Blood Vessels."

DR. SIMON FLEXNER, director of the Rockefeller Institute of Medical Research, who has been chosen by the Association of American Physicians as the lecturer of the Kober Foundation for 1928, will deliver a lecture on "Obvious and Obscure Infections of the Central Nervous System" at Georgetown University.

DR. G. H. PARKER, professor of zoology and director of the zoological laboratory at Harvard University, will give a course of lectures in the graduate school of the Ohio State University from April 9 to 20. The course will consist of six lectures on organic evolution and four lectures on the animal mind.

ON March 17, Dr. C. E. Kenneth Mees, director of the Research Laboratory of the Eastman Kodak Company, Rochester, delivered an address to the Royal Canadian Institute, on the subject "The Formation of a Photographic Image."

DR. CORNELIUS C. WHOLEY delivered an address on "The Nature of Multiple Personality" before the Sigma Xi alumni association of the University of Pittsburgh on March 15. Moving pictures of a person exhibiting multiple personality were shown.

DR. C. DAVISSON, of the Bell Telephone Laboratories, New York, will address the Philosophical Society of Washington, March 31, on "Reflection and Diffraction of Electrons by a Crystal of Nickel."

DR. JEROME ALEXANDER, consulting chemist and chemical engineer of New York, recently lectured on colloid chemistry before the Baltimore section of the American Chemical Society, the Brooklyn Engineers Club and the New York Microscopical Society.

PROFESSOR EDWIN C. KEMBLE, of the Jefferson Physical Laboratory at Harvard University, addressed the Franklin Institute on March 29, when he spoke on "Recent Progress in the Interpretation of Molecular Spectra."

WILLIAM F. M. GOSS, formerly professor of railway engineering and dean of the college of engineering at the University of Illinois, died on March 23 in his sixty-ninth year.

PROFESSOR GAETANO LANZA, emeritus professor of theoretical and applied mechanics at the Massachusetts Institute of Technology, died on March 21, at the age of seventy-nine years.

DR. JOHN P. MUNSON, head of the department of biology at the Washington State Teachers College, died on February 27, aged sixty-eight years.

THE death occurred on March 4, at the age of seventy-five years, of Sir Aubrey Strahan, F.R.S., lately director of the Geological Survey of Great

Britain, and of the Museum of Practical Geology, London.

THE death is announced of Dr. E. J. Lesser, of Mannheim, Germany, known for his work on the carbohydrates, and of Dr. Theodore Curtius, of the University of Heidelberg, author of publications on the hydrazins.

THE sixth annual meeting of the Virginia Academy of Science will be held on May 4 and 5 at the College of William and Mary. A new section, that of geology, is to be organized at this meeting. Other sections of the academy are: astronomy, mathematics and physics, biology, zoology, chemistry, psychology and education and geology. Donald W. Davis, president of the College of William and Mary, is president of the academy.

A NATIONAL meeting on oil and gas power is being planned for June 14, 15 and 16, to be held at Pennsylvania State College. In connection with the meeting will be an exhibition—the first of its kind—of oil and gas engines, parts and accessories. It will be located in the new mechanical laboratory of the college, which is a well-lighted building with 20,000 square feet of floor space. The college is not only providing exhibition space free of charge, but is also supplying light, power, steam and compressed air in limited amount for the use of exhibitors. The technical program calls for a number of sessions on subjects of vital interest to this field of engineering. Such subjects as power economics, fuel, oil specifications, research and specialization in engine manufacturing will be discussed by prominent engineers and executives in the industry. The meeting is held jointly by the oil and gas power division of the American Society of Mechanical Engineers and the Pennsylvania State College.

IN connection with the recent celebration of the twenty-fifth anniversary of the founding of the University of Porto Rico, plans were discussed for the establishment of a school of tropical agriculture. The possibilities of founding a joint school with Cornell University have been considered. Dr. Livingston Farrand, president of Cornell University, who attended the anniversary celebration, is reported to have expressed his approval of the project and has outlined the details of the institution and its requirements, financial as well as scientific and physical, stating that Cornell would need to provide at least $1,000,000 in endowment to carry its share of the burden of the new school. A graduate school of tropical agriculture, Dr. Farrand said, would do more to increase productivity in the tropics and spread prosperity and make better living conditions in backward areas than any one other institution.

THE U. S. Coast and Geodetic Survey will in a short time put into operation at its observatory at Cheltenham, Md., the new seismometer recently developed by Dr. Frank Wenner, of the U. S. Bureau of Standards. This will be its first test at a seismological observatory. It has been operated by Dr. Wenner at the bureau during a period of four months past, during which earthquakes occurring at various parts of the earth have been recorded in a very satisfactory manner. This instrument differs in principle from others as yet in operation in this country in that the shock transmitted by the earth to the instrument is recorded not directly but through a galvanometer. This makes it possible, if desired, to place the instrument in a very small building, or in a cave if necessary, and then have the recording at a convenient building elsewhere.

THE United States government has taken up its option on 22,500 acres of forest land in the Waterville Gap of the White Mountains of New Hampshire. This virtually completes the final step in adding this area to the already extensive forest reservation in that section. With this purchase the government has a total area of nearly 750 square miles of public forest in this part of the White Mountains, which is considered one of the finest scenic sections of New England. The purchase was made at a price of $1,050,000, and became possible through adoption of the McNary-Woodruff bill, which completed its passage through Congress March 14 carrying a $1,000,000 appropriation for the purpose.

A CONFERENCE on racial differences was held in Washington on February 25 and 26 under the auspices of the division of anthropology and psychology of the National Research Council, and the committee on problems and policies of the Social Science Research Council. According to *Eugenical News* the conference was called to consider the coordination and facilitation of research on problems of racial differences and racial changes; such problems as occur in connection with the Negro and the immigrant in relation to Whites and stocks of earlier introduction. The subject was opened by 20 minute addresses by Drs. Fay-Cooper Cole, T. Wingate Todd, Franz Boas, W. I. Thomas, M. J. Herskovits, Joseph Peterson, Thos. Woofter, Jr., and Raymond Pearl.

UNIVERSITY AND EDUCATIONAL NOTES

NEW endowment gifts for the University of Chicago, totaling $208,250, have been announced by President Max Mason. They include $50,000 for scholarships and fellowships in archeology from the estate of

E. L. Ryerson, $50,000 for general endowment from J. J. Dau, of Chicago, $25,000 without limitation as to its use from Edward L. Swift and a number of smaller gifts.

A TOTAL of $96,245 has been received by New York University through gifts and bequests in the last two months. These include the following: From the estate of Margaret Olivia Sage, the university received $45,000; the Nicholas Foundation, Inc., made an additional gift of $23,600 for the William H. Nichols chemistry building fund, and anonymous, through Professor George David Stewart, $10,000 to be used for instruction in surgery in the medical college.

IN recognition of his investigations and experiments on plants, John H. Schaffner, for many years professor of botany and formerly head of the department of botany of the Ohio State University, has been promoted to the rank of research professor of botany.

PROFESSOR GEORGE W. GORRELL has been made head of the department of mathematics at the University of Denver.

DR. BRET RATNER has been appointed clinical professor of pediatrics and lecturer in immunology at New York University and Bellevue Hospital Medical College.

DR. CECIL V. KING, formerly instructor at Columbia University, has joined the staff at Washington Square College of New York University as assistant professor of chemistry.

PROFESSOR WATSON BARTEMUS SELVAGE has been appointed associate professor of education and psychology in Washington and Lee University.

G. ALLEN MAIL has been appointed assistant entomologist at Montana State College, University of Montana, Bozeman, for one year beginning on April 1 and will assist in teaching and conducting mosquito studies in northern Montana.

DR. R. K. BUTCHART, lecturer in mathematics in the University of St. Andrews (University College, Dundee), has been appointed to the chair of mathematics at Raffles College, Singapore.

DR. CHAMPY has been nominated professor of histology in the Paris faculty of medicine in succession to the late Professor Prenant.

DISCUSSION AND CORRESPONDENCE

SCIENCE AND SECRETARIES

THE proposed transfer of the geodetic work of the U. S. Coast and Geodetic Survey to the U. S. Geological Survey, for which provision is made in the bills now before both houses of Congress as noted in SCIENCE for January 13 and as discussed by Dr. Geo. Otis Smith in the number for January 20, involves a principle quite apart from the merits of the proposed administrative change. It is one which should interest all scientists who recognize the very important rôle played by the bureaus of the government in promoting or retarding scientific research.

The question is who should pass upon the conditions affecting the efficiency of research. Are the administrative secretaries in charge of departments competent to do so? It would not be difficult to cite evidence that they commonly are not. Many of them demonstrate abilities of a high order as administrators, but they themselves would disclaim the omniscience requisite to understand the workings of all the scientific bureaus.

The advisers of our secretaries are the heads of the individual bureaus and they naturally have their individual points of view. They are specialists, whose purpose is intensified and narrowed by the responsibility for the development of the work intrusted to each of them separately. They are worthy of all respect, but they can not be credited with a disinterested judgment regarding the relative abilities of their own organization or another's to carry out a particular scientific task.

In any proposal for reorganization of administrative relations two bureaus are commonly involved and often two departments, as in the present case. The two secretaries may agree, but the bureau chiefs may probably differ, as the heads of the respective surveys actually do. It is evident that there is need of independent, unbiased, adequately informed opinion as to the effects of any such transfer upon the efficiency of the research in progress.

The National Academy of Science is by law the adviser of the Government in scientific quesions. It comprises in its membership specialists in all branches of science. Among them are men whose judgment would command the respect of their colleagues at home and abroad and also that of their fellow countrymen who take an intelligent interest in the service our great government bureaus render the people.

Scientists may reasonably claim that research shall be organized according to the recommendations of those most competent to judge its needs and that changes in administration of our government bureaus, where they affect scientific activities shall be referred to the National Academy of Science for an expression of opinion by competent judges before they are made on administrative grounds.

At the Cleveland meeting of the Geological Society of America resolutions were passed recommending that the proposed transfer of the geodetic and seismologic work be referred to the National Academy. Should that be done, as we may hope it will be, a broader proposition will be presented than that which has so far been discussed. The administrative question relates to the economy and convenience of executing primary triangulation in one or another connection. The scientific problems involve the ultimate objects of the triangulation. Will the astronomical and geophysical researches in geodesy be promoted by the change? Will the mathematical-physical investigations pertinent to seismology be advanced? Those are the real questions. And we should not forget that the reputation for work of superior accuracy and penetration which the United States has won during half a century of geodetic work presents a standard not easy to maintain in reorganization; nor that the seismologic studies have as their ultimate purpose the task of educating the American people to a better understanding of earthquakes and to better methods of protecting themselves from disasters such as we have hitherto not escaped. The questions are much broader and of more far reaching significance than the estimated attainment of economy of administration.

Bailey Willis

Stanford University

RE SPECIATION WITHOUT CLIMATIC CHANGE OR GEOGRAPHIC ISOLATION

It is an hypothesis rather generally held, and favored by a certain amount of evidence that speciation is largely dependent on changes of environment. A species moves from its center of abundance into diverse peripheral environments which change it somewhat both in structure and habits. Races are formed which are potential species, and become species by chance or other isolation. A study of races shows that such a process is in fact going forward.

There is per contrast little evidence of speciation in a single uniform circumscribed geographic locality. Nevertheless, certain considerations point to a probability that speciation does take place without environmental change and within the confines of a given locality.

We may conceive that a successful species becomes abundant and quickly reaches its saturation point within its range. Within that range there is, however, one outlet whereby it may still further increase, namely, by specializing in two directions. In due time groups of individuals may arise with such divergent habit tendencies. Slowly to be sure, and in the face of cross-breeding, they would diverge ecologically or physiologically up to that point where sufficient fundamental difference is attained to itself furnish a certain amount of isolation. Then the split might come so quickly, the intergradation period have so short a duration in time as to be seldom noticed. There is evidence, mostly circumstantial to be sure, that such speciation does occur and is of considerable importance. It may well be of primary evolutionary importance, for it is not the peculiar isolated environments most favorable for the differentiation of races which give rise to the successful types which spread and become dominant. It is rather the large, uniform, favorable areas which evolve a strong fauna, hard for weaker forms to penetrate, but whence dominant species spread and radiate to the four corners of the earth. The strong fauna of any given moment has probably corresponded to a distribution center of passing time, and it is from such distribution centers that the animals of succeeding epochs seem to be derived. Correlation of the zoogeographical "fauna" with the paleontological "distribution center" will, in the writer's opinion, clarify the path of both sciences.

It will illustrate the above hypothesis of speciation to cite a few instances where it may have pertained. The pilot-fish (*Naucrates*) seems to be a specialized derivative of the genus *Seriola*. Probably all species of this genus as young fishes have the habit, to a greater or less degree of lurking under some "hover," such as a bit of drift-wood, and of following larger fishes. The pilot-fish does so throughout life, and its generic peculiarities are doubtless correlated with this difference. Furthermore it is logical to suppose that habit and correlated physiological differences in this case preceded structural adaptation, and one may easily conceive the initial habit split to have occurred within some such species as the banded rudderfish, *Seriola zonata*.

Take another case, the well-watered Alleghany mountain region is a center of abundance and variety for salamanders of the genus *Desmognathus*. Various more or less separate or intergrading forms occur here living more or less in and out of the water, and with them is found the more exclusively aquatic derivative genus *Leurognathus* (Dunn, 1926, Salamanders of the family Plethodontidae). It certainly seems as if *Leurognathus* had split off as an ecological adaptation in this optimum region of *Desmognathus* abundance, descendent of those *Desmognathus* with the greatest aquatic tendency.

Among birds, the writer has earlier suggested (1919, *Auk*, p. 225–228) that the numerous related species of Warblers of the genus *Dendroica*, nesting together in the Canadian forest, can be more rationally explained as divergence in one locality to take advantage of special habit niches, than as each the result of past geographic isolation, implying later gathering together and fitting the various forms into the single uniform environment where they now occur.

Again take the case of the flying squirrels (*Glaucomys*, etc.): presumably they arose in a region where there were many arboreal squirrels, descendent from those which did the most jumping, rather than isolated, and as a response to some peculiar environment which made it imperative for squirrels to fly.

J. T. NICHOLS

THE AMERICAN MUSEUM
OF NATURAL HISTORY

WEIGHT AND HUMIDITY

THE article entitled "Weight and Temperature" by Dr. P. G. Nutting, which appeared in SCIENCE of December 30, 1927, states that "a consistent difference of 1.2 mg. was found" between the weight of a lump of gold and the weight of the same lump after it had been rolled into a sheet, and that this difference was "probably due to adsorbed moisture." As there is considerable lack of agreement[1] in the literature regarding the influence of humidity upon weight, it seems desirable to publish the results of an investigation conducted some time ago on this subject.

Since the density of water vapor is less than that of air the hygroscopic condition of the atmosphere may be ascertained by comparing its density with that of dry air. If, therefore, a bulb containing dry air which is in communication with an open vessel containing the drying agent is counterpoised by a pointer, after the fashion of a micro-balance, it is possible to arrange the period of the instrument so that ample sensitiveness for hygrometric work may be assured. This method was tried, using a glass bulb. It was found, however, that the deflections of the instrument were much greater for certain changes in humidity than had been anticipated. An investigation was therefore started to determine whether or not the effect was due to the adsorption of water vapor. The materials used were glass, aluminium, hard rubber, bakelite and quartz. The glass was in the form of a bulb of surface area about 200 sq. cm., the aluminium, hard rubber and bakelite were in sheets of approximately 500 sq. cm. surface, while for the quartz a cup of surface area about 300 sq. cm. was used.

The object to be investigated was placed on the scale-pan of a highly sensitive Becker balance and counterpoised with standard weights. Inside of the balance case were placed two thermometers and two flat dishes which were filled with sulphuric acid of the proper density to assure certain relative humidities inside the balance case. Readings were taken every morning and the acid changed each time. Thus the weight of the object could be determined at relative humidities varying from 10 per cent. to 90 per cent. Care was taken to keep the temperature constant, and the balance was never allowed to oscillate nor was it ever disturbed in any way in the course of the investigation.

It was found that the glass bulb adsorbed 0.5 mg. after having been washed in boiling water and dried over a flame for one hour and 2.3 mg. after having been washed and then dried in air.[2] The quartz cup gained in excess of 1 mg. The gain in weight of the aluminium was about half as much per square centimeter as for quartz. Hard rubber and bakelite were found to be immensely more hygroscopic than these. *But in all cases the amount of water vapor adsorbed varied with the humidity.* Furthermore it was found that the water vapor is adsorbed much more quickly than it is given up. A dry object will adsorb its definite amount of water vapor in an atmosphere of a definite relative humidity in less than two hours; this same object may require a day to lose its water vapor if placed near concentrated sulphuric acid. It was obvious, then, that due to the adsorption of water vapor and this "hysteresis" effect neither the hygrometer mentioned above nor one based on the hygroscopicity of materials is feasible. A successful, continuously indicating, density-difference hygrometer which avoids these disturbing effects was later constructed.[3]

In conclusion we may say that the apparent weight of an object of relatively large surface varies appreciably with humidity and that this fact, as well as the "hysteresis" effect mentioned, should be taken into account in accurate weighings.

ARNOLD ROMBERG
L. W. BLAU

PHYSICAL LABORATORY,
UNIVERSITY OF TEXAS

[1] (a) Warburg and Ihmori, *Ann.*, 27, p. 481, 1886. (b) Trouton, *Proc. Roy. Soc.*, A, 79, p. 383. (c) Kuhn, *Deutsche Chemikerzeitung*, 34, p. 1097, 1910. (d) Scheringa, *Pharm. Weekblad*, 56, p. 94, 1919. (e) Metzger, *Glueckauf*, 60, pp. 39–44, 54–60, 94–97, 112–116, 1924.

[2] *Loc.* 1 (a).

[3] *J. Opt. Soc. Am. & Rev. Sc. Instr.*, 13, p. 717, 1926.

LEPIDOPTERA OF NEW YORK

To users of the "List of the Insects of New York" (Cornell Memoir 101): I much regret that in the circumstances of the compilation of the Lepidoptera records of this list it was not possible to publish many of the authorities for collection or determination of the material gathered before 1916. These data are preserved, however, in our files at Cornell University.

I also regret, although I can not accept personal

blame for them, many obscurities in the credits for records received later, and some errors, resulting from the innumerable changes made in the editorial office of the New York State College of Agriculture. They were made in violation of a definite agreement, and they refused to rectify them in proof. I may say that the proof of the "Lepidoptera of New York" (Memoir 68) had received similar treatment, and that the agreement was made in that connection and reiterated in later letters.

Wm. T. M. Forbes

Cornell University

THE EASTLAND HORNED "TOAD"

Much attention has been attracted recently to a Horned "Toad" (*Phrynosoma cornutum*) which is alleged to have been placed in the corner stone of the Eastland County courthouse, Eastland, Texas, in the year 1897. The animal, it is claimed, remained entombed in the granite corner stone until February 18, 1928, a period of thirty-one years. On the latter date it is said to have been removed from the stone alive, before a large crowd of spectators which had gathered for the occasion.

On February 22, 1928, the writer had the opportunity to go to Eastland and make an examination of the external features of the animal in question. It appeared to be a perfectly normal specimen which had undergone winter hibernation. It was probably an old one for the horns about the head region were considerably worn and the right hind leg had been broken but was healed. Otherwise it appeared no different from a normal Horned "Toad" at this season of the year.

Willis G. Hewatt

Texas Christian University

THE BRASSO FOSSILIFEROUS MIOCENE OF TRINIDAD, WEST INDIES

To avoid any possible future confusion, it seems well to note that the Brasso Miocene clay and Brasso conglomerate described by Mr. Gerald Waring, in his Geology of Trinidad, Johns Hopkins Studies in Geology No. 7, pages 69, 71, and Legend of Map, 1926, are entirely distinct from the fossiliferous Brasso Miocene of my report, Miocene of Trinidad, *Bulletin of American Paleontology,* No. 42, pages 10, 16, 1925. The black clays and conglomerates mentioned by Mr. Waring *underlie* the Manzanilla formation. The fossiliferous beds, typical at Brasso Junction, mentioned in my memoir, *overlie* the Manzanilla, and carry a fauna of Middle Miocene Age, related to the Gurabo and Bowden faunas.

Carlotta J. Maury

Yonkers, N. Y.

SCIENTIFIC BOOKS

THE CEPHALASPIDAE

Paleontologists the world over may justly feel a thrill of pride that one of their number, Erik A: Son Stensiö:, has produced such a splendid publication containing important, new and much needed information on the earliest known vertebrates, those curious mailed Silurian and Devonian chordates, which we have been calling Ostracoderms.[1] The most striking feature is the abundance of data, mostly new, on the nervous and vascular systems, the special sense organs, the finer anatomy of the skeleton, and suggestions as to habits of life. After examining the work one feels that he has been studying a treatise on modern fishes. The author has combined with the usual paleontological methods, those of the anatomical laboratory. His needle dissections under a binocular, the object immersed in a non-refracting medium; his use of the wax-plate method of serial section, invented by Sollas for fossils, his painstaking correlations with refractory material, form welcome and highly useful methods in Paleontology.

Following the first expedition fitted out by Prince Albert I, of Monaco, in 1906, there have been eleven expeditions to Spitsbergen up to 1925. The remains of the Cephalaspidae studied by Stensiö:, 105 specimens in all, were assembled from the collections of these Norwegian expeditions. This forms one of the most important discoveries of fossil vertebrates ever made.

The historical account, covering sixteen pages, itself an undertaking of no small magnitude, reviews the published accounts of the geological occurrence, taxonomy and anatomy of forms known. This is followed by a discussion of the anatomy of the Spitsbergen species; 205 pages being devoted to this phase of the work. Description of the genera and species occupies fifty-one pages. There are five genera, four of which are new, and twenty-four species, *all* new. A brief discussion of the Tremataspidae, and the general relations of other groups of primitive chordates to the *Cephalaspidae,* concludes the text. A reasonable bibliography of ten pages makes no pretense at completeness, but the interested student can safely use these references as a guide to the field. Personally, I should like the references given to be more exact, and to refer specifically to the part of the work which discusses the Cephalaspidae. It would lighten the labor of future workers. The second volume of

[1] "The Downtonian and Devonian Vertebrates of Spitsbergen." Two volumes octavo, pp. 1–391, 1 map, 103 text-figures, 112 plates. Det Norske Videnskaps-Akademi I Oslo. Resultater av de Norske Statsunderstøttede Spitsbergenekspeditioner. Nr. 12, 1927.

112 plates, photographic in large part, leaves little to be desired. One may study these reproductions with a lens or reading glass with great profit. The descriptions of the plates are printed opposite the pictures, and they are given in full in each case—a praiseworthy feature.

Neurologists, especially those dealing with the brain and cranial nerves of fishes, will profit greatly by examining the author's discussion of the brain and adnexa of *Cephalaspis*. Stensiö tells us that he took two months to dissect the endocranial parts shown on plates 49 and 50. He finds the brain to be that of a cyclostome and on this basis as well as others, he says that the creatures we call Ostracoderms are cyclostomes. The differentiation of marginal electric fields will be a surprise, but while he has not defined the electroplaxes, yet it seems reasonable to agree that this neuro-muscular specialization may have taken place as early as the Silurian (Downtonian).

It has taken a long time to extricate the Ostracoderms from the eurypterids, from the arachnoids, from the annelids, but we feel that Stensiö has opened the way for us to believe, with him, that these early Paleozoic fishes are cyclostomes. The importance of this is very great, and if generally accepted will lead to still greater correlations. Our author says:

> It is clear now that the Ostracodermi, though very lowly organized, are true craniate vertebrates which have nothing whatever to do either with the Arthropoda or with the Annelida.
>
> The investigations carried out in this work have thus thrown light not only on the organization of the *Cephalaspidae,* but also on the Ostracodermi as a whole: and we have even been able to establish that the Ostracoderms still persist in the recent *Petromyzontia* and *Myxinoidea,* though they play a much less important part than during the early palaeozoic time.

Those who think the field of vertebrate paleontology is largely exhausted will receive a new stimulus in examining this work of Stensiö. It stirs our ambition to do further work to advance our knowledge of the vertebrates of ancient times. No more worthy scientific piece of work has appeared for decades and Stensiö is to be congratulated on the appearance of this, the most monumental study he has yet made.

ROY L. MOODIE
SANTA MONICA, CALIFORNIA

SCIENTIFIC APPARATUS AND LABORATORY METHODS

A UNIVERSAL MUSCLE LEVER

THE problem of providing a universal muscle lever for the use of students taking their first course in experimental physiology led to the construction of the apparatus here described. The requirements to be filled are not met, to the writer's knowledge, by any instrument on the market—a lever with well insulated "head," so arranged as to allow free adjustment in the horizontal plane, a strong after-loading screw, and, above all, an instrument constructed so sturdily as to withstand rough usage.

A number of attempts were made to modify other muscle levers to suit our requirements but without satisfactory results. Finally, with the assistance of a pattern-maker, a model somewhat like the one sketched in Figure 2 was constructed from soft pine and a few brass castings made. When finished and assembled, the instruments were found to be quite satsifactory.

This instrument consists of a handle, a lever holder or head, and a lever. The handle is made from a 6-inch length of 3/8 inch round bakelite rod which is slipped into the tubular end of a switchboard lug having an opening of that diameter. A hole is then drilled through the lug and the bakelite rod and the rod riveted into place. The flattened portion of the lug is centered and drilled to allow the passage of a number six machine screw.

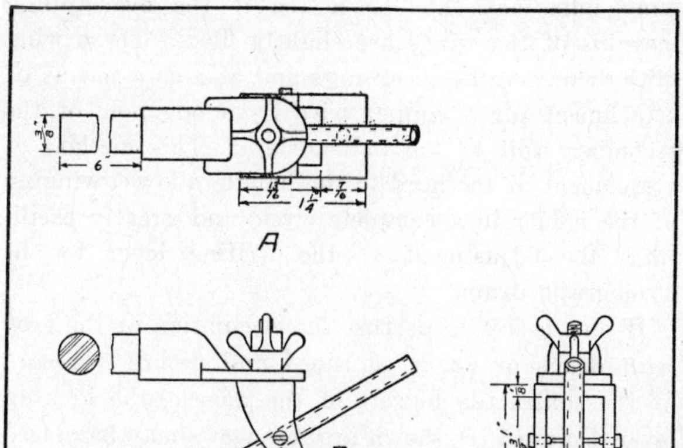

FIG. 1

The holder, the distinctive part of the apparatus, is made according to the dimensions given in Figure 1, A, B, C, showing top, side, and end views, respectively. This holder or head consists of a table, with dimensions as shown in the figure, from two parallel sides of which project downward and parallel to each other, two crescent shaped arms. Across the distal end of these arms is a bar, parallel to the table and 1/8 inch thick in order to support a 6/32 knurled head, brass, machine screw, the after-loading screw. Through the middle portion of the parallel crescents are drilled holes to receive 2-56 cup-pointed machine screws. These cups receive the pointed ends of the lever axle. The lever is made from a 3-inch length of 5/32 inch, outside diameter, brass tubing, which is drilled transversely at its middle point and a small brad soldered in place. Both ends of the brad are then sharpened to make an axle of sufficient length to fit the adjustment limits of the cup-pointed screws. The writing lever is made from a six to eight-inch length of split bamboo rod, about one eighth inch in diameter, and tipped with a small piece of thin brass shim.

The holder is firmly attached to the handle by means of a 6/32 brass machine screw which passes through the center of the table of the holder and whose head is countersunk in and soldered to the lower surface of the table. When assembled, this screw is passed through the hole in the handle and two wing nuts are placed thereon. It has been found that two wing nuts may thus be nested if the overlapping margins of the wings are slightly filed. These wing nuts then serve as check nuts and also as a means of attachment for a copper wire from one pole of the secondary coil of the inductorium. This method of attachment of the head to the handle allows swinging of the holder in a complete circle and greatly facilitates the adjustment of the writing lever to the kymograph drum.

If one desires to perfuse the circulation of the frog with drugs or sugar solutions and secure a record of the contractile powers of the muscle, the kick-up lever, Figure 1, D, shown in three views may be placed in the holder, the frog pinned in dorsal position for perfusion, and the graph made upon a slowly revolving drum.

Nickel- or preferably chromium-plating is useful to protect the brass from the action of sodium chloride and greatly improves the appearance of the apparatus.

Casting of the holders: Reference has been made to the casting of these holders or heads. In Figure 2, A and B, are shown the top and side views, respectively, of the pattern used for casting three holders. It is much more convenient to cast eight or ten holders at a time and partially finish them upon a shaper or milling machine than to cast a lesser number. After partially finishing the castings, they are sawed apart with a machine hack-saw and finished by hand. In all probability jigs could be made which would facilitate this work; but for the number of holders finished, the trouble involved in making jigs was not considered necessary.

In September, 1926, about eighteen of these muscle

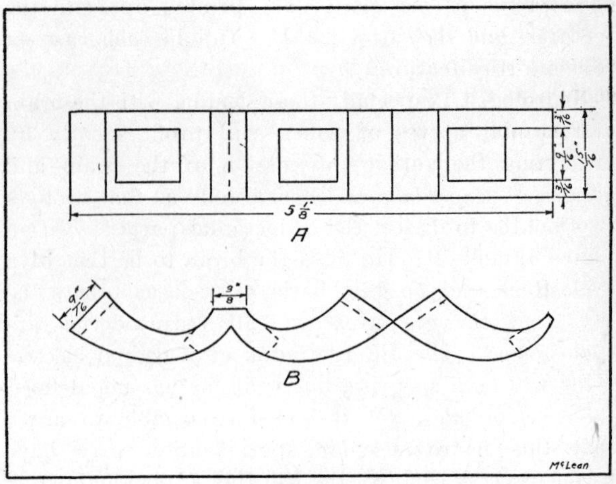

Fig. 2

levers were made and since that time, they have been used by over 600 students working in groups. These levers have been used for recording a simple muscle twitch, for demonstrating the maximum lifting power of a muscle, as well as numerous other experiments, and have given no trouble whatever.

Although this lever is as yet a relatively crude product, finished by hand, it has the following advantages:

1. An insulating handle or support rod;
2. An adjustable head with after-loading screw;
3. It may be used to record the responses of muscles reacting in either the vertical or horizontal plane;
4. It is sufficiently rugged that it will withstand the rough usage of college sophomores who are more accustomed to the manipulation of five-year-old Fords than to the delicate equipment of a physiological laboratory.

A. R. McLaughlin

Michigan State College,
East Lansing

METHOD FOR GROWING SMALL-SEEDED PLANTS UNDER STERILE CONDITIONS

The accompanying figure diagrammatically shows the principal details of a method now being used at the Massachusetts Agricultural Experiment Station for growing tobacco plants under sterile conditions.

In the middle opening of a 3-neck Wolff bottle is placed a plug (H) of absorbent cotton which serves both as a substratum for the plantlet and a wick for the nutrient solution (I). Before seeding, the entire apparatus as shown, with the exception of the layer of nutrient agar (G) and the celluloid cover (D), is set up and sterilized under steam pressure. Then, under aseptic conditions, the thin layer of nutrient agar is added, the seed planted in it, and the cover put on. A glass cover could under some circumstances be advantageously substituted for the celluloid cover.

Sterile non-absorbent cotton is used for protecting exposed openings. After the plantlets grow large enough to fill the cover, it may be removed, all but one plant removed and sterile cotton worked around it, if it be desired to grow it further.

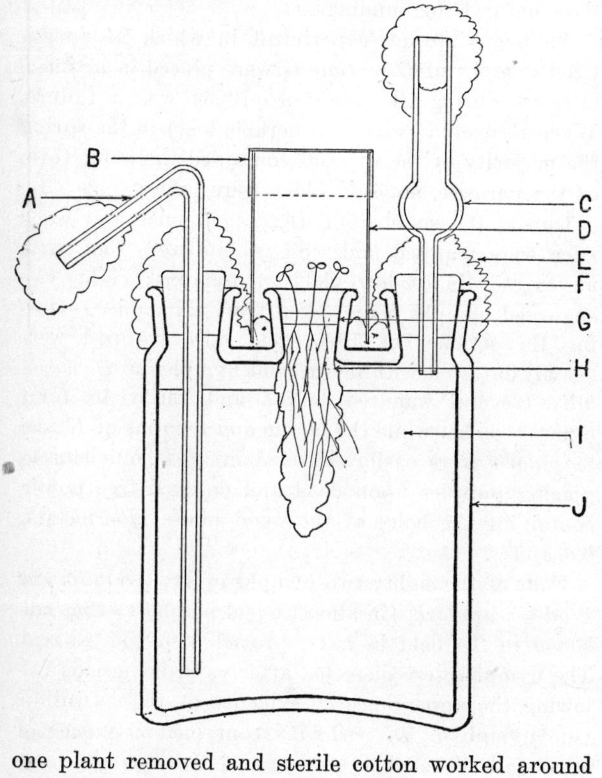

This method was especially worked out for tobacco, but seems applicable to any small-seeded plant whose plantlet is small, slow-growing and difficult to transplant under aseptic conditions. It differs from other proposed methods in that (1) the plantlet remains in the original substratum and (2) that a layer of nutrient agar is introduced to indicate asepticism.

A. B. BEAUMONT
G. J. LARSINOS
MASSACHUSETTS AGRICULTURAL COLLEGE

SPECIAL ARTICLES

THE OVERWINTERING IN MASSACHUSETTS OF IXODIPHAGUS CAUCURTEI

THE purpose of this communication is to record the overwintering of *Ixodiphagus caucurtei*, a hymenopterous chalcidian parasite of ticks, introduced upon the Island of Naushon for the control of *Dermacentor variabilis*, the common dog tick of Eastern Massachusetts.

This fly was discovered by Professor E. Brumpt in nymphs of *Ixodes ricinus* taken in the neighborhood of Paris (Chantilly and Fontainebleau). It was described by M. R. du Buysson in 1912 (*Archives de Parasitologie*, xv, p. 246). Its use for the control of ticks responsible for the transmission of diseases, including Rocky Mountain spotted fever, was proposed by Brumpt in 1913 in a short article "Utilisation des Insectes auxiliares entomophages dans la lutte contre les Insectes pathogénes" (*La Presse Médicale,* No. 36 du 3 Mai 1913). In this article Brumpt records the parasitization by this fly of the following species in addition to *Ixodes ricinus*:

Haemaphysalis concinna
Rhipicephalus sanguineus
Dermacentor andersoni

It is pertinent to recall in connection with this report early work of L. O. Howard. In 1907, he described and figured the first chalcid parasite of a tick and established the genus *Ixodiphagus* in his description of *Ixodiphagus texanus.* (*Ent. News,* xviii (1907), pp. 375–378). His specimens were obtained from nymphs of the rabbit tick *Haemaphysalis leporis-palustris,* Packard, collected in Jackson County, Texas. In 1908 (*Canadian Entomologist,* xl, p. 239–241) he described and figured another chalcid parasite, *Hunterellus hookeri* (tribe Ixodiphagini), obtained from nymphs of *Rhipicephalus texanus,* Banks, taken from a dog at Corpus Christi, Texas.

An unsuccessful attempt to introduce *Hunterellus hookeri* into South Africa is described by C. P. Lounsbury in 1908 (Rept. Govt. Entomologist for 1908, Cape of Good Hope, Appendix iv, p. 65.)

The Naushon experiment is probably the first adequately conducted attempt—apparently successful—involving the introduction and acclimatization of a chalcid parasite of ticks. Dr. S. B. Wolbach had long been interested in the possibilities suggested by Brumpt's brief paper, inasmuch as *Ixodiphagus caucurtei* already existed in a climate not too unlike that of certain Rocky Mountain spotted fever territories to preclude probability of acclimatization. The hope of ultimate utilization of the fly for control of the Rocky Mountain spotted fever ticks was the deciding factor in the decision to try first this method in an attempt to alleviate the heavy tick (*D. variabilis*) infestation of the privately owned island of Naushon, near Woods Hole, Massachusetts. Hence an altruistic spirit as well as a desire for relief from annoyance prompted the owners of the island in their financial support of this experiment. The Department of Pathology of the Harvard Medical School made necessary preparations, provided materials and equipment, and an assistant, Mr. Arthur G. King.

Professor Brumpt received the idea with great enthusiasm and gave permission for his assistant, Dr. F. Larrousse, to undertake the actual conduction of the experiment, which was begun in May, 1926, following the arrival of Dr. Larrousse in this country.

The fly was obtained from the Forest of Fontainebleau. A total of nine deer skins was examined in Professor Brumpt's laboratory between January 12th and March 23rd, 1925, for ticks. In all, 1,205 were collected, the following species being represented: *Ixodes ricinus, Dermacentor reticulatus, Haemaphysalis inermis, Haemaphysalis concinna.* There were 94 nymphs of *Ixodes ricinus,* one of which was parasitized with *Ixodiphagus caucurtei.* From the parasites which emerged from this nymph the strain was propagated in the laboratory.

Dr. Larrousse brought to this country parasitized nymphs of *Dermacentor reticulatus, Rhipicephalus sanguineus* as well as larvae, unparasitized nymphs and adults of both species.

Adults of two species of ticks (*Dermacentor variabilis* and *Rhipicephalus sanguineus*) were collected at Naushon and nymphs raised from these were parasitized in the laboratory of pathology of the Harvard Medical School.

Dermacentor variabilis proved to be easily parasitized by *Ixodiphagus caucurtei,* though difficult to rear in the laboratory as the larvae attached to guinea-pigs and rabbits in small numbers only. Later with Dr. Larrousse's discovery of a natural host of the larvae and nymphs of this species—the common field mouse, *Microtus pennsylvanicus pennsylvanicus,* the rearing and parasitization of nymphs was much facilitated in the field laboratory established at Naushon. Another species of tick, *Ixodes scapularis,* was found in great numbers upon the island and proved also to be easily parasitized by *Ixodiphagus caucurtei.* The normal host of the larvae and nymphs of this tick was found to be the white-footed wood-mouse, *Peromyscus leucopus,* but both larvae and nymphs readily attached to rabbits and guinea-pigs.

Other species of ticks found in smaller numbers upon the island were *Rhipicephalus sanguineus* and *Haemaphysalis leporis-palustris,* the latter found but once.

Experiment proved that nymphs of *Dermacentor variabilis* attached to rabbits become parasitized in the field by flies liberated at distances of 50 and 100 meters, no greater distances being tried in the experiment.

Three methods were used in introducing the parasites.

1. Large numbers of the flies were liberated in situations where nymphs of *Ixodes scapularis* were numerous and in other regions where *Dermacentor variabilis* abounded.

2. Parasitized nymphs of *Ixodes scapularis* were returned to their original situations, mouse holes, etc.

3. Domestic mice (*Mus domesticus*) and field mice (*Microtus pennsylvanicus pennsylvanicus*) with parasitized nymphs still attached were liberated amidst their natural surroundings.

An overwintering experiment in which 34 parasitized nymphs of *D. variabilis* were placed in artificial burrows during the late fall (1926) was a failure. When recovered (with considerable loss) in the spring the majority of the nymphs contained the adult form of the parasite, none of which were living.

During the summer of 1927, field mice and wood mice were trapped and wild rabbits were shot, with an extraordinary low yield of nymphs; eighty-two engorged nymphs being taken from sixty mice. During the summer of 1926, field mice trapped were heavily infested with larvae and nymphs of *D. variabilis* (several hundred larvae and thirty to forty nymphs each), while the larvae and nymphs of *Ixodes scapularis* were easily collected in great numbers by placing puppies upon dead and decayed tree trunks containing the holes of the wood-mouse (*Peromyscus leucopus*).

Four of the eighty-two nymphs of *D. variabilis* and *Ixodes scapularis* (in almost equal numbers) thus collected in the field in 1927, proved to be parasitized. The nymphs were dissected after varying periods following the appearance of evidence of parasitization. One nymph of *D. variabilis* contained a cluster of eggs with developed embryos of *Ixodiphagus caucurtei,* two contained full-grown larvae. One nymph of *Ixodes scapularis* was dissected after the lapse of ample time with failure of the fly to emerge; fully developed adults were found.

These results, though scanty, proved that *Ixodiphagus caucurtei* had survived a New England winter under natural conditions and had propagated itself. It would be perhaps premature to attribute the extraordinary reduction in ticks noticed in 1927 to the parasite alone. Quantitative methods of estimating the tick population were not employed. The difficulty of obtaining larvae and nymphs of *D. variabilis* and *I. scapularis* in 1927 has been noted above. A similar diminution in adult ticks was also noted. Whereas in July, 1926, the ticks, *D. variabilis* in particular, were so numerous that a brief walk through certain places always resulted in the collection of from 30 to 40 ticks upon one's clothing, in July, 1927, the same procedure would yield only an occasional tick, often none at all. Likewise the heavy infestation of domestic animals, cats, dogs, sheep and horses annually experienced disappeared in 1927. This notable decrease of ticks on Naushon was in marked contrast to conditions on the adjacent mainland—Cape Cod, where ticks were unusually numerous at several different points, hence the influence of climatic conditions may be excluded.

Further observations will be made at Naushon during 1928. It is a great source of satisfaction that a similar and more elaborate experiment with the same strain of *Ixodiphagus caucurtei* is under way in Montana, in the Bitter Root Range, under the able direction of Professor R. A. Cooley (*Medical Sentinel*, December, 1927).

Thanks are due to Dr. L. O. Howard for his kindly offices relative to the introduction of the parasite into this country; to Dr. Henry S. Forbes and the owners of Naushon, for their actual participation in the experiment, hospitality and financial support.

F. Larrousse
Arthur G. King
S. B. Wolbach

AN EFFICIENCY FORMULA FOR DAIRY COWS

In 1901 Jordan[1] called attention to the differences in efficiency of the various species of domestic animals as converters of animal feeds into human food materials. He gave the production of pounds of "edible solids" per 100 pounds of "digestible organic matter" in the ration as, in part, follows:

Animal and Product	Edible Solids
Cow, Milk	18.0
Hog, Carcass	15.6
Calf, Carcass	8.1
Fowl, Egg	5.1
Fowl, Carcass	4.2
Steer, Carcass	2.8
Sheep, Carcass	2.6

These figures still pass current as representing the efficiency of the animal producer. Jordan clearly pointed out that the figures given are average values and subject to considerable variation, according to various conditions of management, and as between individual members of the species.

With respect to milk production by the cow it is well known that the efficiency of production depends to a great extent upon the annual yield of milk. This note presents a formula for the estimation of a coefficient of efficiency based on the weight and annual yield of the cow. It is intended further to suggest the significance of milking capacity in the dairy cow from the standpoint of the future of the milk supply. Foods of animal origin are inherently expensive, and their consumption has always become more or less restricted with increasing population. Naturally, the more efficient the animal converter the less such restriction need apply. The significance of the efficient cow to the people at large may be better appreciated when we realize that about 45 per cent. of all animal foods consumed in the United States come from dairy cattle.[2]

The coefficient here proposed is essentially similar to the ratio of Jordan, but with this modification, that digestible nutrients[3] (D. N.) are substituted for his "edible solids" on the one side, and also for his "digestible organic matter" on the other side. Accordingly the coefficient of efficiency (C. E.) is $100 \times$ (digestible nutrients in milk produced) $\div$ (digestible nutrients in food consumed). How is this coefficient related to the annual milk yield and weight of the cow?

The digestible nutrients of the milk will vary with the quantity and quality of the milk. The richness of the milk may be disposed of by expressing the yield in terms of 4-per cent. (fat) milk by use of the formula,[4] F. C. M. = .4M + 15F, where F. C. M. is fat-corrected milk or 4-per cent. milk, M is the actual milk, and F is fat; all in pounds. One pound F. C. M. = .172 pounds of digestible nutrients; and, therefore (digestible nutrients in milk produced) = .172 F. C. M.

The remaining variable factor in the coefficient may be estimated from Haecker's[5] data. His maintenance standard is, Digestible nutrients for maintenance per year = 2.893 W, where W is live weight of the cow in pounds. His data show[6] that, Digestible nutrients for lactation = .327 F. C. M.

By substitution and a simple transformation we have the formula:

$$\text{C. E.} = 52.6 \frac{\text{F. C. M.}}{\text{F. C. M.} + 8.847\ \text{W}}$$

[1] "The Feeding of Animals."

[2] Pearl, "The Nation's Food." This estimate is based on total calories and allows a small but proper credit for the beef and veal derived from dairy stock. Swine supply another forty per cent. It has been often stated, on the basis of the superior efficiency of the cow and hog, that they will be the surviving animals. From the standpoint of food consumption it might be better to say that they *are* the surviving animals.

[3] Protein + carbohydrates + fat × 2.25. It might be better to replace digestible nutrients by net energy if our knowledge of the properties of various feeds in this respect were adequate.

[4] *Bul.* 245, Ill. Agr. Exp. Sta.

[5] *Bul.* 140, Minn. Agr. Exp. Sta.

[6] *Bul.* —, Ill. Agr. Exp. Sta. (in press).

The factor, 52.6, represents the percentage efficiency of the mammary gland itself. The fractional factor shows the proportion of this efficiency which is realized when the additional nutrients required for body maintenance are included. As an example, if the cow weighs 1,000 pounds and her annual yield is 8,847 pounds F. C. M., the maintenance and lactation requirements are equal, and one half of the potential efficiency of the mammary gland is realized by the whole organism; that is, C. E. = 26.3.

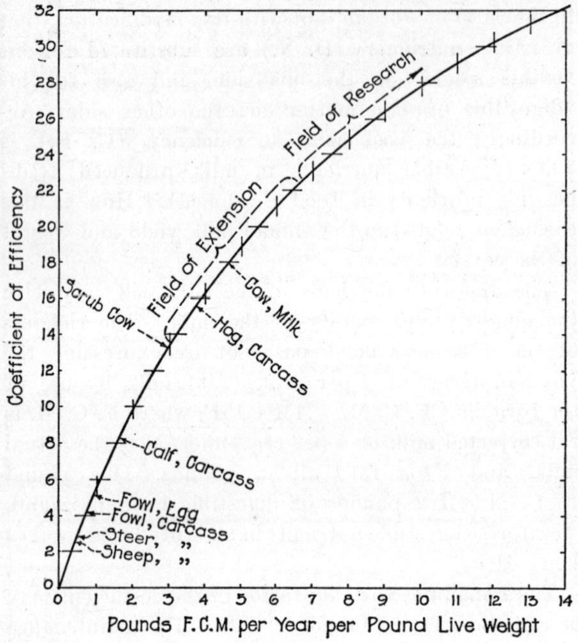

FIG. 1

EFFICIENCY CURVE OF THE COW IN MILK PRODUCTION

The arrows at the right indicate Jordan's average efficiency values for various species. The arrow at the left indicates the average efficiency of the unimproved cow. The first bracket denotes the improvement which may now be readily effected. The second bracket suggests the possibility of still further improvement through the efforts of the breeder and investigator.

Figure 1 illustrates the C. E. curve graphically for yields and weights up to 14,000 pounds F. C. M. per 1,000 pounds live weight. The efficiency values of Jordan, above quoted, are indicated by the arrows at the right of the curve, although they are not strictly comparable with the present formula. It will be noted that the sheep, the steer and the fowl compare in efficiency with a 1,000-pound cow producing 500 to 1,000 pounds F. C. M. per year.

Jordan's efficiency figure for the cow is considerably larger than may be expected of the unimproved animal, whose probable position is indicated by the arrow at the left of the C. E curve. But it is entirely feasible by present known methods of mating and feeding to create and maintain a stock superior in efficiency to Jordan's figure, say up to C. E. = 22 or 23. This may be designated the field of extension, in which so much productive work has been accomplished by the Smith-Lever or corresponding forces of the Land-Grant Colleges, and in which so much still remains to be accomplished. Beyond this there lies the promising field of research in nutrition and in genetics, in which we may possibly hope some day to realize an efficiency of say, C. E. = 30. This, however, is a difficult goal for, according to the formula, C. E. = 30 requires 11,744 pounds of 4-per cent. milk per year per 1,000 pounds live weight, a capacity quite beyond any present certainty of the industry.

Finally, as to the accuracy of the C. E. formula we may consider the very extensive and practical cross-breeding experiments of the Danes. The following figures, adapted from Frederiksen,[7] are the average yearly results for over 1,000 cows during a period of 10 years:

Breed of Cows	Red Danish	Crossbred	Jersey
Weight, lbs.	1021	913	796
Milk, lbs.	7934	6389	5018
Fat, per cent.	3.60	4.28	5.34
Fat, lbs.	286	273	268
F. C. M., lbs.	7458	6657	6027
D. N. in milk, lbs.	1283	1145	1037
D. N. in feed, lbs.	5388	4809	4347
Observed C. E.	23.8	23.8	23.9
Computed C. E.	23.8	23.8	24.3

The C. E. formula is in excellent agreement with these observed average results. As between individual cows we may expect some variability, and the formula may not be expected to apply to some of the advanced registry records of the dairy breeds in this country, where extravagant feeding and delayed breeding have been practiced. But under conservative practices of feeding and breeding (recurrence of conception) it should serve as an index of the relation between yield and efficiency for a given weight.

To determine the milk and fat yields of individual cows is now well recognized as advanced dairy practice. The present formula clearly shows that a record of the weight of the cow as well as her yield is necessary to afford a useful index of her efficiency. Since the weight of dairy cows varies from less than 500 pounds to more than a ton, the weight factor can not be ignored.

W. L. GAINES

AGRICULTURAL EXPERIMENT STATION,
UNIVERSITY OF ILLINOIS

[7] Meddelels 2, Forsøgslaboratoriets Husdyrbrugsafdeling (Copenhagen).

SCIENCE

VOL. LXVII APRIL 6, 1928 No. 1736

CONTENTS

The Physiologic Life: PROFESSOR A. J. CARLSON 355
A Revision of the Fundamental Law of Habit Formation: PROFESSOR KNIGHT DUNLAP 360
Henri Bosmans: PROFESSOR FLORIAN CAJORI 362
Scientific Events:
International Society for the Exploration of the Arctic Regions by Means of the Airship; The Reorganization of the Post-Graduate Medical School and Hospital; The St. Louis Meeting of the American Chemical Society; The Milton Research Awards of Harvard University 363
Scientific Notes and News 365
University and Educational Notes 369
Discussion and Correspondence:
A Periodic Classification of the Hardness and Melting-points of the Elements: DR. S. A. KORFF. *Further Evidence concerning Man's Antiquity in Oklahoma:* HAROLD J. COOK. *The Geology of Sonora:* DR. GRAHAM JOHN MITCHELL. *Threatened Extinction of the Ruffed Grouse:* BIRGER R. HEADSTROM. *What is a Name?* PROFESSOR WM. T. M. FORBES 370
Scientific Books:
West's Treatise on the British Freshwater Algae: PROFESSOR CHARLES A. KOFOID. *Fischer's Gewebezellen:* ALBERT H. EBELING 373
Scientific Apparatus and Laboratory Methods:
Method for Demonstrating the Diffusion of Oxygen through Rubber: SAMUEL E. HILL 374
Special Articles:
The Production of Mutations and Rearrangements of Genes by X-Rays: DR. ALEXANDER WEINSTEIN. *A Determination of the Newtonian Constant of Gravitation by a Study of the Vibrations of a Torsion Pendulum:* T. E. STERN 376
Science News x

SCIENCE: A Weekly Journal devoted to the Advancement of Science, edited by J. McKeen Cattell and published every Friday by

THE SCIENCE PRESS

New York City: Grand Central Terminal.

Lancaster, Pa. Garrison, N. Y.

Annual Subscription, $6.00. Single Copies, 15 Cts.

SCIENCE is the official organ of the American Association for the Advancement of Science. Information regarding membership in the Association may be secured from the office of the permanent secretary, in the Smithsonian Institution Building, Washington, D. C.

THE PHYSIOLOGIC LIFE[1]

WE know to-day many factors that injure the individual, and a few that seem to injure the race. But in our almost complete ignorance of the mechanisms of race improvement, we seem impotent on the positive side, except that by eliminating those who deviate markedly from the average we may give the latter group more elbow room. By selection and controlled breeding we seem to be able to secure a fatter hog and a faster horse. Have we thereby secured a better hog and a better horse?

Assuming that we know how to achieve fundamental race improvement, is there any agreement as to the goal? Is the super model of *homo sapiens* to be constructed on the line of a Mussolini, a Gandhi, an Einstein, a Dempsey, a Darwin or a Henry Ford? Is he to be "wet" or "dry"? Should he be white, black, yellow, brown, pink or gray? Should he be six or sixty feet tall? Should he be a more rational or a more emotional machine? Is he to be a pacifist or a man fitted to wage bigger and better wars? Are we to aim at a better coordinated society of masters and slaves or a democracy?

The present state of development of man and his fellow animals has come about through the forces of heredity and environment, practically without an iota of conscious direction based on accumulated experience. The time during which we have had even an approximate understanding of our physiological processes, and the factors that favor or impede the same, is so short that it may virtually be ignored in the total time span that man and other animals have existed upon the earth. If we knew what our forebears ate and drank (and how much); if we knew how they worked, rested, loved, we could with greater certainty put the labels "favorable" and "unfavorable" on the manner of living and on the man-made environment of to-day.

We may assume that the present man is the best possible product of past conditions. In what respects do conditions of human life to-day differ from those of yesterday, and do any of the new conditions bode ill for to-morrow?

1. Modern man cooks, preserves, sterilizes and denatures his food to a greater extent than his forebears.

2. Modern man lives under more uniform climatic

[1] Address given at the third Race Betterment Conference, Battle Creek, Michigan, January, 1928.

conditions because of clothes, houses and fire. Also, in consequence of these, he lives less in the open and farther from the sun than did the primitive man.

3. As a consequence of industrial developments and growth of cities a large proportion of men of to-day are more crowded, more subject to polluted air, polluted drinking water and industrial poisoning than our ancestors.

4. As a consequence of the growth of knowledge, particularly of chemistry and medicine, man of to-day is being subjected to a greater variety and quantity of stimulants and drugs.

5. Because of greater knowledge of nature modern man has less fear, but probably more anxiety than the man of the past.

6. The sex life of modern man seems ill-adjusted to prevailing social theory and practice. We do not know, but it seems probable, that the very ancients lived a more biological sex life.

7. In consequence of the growth of knowledge, art, industry and invention, man of to-day is probably subjected to a more continuous, if not more varied, nerve strain than in the remote past. We have accumulating evidence that excessive brain activity may interfere with some fundamental physiological processes, as a powerful gas engine may shake to pieces a less solidly built chassis.

Foods

We may assume that our forebears (as well as all other animals in all ages) have from time to time been subjected to quantitative under-nutrition, that is, starvation. In tropical climates this is merely a question of the number of animals and quantity of available food. In temperate climates it is also a question of seasons. To be sure, many animals have become adapted in relation to the second factor, they have become accustomed to prolonged inactivity and starvation (hibernation). We have no evidence that man himself ever was a hibernating animal. But we think it is safe to assume that modern man has reached his present stage of perfection (or imperfection) through periods of quantitative under-nutrition as well as periods of gorging in the presence of plenty. There is no reason to think that our ancestors, any more than their fellow animals or modern man refrained from eating far above their actual physiological needs if plenty of food was available. It seems probable that qualitative under-nutrition, that is, diets lacking for a long time in essential salts, essential vitamins, essential proteins and in essential roughage, was probably less prevalent among our primitive ancestors, because cooking and food refining is a late acquisition. If this is correct, it follows that most of our food-deficiency diseases, excepting, of course, those that are brought on as a result of quantitative starvation, are man-made diseases. I refer to the various pathological processes induced by lack of vitamins, by lack of adequate proteins, by lack of roughage in the food and by lack of proper salts in the food. Man has brought these on himself largely through misguided esthetics and perverted taste, and by commercialism not controlled by physiologic knowledge.

We should add in all fairness that as man is now distributed on the earth various types of food preservation or sterilization is a necessity, not only preservation from season to season, but such preservation that food can be shipped long distances from one country to another where the density of population is in excess of the ability of the country to feed it. The problem of food preservation and a food purification is one of commanding importance to our race to-day, because in this respect industrial processes and dietary habits of long standing are only slowly brought under control of physiologic knowledge. We still mill our grain and feed the bran to hogs and cattle. This may help to develop super hogs and super cattle, but it is no aid to the physiologic life of man.

On the basis of our present knowledge of the physiology of man, the old question of vegetarianism *vs.* foods of animal origin has little or no merit in fact. There is no doubt that the individual man can injure himself temporarily and possibly permanently by the overeating of meat. Possibly our very remote ancestors were strictly herbivorous; the earliest animals must, perforce, until they turned cannibals, have been herbivorous, but man, as we know him to-day, can use food of animal origin with impunity and physiological profit. We should say that the more nearly omnivorous the human individual is, the more certain he is to avoid diseases due to faulty diets. Indeed, it would be more conducive to the physiologic life if we set about, through education, to remove the present human prejudices against certain species of animals as sources of food than to keep alive the "religious" superstitions that some or all foods of animal origin are taboo. I refer to such notions as "clean" and "unclean" animals handed down to us by the laws of Moses, the abstaining from meat on the basis of "transmigration of souls," the eschewing of certain animals as food because they look repulsive or disagreeable or because they are friends of man. Almost any species of animals, by proper training, can be made the apparent friend of man. If the present rapid increase in population continues we should contribute more to the physiologic life by teaching universal omnivorousness than by clinging to ideas handed down to us by the ignorant past or dictated by the whims of imagination. The eel is not a poisonous article of food merely because it has the body form of a snake; the snake itself is not bad eating despite the alleged rôle of the snake in the "fall of man." By omnivorous I do not mean food of animal origin alone; I mean also a much greater extension of the use of the vegetable kingdom. Sailors learned to cure scurvy by a decoction of pine needles when nothing else was at hand. It is hinted that the eating of grass by Nebuchadnezzar was a "curse of God," while, as a matter of fact, it was part of wisdom.

With every new advance in the knowledge of the specific rôle or of specific needs for food elements, there blossom forth commercial enterprises whose advertising tends to confuse the public mind. Thus, we are urged to buy vitamin concentrates over the drug counter instead of natural foods at the grocery store. We eliminate roughage from the food and try to palliate constipation by mineral oils. We are made to believe by persistent advertising that we are on the brink of an abyss unless cod-liver oil, yeast or nuxated iron is ingested daily. We are taught to identify whiteness or absence of color in many foods with purity and, by inference, wholesomeness of such food articles.

The problem of obesity in the human individual is largely a question of overeating and under-exercising. To what extent overeating may contribute to race deterioration it is difficult to say, because that implies injury to the germ plasm; the possible injury to the individual is of little racial significance.

Work

If we survey the animal kingdom as it exists today it seems, by and large, that except for the play of the young, the only exercise taken is that rendered necessary for the securing of food, the propagation of the species and escape from pain. Of course, in all animals living in temperate or colder climates, cold itself, for the warm-blooded animal like man, is efficient physical exercise. But when not driven by hunger or sex most animals (including man) are lazy. It is highly probable therefore that man has reached his present state of development on the basis of exercise largely determined by physical necessities. This rule still applies to the majority of humans the world over. The majority have no accumulated food reserves. Most of us have to do physical work every day for a living. The problem of race deterioration from physical inactivity applies therefore only to a small portion of society, the so-called well-to-do, who can through their wealth command the satisfaction of most needs without individual physical exertion. There is no question in the case of many of the body organs that a certain amount of atrophy and deterioration follows in the wake of disuse, and consequently, activity, however caused, is within limits beneficial. But does such physical inactivity cause deterioration of the germ-plasm? And at what point does excess of physical work lead to germ-plasm degeneration? Biology has as yet no clear answer to these questions.

Housing

The only abodes of our most ancient forebears that have survived to historic time are natural caves, but even assuming that humans were not very numerous in those days, I doubt whether there were caves enough to house them all. And it is not unlikely that our forebears lived in trees for some time before they stepped down into caves. The caves of our forebears were probably no healthier than modern apartments. Some type of hole in the ground, or on the ground, seems necessary as a protection against the rigors of climate. But modern industry demands and creates these holes in ever-increasing numbers of horizontal layers. The influence of city life on the race is a large problem, without an answer as yet. It is a question not only of sunlight and pure air, but of crowding, of infections, of immunity, noise, glare, mimicry and exhaustion. A place under the ultraviolet lamp may be a safe substitute for the place in the sun. Many species of animals have not only survived but apparently made continued progress in almost total absence of sunlight. I do not refer to animals living permanently in caves, because in many of these we see some signs of degeneration, probably because the cave of life has been adopted too suddenly, but I refer to animals that during the day live in caves or holes in the ground and hunt for their food during the night. Pollution of air and water by modern cities and modern industry is on the increase, and the probable danger from these conditions seems only partly appreciated by society. Formerly, lead poisoning was largely confined to workers in lead industries. Now lead is blown into the air from the exhaust of nearly every automobile. Lead and arsenic are taken into our system with the apple and the pear. We may not inhale enough lead in our breathing or consume enough lead and arsenic in our fruit to produce acute poisoning and tissue injury, but who is there to say that this slow assimilation of metallic poisons brought about by modern industry is without danger and ultimate injury? The only factor of safety that I can see in this situation is the phenomenon of tolerance, that is, the capacity of the living organism, if it is not seriously wrecked by the poisons, to so adjust the internal processes as to render the poisons less and less injurious. Tolerance means physiologic compromise, but such continued existence does not necessarily mean the higher life. Continued increase of population means increased growth of cities, increased industrial concentration and increased industrial poisoning, despite all measures to eliminate the latter.

The Sex Life

One of the fundamental physiologic processes that at present seems to be out of adjustment to a greater extent in man than in our fellow animals is sex life. We are not agreed as to what is the normal sex life of modern man, but ethical leaders in all races have on the whole tended to the view that sex activity should and can be repressed or consciously controlled by the individual or society to a greater extent than the urge of hunger and thirst or the call for evacuation of the bowels. In many if not most animals the essential sex urge is seasonal and closely associated with reproduction, and, as a rule, the reproductive processes in animals start with sexual maturity and continue throughout the sex life of the individual. In most parts of the world human society is now so organized and human habits fixed in such a way that approved sexual intercourse can not start with sexual maturity in our children. This means a long period of sex repression, "illegitimate" sexual intercourse, or perverted sex practices. It is held by many, though in most cases physiologically unproved, that these three sequelae of our modern social orders as related to sex life are injurious to body and brain. The physiologist may view the mental gymnastics of the Freudians with wonder, but he is not in position to state that the present social practices as to sex are the best possible for the present or future of the race. The physiologist is puzzled by the evidence in modern man of a sex drive in excess of the need of reproduction. He is aware of the speculation that the sex drive means more than reproduction, that it is the basis of all progress in inventions, in art, in warfare, in practically everything in which modern man seems to have exceeded the ancients. If this is the case, the physiologist should not concern himself with the means of controlling or delaying the sex urge. The solution is birth control. The greater continuity and persistence of the sex urge in man than in most of the other animals may be related to the greater brain development (memory, imagination). If this is correct we have here an instance of uncorrelated development, that is, development of one organ or process leading to discoordination or injury of another.

Stimulants and Narcotics

The indulgence in narcotics and stimulants antedates chemical knowledge, but chemistry and commerce have greatly enlarged the field. We not only isolate and concentrate new drugs from plant and animal tissues, but almost every day records the synthesis of new drugs in the laboratory. Individual and organized greed extends the facilities for drug addiction.

Do not expect me to say anything new and true on the alcohol question as related to race betterment. People have imbibed alcohol in the past, have lived and reproduced. It is not difficult to prove the deterioration of the individual, and in some cases the offspring, by excessive alcoholic indulgence. Man appears, by and large, to be the only animal with the alcohol habit. All human races can become alcohol addicts unless checked by ethical considerations. "Tolerance" to alcohol has not yet been acquired by the race as a whole. Alcohol may be indifferent in race improvement, but if the issue is forced to-day, the physiologists must vote against alcohol on the basis of probable injury.

No word can be said in defense of the other narcotic drugs. Their influence on normal life seems to be uniformly injurious, except possibly in the direction of protection of the brain against the over-stimulation and over-fatigue of the modern man-made environment. There are instances from experimental laboratories of morphine, barbital or ether protecting the brain or parts of the brain from fatal effects of such stimulation or from otherwise fatal effects of acute poisoning.

I know of no evidence that the alkaloids of coffee, tea and tobacco improve the individual or the species. Whether they are factors leading to race deterioration is an open question. Many people believe that this is the case, but belief is not knowledge. Some weight should be given to the fact that during the period that many humans have indulged in these substances, man has made rapid progress in externals, but this progress has probably been made despite this indulgence rather than because of it.

Modern chemistry has opened up another avenue of poisoning the human system through the field of food preservatives and food substitutes. We have the problem of the harmfulness or the harmlessness of the various baking powders, of benzoic acid as a permissible food preservative, of saccharine as a substitute for sugar, etc. Many of the experiments purporting to prove the permissibility or harmlessness of the substance or preservative, even those carried out by competent scientists, seem to me wholly inadequate. I have in mind, as an example, the experiments and finding of the Remsen Consulting Board, on the question of saccharine in foods. Under the direction of this board, composed of leading biochemists and chemists, varying quantities of saccharine were fed to a small number of healthy young men, daily, for periods up to nine months. The board concluded that the daily ingestion of this food substitute below a certain quantity (.3 gram per day) is without injurious effects; above this saccharine produces injury. This conclusion became guide to federal legislation and regulation. Was the above conclusion warranted by the experiments performed? We think not. All the experiments proved was that the substance (saccharine) when taken by healthy young men over this period did not produce any injury that the commission could detect by the tests used. Society is composed of individuals other than healthy young men, and nine months is a short period in the span of human life. There are many deviations of physiological processes that can not be detected by body weight, food intake, or the chemical examination of the urine. Most of the organs in the body can be injured a great deal before we become actually sick. It would seem a safer principle for governments and society to insist that the burden of proof of harmlessness falls on the manufacturer or the introducer of the new food substitutes rather than on society, and the test of the harmfulness or harmlessness should involve all physiological processes of man.

THE INVISIBLE ENEMIES

There are people who believe that the future progress of the human race will be measured by our success in eradicating infectious organisms (preventive medicine), and in such complete understanding of physiological processes as to enable us to control the processes of immunity. Paleopathology furnishes no conclusive evidence that races or species now extinct were slain by infectious diseases. Far be it from me, as a worker in one corner of the medical garden, to minimize the importance of medical science both in the preservative and in the curative aspect of race betterment. But I can not see how mere prolongation of the individual life span or mere multiplication of human individuals will enhance human evolution. Indeed the reverse argument is not easily met, namely, that medical science to-day helps to deteriorate the race by helping the biologically weak to survive and reproduce. Knowledge of the processes of immunity sufficient to enable us to augment this factor in the individual, apart from what we already know in a general way of hereditary strain, improved nutrition and hygienic surroundings, seems far afield; but, again, it may come faster than the most optimistic prediction.

Eradication of infectious organisms or complete control of the individual infection by chemotherapy seems Utopian. The scientist who ventures to prophesy to-day has a good prospect of being shown up a fool to-morrow. But it seems likely that the human race will survive (and in fair if not improved shape) all now known infectious organisms, not by the process of eradication or scientifically controlled immunity, but by the process of tolerance and symbiosis. Whether this prospect is cheerful or abhorrent depends on whether the symbiosis involves the loss of any essential element of further evolution of our species.

CLIMATE AND HUMAN EVOLUTION

Some one has remarked that our planet is better fitted for pisciculture than for human culture, since water covers the greater area of the earth's surface. The cradle (or cradles) of the human race is not yet located, hence the climatic conditions of early human evolution is one of the many unknowns in the process. But to-day, man (as well as the rat, the body louse and the English sparrow) covers practically all of the land, so that we have all the possibilities for favorable and unfavorable evolution so far as evolution is conditioned by climatic factors alone. This gigantic experiment in human ecology is, however, becoming increasingly complicated by man-made modifications of his environment. We have scarcely made a beginning in the study of the influence of climate on human physiology. The sporadic appearance of the externals of human culture in diverse places of the earth in the past is probably not primarily a matter of climate. Heat and humidity can be depressing on some physiologic processes. Because of the factor of basal metabolic rate man is less able to adjust to the extremes of heat and humidity than to extreme cold. We know some of the favorable effects of sunlight (*e.g.*, bone growth, killing of bacteria, etc.); we have hints of unfavorable effects on the blood, the blood pressure and the retina, and the skin. The latter may not be fundamental and there is no evidence that the germ plasm is unfavorably influenced.

We know something of the favorable and unfavorable influence of diets, work, behavior, natural and man-made environments, poisons, etc., on the physiologic processes of the individual. But this is merely limiting or permitting full development of individual growth and functions. Unless these factors modify the germ plasm (rapidly or slowly) they are not significant in relation to race betterment. The only clear instances we have of rapid modification of the germ plasm by experimental (drugs) or environmental means seem to be injurious or destructive. Man to-day is like a curious and clumsy and very ignorant child tinkering with the watch; will he to-morrow contrive a superior mechanism? The lesson for the present seems clear: *The germ plasm can be injured; some phases of the present man-made environment seem to enhance such injury.* Are the ablest the strongest, the wisest men merely grave-diggers in disguise? Is it possible to detect the factors and abort the danger so that man himself may not deflect or impede the river of life?

A. J. CARLSON
UNIVERSITY OF CHICAGO

A REVISION OF THE FUNDAMENTAL LAW OF HABIT FORMATION[1]

THE principles of learning, or habit formation, as they are taught by contemporary psychologists, include as fundamental the principles of recency and frequency. It is true that there are considerable differences in the relative emphasis placed on these principles by different authors—few, for example, going as far as Watson and the present writer have gone in the past in the ascription of importance to frequency. Nevertheless, the importance of these factors has been emphasized by almost all contemporary psychologists (with the possible exception of Carr), who seem to have assumed that they are of some positive value in the fixation of a response into a habit.

Behind these principles, however, there is a more fundamental assumption, which was sharply indicated by William James, but which has seemed too obvious to need statement by those of us who have nevertheless continued in the Jimmian philosophy. This assumption is as follows: *A response* (that is, even a single response) *to a given stimulus pattern definitely increases the probability that on the reoccurrence of the same, or substantially the same, stimulus pattern, the same, or approximately the same, response will occur.* This principle I shall call the *alpha-postulate* of learning.

That this principle underlies the "law of frequency" is obvious, for if one response had no positive effect, then the summation of an indefinite number would have no effect, the sum of zeros being zero. The pictorial statement of this assumption is to be found in the formulations of the old "brain path" superstition, with its analogies to the flow of water eroding a channel, the fold in a coat sleeve, etc.

It has not been denied by any one, so far as I know, that the positive effects of repetition might not be neutralized by other factors, nor that certain other factors may be, in some cases at least, more potent positively. But running through all our disquisitions on learning has been the implication that repetition itself, aside from other factors, has a positive effect; and in our practical work with adjustment cases, this implication has always been respected.

For nearly twenty-five years the present writer has been teaching, explicitly and implicitly, this orthodox doctrine, and attempting to fit the facts somehow to the theory. Even the contradictory results of the Pavlovians failed to shake his faith, because obviously (at least, so far as references in English indicate) neither Pavloff nor his students have ever performed the critical experiment of feeding the dog by stomach injection, without odor or other "conditioning" stimulation, during the period during which the newly formed associative response ("conditioned response") is being tested. The Russian work on this particular point (of the effect of repetition) is therefore beside the mark, and did not even suggest to the present writer a revision of the laws of learning. Psychologists, in fact, have long been acquainted with cases in which habit-tendency disappears in spite of repetition of the stimulus, and this phenomenon has offered no difficulties to the orthodox theory.

The cumulative effect of the difficulty of fitting facts to the theory, however, has, although no longer ago than last summer, suggested that it would be much simpler to fit the theory to the facts. It has seemed well, therefore, to question the fundamental assumption on which we have proceeded.

If we no longer take the assumption of the positive effect of response as a divinely revealed truth, but as a mere postulate, it is at once seen that there are two other postulates possible. One of these, the *beta-postulate,* as I shall call it, is that response, in itself, has *no* effect on the future probability of the same stimulus pattern producing the same response; the other, the *gamma-postulate,* is that response *decreases* the probability. Although the latter of these postulates is more consonant with our present-day neurological theories, and, as I shall show later, has interesting applications to a difficult psychological problem, a certain conservatism, which I think is intelligent, leads me to consider seriously the beta-postulate first.

If "repetition" has in itself no effect, but is important merely in that through it certain positive factors have their chance to operate, then it at once becomes a live possibility that negative factors also may be allowed to operate through repetition. Thus would be explained the apparent "neutralizing" of the effects of repetition, not as actual neutralization in this sense, but as either the operation of negative factors in the absence of positive, or the prevalence of the negative over the positive.[2]

[1] Read before the Section on Psychology, the American Association for the Advancement of Science, Nashville, December 27, 1928.

[2] I am informed by Dr. T. V. Moore that Thomas Aquinas enunciated this doctrine. I should certainly feel honored if I am in any wise treading in the footsteps of the *Doctor Universalis.*

The deductions from our postulate are still more interesting. If the negative factors, those which decrease the probability of the recurrence of the response, can be discovered, repetition may be used practically for the abolition of a habit already formed. This is, I think, a new idea, and worth trying, even aside from the possible light the results may throw on our postulate. Can we, for example, cure stammering, through causing the patient to stammer voluntarily in as nearly as possible the same way in which he ordinarily stammers? Can we abolish tics through causing the tic to occur? If so, we should have a method of "catharsis" of enormous value, and the method should be applicable to a host of minor defects of response and conduct, as well as to such major troubles.

The first question which arises is as to the negative factors which may be called into operation. Consideration of the experimental techniques such as dart-throwing and other practice work which had led to my scepticism concerning the orthodox postulate brought out conventional factors of *"interest," "anticipatory idea,"*[3] and *satisfaction.* It seemed useful, therefore, to proceed tentatively on the assumption that the satisfaction of abolishing an annoying process (and perhaps the futuric interest and expectation of such satisfaction), together with the expectation of attaining an end definitely thought of (anticipatory idea), and, where possible, the desire of this end, would be useful negating factors, and to see what could be done with the aid of these.

The first opportunity which occurred for the testing of this method lay in an idiosyncrasy of my own in typewriting. For some years I have been annoyed, when typing rapidly, by an occasional transposition of the letters of a word, the word "the" being especially troublesome, so that in reading over a manuscript of my own typing I would sometimes find two, three or more of these transpositions into "hte." Several times I have attempted, by careful practice, to train myself out of the habit. The fact that in the majority of cases I actually wrote "the," exchanging it for "hte" only in a minority of cases and when typing rapidly, in itself indicates the futility of increased repetition of the "right" spelling.

On the basis of the neutral postulate, I now proceeded to try the typing of "hte" voluntarily, as a means of destroying it. I set to work deliberately and wrote about a half page, single spaced, of the "hte" combination, with the futuric thought that this was a "word" that I would *not* write in the future (unless deliberately and voluntarily). Somewhat over a week later, I followed this with a second "practice period," writing less than a third of a page. This was over three months ago. Since that time I have typed many pages, some rapidly, but have not found on reading them over a single case of "hte"! This may sound too easy to be true, but as a matter of fact a long-standing and troublesome habit has disappeared.

Having just changed from driving a Ford to operating a gear-shift car, certain minor vices of technique, such as a tendency to step on the accelerator, when meaning to apply the brake, manifested themselves. The application of the catharsis method seems to have overcome these faults very quickly. Such trials on myself have, of course, no scientific value, but served merely as encouragement in the application to more critical cases.

The application of the method to speech defects offers an interesting field. In the case of stammerers, the vital point of proceeding here is to study the specific type of stammering and then induce the patient to reproduce voluntarily his characteristic verbal performance, criticizing and assisting him until his voluntary stammering is as nearly as possible like his involuntary. From that point on, the technique is complicated, and we do not expect to have it perfected until many cases have been experimentally subjected to it. In the meantime, the results even with the crude preliminary method are very favorable.

Tics offer another interesting field of application, where methods are being developed. Thumb-sucking and similar wrong habits of two or three year old children have been treated with results that apparently show that the method is useful at these ages, where I feared it could not be applied. There are many other directions of application, such as bed-wetting and masturbation, where the method can probably be applied as soon as the technique is better developed. It has already been applied to a case of homosexuality, with astonishingly rapid results. It is hard to set the limits of possible application, and from present indications a vast number of hitherto insoluble problems may be solved in this way.

So far, in all applications, we have assumed the importance of anticipatory ideas and desire as elementary factors. The patients are (1) selected on the basis of their desiring, for one reason or another, to cure the habit, and (2) are carefully instructed that the voluntary performance, under the experimenter's control, is something which will assist in the abolition of the behavior at other times.

One of the most important applications of the new postulate, and one of its most interesting points theoretically, is in the explanation of dreams. So

[3] I can't well use the term ''purpose'' in this connection, because ''purpose'' has been given an anti-mechanistic, *i.e.,* mystical, interpretation, and I wish to discuss and investigate this problem on the plane of strict mechanism.

far, dreaming has been assumed to be a pathological function, although of minor importance in most cases, or else has been assumed to be a mere by-product of mental life, in itself of no value. It has long seemed to me, however, that the development and retention of function, generation after generation, indicates a strong probability that the function is not pathological, but has some important value for practical life. The difficulty has been in discovering the practical value of dreams.

As soon as we reject the old alpha-postulate of learning, however, and assume either the beta-postulate or the gamma-postulate, the function of the dream becomes apparent. The dream is a process of eliminating, or "forgetting," details of mental performance which it is useful to take out of the habit-systems, either because of their irrelevancy, or perhaps because of their interference with orderly mental life. The importance of forgetting as compared with remembering, or, in a more comprehensive way, of elimination of habit tendencies, as compared with their fixation and retention, has long been recognized. The greater part of daily experience must be forgotten, and removed from the danger of associative recall, if the remaining small parts of the experiences are to be effectively utilized. The greater part of our daily activities of all sorts, also, must be prevented from becoming response habits. Ideational retention, that is, the tendency to reproduce in thought the contents of preceding perception and thoughts, is of especial importance. If one should retain, subject to complete recall, all the experiences of a single day, his mental efficiency would be sadly reduced thereby. One aspect of this incompetence is nicely portrayed by James in his account of "total redintegration," characteristic of many women and some men.

Many experiences, we may well assume (if we reject the alpha-postulate), leave no tendencies to recall, or towards partial recall which would interfere with other processes. Others, however, because of the operation of favorable fixation factors, tend to persist, and require some help in their elimination.

The known peculiarities of dreams fit in very well with this hypothesis, and with general suspicions regarding important fixation-factors. Dreams are most characteristically about trivial and unimportant matters—just the sort of things which need to be eliminated. In other cases, they are reproductions of emotionally stressed factors of working life, which especially need elimination. In many of these cases, it is obvious that an unsuccessful effort is being made to eliminate, and this effort may be repeated in many successive dreams. It is to be expected, too, that not only will repetition fail to eliminate in some cases, but that even the repetitive process will itself partially fail, and the dream be composed of factors associated with the factors which ought to be eliminated, rather than of those factors themselves. The importance of the problem of *improving* dreams, of making dreams more effective and of the *production* of dreams to assist in eliminating disturbing factors of daily life is at once seen. Much research needs to be done here. As I have earlier pointed out, dreams consist mainly of, or center about, experiences in which a futuric factor has been a feature. That is to say, anticipatory ideas, centered often in hopes, fears, expectations and desires, are the chief causal factors in dreams. This agrees with the supposition, made on other grounds, that an important fixation factor in habit formation is expectation, or anticipatory ideas of the result to be obtained.

In considering the dream situation, one might perhaps incline to the adoption of the gamma-hypothesis instead of the beta-hypothesis, were it not for the consideration that even here it is not, as yet, necessary to make the assumption that repetition has, in itself, an eliminative effect. All we need to assume, for the present, is that conditions are favorable, during sleep, for the operation of eliminative factors, whatever these may be. If, later, we have to assume that repetition itself is the factor, that is a matter to be faced then. For the present, we may follow the principle of parsimony, and make the simpler assumption; namely, the beta-postulate.

The same consideration appears in the problem of the ancient confessional as utilized in the "psychoanalytic" method. The expression of troublesome thoughts need not be assumed to be cathartic in itself; the conditions of the confessional may introduce eliminative factors which are not operative in other phases of the patient's repetitions. Many other factors need to be investigated in these cases, including the relation of speech formulation in processes which have previously been internal (cerebro-cerebellar, according to my own hypotheses).

In conclusion, it may be pointed out that the successful eventuation of methods of therapy deduced from the beta-postulate do not prove the final truth of the postulate. But its value is certainly demonstrated by the practical benefits derived from these deductions.

KNIGHT DUNLAP
JOHNS HOPKINS UNIVERSITY

HENRI BOSMANS

WITH the death of Henri Bosmans, of the Jesuit College of Saint-Michel, at Brussels, there passed away one of the most active men of the present century in the field of the history of mathematics. Bosmans died on February 3 of the present year, at the advanced age of seventy-six and in the fifty-seventh year of his religious life as a Jesuit. His first historical paper published in 1900 related to Snell's measurement of the earth's meridian; his last contribution which has reached us is a Preface to Gillain's Arithmétique Egyptienne, dated October, 1927. Between 1900 and 1928, Bosmans issued a steady flow of papers relating mainly to fifteenth, sixteenth and seventeenth century mathematicians, most of whose works are not generally accessible. He remained active to the last, notwithstanding his partial blindness in later years. A noteworthy incident was his borrowing from the Louvain Library one of the very few copies still extant of Simon Stevin's book, Le Thiende, on decimal fractions, and thereby saving it from destruction, for while the book was in his possession the Louvain Library was burned. Bosmans was of a kindly disposition. Some years ago, when the present writer happened to state in a letter that he was working on the evolution of the theory of limits, and ought to have access to Gregory St. Vincent's geometry, Bosmans had passages in that work photographed which he sent with his compliments. His keenness of mind as well as his sympathetic and appreciative nature are seen in his numerous book reviews.

FLORIAN CAJORI
UNIVERSITY OF CALIFORNIA

SCIENTIFIC EVENTS

INTERNATIONAL SOCIETY FOR THE EXPLORATION OF THE ARCTIC REGIONS BY MEANS OF THE AIRSHIP (AEROARCTIC)

MORE than three years ago the society under consideration was organized in Germany. It attracted a number of people of different countries interested in the investigation of the Arctic regions, and, so far as Europe and Asia are concerned, it has a good representation in nearly all the countries of the Old World. The society was well represented at its first international meeting, which was held in Berlin from November 9 to 13, 1926. The second meeting will be held in June of this year at Leningrad, U. S. S. R. Beginning in 1928 the society will publish a quarterly journal, *Arctis,* under the editorship of Dr. Fr. Nansen, president. Among the collaborators of the journal in the United States are Dr. L. A. Bauer, director of the Department of Terrestrial Magnetism of the Carnegie Institution of Washington, V. Stefansson, and the writer. Besides Dr. Nansen, the membership list of the society contains a number of people well-known in connection with the exploration of Arctic regions in their respective countries as well as internationally.

The epic heroic period of Arctic travels might be considered finished with the last memorable Peary expedition, but Arctic regions are still very little known and much less explored and investigated. The new international society attacks the problem from different points of view. Being ready to send Arctic expeditions in an airship and already preparing them, the society puts the greatest weight on the conquering of Arctic regions by means of a regular siege, which will be possible only if all the countries bordering the Arctic will cooperate in carrying on systematic work within their national borders. The program of the society can not be accomplished by any one country alone, but is an international enterprise which has to be worked out in national frames.

The United States and Canada, the countries of the New World having Arctic possessions, have not been represented previously in this international organization. However, the Canadian branch is now being organized, and the American branch for the United States has come into life during this year. The officers of the American branch are: *President,* Dr. L. A. Bauer; *vice-president,* Dr. J. A. Fleming, of the Carnegie Institution of Washington; *secretary,* I. P. Tolmachoff, of the Carnegie Museum of Pittsburgh. Any information concerning the new organization can be obtained from the secretary.

Dr. Fr. Nansen in May of this year is expected in this country to attend the meeting of the American Peace Society at Cleveland, Ohio, and it may be also possible for him to give some lectures on the activity of the International Society for the Exploration of the Arctic regions, its achievements and the program of the future work.

I. TOLMACHOFF
CARNEGIE MUSEUM,
PITTSBURGH, PA.

THE REORGANIZATION OF THE POST-GRADUATE MEDICAL SCHOOL AND HOSPITAL

THE appointment of Dr. Edward Hicks Hume, former president of the Colleges of Yale-in-China and for many years identified with national and international hospital and medical educational work, director of the New York Post-Graduate Medical School and Hospital, recently recorded in SCIENCE, marks a change in the policies of the institution. It follows a survey made of the personnel and resources of the institution, which Dr. Hume has been working on since May, 1927, which proposes certain administrative and teaching rearrangements, and makes recommendations regarding a new building program and better integration with the nation-wide plans for graduate medical teaching. Under the new régime, responsibility will be centralized, so that the various departments of the institution, as well as the three officers directly concerned with administration, namely, the dean of the medical school, the superintendent of the hospital and the principal of the school of nursing, will be responsible to the board of directors through the newly appointed executive officer.

The New York Post-Graduate Medical School and Hospital, founded by Dr. D. B. St. John Roosa in 1882, was incorporated on May 25, 1886, the object of the incorporation being the establishment of a school for the further instruction of persons already possessing the degree of doctor in medicine, and a hospital for the treatment of diseased and injured persons.

During the 42 years since its incorporation, over 25,000 physicians have matriculated at the medical school, coming from every state in the union and from many foreign countries to take graduate courses here.

The directors of the institution, appreciating the need of a new program adequate to the demands of advancing medical practice, have determined to build up for the institution such a program of medical opportunity in teaching and research, and such a financial foundation as will enable it more adequately to serve the field. In this connection it is significant that the New York Academy of Medicine has just completed a series of studies on the past, present and future of graduate medicine in the vicinity of New York. The study on the future of graduate medicine was prepared by a member of the staff of the New York Post-Graduate Medical School and lays chief emphasis on the fact that graduate medical teaching, like undergraduate teaching, is a part of the national health service.

THE ST. LOUIS MEETING OF THE AMERICAN CHEMICAL SOCIETY

A SYMPOSIUM on atomic structure and valence has been arranged in connection with the seventy-fifth meeting of the American Chemical Society which meets in St. Louis, from April 16 to 19. The underlying purpose of the symposium, according to a statement made by Professor George L. Clark, of the University of Illinois, chairman of the division of physical and inorganic chemistry, is to acquaint physicists and chemists with each other's points of view and each other's demands which must be satisfied by any comprehensive theory of atomic structure in the effort to arrive at some common basis of understanding.

Speakers will include: Professor M. S. Kharasch, University of Maryland; Professor William D. Harkins, University of Chicago; Professor Samuel C. Lind, University of Minnesota; Professor C. E. M. Jauncey, Washington University, St. Louis; Karl K. Darrow, Bell Telephone Company; Professor W. H. Rodebush, University of Illinois; Professor J. H. VanVleck, University of Minnesota; Professor W. A. Noyes, University of Illinois; Professor H. Shipley Fry, University of Cincinnati; Professor Donald H. Andrews, the Johns Hopkins University; Victor Cofman, E. I. duPont de Nemours and Company.

All divisions of the society except the colloid, fertilizer, and leather and gelatin chemistry divisions will meet at St. Louis. A preliminary report of the section programs was printed in SCIENCE for March 2, page 235.

Following the registration of delegates at the Hotel Chase, the opening event will be a meeting at 2:00 p. m., on Monday, April 16, of the society's Council, presided over by the president of the society, Dr. S. W. Parr, professor emeritus of industrial chemistry in the University of Illinois.

G. S. Robins, of the G. S. Robins and Company, 316 South Commercial Street, St. Louis, has been appointed chairman of the executive committee in charge of arrangements for the convention. Other St. Louis committee chairmen have been named as follows: *Finance,* H. A. Carlton, Mallinckrodt Chemical Works; *divisional meetings,* L. A. Watt, Monsanto Chemical Works; *hotel arrangements,* Eugene S. Weil, G. S. Robins and Company; *registration,* T. R. Ball, Washington University; *transportation and plant visits,* J. R. Hoff, Anheuser-Busch; *entertainment,* Ralph R. Matthews, Roxana Petroleum Company; *ladies' entertainment,* Mrs. R. R. Matthews; *speakers' committee,* F. W. Russe, Mallinckrodt Chemical Works; *program,* A. F. Schlichting, St. Louis College of Pharmacy; *publicity,* Chas. W. Rodewald, Washington University.

THE MILTON RESEARCH AWARDS OF HARVARD UNIVERSITY

ANNOUNCEMENT is made of thirty-seven awards to teachers in Harvard University, in accordance with the provisions of the Milton Fund for Research. This fund, which Harvard received in 1924, yields about $50,000 a year.

After the death of his wife the bulk of the estate of the late William F. Milton, '58, was to go to Harvard University for the building of a university library, or, if the university had a suitable library building, to defray the expenses of any special investigation of a medical, geographical, historical or scientific nature. It was further stated that such investigation should be "in the interests of, or for promoting the physical and material welfare and prosperity of the human race, or to assist in the discovery and perfecting of any special means of alleviating or curing human disease, or to investigate and determine the value or importance of any discovery or invention, or any other special or temporary object of the nature above stated."

A committee was appointed, consisting of Mr. Frank B. Jewett, electrical engineer of New York, *chairman;* Professor Edwin F. Gay, of Harvard's Economics Department, and Dr. W. J. V. Osterhout, botanist of the Rockefeller Foundation; to advise the president and fellows of Harvard College in making a selection among the investigations proposed by any member of the instructing, scientific or administrative staff of the university. Requests for aid in such research were received by the committee this year up to January 10.

The grants from the Milton Fund for next year include the following:

Thomas Barbour, director of the University Museum, and Dr. Afranio Do Amaral, lecturer on ophiology, to enable them to collect neotropical snake venom for use in experimentation concerning the nature of snake venom and in preparing the curative antivenin.

Percy W. Bridgman, Hollis professor of mathematics and natural philosophy, to pay for the salaries of assistants and the purchase of apparatus to continue his work on high pressure studies and on an investigation on the properties of single crystals.

Edward S. Castle, assistant in physiology, to pay for the services of a technician in constructing apparatus for the study of the growth of plants in relation to light and temperature.

William J. Crozier, professor of general physiology, for the study of the nature of central nervous processes.

Walter F. Dearborn, professor of education, for the study of the mental and physical development of school children.

William Duane, professor of biophysics, for research in X-radiation.

Robert Emerson, research fellow in general physiology, for the services of a technician to set up and calibrate precision apparatus to study the formation of chlorophyll and development of its photosynthetic activity.

George S. Forbes, professor of chemistry, for chemicals, supplies and apparatus to be used in an investigation of conditions for electrochemical equilibrium.

Worthington C. Ford, lecturer on historical manuscripts, to complete his research in the sources of American history.

Charles Hartshorne, instructor in philosophy, to complete the preparation for publication of five volumes of the Charles S. Peirce manuscripts on philosophy.

Leigh Hoadley, assistant professor of zoology, for supplies, apparatus, expenses, etc., for an assistant in an investigation of the embryonic segregation preceding primitive streak formation in the vertebrate embryo.

Hudson Hoagland, research fellow in general physiology, for the services of an assistant to examine the underlying mechanism of tonic immobility in vertebrates.

Earnest A. Hooton, associate professor of anthropology, to continue his study of race and nationality in their relation to crime in the United States.

Grinnell Jones, associate professor of chemistry, for chemicals and apparatus, etc., in an investigation of properties of solutions of electrolytes.

Edwin C. Kemble, associate professor of physics, for the purchase of a Kipp thermo-relay amplifier and galvanometer for use in determining infra-red absorption spectra of gases.

Arthur B. Lamb, Sheldon Emory professor of organic chemistry and director of the chemical laboratory, to continue research on crystalline adsorbents.

Albert E. Navez, lecturer on physiology, for the services of an assistant to build apparatus and make experimental observations in connection with a research of geotropism in plants.

Ralph B. Perry, professor of philosophy, to prepare a volume on William James, philosopher and psychologist, from his unpublished correspondence, lecture notes, etc., in the Widener Library.

Harlow Shapley, Paine professor of practical astronomy and director of the Harvard College Observatory, to continue his research on variable stars and the dimensions of the Galaxy.

Theodore J. B. Stier, assistant in the division of biology, for the part-time services of an assistant to construct apparatus to be used in an investigation of the effects of temperature on the spontaneous activity of mice.

Robert DeC. Ward, professor of climatology, to study climatology of North America and of the West Indies for inclusion in a volume on the world's climates edited by Professor W. Köppen.

Jeffries Wyman, Jr., instructor in zoology, for expense of apparatus and materials for a study of the physical chemistry of the proteins.

SCIENTIFIC NOTES AND NEWS

Theodore William Richards, professor of chemistry at Harvard University since 1894, director of the Gibbs Memorial Laboratory since 1912, died on April 2, at the age of sixty years.

The sixty-fourth annual meeting of the National Academy of Sciences will be held in its building in Washington, D. C., on April 23, 24 and 25.

The annual meeting of the American Philosophical Society will be held in the hall of the society at Independence Square, Philadelphia, on April 19, 20 and 21, under the presidency of Dr. Francis X. Dercum.

The regular spring meeting of the executive committee of the American Association for the Advancement of Science will be held in Washington on Sunday, April 22. Matters to be considered by the committee should be in the hands of the permanent secretary a few days before the meeting.

The coinage of a medal commemorating the achievements of Thomas A. Edison was approved on March 29 by the house coinage committee in reporting a bill by Representative Perkins. An appropriation of $1,000 would be made to enable the secretary of the treasury to prepare a suitable medal.

Dr. Elihu Thomson, consulting engineer for the General Electric Company at its Lynn works, celebrated his seventy-fifth birthday on March 29. On that date a special resolution in honor of Dr. Thomson was passed by the executive committee of the National Electric Light Association.

The Halley lecture at Oxford University will be delivered on June 18 by Dr. Harlow Shapley, director of the Harvard College Observatory, on "The Extent and Structure of the Milky Way."

Dr. Ernest W. Brown, Sterling professor of mathematics at Yale University, has been elected to membership in the Royal Academy of Science of Belgium, "because of his eminent contributions to the science of mathematics."

The cross of the Commander of the Order of the White Rose has been conferred by the Republic of Finland on Dean Albert R. Mann, of the New York State College of Agriculture, in recognition of his services in connection with the development of agricultural education. The award is the highest honorary decoration of Finland.

Henry F. Schmidt, consulting engineer of the Westinghouse Electric and Manufacturing Company, has been awarded the medal of the American Society of Naval Engineers for the best article submitted during the year 1927. Mr. Schmidt, besides being awarded a gold medal, was given an honorary life membership in the society and a cash prize for his paper entitled "Some Screw Propeller Experiments with particular reference to Pumps and Blowers."

On March 8 the University of Oxford conferred the honorary degree of M.A. on Mrs. Florence Joy Weldon, widow of the late Dr. W. F. R. Weldon, professor of zoology, who has given many valuable pictures to the university galleries.

The German Academy of Sciences in Halle has elected Dr. M. Guggenheim, director of the F. Hoffman-La Roche and Company, Basle, to membership in recognition of his contributions to the biological sciences.

Professor Jolly, who holds the chair of histophysiology at the Collège de France, has been elected a member of the French Academy of Medicine.

Professors Nicolas and Pierre Duval, of Paris, have been elected foreign corresponding members of the Royal Academy of Medicine of Belgium.

Dr. Ephraim P. Felt, New York state entomologist, retired on March 31 to become adviser on shade tree and forest insect problems with the Bartlett Research Laboratories at Stamford, Conn.

Dr. George R. Minot, who was recently made director of the Thorndike memorial laboratory at the Boston City Hospital and professor of medicine at Harvard University, has been appointed consulting physician at the Peter Bent Brigham Hospital.

Professor G. S. Parks, of the department of chemistry at Stanford University, has been elected chairman of the California section of the American Chemical Society for 1928.

Dr. Joseph S. Illick, state forester of Pennsylvania, was elected chairman of the Allegheny section of the Society of American Foresters at its annual winter meeting.

At the annual meeting of the American Heart Association, Boston, on February 6, the following officers were reelected for the ensuing year: Drs. James B. Herrick, Chicago, *president;* William H. Robey, *vice-president;* Haven Emerson, New York, *secretary,* and Paul D. White, Boston, *treasurer.*

Dr. Ernest J. Hoffman, research chemist, recently with W. B. Pratt, Boston, has been appointed associate chemist in the chemical engineering division, chemical and technological research, Bureau of Chemistry and Soils, to conduct research studies on farm fires with special attention to the causes of the spontaneous combustion of hay and other agricultural products.

In the U. S. Department of Agriculture Dr. A. E. Wight has been appointed to succeed the late Dr. John A. Kiernan as chief of the tuberculosis eradication division. Dr. George W. Pope has been appointed chief of the field inspection division, succeeding Dr. A. W. Miller, who is now chief of the packers and stockyards division. Dr. Miller succeeds John T. Caine, resigned. Dr. W. E. Cotton has been designated as acting superintendent of the bureau's experiment station at Bethesda, Md., succeeding the late Dr. E. C. Schroeder. The administrative changes have also provided for two new positions, designated as associate chief of the bureau and assistant chief. Dr. U. G. Houck, who continues as chief of the division of hog-cholera control, also holds the title of associate chief of bureau. Dr. A. W. Miller, besides being chief of the packers and stockyards division, is assistant chief of bureau.

The sixth Harvey lecture, by E. J. London, director of physiology at the University of Leningrad, on "Experimental Fistulae of Blood Vessels," which was announced for April 13, has been postponed until April 20 at 8:30 o'clock.

DR. J. J. R. MACLEOD, of the University of Toronto, lecturer for 1928 under the Louis Clark Vanuxem foundation at Princeton University, gave four lectures during March under the general title "The Fuel Used for Energy Production in Animals." These recent investigations in animal metabolism are to be published in book form.

DR. DAVID RIESMAN, of the University of Pennsylvania, gave an illustrated lecture at the annual meeting of the George Washington University Medical Society in Washington, March 17, on "Man before the Dawn of History."

EDWARD W. BERRY, professor of paleontology at the Johns Hopkins University, delivered an address entitled "Idols of the Market Place" before the Yale University geology club on March 29.

DR. W. H. EMMONS, professor of geology at the University of Minnesota and state geologist of Minnesota, delivered a lecture on March 22 to the students in geology at the University of Toronto, on "The Relation of Metalliferous Lodes to Igneous Intrusions."

DR. BORIS SOKOLOSS, a former deputy in the North Russian government, who has paid especial attention to cancer research, is in this country and will work in the Rockefeller Institute.

PROFESSOR MARGARET C. FERGUSON, of the department of botany at Wellesley College, is giving a series of six lectures, under the auspices of the Ropes memorial organization of Salem. The lectures center around the subject of plants and advancing civilization and are being given in Salem at the Ropes memorial building on consecutive Wednesday afternoons in March and April.

LIEUTENANT-COLONEL CHAS. F. CRAIG, of the Army Medical School, Washington, D. C., lectured to the research club of the department of medical zoology of the Johns Hopkins School of Hygiene and Public Health on March 30 on the subject of "Complement Fixation in Amoebiasis."

GERRIT S. MILLER, JR., curator of the division of mammals in the U. S. National Museum, has arrived in Sanchez, Dominican Republic, where he will spend the next few months investigating the caves of the region for bones of the extinct fauna of the island. A. J. Poole was expected to return to the museum early in April, having spent about four months in the same kind of work in Haiti, on the opposite side of the island.

PROFESSOR YOSHINORI TAKEZAKI, in charge of the plant-breeding work of the department of agriculture, Kyoto Imperial University, Japan, is visiting the United States.

RICHARD S. SCHONLAND, of the forest service of the Union of South Africa, has been in the United States for a year studying forest conditions and practices and the organization of forest experiment stations.

PROFESSOR JIRI V. DANES, of Charles University, Prague, who is in this country as an official lecturer under the auspices of the International Institute of Education, lecturing at various colleges and universities, is taking the opportunity to study some of the karst areas of the United States.

DR. ALFONS JACOB, lecturer in psychiatry at Hamburg, has been invited by the Brazilian government to undertake the establishment of an institute for the study of the anatomy of the brain at Rio de Janeiro, and to deliver a course of lectures on nervous and mental diseases from May to July.

BEGINNING May 14 and continuing until June 24, E. O. Essig will conduct a University of California course in field entomology in the Yosemite National Park, with headquarters at the new Yosemite Park Museum. From July 1 to August 1 of the same season he will be at his permanent summer camp at Echo Lake, in the High Sierras, 7,500 feet altitude, eleven miles from Lake Tahoe. Entomologists visiting California are invited to call on Professor Essig at either of the above places and he will be very glad to assist them in the various types of entomological work in those regions.

DR. R. A. MILLIKAN, director of the Norman Bridge laboratory of physics of the California Institute of Technology, gave one of the Proctor Foundation lectures at the Brooklyn Institute of Arts and Sciences on April 5. His subject will be "Recent Advances in Spectroscopy."

DR. WILLIS R. WHITNEY, director of research of the General Electric Company, has been selected by Midwest Association of Sigma Xi to deliver its inaugural addresses on April 12, in Chicago. The midwest association is an affiliation of the three university chapters of the national honorary research fraternity in Cook County, Illinois, with about five hundred other members in the Chicago district engaged in professional work outside university circles. The address will be preceded by a banquet.

DR. ARTHUR D. LITTLE, president of Arthur D. Little, Inc., delivered the Aldred lecture at the Massachusetts Institute of Technology, March 23, on "Chemical Industry."

PROFESSOR WILLIAM L. BRAGG, of the University of

Manchester, addressed the physics colloquium at Harvard University, March 26, on "A Direct Determination of Zero Point Energy."

Professor A. S. Eddington, F.R.S., Plumian professor of astronomy at the University of Cambridge, has accepted an invitation to deliver the Adamson memorial lecture. His subject will be "Philosophical Tendencies in Modern Science," and the lecture will be delivered in the university on May 4.

E. W. Maunder, who was for many years superintendent of the solar department at Greenwich Observatory, died on March 21 at the age of seventy-six years.

Sir David Ferrier, the distinguished English neurologist, died on March 19 in his eighty-sixth year.

The diamond anniversary of the founding of the California Academy of Sciences was celebrated in the building of the academy on April 4. After a formal reception, brief addresses were given by the Honorable William H. Crocker, president of the board of trustees; Dr. C. E. Grunsky, president of the academy, and Dr. Barton Warren Evermann, director of the museum.

The annual meeting of the Federation of the American Societies for Experimental Biology will take place at Ann Arbor, Michigan, on April 12, 13 and 14. The federation includes the American Physiological Society, the Society of Biological Chemistry, the Society of Pharmacology and Experimental Therapeutics and the Society of Experimental Pathology. The annual Conference of Biological Chemists will be held in connection with this meeting; the main topic for discussion this year is the proposed changes in the biochemical curriculum in the medical schools.

The Society of Experimental Biology and Medicine during the past few years has established branch sections in several institutions in the United States. Recently the question has been raised as to whether a branch should be established in Rochester, Minn. There are at present sixteen members of the national organization in Rochester. At a meeting of this group it was decided to form a local society and to hold meetings at which the results of experimental work could be presented and discussed. Final decision in regard to affiliation with the national organization was postponed until after the organization of the local group has been perfected.

The National Colloid Symposium has accepted the invitation of the University of Toronto to hold the Sixth Symposium there on June 14, 15 and 16. The guest of honor at this meeting will be Sir William Hardy, of Cambridge, England. Arrangements have been made for an exhibition of experimental methods in colloidal work; a large hall has been secured adjoining the building in which the symposium will be held, and space will be offered free for exhibits accepted by the local committee. It is thought that in this way workers in colloids may be enabled to bring to the attention of their colleagues many details of experimental arrangement and technique which are necessarily crowded out of the limited program of papers; it is hoped that those presenting papers at the symposium will accept this opportunity of displaying the apparatus used in their work and that others with novel types of apparatus will take advantage of the opportunity to exhibit them.

One of the features of the second session of the Institute of Chemistry of the American Chemical Society, to be held at Northwestern University, Evanston, Ill., from July 23 to August 18, will be a series of lectures, specialized in character and treating thoroughly a variety of topics of interest alike to academic and industrial men. Those taking part include Harry N. Holmes, head of the department of chemistry of Oberlin College, who will take for his subject "Colloids." B. S. Hopkins, of the University of Illinois, will lecture on "Modern Inorganic Chemistry." Arthur I. Kendall, of the Washington University School of Medicine at St. Louis, will lecture on "The Chemistry of Bacteria." Victor K. La Mer, of Columbia University, will present a series of lectures on "Modern Physical Chemistry." W. T. Read, now of the Texas Technological College and formerly at Yale University, will discuss "Modern Industrial Chemistry." G. L. Wendt, at present dean of chemistry and physics at Pennsylvania State College and director of the Battelle Memorial Institute, will lecture on "Industrial Research." F. C. Whitmore, the director of the second session of the Institute of Chemistry and professor of chemistry at Northwestern University, will lecture on the subject of "Modern Organic Chemistry."

The former section of history of chemistry of the American Chemical Society is now a division, and members who wish to be enrolled in this division are invited to send their names to Dr. Tenney L. Davis, Massachusetts Institute of Technology.

The first convention of Sigma Pi Sigma, national physics fraternity, will be held at Davidson College, Davidson, N. C., on April 10 and 11. Dr. Marsh W. White, of Pennsylvania State College, will be the principal speaker.

At a meeting of the chemistry research club of Columbia University on March 29, papers were presented on "The Hydrolysis of Sucrose by Invertase," by Maxwell Schubert, and "Activity Coefficients of High Valence Ions and a Simple Method of Handling the General Solution of the Debye Theory of Electrolytes," by Victor K. La Mer.

THE National Park Service announces plans for the fourth summer school for the training of naturalists, nature guides and teachers of natural history, to be opened on June 25 in the Yosemite National Park. The work was inaugurated by the California Fish and Game Commission and is also participated in by the Yosemite Natural History Association. The school has a faculty of seven, under the leadership of Ansel F. Hall, chief naturalist.

THE Whiting Corporation, Harvey, Ill., has established in the Mellon Institute of Industrial Research an industrial fellowship, whose holder, Dr. Edward E. Marbaker, will conduct research on cast iron. The results of these investigations will be published for the general benefit of the foundry industry.

JEFFERSON MEDICAL COLLEGE has given notice in Orphans Court of an intention to claim a $67,000 trust fund left by Dr. James Ewing Mears to Harvard University for the study of eugenics, which that university rejected a year ago.

PROFESSOR R. P. COWLES has presented to the department of zoology of the Johns Hopkins University his collection of gastropod shells, marine and terrestrial. These shells were collected at the Marine Biological Station in the Philippine Islands, located at Puerta Galera, on the Island of Mindoro.

THE United Engineering Society has received a bequest of $1,000 through the will of the late Oberlin Smith, president of The American Society of Mechanical Engineers in 1890.

WITH the aid of students now in residence, the Brooks research fund, designed to aid students in botany and zoology at the Johns Hopkins University, has now passed the ten thousand dollar mark.

ADDITIONAL funds have been received by the Fitzwilliam Museum, of the University of Cambridge, completing the fund of £100,000 required for the proposed extension.

THE widow of the late Professor Emanuel Kayser, paleontologist and geologist, of Munich, desires to sell his library. It has about 11,000 pamphlets and 500 to 600 books. Those interested should address his daughter, Frau Cilly Engelmann, Weissenburgstrasse 3, Marburg, Germany.

THE Comitè National Belge de l'Eclairage has accepted the task entrusted to it by the International Commission on Lighting of establishing in Brussels an international research department on the distribution of electrical illumination with the view of drawing up a series of standards.

THE British National Institute of Industrial Psychology, London, which was founded seven years ago for the application of the human sciences to the everyday needs of industry, has received an anonymous gift of £4,000 towards the cost of new premises.

THE Martin Johnson African Expedition Corporation, through its president, Daniel E. Pomeroy, has presented to the American Museum of Natural History 200,000 feet of film taken by Mr. and Mrs. Martin Johnson during their four years in Africa. The museum has placed the 8,000 feet of this film, which made up the motion picture "Simba," in a vacuum sealed container, which will not be opened for fifty years, when it is believed that a majority of the animals now constituting the wild life of Africa will have disappeared.

UNIVERSITY AND EDUCATIONAL NOTES

PRINCETON UNIVERSITY has received a quarter of a million dollars in pledges toward the alumni fund to raise teachers' salaries as the result of the first month of the canvassing for a $2,000,000 endowment.

BEQUESTS of the late James Ward Packard include $20,000 to Lehigh University. After Mrs. Packard's death one third of the residuary estate will go to the university.

THE University of Buffalo has received a gift of $100,000 from Mr. Darwin D. Martin to establish the Martin professorship of mathematics.

GEORGETOWN UNIVERSITY has received $250,000 from Mr. and Mrs. Thomas J. Maloney, of Waldwick, N. J., for the Chemo-Medical Research Institute to be built on the university grounds.

DR. ARTHUR L. TATUM, of the University of Chicago, has been appointed professor of pharmacology at the University of Wisconsin, in association with Dr. A. S. Loevenhart. He will assume his duties at Madison on September 15.

PROFESSOR H. B. WALKER, head of the department of agricultural engineering at Kansas State Agricultural College, has resigned to accept a similar position with the agricultural branch of the University of California at Davis.

AT Yale University, Professor William R. Longley, professor of mathematics, has been appointed to the Colgate professorship in place of Professor Luquiens. The following assistant professors were promoted to the rank of associate professors: Dr. Oystein Ore, mathematics; Dr. Stuart R. Brinkley, chemistry; Roscoe H. Suttie, civil engineering; Archer E. Knowlton, electrical engineering; Everett O. Waters, mechanical engineering; Arthur Phillips, metallurgy, and Dr. Blair Saxton, chemistry. Instructors who were promoted to assistant professorships are: Dr. Robert De W. Coghill, chemistry; Lauren E. Seeley, mechanical engineering; Dr. Richard F. Flint, geology; Dr. Lucius T. Moore, mathematics; Dr. Jesse W. Beams, physics. Dr. Dirk Brouwer has been appointed research assistant in mathematical astronomy.

AMONG those who will give courses at the summer quarter of Stanford University are: Dr. Harry Clark, associate member of the Rockefeller Institute, in physics; Dr. Alfred Errera, of the University of Brussels, and Dr. Carl Einar Hille, of Princeton University, in mathematics; Dr. J. J. Runner, assistant professor at the University of Iowa, in geology, and Professor Edward A. Bott, of the University of Toronto, in psychology.

DR. ROBERT ROBINSON, professor of organic chemistry at the University of Manchester, has been appointed to the chair of organic chemistry in University College, London.

DR. GEORGES FONTÈS has been appointed professor of biological chemistry at Strasbourg, and Dr. Arnt Kohlrausch, of Greifswald, professor of physiology at Tübingen.

DISCUSSION AND CORRESPONDENCE

A PERIODIC CLASSIFICATION OF THE HARDNESS AND MELTING-POINTS OF THE ELEMENTS

IT is possible to classify the elements according to hardness and melting-point, and this classification fits with considerable precision into an eighteen-period table based on spectroscopic similarities.

The table (see Fig. 1) represents the elements arranged according to atomic number, with those of similar spectra in columns. The columns under H and He represent the first stage in the building-up of the electron structures of the atom, that of building on the two "s" electrons; the six following columns add the "p" electrons, while the long group from Sc to Zn all contain elements to which the "d" electrons are being added. Thus at the end of each column we have the complete shells; the "s" shells under He, the "p" shells under the rare gases, and the "d" shell under Zn. Lanthanum and the 14 Rare Earths come under Y. These represent the "f" electron being built on.

Let us first consider the melting-points. If we examine the table, we find some striking characteristics. In the first place, all the elements with high-melting points are at one end of the table, while those with low melting points are at the other. Then let us examine the columns. For each column under Sc, Ti, V, Cr, Mn, Fe, Co, Ni, the melting-points increase down the column. Under Cu all are nearly equal. Under Zn, B, C, there are minima at Hg, Ga, Sn, respectively. The N column has a maximum at As. The melting-points under O, F, Ne, all increase down the column. It is interesting to note that the permanent gases conform to this periodicity as well as the non-gases. The alkali metals decrease in melting-point down the column. Under Be there is a minimum at Mg. The only discrepancy is Ti, whose melting-point is slightly above what we should expect.

Another interesting characteristic is that the whole first long period row (Sc–Cu) have similar melting-points, falling off slightly at either end. The same is true for the next two rows.

Turning to the subject of hardness, we find that this in general varies as the height of the melting-point. It is of course difficult to obtain accurate values for absolute hardness but considering some recently obtained by A. Mallock,[1] and others, we note that all the hard metals are bunched, as are the soft ones. The maxima and minima are in the same places, and the runs follow the same sequences as do the melting-points. The discrepancies are, V, and Pd; but Mallock claims the V was not obtainable pure in the proper form for the test, and Rydberg[2] claims that

[1] A. Mallock, *Nature*, Feb. 19, 1927, p. 276.

[2] Rydberg, *Zeits. f. Physikalische Chemie*, 33 (1900) 353–9.

																	H	He
																	Li	Be
											B	C	N	O	F	Ne	Na	Mg
											Al	Si	P	S	Cl	A	K	Ca
	Sc	Ti	V	Cr	Mn	Fe	Co	Ni	Cu	Zn	Ga	Ge	As	Se	Br	Kr	Rb	Sr
	Y	Zr	Cb	Mo	Ma	Ru	Rh	Pd	Ag	Cd	In	Sn	Sb	Te	I	Xe	Cs	Ba
La and 14)		Hf	Ta	W	Re	Os	Ir	Pt	Au	Hg	Tl	Pb	Bi	Po	85	Rn	87	Ra
Rare Earths)		Th	Ux	U	93													

FIG. 1. Table of the elements, arranged with regard to spectroscopic similarities, in order of atomic number. Inspection will show how hardness and melting-point fit in, the harder ones being at the middle of the (left) long period.

Pd and Fe are about equally hard, as we should expect. That C, B, Be, and others are hard, while Cs, Rb and P are soft is well known. We see, therefore, that hardness is quite well expressible in the same curve as melting-point.

We have, then, an interesting correlation. The spectroscopic properties and the melting-points and hardnesses are expressible in the same table. And as the agreements on the whole are so good, holding not only for metals, but for non-metals and gases, we might venture to predict the characteristics of those whose melting-points and hardnesses have not yet been determined. Thus we suggest that 85 (Eka-Iodine) will melt at about 250° C. and be fairly soft, and that 87 (Eka-Caesium) will melt at about 18° C., and be very soft. Number 93 will be hard and of high melting-point, coming as it will below Re. We also suggest that the value of Masurium, assumed in the International Critical Tables to be 2,300° C., will be nearer 2,500° C.

It is evident from the foregoing that there exists a relation between the electronic configuration and the melting-point and hardness. We notice that the atoms with the complete shells have the lowest melting-point. Those with a partial shell, such as W, Re, and Os, where about half the "d" shell is on, have high melting-points, and are hard. The "irregular" atoms, whose electron shell structure, and in particular, whose outer shell is incomplete, thus have greater mutual attraction, and less yielding to deformation of the solid configuration than those with complete shells. The deformation of a substance by shear and compression forces (the method of testing hardness) is thus quite similar in its fundamental effect on the atoms of the substance to the deformation in melting; atoms sliding on atoms more readily if the atoms have complete shells. There is evidently less stray field holding these complete shells together. Hence in the central part of each period we find the harder elements and the soft ones at the ends. This, according to our interpretation of the table, means that the elements increase in hardness as more electrons are built on, attain a maximum somewhere before half the shell is completed, and fall off in hardness as the shell nears completion to a minimum at the complete shell.

S. A. Korff

Princeton University

FURTHER EVIDENCE CONCERNING MAN'S ANTIQUITY AT FREDERICK, OKLAHOMA

In Science of February 10 appears a note by Dr. Leslie Spier, of the University of Oklahoma, questioning certain phases of the evidence bearing on man's antiquity at Frederick, Oklahoma. The geological age of the deposits, their nature and occurrence, are well established and not questioned. He states however, "The artifacts themselves are equivocal," and questions their occurrence and contemporaneity with the fossils; and their Pleistocene age.

In relation to their authenticity as human implements, according to his own statement therein, *i.e.*, "— I have not seen the originals," he is hardly in a position to speak with authority on the matter, especially in the face of the fact that no one who *has* seen them has questioned their authenticity as human artifacts.

Dr. Spier particularly questions the grinding stones to which we have referred as "metates," in describing them. It would appear that his objection may be based on our choice of name for them, or upon a misunderstanding as to how such grinding stones were used by nomadic, non-agricultural Indians,—uses to which his published remarks would indicate a lack of familiarity. In regard to this matter, the writer has in his personal collection a number of such grinding stones from the region near the Black Hills, South Dakota, which were used by the Sioux Indians of that region when the writer first knew them as a boy. These Indians did not raise or use any sort of grain or cereal, and were a nomadic, hunting race; yet they did use, until they secured better implements and food from the white man, "metates," or grinding stones, of the type found at Frederick, Oklahoma. They used these at semi-permanent camp sites for crushing and breaking up dried fruits, (such as cherries and plums), dried meat, "Indian 'turnips,'" and other dried roots and plants which they dried and cured for winter use, much of which dried exceedingly hard.

It is entirely probable that in this, as in many other instances, need and a similar environment have caused different peoples at widely separated times and places to do similar things independently and reach similar results; and it certainly is not, in itself, and unsupported, evidence of racial homogeneity. It can equally well be, and probably is, another case of parallelism. I have personally seen these stones so used many times, and now have some of their dried foods as well as grinding implements in my private collection. Therefore, the argument that such could not have great antiquity, because, "All Americanists are agreed that cereal raising is not one of the original constituents of Indian culture" is without value. Beyond this, what "Americanist," or anyone else, for that matter, is in a position at this time to speak with authority of the habits or customs of any race of men in early Pleistocene times in America—beyond that offered by the limited evidence of this Frederick discovery, and one or two others.

Dr. Spier's reference to determination of age by the type of artifacts characteristic of certain cultural stages in Europe is also assuming something, when applied to North America, that no one yet knows. It is well to bear in mind that the well known stages of Europe are *terminals,* and may have diverged widely from what was going on in America in Pleistocene times. Granting man's presence here, it is not safe to draw *a priori* conclusions on circumstantial inference, until they are supported by clean-cut evidence in North America. Our archeologists have studied, almost wholly, the cultures of comparatively recent times on this continent, and have not, in conjunction with geologists, (as has been done in Europe), worked out the sequence of Pleistocene events in this country, in relation to mankind. Until this is done, evidence based on type of workmanship in stone found here, is mere guesswork, outside of comparatively modern cultures. There is crying need for much to be done in this direction at this time, in America. The conviction in the minds of some men that no such evidence would ever be found in America, has, beyond doubt, gone far to retard such research.

As to the authenticity of these grinding stones, as such: Professor E. B. Renaud, internationally known archeologist, now of the University of Denver, is the last specialist who has examined these artifacts, and has just measured and examined them critically with the writer, since Dr. Spier's article appeared. He, like all others who have seen them, gives them his unqualified indorsement as human artifacts. We find all three artifacts figured in the original accounts to bear unmistakable evidence of human workmanship. The edges show distinctly the coarse chipping done in shaping them with "hammer stones" or other implements, on all sides. All three show clearly evidences of abrasion and wear *in the center on both sides.* The larger grinding stone has had the most wear, and is abraded in an oblong basin to a depth of twenty-three millimeters on one side, by about three hundred and eighty millimeters long; and eight millimeters deep on the reverse side, in a depression two hundred and seventy millimeters long. Distinct striæ from abrasion, "pecking marks," and other usual evidences of such use and wear, with which any one who knows such stones is familiar, are clear cut and abundant. There is no mistake. They are real, humanly formed artifacts, as may be observed by any one who cares to examine them, and, not merely "selected as metates because of their close resemblance to such forms."

As to their being contemporaneous with the fossil mammals of that deposit, (which Dr. O. P. Hay and the writer are describing elsewhere, in joint papers), we have rather definite, unpublished evidence to offer.

During a recent visit to Frederick, (December, 1927), the writer took occasion to examine much more carefully the upper bed in that section, (Bed C. of our published diagrams)[1] and secured evidence that we had overlooked in the early examinations. This upper bed, three to five feet in thickness, with columnar structures when dry, is composed largely of fine clays and silts, the shrinkage of which is responsible for such structure, as it dehydrates. But mingled through this bed irregularly are considerable quantities of granitic gravels, some very coarse. Being situated on a hilltop, it is obvious that this gravel must have been washed there from higher levels before it *was* a hilltop, and while the surrounding surface levels were at least as high or higher than this hill is to-day. As the hill is about one hundred feet above local valleys, and in the light of correlated evidence on this erosion, previously published, it becomes obvious and certain that Bed C, as well as the underlying cross bedded sands and gravels, is of Pleistocene age. Only in its very surface, and a few inches down, are recent deposits possible, save by intrusive burial of some sort. Now, Bed C is very dark red in color, heavily permeated with stains of hematite, so that all included gravels and anything it may contain are stained a deep, muddy red, so dark that even photographs of the deposit sharply outline it from the underlying Bed B. Obviously any implement which came from these surface deposits, or any such wash-filled basin as Dr. Spier imagines as possible or even from any stage of the Pleistocene Bed C, would certainly bear unmistakable evidence of its origin from this stain.

Re-examining with this in mind, with Dr. Renaud, we note that these grinding stones are *not* so stained, but bear only a slight, much lighter colored stain, such as characterizes Beds A and B in local lenses. Beyond this, in the rough surfaces of the stone, and adhering to their surfaces in many places, are still many areas of matrix, still cemented to the stones and unmistakably undisturbed, as found by Mr. Holloman. This matrix is that most characteristic of Bed B, but also occurs in the upper part of Bed A, where Mr. Holloman reported finding the implements; and, by no chance could it pertain to a level as high as Bed C.

I believe that no further authentication of the accuracy of Mr. Holloman's statement as to their

[1] *Natural History,* Vol. XXVII, No. 3, 1927.

actual occurrence in these Pleistocene beds is necessary. Mr. Holloman is now keenly alive to the importance of these discoveries, as he was not when we first talked to him; and, as he had previously found and discarded other similar implements before we saw him, he is confident of eventually finding more, as commercial quarrying continues in this deposit. When it is found, he told the writer that he would do all in his power to protect it *in situ,* and wire for authorities to come and view it for themselves. Consequently, as the quarry is now being actively developed, further discoveries are to be expected in this great deposit.

HAROLD J. COOK

COLORADO MUSEUM OF
NATURAL HISTORY

THE GEOLOGY OF SONORA

WHILE making a study of the sedimentary rocks in the Cananea Mining District, Cananea, Sonora, Mexico, I found some fossils which Dr. G. H. Girty, of the U. S. Geological Survey, has determined as belonging to the Carboniferous Age. The limestone in which the fossils occur was formerly considered to be Cambrian.[1]

Dr. Girty says: "The fossils from Cananea accompanying the letter of February 19 from Dr. Graham John Mitchell are, without much question, of Carboniferous Age, but to assign them within the Carboniferous System with any degree of certainty is impossible. The specimens, all very fragmentary, include cup corals (*Triplophyllum?* and *Lithostrotion?*), a strophomenoid (*Schuchertella* or *Derbya*), a *Spirifer* (apparently of the *Rockymontanus* group), and *Hustedia*."

GRAHAM JOHN MITCHELL

THREATENED EXTINCTION OF THE RUFFED GROUSE

ACCORDING to a recent report of the Department of Fisheries and Game, the ruffed grouse is facing extinction in the state of Massachusetts. Only a few of these magnificent upland game birds have been seen within the past year; and why this is so is not fully known, though it is believed that they have succumbed to a periodic visit of the partridge sickness. The winter and spring of 1926–27 were not sufficiently severe so as to decimate any large numbers of them, nor was the toll of the hunting season unusually large. But with the present mild winter, and a good breeding season, it is hoped that this once common game bird will be able to make sufficient numbers to withstand successfully the depredations of its natural enemies during the coming year. And with a closed season next fall, which the legislature is at present considering, to assist in their fight, it is believed that within a year or two they will be back on a fairly sound basis. It is to be regretted should this bird have to be added to the already long list of vanishing species.

BIRGER R. HEADSTROM

MEDFORD HILLSIDE,
MASSACHUSETTS

[1] *Ec. Geology,* vol. 5, No. 4, June, 1910, page 317.

WHAT IS A NAME?

SINCE Dr. Holland's recent fatherly note (SCIENCE, Feb. 10, p. 161) the differences between us seem reduced to one (I will not quarrel over the word "binomial"):

Is Limnas ferruginea Chrysippus (Hübner) as good a name as Papilio Danaus Festivus Chrysippus (Linnaeus) or Sphinx Adscita Phegea, which every one accepts?

The idea will be expanded in *Entomological News.*

WM. T. M. FORBES

CORNELL UNIVERSITY

SCIENTIFIC BOOKS

A treatise on the British Freshwater Algae in which are included all the pigmented Protophyta hitherto found in British freshwaters, by the late G. S. West, M. A., D.Sc., F. L. S., A. R. C. S., professor of botany at the University of Birmingham. New and Revised Edition in great part rewritten by F. E. FRITSCH, Professor of Botany in the University of London. (Cambridge, The University Press) xviii+534 pp., 207 figs. in text. Price 21 shillings. 1927.

THE first edition of this highly valued treatise, issued nearly twenty-five years ago, has been so long out of print that this new and up-to-date edition will be doubly welcome. Since the microscopic freshwater flora is so cosmopolitan in its distribution this handbook will serve others than British investigators. It will also be useful to zoologists as well as to botanists, since the reviser has included all pigmented or colored flagellates within the Algae. The first fifty pages are given to generalities, such as the ecology, distribution, collection, cultivation, structure, cytology and reproductive processes of the Algae. The author is inclined to minimize the significance of the polymorphism of the unicellular Algae brought about in cultures because of the lack of correlation of such results with the same species in their natural environments. Certain normal well established instances of polymorphic life cycles of both unicellular and multicellular stages do not justify sweeping general conclusions at present as to the extent of comparable polymorphism elsewhere among the Algae.

A very useful list of the algae of typical associations is given for various habitats such as ponds and ditches, rainpools, lakes, mountain tarns, flowing waters, bogs, salt marshes, wet rocks, damp ground, subterranean soil and tree trunks.

The greater part of the book is concerned with a systematic discussion of the eleven classes of freshwater Algae as follows: Isokontae, Heterokontae, Chrysophyceae, Bacillariales (Diatomales,) Cryptophyceae, Dinophyceae (Peridinieae,) Chloromonadales, Euglenineae, Rhodophyceae, Myxophyceae (Cyanophyceae.)

The author accepts the view of Luther, Borzi, Bohlin and others that the various classes of algae have had their origin from unicellular flagellates with similar pigments and storage products. He accordingly includes such flagellates in these respective algal classes. Zoologists will be interested in the bearings of these segregations on current classifications by protozoologists. The desirability of some sort of protistological organization of this common ground of the two biological disciplines and jurisdictions is rapidly becoming more evident.

The author uses the term Dinophyceae in lieu of Dinoflagellata. This is to be regretted, since the latter has been so widely used for many years, and the scope of the former strictly speaking can not be legitimately extended to include the Gymnodiniaceae and Peridiniaceae. The citation of Woloszynska's observations of polygonal plates on *Gymnodinium* without criticism might lead the reader to accept the idea that the structures thus detected really belonged to a true *Gymnodinium* instead of to a young or recently exuviated member of some armored genus such as *Peridinium*.

The illustrations are mainly old, but well selected and well executed. One might wish there were more of them, especially in a systematic treatise of this sort, but the author had to choose between the Scylla of condensation and the Charybdis of expense. A brief list of important works and a full index add to the usefulness of this excellent revision of a highly valued handbook.

CHARLES A. KOFOID

Gewebezüchtung. Handbuch der Biologie der Gewebezellen in Vitro. 2 vermehrete Auflage. By ALBERT FISCHER. München: Rudolf Müller und Steinicke, 1927. 508 pages, and 151 illustrations.

THIS volume is a German edition of Albert Fischer's "Tissue Culture," which was published in 1925 by Levin and Munksgaard, Copenhagen. Fischer may well be regarded as the most successful research worker in all Europe in this particular field. The excellent introduction was written by Dr. Alexis Carrel, the eminent authority on the subject of tissue cultivation. The book is really an entirely new edition of the first, fully revised and enlarged. A thorough description of the technique of tissue culture renders the book especially valuable for investigators in this field, which is rapidly becoming more and more important. In addition, the value of his work is greatly enhanced by the comprehensive and critical presentation of the very significant results and numerous new formulations of biological questions brought out by this method.

An historical review is followed by chapters on: (1) Media employed in the cultivation of tissues *in vitro;* (2) technique covering the preparation of culture media and the various substances now used; cover-glass preparations; measurement of the rate of growth; flask culture method; application of the microdissection method; photography and microscopic examination of cultures; (3) pure strains of cells; (4) tissue culture as a physiological method; (5) morphology; (6) tissue culture as a pathological method, and lastly, a most important chapter on the behavior of tumor cells *in vitro*. An excellent bibliography is appended.

The author's success in the cultivation of tumor cells is outstanding. He devised a technique whereby strains of malignant cells are made to grow permanently outside of the organism. The tumor cells do not lose their malignancy during their life *in vitro*. Even after many passages, a culture when transplanted to an animal gives rise to a tumor with metastases. This is true not only of Rous sarcoma, but also of different epithelial tumors which have been cultivated; for example, the carcinomata of mice.

The results obtained by the method of tissue culture have widened our scientific outlook and have correspondingly increased our knowledge of cell physiology, and Albert Fischer is to be highly congratulated upon his book on this subject.

ALBERT H. EBELING

ROCKEFELLER INSTITUTE FOR
MEDICAL RESEARCH

SCIENTIFIC APPARATUS AND LABORATORY METHODS

A SIMPLE VISUAL METHOD FOR DEMONSTRATING THE DIFFUSION OF OXYGEN THROUGH RUBBER AND VARIOUS OTHER SUBSTANCES

IN experimental work in which small quantities of oxygen are to be measured, rubber connections must be avoided because of the error introduced by the diffusion of oxygen through rubber. Coating such connections with paraffine, as is sometimes done, is of negligible value, as is shown by the following experiments. A simple visual demonstration of the diffusion of oxygen may be made by using luminous bacteria as an indicator. It has been shown by Harvey and Morrison (1923)[1] that these bacteria will give a just perceptible glow when the partial pressure of oxygen is only .0053 mm Hg.

A test tube is completely filled with a dilute suspension of luminous bacteria and closed with a rubber dam, care being taken to see that no air bubbles are included. The suspension will glow brightly until practically all the oxygen has been consumed. The light then disappears except in contact with the membrane and for a short distance from it. If a suspension of the proper concentration has been chosen a gradient of brightness is obtained, most brilliant in contact with the membrane and fading out toward the other end of the tube. The critical worker who desires a control may use for the purpose a glass-stoppered tube or graduate of the same diameter as the experimental tube. This becomes completely dark.

If it is desired to form a rough estimate of the relative amounts of oxygen diffusing through various substances, this may be done by comparing the length of the luminescent columns, provided that all the tubes are filled with a suspension of the same concentration and that convection currents are reduced to a minimum. In a recent experiment, the results shown in the table were obtained. The thermostat was kept at 24.6 ± .3° C., and top and bottom temperatures of the double walled box in which the apparatus was set up were recorded by Beckmann thermometers. The maximum difference between top and bottom was .054° C., and the average difference for the time of the experiment was .024° C. It is not believed that this difference was sufficient to set up disturbing convection currents.

It will be apparent from a glance at the table that for detecting the presence of minute quantities of oxygen very dilute suspensions are best, while for estimating relative quantities, suspensions somewhat more concentrated must be used. There is then established a mobile equilibrium, oxygen diffusing in at a definite rate, and being consumed at a definite rate, the ratio of the two rates determining the length of the luminescent column.

The long-continued luminescence under kerosene and xylol is surprising, as both of these are cytolyzing agents. On pouring off the oils at the end of the sixth hour, those under these two substances were found to be somewhat injured, as they did not exhibit full brilliance. Small quantities of all the substances used were shaken with bacterial suspensions, and all

[1] Harvey, E. Newton, and Morrison, Thos. F., "The Minimum Concentration of Oxygen for Luminescence by Luminous Bacteria," *J. G. P.*, 6, 13, 1923.

	Suspension 1		Suspension 2
	2 hours	6 hours	3 hours
Open control	10 cm.	10 cm.	10 cm.
Glass stoppered control	(Dark in 45 min.)		(Dark in 3 hours)
Wet collodion	4 cm.	4 cm.	10 cm.
Kerosene	4 cm.	3 cm. (dim)	10 cm. (dim)
Paraffined cork	3 cm.	3 cm.	10 cm.
Paraffine oil	3 cm.	3 cm.	10 cm.
Paraffine (52°)	3 cm.	3 cm.	10 cm.
White vaseline	3 cm.	3 cm.	10 cm.
Amber vaseline	2 cm.	2 cm.	10 cm.
Wet parchment	2 cm.	2 cm.	10 cm.
Paraffined parchment	2 cm.	2 cm.	10 cm.
Olive oil	1.5 cm.	1.5 cm. (dim)	10 cm. (dim)
Thin lubricating oil	1.5 cm.	1.5 cm.	10 cm.
Xylol	1.5 cm.	1.5 cm. (dim)	10 cm. (dim)
Rubber dam	.5 cm.	.5 cm.	4 cm.
Paraffined rubber stopper	Trace	0	trace
Medium motor oil	0	0	.5 cm.
DeKhotinsky on rubber dam	0	0	0
DeKhotinsky on cork	0	0	0
Dried collodion on linen	0	0	trace

Length of luminescent columns of bacteria under various oils, etc. The tubes used contained 10 cm. of the bacterial suspension.

were found harmless except olive oil, kerosene and xylol, each of which caused a considerable diminution of brilliance. Evidently the slight solubility and slow diffusion downward of these substances saved the bacteria from cytolyzing effects.

The impermeability or very slight permeability of viscous motor oil to oxygen is in agreement with the finding of Kruse (1926)[2] that alkaline pyrogallate solutions under medium motor oils were not perceptibly oxidized after eight weeks, while those covered with kerosene and mineral oil were oxidized 30 per cent. and less than 5 per cent., respectively. This difference Kruse ascribes to the greater viscosity of the motor oils.

It will be noted that of the liquids used the medium motor oil is by far the best for exclusion of oxygen. Heavy rubber stoppers and thick tubing, if time is allowed for diffusion out of the oxygen dissolved in the surface, will introduce only small errors, the diffusion of oxygen through rubber as thick as 1 cm. being slight.

SAMUEL E. HILL

PHYSIOLOGICAL LABORATORY,
PRINCETON UNIVERSITY

SPECIAL ARTICLES

THE PRODUCTION OF MUTATIONS AND REARRANGEMENTS OF GENES BY X-RAYS

MUTATIONS and rearrangements of genes have been produced by Muller by subjecting *Drosophila melanogaster* to the action of X-rays.[1] Similar experiments have since been performed by the writer; and these, while not so extensive, are in entire agreement with those of Muller. As a result of X-ray treatment, there have been obtained mutations producing visible and lethal effects, as well as genetic modifications of the frequency of crossing over, and attachments between genes of different chromosomes.

Males of *Drosophila melanogaster* were exposed to X-rays in dosages corresponding approximately to those designated by Muller as T4 and T2, the former being about twice the latter. The treated males and untreated brothers used as controls were mated to untreated females. The fertility of the irradiated males and of their offspring was reduced, the stronger treatment being the more effective in each case. As has been suggested by Muller, sterility might be produced in the treated males by mutations resulting in dominant lethal genes, and it might be produced in the offspring by mutations resulting in dominant genes for sterility.

The experiment was designed primarily to test the effect of the treatment on the X-chromosome. In order that the treated and control X-chromosomes might be recognized in subsequent generations, the males were mated to females that differed from them in certain sex-linked genes. Since every daughter received a treated or control X, any change in this chromosome would be inherited by half her sons and would be detected if it produced a visible or lethal effect.

Nine of the thirty-seven F_1 females in the T4 series and ten of the forty-seven F_1 females in the T2 series were found to have inherited altered X-chromosomes from their fathers. No changes in the X were observed in the fifty-six F_1 females of the controls. (Only the fertile females are included in the reckoning.) In X's of the T4 series there were three mutant genes (one dominant, two recessive) producing visible effects, and six lethals. In X's of the T2 series there were two genes (both recessive) producing visible effects, and eight lethals. Of the non-lethal mutant genes, three recessives are allelomorphs of genes already known (deltex, furrowed, uneven); the others seem to be changes in hitherto unknown loci.

The experiment was not designed to detect mutations in the autosomes; and such changes resulting in recessive genes would, for several reasons, have escaped discovery. (One autosomal recessive was found in an F_2 culture in the control series, but it must have been present in heterozygous form in either the male or the female of the P_1 generation.) New autosomal dominants, however, could be recognized; and three were found, all in the T2 series. One of these (an eye color—the only dominant mutant eye color known in *D. melanogaster*) arose in a treated male; the two others (probably allelomorphs of Star and Hairless, respectively) may have originated in either the males or the females of the P_1 generation.

In the offspring of the treated flies there were found six translocations in which genes of the second chromosome behave as if attached to the X; that is, they are inherited in sex-linked fashion. In at least some of these cases, genes along the entire length of the second chromosome behave in this way. The point of attachment in the X differs in different cases; whether or not the point of attachment in the second chromosome differs is not known. The results would

[2] Kruse, T. K., "The Relative Efficiency of Several Oils for the Exclusion of Oxygen," *J. Phar. and Exp. Ther.*, *27*, No. 3, April, 1926.

[1] Muller, H. J., "Artificial Transmutation of the Gene," SCIENCE, Vol. 66, pp. 84–87 (1927); "The Problem of Genic Modification," *Proc. Fifth Int. Congress of Genetics* (in press); "The Effects of X Radiation on Genes and Chromosomes," abstracts in *Anat. Record*, Vol. 37, p. 174, and SCIENCE, Vol. 67, p. 82.

seem at first sight to imply attachments between entire chromosomes; but they might also be produced by the attachment to one chromosome of a piece of another, provided that individuals receiving more or less than the normal complement of genes did not survive. Tests are being made to decide between these alternatives and to discover (if fragmentation is involved) which chromosome is broken. Three of the translocations occurred in the T4 series (where such changes could have been detected in seventeen cases), and three in the T2 series (where they could have been detected in forty-three cases). None were observed in the controls, although here they could have been detected in fifty-five cases. It seems probable that in the irradiated flies there occurred in addition to the translocations observed others involving genes not followed in the experiment. (No genes of the third or fourth chromosome were followed.)

Eight cases of genetic reduction of crossing over in the X-chromosome were observed; some prevent crossing over almost entirely, others affect only part of the chromosome. Five were in the T4 series and three in the T2 series; but this does not represent the total frequency of such modifications, since they could have been recognized in only twenty-two cases in the former and thirteen in the latter. In the controls no such changes would have been detected; but it is very unlikely that they occurred, for in all the *Drosophila* work in which X-rays have not been used only five genetic modifications affecting crossing over in the X-chromosome have been found. In the present experiment one of the modifiers is associated with no other effect, one is associated with a non-lethal mutant gene, the others with lethals or translocations.

The dominant eye-color gene behaves as if it were continually mutating in both germ and somatic cells. It is not yet certain, however, that the behavior is to be ascribed to mutation.

Apart from this, the new genes (they have all, with the exception of one lethal in the T2 series, been followed through several generations) seem to behave like ordinary mutant genes. It is possible that some of the lethals are not due to point-mutations. Six of them are associated with crossover modifiers or with translocations; and this suggests that the same disturbance may be responsible for all the effects in each case. There is also a possibility that some of the other lethals are due to translocations involving genes not followed in the experiment. Nevertheless, it is probable that at least some of the lethals are due to changes in single genes. One of the lethals apparently crosses over from the translocated genes with which it is associated. And all the non-lethal genes behave like point-mutations—some of them are, in fact, allelomorphic to, if not identical with, genes produced by ordinary mutations. The nature of the crossover modifiers has not yet been ascertained.

A comparison of the mutation rates is best made on the basis of the changes in the X-chromosomes. If we include the visible mutants and the lethals, about one X-chromosome in four mutated in the T4 series, about one in five in the T2 series, and none in the controls. The figures suggest that a greater effect was produced by the stronger treatment (and the same is true of the translocations). But the numbers are not large enough to decide whether the effect is proportional to the dosage or to some function of it. Moreover, it may be that the effect of the stronger treatment is relatively underestimated. For there was more sterility in the T4 series; and if the frequency of mutation was correlated with sterility (quite apart from whether sterility was produced by mutations), then the individuals in which the greatest number of mutations occurred were the very ones that could not be tested.

But if the results do not show precisely how the mutation rate varies with the strength of the treatment, they demonstrate the effectiveness of the treatment itself. There were eight (possibly ten) mutant genes producing visible effects and fourteen lethals in the eighty-four treated individuals, and none in the fifty-six controls. The results are being subjected to further analysis; but the work has gone far enough to show that, as in the experiments of Muller, genes can be modified and rearranged as a result of treatment with X-rays.

The writer desires to thank Dr. L. A. Milkman for his cooperation in administering the X-ray treatments.

ALEXANDER WEINSTEIN
COLUMBIA UNIVERSITY

A DETERMINATION OF THE NEWTONIAN CONSTANT OF GRAVITATION BY A STUDY OF THE VIBRATIONS OF A TORSION PENDULUM

CONSIDER the result of suspending an enclosed torsion pendulum, supposed for simplicity to consist only of two massive particles m, m at distances b from the axis of suspension, in the vicinity of the spherical bob of a common pendulum; the latter being symmetrically placed with respect to the torsion pendulum and executing vibrations of amplitude b in a plane parallel to m, m. If the two periods are nearly equal, the alternate gravitational attractions of the large mass upon the two particles m, m will cause the torsion pendulum to vibrate about its axis of suspension. Besides the torsional oscillations there will be forced

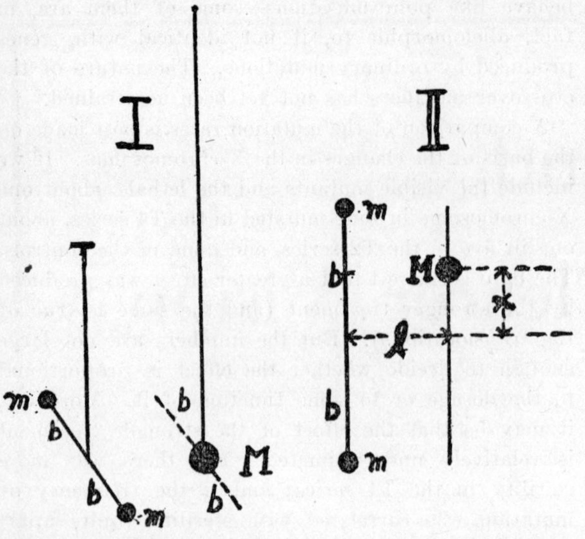

pendular vibrations; but these may be neglected. Let I be the moment of inertia of the torsion pendulum; k the couple due to damping for unit angular velocity; and μ the moment of torsion of the suspension. Let the displacement $\varkappa$ of M at time t be $\varkappa = b \sin \varrho t$. Set

$$2a = \frac{k}{I};\quad n^2 = \frac{\mu}{I}.$$

Then the differential equation of motion of the torsion pendulum is

$$(1). \; . \; . \frac{d^2\vartheta}{dt^2} + 2a\frac{d\vartheta}{dt} + n^2\vartheta = \frac{GMmb}{I\,l^2}\left[\frac{1}{\left\{1+\frac{1}{l^2}(b-\varkappa)^2\right\}^{3/2}} - \frac{1}{\left\{1+\frac{1}{l^2}(b+\varkappa)^2\right\}^{3/2}}\right]$$

where G is the constant of gravitation. The right hand member of (1) may be replaced by the first term of its Fourier sine series (suggested by E. P. Adams), which it very nearly equals:

$$(2) \; . \; . \; . \; . \frac{GbMm}{I\,l^2}\left(1 - \frac{1}{\left(1+\frac{4b^2}{l^2}\right)^{3/2}}\right)\sin \varrho t = B \sin \varrho t.$$

The solution of (1) which satisfies the initial conditions is

$$(3) \; . \; . \; . \vartheta = \frac{B}{\left\{(n^{1 2} - \varrho^2)^2 + a^2(a^2 + 2n^{1 2} + 2\varrho^2)\right\}^{1/2}}\left\{e^{-at}\frac{\varrho}{n^1}\sin(n^1 t + \varepsilon^1) + \sin(\varrho t - \varepsilon)\right\}$$

where $n^{1 2} = n^2 - a^2$; $\tan \varepsilon = \frac{2a\varrho}{n^{1 2} - \varrho^2 + a^2}$;

and $\tan \varepsilon^1 = \frac{2an^1}{\varrho^2 - n^{1 2} + a^2}$.

The period of free torsional oscillation $T = \frac{2\pi}{n^1}$; and $aT = \log \eta$, the logarithmic decrement of the torsion pendulum for complete swings.

Suppose that we make the periods equal, so that $n^1 = \varrho$: Then

$$(4) \; . \; . \; . \; . \vartheta = \frac{B}{a(4\varrho^2 + a^2)^{1/2}}\left\{e^{-at}\cos(\varrho t + \varepsilon^1) + \sin(\varrho t - \varepsilon)\right\}$$

where $\varepsilon = \varepsilon^1 = \tan^{-1}\frac{2\varrho}{a} = \frac{\pi}{2}$ nearly.

As $t \rightarrow \infty$, the amplitude approaches a maximum $\vartheta_m = \frac{B}{2\varrho a}$ nearly. Substituting for B its value from (2), $\varrho = \frac{2\pi}{T}$, $a = \frac{1}{T}\log \eta$, $I = 2mb^2$, and solving for G, we find:

$$(5) \; . \; . \; . \; . G = \frac{8\pi b\, l^2 \log \eta.}{MT^2\left(1 - \frac{1}{\left(1+\frac{4b^2}{l^2}\right)^{3/2}}\right)}\vartheta_m.$$

In the writer's experiments the torsion pendulum was adjusted until its period was 7.4485 sec. That of the common pendulum was 7.4508 sec. M was the bob of a Foucault pendulum, and weighed 5.5×10^5 grams. In one particular experiment b was 38.5 cm., l was 29.7 cm., and $\log \eta$ was found by an auxiliary experiment to be .00603. The only effect of convection currents in the torsion pendulum box could have been to hasten the approach of the amplitude to ϑ_m (which might otherwise be asymptotically approached). After about fifty minutes, ϑ_m was reached; and by a set of readings by mirror and scale was found to be 3.8×10^{-4} radians. By (5) G was found to be 6.75×10^{-8} C.G.S. units. The average of the results of several such experiments was

$$G = 6.6_5 \times 10^{-8} \text{ C.G.S. units.}$$
$$(\text{True value } G = 6.6576 \times 10^{-8})^1$$

Though not as accurate as the refined Cavendish method, this experiment is a simple one to perform. The writer's apparatus was assembled in about six hours' time, since he was aided by the presence of a large Foucault pendulum. In case no great accuracy is desired, the method presents the advantage that it is free from errors due to non-periodic convection currents, so troublesome in the Cavendish form of the experiment.

T. E. STERN

PALMER PHYSICAL LABORATORY,
PRINCETON UNIVERSITY

[1] C. V. Boys, Phil. Trans. A, 1895, part 1.

SCIENCE

VOL. LXVII APRIL 13, 1928 No. 1737

CONTENTS

The American Association for the Advancement of Science:
Contributions of the Chemist to our Knowledge of Biological Oxidations: DR. EDWARD C. KENDALL ... 379
Contributions of Anthropology to Medicine: DR. ALEŠ HRDLIČKA ... 385
Edward Sandford Burgess: THEODORE E. HAMILTON 388
Scientific Events:
A New Edition of Willard Gibbs's Works; Barro Colorado Island Station; Appropriations of the General Education Board; Annual Meeting of the American Geophysical Union ... 389
Scientific Notes and News ... 391
University and Educational Notes ... 394
Discussion and Correspondence:
The Aurora of March 28, 1928: DR. H. T. STETSON. *The Washboard or ''Corduroy'' Effect in Dirt Roads:* RAY C. TREASHER, ELLWOOD WILSON. *Ovarian Secretion and Cancer:* WILLIAM S. MURRAY. *Relation of the Sun's Activity to some Biological Factors:* DR. G. I. POKROWSKI. *The Sharp Rattling in Steam Pipes:* PROFESSOR R. C. COLWELL. *Scientific Obscurity:* DR. EDWIN E. SLOSSON ... 394
Scientific Books:
Hoffmann's Birds of the Pacific States: DR. TRACY I. STORER. *Rogers's Text-Book of Comparative Physiology:* PROFESSOR C. W. GREENE ... 398
Scientific Apparatus and Laboratory Methods:
The Collodion Method and Serial Sections: DR. E. E. CAROTHERS ... 400
Special Articles:
Direct Evidence of Atom Building: DR. R. A. MILLIKAN and DR. G. H. CAMERON. *Water Soluble Phosphorus in Soils:* DR. F. W. PARKER ... 401
The American Philosophical Society ... 403
Science News ... x

SCIENCE: A Weekly Journal devoted to the Advancement of Science, edited by J. McKeen Cattell and published every Friday by

THE SCIENCE PRESS

New York City: Grand Central Terminal.
Lancaster, Pa. Garrison, N. Y.
Annual Subscription, $6.00. Single Copies, 15 Cts.

SCIENCE is the official organ of the American Association for the Advancement of Science. Information regarding membership in the Association may be secured from the office of the permanent secretary, in the Smithsonian Institution Building, Washington, D. C.

CONTRIBUTIONS OF THE CHEMIST TO OUR KNOWLEDGE OF BIOLOGICAL OXIDATIONS[1]

THE contributions of the chemist to our knowledge of biological oxidations are today of such magnitude that they constitute a subdivision of biochemistry. A mere enumeration of the problems which have been solved would be of little purpose; on the other hand, to speak at length on a few interesting details would be evidence of lack of appreciation of the great contributions which have been made. I shall therefore try to point out the methods by which the various types of investigation have been carried out rather than give great detail concerning any one investigation.

CALORIGENIC RELATIONSHIPS

The problem of the oxidation of foodstuffs may be considered from the standpoint of the three classes of compounds, carbohydrates, fats and proteins. The calorigenic relationships were placed on a firm basis when it was shown that the same amount of heat was produced whether glucose was burned in the body or in a bomb calorimeter. Studies in the complicated apparatus necessary for direct calorimetry have now given way to the analysis of expired air, and for most work all the essential data may be obtained by indirect calorimetry.

After it had been shown that 1 gm. of glucose, 1 gm. of fat and 1 gm. of protein furnish to the animal organism 4.2 calories, 9.46 calories and 4.3 calories, respectively, it was realized that all the essential data required to estimate the diet requirements of an animal organism were at hand. These data, however, furnished no information concerning the mechanism by which glucose, fats and proteins were burned in the animal organism.

INTERMEDIARY METABOLISM

Despite the large amount of work carried out in the field of intermediary metabolism many important questions remain unanswered. Embden and Meyerhof have shown that glucose apparently is utilized through the decomposition of a hexose phosphate, and the work of Hill and Meyerhof is very suggestive that at least a portion of the lactic acid is burned to

[1] Presented as part of a symposium on ''The Contributions of Other Sciences to Medicine'' at the annual meeting of the American Association for the Advancement of Science, Nashville, December 28, 1927.

carbon dioxide and water. This detail of the combustion of glucose has not, however, been proved, and Lusk has placed an interrogation point after this portion of the Hill-Meyerhof theory. It is possible that other substances are burned in place of lactic acid.

There is also the question whether glucose can be burned by any mechanism in the animal organism other than through the course of phosphoric acid ester, lactic acid, carbon dioxide.

Thunberg has shown that succinic acid is readily attacked by enzymes in the muscle, and the significance of this observation in relation to the combustion of sugars, proteins and fats is not clear.

Other problems relating to the oxidation of glucose deal with the phenomenon of antiketogenesis. Is sugar necessary for the proper combustion of fat in the animal organism? Shaffer and coworkers and others have indicated that it is, and have suggested a stoichiometric relationship. On the other hand, it has been suggested that ketone bodies are formed when the quantity of fat utilized is raised above a certain level. If glucose is burned in preference to fat the addition of carbohydrate to the diet would relieve the ketogenesis, but by a different mechanism than that suggested by Shaffer.

Still another problem in the oxidation of glucose is the specific dynamic action of this material. Lusk has shown that a plethora of glucose produces an increased rate of utilization of this sugar, and Woodyatt has shown that continuous injection of glucose results in an increased rate of the oxidation of this material.

The combustion of fats is still shrouded with mystery. The one most important fact in the oxidation of fat is the evidence concerning the point of attack in a fatty acid; this was shown by Knoop. A long chain of carbon atoms terminating in a carboxyl group can be burned in the animal organism by the successive breaking off of groups of two carbon atoms at a time, but the details of this decomposition and the fate of the two carbon atoms is still unknown. Meissl and Strohmer, Voit and Lehmann and Lusk have shown that glucose can be converted into fat and it seems probable that the combustion of fat can be utilized for the production of mechanical energy in the body, but no one has yet conclusively shown that fat can be converted into glucose. The problems to be answered in this field are closely bound up with the fatty-acid-containing substances of the body, such as lecithin, cephalin, fatty-acid esters of cholesterol and other substances, some of which are insoluble in water, and yet are absorbed through the intestine and transported in the blood.

The combustion of the proteins involves the added problem of the fate of the nitrogen-containing substances. Some of the amino acids in protein can be converted into sugar and are probably burned as glucose; some apparently can not be converted into glucose but follow a separate path. Knoop has suggested that ketone acids and ammonia can interact with the formation of amino acids through the aid of the sulphydryl group of glutathione which functions as a reducing agent.

The influence of proteins on cellular activity has been investigated for many years. Through the work of Voit, Rübner, Lusk and many others it has been shown that the administration of proteins and certain of the amino acids results not only in the combustion of these substances but also in an increased rate of oxidation of other metabolites. This occurs in the phlorizinized dog, even though the carbon content of the amino acid is quantitatively excreted as glucose. The specific dynamic action of proteins is one of the most interesting and important phases of oxidation in the animal organism.

Probably the most important problem in the oxidation of glucose, fats and proteins is the relationship of glucose to other carbon compounds. It is hoped that the investigation of intermediary metabolism will eventually explain the conversion of glucose-forming substances to sugar and bring into harmony the theories concerning the utilization of carbohydrates, fats and proteins for the production of heat and energy.

Food Accessories

After it had been shown that a diet should contain carbohydrate, fat and protein, it was assumed that any normal animal organism would grow to maturity and enjoy normal health provided a sufficient number of calories of a well-balanced diet was furnished. The satisfied feeling which accompanied this conclusion was rudely jarred about fifteen years ago by the discovery of a group of substances which were termed food accessories, or vitamins, that appeared to be essential for the proper growth and maintenance of health in the normal animal organism.

This problem is with us to-day and one receives at least an introduction to these substances through the columns of the daily newspaper or the popular weeklies. I shall not discuss in detail the influence of the vitamins on the oxidation in the animal organism, but shall call attention to three substances which appear to be related, at least in their action, to the so-called food accessories.

Throughout the period during which biological oxidations have been investigated each successive decade has given its own peculiar contribution to the problem, and the investigators who have taken up this work in turn have doubtless felt that until some unsuspected door was opened, further progress with the problem would be but meager.

The physicist of 1895 could not visualize the magnitude of the regeneration which would follow the discovery of radioactivity and the better understanding of electromagnetic vibrations. The biochemist in 1895 did not realize that he would soon look down a long avenue through a door which had just been opened to permit a partial view of the problems and triumphs which were to come.

During the few years preceding 1895, the attention of clinicians was strongly attracted to the striking results obtained by feeding the thyroid gland to human beings and experimental animals deficient in thyroid function, and in December of that year Baumann published the important discovery that iodine was a normal constituent of the thyroid gland. Because of the clinical importance of this work it was soon followed by a more detailed investigation and in a relatively short time Magnus-Levy showed that administration of the thyroid gland increased the rate of oxidative processes in the body. I shall not at this time outline the isolation of thyroxine and the subsequent developments in this field.

About twenty-five years ago through the efforts of Abel, Takamine, Aldrich, Lucius, Brüning and Flächer, the first crystalline compound from a gland of internal secretion was isolated, identified and synthesized and it was soon shown that epinephrin or adrenaline affected physiological processes to a marked degree. Many years passed, however, before Boothby, Marine, Means, Soskin and others showed that in this case also at least a portion of the effect is due to a change in the rate of oxidation.

Through the efforts of still a third group of investigators, Hottinger, Thunberg, Meyerhof, Hopkins, Dixon, Tunnicliffe, Voegtlin and others, another agent of great significance in biological oxidations was recognized and finally isolated, identified and synthesized, glutathione.

The isolation and identification of these compounds, however, did not mark the completion of the problem. The chemical properties and effects of these three compounds and related substances will occupy the attention of investigators for many years.

The first step necessary was to determine the end results brought about by the administration of these compounds. Careful determinations of the basal metabolic rate and of the intake and output of nitrogen, sulfur, calcium, etc., have been made and quantitative relationships have been determined concerning the effect of thyroxine.

The influence of adrenaline on blood sugar, carbon dioxide output and oxygen consumption has been shown, and the influence of glutathione on oxidation in vitro and on muscle tone has been studied. These results deal only with the end products of reactions which are irreversible within the animal organism. It was recognized that energy had been generated by a combination of the oxygen of the air with hydrogen and carbon of the food, but the mechanism by which thyroxine, adrenaline or glutathione brought about a change in the velocity of oxidative processes has remained up to the present time an unsolved problem.

The problem is complex and must be approached through the efforts of investigators from many different points of view. The processes influenced by these agents take place in a colloidal medium where surface tension, phenomena of adsorption, the selective action dependent on stereoisomerism—and the commanding influence of hydrogen-ion concentration affect the mechanism involved. The equilibrium which exists is delicately balanced.

It is obvious that the tissues can not be in a state of static equilibrium. Even at rest chemical processes are continually occurring and the problem involves a kinetic equilibrium which is influenced by innumerable factors.

OXIDATION-REDUCTION POTENTIALS

Before the work of van't Hoff, Arrhenius, Ostwald, Sorenson, Clark and others the relations between amphoteric substances and hydrogen-ion concentration in biological phenomena were not appreciated. The early workers in the field of biological oxidations were not cognizant of the static and kinetic equilibriums which exist between oxidizing and reducing agents and the velocity of the reactions associated with life processes. By the use of oxidizing dyes many qualitative results were obtained and attempts were made to determine the intensity of oxidation in the animal organism, but the actual progress made toward this objective was but meager until still another avenue of approach for a quantitative study of the oxidation-reduction intensity was opened by Clark and coworkers.

This group of investigators has made a great contribution to our knowledge of oxidation-reduction potentials, and now for the first time the investigator in oxidation-reduction processes is equipped not only with an adequate theory concerning the mechanism involved but furthermore with a series of dyes which have been studied with precision so that the intensity of oxidation of any given solution can be determined within narrow limits.

This painstaking investigation has opened for the biochemist of 1927 a wide entrance to a fertile field; before the end is reached biological oxidation will be intimately linked with simpler systems by means of a fuller understanding of the physico-chemical principles involved. The processes occurring in the tissues, which are described to-day as enzyme action, will be explained in terms of thermodynamics to a degree which has been up to the present wholly unattainable.

The problem of biological oxidation was presented by Hopkins in 1926 at the International Congress of Physiologists. He reviewed the two theories: activation of oxygen suggested by Warburg and others, and primary dehydrogenation suggested by Wieland and others. The dehydrogenation theory of Wieland was favored by the essayist, although it was evident that probably a middle ground would eventually afford the correct interpretation of the phenomena.

Clark has shown that the intensity of oxidation or reduction of organic dyes is related to the structure of the dye and he has proposed a theory of the mechanism of oxidation-reduction processes which is broad enough to include the essential features of both those of Wieland and of Warburg. This theory expresses the oxidation and reduction of complex organic dyes in the same terms employed to describe the reaction involved in the oxidation or reduction of inorganic compounds such as ferrous and ferric salts. In the words of Clark:

> Oxidation may be regarded as the withdrawal of electrons from a substance with or without the addition of oxygen or elements analogous to oxygen or as a withdrawal of electrons with or without the withdrawal of hydrogen or elements analogous to hydrogen. Reduction is the reverse of oxidation as defined above.

This definition meets on common ground with the definition of an acid and a base given by Lewis:

> A basic substance is one which has a lone pair of electrons which may be used to complete the stable group of another atom, and that an acid substance is one which can employ a lone pair from another molecule in completing the stable group of one of its own atoms. In other words, the basic substance furnishes a pair of electrons for a chemical bond, the acid substance accepts such a pair.

When the phenomena of biological oxidation are investigated with this broad viewpoint, both in respect to the nature of oxidizing and reducing substances as well as acid and basic compounds, the nomenclature and the significance of the chemical reactions involved form a continuous pathway from the complex field of biological oxidation through to the realm of simple water solutions containing only inorganic substances. Such a theory has proved adequate up to the present and, by excluding the question of whether or not hydrogen is added or removed during the processes of oxidation and reduction, has eliminated an unnecessary and superfluous detail.

To insist upon the addition or removal of hydrogen but complicates the problem. Clark has pointed out that because hydrogen is associated with a reductant when removed from solution is not evidence that the hydrogen is actually a component part of the compound as it exists in solution. However, the theory that the reactions are dependent on the transfer of electrons from those substances which can furnish electrons, or the acceptance of electrons by compounds that can accept them furnishes a viewpoint which will satisfy the broadest requirements of the problem, at least for many years.

Oxidation Characteristics of Adrenaline and its Derivatives

The beautiful experiments of Gesell on control of respiration have been made possible by the development of methods for the determination of the relationship between oxygen, the oxidative rate in the tissues and the hydrogen-ion concentration in the living animal organism. Means has also reported the effect on the circulation of changes in the basal metabolic rate due to the administration of thyroxine and adrenaline. An investigation has been carried out in my laboratory, with E. J. Witzemann, which carries our knowledge of the chemical reaction involved back one step further and has brought to light some chemical characteristics of adrenaline and glutathione which have been demonstrated in simple buffer solutions.

Throughout this work it was assumed that the surface of the platinum electrode indicated the concentration of electrons from the substances in the solution which could be regarded as reducing agents, and that the oxidation-reduction potential indicated by the platinum was the algebraic sum of the influence of available electrons and the effect of the total oxidant in the solution. The compounds related to adrenaline can be divided into three groups: (1) ephedrin, (2) adrenalone, and amino and dimethylaminoacetopyrocatechol, (3) adrenaline, the methyl and ethyl ethers of adrenaline and the anhydride of adrenaline.

The first problem investigated was whether these substances can be reversibly oxidized. It was quantitatively shown that ephedrin could be neither oxidized nor reduced at a pH 7.4 with any of the oxidizing dyes used, with or without the presence of molecular oxygen or hydrogen peroxide. Adrenalone and its two derivatives act as reducing agents toward dibromophenolindophenol and indigo carmine and can be reversibly oxidized; adrenaline and its three ether derivatives are all oxidized by dibromophenolindophenol, but are not oxidized by indigo carmine. However, when the compounds in Group 3 are oxidized, the molecule is so altered that the solution does not contain any oxidizing substances. The end products of mild oxidation of adrenaline, therefore, may be described as irreversible.

The results of this part of the investigation have established certain characteristics of these substances which are of the greatest significance: first: the velocity of oxidation and the degree of oxidation are not determined by the intensity of the oxidizing agent used; and, second, before adrenalone and its derivatives can act as reducing agents some intermediate addition complex must be formed which activates the compound and permits it to function as a reducing agent.

The first conclusion is clearly shown by the velocity of oxidation of adrenalone and its derivatives with dibromophenolindophenol, methylene blue and indigo carmine. Indigo carmine has an almost specific effect on the molecule and the presence of 5 per cent. of one equivalent of indigo carmine markedly increases the velocity of oxidation with dibromophenolindophenol. Such a result is contrary to the usual velocity of oxidation induced by these dyes.

When molecular oxygen is passed through a solution of adrenalone dissolved in phosphate buffer, pH 7.4, no oxidation of the adrenalone occurs. If, as assumed by Wieland, hydrogen is first removed from the molecule then adrenalone can not spontaneously act as a hydrogen donator in the presence of molecular oxygen, or in the terms of Clark we can conclude that electrons can not be withdrawn from the adrenalone molecular with molecular oxygen. The same stability of the molecule is exhibited toward hydrogen peroxide. Furthermore, adrenalone does not appreciably affect the platinum electrode, which indicates that adrenalone can not affect the concentration of electrons in a solution at pH 7.4. However, if to such a solution 5 per cent of one equivalent of indigo carmine is added, the dye is rapidly reduced, and the platinum electrode indicates a marked reduction potential. If, as well as the indigo carmine, molecular oxygen or hydrogen peroxide is added there is a cyclic oxidation and reduction of the indigo carmine resulting in the oxidation of the adrenalone. This effect of adrenalone is evidence for the second characteristic which I have attributed to this substance and can be explained on the assumption that some type of addition compound is formed between indigo carmine and adrenalone: the result of this reaction is the liberation of available electrons.

Two other observations were made: (1) Indigo carmine is reduced by adrenalone even in the presence of an excess of hydrogen peroxide. Hydrogen peroxide added to a solution of reduced indigo carmine results in the rapid oxidation of the dye, but in the presence of adrenalone oxidation of the reduced indigo carmine occurs but slowly.

(2) The formation of some addition complex between adrenalone and the oxidizing dye is indicated by the addition to the solution of a compound which does not have oxidation-reduction power itself, but which inhibits the oxidation of adrenalone by the oxidizing dye. Such a substance is tungstic acid. If but a small percentage of one equivalent of tungstic acid is added to a solution of adrenalone in phosphate buffer, pH 7.4, there is no change in hydrogen-ion concentration, but the velocity of oxidation with dibromophenolindophenol or with indigo carmine is reduced almost to zero. It can not be assumed that the amount of tungstic acid in the solution caused an oxidation of the reduced form of the dye, and the reaction is adequately explained by the assumption that the formation of an addition complex between adrenalone and the dye is prevented by the presence of the small amount of tungstic acid. No precipitate is formed in the solution.

The effect of oxidizing dyes on adrenalone is similar to the effects of oxidizing dyes on other biological products. As Oppenheimer points out, nothing occurs in these cases except that the hydrogen is taken up by the acceptor and then the leuco dye formed turns it over to the oxygen. He concludes by saying, "This is the fact, the explanation is not available."

The results which I have outlined indicate that actual addition products are formed in the solution.

The necessity for a consideration of the chemical configuration of an oxidizing dye is strikingly shown by the influence of dibromophenolindophenol, methylene blue and indigo carmine on dimethylaminoacetopyrocatechol. This compound reacts sluggishly with dibromophenolindophenol, but if indigo carmine is added to the solution the velocity of oxidation is markedly increased. The discrepancy reaches its maximal proportions when methylene blue is used. This dye is not reduced by dimethylaminoacetopyrocatechol, but if a small percentage of one equivalent of indigo carmine is added to the solution prompt reduction of both dyes occurs. This is evidence that the formation of an addition complex is essential for the interaction of this group of compounds with oxidizing dyes.

If addition complexes between adrenalone and metabolites can be formed in the animal organism, it is possible that this reaction explains in part the marked effect of this series of compounds on the oxidative process in the animal organism. It therefore became desirable to show that a similar reaction occurs with adrenaline. Toward oxidizing dyes adrenaline reacts in a manner closely simulating that of adrenalone, except that it is entirely stable toward indigo carmine.

Experiments showed, however, that adrenaline does not function as an oxidizing agent after it has been partially oxidized with a dye. This was eventually shown to be due to the fact that one portion of the adrenaline molecule is too unstable to remain unaffected by the oxidized portion of the molecule. The result of the interaction of the two portions of the adrenaline molecule is the loss of all oxidizing power which can be transferred subsequently to another substance. This suggested the possibility of demonstrating the cyclic oxidation and reduction of adrenaline, provided some substance was present which would reduce oxidized adrenaline before one portion of the adrenaline molecule reacted with the oxidizing group. Adrenalone will serve this purpose. If air is passed through a solution of adrenaline the adrenaline is oxidized. If air is passed through a solution of adrenalone there is no effect. If air is passed through a solution of adrenalone containing a small amount of adrenaline the adrenalone is oxidized and then, and only then, will the molecular oxygen destroy the adrenaline. The presence of adrenalone, therefore, prevents the adrenaline molecule from reacting with itself, and the net result of the reaction is the oxidation of adrenalone.

This reaction, however, is not quite so simple. It will occur provided a fourth compound is present in the solution, but the presence of such a substance is essential. Such a compound is present in a solution of glucose which has been oxidized with molecular oxygen in the presence of alkali and indigo. The chemical groups which are necessary are unknown, but, in the presence of this compound, molecular oxygen will oxidize adrenalone provided adrenaline is also present. The results are quantitative and striking, and emphasize the necessity for the presence of these four substances before this reaction can take place.

This indicates the delicately balanced equilibrium which must be present, and further indicates the necessity of the formation of addition products before oxidation can occur.

Oxidation-Reduction Potentials of Glutathione

Still further evidence concerning the formation of addition complexes has been secured by Nord in the oxidation of glutathione. In the absence of oxygen or sulfur, glutathione and cysteine can not reduce indigo carmine; if, however, oxygen is admitted to a solution containing cysteine and indigo carmine or if a small percentage of one equivalent of sodium disulfide is added to such a solution, prompt reduction of the indigo carmine occurs; moreover, the solution is capable of reducing further additions of indigo carmine.

If such a solution is boiled the cysteine or glutathione present can no longer reduce indigo carmine, and finally the actual oxidation-reduction intensity of the solution is determined by the ratio of –SH to the –SS groups which are present in the solution. These results are explained by the formation in the solution of thermolabile oxygen or sulfur addition products between indigo carmine and cysteine which activate both the –SH and –SS groupings.

These results indicate that the –SS grouping is capable of exerting an oxidizing influence, and, although such power of the –SS grouping is absent in a simple phosphate buffer solution, in the presence of the oxygen addition product the –SS grouping of cystine or oxidized glutathione will oxidize reduced indigo or reduced indigo carmine.

The demonstration that the activity of glutathione is dependent on the presence of thermolabile unstable addition products containing oxygen and sulfur suggests that the biological significance of these compounds depends upon the presence of similar substances in the animal organism. Investigation of the activity of the –SH and –SS forms of glutathione in vivo has shown that the condition in which these substances exist depends on the metabolic changes occurring in the muscles, liver and kidneys.

The potentiometric investigation of the activity of these compounds furnishes a glimpse of that complex, ever-changing series of reactions which is occurring in vivo and upon which physiological processes are dependent.

Necessity for Activation

The determination of the oxidation-reduction potentials of the derivatives of adrenaline is conclusive evidence that these substances are not of themselves powerful reducing or oxidizing agents and that they must be activated by other substances in the tissues of the animal organism before they can influence the intensity of the oxidation-reduction processes involved.

Dixon has suggested that the –SH group of cysteine dissociates even in a simple phosphate buffer with the liberation of hydrogen and the formation of cystine. The results reported in this communication indicate that before the –SH group can function as a reducing agent with sufficient intensity to reduce indigo carmine the sulphydryl grouping must be activated by the presence of some type of oxygen addition product.

These results emphasize the importance, in biological processes of oxidation, of addition complexes which appear to be essential for the functioning of at least adrenaline and glutathione. The activating influence of oxygen or its chemical equivalent has not been appreciated, largely because the experimental methods employed have not adequately excluded oxygen from the sphere of reaction. With properly controlled experimental technic it can be shown that oxygen occupies a unique position concerning the oxidation-reduction power of cysteine and glutathione. This action is not concerned with the oxidizing power of oxygen but with the activation of the sulfur atom in the presence of thermolabile oxygen addition products so that the -SS and -SH groups can manifest their latent powers of oxidation and reduction.

Edward C. Kendall

Mayo Foundation

CONTRIBUTIONS OF ANTHROPOLOGY TO MEDICINE[1]

In the first number of the *American Journal of Physical Anthropology* for this year, I had occasion to point out the intimate and direct relations of anthropology with medicine and to show, briefly, what medical men, more particularly the anatomists, have done for anthropology. On the present occasion I want to call attention, equally briefly, to what anthropology has done for medicine.

The subject will, I think, be at once clearer and more sympathetic to you when I remind you that anthropology, in a large measure, is merely the daughter and a continuation of the medical sciences. The best and briefest definition of physical anthropology that we are able to arrive at to-day is that it is the human *phylology* of the past, the present and the future. More in detail it is, first, the science of human origin and evolution, or of human phylogeny; second, it is the comparative science of the human life cycle from its inception to its end or human ontogeny; and third, it is the science of human variation. All of which means merely that it is human biology, and advanced, comparative, human anatomy, physiology, chemistry and even pathology.

The distinctive feature of anthropology and the one that separates it most from the regular medical sciences is its *comparative* nature. It deals not with the characters and manifestations of an abstract or average human being, as do the medical branches, but studies human groups, whether they be age, sex, racial, social, occupational or even abnormal groups, comparing them with others. As to "practical" application there is the difference that medicine tries essentially to restore the damaged or diseased goods, while anthropology endeavors to find and to show the harmful as well as the favorable means for further human evolution. Anthropology, with much justice, could be called the medicine of human groups.

Being what it is, it must be quite plain to all of us that indirectly or directly the bulk of the research in physical anthropology is of more or less value to medicine. That medicine does not or can not as yet make fuller use of anthropological knowledge is quite another matter, related to its similar inabilities in respect to biology, physics and even chemistry; it is the difficulty of assimilation. It may be said at once, however, that medicine is already using many results of anthropological research without being always conscious of the source.

Let us approach the concrete facts. Research in physical anthropology began materially in the fifties of the last century. The register of printed anthropological articles and books since then reaches many thousands.

Taking the card catalogue of these publications in my division, I find that over 50 per cent. of the titles are direct contributions to comparative human anatomy, physiology or pathology. A few examples may elucidate this further. Let us take, quite at random, the three items of "skull," child" and "pelvis," and see the nature of the anthropological studies under these heads:

Skull	Children	Pelvis
Anomalies	Abnormalities	Age changes
Architecture	Backward	Anomalies and abnormalities
Asymmetries	Births, multiple, etc.	Anthropological differences
Capacity	Brains of defective	Deformations
Capacity vs. stature in defectives	Development	Dimensions
Deformations	Dimensions	Evolution in fetus and child
Development and growth of distinguished men and women	Infanticide	Ossification
Evolution	Pathology, comparative	Sexual characters
	Pulse, respiration, temperature	Variation

Practically every more civilized country has already one or more periodicals devoted largely or entirely to physical anthropology. Let us take the first page or two of the index of the oldest of these journals, the *Bulletin* of the Anthropological Society in Paris, and we find such items as these:

Abdomen: (racial differences in the muscles of);
Acclimatization;
Accouchement (childbirth), among different peoples;
Achondroplasia;
Acrocephaly;
Acromegaly;
Agraphy;
Albinism;
Alcoholism, and depopulation, criminals, suicides;
Algiers—demography, psychology;
Alienation, mental, and the brain, etc.

[1] Presented as part of a symposium on "The Contributions of Other Sciences to Medicine" at the annual meeting of the American Association for the Advancement of Science, Nashville, December 28, 1927.

A still better illustration, perhaps, may be furnished by our own journal of physical anthropology (*The American Journal of Physical Anthropology*, Wistar Institute) which I had the privilege of founding in 1918. Taking the more formal communications alone, we have the following record for the first ten volumes:

Human Evolution Early man Origin of races	Embryology Childhood and Adolescence Senility Elimination General body proportions	Human Variations; Racial; Individual parts and organs (External parts, internal organs, brain, skeleton, etc.) Teeth	Heredity Eugenics Demography Abnormal Classes	Comparative human physiology Chemistry Pathology Teratology Primitive surgery	The characteristics, morphological, physiological, etc., of the people of the U. S. A.	General, Historical, Methods, Instruments.
(23)	(20)	(75)	(6)	(19)	(6)	(23)
Per cent. *13.4*	*11.6*	*43.6*	*3.5*	*11*	*3.5*	*13.4*
						Total: 172

Another illustration, and one of some interest also to the chemists, may be had by reading the titles of papers published in the first three numbers of the journal just named, of the current year. They are:

Hrdlička (Aleš): Anthropology and Medicine.

Manoiloff (E. O.): Discernment of Human Races by Blood.

Poliakowa (Anna T.): Manoiloff's "Race" Reaction and its Application to the Determination of Paternity.

Suk (V.): Anthropological and Physiological Observations on the Negroes of Natal and Zululand.

Davenport (C. B.): Measurement of Men.

Connolly (C. J.): Relation of the Orbital Plane to Position of Teeth.

Hirsch (N. D. M.): Cephalic Index of American-born Children of Three Foreign Groups.

Cummins (Harold) and Midlo (Charles): Dermatoglyphics in Jews.

McMurrich (J. Playfair): The Evolution of the Human Foot.

Morton (D. J.): Human Origin.

Hrdlička (Aleš): Anthropology of the American Negro.

Appleton (Vivia B.): Growth of Chinese Children in Hawaii and in China.

Larsen (Nils Paul) and Godfrey (Lois Stewart): Sacral Pigment Spots.

Cameron (John): Cranial Studies.

Ingalls (N. W.): Studies on the Femur.

Manoiloff (E. O.): Blood: Species Reaction.

Scammon (R. E.): The First Seriatum Study of Human Growth.

Dodge (C. T. J.): Weight of Colored Infants.

Hrdlička (Aleš): Quadruped Progression in the Human Child.

Bushkovitch (V. J.): An Automatic Apparatus for the Measurements of Cranial Capacity.

Slome (D.): The Curvature of the Bushman Calvarium.

Bernstein (Morris) and Robertson (Sylvan): Racial and Sexual Differences in Hair Weight.

Cady (Lee D.) and Francis (Byron F.): The Supracondyloid Process in the Feeble-minded.

Ingalls (N. W.): Studies on the Femur in the White and the Negro.

Among the more noteworthy individual contributions of anthropology to medicine may be mentioned—to select only a few of the older names—those of Paul Broca and Gustaf Retzius on the brain; of Manouvrier on brain physiology; of Rudolf Virchow on deformities of the skull; of Quetelet and Vierordt on human proportions; of Galton, Lombroso on human heredity, on men of genius and on the defective classes; those of Sir Armand Ruffer on prehistoric pathology, etc., etc.

Taking the older American anthropologists,[1] we see Samuel D. Morton, as early as 1850, contributing on "the size of the brain in various races and families of man"; Joseph Leidy, in his anthropological work, contributes on acephaly; blood crystals; causes of monstrosities; senile changes in the jaw; reversed viscera in man, and the anomalies of the human skull. J. C. Nott, in 1857, writes on "Acclimatization," or the comparative influence of climate and disease on the races of man; Jeffries Wyman, in 1849, publishes "Twelve Lectures on Comparative Physiology"; in 1854–1862, "Dissections of a Human Fetus, a Chimpanzee, a Hottentot"; in 1864–68, on "Symmetry and Homology in Limbs," and on "Malformations." Henry P. Bowditch, beginning to publish in 1877, gives us valuable papers and memoirs on the growth of children; relations between growth and disease,

[1] See full bibliographies in Hrdlička, A., "Physical Anthropology: Its Scope and Aims; its History and Present Status in the U. S. A." 8°, 1919 (Wistar Inst., Phila.).

and the physique of women in Massachusetts. Harrison Allen publishes (1867–97) on the effect of the bipedal position in man; the Siamese twins (autopsy); edentulous jaws in man; congenital defects of the face; hyperostosis of lower jaw; effects of cretinism on the nasal chambers, and the effects of senility and disease on the teeth. Thomas Dwight, Burt G. Wilder, Dudley A. Sargent, the two Spitzkas, A. F. Chamberlin, Geo. S. Huntington, F. P. Mall left us studies of value on the spine, the appendix and viscera, the brain, the embryo, the child, the college boy and girl. And this by no means exhausts the lists.

Coming to the still living American anthropologists, we find Bean contributing to our knowledge of the weight and size of the internal organs, in health and disease, and to the relation of man's build to pathology. Boas has dealt with growth of children, effects of hybridism and race mentality. Davenport deals with human heredity and the defectives. Hooton has published, among other works, on herbivorous and carnivorous types of man; on the evolution of the human face, and on surgery in ancient Egypt. Terry and his associates, and Danforth, are contributing to our knowledge of the human hair, bone variation, anomalies, and human variation in general. Todd and his students have published on age changes in human bones (pelvis, scapula), on the femur, on structural differences between the white and negro. The anthropologists of the Smithsonian Institution have or are still carrying on researches on prehistoric trephining; on physiological and medical observations on the Indians; on tuberculosis in the Indians; on brain weight, brain preservation, racial brains; on the dental arches and teeth; on the physical and physiological characteristics of the adult white Americans; on ear tumors and other ear abnormalities in prehistoric Indians, etc., etc.

Taking all this impersonally and from a wider angle, we see that anthropology has given medicine, and is now giving, three lines of contributions of both weight and value. The first of these is the ever-growing light on human evolution, and that both in the past and at the present; the second comprises the results of our studies on human variation; and the third is the furnishing to medicine of normal standards.

A knowledge of human evolution, past, present and with indications for the future, is indispensable to medicine if this is to fathom the deeper causes, and the trends, of a large part of human pathology, with its differences according to race and type and group.

Equally indispensable to scientific medicine of the future will be a sound knowledge of human variation. For this teaches that even under the most "normal" or uncomplicated conditions, everything, in our frame, organs, functions, and even the causes of disease, and the process of the same, is subject to an important range of variation. The medical text-books, your anatomies, physiologies and pathologies, deal not with the realities as they are, but with "workable" abstracts or gists of these realities. Yet without the understanding of the normal variation of every feature, every process, every manifestation of man, normal and abnormal, a true understanding of any part of medicine is not possible.

Here anthropology has been and continues to be a veritable handmaid of medicine. It shows that, for example, the normal weight of the child, at any age, is not just *that*, but between so much and so much. The normal stature of an adult American male is not 5 feet 7½ inches, but anywhere between, say, 5 feet 4 inches and 6 feet 3 inches. The normal male pulse is not invariably 71.5, but ranges between 66 and 78 per minute. The normal pelvis, head, any part or organ may show as much as 10 to 16 per cent. normal variation in size, with a considerable variation in form. The "normal" course of lobar pneumonia or any other affection is not "just so," but will oscillate between such and such limits.

The third main service of anthropology to medicine, the determination of standards, is connected with the preceding. It is self-evident that the medical man to judge properly must have normal standards of the parts in which he is interested at the time, in the particular people with whom he is dealing. And to find these standards (or averages), with their range of normal (non-pathological) variation, is the peculiar function of anthropological endeavor. A concrete example of this may be found in the recently published work, the "Old Americans,"[2] which brings such data on the principal morphological or physiological characters of the older white American population.

The value of anthropology to medicine is much better appreciated in the Old World, and even in such countries as Japan and China, than it is as yet in this country. There is not a first-class medical school abroad in which anthropology would not have more or less of a part. One of the best examples of this is Great Britain. In our own country, more or less anthropological instruction is given in the medical schools of Johns Hopkins, Harvard, University of Virginia, Western Reserve, Washington University (St. Louis), the University of Chicago and Stanford; the only regular course with a special lecturer in the subject (Professor A. Schultz) being that of the Johns Hopkins.

Many of our medical colleges and graduates, regrettably, do not as yet know sufficiently of this source of

[2] Large 8°, 1926, Williams and Wilkins, Baltimore, Md.

helpful knowledge. Our anthropological journals have less subscribers and readers among the medical men, even the medical teachers, than they have among, for instance, the dentists, and the vast collections of both normal and pathological material in our osteological, brain and other collections are not used nearly so much as they should be by the medical man and the surgeon. All of which is due essentially to a lack of mutual contact and understanding. An improvement in these conditions is not merely desirable but necessary, and the anthropologist therefore welcomes the occasion of this symposium where he may point out some at least of the advantages of medicine and anthropology getting closer together.

Aleš Hrdlička

U. S. National Museum

EDWARD SANDFORD BURGESS

Dr. Edward Sandford Burgess, for thirty years professor and head of the department of biological sciences and for a time acting president of Hunter College, New York City, died after a brief illness on February twenty-third. He was born in 1855 at Little Valley, New York. His father, the Reverend Chalon Burgess, D.D., was long the pastor of the Presbyterian church at Silver Creek and was one of the most scholarly of the clergymen of western New York. His mother was Emma Johnston, daughter of the Reverend Charles Johnston, of Ovid, Seneca County.

Professor Burgess graduated from the State Normal School at Fredonia and later in 1879 with high distinction from Hamilton College. For two years he held a graduate fellowship in Greek, under the eminent scholar, Professor Gildersleeve, at Johns Hopkins. But because of his ardent love of nature and his habit from early boyhood of scientific observation, he decided to make the teaching of science his life work. In 1899 he received the degree of doctor of philosophy at Columbia University. Hamilton College, wishing to honor him for his distinguished work as a teacher and his contributions to scientific research, conferred upon him, in 1904, the degree of doctor of science.

He was for thirteen years professor of botany in the Central High School of Washington, D. C., and, during the same period, at the Martha's Vineyard Summer Institute. He taught also at Johns Hopkins (1885) University. In 1895 he was called to the professorship in biological sciences at Hunter College. His special spheres of labor were: (1) Botany, especially in asters; (2) botanical names, Indian names; (3) paleontology, anthropology, evidences of human descent.

Among his published works are the Chautauqua Flora (1877); botanical descriptions in the Century dictionary; the asters of the northern United States (in Britton and Brown's "Illustrated Flora"—with Dr. N. L. Britton (1898)); the asters of the southern United States (in Small's Southeastern Flora (1903)); history of Pre-Clusian botany (1902); species and variations of biotian asters (1906); essays on Indian lore, and poems. His unpublished manuscripts include a work on anthropology and research material in several fields.

Dr. Burgess was a member of Phi Beta Kappa; the American Association for the Advancement of Science; the New York Academy of Sciences; the Torrey Botanical Club, of which he was at one time the president; American Anthropological Society and American Folklore Society.

Professor Burgess is survived by Mrs. Burgess and his sister, Miss Julia Burgess, professor of English in the University of Oregon. His brother, Dr. Theodore C. Burgess, was for many years professor of Latin and Greek at the State Normal School at Fredonia and later the president of Bradley Institute, Peoria, Illinois.

At the time of his retirement from the professorship the following tribute was offered to him:

A TRIBUTE

In grateful recognition of thirty years of distinguished service to science, to the cause of higher education, and in particular to Hunter College, New York City, and to the thousands of young women who have studied there, this tribute is offered to

DOCTOR EDWARD SANDFORD BURGESS

PROFESSOR AND HEAD OF THE DEPARTMENT OF BIOLOGY AND SOME TIME ACTING PRESIDENT.

An organizer and executive of marked ability, a gifted and inspiring teacher, a model of devotion to duty, a master of his subject and a thorough scholar in many other fields, a man inspired by the highest ideals and responsive to all the finer and nobler things of life, beloved and admired by his pupils and associates, his services can not be measured, for they have become a part of the lives of all who know him. He has given of his best, and a best far above the average, and he also receives of the best—the consciousness of high service nobly done. Could all those who have been made better by his presence, influence, and example give adequate expression to their appreciation, it would be as a fadeless garland in which the laurel of victory is entwined with the roses of love.

Theodore E. Hamilton

SCIENTIFIC EVENTS

A NEW EDITION OF WILLARD GIBBS'S WORKS AND PROPOSED COMMENTARY

IN 1906 the writings of Willard Gibbs were printed in a collected edition of two volumes entitled, "The Scientific Papers of J. Willard Gibbs." Volume I contained all his papers on thermodynamics, and volume II the remainder of his published writings, with the exception of the book "Elementary Principles in Statistical Mechanics," which had been published only five years earlier and was at that time still available. At the present time both volume I of the "Scientific Papers" and the volume on "Statistical Mechanics" are out of print.

In connection with a movement started last winter to establish at Yale University a memorial in honor of Willard Gibbs, provision has been made, through the generosity of a donor who prefers to remain anonymous, for a new and complete edition of Willard Gibbs's writings. This will consist of either two or three volumes, well printed and bound, and will be sold at a very moderate price to encourage a wide distribution. It will probably be published during 1928.

In addition to this reprinting of the original text of Gibbs's works, it is proposed to publish, at some later date, a volume or volumes designed to aid the reader to bridge the well-recognized gap between Gibbs's theorems on the one hand and the actual experimental data of the chemist and physicist on the other. This supplementary material, to be written by competent authorities in the several fields, would aim (a) to explain the philosophical background of Gibbs's method; (b) to amplify the treatment of points of special difficulty; (c) to discuss the evaluation of Gibbs's functions in terms of directly measurable quantities, and (d) to furnish a variety of illustrative examples from the literature now available. Such treatment is most needed in the case of the thermodynamic papers, but the plan may be extended to cover Gibbs's writings on other subjects if it seems expedient. The financial support of the undertaking has been liberally provided for, and suitable honoraria will be paid to the authors of the new material.

The undersigned committee, appointed to study this plan, earnestly solicits suggestions and comments from all persons interested, especially with respect to any or all of the following questions:

I. Which of the aims outlined above are the most important?

II. How should the subject-matter be subdivided into parts which can be handled by a single author?

III. What persons, irrespective of nationality, are best fitted by ability and training to undertake these different parts?

Letters containing suggestions or criticisms will be welcomed and may be addressed to the Gibbs Committee, Sterling Chemistry Laboratory, New Haven, Conn.

JOHN JOHNSTON,
WILLIAM F. G. SWANN,
RALPH G. VAN NAME, *Chairman*
YALE UNIVERSITY

BARRO COLORADO ISLAND STATION

DR. THOMAS BARBOUR, chairman of the executive committee of the Institute for Research in Tropical America, has made his fourth annual report on Barro Colorado Island Station. It is a report of encouraging progress in the work and material development of the station.

"Redwood House," at the end of Armour trail, has been built of redwood lumber sent from California in order to test this lumber for resistance to termites. The new house is now completed and provided with everything necessary for a stay of several days. A new storeroom 28 feet long and 9 feet wide has also been built of redwood. An observation tower 28 feet high has been erected on the highest point of the island. Old trails have been extended and new ones laid out. Bridges have been made across some of the steepest ravines.

Among those who have carried on studies at the station during the year may be mentioned Dr. Frank M. Chapman, of the American Museum of Natural History; Dr. L. A. Kenoyer, head of the department of biology of Western State Normal School at Kalamazoo, Michigan; Dr. Josselyn Van Tyne, of the museum of zoology of the University of Michigan; Dr. Alfred O. Gross, professor of biology at Bowdoin College; Dr. George B. Wislocki, of the department of anatomy of the Johns Hopkins University; Dr. Curt P. Richter, of the Johns Hopkins Hospital; Miss Walburga A. Petersen, of the University of Wisconsin; Dr. Howard E. Enders, head of the biology department of Purdue University; Dr. Herbert Osborn, director of the Ohio Biological Survey; Dr. Thornton W. Burgess, of Springfield, Mass.; Dr. W. E. Hastings, of the conservation commission of Michigan, and Messrs. Ludlow Griscom and Maunsell S. Crosby, of the Museum of Comparative Zoology.

During the year a number of technical papers of importance have been published by various workers embodying the results of work on the Island and Isthmus.

The financial support of the station has continued to come from the University of Michigan, American Museum of Natural History, Harvard University, the Johns Hopkins University and Missouri Botanical Garden; from fees from scientific workers, and from private sources, notably from Dr. Barbour and Mr. Allison V. Armour.

The station is in much need of larger financial support than it now has. Other institutions like those mentioned should make annual subscriptions. Any subscribing institution has the privilege of having its members given preferential treatment when there are more applicants for place than is available.

Applications for space should be made as far in advance as possible to Dr. Thomas Barbour, Museum of Comparative Zoology, Cambridge, Mass. Dr. Barbour will supply intending workers with all necessary information.

VERNON KELLOGG

NATIONAL RESEARCH COUNCIL

APPROPRIATIONS OF THE GENERAL EDUCATION BOARD

THE General Education Board has issued its annual report giving an account of its activities during the year July 1, 1926, to June 30, 1927. Previous reports have called attention to the fact that the board has decided to transfer its main interest from college to university development. At the college level the general public, alumni, local communities and denominational agencies must mainly deal with the financial situation. The same can not be said of research and teaching at the research level. Men are relatively few; facilities are relatively undeveloped; public interest is still to be aroused.

In the field of science, exclusive of medical education, appropriations have been made as follows:

California Institute of Technology

The General Education Board has already cooperated with the California Institute of Technology in the development of its facilities for advanced work in physics, chemistry and mathematics. The authorities now plan further extensions in mathematical physics, biophysics and organic chemistry, and around these strengthened departments they hope to develop geology and biology, the former already established two years ago. The entire program, as now outlined, calls for additional endowment to the extent of $4,000,000. In view, however, of the difficulty of procuring personnel, the program has been divided into two parts, and the institute is now undertaking to raise $2,100,000. Towards this sum, the General Education Board appropriated $1,050,000.

Harvard University

Harvard University, long eminent in respect to its personnel in the physical, biological and mathematical sciences, has only recently begun to procure adequate facilities for graduate studies. A new laboratory for chemistry is now in process of construction; the biological laboratories and collections, now scattered, need to be brought together in as close proximity as possible to other sciences. It is proposed at this time to procure funds which will enable the university to devote the Jefferson Laboratory to undergraduate work and to construct and equip a fireproof building to be used for research and graduate instruction. To accomplish this improvement in the department of physics, the sum of $1,100,000 is required. Towards this total, the General Education Board appropriated $400,000.

University of Chicago

At the time of its foundation, the University of Chicago occupied an advanced position in respect to the physical and biological sciences. It is still eminent; but its accommodations remain practically what they were thirty years ago. With the exception of zoology, none of the physical and biological sciences possesses adequate space and equipment for research and the training of advanced students. The university has now undertaken to raise $2,790,000, to be apportioned approximately as follows: botany, $250,000; mathematics, physics and astronomy, $1,600,000; chemistry, $940,000.

Towards the total sum thus required, the General Education Board appropriated $1,500,000.

Vanderbilt University

A few years ago Vanderbilt University established a school of medicine with ideals as exacting as those elsewhere in the country. This step rendered imperative an effort to lift the entire institution to a corresponding level. To achieve this end, an initial campaign was planned, calling for the sum of $4,100,000 in three distinct portions—$1,300,000 to be devoted to improving facilities in science, $1,300,000 for improvement of work in the humanities and social sciences, $1,500,000 for general endowment, the income to be utilized mainly in graduate work.

The first step has already been taken, and pledges amounting to the requisite sum have been secured. Towards the second and third steps the General Education Board has appropriated $900,000.

ANNUAL MEETING OF THE AMERICAN GEOPHYSICAL UNION

THE ninth annual meetings of the American Geophysical Union and of its sections will be held in Washington on April 26 and 27. A joint meeting of the sections of meteorology and oceanography will be held on both the morning and afternoon of April 26 and will be devoted to a symposium and discussion on interrelations between the sea and the atmosphere and the effect of these relations on weather and climate;

the 15 papers to be presented at this symposium will be grouped into (1) problems related to solar radiation, (2) problems related to surface-water temperature and (3) problems related to atmospheric circulation. The joint meeting of the sections of terrestrial magnetism and electricity, seismology and geodesy, to be held on the morning of April 26, will be devoted to a symposium and discussion on geophysical methods as applied in the study of geological structure; the program for the symposium will consist of six papers. The section of geodesy will hold a meeting on the morning of April 27 to hear reports of progress from representatives from Mexico, Canada and the United States, to be followed by a symposium on the figure of the earth. The section of volcanology will also meet on the morning of April 27, the program of scientific papers and discussion being devoted largely to questions of volcanic activity, the year's volcanologic publications and volcanologic work of the U. S. Geological Survey. The general assembly of the union is scheduled for the afternoon of April 27; in addition to business matters and reports concerned with the union's activities for the year, there will be reports of the delegates to the third general assembly of the International Geodetic and Geophysical Union at Prague and a general discussion with reference to the proposed publications of bulletins on geophysical methods, instruments, results, etc., under the auspices of the division of physical sciences of the National Research Council.

SCIENTIFIC NOTES AND NEWS

A CELEBRATION in honor of the fiftieth anniversary of the invention of the dynamo will take place at the Franklin Institute, Philadelphia, on April 18, where the first tests were made in 1878 by Dr. Elihu Thomson and Professor E. J. Houston. Dr. Thomson and Dr. Charles F. Brush, who invented the type of dynamo finally recommended, will be the guests of honor and will present papers.

THE Frank Nelson Cole prize of $200 for original work in algebra was awarded to Professor L. E. Dickson, of the University of Chicago, at a meeting of the American Mathematical Society at Columbia University on March 7. The prize, which is awarded every five years, was established in honor of Frank Nelson Cole, who was secretary of the society for twenty-five years.

THE University of Dublin will confer the honorary degree of D.Sc. on Dr. G. L. Streeter, director of the department of embryology, Carnegie Institution of Washington, Baltimore, and Professor A. S. Eddington, Plumian professor of astronomy and experimental philosophy in the University of Cambridge.

DR. CARL STUMPF, the distinguished psychologist, celebrates his eightieth birthday on April 21. On that occasion a bronze bust of him by Georg Kolbe will be unveiled in one of the rooms of the University of Berlin.

DR. ADOLPH ENGLER, professor of botany in the University of Berlin, has been elected an honorary member of the Russian Academy of Sciences.

DR. ALFRED DENKES, professor of medicine at the University of Halle, has been elected a corresponding member of the Royal Society of Medicine, London.

DR. PAUL ALEXANDDROFF, professor of mathematics at Moscow, has been elected a corresponding member of the Göttingen Scientific Society.

THE gold medal of the British Institution of Mining and Metallurgy has been awarded to Sir Alfred Mond, "in recognition of his scientific and industrial services in the development of the mineral resources and metallurgical industries of the British Empire."

THE Frank N. Meyer medal for distinguished service in plant introduction has been presented to H. N. Ridley, in recognition of the important part he played in establishing plantations of the Para rubber tree in the Oriental tropics. The presentation was made by the American consul-general on behalf of Mr. David Fairchild, president of the American Genetic Association, to whom the award is entrusted by the staff of the office of foreign plant introduction of the United States Department of Agriculture.

WE learn from *Nature* that elections to the following offices in the British Chemical Society have been made: *President,* Professor J. F. Thorpe; *Treasurer,* Dr. T. Slater Price; *Secretary,* Professor T. S. Moore. The retiring president, Professor H. Brereton Baker, delivered his presidential address, entitled "Constitution of Liquids: Some New Experiments," at the annual general meeting on March 22.

DR. JOSEPH S. ILLICK, state forester of Pennsylvania, was elected chairman of the Allegheny section of The Society of American Foresters at the annual meeting held at Harrisburg. The Allegheny Section comprises the states of New Jersey, Delaware, Maryland, West Virginia and Pennsylvania.

BY the operation of the age limitation law, Edward Howe Forbush will retire on April 24 from his position as director of the division of ornithology of the Massachusetts State Department of Agriculture. His work will be taken up temporarily by Dr. John B. May, who has been his assistant for some years.

PROFESSOR F. O. DUFOUR, head of the civil engineering department of Lafayette College, has resigned to accept a position as engineer in charge of structural work with the United Engineers and Constructors Company, of New York and Philadelphia.

Dr. Joseph Francis Merrill, after an official connection of thirty-five years with the University of Utah, thirty years of which time he served as director of the school of mines and engineering and professor of electrophysics, has accepted the position of commissioner of education of the Church of Jesus Christ of Latter-day Saints.

Dr. James F. Norris, director of the research laboratory of organic chemistry of the Massachusetts Institute of Technology, has undertaken the consulting editorship of the International Chemical Series, published by the McGraw-Hill Book Company. Dr. Norris succeeds the late Dr. H. P. Talbot.

The managers of the Royal Institution have appointed Dr. Alex. Muller, known for his work on crystals, to be assistant director of the Davy Faraday Research Laboratory.

According to *Nature* the appointments made by the British secretary of state for the colonies during the month of February, in addition to those for the East African Agricultural Research Institute, Tanganyika Territory, include the following: Dr. H. Scott, entomologist, Iraq; J. L. Illingworth, curator and agricultural superintendent, Virgin Islands; C. B. C. Handley, assistant agricultural officer, Kenya; Mr. H. Marsland, cotton investigator, Agricultural Department, Tanganyika Territory; R. S. Kyle, veterinary officer, Tanganyika Territory.

The annual medical clinic of the State University of Iowa College of Medicine will be held at Iowa City from April 10 to 11. Dr. Dallas B. Phemister, professor of surgery, University of Chicago, will give an address, Tuesday evening, April 10, and Dr. Louis B. Wilson, Rochester, Minn., will give an address on Wednesday.

Dr. Harry B. Weiser, head of the department of chemistry of Rice Institute, Houston, Texas, will give two courses of thirty lectures each in the field of colloid chemistry in the forthcoming summer session at Western Reserve University, beginning on June 18.

Dr. C.-E. A. Winslow, professor of public health at Yale University, has been appointed Cutter lecturer on preventive medicine for 1928–29 at Harvard University.

Dr. George Otis Smith, director of the U. S. Geological Survey and newly elected president of the American Institute of Mining and Metallurgical Engineers, will deliver the commencement day address at the Colorado School of Mines.

Dr. Thomas Addis, professor of medicine at the Stanford University school of medicine, will deliver the seventh Harvey Society lecture at the New York Academy of Medicine, on Friday evening, April 27. His subject will be "The Renal Lesion in Bright's Disease."

Dr. Robert Balk, of New York, addressed the Boston Geological Society, on March 23, on "Movements in Rocks."

On March 31 Dr. Ralph Linton, of the Field Museum of Natural History, Chicago, delivered an address to the Royal Canadian Institute, on the subject "Two Years in Madagascar."

L. W. Kephart, of the U. S. Department of Agriculture, will address the Philosophical Society of Washington, on April 14, on "Plant Hunting through East Africa."

Dr. W. J. V. Osterhout, of the Rockefeller Institute for Medical Research, has sailed for Bermuda, to spend three weeks at the biological laboratory.

Dr. William Beebe, of the New York Zoological Society, has returned from a month's photographic expedition to the Florida Keys.

R. A. Cushman, assistant custodian of hymenoptera at the U. S. National Museum, who went to the Philippines last fall to attend to the packing and shipment of the C. F. Baker collection of insects, which had been bequeathed to the museum, returned to Washington on March 27. The collection is now on its way to the museum.

Sir John Russell, director of the Rothamsted Experimental Station, will soon leave England to visit Australia, where he is going at the invitation of the Australian universities to lecture on the applications of science to agriculture.

Dr. J. Brace Chittenden, professor of mathematics at the Brooklyn Polytechnic Institute, died on March 20, aged sixty-four years.

Dr. Charles H. Viol, director of the radium research laboratory of the Standard Chemical Company of Pittsburgh, died on April 6 at the age of forty-one years.

Sir Aubrey Strahan, formerly director of the Geological Survey of Great Britain and the Museum of Practical Geology, died at the age of seventy-five on March 4.

Professor Antonio Abetti, director of the Astrophysical Observatory of the Royal University of Florence from 1894 to 1922, died at his home in Florence on February 20, in his eighty-second year.

ACCORDING to an Associated Press dispatch, Dr. Alexander A. Bogdanoff, director of the State Scientific Institute for Blood Transfusion at Moscow, died on April 8. It is reported that his death was caused by the effects of a transfusion experiment made on himself.

THE colleagues of the late dean of the Stanford University School of Medicine, Dr. Albion W. Hewlett, who died in 1925, have revised his book "Pathological Physiology of Internal Diseases—Functional Pathology," as a memorial. In the foreword the president of the university, Dr. Ray Lyman Wilbur, says: "Dr. Albion Walter Hewlett, the author of this book, was primarily a trained physiologist who developed into a skilled practitioner. No one in America was better fitted to present the various subjects covered."

ACCORDING to the will of Dr. William Charles Lawson Eglin, his collection of books, pamphlets and manuscripts relating to science and technology, one of the largest and most valuable privately owned collections of its kind in this country, will go to the Franklin Institute. Prior to his death on February 8, Dr. Eglin had given much of the collection to the institute, of which he was president.

THE Maryland chapter of Sigma Xi was installed at the University of Maryland on Friday afternoon, March 2, by the national treasurer, Dr. G. B. Pegram, of Columbia University. There were twenty-three charter members. After the installation ceremony there was a banquet. In the evening, addresses were given by Dr. Pegram and Dr. A. F. Woods, ex-president of the university. The chapter officers are: Dr. C. O. Appleman, dean of the graduate school, *president,* Dr. E. C. Auchter, *vice-president,* and Dr. M. M. Haring, *secretary-treasurer.*

A NEW organization, composed for the present of those interested in bacteriology in central California, to be known as the Society of Bacteriologists (geographically qualified by terms not yet defined), was organized in San Francisco on March 27. Dr. J. Russell Esty was elected *president;* Dr. William V. Cruess, *vice-president;* Dr. M. S. Marshall, *secretary-treasurer,* and Captain V. H. Cornell, M.C., U.S.A., and Dr. Harry E. Foster, *councillors.* Dr. Karl F. Meyer, director of the George Williams Hooper Foundation for Medical Research and professor of bacteriology of the University of California, addressed the meeting, giving his recent observations of research work being performed in various eastern institutions. At the close of the meeting 78 were definitely enrolled in the organization.

THE House Committee on Foreign Affairs on March 31 voted a favorable report on a resolution to extend invitations to foreign nations to participate in the International Congress on Entomology to be held in the United States in 1928.

NEXT September a meeting of the International Illumination Commission, which was formed in 1900 and includes both gas and electrical interests, is to be held in the United States. The objects of the commission are the study of all subjects bearing on illumination and the cognate sciences and the establishment of international agreements in illumination matters. There are at present National Illumination Committees in Austria, Belgium, France, Germany, Great Britain, Holland, Italy, Japan, Switzerland and the United States. C. C. Paterson, director of the research laboratories of the General Electric Co., Ltd., Wembley, was unanimously voted president at the Bellagio meeting in September, 1927.

A NATIONAL agricultural museum and a research institute on rural affairs, both planned as centers of international interpretation and research, are being advocated by Dr. Nicholas Murray Butler, president of Columbia University. Dr. Butler estimates that $50,000 would be needed to effect a realization of the institutions to work cooperatively with the present research work at Columbia.

A GIFT of $180,000 by Eversley Childs, of New York, to establish a treatment station for the milder cases of leprosy at Cebu, in the Philippine Islands, has been announced by General James G. Harbord, national chairman of the Leonard Wood memorial for the eradication of leprosy. The new station will consist of laboratories, a medical center, clinics, wards, a pharmacy, a dispensary for out-patients, cottages for the staff and all necessary equipment.

NEW appropriations by the Kentucky legislature for research, topographic mapping and administration for the oncoming biennial budget of the Kentucky Geological Survey, amounting to $264,000, are announced by Dr. Willard Rouse Jillson, state geologist. To this amount an additional $30,000 has been added from the state highway revenues, making a sum of $294,000 of state money available for the various activities during the coming biennium. Federal mapping funds to match a portion of this will be secured.

THE University of California College of Dentistry Alumni Association have announced plans for accumulating a $50,000 fund, the interest of which will be used as a traveling fellowship to carry students of dentistry or allied subjects to other countries to study, or to bring students of other countries to California.

THE United States Department of Agriculture has organized an expedition, under the leadership of Dr.

E. W. Brandes, sugar plant specialist, which will use an airplane in searching the unexplored wilds of New Guinea for disease-resistant varieties of sugar cane that may prove valuable to the industry in Louisiana and other parts of the South. Dr. Brandes will sail from San Francisco April 12, accompanied by Dr. Jakob Jesweit, who was formerly chief of sugar-plant breeding work in Java and now of the University of Wageningen, Holland, and Richard K. Peck, who will pilot the plane. They will be joined at Honolulu by C. E. Pemberton, entomologist of the Hawaiian Sugar Plant Association Experiment Station, and proceed to Port Moresby, the base of the expedition on the southeast coast of New Guinea.

LECTURES will be given during April and May at the New York Botanical Garden on Saturday afternoons at 4:00 P. M. as follows: April 7, "Beauties from the Flower Shows," Kenneth R. Boynton; April 14, "On the Long's Peak Trail," Howard H. Cleaves; April 21, "Gladiolus, Wild and Cultivated," Dr. Forman T. McLean; April 28, "Insects of Shade Trees and Ornamentals," Dr. E. P. Felt; May 5, "Daffodils," B. Y. Morrison; May 12, "Farming for Bouquets on the Cote d'Azur," Mrs. Wheeler H. Peckham; May 19, "How to Study Ferns," Professor Henry J. Fry, and May 26, "Chinese Asters," Professor Roland H. Patch.

THE summer school for engineering teachers which was established by the Society for the Promotion of Engineering Education in 1927 is to continue its sessions during the coming summer. Two schools will be held: one for teachers of physics and the other for teachers of electrical engineering. As in 1927, when mechanics was the subject studied, the purpose will be to study the principles and methods of teaching rather than to review actual content of subject-matter. The session on the teaching of physics will be held at the Massachusetts Institute of Technology, under the directorship of Dr. S. W. Stratton, president of the institute. The session on electrical engineering will be held at Pittsburgh, under the joint auspices of the University of Pittsburgh and the Westinghouse Electric and Manufacturing Company. Dr. F. L. Bishop, of the University of Pittsburgh, secretary of the Society for the Promotion of Engineering Education, and Professor Charles F. Scott, of Yale University, chairman of the society's board of investigation and coordination, will serve as codirectors of the Pittsburgh session of the school. Professor H. P. Hammond, associate director of the society's investigation of engineering education, is in general charge of the school. Both sessions will be of three weeks' duration and will begin shortly after July 4.

THE Rockefeller Foundation has taken action converting its previously made pledge to an appropriation of $312,500 for the support of fellowships in physics, chemistry and mathematics by the National Research Council during the years 1928 to 1930, inclusive, at the rate of $125,000 a year for 1928 and 1929, and $62,500 for the year 1930.

UNIVERSITY AND EDUCATIONAL NOTES

DARTMOUTH COLLEGE will receive about $1,500,000 from the estate of the late Edwin Webster Sanborn.

PHILIP S. BIEGLER, professor of electrical engineering at the University of Southern California, has been appointed acting dean of the college of engineering just created at that institution.

PROFESSOR LESTER S. GRANT, dean of the faculty and professor of mining engineering at the Colorado School of Mines, has resigned.

PROFESSOR A. I. KENDALL has left the medical school of Washington University to become research professor of bacteriology at Northwestern University.

DR. CLARENCE ERROL FERREE, of Bryn Mawr College, has been appointed resident lecturer at Wilmer Institute at the Hopkins Medical School and director of the research laboratory in physiological optics.

DR. ERICH BRENNECKE, of the Geodetic Institute in Potsdam, has been called to the professorship of geodesy at the Berlin Institute of Technology.

DISCUSSION AND CORRESPONDENCE

THE AURORA OF MARCH 28, 1928

THE peculiar combination of an aurora with a lunar halo as visible in Cambridge on the night of March 28 is such an unusual occurrence that the event seems deserving of more than passing mention.

The lunar halo first attracted my attention about 11 P. M., Eastern Standard Time. A few minutes later the halo bore a fringe strikingly suggestive of a solar corona. By 11:30 a well-defined auroral fan was centered at a point on the horizon directly under the moon (at first quarter) with a streamer extending from the horizon directly past the moon and vertically upward. Oblique streamers arranged themselves approximately symmetrically about this line. One of these passed above Capella and at 11:50 P. M. extended across Polaris, and between Vega and Hercules to the eastern horizon.

A similar brilliant streamer mounting from the auroral center extended southward, passing Procyon and Regulus in Leo. These two streamers crossed the lunar halo very nearly on the same circle of altitude as the moon and the crossing points were marked by exceptionally brilliant patches of auroral light. The outstanding feature of the phenomenon was the existence of horizontal streamers extending several degrees through the patches and diverted away from the moon as an apparent radiant point. These horizontal streamers with an apparent radiant at the center of the halo made angles of 20°–30° with the long auroral streamers but gave every appearance of a true auroral effect. The distance of one of the bright patches from the moon was observed with a sextant and found to be 25°, thus fixing the radius of the lunar halo. The large halo vanished at 11:50 P. M., whereupon a smaller ring of 4° radius appeared about the moon. This in turn vanished at midnight. At 12:10 A. M. the large 25° halo returned for about five minutes and at 12:20 A. M. a symmetrical cross with horizontal and vertical beams appeared across the moon's disk. Shortly after 1 A. M. a light cirrus stratus had developed and the aurora faded. The temperature was 30° F. There had been a fall of 33° F. since the day previous.

The combination of the optical effects in an all but invisible cirrus stratus with a true auroral glow gave a suggestion of the problem encountered in a study of the solar corona, where we may very well have light from electrical excitation mixed with an optical corona formed from minute particles comprising a circulating circumsolar cloud.

The effect of the auroral streamers at presumably an altitude of four or five hundred miles, combined with optical phenomena in a layer of cirrus at an altitude of four or five miles gives one food for thought.

On examining our sunspot photograms the following day a spot of marked intensity passed within 5° of the sun-earth line on midnight, Eastern Standard Time, March 28–29. The field strength of WBBM as measured on the automatic radio recorder 9–10 P. M., March 28, was exceptionally low and the static heavy.

H. T. STETSON

ASTRONOMICAL LABORATORY,
HARVARD UNIVERSITY

"WASHBOARD" OR "CORDUROY" EFFECT DUE TO THE TRAVEL OF AUTOMOBILES OVER DIRT AND GRAVELED ROADS

SEVERAL articles have appeared in SCIENCE[1] dealing with the subject of washboarding of highways and there are some confirmations and some new ideas I would like to present.

In regard to the washboards themselves, the term is in common use in the Pacific Northwest where practically every graveled road is inflicted with them. In the semiarid regions, during the drier seasons, these corrugations develop to considerable size and the maintenance of roads is a very difficult problem. No sooner is a newly graveled road opened to traffic than the washboards develop and there they stay, increasing in size until the grading crew removes them, temporarily.

It should be noted that it is the high-speed traffic that causes the washboarding. Horse-drawn vehicles do not develop these road-waves, nor do heavy trucks, which pound a road into many spring-breaking chuckholes. It is the pleasure car with its pneumatic tires and high rate of speed that appears to do the damage. Tires with new treads can throw loose pieces of road metal with considerable violence, in fact the writer was recently in a car which had its windshield broken by a passing car throwing a small pebble.

Loose gravel does not appear to develop washboarding until a portion of the surface has become hard enough to wave. This is of importance in road maintenance, for dirt binders are frequently added to pack the crushed rock, and thus automatically increase the liability of washboarding.

The writer was employed by the Washington State Highway for some time. Washboarding was an important maintenance problem, in fact one of the biggest. The opinion was reached that when the rear wheels of the car hit a small bump they begin vibrating. The resultant spin of the wheels while they are in the air digs out small depressions when they hit, and the corrugations grow in the line of travel with each succeeding car. On roads covered with loose gravel, an experienced driver can frequently find relief by driving a few inches to one side of the well-packed rut and thus escape part of the vicious, neck-breaking vibrations. However, he simply widens the washboarding and soon they extend across the road.

With this idea in mind, the following experiment was performed on a newly graded and graveled road between Yakima and Ellensburg, Washington, under the direction of Max L. Mook, District Engineer for the state highway department. The road grade had been allowed to settle for a year, then dragged and graded and treated with fine crushed basaltic rock to which a small amount of dirt binder had been added. The road was opened in perfect condition. The in-

[1] Dodd, L. E., "'Washboard' or 'Corduroy' Effect due to the Travel of Automobiles over Dirt Roads," SCIENCE, September 2, 1927, 214–16.

Ruckmick, Christian A., "'Washboard' or 'Corduroy' Effect due to the Travel of Automobiles over Dirt Roads," SCIENCE, November 18, 1927, 481–82.

spection party stationed themselves on either side of a fill with the level of their eyes at the road grade, and a three-fourths-inch rope was stretched across the grade. As the cars hit the rope, the rear wheels were set into vibrations which continued for some distance, and each time the wheels hit the road grade they were observed to throw small amounts of gravel. Within a short time a beautiful set of washboards extended away from the rope but on the approach side little or no corrugations were observed. It might be added that in two weeks' time the road was so badly washboarded that it was necessary to put on a grading crew to resurface the road.

In this semiarid country, the driver's chief object is to get over the road just as quickly as the uniformed motorcycle patrol will allow him. Washboards will develop. It is hoped that road oil, used to reduce the dust menace, will alleviate the damage somewhat. Even the widely praised black-top or bithulitic pavements washboard in hot weather. It appears that the solution is to be found in either leaving the car at home, or in paving with concrete.

Ray C. Treasher

Livingston, Montana

Following the discussion and correspondence on the "Washboarding" or corduroy effect on roads traveled by automobiles by L. E. Dodd and Christian A. Ruckmick in the issues of September 2 and November 18, I have a version to contribute. Mr. Dodd's physics is beyond dispute, but my addition is to the road scraper theory. I have seen this sort of ripple on tar and macadam roads. Scrapers are not used on the surfaces of these, although they may be used in leveling the work before the hard surface is put on, and any initial roughness may be imparted up to the surface. Again, in leveling off the surface of macadam a straight edge board is often used, a man on each end pushing it along, but any waviness here would be very minute.

Last summer I was returning by motor from a trip into the Province of Quebec. All the crushed rock and gravel surface roads between the St. Lawrence River and the New England line are very "washboardy." Canada has some very good roads and some very poor ones, concrete and macadam in proportion to the size of the country with the United States, but in this eastern township's part of Quebec the main route north from New England is not yet all hard surface across the line, although roads are very good. You see a great many more horses belonging to the farmers, perhaps one Ford to each farm and a lot of auto tourist cars.

Having crossed back down into Vermont where the macadam began again, I was driving along, when there turned into the highway ahead of me a team of horses drawing a load of hay. It was a warm day, and as is the case when macadam becomes soft with the heat of the day, the heels of a man's shoe or the shoes on the horses sank into the tar slightly, leaving a small mark or hole. A team of horses, walking along a road as I could watch these walking, leave their hoof prints at regular spaces. As I drove along behind, before passing, I noticed how evenly, and, as near as I could judge by eye, this spacing was the same as the wave-lengths of the washboarding. After a team has gone along like this, the automobiles, coming along afterward, will pick up the little loose bits of tar dug up by the calks of the shoes, and by the friction, suction and so forth of the tire treads, hollow out the depression more and more.

The large number of these roads in Canada, as it may be in the West, corresponded, I thought, with the greater number of horses still there. I should say there were fifty per cent. more horses than in New England and New York, where farming is in many places on the decline.

The reason why the concrete roads do not washboard is because they have too hard a surface for the horses' iron to indent. Because, even though the concrete is so much harder, if there were any initial unsmoothness in the construction, either in using a scraper in the leveling of the bed above the subbase or in smoothing off the newly poured cement, in time, heavy automobile or truck tires would cause this effect. Often you do see a certain slight roughness in a concrete road (I mean aside from the cracking), which has come there by the hand smoothing of the men pushing the smoothing board over it, and a slight vibration results, but this never enlarges to the common washboard size.

Ellwood Wilson

Cambridge, Mass.

A NOTE ON OVARIAN SECRETION AND CANCER

In an article published in the issue of Science, for December 16, 1927, I gave a short preliminary report of work done upon the effect of ovarian secretions on the incidence of mammary cancer in a stock of dilute brown mice. One of the primary objects of the paper was to report the successful feminization of castrated males, by means of ovarian transplants, to the extent that they developed, spontaneously, mammary tumors; a thing which thousands of unoperated male mice of this stock have not done.

In Science of January 27, 1928, Dr. Leo Loeb calls me to task for not quoting him exhaustively in my bibliography and lists two "extensive" reports of his which I did not mention, thus creating in his opinion, an "erroneous impression as to the development of our knowledge of this problem."

In a brief report such as mine, it is obvious that an extended bibliography would have been out of place. It seemed, moreover, advisable not to make any further reference to Dr. Loeb's work because of the following facts:

(a) The mixed stocks used in his experiments were raised outside of his own laboratory and their ages were only approximately recorded, while the mice which I used have been inbred brother to sister under constant observation since 1909, the exact date of birth of each animal being recorded.

(b) Loeb's youngest class of spayed animals was three to six months old at castration; they may or may not have been bred previous to this. He makes no statement regarding this point, whereas my female mice were all castrated within the 28 to 35-day period and were virgins.

(c) In his total of 133 castrated animals, 98 were non-tumorous, while 35, or 26.3 per cent., were tumorous. These findings he considers significantly different from his 63 non-breeding animals (virgins), 44 of which were non-tumorous and 19, or 30.1 per cent., of which were tumorous. It seems that should a probable error be applied to these figures, there would be no significant difference between them. This fact is shown more conclusively if the totals for my experiment, shown below, are compared with his, mentioned above.

Virgin females, 207; Cancerous 20, or 9.6 per cent.; Non-cancerous 187.

Spayed females, 210; Cancerous 21, or 10 per cent.; Non-cancerous 189.

This provides clear evidence that his statement "prevention of breeding has some influence on the cancer incidence in mice but to a much less extent than castration" is entirely unconfirmed by experiments more than twice as extensive as were his.

(d) In that part of his experiment in which he attempted to "feminize" castrated males by implanting ovaries, he used a grand total of 19 animals, none of which developed mammary tumors.

In my experiment 210 animals were used for operation and four developed mammary tumors.[1]

This in turn provides clear evidence that his conclusion that the "transplanted ovaries are probably not able to call forth rhythmic growth changes in the mammary gland . . . and consequently cancer is not induced in such animals as the result of the experimental procedure" is totally contrary to the fact obtained in a series more than ten times as extensive as his own.

Without the positive evidence that it is possible to cause mammary tumors by transplanting ovaries to the bodies of castrated males, the statement that ovarian hormones are one of the factors in the etiology of mammary cancer seems to lack final confirmation. Such proof was not provided by Loeb's work.

In view of these facts, it still seems that it would have been better had Dr. Loeb not forced a consideration of the earlier papers to which he referred.

WILLIAM S. MURRAY
LABORATORY OF MAMMAL GENETICS,
UNIVERSITY OF MICHIGAN

[1] Since my paper was published, seven additional males in this experiment have developed mammary tumors and many of the animals are yet alive.

ON A RELATION OF THE SUN'S ACTIVITY TO SOME BIOLOGICAL FACTORS

THE relation between the activity of the sun and different physical and biological factors on the earth can be illustrated by the following curves. The curve S gives the number of sun spots as a measure of the sun's activity (*Wolf*). Curve L_1 gives the relative

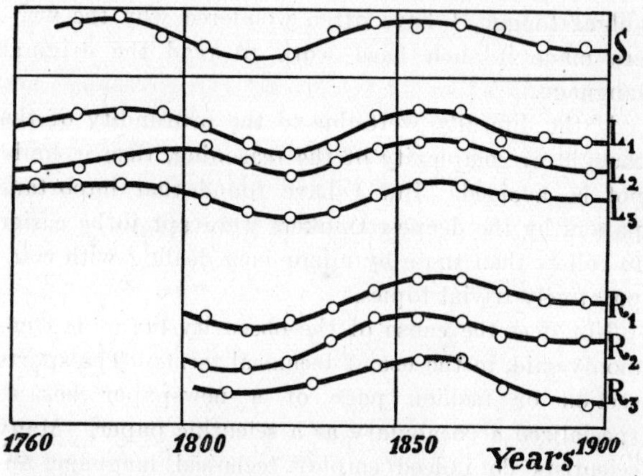

numbers of births, L_2—deaths and L_3—marriages for Leningrad and the curves R_1, R_2, R_3 give the same numbers for all the territory of Russia. In all cases there are given *means for ten years.* It would be of interest to find the same relations for other countries.

G. I. POKROWSKI
PHYSICAL INSTITUTE OF THE SCHOOL
OF TECHNOLOGY, MOSCOW

THE SHARP RATTLING IN STEAM-PIPES

WHEN the water in a cryophorus is at a temperature somewhat above freezing, it is possible to trap bubbles of water vapor in the liquid column by holding the cryophorus horizontally. Under the proper conditions of pressure due to motion of the liquid column, the bubble of water vapor will *suddenly* condense, causing the water surfaces of the bubble to come together with a sharp click.

This observation is at once applicable to the steam in radiator pipes. Most text-books in physics give the following explanation: "The sharp rattling noise in steam pipes is due to the water hammer. A column of condensed water is driven along the pipe by the steam, the cooler steam ahead of the column condenses, and the column of water hammers against the end of the pipe or against a stationary body of water in the pipe." This description of the phenomenon is correct as far as it goes, but it fails to emphasize the fact that for the sharp clicks the whole mass of water vapor between the two surfaces of water (that is, the bubble) *condenses into water instantaneously.*

The observations upon the bubbles in the cryophorus were made by my assistant, Mr. Lee Fullmer, who also differentiated the sharp clicks in the steam-pipes from the duller thud of the water hammer.

R. C. COLWELL

WEST VIRGINIA UNIVERSITY

SCIENTIFIC OBSCURITY

SINCE it has been my lot for many years to earn my living by translating scientific literature into the vulgar tongue, I have often wondered why the writers made it such hard work to read the original language.

If the difficulty were due to the profundity of the thought or complexity of the reasoning, then it could not be avoided. But I have found that important papers by the deepest thinkers were apt to be easier to follow than those by minor men dealing with comparatively trivial topics.

Nor does the cause of the obscurity lie, as is commonly said, in the use of technical terms. The sports section or fashion page of a newspaper has as specialized a vocabulary as a scientific paper. Many scientists do indeed employ technical language unnecessarily in writing for the outside public, but even where the words are all familiar the meaning may still be obscure.

I have come to the conclusion that the chief reason why scientific literature offers such high resistance to reading is the use of the alternating current instead of the direct in conveying the thought. The writer interposes a negative every few words that reverses the meaning of the sentence. This keeps the reader on the jump.

The asymptotic ideal toward which scientific writing tends is a sentence structure something like this:

> The present writer is indisposed to deny that he is unconvinced of the necessity of refusing to accept the infrequency of negative reactions as a not insuperable argument in disproof of the theory.

Such sentences may be quite logical and free from technical terms. They can be disentangled in time and when straightened out the meaning may turn out to be something simpler than it sounds. But they are constructed like the Chinese boxes, when you get one opened you come on to another. The process of extracting the meaning is like the simplification of a complicated algebraic equation, and in extricating the internested parentheses you are likely to come out with the plus and minus signs mixed.

In conclusion, the present writer is indisposed to deny that he put the wrong title at the top of the letter. It should be, not "Scientific Obscurity" but "Unscientific Obscurity in Writing on Scientific Subjects."

EDWIN E. SLOSSON

SCIENCE SERVICE,
WASHINGTON, D. C.

SCIENTIFIC BOOKS

Birds of the Pacific States. By RALPH HOFFMANN. Boston, Houghton Mifflin Co., xix + 1–353 pp., with 10 color plates, and over 200 black and white illustrations, by Major Allan Brooks. 1927.

THE diversity of native animal and plant life in the Pacific states has long been a source of attraction for students of biology, but beginning acquaintance with the fauna and flora has heretofore been hampered by the lack of suitable manuals. This need is now in process of being satisfied, as during the past three years there have appeared four important keys which will help to unlock the doors leading to accurate knowledge of the western biota. Jepson's "Manual of the Flowering Plants of California" is the first statewide botanical key for California; Essig's "Insects of western North America" is the very first comprehensive western volume in entomology; Johnson and Snook's "Seashore Animals of the Pacific Coast" is the pioneer volume in the popularizing of western marine biology; and Hoffmann's "Birds of the Pacific States," while preceded by other volumes dealing with birds, easily stands premier as a manual for field ornithology in the west.

Most bird students are interested in the living bird, and in the early stages of their interest they are concerned chiefly with the problem of identification in the field. Despite this obvious fact, a majority of the bird books heretofore issued have ignored or given but minor attention to this phase of the subject. Mr. Hoffmann was, and still is, a pioneer in the production of workable field manuals. In 1904 there appeared his "Guide to the Birds of New England and eastern New York" which dealt with "over two hundred and fifty species with particular reference to their appearance in the field." For the novice this volume is still the best field book of birds for the area indicated. The present contribution treats of more than four hundred western species from the standpoint of their field appearance and behavior.

"Birds of the Pacific States" is a compact volume (one and one-eighth by five and three-eighths by seven and five-eighths inches) substantially bound in green buckram, and hence suited for actual field use. The style is terse, an element of the contract which produced a volume useful from Vancouver Island to San Diego and from the Pacific Ocean to the Great Basin. The appearance, voice and movements of the bird, its habitat preference and the ways in which it may be differentiated from other species of similar appearance constitute the principal parts of the text of the species chapters. The plumage, geographic range and nesting habits are set forth briefly, following the paragraphs dealing with identification. The *species* is (with one or two exceptions) the unit of consideration; subspecies are listed with their respective ranges but without reference to their characters. The book follows the "new" or revised classification and sequence which will be used in the forthcoming Fourth Edition of the American Ornithologists' Union check-list and which American bird students will soon be forced to learn.

The illustrations merit special mention. All are by Allan Brooks and all are *new*. There are ten plates in color, showing in all forty-seven species. In several instances both males and females are figured. The plates are not quite right in this impression; either the etching or inking is slightly in error, giving too much red in several figures, a fault which can be corrected in future printings. The black-and-white illustrations are from pen-and-ink sketches, a medium seldom used heretofore by Brooks, but one which he has handled exceedingly well. Differences in color are indicated by different types of line treatment so that the student obtains a very good idea of the distribution of color masses on the bird. Here again some of the figures are of groups of two or three species or exhibit differences in plumage due to sex or season so that, in all, upwards of 60 per cent. of the species are shown either in color or line. The reviewer is of the impression that, in general, black and white illustrations are better than color for the beginning student, although the novice will probably believe the contrary to be true. The element of conservation in identification is involved here, an item which also is stressed by our author.

Among the thousands of items of record in the volume under discussion a few—a very few—catch the eye as errors or omissions. The iris of the barn owl is dark, not yellow (p. 161), the pileated woodpecker resides in the Coast Ranges from Lake and Mendocino counties northward as well as in the Sierra Nevada (p. 193), the breeding range of the robin scarcely includes the Sierran foothills (p. 259) but begins with the yellow pine forest; it also nests at various places in the Coast Ranges and locally in the lowlands of California. The ecologic preferences of certain species are even more restricted than indicated. The Bell sparrow (p. 326) is a bird of the greasewood (*Adenostoma*) chaparral, the rufous-crowned sparrow (p. 327) chiefly of the "old-man" sage (*Adenostoma californica*). It would have been helpful to indicate (for the beginner) the meaning of the few abbreviations used, and dimensions for nests and eggs would have aided in field identification of accessories.

This volume is built upon the principle that the habits of birds are, in general, so stable that we can predict their behavior and can use behavior as a means of field identification. This point, although well known to critical teachers of ornithology, has not found adequate expression heretofore in field manuals. The habits of birds are specific characters no less than the details of skeletal structure, soft parts and feather architecture. Mr. Hoffmann has written his book largely upon this basis and has produced a "comparative field ornithology" or a "manual of comparative behavior of birds" which we can rank with our manuals of comparative anatomy.

The quality of the present volume rests, among other things, upon the author's energetic field work; during his seven years of residence on the Pacific coast he has succeeded in observing alive upwards of 95 per cent. of the species described. First-hand impressions, written on the spot, and, with many species, tested by repeated contact, are the firm foundation on which this outstanding manual is constructed.

Tracy I. Storer

University of California

Textbook of Comparative Physiology. By Charles Garner Rogers. McGraw-Hill Co., N. Y., 1927.

Rogers' book on comparative physiology of animals is the most comprehensive discussion in this neglected field that has yet appeared in a single volume in the English language. Emphasis in recent years on the teaching of physiology under pressure for direct training in subject-matter for immediate practical application in the arts of medicine and of agriculture has led to the extreme development of human and mammalian physiology to the exclusion of that degree of comparative training which we accept without question as necessary for cytology and for anatomy.

There are twenty-nine chapters on the subjects of properties of protoplasm, the cell, general phenomena of life, organ systems, the transport system, the blood as an oxygen carrier, catalytic actions of animals, and the more conventional topics on secretion, nutrition of animals, circulatory mechanisms, physiology of the heart, etc. The chapter on the nervous system has eighty odd pages of an exceptionally able discussion of the origin and development of the nervous system as a coordinating mechanism. It is illustrated by examples drawn from a great variety of nervous organizations from the neuromuscular apparatus of the protozoa and the nerve net of the coelenterates to the neurone and the synaptic systems of a wide range of invertebrate and vertebrate nervous systems. The segmental nature of the nervous system is presented by discussion of the functional behavior of a well-chosen series of invertebrates in which the chain ganglia are still distinct.

There are able discussions of several topics peculiar to comparative physiology, for example, the functions of the swim bladder as a static organ. However, the important problem of animal luminescence seems to be wholly neglected.

At the close of the volume are references to selected literature of value to the investigator in the field.

This volume should have a distinct influence in rescuing the subject of physiology from the restrictive dominance of the arts and to that extent should give back to practical medicine and to agriculture correspondingly broader training in the basic physiological sciences.

C. W. GREENE

SCIENTIFIC APPARATUS AND LABORATORY METHODS

THE COLLODION METHOD AND SERIAL SECTIONS

THE collodion (celloidin) method is admitted to give better effects than can be secured by the use of paraffin on a number of tissues, while for certain material, *e.g.*, grasshopper eggs, it is the only known means of securing satisfactory results. Nevertheless, there is a general reluctance to use collodion due chiefly to the belief that it is difficult to preserve the serial order of the sections by this method. In reality, mounting in serial order is very easily accomplished and, while the collodion method is slightly slower than the paraffin method, with some simplification of details it is easier, in many respects, to handle. This article contains little that is new, but the various points are so scattered through scientific papers that it seems desirable to make the whole procedure available.

Preliminary steps. The first part of the process is the same as for the paraffin method. Dehydration must be completed by the use of absolute alcohol since "clearing" oil is not used. The principle involved in clearing, however, is employed, *e.g.*, the tissue is saturated with a solution which is miscible with the infiltrating substance, namely, a mixture of equal parts of absolute alcohol and ether.

Infiltration and embedding. The usual method of accomplishing these processes by two distinct steps is largely responsible for the prevalent idea that the collodion method is necessarily cumbersome. However, they may be combined in a very simple way by using a shell-vial or a similar vessel of suitable size as a container. It is desirable that the container should not have a neck in order to facilitate the later removal of the hardened mass.

Tri-nitro-cellulose under some of its trade names (collodion, celloidin, parlodion, etc.) is dissolved in equal parts of absolute alcohol and ether and used as the infiltrating medium. The solution, which ordinarily should be fairly thin, readily penetrates without heat tissues which are already saturated with the solvents. The time required varies widely. Usually the container is kept tightly closed for several days or in some cases even weeks or months. The cover is then slightly loosened to permit a very gradual evaporation of the solvents with a corresponding concentration of the collodion in the tissue. When the solution has become fairly viscous the tissue is oriented as desired. After the mass becomes firm it should be loosened about the edge so that it will contract away from the vial. When it has become sufficiently solid it can be removed easily. Evaporation should occupy several days; if sufficient time is not given the mass will not be of uniform density.

Hardening and blocking. The mass is trimmed, leaving about 1 mm. of collodion about the tissue and a flat base for mounting. It is then returned to the vial together with a piece of cotton saturated with chloroform for further hardening. The block may be stored in 70 per cent. or 80 per cent. alcohol indefinitely, but it should be hard enough for sectioning before it is placed in the alcohol. The necessity for again dehydrating, however, is obviated if the block containing the tissue is mounted on a proper support before placing in alcohol. The simplest procedure is to take the block directly from the chloroform vapor, stand the base for a moment in alcohol and ether to soften it, then transfer quickly to a fiberoid block, the top side of which has just received two or three drops of thick collodion. After not more than ten minutes' exposure to the air, in order that the collodion may set, the whole is placed either in chloroform vapor for further hardening, or, if the mount is small, directly in 70 per cent. alcohol, where it should remain for several hours before sectioning in order that the entire mount may become very firm.

Cutting and mounting of sections. Collodion sections are cut with the knife placed at the least possible angle to the direction of movement. The knife is kept wet during the process, usually with 65 per cent. to 70 per cent. alcohol. This may conveniently be accomplished by arranging an automatic oil cup so that it will drop the alcohol on the knife at the desired rate. The cutting should be done with a quick, firm motion. If the block has been sufficiently hardened and the knife edge is in good condition every section should be perfect and the thickness of successive sections uniform. A small sable brush is best for handling the sections. The brush is kept wet in the alcohol on the knife and if the sections are to be mounted serially they are arranged near the back of the knife from right to left as they are cut, always keeping them moist. Several rows of the proper length to fit under the cover-glass may be so arranged in the relation to each other which they are to occupy on the slide. A thin piece of tissue paper is placed smoothly over the sections, being sure that there is sufficient alcohol to wet through the paper. With a uniform downward motion the paper is pulled off the knife, preferably over the back. The sections sticking flat to the paper are carried across to a chemically *clean* slip on which the paper is laid reversed so that the first section cut occupies the upper left hand corner and so that the sections are properly centered. The paper may be smoothed out with the addition of a small amount of alcohol if necessary. Several layers of absorbent paper are placed on top and the whole rolled lightly but firmly with some cylindrical object for about ten seconds. This, in addition to pressing the sections tightly against the glass, removes the 70 per cent. alcohol. The paper is then quickly peeled off, leaving the sections on the slide where they are instantly flooded with clove oil, which should remain until the sections are perfectly translucent. The clove oil will dissolve sufficient of the collodion to fasten the sections to the slip; after about eight minutes the surplus oil is drained off and the slide placed in 95 per cent. alcohol. After ten or fifteen minutes it is changed to fresh 95 per cent. alcohol to insure the complete removal of the clove oil. From this point on the preparation is treated the same as if it contained paraffin sections except that the collodion is not removed. Dr. Miriam J. Scott is authority for the statement that some of her slides, so prepared, were kept in 70 per cent. alcohol for two months without the loss of a section. An equally satisfactory method, if properly used, is to smear the surface of the chemically clean slip with a film of Mayer's albumen, place the sections on it as directed above, and, omitting the clove oil, immerse quickly in 95 per cent. alcohol for at least ten minutes. One small drop of Mayer's albumen is sufficient to prepare 25 or 30 slips. Any considerable amount of albumen precipitated under the sections impairs the stain and lessens the probability of the sections remaining on the slip.

Cautions. (1) The block must be sufficiently hard to be quite rigid, otherwise its elasticity will interfere with cutting perfect sections such as are necessary for serial preparations. The proper degree of hardness should be obtained before placing in 70 per cent. alcohol.

(2) The slip must be chemically clean. It may be tested in this respect by placing a drop of distilled water on its surface. It is satisfactory if the water spreads uniformily and does not roll off when the slip is tilted without wetting the glass. (This is the most important of the precautions.)

(3) Just after the sections have been placed on the slide there is a moment when very precise work is necessary. After they are covered with the absorbent paper, they must be rolled long enough to remove practically all of the 70 per cent. alcohol except what is actually in the sections; when this condition has been obtained, speed is necessary in order to remove the paper and get the sections covered with the next medium before air gets between them and the slip, owing to the evaporation of the alcohol which is in the sections.

E. Eleanor Carothers
University of Pennsylvania

SPECIAL ARTICLES

DIRECT EVIDENCE OF ATOM BUILDING[1]

Through new and more precise measurements on cosmic rays than those heretofore made, Millikan and Cameron have just succeeded in bringing forth quantitative evidence that those rays represent the precise amount of energy which should, according to Einstein's equation showing the relation of mass to energy, be emitted in the form of ether waves when the primordial positive and negative electrons unite to create helium atoms and other light atoms such as oxygen and silicon, magnesium and iron.

Millikan and Cameron have investigated these rays through experiments in high mountain lakes, both in California and in Bolivia, and Millikan and Bowen have studied them with the aid of self-recording electroscopes sent up by sounding balloons which reached nine tenths of the way to the top of the earth's atmosphere.

The results obtained in such investigations during the past eight months constitute the first indubitable evidence that the cosmic rays on which they have been experimenting, instead of being spread like white light

[1] A report made in Pasadena to the California Institute Association on March 16.

over a considerable spectral region, consist of bands of definite frequency, or color, like the light from a neon lamp or from a Cooper-Hewitt mercury arc.

The general spectral region, however, in which these bands are found, corresponds to frequencies 100,000,000,000 times greater than those emitted by the aforementioned lamps. This is why these cosmic radiations are powerful enough to penetrate 200 feet down into a mountain lake before they are completely absorbed.

The rays brought to light by this most recent work correspond to four main radiations extending over a spectral region three octaves wide and having frequencies identical with those which are computed theoretically from the loss of mass which would occur in accordance with the foregoing equation of Einstein, first, when the helium atom is created out of the nucleus of the hydrogen atom (the positive electron) two negative electrons acting as the binding agents; second, when oxygen and nitrogen atoms are similarly created out of hydrogen; third, when silicon and magnesium are so produced, and, fourth, when the atom of iron is born.

Hydrogen and helium are extraordinarily abundant gases, while the four elements—oxygen, magnesium, silicon and iron—are the most abundant elements found in meteorites and constitute a not unlike percentage of the earth. The agreement between the observed and computed frequencies is so good as to make it highly improbable that it represents an accidental coincidence.

The quantitative nature of the agreements obtained is illustrated as follows: While the atomic weight of hydrogen is 1.00778, the atomic weight of helium is 4.00054; when helium is created by the union of four hydrogen atoms an amount of matter disappears which is equal to four times 0.00778.

The difference—namely, .03058 grams—must, according to Einstein's equation (MC^2-E), go off in the form of radiant energy when the helium atom is formed, and the appearance of this amount of energy in the form of a monochromatic ether wave would give that ether wave the penetrating power which is represented by an absorption coefficient numerically equal to .305.

This is within a few per cent. of the absorption coefficient directly observed by Millikan and Cameron for the most conspicuous band in their cosmic ray spectrum.

There is, further, a philosophic argument which supports the results of this observation. We have long known that all elements have a structure which indicates that they are exact multiples of the mass of the positive electron, which is the nucleus of the hydrogen atom.

We have also known for thirty years that in the radio-active process the heavier atoms are disintegrating into lighter ones. It is, therefore, to be expected that somewhere in the universe the building-up process is going on to replace the tearing-down process represented by radio activity.

Up to the present, however, no evidence had ever been found that this building-up or creative process is going on now. The present experiments constitute the first discovery of such evidence.

It must be taken with some reserve and must be subjected to further critical analysis and further experimental tests. But, so far as they go, these experiments are at least indications, and the first direct indications, that all about us, either in the stars, the nebulae or in the depths of space, the creative process is going on, and that the cosmic rays which have been studied for the past few years constitute the announcements broadcast through the heavens of the birth of the ordinary elements out of positive and negative electrons.

When it is remembered that the positive electron is the nucleus of the hydrogen atom, and that the spectroscopic survey of the heavens shows the extraordinary abundance everywhere of hydrogen; and when we reflect that we have known for fifteen years that all the elements have weights that are practically exact multiples of the weight of the hydrogen atom as it appears in the structure of helium, the foregoing conclusion that the process of atom-building out of positive and negative electrons (the latter have a mass that is negligible in comparison with the former) is now going on gains additional plausibility.

If it is confirmed it will constitute new proof that this is a changing, dynamic and continuously evolving world instead of a static or a merely disintegrating one.

Further qualitative support for the validity of the foregoing evidence is derived from the fact that so far as we can now see there are no sorts of nuclear changes which could take place powerful enough to produce the observed cosmic rays except those herewith suggested.

Putting together, then, the quantitative and the qualitative evidence, we may have some confidence in the conclusion that the heretofore mysterious cosmic rays, which unceasingly shoot through space in all directions, are the announcements sent out through the ether of the birth of the elements.

R. A. MILLIKAN,
G. H. CAMERON

FORMS AND PROPERTIES OF WATER SOLUBLE PHOSPHORUS IN SOILS

A RECENT publication from this laboratory gave a method for the quantitative determination of organic and inorganic phosphorus in soil solutions and extracts. Another paper gave data showing the amounts of each form of phosphate in the displaced solutions and 1:5 water extracts and also presented results showing that the organic phosphate was not absorbed by plants. Subsequent studies have given additional data on the forms and properties of the water soluble phosphorus in soils.

While studying the decolorization of soil solutions by the use of carbon black, it was noted that the carbon absorbed a considerable portion of the organic phosphate but very little of the inorganic phosphate. Further studies showed that while a considerable part of the organic phosphate was readily absorbed by the carbon black, another portion was not easily removed by the use of carbon black. This is evident from the results of an experiment in which 100 cc. portions of two soil extracts were treated with 0.20, 0.50, and 2.00 gms. of carbon black. The results of the experiment are given in table 1.

TABLE 1

AMOUNTS OF INORGANIC AND ORGANIC PHOSPHATE IN SOIL EXTRACTS RECEIVING THE CARBON BLACK TREATMENTS INDICATED.

Treatment per 100 cc. extract	Extract 449		Extract 561	
	Inorganic PO_4	Organic PO_4	Inorganic PO_4	Organic PO_4
	p.p.m.	p.p.m.	p.p.m.	p.p.m.
None	0.58	0.38	Trace	0.24
0.20 gm. carbon..	0.61	0.23	Trace	0.12
0.50 gm. carbon..	0.61	0.23	Trace	0.12
2.00 gm. carbon..	0.51	0.21	Trace	0.12

The treatment with 0.20 grams resulted in the adsorption of 0.15 p.p.m. and 0.12 p.p.m. organic phosphate. Increasing the amount of carbon black to 2.0 gms. did not increase the amount of organic phosphate adsorbed. Similar results have been secured with extracts of other soils and with some displaced soil solutions.

In another experiment two soil extracts and a soil solution were treated one, two and three times with 0.50 gms. of carbon black. In all cases the first treatment resulted in the adsorption of considerable organic phosphate while the second and third treatments removed very little additional phosphate.

These results seem to indicate the presence of at least two forms of organic phosphate in soil extracts and solutions. One form is very readily adsorbed by carbon black while the other form is adsorbed in small amounts if at all. The relative amounts of the two forms seem to vary somewhat in the extracts and solutions from different soils. In general, however, they are usually present in approximately equal amounts. Neither form seems to be associated with the coloring matter of the extract or solution as many extracts that are practically colorless contain considerable amounts of both forms.

All the organic phosphate is apparently rather stable toward heat. Soil extracts and a soil solution were boiled two hours under a reflux condenser without materially increasing their content of inorganic phosphate.

Experiments with aluminum hydrate, prepared by the method of Emerson, as a decolorizing reagent have shown that it removes all of the inorganic phosphorus from solution but does not adsorb all of the organic phosphate. It does, however, adsorb some organic phosphate, probably the same portion that is readily adsorbed by carbon black. Increasing the amount of aluminum hydrate ten times did not increase the adsorption of organic phosphate.

These results confirm those previously reported showing that soil solutions and extracts contain considerable quantities of organic phosphate as well as inorganic phosphate. They further indicate that there are at least two forms of organic phosphate. Additional studies should be made to determine other properties of the organic phosphate including its rate of decomposition by biological action.

F. W. PARKER

SOILS LABORATORY,
ALABAMA AGRICULTURAL EXPERIMENT STATION

THE AMERICAN PHILOSOPHICAL SOCIETY

THE annual general meeting of the American Philosophical Society will take place in Philadelphia on April 19, 20 and 21. Following is the preliminary program of the sessions for the reading of scientific papers:

Thursday, April 19, at 2:00 P. M.

Francis X. Dercum, president, in the chair

Tundra vegetation of Central Alaska: JOHN W. HARSHBERGER, professor of botany, University of Pennsylvania.

Features of cells that live long: DANIEL T. MACDOUGAL, director of the laboratory of plant physiology, Carnegie Institution of Washington.

A geno-geographical study of the genus Bursa: GEORGE H. SHULL, professor of botany and genetics, Princeton University.

Trianaeopiper, a new genus of Piperaceae: WILLIAM TRELEASE, professor of botany, University of Illinois.

Cell division and differentiation: EDWIN G. CONKLIN, professor of biology, Princeton University.

Probable rôle of internal secretions in structure and growth as illustrated by breeds of dogs and peculiar types in man: CHARLES R. STOCKARD, professor of anatomy, Cornell University.

Functions of the internal secretions or endocrine organs that scientific progress has sanctioned: Charles E. de M. Sajous, professor of endocrinology, University of Pennsylvania, Graduate School of Medicine.

Cod-liver oil and the cod: Alfred F. Hess, clinical professor of pediatrics, University and Bellevue Hospital Medical College, New York City. (Introduced by Dr. Dercum.)

Different rates of growth among animals: Philip P. Calvert, professor of zoology, University of Pennsylvania.

Friday, April 20, at 10 A. M.

Henry Fairfield Osborn, vice-president, in the chair

Omorphamphus, a new flightless bird from the Eocene of Wyoming: William J. Sinclair, associate professor and curator, Princeton University.

The reports of the Princeton University expeditions to Patagonia: William B. Scott, professor of geology, Princeton University.

The astrapotheria of the Miocene of Patagonia: William B. Scott, professor of geology, Princeton University.

Were the ancestors of man primitive brachiators? William K. Gregory, professor of paleontology, Columbia University. (To be read by Francis Montague Ashley-Montagu.)

Racial characters in human dentition: Milo Hellman, New York City. (Introduced by Dr. Osborn.)

Present status of the problem of human ancestry: Henry Fairfield Osborn, American Museum of Natural History.

Flood control: Arthur E. Morgan, president of Antioch College. (Introduced by Dr. Conklin.)

Storms which issue from the inland-ice of Greenland: William H. Hobbs, professor of geology, University of Michigan.

A guide book to the world's weather and climates: Robert DeC. Ward, professor of climatology, Harvard University.

Friday afternoon at 2:00 P. M.

Cyrus Adler in the chair

Symposium on Aviation

Commercial aspects of aviation: William P. MacCracken, Jr., assistant secretary of commerce for aeronautics.

The application of aerodynamics: Edward P. Warner, assistant secretary of the Navy for aeronautics.

Lighter than air machines: C. E. Rosendahl, lieutenant commander, U. S. Navy.

Heavier than air machines: C. H. Biddlecomb, New York City (formerly major in the Royal Air Force).

Meteorology for aviation: William R. Blair, major, Signal Corps, U. S. Army.

Friday evening

Reception from 8 to 11 o'clock in the Hall of the Historical Society of Pennsylvania.

Richard P. Strong, professor of tropical medicine in Harvard University, will speak on "Studies of Human and Animal Diseases made during the Recent African Expedition."

Saturday morning, April 21, at 10:00 A. M.

William W. Campbell, vice-president, in the chair

Can business be made a science? Emory R. Johnson, professor of transportation and commerce, University of Pennsylvania.

Some economic implications in America's changing world status: Ernest M. Patterson, University of Pennsylvania. (Introduced by Dr. Johnson.)

An enactment of fundamental constitutional law in old South Arabia: James A. Montgomery, professor of Hebrew and Aramaic, University of Pennsylvania.

Textual criticism of the Greek Old Testament: Max L. Margolis, professor of biblical philology, Dropsie College for Hebrew and Cognate Learning.

Research in education: Frank Pierrepont Graves, president of the University of the State of New York.

An early Colonel House: Unofficial missions to England in 1842 and 1843 of General Duff Green: St. George Leakin Sioussat, professor of American history, University of Pennsylvania. (Introduced by Dr. Lingelbach.)

Fact: Henry Osborn Taylor, New York City.

Noah, a suggestion: Robert P. Field, Philadelphia.

Saturday afternoon at 2 P. M.

Francis X. Dercum, president, in the chair

Metabolism in the tropics: A study on some browns and blacks in Jamaica: Francis G. Benedict, director of Nutrition Laboratory, Carnegie Institution of Washington, and Morris Steggerda.

Racial chromosomal differences in Datura and their bearing on differentiation of species: Albert F. Blakeslee, assistant director in plant genetics, Carnegie Station for Experimental Evolution, Cold Spring Harbor.

Influence of groups containing sulphur on the color of azo dyes: E. Emmet Reid, profesor of chemistry, Johns Hopkins University. (Introduced by Dr. Smith.)

A method for determining the constants of electrical engineering, Harvard University: Arthur E. Kennelly, professor of electrical engineering, Harvard University.

Discussion of the kinetic theory of gravitation IV: Correlation of continual generation of heat in some substances, and impairment of their gravitational acceleration: Charles F. Brush, president of the Cleveland Chamber of Commerce.

A search for the galactic center: Harlow Shapley, director of the Harvard Observatory.

The distances of the stars: Samuel A. Mitchell, professor of astronomy and director of the Leander McCormick Observatory, University of Virginia.

Saturday evening, April 21, at 7:30 P. M.

Annual dinner in the north room of the Bellevue-Stratford Hotel.

SCIENCE

VOL. LXVII APRIL 20, 1928 No. 1738

CONTENTS

International Relations in Science: PROFESSOR GEORGE BARGER 405

Science Week in New York: DR. HENRY FAIRFIELD OSBORN 411

Walter Le Conte Stevens: PROFESSOR BENJAMIN A. WOOTEN 413

Scientific Events:

Proposed Memorial to the Late Professors Sir William M. Bayliss and Ernest H. Starling; The Yale School of Forestry; Increase of Salaries at Columbia University; American Medical Association Grants for Research 414

Scientific Notes and News 416

University and Educational Notes 420

Discussion and Correspondence:

The Instability of Condensed Substances near Absolute Zero: DR. R. D. KLEEMAN. *Ethylene as a Ripener of Fruits:* DR. R. B. HARVEY. *Banana Stowaways:* PROFESSOR GEORGE WAGNER, EDWARD R. WARREN. *Galilei or Galileo?* A. KAMPMEIER. *A Memorial to Laplace:* G. W. LITTLEHALES 420

Scientific Books:

Standley's Flora of the Panama Canal Zone: DR. JOHN M. COULTER 423

Special Articles:

Vitamins and the Oxidation of Fats and Oils: DR. GEORGE E. HOLM. *Modifications in Chilodon by Ultra-violet Light:* PROFESSOR MARY S. MACDOUGALL 424

The National Academy of Sciences 425

Science News x

SCIENCE: A Weekly Journal devoted to the Advancement of Science, edited by J. McKeen Cattell and published every Friday by

THE SCIENCE PRESS

New York City: Grand Central Terminal.

Lancaster, Pa. Garrison, N. Y.

Annual Subscription, $6.00. Single Copies, 15 Cts.

SCIENCE is the official organ of the American Association for the Advancement of Science. Information regarding membership in the Association may be secured from the office of the permanent secretary, in the Smithsonian Institution Building, Washington, D. C.

INTERNATIONAL RELATIONS IN SCIENCE[1]

IN this my introductory lecture, I take pleasure, at the very outset, in expressing my gratitude to the president of your university, to Professor Dennis and to the other authorities responsible for having addressed to me an invitation to come to you as lecturer on the Baker Foundation. I regard this invitation as a great honor, altogether beyond what I have deserved, and it will be my earnest endeavor, during my stay in your midst, to discharge the duties of this lectureship to the utmost of my ability.

The first of these duties in point of time is to deliver an introductory lecture on a non-technical subject. The choice of such a subject for the present occasion has caused me not a little difficulty. At the outset it seemed to me that since the purpose of the Baker Foundation is to bring over lecturers from other lands and thus facilitate intercourse between workers of different nationalities, I might perhaps suitably discuss the nature and extent of the intercourse between scientific men in different countries, both in the past and in the present. When I mentioned my plan to a friend who had lectured in a western university, he told me that the relations between European scientists would not be of any particular interest here, where a single nation stretches right across a continent. He further suggested that Americans are not so well informed about the national peculiarities of Europeans as I imagined, that they have no sympathy for our difficulties and are indeed somewhat impatient of European squabbles and jealousies. I was advised to discuss instead some more concrete chapter in scientific research and to treat it in a popular fashion. This suggestion, that America stands aloof from European affairs, did not, however, agree with my own impressions, previously gathered from American colleagues visiting Europe. The very fact that your university makes a practice of inviting foreign lecturers and the assurances of two of my predecessors in the Baker lectureship, convinced me that here in the east, at any rate, you are not only well acquainted with conditions in Europe, but also understand our difficulties, so that I still hope I may bring before you certain general considerations affecting scientific progress, and thus discharge my obliga-

[1] Introductory public lecture by Professor George Barger, of the University of Edinburgh, non-resident lecturer in chemistry at Cornell University.

tion, without discussing in detail any particular line of research.

Apart from its effect on the progress of science, the intercourse which I propose to discuss may contribute largely to the mutual understanding of nations. If the consent of scientific men, instead of that of parliaments, were required for the making of wars, the peace of the world would not indeed be assured, but I venture to think—I certainly hope—that it would be less precarious than it is at present. Scientific research is one of the most international forms of human endeavor. Perhaps it might be considered second to music in this respect, since music is independent of human speech; we can enjoy the compositions of foreign composers without knowing their mother tongue. Yet for this very reason music does not greatly help us to understand other nations and the music of the east may even be unintelligible to the west. Athletic contests and games like chess bring about the meeting of competitors from distant lands, but these international competitions affect only a handful of champions. The Olympic games no longer bring together the nations of the modern world as they united the communities of ancient Greece. But scientific phenomena are universal; they are the same all the world over. How often does the specialist worker remain isolated in his own country and find that his particular field is only cultivated by workers abroad! My further lectures will furnish many examples of this, as indeed all scientific lectures are apt to do. Let me, for the purposes of the present occasion, anticipate. The intense physiological action of extracts of the adrenal gland was discovered by two Englishmen and practically at the same time by two Poles. The isolation of epinephrin was then attempted by an Irishman and by an Austrian; it was accomplished in the United States by one of your countrymen and by a Japanese. The substance was next investigated by a Frenchman, an Englishman and by several Germans, one of whom synthesized it; it was also synthesized by an Englishman. Allusion to this chain of researches, extending over less than a decade, has already involved me in the mention of eight nationalities. Hence it is clear that international relations play a considerable part in scientific research.

Western science originated with the Greeks and in the Hellenistic period became concentrated at Alexandria; other civilizations, such as that of the Chinese, remained isolated, and facts known to them were rediscovered later in the west. In ancient times there was a good deal of intercourse among philosophers all round the eastern half of the Mediterranean. Already the Ionian Greeks of the fifth century B. C. were characterized by a love of travel for the sake of the "wonders" to be seen in strange lands. Thales (624–547 B. C.), the founder of Greek geometry and of Greek astronomy, traveled in Egypt, and Pythagoras also undertook extensive journeys. Mathematical discoveries, whether made in Asia Minor, in the east or in Magna Graecia in the west, became widely known by an intercourse facilitated by a common language and apparently not hampered greatly by political differences or even by wars; yet the harmful effect of war on scientific progress was early illustrated by the killing of Archimedes by a Roman soldier at the sack of Syracuse in 212 B. C.

The decay of the Roman empire was accompanied by that of Greek science, which passed at a later period to the Moors. Not until the Renaissance did the pursuit of science spread to the nations of the west, and then, for a time, it would seem to have been more international than other forms of human activity. In the school of medicine at Salerno and the earliest universities of Bologna, Padua and Paris, the universal use of Latin established a freemasonry among the learned, where accidents of nationality did not count and difficulties of communication were overcome. Vesalius, a Belgian, taught anatomy at Padua, Paracelsus traveled widely in troublous times, and science appeared wholly dissociated from politics. Although Spain was the chief nation concerned in the discovery of America, Columbus was an Italian, and the name of your continent is likewise of Italian origin.

The number of foreign students in medieval universities was great. A document of the year 1228, exactly seven hundred years ago, records the presence at Padua of French, English, Norman, Provençal, Spanish and Catalan students. This was only six years after the foundation of that university. Later the number of foreigners increased still further. They came "non ex propinquis tantum regionibus, non ex ultima solum Italia, sed . . . ex toto prope terrarum orbe." Ultimately twenty-two "nations" were represented, ten from beyond the Alps, twelve from various regions of Italy. Each "nation" elected one or more councilors who assisted the rector in the government of the university. Traces of this divisional arrangement of the students survive in certain Scottish universities. In the fifteenth century there were about a hundred French students at Padua, nearly as many English and Scottish, and over three hundred German. Even now the crests of students from many nations (that of Harvey among the number) may be seen in the old loggia and aula of Padua University and afford interesting testimony to the international character of medieval learning. Professorships were not infrequently held by foreigners;

it is early recorded that the highest office of the university, the rectorship, was held by a Pole in 1271.

At first the study of science was the work of a few devotees who communicated their discoveries by personal intercourse or in the form of books. To these men science was a passion or an obsession, in any case their main interest in life. In course of time the amateur also made himself felt. Otto von Guericke, burgomaster of Magdeburg, was presumably as much occupied with civic affairs as with his air pump; although King Charles II of England founded the Royal Society and sometimes attended its meetings, his main interest can not be said to have been scientific. The diaries of Pepys and of Evelyn give an interesting sidelight on the attitude towards science of the amateur of that period. One of your earliest statesmen, Benjamin Franklin, was distinguished for his important contributions to natural knowledge. Priestley, one of the discoverers of oxygen, was in later life much more interested in theology than in the constituents of the atmosphere. The importance of the work of amateurs, or at least of men not holding official positions, seems to me to have been specially characteristic of British science; I need only mention the names of Boyle and of Cavendish, both scions of noble houses, and of Joule, a brewer.

The growing interest in science led, in the second half of the seventeenth century, to the foundation of societies and academies, who published short communications in their proceedings. The Royal Society of London received its charter in 1662 and arose out of informal earlier meetings at Oxford. Its "Philosophical Transactions" were first published in 1665. About the same time were founded the Accademia del Cimento of Florence (1657), the Academy of Vienna (1652) and the Académie Royale of Paris (1666); the memoirs of the latter began in 1699; in 1700 the Berlin Academy was founded. At first the publications of these various societies preserved the appearance of private intercourse, for they frequently were in the form of letters addressed to the secretary. As an example I may refer to the important microscopic discoveries of Anthoni van Leeuwenhoek, who during the latter years of the seventeenth century wrote several hundred letters from his sleepy little town of Delft to the secretary of the newly founded Royal Society of London; a portion of these letters, published in Dutch, occupies four large volumes. Leeuwenhoek, employed as janitor at the town hall, became, in his spare time, an expert in the grinding of lenses and made his own very powerful simple microscopes, tiny instruments compared with the compound microscopes of a later date. His equipment was indeed in strange contrast to that of the chemical laboratory of this university, which, I understand, has a special section devoted to the application of the microscope to chemistry. Yet Leeuwenhoek's discoveries were of a fundamental kind; thus he first saw and figured infusoria and spermatozoa, and investigated the process of reproduction in various animals. Another famous microscopist of that time, Malpighi, an Italian, also communicated his discoveries to the Royal Society; his original letters, with those of Leeuwenhoek, form an interesting part of the archives of the society.

One of the effects of the foundation of national academies was an increased use of the native tongue in scientific communications, and instead of, or in addition to Latin, it has now become necessary for the man of science to know several modern languages. The abandonment of Latin as the universal language proved an obstacle to scientific intercourse. When lectures at the universities were no longer given in Latin, it became more difficult to obtain teachers from abroad. The change made itself felt in the beginning of the eighteenth century. In the middle of the previous one it was still possible to call to Leiden a Hanoverian physician, Franciscus Sylvius, to teach chemistry and medicine; he indeed founded there the first university chemical laboratory, a humble precursor of the magnificent building in which we are now assembled. When later, early in the eighteenth century, the school of medicine, to which I myself belong, was developed at Edinburgh, the use of spoken Latin, which, as we have seen, had done so much for the medieval universities, had declined, the teachers were all Scotsmen, who had indeed been influenced by the great Boerhaave, of Leiden, but did not use Latin to any large extent in their own lectures. As a written language Latin survived to a much later date, particularly in academic publications, such as doctoral theses which at Edinburgh, for instance, continued to be in Latin until about one hundred years ago; in Germany Latin was still employed for this purpose until about the middle of the last century. To-day the use of Latin in scientific publications is rare and almost restricted to a few botanical and zoological works of reference chiefly of interest to the systematist. Its use as a spoken language is extremely rare; apart from ceremonial occasions at the older English universities, I have myself heard it only twice at international gatherings; on both occasions it was used by Swedes.

The use of the vernacular instead of Latin caused at least a relative setback in the intercourse between the scientific men of various nations. The growth of nationalism in the nineteenth century acted in the same direction, and it was not until travel had been facilitated through the spread of railways that the abandonment of Latin as a universal language was compensated for by the greater ease of communication.

In giving facilities to advanced students from abroad, for some time Paris and later on the German universities took a leading part and thus contributed greatly to the furtherance of international relations, not the least by spreading a knowledge of French and German among scientific men. Thus the laboratory of Wurtz attracted many foreign chemists to Paris, as did that of Liebig to Giessen. The Pasteur Institute later drew bacteriologists to Paris and towards the end of the century it became comparatively common, particularly for American and English scientific men, to spend a year or so in research at a foreign university. They thus acquired a knowledge of the spoken language, which sometimes proved useful in strange circumstances. When, as the result of the Armistice, the allied chemical experts inspected certain German chemical factories, which had been used for the production of munitions of war, there was at least one occasion when an English and a French chemist met a German expert and the victors had to speak the language of the vanquished, for German was the only language known to all. Personally, I remember a chemical congress held a few years after the war, at Cambridge. England and France were largely represented; there were no Germans; there was a distinguished chemist from Japan who had studied in Germany and spoke its language fluently, but did not speak French. I took pleasure in introducing him in German to his French colleagues who too spoke that language fluently, and later admitted to me privately that it was a very useful one.

Among the advantages of foreign study may therefore be counted the acquisition of a thorough knowledge of a foreign language and some insight into the character of another nation. For various reasons residence abroad has however of late become less frequent, at least relatively so. The great development of your own universities has diminished the inducement to your students to spend some years in Europe, when they find at home an extensive choice of distinguished teachers and of excellent laboratories. The late war has had a great effect in the same direction, particularly on the younger workers in my own country. Formerly it was common for British students to spend a year or two at a German university, in order to obtain the degree of doctor of philosophy, but as a result of the late war practically all British universities have copied Germany in instituting such a degree; the effect has certainly been good in stimulating research among British students at home, but it has also tended to make the younger generation more insular and less acquainted with foreign life and thought. To some extent this is compensated for by the increased number of traveling fellowships, mostly founded by Americans; to these I will refer later.

We have seen that the disuse of Latin as a vehicle of instruction made the occupation of teaching posts by foreigners more difficult, but the practice has never died out. Thus in 1845 Prince Albert, the Consort of Queen Victoria, and a German who did much to stimulate scientific research in his adopted country, secured the migration to London of A. W. Hofmann. The nineteen years which Hofmann spent in England not only saw the production on a commercial scale of mauve, the first aniline dye, by his pupil Perkin, but Hofmann's stay in England did also much to further Anglo-German chemical relations. A number of German chemists settled in England, and Hofmann, after he had returned to his native country to occupy the chair of chemistry at Berlin, brought about the foundation of the German Chemical Society on the model of the English society, with which he became familiar during his years in London. While Hofmann was in England, another German organic chemist, Kekulé, was professor in Belgium, at the University of Ghent, and there worked out his famous benzene formula; he soon afterwards returned to Germany, but yet another German, Körner, migrated permanently to Italy, where he had many pupils and died only a few years ago. Such examples of migration are most frequent in the smaller European countries whose size restricts their choice of native candidates. Moreover, in a country such as Holland every university student knows English, French and German, so that there is no difficulty about a foreigner lecturing in one of these languages until he has learned the vernacular. There are always a few Germans among the professoriate of the Dutch universities. About thirty years ago an Englishman was appointed to a theological professorship at Leiden, and when he migrated to the United States, he was succeeded by a Norwegian; in this way the Dutch government attempted to avoid the *odium theologicum* which would have resulted from the appointment of a native. Dutchmen have from time to time occupied chairs abroad; thus van't Hoff left Amsterdam for Berlin, and within recent years Holland has supplied a professor of physics to Scotland, one to Germany and a professor of medicine to Vienna. Sweden has a German professor of chemistry, and an English professor of pharmacology, who came there after holding a chair in Switzerland. This latter country is, of all, the most ready to appoint foreigners; indeed, at one time a Swiss chair was frequently a stepping-stone to a more important one in Germany. Besides quite a number of Germans I can think of one or two Frenchmen, several Poles and Russians, two Americans, an Englishman, a Dutchman and an Austrian, who have in recent times held Swiss professorships. Such a lively interchange would however offend the nationalism of the larger countries, where there is moreover a larger choice of native candidates and where the wars of 1870 and 1914 have produced a serious setback in international exchanges.

After 1870 politics entered into science as never before. French science became national, almost insular. Germans no longer studied in Paris, and for many years no French workers came to German laboratories; by slow degrees formal relations were ultimately resumed, more readily perhaps by the victors than by the vanquished. Franco-German susceptibilities became the chief stumbling-block in any international organization, as they did in European politics. Among the most noteworthy of these organizations are various congresses at which devotees of the same branch of science meet periodically for communication and discussion of their researches. One of the oldest and most successful of these is the congress of physiologists, started in 1889 on the initiative of Michael Foster and, except during the late war, held at intervals of three years. In a gathering of this kind the very choice of a meeting place is already influenced by politics. Just as the International Postal Union and the League of Nations meet in Switzerland and the International Court of Justice in Holland, so the congress of physiology began by meeting in small countries to avoid the jealousies of the larger ones. The first six meetings were held in Switzerland, in Belgium, again in Switzerland, in England, in Italy and again in Belgium. Although Germany has important physiological laboratories, it took eighteen years for the congress to come to that country (Heidelberg, 1907). In Paris, in 1920, no Germans were present, and in 1923 at Edinburgh, the great problem was to bring the late belligerents together again. The organizer of the latter congress received strong expressions of opinion from American and English physiologists that they would welcome the presence of German and Austrian colleagues, and invitations were accordingly sent to them, but this very fact kept away many Frenchmen and Belgians. Those who were present realized, however, how the restoration to the congress of its truly international character increased its scientific value, and three years later at Stockholm, it was generally agreed that the Franco-German difficulty was at an end among the physiologists. The next meeting is to be held in 1929 at Boston, and this decision illustrates yet another problem, not political, but geographic and financial, for it will have taken the congress exactly forty years to come to America.

This is far from satisfactory. American physiologists have attended previous meetings in large numbers, they have enhanced the scientific value of the congress by their communications, yet many of them could ill afford the expenses of a journey to Europe. Of course many European university teachers are even less able to defray the cost of transatlantic travel. There is here a difficulty inherent in the spread of science over two continents. Yet it is to be hoped that, in spite of this difficulty, a numerous contingent from Europe may find it possible to accept the warm invitation of their American colleagues. Thus the visitors will be able to learn at first hand about divisions of their subject which have been developed by American pioneer work and have as yet hardly been studied on the continent of Europe.

The political difficulties in other departments of knowledge have varied. It would seem that after the war international relations were most readily resumed in those sciences which are most remote from practical considerations. Where, as in chemistry, industrial or military applications interfere, progress has been less rapid.

Thus the late war had very little effect on astronomers, but industrial rivalry and chemical warfare have delayed a *rapprochement* among the chemists. Yet here also progress may be recorded. Thus, Professor Richard Willstätter, a leader of German chemistry, who, you may recall, visited this university less than a year ago, was invited to give the Faraday lecture to the Chemical Society of London, and generously allowed himself to be reelected an honorary fellow of that society. The celebration of the Berthelot Centenary in Paris last October, the most distinguished chemical gathering in which it has been my privilege to take part, was attended by nine German and by two Austrian delegates.

Mention should also be made of the International Research Council formed as a result of meetings in London and Paris in 1918 and at Brussels in 1919. It is practically a union of academies formed for the purpose of facilitating international cooperation in scientific work, and promoting the formation of international unions in different branches of science. The statutes of the Research Council were so framed that the central powers were excluded; their inclusion immediately after the great war would indeed have been surprising. Seven years later, however, at Brussels, in 1926, the Royal Society of London, at the instigation of Holland and Denmark, proposed that the five German academies should be invited to join the International Research Council, an invitation which has not yet been accepted. Its non-acceptance must be a disappointment to the Dutch and Danish academies, and to all who wish to see science dissociated from politics. The accession of the German academies might not be very important in itself, but it would bring with it membership of the various unions. One of these is the "Union internationale de la chimie pure et appliquée." I purposely quote its French title, for since its inception it has been largely under French influence, and at its first four annual meetings there was no question of admitting German chemists. Any one acquainted with the magnitude of the contribution which Germany has made to chemical science will realize that the union thereby greatly handicapped itself. At the sixth meeting at Bucharest in 1925, a motion was finally carried expressing the wish that the International Research Council should modify its statutes, so as to permit the entry into the affiliated unions of all countries who are members of the League of Nations. Apart from the furtherance of individual scientific intercourse, which may be secured in other ways, this entry would bring about the cooperation of the Germans in the attempt to secure a uniform chemical nomenclature, which without them is a somewhat sterile labor, since the chief exhaustive chemical dictionaries and cyclopedias have been published as the result of German enterprise and diligence. For the advance of science in general, and of chemistry in particular, it is very much to be hoped that the German academicians will accept the invitation to join the International Research Council and thereby facilitate cooperation among the younger men.

On the whole the setback in scientific intercourse produced by the late war seems to me not so great as the magnitude of the struggle might lead one to fear; the cleavage between France and Germany is no greater than it was after 1870. Moreover, we can record the beneficent effect of certain agencies which have only come into being during recent years. Thus the League of Nations, in its public health work, has incidentally brought medical men together, and from the outset German delegates have taken part. For instance, international standards have been adopted for the strength of certain drugs, and the biological methods used in testing them have formed a subject of research by pharmacologists of various nations. While this country of yours is so remote from the turmoil of European affairs that it has remained outside the League of Nations, I need hardly say that American delegates have heartily cooperated in the health work of the league, as in some other of its activities. The attitude of your government has not prevented private individuals and foundations from exercising a powerful influence in favor of the resumption of international intercourse and the furtherance of scientific cooperation. It is peculiarly appropriate that in addressing you I should record here in the first place the work of the distinguished president of this great university, who was the first chairman of the League of Red Cross Societies, at Geneva and Paris. Then I would mention the work of the Rockefeller Foundation, particularly in regard to medical education. I well remember the impression produced by a large gift to the medical school of University College, London, a few years after the war. The idealism, shown by giving so large a sum to a foreign institution, aroused feelings of enthusiasm and admiration among British men of science, and since then medical education has benefited in other countries, regardless of politics. I take pleasure in recording that the medical school with which I am myself associated has received several benefactions from the Rockefeller Foundation. Moreover, by giving traveling fellowships regardless of nationality, the foundation has done much to further scientific intercourse, particularly by enabling the younger men to visit foreign laboratories. Thus the first visitor from Central Europe to work in my laboratory after the war was enabled to do so by a Rockefeller Traveling Fellowship, and several of my pupils owe experience gained in American laboratories to the same endowment. The annual review of the work of the foundation gives an idea of its world-wide activities. Thus in 1925, in addition to taking measures for the combating of hookworm disease, yellow fever and malaria, the foundation contributed to the progress of medical education in many countries, maintained a modern medical school in Peking, provided, directly or indirectly, fellowships for 842 men and women from forty-four different countries and financed the travel of fifty other persons, officials and professors. Such activities are indeed a powerful and beneficent factor in international scientific intercourse. The International Education Board, established in 1923 by Mr. John D. Rockefeller, Jr., is an agency working in the same direction. In theory it may include the United States in its field of work. In practice, however, its interests lie mainly in other countries, since the General Education Board, founded by Mr. John D. Rockefeller, Sr., in 1902, is limited by its charter to the advancement of education in the United States. During the year 1925–1926 the International Education Board made ninety-seven first awards of fellowships and twenty-nine renewals; the holders came from twenty-five different countries. The voluntary migration of three hundred or more young scientists under the auspices of the board since its foundation provides interesting indications where, in the opinion of the European and American sponsors, the more favorable conditions for research may be found at the moment. Thus in mathematics there is a marked migration toward France, Germany and Italy, in physics the trend is definitely toward England, the United States, Denmark and Germany.

The primary object of the Rockefeller Foundation the improvement of health and of education; a valuable secondary result of their activities is the promotion of international amity. This latter object is the primary one in the case of certain other benefactions, such as that of the thirty-two scholarships for American students, founded a generation ago by an Englishman, Cecil Rhodes, in his own University of Oxford. In this, as in other matters, Rhodes was a pioneer. His foundation has now a counterpart in the Commonwealth Fund, supported by gifts from the late Mrs. Stephen V. Harkness, which fund has established a number of fellowships for British graduates, tenable at American universities. I may perhaps quote from the official memorandum: "In creating these Commonwealth Fund Fellowships the Directors of the Fund have been impelled by a belief in the value of international opportunities for education and travel to young men and women of character and ability, and by a conviction that such opportunities offered to British students will promote the mutual amity and understanding of Great Britain and the United States." The John Simon Guggenheim Memorial Foundation indirectly furthers the same object by giving fellowships to American graduates for study abroad. All these factors are bound to have a favorable effect on the outlook of the younger generation of scientific workers; half a century ago they did not exist; in the main we owe them to your country.

National characteristics have an interest, comparable to that which the student of natural history takes in the various species of animals and plants. National psychology may be as interesting as the nesting habits of birds. Each nation has its own particular genius, without which the world would be the poorer. It is interesting to inquire which nations show the greatest aptitude for scientific research, and why they do so. I feel convinced, as a result of a statistical inquiry, into which I can not enter here, that the small nations are preeminent in this respect. Per million of population Holland, Switzerland and the Scandinavian countries at present seem to contribute more to the progress of science than any of the larger nations. Why this is so it is difficult to say. It is also interesting to speculate on the reasons which make pure mathematics flourish in Italy and in Sweden, music and organic chemistry in Germany, biochemistry and psychology in the United States, physiology in Britain. Whilst we need not agree wholly with the opening words of Wurtz's dictionary of chemistry, which claims this science as French, and Lavoisier as its founder, we must recognize that we owe bacteriology to Pasteur and to France. The various nations have each their peculiar aptitude which by itself constitutes a reason for furthering international relations in science; my main reason for having brought this subject before you is, however, a desire to promote, in the words of the Commonwealth Fund Memorandum, "mutual amity and understanding." This object has already appealed to a number of your citizens; with the westward trend of civilization it is all the more desirable that the difficulties of an enfeebled Europe should be understood by America, which has become the economic mistress of the modern world, just as Rome in the third century B. C. became the political mistress of the Mediterranean. Europe, like Greece, has suffered from internal strife, yet the influence of Greece was not extinguished by the loss of political independence; the Academy survived for seven centuries, and the migration of Greek scholars began the Renaissance. Similarly, the influence of Europe will survive her economic adversity; America will doubtless become even more interested in European affairs, just as Rome looked more and more to Greek civilization.

I hope I have not wearied you with the dissensions of European men of science. In discussing them I have had in mind the words which mark so impressively the tomb of your great countryman, Grant, on the bank of the Hudson River. These words, used after a great crisis in your political history, I would apply to scientific affairs of to-day: "Let us have peace."

GEORGE BARGER

CORNELL UNIVERSITY

SCIENCE WEEK IN NEW YORK

DECEMBER 27, 1928, TO JANUARY 2, 1929

THOSE who are engaged in the preparation for the coming eighty-fifth meeting of the American Association for the Advancement of Science and Associated Societies, which will be held in New York City from December 27, 1928, to January 2, 1929, are endeavoring to arrange a week's program so attractive and interesting that the members of the association and the societies will be more than usually tempted to extend their individual visits to New York over the entire week from Thursday evening, December 27, to Wednesday evening, January 2.

With the commodious facilities afforded by several new, large, medium-priced hotels, recently constructed in the city, the local committee hopes to secure favorable weekly—and, if possible, half-weekly—rates. The American Association program will begin with the opening session on Thursday evening, December 27, and will conclude with a very interesting general address on Wednesday evening, January 2. Thus ample time will be afforded the members of the association and of the societies to visit personally the remarkable group of scientific institutions which have been springing up in various parts of New York City during the last twenty-five years and which have transformed the city from a merely social, economic and artistic municipality into one of the most interesting centers of scientific activity in the world. Every branch of science represented in the American Association and Associated Societies has been affected by this astonishing expansion, which, in itself, is due to the intelligence and energy of the scientific men and women who have been attracted to the city, and also to the unprecedented inflow of wealth and beneficence that has touched and enriched every branch.

In geology and geography, in physics and chemistry, in mathematics and engineering, in all the botanical and zoological sciences—including biophysics and biochemistry—finally in anthropology, psychology and education, as well as in the medical sciences, the City of New York has made wonderful progress. Its laboratories and museums, the rapidly extending exhibition halls and scientific collections connected with its leading institutions of learning and culture, are in themselves worthy of prolonged study; because many of them represent the last word in the technique of scientific research. The governing officials of all the sixty institutions where various new facilities for research and education are to be seen have united in extending a cordial welcome to the visitors who will come to New York for the approach of Science Week. It will be a great loss, especially for those coming from a distance, if their plans are made for so short a visit that they will be obliged to spend all their time in the scientific sessions, thus making it impossible or difficult to take advantage of the opportunity of accepting the hospitality of these numerous institutions. It is planned that the week's program will include one special day for each of the most interesting organizations, on which day these organizations will be specially prepared for the reception of those who are in attendance at the great science convention.

The American Museum of Natural History—with its fifty exhibition halls covering every branch of natural history and anthropology—will itself fill a great deal of the time most advantageously. Visitors will be surprised to find in this institution a finely equipped laboratory for experimental zoology and will be pleased with the beginnings of the new extension of its exhibitions and researches into other fields of biology, ichthyology and oceanography, as well as with the foundations of the future great Hall of Astronomy.

Columbia University has offered its hospitality to the association and the societies; Dean George Braxton Pegram, of the Faculty of Science, is in charge of the university's arrangements, as well as the general arrangements for the meeting, and all inquiries for meeting places—whether at Columbia, the American Museum, the Engineering Building, the Rockefeller Institute or the Cornell Medical College—should be addressed to him. Of especial interest to the members of both the association and the societies are the superb buildings erected in the various departments of science since the association last met at Columbia, in 1916. Foremost among these buildings is the new Chemistry Hall, planned under the direction of the late Professor Charles F. Chandler and embodying all the newest ideas in the construction of a chemistry building, both for practical and experimental laboratories, and the encouragement of various branches of research. It is expected that many of the sections of the association and the societies associated with it will find ample accommodation in the numerous lecture halls and laboratories of the university. The adjacent Teachers College, with its large auditoriums and lecture halls will especially welcome the various meetings devoted to education; while Barnard College, Horace Mann School, International House and Casa Italiana, on the university grounds, stand ready to open hospitable halls. The New York Historical Society, adjacent to the American Museum, offers further accommodations at that part of town, while the medical and engineering sections will be magnificently provided for.

Special efforts are being made to have the scientific sessions of the association and the societies distributed as satisfactorily as possible in Science Week. It is hoped that the majority of the society meetings may not be crowded into the first half-week (December 27 to 29) but that many of the societies will arrange to hold their meetings, receptions and dinners from Sunday, December 30 to Wednesday, January 2, the date on which the last general session of the American Association will be held, followed by the closing general reception.

Evening addresses of general interest in the several science fields are being planned for every evening of the week, which are to be announced later. These will be delivered in the great Hall of the American Museum of Natural History (77th St., and Central Park West) and each is to be followed by a reception for those interested in the field of science represented by the address. The receptions will be held in the new education hall of the museum and the appropriate exhibition halls will be open during the evening, with special arrangements of exhibits planned particularly for these occasions.

Registration offices for the convention will be in education hall at the museum, also at Columbia University, where many of the scientific sessions are to be held, and probably at the Engineering Societies Building (29 West 39th St.) and at Cornell Medical College (28th St. and Avenue A). Arrangements are in progress by which those who register may be subject to just as little inconvenience as possible, especially with reference to the validation of reduced-rate railway certificates and other features of registration. These arrangements will be announced later from the Washington office of Dr. Burton E. Livingston, permanent secretary of the association, in the Smithsonian Institution Building.

The local arrangements for meeting places and equipment and for the general sessions, receptions, etc., are, as usual, in the hands of the local committees for the meeting, with a local executive committee consisting of the following members, as thus far appointed:

Henry Fairfield Osborn, president of the American Association.

Michael I. Pupin, honorary chairman of the local committee.

George Braxton Pegram, general chairman of the local committees.

J. McKeen Cattell, chairman of the executive committee of the American Association and editor of SCIENCE.

Sam F. Trelease, secretary of the local committees.

Communications regarding arrangements for the meeting should be addressed to Dr. Sam F. Trelease, secretary, American Association office, American Museum of Natural History, West 77th St., New York City, and a copy of each communication should be simultaneously sent also to Dr. Burton E. Livingston, permanent secretary, American Association for the Advancement of Science, Smithsonian Institution Building, Washington, D. C.

The chief purpose of the newly elected president is to make the coming eighty-fifth meeting of real scientific significance in the advancement of science in this country, as is done, year by year, in the splendidly organized meetings of the British Association for the Advancement of Science. Accordingly, invitations are being sent to the leading scientific representatives of New York, Princeton and New Haven, to serve as members of local advisory committees for the several sections of the Association and their associated societies. Names of the members of these advisory committees will be published in the near future. It is hoped that they will lend their influence and scientific prestige to the meeting and aid in making the New York programs much more valuable than usual.

The president is also suggesting to the vice-presidents for the sections that they choose for their addresses subjects of current popular interest, and that they prepare their manuscripts, with summaries, well in advance, so that these may be released to the press in distant cities on the respective days when the addresses are delivered.

It fortunately happens that many of the most distinguished men of American science are going to be in New York during this Science Week, so the principal general addresses will be very important. The plan of extending an invitation abroad to at least one great public lecturer is also under consideration. Another very important feature of the coming meeting will be the symposia on topics of present interest, some of which may be suggested by the president of the association. It is, moreover, eminently desirable that the section officers and the officers of the associated societies join forces in avoiding conflicts of program so as to successfully amplify each other.

Later issues of SCIENCE will contain further announcements of preparations for this really notable event in American scientific history.

HENRY FAIRFIELD OSBORN,
President of the American Association for the Advancement of Science.

WALTER LE CONTE STEVENS

WALTER LE CONTE STEVENS was born in Gordon County, Georgia, on June 17, 1847.

His early education was obtained from tutors in his father's home and from local private schools near Walthourville. He entered the University School at Athens in 1862 and studied there for two years. During this time, though only sixteen years of age, he taught Latin and Greek in addition to his regular work as a student.

In 1864 he entered the Confederate army and was stationed with the field artillery at Fort McAllister, Georgia. He was transferred to the Signal Corps and served as a telegraph operator until stricken by malaria. He spent most of his time while a soldier as an invalid.

He entered the University of South Carolina in 1866, just as that institution was changing from a college to a university, and received the degree of A.B. in 1868. His graduating essay was on "Physics and Metaphysics," showing, in spite of almost exclusively classical training, a leaning toward scientific subjects. This leaning was, no doubt, fostered by his early association with his father, who was a country physician, and with his uncles, the famous Le Conte brothers.

After graduation he clerked for a short time in a drug store in Columbia and he tutored and taught in local schools for about two years. It was during this time that his first paper, "Mutes and Liquids," appeared in *The Virginia Educational Journal*.

He was elected professor of chemistry and modern languages in Oglethorpe College and he spent the year of 1870–71 at the University of Virginia studying chemistry. After Oglethorpe College was closed in 1873 he taught science in the high schools of Savannah, Georgia, until 1876. In 1876–77 he again attended the University of Virginia, this time studying mathematics.

Feeling that his chances for further development were small in the south he went to New York in 1878 and taught as a special lecturer for five years, attending night classes at Cooper Union. He spent much of his spare time in research on binocular perspective during this period. Several papers on this and related subjects appeared at about this time. Largely as a result of this work, the University of Georgia granted him an honorary Ph.D. in 1882.

He was elected professor of physics (and of course many other things as well) in the Packer Collegiate Institute in Brooklyn in 1882, which position he held until 1890. During this professorship he published a number of articles on sound. On resigning this position Dr. Stevens spent about two years in Europe, studying in Strassburg, Berlin and Zurich, returning to America in 1892 to accept a professorship of physics at the Rensselaer Polytechnic Institute.

In 1892 he was elected secretary of Section B of the American Association for the Advancement of Science and in 1894 he became vice-president of this section.

He came to Washington and Lee University in 1898 as McCormick professor of physics, which position he held until his retirement as emeritus professor in 1922.

His training and experience were broad and his interests were many. Music was his chief delight and he accumulated a most unusual library of graphophone records. He wrote many essays on cultural as well as scientific subjects, and his condensed reviews of operatic librettos were of the greatest interest and use to his friends.

His death in Lexington, Virginia, on December 28, 1927, removed one of the few remaining scientists of the old school. He was an accurate thinker and a powerful teacher, and his personality showed a most pleasing blend of classical polish and scientific precision. He never allowed himself to specialize, but remained broad in tastes and interests. He felt that all the fields of physics were his own.

His long life of hard work and valuable accomplishment was ended quietly and peacefully in his home in Lexington, and his interest in current happenings and affairs continued practically to the end.

He is survived by his wife, Mrs. Virginia Lee Letcher Stevens, of Lexington, Virginia, and by his brother, J. Percy Stevens, of Atlanta, Georgia.

BENJAMIN ALLEN WOOTEN

SCIENTIFIC EVENTS

PROPOSED MEMORIAL TO THE LATE PROFESSORS SIR WILLIAM M. BAYLISS AND ERNEST H. STARLING

A COMMITTEE has been formed to raise funds wherewith to commemorate the work of the late Professors Sir William M. Bayliss and Ernest H. Starling. This committee has issued the following memorandum:

The opinion has been frequently and widely expressed that some fitting memorial should be made to record the great services rendered, both to the science of physiology and to its applications in the practical problems of medicine, by the labors of Bayliss and Starling, who were intimately connected for so many fruitful years. That they contributed greatly to the progress of physiology is too well recognized to need emphasis. The patient zeal of the one, the fire and enthusiasm of the other and the eagerness of both on all occasions to place their knowledge and experience at the disposal of other workers from any part of the world, have led to a universal appreciation of their services. The number of individuals in all countries who have profited directly from their help or indirectly by their influence is very great, and their writings stand as monuments to their industry and learning.

A committee, the constitution of which is given below, has been formed to issue an appeal for funds wherewith to commemorate the connection with physiology of these great partners in a manner of which they themselves would have approved: a material memorial or an annual lecture would have seemed a smaller thing to them than the provision of means whereby young workers of suitable training and ability might be attracted into their chosen subject. The committee, therefore, is of opinion that the most fitting memorial would be the creation at University College of a Bayliss and Starling studentship, open to any graduate in science of any university, or any graduate or undergraduate in medicine of suitable standing, to enable him to spend a year or more in such training in physiology and biochemistry as would fit him for research. A small part of the funds collected might be employed in the erection of a simple memorial tablet in the entrance hall of the Institute of Physiology.

Subscriptions may be sent to Professor Lovatt Evans at the Institute of Physiology, University College, Gower Street, London.

Members of the Committee: Professor J. Barcroft, Cambridge; Samuel Bayliss, Wolverhampton; Sir J. Rose Bradford, president of the Royal College of Physicians; Professor W. B. Cannon, Harvard Medical School; Professor E. P. Cathcart, Glasgow; Dr.

H. H. Dale, National Institute for Medical Research; Professor J. C. Drummond, University College, London; Professor C. Lovatt Evans, University College, London; Dr. J. Fawcett, Guy's Hospital; Sir Gregory Foster, provost of University College, London; Sir J. Kingston Fowler, London; Professor A. V. Hill, Foulerton professor, Royal Society; Sir F. G. Hopkins, Cambridge; Professor J. B. Leathes, Sheffield; Sir T. Lewis, University College Hospital, London; Professor Graham Lusk, Cornell Medical College, New York; Professor Sir C. J. Martin, director, Lister Institute; Professor M. S. Pembrey, Guy's Hospital Medical School; Professor Sir E. Sharpey-Shafer, Edinburgh; Sir C. Sherrington, Oxford; Professor G. Elliot Smith, University College, London; Dr. Hubert Starling, Norwich; Professor J. F. Stenning, warden of Wadham College.

THE YALE SCHOOL OF FORESTRY

THE Yale School of Forestry has announced certain changes in policy designed to strengthen its course of study and broaden the opportunities for work of an advanced and specialized character. These changes involve first a modification of the requirements for the degree of master of forestry, second the recognition of forestry by the graduate school of the university as an appropriate field of study for the degree of doctor of philosophy and third the enlargement and enrichment of the courses offered in a number of subjects. The new educational policy aims to provide, as formerly, a training for the general practice of forestry and, in addition, to afford special opportunities for the advanced student who desires to specialize in some branch of forestry. This will strengthen the present curriculum and enable the school to fulfil its fundamental objective of offering to the individual student a type of training which best meets his special educational needs. Under the new plan the requirements for the degree of master of forestry include: two years' work in technical forestry, one year of which must be in residence at Yale; a thesis representing work of an individual character, and an examination covering the general field of forestry.

The degree of doctor of philosophy is conferred by the graduate school of the university. The work of the student is under the direction of the faculty of forestry of the graduate school, which includes the professors of the school of forestry giving instruction in the graduate school and representatives from other departments whose work is affiliated with forestry.

A number of the courses offered by the school will be enlarged and made more comprehensive. The former plan of a prescribed curriculum necessitated the curtailment of certain courses in order that each student might be able to cover the field of forestry in a specified period of time. In consequence these courses could not be given with the degree of thoroughness compatible with sound education.

Of special importance is the extension of work in soils. Through a cooperative arrangement with the Connecticut Agricultural Experiment Station, the school has secured the services of Mr. M. Francis Morgan to conduct the instruction in this subject. He will offer a foundation course especially designed for forestry students and also will direct the work of advanced students.

The course in forest entomology will also be enlarged. The instruction in this subject will be given by Dr. Roger Boynton Friend. He will offer a foundational course in entomology and direct the work of those specializing in forest entomology.

Larger opportunities for the graduate student will be afforded in the fields of forest products, forest policy, economics and forest pathology.

INCREASE OF SALARIES AT COLUMBIA UNIVERSITY

A RISE in salaries of teachers and administration officers of Columbia University, effective on July 1, has been authorized by the board of trustees. The increases will affect all the 450 members of the teaching and administrative staff appointed directly by the trustees for full-time service, except for two small groups for whom provision has already been made, either by special salary rises or by appropriations in the 1928–29 budget.

The new salary schedule will increase the present minimum scale for full professors to $7,500 a year, instead of $6,000 as heretofore, and will provide three groups—one at $9,000, one at $10,000 and one at $12,000—to which individual professors of exceptional service or distinction may be advanced or appointed. Sixty-eight professors have now been placed in these groups.

The new normal minimum for associate professors will be $5,000, instead of $4,500, with a $6,000 classification for individuals of exceptional service or distinction, fifteen having already been placed in this category.

Assistant professors will receive a normal minimum of $3,600, instead of $3,000 as heretofore, and there will be groups at $4,000, $4,500 and $5,000 for those of exceptional distinction or service. Fifty are already allotted to these groups.

The new minimum for instructors has been set at $2,400, replacing the old minimum of $2,000, with advancement in the following years, if reappointed, to $2,700 and $3,000. Additional compensation has been provided also for fourteen officers of the university administration, seventeen members of the library staff and five members of the business administration. The new schedule will not apply to services given in the summer session or in extension work.

Remarking that the action of the trustees was consistent with a liberal policy adopted as far back as 1875, President Butler said:

They have now, through their careful husbanding of the university's resources, and by reason of recent benefactions, been able to take action which will add greatly to the satisfaction and material rewards of academic service at Columbia University. It is greatly hoped that this action will set an example to be followed at other institutions to the well-deserved advantage and comfort of the great body of American scholars engaged in the world of university teaching and research.

AMERICAN MEDICAL ASSOCIATION GRANTS FOR RESEARCH

The committee on scientific research of the American Medical Association has made a grant of $250 to Dr. O. Larsell, of the University of Oregon Medical School, Portland, in aid of his studies on the hemopoietic effect of nuclear extractives.

Dr. A. A. Maximow, professor of anatomy at the University of Chicago, has received $1,000 from the association for paying skilled technical help.

Dr. G. A. Talbert and his collaborators of the physiological department of the University of North Dakota have received a third grant of $300 for continuing the research on the "Constituents Common to the Sweat, Urine and Blood."

A substantial grant has been made to the department of agricultural chemistry of the University of Wisconsin for a quantitative study of the distribution in foodstuffs of copper which, from recent researches in that department, is now known to supplement iron in the building of hemoglobin in the mammal.

SCIENTIFIC NOTES AND NEWS

Dr. William D. Harkins, professor of chemistry at the University of Chicago, has been awarded the Willard Gibbs gold medal of the Chicago section of the American Chemical Society.

The Louis Edward Levy medal of the Franklin Institute of Philadelphia has been awarded to Dr. Vannevar Bush, professor of electric power transmission at the Massachusetts Institute of Technology, for two papers on the Product Integraph, a mathematical instrument developed under Dr. Bush's direction. The medal will be presented at the annual medal day exercises of the Franklin Institute on May 16.

At the annual general meeting of the Institute of Chemistry, held on March 1, the Meldola medal for 1927 was presented to Dr. J. H. Quastel, fellow of Trinity College, Cambridge.

The editors of the *Journal de Mathématiques* announce that the volumes for 1928 and 1929 will be dedicated to the eminent mathematicians Paul Appell and Émile Picard, as a tribute upon the occasion of their scientific jubilees. The edition will be limited, and the volumes will not be reprinted.

Dr. Weber, professor in the University of Geneva, presided over the Congress of the Anatomists' Association which opened on April 3 in Prague. The vice-president is Dr. J. P. Hill, professor of embryology in the University of London.

Waldemar Kaempffert, of New York, the editorial and scientific writer, has been appointed director of the Rosenwald Industrial Museum, Chicago.

Professor Dr. C. Ramsauer, director of the Physical Institute of the Technical High School of Dantzig, Germany, has been appointed head of the new research laboratory which the Allgemeine Elektricitäts Gesellschaft is establishing in Berlin.

Dr. George T. Pack, for five years professor and head of the department of pathology, University of Alabama School of Medicine, has accepted an appointment at the Memorial Hospital for Malignant Diseases, New York.

Dr. B. Youngblood has resigned as director of the Texas Agricultural Experiment Station, effective on April 30, to continue the development of the cotton utilization research program of the U. S. Bureau of Agricultural Economics. He is succeeded as director of the station by A. B. Conner, who has been connected with the Texas station since 1904, as agronomist, vice-director and acting director.

Edgar S. Ross, senior fellow at the Mellon Institute, has resigned to become manager of research and development for the Headly Good Roads Company, of Philadelphia.

Dr. George T. Moore, director of the Missouri Botanical Garden, is making an extended trip abroad, during which he will visit the leading botanical gardens and experiment stations of Europe, as well as the principal bulb and orchid growers.

Professor and Mrs. T. D. A. Cockerell have left Siam for Australia after conference with Dr. Kerr on the Siamese flora and with Dr. Hugh M. Smith on Siamese fishes.

DR. WILLIAM H. F. ADDISON, of the University of Pennsylvania, who has been at the Instituto Cajal, Madrid, for the past two months, will go to London about the first of May to attend the Harvey tercentenary celebration.

DR. H. A. GLEASON, of the New York Botanical Garden, sailed on March 22 for Europe, where he will devote the ensuing six months to a continuation of his studies on the plant life of British Guiana. His work will be done mainly at the Royal Botanic Gardens, Kew, England, where the most important collections of Guiana plants are conserved.

DR. THOMAS A. JAGGAR, seismologist of the United States Geological Survey in charge of the Hawaiian Volcano Observatory, has left Washington to head the National Geographic Society's expedition to explore the Mount Pavlof sector of the Alaskan peninsula and Aleutian Islands volcanic chain.

ERNEST G. HOLT will head an expedition to South America to study bird life, which is being organized under the auspices of the Carnegie Museum and the National Geographic Society.

T. H. C. TAYLOR, entomologist of the Department of Agriculture of Fiji, recently visited the fruit-fly laboratory of the U. S. Bureau of Entomology at Ancon, Canal Zone, on his way from Trinidad to Fiji.

ACCORDING to the *Electrical World*, P. A. Maximov, president of the Soviet Electrotechnical Trust, has arrived in this country, accompanied by B. I. Bukhovtsev, production manager of the trust, to make a study of the electrical industry.

HARRY A. CURTIS, professor of chemical engineering at Yale University, sailed on April 11 as a representative of the U. S. Department of Agriculture to the International Nitrogen Conference which begins April 30. This is the conference to be held aboard the North German Lloyd steamer *Lutzow* in the Adriatic. Dr. Curtis expects to return early in June.

DR. SOLOMON KATZENELLENBOGEN, former chief resident physician at the Hospital Canton, Geneva, Switzerland, and lecturer in internal medicine at the University of Geneva, has arrived in Baltimore to take over his new duties as associate professor in psychiatry at the Johns Hopkins University School of Medicine.

DR. SERGIUS MORGULIS, professor of biochemistry in the University of Nebraska College of Medicine, has been invited to deliver the introductory lecture at the meeting of the congress of the Gesellschaft für Verdauungs- und Stoffwechselkrankheiten. The congress will hold its session in Amsterdam from September 12 to 15.

PROFESSOR SAMUEL J. BARNETT, of the physics department of the University of California at Los Angeles, has been selected to deliver the fourth annual research lecture at the university on April 20. His subject will be "The Elementary Magnet as a Spinning Top" and will be a popular treatment of the subject of gyro-magnetic phenomenon.

DR. COLIN G. FINK, head of the division of electrochemistry of Columbia University, has addressed the Maryland section of the American Chemical Society on "Corrosion, its Prevention and the Restoration of Ancient Bronzes."

D. MCFARLAN MOORE, of the Edison Lamp Works, recently addressed the chemical engineering students of Columbia University on "Neon and the Electric Conduction of Gases."

DR. W. W. LEPESCHKIN, professor of plant physiology, University of Prague, Czechoslovakia, will give an address at the Michigan State College on April 20, under the auspices of the Phi Sigma Society. The subject of the address is "Colloidal State of Substances as a Necessary Condition of Life."

PROFESSOR JAMES FRANCK, of the University of Göttingen, Germany, recently gave at Cornell University a series of five lectures on "Quantum Jumps of Electrons."

PROFESSOR BRUNO BLOCH, director of the dermatological clinic of the University of Zurich at Strasbourg, lectured at the Harvard Medical School on April 16. His subject was "Formation of Pigment in the Skin."

UNDER the joint auspices of the University of Chicago and the Institute of Medicine, the third John M. Dodson lecture of the Rush Alumni Association was given on April 16, at the University of Chicago clinics, by George Barger, professor of biologic chemistry, University of Edinburgh, on "The Thyroid Hormone."

ISAAC PHILLIPS ROBERTS, emeritus professor of agriculture in Cornell University and formerly dean of the College of Agriculture, died on March 17 at Palo Alto, California, in his ninety-fifth year.

THE ninth annual meeting of the Southwestern division of the American Association for the Advancement of Science will be held in conjunction with the first special joint meeting of the Pacific division at Flagstaff, Arizona, from April 23 to 26, inclusive. A feature of the meeting will be the attendance and participation in the programs of a number of members of the Pacific division. Under tentative plans each division will designate the regular annual meeting of the other as a special meeting of its own.

THE fifth annual meeting of the West Virginia Academy of Science will be held on May 18 and 19 at Davis and Elkins College, Elkins, West Virginia. On Friday evening an illustrated lecture on "South America and its Mineral Resources" will be given by Dr. Benjamin L. Miller, professor of geology in Lehigh University. The sections of the academy are: Biology, chemistry, geology and mining, mathematics and physics and social science. Dr. John L. Tilton, professor of geology in West Virginia University, is the president of the academy.

THE North Dakota Academy of Science will hold its twentieth annual meeting at the North Dakota Agricultural College, Fargo, on May 4 and 5. Dr. H. L. Walster, dean of agriculture at the North Dakota Agricultural College and agronomist at the experiment station, will preside. Professor J. Arthur Harris, head of the botany department of the University of Minnesota, will make the invitation address on the topic "The Biological Application of Practical Agricultural Experimentation."

THE Rocky Mountain Section of the Mathematical Association of America will meet at the Colorado School of Mines on April 20 and 21. The outside speaker will be Dr. E. B. Stouffer, dean of the graduate school and professor of mathematics at the University of Kansas.

THE fifty-seventh annual meeting of the American Public Health Association will be held in Chicago, from October 15 to 19, with headquarters at Hotel Stevens. The American Child Health Association and the American Social Hygiene Association will meet with this organization. Dr. Louis E. Schmidt is chairman of the local committee and Arthur E. Gorman is secretary. Sessions are being arranged for health officers, child hygienists, public-health nurses, laboratory technicians, vital statisticians, health education directors, food and drug experts, industrial hygienists and public-health engineers.

THE sixteenth annual meeting of the Eugenics Research Association will be held at the American Museum of Natural History in New York City on Saturday, June 2. This will be a joint meeting of the Eugenics Research Association and the American Eugenics Society.

DR. MARK H. INGRAHAM, associate secretary of the American Mathematical Society, writes that the society held its spring meeting in the west at the University of Chicago on April 6 and 7. The attendance was about 120, including approximately 100 members. There were 49 papers presented to the society: 15 in geometry, 7 in applied mathematics, 10 in algebra and 17 in analysis. On Friday afternoon Professors E. B. Stouffer and E. P. Lane gave symposium addresses on "Recent Developments in Projective Differential Geometry." At the dinner held Friday evening Professor L. E. Dickson was presented with the first award of the Frank Nelson Cole prize. This was presented for his book "Algebren und ihre Zahlentheorie" and other works. These works are a continuation of the work in linear algebras for which he was presented with the thousand-dollar prize at the meeting of the American Association for the Advancement of Science in Cincinnati.

A CONFERENCE on the improvement of hard spring wheat was held at Fargo, North Dakota, on March 27, at the North Dakota Agricultural College, with Dr. J. L. Coulter, president of the institution, presiding. The aim of the conference was to discuss the development of wheats more resistant to disease, especially to stem rust, and possessing better quality. There were sixty-five in attendance at the conference. Addresses were made by plant breeders, plant pathologists and agronomists, and by men representing commercial interests. In addition to the addresses, committees were appointed to formulate a program of wheat improvement, to discuss the organization and cooperation of the program and the financing of it. The conference adjourned after having elected Dr. J. L. Coulter, *president;* Dr. Andrew Boss, *vice-president,* and Dr. L. R. Waldron, *secretary-treasurer,* and after appointing a program committee of eighteen and a finance committee of five.

A CONFERENCE on industrial gas and coke heat was recently held at the Mason laboratory of mechanical engineering at Yale University, under the auspices of the mechanical engineering department, cooperating with the Manufacturers' Association of Connecticut. Over two hundred and fifty engineering executives attended, from not only Connecticut, but from other eastern states. This was the second of a series of similar meetings on heat and heat treating inaugurated by the university and the Manufacturers' Association as a service to Connecticut industries, the first conference dealing with electrical heat-treating.

THE United States Civil Service Commission announces competitive examinations for men for biochemist (soil fertility), $3,800 to $5,000; associate soil technologist, $3,000 to $3,600, and assistant soil technologist, $2,400 to $3,000. Applications for these positions must be on file with the commission at Washington, D. C., not later than May 8. The examinations are to fill vacancies in the Bureau of Chemistry and Soils, Department of Agriculture, for duty in Washington, D. C., or in the field.

IT is announced by Dr. Howard McClenahan, secretary of the Franklin Institute, that the institute now has money and property in hand amounting to $2,000,000, which it proposes to apply toward building on the Parkway a great museum of industry and physical science.

ENDOWMENT of $7,000,000 is being sought for the Engineering Foundation and the Engineering Societies Library, according to an announcement by the board of trustees of the United Engineering Society, representing the national societies of civil, mining and metallurgical, mechanical and electrical engineers. One fund of $5,000,000, it is planned, will be applied to the research projects of the foundation, and a second fund of $2,000,000 to the maintenance of the library. The foundation was established thirteen years ago with a gift of $500,000 from Ambrose Swasey, engineer and manufacturer of Cleveland, Ohio. This amount has been increased to about $625,000.

AN appropriation of $300 each year for a period of five years for the International Society for the Exploration of the Arctic Regions by Means of the Airship (see SCIENCE for April 6, page 363) will be recommended to the House by the Committee on Foreign Affairs. The committee, on March 31, voted a favorable report on the Porter resolution, designed to carry out the recommendations of President Coolidge on the subject. The 19 nations which are expected to contribute to the work of the society, of which Fridtjof Nansen is the president, are: Bulgaria, Denmark, Germany, England, Estonia, Finland, France, Italy, Japan, Latvia, the Netherlands, Norway, Austria, Sweden, Switzerland, Spain, Czechoslovakia, Russia and the United States.

THE final closing of a contract with the Amarillo Oil Company, of Amarillo, Texas, which, it is thought, will greatly increase the available supply of helium required for the operation of dirigibles, is announced by the U. S. Bureau of Mines. Under the terms of the contract, the bureau will undertake the extraction of the helium from natural gas from the company's leases on the Cliffside Structure in Potter County, Texas, at a new helium plant to be constructed by the government at Amarillo.

PURCHASE of a property at 135 North 19th Street, which will complete the site for the proposed building group of the Franklin Institute, was approved at a meeting of the institute on March 15. Henry Howson, senior vice-president of the institute, announced that the purchase gave that body title to the entire plot, 288 by 110 feet, along 19th Street, between Cherry and Race Streets. At the lecture which followed the meeting a report on the work of the Bartol Research Laboratories was submitted by Dr. W. F. G. Swann, director. Dr. Swann discussed the more important researches which have been completed or are being carried on at this time.

THE Canadian correspondent of *Engineering and Industrial Chemistry* writes that the Dominion Government will proceed during 1928 with the establishment of National Research Laboratories for Canada at Ottawa. In the government estimates for the year, just made public by the minister of finance, the sum of $750,000 is provided for the construction of the first unit of a series of laboratories for the conduct of industrial research and the determination of standards. This combines, in a way, the functions of such institutions as the Bureau of Standards at Washington and Mellon Institute of Industrial Research at Pittsburgh. The project has been under consideration for several years. With the necessary money voted for a building and equipment, the National Research Council will be able to make definite progress this year. Two other items in the government estimates are of interest to chemists. In the Mines Department appropriations, there is the sum of $12,000 for the Explosives Division for organization and equipment purposes, and there is another item—$50,000—for new laboratories in connection with the Fuel Testing Division. There are also increased appropriations for dairying, feed and fertilizer control and experimental farms. Canada's main estimates for the year are $373,796,856, an increase of $7,725,542 over the total provided for the current fiscal year. Supplementary estimates will be tabled towards the close of the parliamentary session.

THE Russian Academy of Sciences has decided to organize a joint expedition with German scientists for the purpose of exploring the Pamir. Among the members of the expedition will be geologists, meteorologists, botanists, geographers, etc. The Academy of Sciences will be represented in the expedition by Professor Korzhenevsky, of Tashkent University, the geologist Stcherbakov, and Professor Belayev, while the Germans will include Professor Ficker, of the Berlin Meteorological Institute, the geologist Rickmers and others. The expedition is to take place in May.

THE request of the Stoll-McCracken expedition for permission to explore northeast Siberia and study mammals and birds has been approved by the All Union Society for Cultural Relations. Members of the expedition include Harold McCracken, associate editor of *Field and Stream;* Dr. H. E. Anthony, mammalogist of the American Museum of Natural History; Charles H. Stoll, New York financier; John Burnham, president of the American Game Protection Association; Carl Fredericks, president of the Campfire Club of America; George Potter, taxidermist, and

Mrs. Charles H. Stoll, photographer. The party proposes, after exploring Alaska and the Aleutian Islands, to arrive at Petropavlovsk, Kamchatka, on June 1, on board the ship *Morrissey,* commanded by Captain Bartlett. After Kamchatka the party will proceed to the Gulf of Anadir and then through Bering Strait to the mouth of the Kolymia River.

ACCORDING to *Industrial and Engineering Chemistry,* invitations have been received by the executives of large American chemical companies to attend an international nitrogen conference in the Adriatic, beginning April 30. The invitations were issued by the following, who comprise the largest nitrogen producers of Europe: Comptoir Français de l'Azote, Paris; Montecatini Societa Generale, Milan; Nitram, Ltd., London; Norsk Hydroelektrisk Kvaelstofaktieselskab, Oslo, and Stickstoff-Syndikat, G. M. B. H., Berlin. The scope and objects of the meeting will be to put on record the knowledge which has been gained since the conference held at Biarritz last year in regard to fertilizers in their relation to agriculture and to afford opportunity for discussion. Papers will be presented by J. Bueb, F. C. O. Speyer, L. Bretigniere, H. Warmbold, Sir Frederick Keeble, A. Demolon, Erwin Baur, H. J. Paige, T. H. J. Carroll and J. Galland.

UNIVERSITY AND EDUCATIONAL NOTES

THE cornerstone of the William H. Welch medical library at the Johns Hopkins University School of Medicine has been laid by the president of the university, Dr. Frank J. Goodnow, who placed in the stone a copper box containing correspondence between Dr. Welch, the university and the General Education Board, whose financial help made the library possible.

IMMEDIATE construction of a new chemistry building to cost $350,000 has been authorized by the board of trustees of the University of New Hampshire. The establishment of a department of agricultural economics in charge of M. Gale Eastman has also been authorized.

THE *Journal* of the American Medical Association records the appointment of Dr. Stuart Graves, of Louisville, Ky., as dean of the school of medicine of the University of Alabama to succeed Dr. Clyde Brooks, who has been appointed chairman of a newly created faculty committee on research, for which the last legislature made a special appropriation. The appointment of Dr. Graves is said to be the first step in a program to establish a four-year medical course at the university.

PROFESSOR A. B. COBLE, of the Johns Hopkins University, recently accepted a professorship of mathematics at the University of Illinois, where he had been prior to the present academic year.

DR. WILLIAM W. WATSON, assistant professor of physics at the University of Chicago, has been appointed assistant professor of physics at Yale University.

AT Princeton University, Dr. Herman Weyl, professor of high mathematics at the Eidenossischen Technischen Hochschule in Zurich, Switzerland, has been appointed to the Thomas D. Jones research professorship of mathematical physics. The following three members of the department of mathematics have been promoted from associate professor to full professor: James Waddell Alexander, Solomon Lefschetz and Joseph H. M. Wedderburn.

IN place of the existing department of philosophy and psychology at University College, London, a department of philosophy and a department of psychology have been instituted. Professor C. E. Spearman, now Grote professor of philosophy of mind and logic, will be head of the department of psychology, his title being changed to professor of psychology in the University of London.

DR. WERNER HEISENBERG, of the University of Copenhagen, has been appointed professor of theoretical physics at the University of Leipzig.

DR. DEBEYRE has been appointed successor to the late Professor Lanesse in the chair of histology at the University of Lille.

DISCUSSION AND CORRESPONDENCE

THE APPEARANCE OF INSTABILITY OF CONDENSED SUBSTANCES NEAR THE ABSOLUTE ZERO OF TEMPERATURE

IN a previous article in SCIENCE,[1] the writer called attention to the possibility of condensed substances becoming unstable and exploding under a high pressure at or near the absolute zero of temperature, and mentioned that *white* tin should behave in this manner. The criterion for the existence of such an instability is that if from external evidence it appears that the controllable internal energy of a substance can not lie below a certain value, and this can not be accounted for by integration of the specific heat down to the absolute zero of temperature, the substance

[1] LXVII, 1725, p. 69, 1928.

must become unstable at or near this zero and explode. Thus, for example, the heats of formation of mols of the substances H_2O, CH_4, NH_4 and CO_2 in the gaseous state from the elements C (graphite), H_2, O_2, N_2 are about 57,880, 18,300, 9,500 and 97,000 cal's, respectively, at room temperature. These heat energies are derived from the internal energies of the elements, which, if no instability occurs, are given by the integration of the specific heats down to the absolute zero of temperature with the final state being solid. But the internal energies of the foregoing elements obtained in this way by the writer (May number of the *J. Franklin Inst.*) are 45, 1,100, 2,980, 3,090 cal's, respectively, and are thus not sufficiently large to account for the heats of formation. It was also shown in this paper that the temperature at which instability begins is always above the absolute zero. Thus one of the elements of each of the foregoing compounds becomes unstable at a low temperature. But since the heat of formation of a compound is not likely to be derived from the internal energy of one of its elements only, each of the foregoing elements very probably becomes unstable at a certain temperature. Thus frozen solid masses of these elements in interstellar space are likely to explode when their temperatures have fallen below certain values.

If an external pressure is applied to such a substance to prevent the explosion, and the substance is then allowed to expand doing external work, a state will eventually be reached at which the pressure and the internal energy is zero.[2] The substance is now a modification of the original substance. In the case of *white* tin we have already seen that the modified form is *gray* tin. Such modifications at low temperatures of the elements mentioned should exist, but at present they are not known. The vapors of such elements in interstellar space near the absolute zero of temperature would tend to condense into the stable modifications, but the process would take place almost infinitely slowly.

R. D. KLEEMAN

SCHENECTADY, N. Y.

[2] *J. Phys. Chem.*, 31, 1669–1673, 1927.

ETHYLENE IS A RIPENER OF FRUITS AND VEGETABLES

IN an article published in the *Journal of Industrial and Engineering Chemistry* (Vol. 19, p. 1135, 1927), Chace and Church decry the "wide publicity of the alleged ripening effect" of ethylene on certain green fruits. They state that the treatment of green bananas with ethylene in a concentration of 1–5,000 produced no acceleration of color or respiration increase, in opposition to the data which I have reported. It should be noticed that Chace and Church and Denny recommended concentrations less than 1 part of ethylene to 5,000 of air in the coloration of citrus fruits, whereas I have recommended 1 to 1,000 for the ripening of fruits at temperatures above 65° F. Chace and Church report no effect of ethylene upon the ripening of dates, and state there occurred "no material difference in composition between the treated and untreated fruits" of lemon. Denny had previously reported a marked action on the stimulation of respiration in lemons under ethylene treatment to produce coloration. It seems unreasonable that the respiration can increase and still produce no effect on composition of the fruits. The data reported by the authors simply show that these workers in the U. S. Department of Agriculture do not know the proper conditions for ripening fruits with ethylene.

An editorial in the *Scientific American* hastens to state that "the investigations carried out by Messrs. Chace and Church tend to disprove Dr. Harvey's conclusions." The statement that "these investigators have carefully studied the effect of ethylene on citrus fruits, dates, persimmons, bananas, tomatoes, pomegranates and avocadoes and find that while the color of the fruit is affected, none of the changes ordinarily connected with ripening are observable" is unjustified even by the article referred to. The effect of these publications is to bring under suspicion unjustly the process of ripening fruits with ethylene gas, a process which has been successfully used by hundreds of fruit jobbers to produce quicker ripening and a product of superior flavor.

The statement by Chace and Church that the use of ethylene on persimmons "will be of no use to the grower because they could not be shipped after ripening" is not to the point, for every fruit jobber knows the advantage of shipping fruits in the firm condition. The difficulty of ripening such fruits after shipment has been removed by the discovery of this process whereby they may be quickly ripened at destination. We should be able now to import fruits from the tropics which were not available before.

The ripening effect of ethylene on fruits and vegetables can be demonstrated easily by any one who is willing to carry out the simple instructions for the process, namely: the green fruit should be put into a reasonably tight chamber, the temperature should be preferably at 65° F. but may be higher in some cases, and the concentration of ethylene should be established at 1 cu. ft. for each 1,000 cu. ft. of air space. The gas may be renewed each day. The fruit should be so packed into the space that there is free air circulation and an abundant supply of oxygen to care for a rate of respiration which is much increased.

Ethylene causes an increased rate of digestion of starch, which may make fruits sweeter, it causes changes in the cell wall materials just as in ripening fruits, it causes the disappearance of tannins and of organic acids to some degree, and increases protein cleavage. These same changes when occurring in fruits on the tree may be taken as evidences of ripening.

The work of E. M. Harvey, J. T. Rosa, R. P. Hibbard, W. A. Gardiner, and others than the parties to this controversy has proven that ethylene and some related compounds have remarkable effect on stimulating enzyme actions. These compounds act as coenzymes, if such a blanket term is permitted, for the hydrolytic enzymes and may act as hydrolytic catalysts themselves according to data by Rhea and Mullinix. The triple bond as in acetylene has a different action from the double bond of ethylene and propylene. The addition of elements at the double bond seems to destroy the action, except in some compounds which may yield ethylene. The formation of the oxide from ethylene destroys the effect. One is inclined to wonder if this catalytic action on hydrolyses is not a function of the double bond which may take on hydrogen and hydroxyl ions and again yield them easily to anhydrides. The surface tension effects, solubility in aqueous and lipoid phases, as well as the low molecular weight may give these double bond compounds properties not possessed by other such compounds found in plants.

I had been asked by two journals which have published articles in this controversy to write articles for them on the ethylene process. The data of value for commercial application had already been published sufficiently, and explicitly. I can see no reason why one should be required to publish before he is ready to do so. Charles Darwin would have had a slim chance of accumulating data for eighteen years if he had lived under our present system of reporting scientific results.

R. B. Harvey

Cambridge, England

BANANA STOWAWAYS

In reference to the note of Mr. L. A. Adams in Science of February 24, 1928, it may be of interest to record that in the summer of 1909 a laborer engaged in carrying bananas from a refrigerator car to a warehouse in Madison, Wisconsin, was terrified by having an animal leap from a bunch he had just placed on his shoulder, and attack his throat. The creature was captured and brought to our laboratory. It proved to be a female Marmosa, probably *M. murina,* and carried a litter of young on her back. The whole family was kept alive for some days, but eventually died of malnutrition. Twice in the last twelve years we have received specimens of a small boa snake, taken from banana bunches, one at Madison, and one at St. Croix Falls, Wisconsin.

George Wagner

University of Wisconsin

Under the above caption in Science for February 24, L. A. Adams mentions the finding of opossums of some species of the genus Marmosa in a bunch of bananas at Urbana, Ill.

I have in my collection two specimens of small opossums, each taken in Colorado Springs. One is *Marmosa cinerea,* and was found in a bunch of bananas about August 2, 1905. I saw an account of the capture in a local paper and secured the animal, keeping it alive for several days. Like Mr. Adams' animals it ate grasshoppers as well as other food. I was told that when caught it had a young one clinging to it, but that had disappeared before the animal came into my possession. The specimen was a female.

The other example, *Marmosa zeledoni,* is a skin given me by C. E. Aiken, October 5, 1912. He told me the animal was given him in the flesh by a man who had killed it in a commission warehouse, thinking that it was a rat. The type locality of this species is Navarro, Costa Rica, and doubtless the animal reached here with bananas. Both of these specimens were identified by the Bureau of the Biological Survey.

If my memory does not play me false, Victor Borcherdt, of Denver, told me that he had known of several instances of small tropical opossums being found in bananas in the city.

Edward R. Warren

Colorado Springs, Colo.

GALILEI OR GALILEO?

Would it not be time to call the great Italian by his right name? He is always referred to as *Galileo.* But *Galileo* was his given name, while *Galilei* was his family name. The French and Germans have always referred to him as *Galilei.* Of course the objection will be made that this is a paltry matter and that the usage *Galileo* is time honored. Still it is wrong. How would it do, if we referred to noted men bearing the names William Williams or Samuel Samuels as William or Samuel?

A. Kampmeier

Davenport, Iowa

CONTRIBUTIONS ASKED FOR MEMORIAL TO LAPLACE

From the Philosophical Society of Washington, accompanying its subscription to the fund for the erection of a monument to the memory of the illustrious Laplace, comes the suggestion that a place should be requested for the publication in Science of the aspiration on the part of the Municipal Council of Beaumont-en-Auge, where Laplace was born, to proceed with the project formed before the World War to erect a memorial to Pierre Simon Laplace, author of "La Mécanique Céleste" and "L'Exposition du Système du Monde."

A committee has been organized in France of the most distinguished members of the Academy of Sciences and affiliated bodies, whose resolve to make the intended monument an international tribute, worthy of the universal service performed by Laplace in the advancement of civilization, extends a call to scientists and scientific bodies of the United States, as well as those of other foreign countries, to hear this appeal for contributions toward the sum of $3,000 which has been apportioned to be raised here.

Checks drawn to the order of Monsieur Pierre Leger, treasurer of the Committee of Initiative, Paris, and sent to Monsieur Maxime Mongendre, Consul-General of France in New York, at 9 East Fortieth Street, New York City, will be forwarded to M. Leger.

G. W. Littlehales

Hydrographic Office,
Washington, D. C.

SCIENTIFIC BOOKS

Flora of the Panama Canal Zone. By Paul C. Standley. Contribution U. S. Nat. Herbarium. Vol. 27. 1928.

Standley has published a very important contribution to our knowledge of the flora of the Panama Canal region. In 1921 the governor of the Canal Zone asked the assistance of the Department of Agriculture in the preparation of an illustrated flora of the region. Standley was selected to prepare the flora, and the results of his investigations are now published. The purpose of the investigation was not only to contribute to our scientific knowledge of the region, but also to develop our knowledge of tropical agriculture. Some idea of the method of presentation may be obtained from the statement that "with the aid of the many English and Spanish common names, it should not be difficult for the casual visitor to identify most of the important plants of the Canal Zone."

The flowering plants of the region number about two thousand species. Besides the native plants, the keys include also the cultivated plants. The work is based on the collections of the United States National Herbarium, which for many years has been receiving a wealth of material from collectors. Standley himself visited the Canal Zone twice, studying the flora and making collections. He gave special attention to the common names in use and also to the local uses of plants. The publication, therefore, is not merely a taxonomic account of the flora, but includes also much material of more general interest.

An interesting account is given of the contrasts in physiography and flora of the Atlantic and Pacific slopes. About two thirds of the Canal Zone lies on the Atlantic slope and has a highly diversified flora, very little of the pioneer vegetation remaining. The Pacific slope is comparatively arid, and the vegetation is very different in type from that of the Atlantic slope. This difference in the two floras consists not only in the general appearance, but also in the genera and species represented. The most conspicuous element of the Atlantic slope flora is the great number and variety of palms. The author also includes a very interesting account of the history of botany exploration in Panama. In short, the publication assembles in a single volume all the available information in reference to the development of our knowledge of a very interesting region. It will also make possible to appreciate and investigate more intelligently the closeness of the relationship of this flora to that of South America. The sixty-six remarkably fine plates picture some of the outstanding features of the flora.

Only about fifty pages are taken up with the general presentation of the region, its history and its outstanding features. The bulk of the volume is made up of the taxonomic presentation of the flora. It is not written in ordinary taxonomic style, but presents the taxonomic facts in simpler and more readable form. Detailed descriptions are not given, but there are keys for identification that will help the taxonomist. These keys include not only the native or naturalized species, but most of the introduced plants grown for ornament or for economic purposes. In the case of the more important plants, those likely to prove of the greatest interest to the public, more extensive accounts are given which will assist in recognizing the species. It is not a rigidly taxonomic work in the usual sense, therefore, but a general introduction to the flora of an interesting region, which may be of service not only to botanists, but also to all who may be interested in the region.

John M. Coulter

Boyce Thompson Institute

SPECIAL ARTICLES

VITAMINS A, D AND E AND THE OXIDATION OF FATS AND OILS

THE potency of oils and fats in vitamin deficiency work is closely related to their unsaturation. Evans and Burr[1] have shown that the compound concerned in vitamin E contains double bonds; and Hess and coworkers,[2] Rosenheim and Webster[3] and Holtz[4] have shown that the compound concerned in vitamin D formation is associated with ergosterol—a triunsaturated sterol. Vitamin A is known to be similar to some degree in this respect.

Beyond the knowledge of association of unsaturation with the vitamins little is known. Nothing is known concerning the activating mechanism. The works of Mattill,[5] Hess and coworkers,[2] Anderegg and Nelson,[6] Evans and Burr[7] and others show, however, that oxidation is a serious factor in vitamin destruction. This is of natural consequence since when active oxidation begins in the oil or fat the unsaturated compounds associated with vitamin activity, like all the unsaturated compounds present, would themselves be involved.

Irradiation catalyzes autoxidation[8] and hence promotes the onset of the active oxidation period. However, with irradiation, active oxidation does not begin immediately but passes through an induction period during which there is practically no oxygen absorption.[8] One must not assume, however, that during this period no reaction occurs. Some reaction must occur to increase the oxidizing intensity to the point where the double bonds are attacked, and then active autoxidation begins.

The ease with which fats are attacked depends upon the type of unsaturated compound present as well as upon the presence of compounds containing hydroxy groups.[8] Ergosterol, a highly unsaturated compound, should respond readily to any treatment tending to alter its susceptibility to oxidation. Cholesterol, on the other hand, is very resistant to oxidation and responds to irradiation only when this treatment is prolonged at higher temperatures.[9]

The induction period is of special interest in susceptibility studies and from the author's point of view should be of interest to workers in the field of nutrition. Irradiation shortens the induction period,[8] or increases susceptibility to oxidation, and during this irradiation the vitamin D content increases. Prolonged irradiation induces active oxidation with simultaneous destruction of vitamins A, D and E.

A correlation of published data of work in nutrition and fat oxidation suggests that vitamin D and perhaps also vitamins A and E may be closely allied with changes occurring to vary susceptibilities to oxidation, or, in other words, may be allied with intermediate oxidation reactions. If slight oxidation is involved it should be possible to obtain vitamin D activity with other unsaturated compounds very similar in their chemical nature to ergosterol and stabilized by the presence of hydroxy groups, but as heretofore suggested irradiation would have to be adjusted to the stability of the compounds to oxidation.

Rosenheim and Webster[3] assert that the OH group is necessary to the mechanism concerned in vitamin D formation. It seems unnecessary to assume at present that it actually enters into combination to form the active (vitamin) compound. Unsaturated compounds containing OH groups (ricinoleic acid) oxidize slowly[8] and it is probable that the action of these groups is merely one of retarding the oxidation which destroys the "vitamin." The hydroxy groups may, therefore, be present as part of the compound concerned or as a constituent group of another compound. The latter case seems to have been shown by the experiments of Mattill,[5] who postulates also that the OH group is perhaps an important constituent of a fat in the prevention of the destruction of vitamins A and E by oxidation.

Another explanation of protection seems possible. If the constituents of an admixed oil or fat oxidize at a lower intensity level than do the compounds responsible for vitamin activity, it seems probable that oxidation may in some cases, especially those wherein water is present, proceed to some extent without involving the "vitamin" parent substance.

That *vitamins are labile states and not stable entities* seems to follow from a consideration of their properties. *Oxidation may, however, be involved in their formation.* Hart, Steenbock, Kleitzein and Scott's[10] experiments upon vitamin D may bear directly upon this point. Corn oil and the non-saponifiable fraction of cod-liver oil, neither potent when fed to goats, showed potency when mixed and fed.

Irradiation may be viewed as a promoter of oxidation and the extent to which it can be carried depends

1 Evans, H. M., and Burr, G. O., Univ. of California Memoir No. 8 (1927).

2 Hess, A. F., *J. Am. Med. Assn.*, 1927, LXXXIX, 337.

3 Rosenheim, O., and Webster, T. A., *Biochem. J.*, 1927, XXI, 389.

4 Holtz, F., *Klin. Wochenschr.*, 1927, VI, 535.

5 Mattill, H. A., *J. Am. Med. Assn.*, 1927, LXXXIX, 1505.

6 Anderegg, L. T., and Nelson, V. E., *Ind. and Eng. Chem.*, 1926, XVIII, 620.

7 Evans, H. M., and Burr, G. O., *J. Am. Med. Assn.*, 1927, LXXXIX, 1587.

upon the resistance of the oil used to oxidation. Irradiation in vacuum must be carefully controlled in order to yield infallible results. Few oils are entirely free from loosely bound oxygen and even after exhaustive evacuation at low pressures they contain enough oxygen to autoxidize actively when sealed in vacuum.[8] Ethyl ether, due to the presence of peroxides, is not a safe reagent to use in work upon vitamins. Water and alcohols have a protective action to autoxidation[11, 12] and have been shown to have a protective action upon vitamins in diets.[6]

In view of vitamin destruction through oxidation the practice of administering materials to be tested admixed with easily oxidizable oils is apt to yield inconsistent and unreliable results.

GEORGE E. HOLM

BUREAU OF DAIRY INDUSTRY,
U. S. DEPARTMENT OF AGRICULTURE

MODIFICATIONS IN CHILODON UNCINATUS PRODUCED BY ULTRA-VIOLET LIGHT

USING a Cooper-Hewitt mercury vapor quartz lamp, run on three and a half amperes, rapidly dividing and conjugating cultures of *Chilodon uncinatus* were exposed to ultra-violet light. The distance from the light to the top of the cultures was twenty-two centimeters. The cultures were exposed for two minutes at intervals of two and three days, depending upon the state of the cultures. There were eight exposures in all.

One ex-conjugant, not fully reorganized, was used to start a culture, and eight subcultures were made from this, two being used as controls, and six exposed to ultra-violet light.

In five of the cultures, no important changes were observed. In the sixth, a culture in which an epidemic of conjugation was occurring at the time of the last two exposures, many abnormalities were found, and three distinctly different types of animals.

(1) The normal *Chilodon uncinatus*. This type has four chromosomes in the diploid count, easily determined during conjugation. The controls show this same number.

(2) A larger animal having the same features as the controls, but which, when isolated and cultivated, was found to have eight chromosomes. This has been checked up through three conjugation epidemics. The form is, therefore, a tetraploid form.

(3) The third type of animal is very different from the other two, as it shows characteristics of both *C. uncinatus* and *C. cucullulus*. The macronucleus has moved from the posterior end of the animal to the middle. In appearance, this macronucleus is much more like that of *C. cucullulus* than *C. uncinatus*, the shape being elliptical, and the portion surrounding the endosome is much less granular. The micronucleus, as in *C. cucullulus*, is not in the posterior portion of the macronucleus, but on the left side near the anterior end.

One vacuole has changed position. In *C. uncinatus*, there is a vacuole on the left side near the margin at the anterior end, and one on the right side near the margin about one fourth of the distance from the posterior end. In the new form, this last vacuole has moved to the posterior end in the center.

The pharyngeal basket is shorter, and is more anterior. The average number of trichites seems to be twelve.

In general shape, the animal looks more like *C. cucullulus*, but the ciliation is more like *C. uncinatus*, the only difference being that here the usual short marginal rows are a little longer than in the original.

Though this animal has been kept alive in pure cultures since the last week of August, 1927, it has never conjugated. In cultures where the animals are fairly abundant, encystment has occurred regularly, the whole culture sometimes encysting within a few hours. The length of time elapsing before animals are recovered from the cysts is very variable. Seven days is the shortest time in which they have been observed to emerge, and three to four weeks is more usual.

A more detailed description, with figures, will appear in a later paper.

MARY STUART MACDOUGALL

AGNES SCOTT COLLEGE

THE NATIONAL ACADEMY OF SCIENCES

THE National Academy of Sciences will hold its annual meeting in Washington on April 23 and 24. The following papers will be presented:

MONDAY, APRIL 23

Morning, 10:00

WILLIAM DUANE: *X-radiation from Mercury Vapor* (illustrated).

EDWIN H. HALL: *Electron Free Path and Supra-conductivity in Metals* (illustrated).

W. A. NOYES: *Reactions of Compounds having Odd Electrons; Nitric Oxide and Nitrogen Trichloride.*

R. M. LANGER and GERALDINE K. WALKER (introduced by

[8] Holm, G. E., Greenbank, G. R., and Deysher, E. F., *Ind. and Eng. Chem.*, 1927, XIX, 156.

[9] Striteskey, J., *Biochem. Z.*, 1927, CLXXXVII, 388.

[10] Hart, E. B., Steenbock, H., Kleitzein, S. W., and Scott, H., *J. Biol. Chem.*, 1927, LXXI, 271.

[11] Holm, G. E., and Greenbank, G. R., Proc. World's Dairy Congress, 1923, II, 1253.

[12] Greenbank, G. R., and Holm, G. E., *Ind. and Eng. Chem.*, 1924, XVI, 598.

George K. Burgess): *Models of the Schrödinger Atom* (illustrated).

E. O. HULBERT (introduced by J. S. Ames): *Ionization in the Upper Atmosphere of the Earth* (illustrated).

C. J. DAVISSON and L. H. GERMER (introduced by F. B. Jewett): *Reflection and Refraction of Electrons by a Crystal of Nickel* (illustrated).

LEON BRILLOUIN (introduced by C. E. Mendenhall): *A Possible Direct Experimental Test of the Existence of the Spinning Electron* (illustrated).

EDWIN H. HALL: *Comments on Sommerfeld's Electron Theory of Metals.*

FRANK WENNER (introduced by George K. Burgess): *A Seismometer Employing Electromagnetic and Optical Magnification and Electromagnetic Damping* (illustrated).

WALTER S. ADAMS and HENRY NORRIS RUSSELL: *Preliminary Results of a New Method for the Analysis of Stellar Spectra* (illustrated).

W. H. WRIGHT: *Photography of the Planets, Saturn, Jupiter, Mars and Venus, by Light of Different Colors* (illustrated).

Afternoon, 2:00

R. C. GIBBS and H. E. WHITE (introduced by Ernest Merritt): *Some Recently Discovered Spectroscopic Relationships* (illustrated).

R. W. WOOD: *Recent Results of the Fluorescence of Iodine and Mercury Vapor with Especial Reference to the Infra-red* (illustrated).

R. W. WOOD and R. CANFIELD: *Exhibition of Echelette Diffraction Grating in the Infra-red* (illustrated).

W. F. DURAND: *New Methods for Treating the Problem of the Surge Chamber* (illustrated).

ELMER A. SPERRY: *The Reaction of the Gyroscope to the Rotation of the Earth, and the Relative Value of the Gyro as a Torque Producer* (illustrated).

GEORGE F. MCEWEN (introduced by T. Wayland Vaughan): *An Analysis of Temperature Changes in Lake Mendota regarded as Effects of Penetrating Radiation, Surface Loss of Heat and Turbulence* (illustrated).

MARSHALL A. HOWE: *Algae as Reef-builders and Land-formers* (illustrated).

DAVID WHITE: *Algal Deposits of Unkar Proterozoic Age in the Grand Canyon, Arizona* (illustrated).

HENRY S. WASHINGTON: *The Bearing of the Pacific Lavas on the Question of the Atlantic and Pacific Rock Clans.*

EDWARD KASNER: *Geodesic Families of Curves.*

FRANCIS D. MURNAGHAN (introduced by J. S. Ames): *On a Symmetrical Presentation of Dynamical Theory* (illustrated).

Evening, 8:15, in the Central Hall

JAMES FRANCK (by invitation): *Molecular Collisions* (illustrated).

I. S. BOWEN (by invitation): *The Story of Nebulium* (illustrated).

R. A. MILLIKAN: *The Origin of the Cosmic Rays* (illustrated).

Following these addresses, to which the members of the scientific societies of Washington are invited, the rooms adjacent to the central hall will be open for the inspection of scientific exhibits.

TUESDAY, APRIL 24

Morning, 9:00

WILLIAM TRELEASE: *Biographical Memoir of Charles Sprague Sargent.* (To be read by title.)

ALEŠ HRDLIČKA: *Traces of Prehistoric Man in Alaska* (with demonstration of specimens).

TRUMAN G. YUNCKER (introduced by William Trelease): *A Monograph of the Genus Cuscuta.*

CHARLES P. BERKEY: *Evidences of Changes of Climate in the Gobi Region of Central Asia* (illustrated).

JAMES W. GIDLEY (introduced by C. G. Abbot): *Additional Evidence on Pleistocene Man in Florida* (illustrated).

H. L. SHANTZ (introduced by L. O. Howard): *World Vegetation and Potential Agricultural Land* (illustrated).

S. A. COURTIS (introduced by Raymond Pearl): *The Factors Determining Growth* (illustrated).

FRANCIS G. BENEDICT and G. D. WILLIAMS: *The Racial Factor in Basal Metabolism: a Study of Maya Indians in Yucatan* (illustrated).

J. C. WALKER (introduced by L. R. Jones): *Inheritance of Fusarium-resistance in Brassica oleracea* (illustrated).

WALTER T. SWINGLE (introduced by R. A. Harper): *Metazenia in the Date Palm, Possibly a Hormone Action Exerted by the Endosperm* (illustrated).

JOHN M. ARTHUR (introduced by John M. Coulter): *Plant Growth in Artificial Climates* (illustrated).

H. J. MULLER (by invitation): *The Production of Mutations by X-rays* (illustrated).

HENRY FAIRFIELD OSBORN: *Recent Discoveries Relating to the Tertiary Ancestry of Man* (illustrated).

Afternoon, 2:00

E. H. MORRIS (introduced by W. H. Holmes): *Discovery of Extraordinary Turquoise Mosaic in the Buried Temple at Chichen Itza, Yucatan* (illustrated).

W. J. V. OSTERHOUT and E. S. HARRIS: *Positive and Negative Currents of Injury* (illustrated).

HENRY H. DONALDSON: *A Study of the Brains of Three Scholars* (illustrated).

GEORGE W. CRILE (introduced by Dayton C. Miller): *An Interpretation of Excitation, Exhaustion and Death in Terms of Physical Constants* (illustrated).

L. A. ROGERS and E. O. WHITTIER (introduced by Ludwig Hektoen): *The Limitation of Population in Bacterial Cultures* (illustrated).

C. R. STOCKARD: *Type Hybrids in Dogs and Development of Female Genitalia in Male Individuals* (illustrated).

CHARLES F. CRAIG (introduced by W. G. McCallum): *Observations upon Complement Fixation in Infections with Endamoeba hystolytica* (illustrated).

H. M. JOHNSON (introduced by Aleš Hrdlička): *The So-called "Depth of Sleep"* (illustrated).

SCIENCE

Vol. LXVII | April 27, 1928 | No. 1739

CONTENTS

Research, an Educational Asset: Professor B. S. Hopkins ... 427

The Need for Training Taxonomic Botanists: Dr. A. S. Hitchcock ... 431

The Fifth New York Meeting of the American Association and Associated Societies: Dr. Burton E. Livingston ... 432

Scientific Events:
The International Population Union; International Conferences in 1928; Forestry Advances in the United States; Dr. B. L. Hartwell and the Rhode Island Agricultural Experiment Station ... 435

Scientific Notes and News ... 437

University and Educational Notes ... 441

Discussion and Correspondence:
A Note on the Fluorescence of Teeth in Ultra-Violet Rays: Dr. H. C. Benedict. *On the Antiquity of Relics of Man at Frederick, Oklahoma:* Dr. Oliver P. Hay. *One Hundred Per Cent. Hatch:* Ralph C. Jackson. *More Data:* Dr. Christine Ladd-Franklin ... 442

Scientific Books:
Proctor's Romance of the Sun: Dr. Ida Barney 444

Scientific Apparatus and Laboratory Methods:
Mounting Chick Embryos: Professor James W. Mavor. *Color Discs Used in Soil Color Analysis:* G. B. Bodman ... 445

Special Articles:
Living Cells Two and a Half Centuries Old: Professor D. T. MacDougal and J. G. Brown ... 447

Science News ... x

SCIENCE: A Weekly Journal devoted to the Advancement of Science, edited by J. McKeen Cattell and published every Friday by

THE SCIENCE PRESS

New York City: Grand Central Terminal.

Lancaster, Pa. **Garrison, N. Y.**

Annual Subscription, $6.00. **Single Copies, 15 Cts.**

SCIENCE is the official organ of the American Association for the Advancement of Science. Information regarding membership in the Association may be secured from the office of the permanent secretary, in the Smithsonian Institution Building, Washington, D. C.

RESEARCH, AN EDUCATIONAL ASSET[1]

It is eminently fitting that the university should pause in the midst of its busy life to do honor to those students who have won distinction by their scholarly achievements. Educators of our day have complained that the "side shows" of our educational system are attracting more attention and receiving more generous support than the main purposes for which the system itself was established. Many a bitter complaint has been registered against the custom of lionizing the athletic hero and ignoring the student who has outstripped his fellows in the intellectual pursuits of the classroom. That such a tendency exists few will deny, but the evil, if such it be, can never be corrected by complaint nor by eulogizing the intellectual giants of the good old days when higher education was the privilege of the select few and the masses of the people were denied the educational advantages of which our modern democratic civilization is so proud. The purposes of Honor's Day and its associations are to recognize excellence in scholarship and to furnish in some tangible fashion a reward for leadership in the intellectual pursuits of college life.

There have been many definitions of the term education, but the ones that appeal most to me are those which take into account the development of the human mind as a preparation for better living. That person may be considered educated who has learned to adjust himself to his surroundings, who can live comfortably and successfully under unusual conditions, who can turn defeat into victory and use obstacles as stepping stones to success. We may consider any one undeveloped educationally who has not learned to accommodate himself to the conditions under which he must live and to meet the problems of life with a stout heart and firm determination to do his part in making the world a better place in which to live. It is to one of these factors in mental development that I desire to call your attention for a few minutes this morning.

Much has been written concerning the value of research and its place in a modern educational system. There seems to be little doubt concerning the value of investigations which have to do with the control of diseases, the utilization of by-products or the increase of food production. The successful completion of such a project prolongs life, decreases the cost of living or tends to increase human happiness and so

[1] Honor's Day address at the University of Illinois.

they have a practical aspect which presents a strong appeal. But any undertaking which can not point in advance to a practical application, which will not fill a long-felt want or which can not be immediately commercialized in figures of astonishing size is frequently looked upon as a useless expenditure of time and money. Any discovery of which it must be said "it is of scientific interest only" has little interest for the practical man who wants results and who insists that our educational system must be so constructed and operated that it will turn out practical men and women of the everyday world.

But the value of research is not always easily determined, since its bearing upon life is usually not evident at first. When Newton discovered the law of gravitation its value was not appreciated; when Dr. Morton first used the principle of anesthesia it must have been regarded as a useless curiosity; when Lavoisier discovered the element, oxygen, the practical men of his day probably asked "What of it?"; when Pasteur announced his germ theory of disease, no one realized its importance. Yet from each of these investigations there has sprung a modern science which is contributing in a large way to the comfort, safety and well-being of the human race. These have been discoveries of basic importance, yet in their infancy they seemed impractical, visionary and of scientific interest only.

Previous to 1860 the methods of identification of new substances required tedious and painstaking work upon the physical and chemical properties of the material under examination. The invention of the spectroscope by Robert Bunsen permitted the study of gases and incandescent solids by noting the wave length of the light which each absorbed or emitted. Soon this instrument was recognized as furnishing an efficient means of detecting the presence of new elements, and in its various modifications, spectrum analysis has been directly responsible for the discovery of nearly all the elements since the spectroscope first became available. It was first used in studying the atmosphere of the sun in a total eclipse which was visible in India in 1868. As a result of this study, the eminent British astronomer Lockyer reported a bright yellow line whose wave length did not agree with that produced by any known substance. Accordingly it was concluded that there must be a substance in the sun's atmosphere which did not exist upon the earth. The name helium—the sun element—was given to this substance and for twenty-seven years scientists speculated about its nature and its relationship to the earth. In 1895 Sir William Ramsay discovered that helium could be extracted from certain minerals and in 1903 Cady and McFarland reported that certain natural gas supplies in southern Kansas contained appreciable quantities of helium. Here was a succession of discoveries of great interest to scientists, but of so little practical application that they attracted little or no attention, and so they were all but forgotten. But when the Great War broke out and modern methods of military operation demanded the use of innumerable balloons for observation work, a new and serious problem arose. The gas hydrogen is inexpensive and efficient for the inflation of balloons, but it has one serious handicap—it is highly inflammable. A flash of lightning from a passing cloud, a flaming bullet from an enemy aeroplane or a spark from the dirigible's own motor and the balloon instantly becomes a roaring furnace with an appalling loss of life and property. An immediate and urgent demand arose for a light gas which would not burn and the only gas of that type known is helium. It was a courageous suggestion, for the largest quantity of helium which had been collected at that time was probably less than one hundred cubic feet and the cost was about $1,700 per cubic foot. At that rate the value of the helium required to lift the simple weight of an average man would be over three and one half million dollars. The application of modern scientific methods to the purification of helium has decreased its cost thirty thousand fold and permitted the United States government to prepare enough of the gas to fill four of the ordinary type of kite balloons before the signing of the armistice. While the development of this project did not come soon enough to aid in saving life during the war, it has contributed much to the safety of aviation in lighter-than-air craft, and the generous supply of helium in this country is to be regarded as one of the most important items of defense at our command.

While we are proud of these developments and watch with interest the growing importance of helium in aviation and in scientific pursuits, we should not forget that the discovery of the element, the finding of commercial quantities, the methods of extraction, purification and use are all due to the culmination of problems of research in pure science, which at first seemed wholly impractical and without useful application.

But it should not be necessary at this time and in this place to multiply examples of this kind to prove the point that research frequently has an importance greatly in excess of the expectations of its promoters. Even if we admit that nine out of every ten research problems fail to benefit the human race directly, it is clear that the tenth is sufficiently important to overbalance the cost of all ten.

But why should business be interested in research? It is doubtless unnecessary to argue in favor of any investigation on such problems as the methods of increasing sales, improving manufacturing processes or utilization of waste materials. The value of such undertakings is evident to all. But in what way is the American business man interested in problems of pure science which may have no apparent bearing at all upon his business? The history of American business has shown that all too frequently the value of scientific research is ignored with disastrous results to a business which seemed to be as well established as Gibraltar itself. Let us look for illustrations to prove this statement.

Several years ago a firm was organized to put on the market a new variety of food products. The process was original, the product attractive and soon a thriving business was established. The process involved many chemical steps and the firm employed a chemist to develop the details of the work. When the business had become well established and the profits were coming in nicely, the manager summoned the chemist to his office and said: "We are now well established, our process is working satisfactorily and we are satisfied with our products. We appreciate the help you have given us but after the end of this month we shall not need your services any longer." Shortly after this interview, the chemist removed to another state and lost contact with his former associates. After several years he returned for a visit, expecting to see a greatly enlarged and thriving factory. Imagine his disappointment when he found the doors nailed up and the windows bearing mute testimony to the unerring accuracy of missiles from the hand of the small boy. As he looked upon the scene of desolation there appeared above the door an inscription, invisible to all save him, in these familiar words: "We are satisfied with our product."

In January, 1925, there was a thriving industry in this country producing wood alcohol or methanol and its by-products by the distillation of wood. The total investment in this industry was more than $100,000,000, while its annual production was about $35,000,000. The industry was one of our most flourishing enterprises, securely entrenched and supplying an essential basic material to several important industries. Two months later this prosperous industry was seemingly on the verge of complete wreck with almost a complete loss of the invested capital. What had happened to produce so sudden and so complete a change? Methanol was being manufactured in Europe from cheap raw material and the product was being imported by the United States at a price much below the cost of manufacture from wood. The American manufacturers, feeling secure in their position as producers of an essential basic material, had failed to remember that chemists are able to make rapid strides in the development of chemical manufactures. Failing to appreciate the importance of fundamental research, they had allowed the chemists of both France and Germany to develop a new process which means the entire remaking of their industry. It not only appeared certain that our wood distillation industry was doomed, but it also seemed likely that we would be compelled to manufacture our methanol under license from the German patentee. during the fifteen-year life of the patent. It is not to our credit to know that we are saved from such humiliation by a technicality of our own patent laws.

In one of our thriving mid-western cities there is a firm which may be called The People's Ice Company. Recently it enjoyed a practical monopoly in supplying ice to the homes, stores and factories in the entire community. Business was good and the future looked promising since growth was substantial and refrigeration is essential in the handling of food products. But in spite of optimism the sales began to drop off and the businesss was very evidently losing ground. Upon inquiry it was found that more and more the stores and homes were installing individual refrigerating plants which were operated by electric motor. It was evident that something must be done to save the business, for the days of the ice wagon seemed to be numbered. Investigation showed that the electric refrigerating process was based on well-known principles of physics and chemistry, so a group of scientific men was set at work to build an equipment which could compete with other devices of the sort. The experiment was successful and now The People's Ice Company is introducing its own appliances throughout the length and breadth of the land. By the time the ice wagon has disappeared from the city streets the business activities of the firm will be so completely adjusted to the new situation that the change will be welcome. In this case research has built a larger and broader business to meet the changing demands of a scientific age.

These illustrations are sufficient to indicate that research is a vital part of business if success is to continue in this rapidly advancing age of ours. Few industries are safe from the revolutionizing influences of scientific achievement unless they are constantly on the alert for the latest developments in their fields of endeavor. To discontinue research, to feel satisfied with the product, to fail to advance is to drop behind in the procession of modern scientific accomplishment. To attempt to stand still is to invite disaster in the rush of modern traffic.

Do these statements seem extravagant or over-enthusiastic? Is a scientist getting out of his field when he attempts to emphasize the importance of science in the business world? If so, then listen to a few sentences taken at randon from an article on "Science and the Investor" published in a recent number of one of our leading metropolitan commercial journals:

> There is no business to-day whose welfare and interest are not bound up with chemistry. . . .
>
> There is no industry that is not in danger of waking up to-morrow and finding that the chemist has made a discovery that might revolutionize it. . . .
>
> No industry which does not command the resources of scientific laboratories can be regarded as secure. . . .
>
> No investor or banker can feel sure that his interest in any security is secure in the absence of the assurance given by the knowledge that science is on guard. . . .

These quotations sound like the enthusiastic endorsement of an over-zealous chemist, but it must be remembered that they were written by a man who is not primarily a scientist, but the financial editor of one of our greatest business journals. His best advice to prospective investors in any business undertaking might be epitomized thus: "Be sure the institution is keenly alive to the importance of scientific research before investing in its securities."

Similar testimony has recently been given by the vice-president of one of the largest banking institutions in New York City. He was quoted as saying in substance:

> When any New York banker is called upon to finance any corporation or business especially one based directly or indirectly upon scientific pursuits, the first investigation made is in regard to the attitude of the institution toward the advancement of scientific knowledge. If there is maintained a scientific laboratory with a generous regard for the advances in pure science, the security is, to that extent, considered good. But if no attempt is being made to keep up with, or a little in advance of the developments in science, then no considerable loan will be risked upon such a venture. Permanent business success is too intimately linked with scientific attainment to make any other attitude safe.

It is not to be presumed that these students of economic conditions had in mind any particular branch of science to the exclusion of others. For what is true in this respect concerning chemistry is true with equal force of physics, of engineering, of the social sciences, of business relations and many other lines of human endeavor which are touched by the advances of our modern civilization.

Perhaps all this seems far removed from the everyday problems of life. We might have little difficulty in reaching an agreement as to how research should be used to improve and stabilize big business, but how may it be applied to the everyday events and activities of our own existence? I believe the training received in investigational work and the mental attitude developed by it may be made a very potent factor in education, which should after all be a training for a useful and full-rounded life.

Research has been defined as a careful or critical inquiry or examination in seeking facts or principles; a systematic investigation of phenomena by the experimental method, to discover facts or to coordinate them into laws; a critical examination of conditions as we find them with the desire to improve whenever possible. In simple language research may be regarded as childish curiosity, grown to maturity and given a college education. The term "pure research" is sometimes used to refer to pursuit of knowledge for its own sake, to a search after truth for truth's sake, without a thought of the present or future value of the results. Consequently, there is an element of unselfishness in pure research, and the seeker after truth has no concern in the practical value of his discoveries. Many of civilization's most notable achievements have resulted from this unselfish spirit of research workers; this spirit has blessed the world thousands of times and it is still the actuating motive of a very large army of workers in various fields of human endeavor.

One of the most valuable assets to be obtained through the medium of education is the ability to think clearly and to analyze a complicated problem, putting the various factors into their proper relationship and value. Such a process is as truly research as the discovery of unknown lands in the polar seas, the perfecting of a new method of combating disease or the building of a new chemical compound. If we can subject the ordinary problems of our life to the careful scrutiny of critical examination; if then we can apply to these everyday matters the spirit of pure research with the unselfish desire to improve, to benefit and to serve, then we shall in some small measure justify the existence of the system of education of which we are a part. Study your job intently, whether it be the running of a great railway system or of a disc harrow; whether you are called upon to preside over a legislature or a country school; whether you wield a scepter or a broom. Bring to your task the spirit of research, of improvement, of service and of devotion; for by so doing work becomes a joy, a blessing, a benediction.

I congratulate the honor students of the University of Illinois for the excellent accomplishments of the past. It is no small achievement to be selected from so large a student body for the distinction of Honor's Day. You are to be congratulated upon your ability to keep in mind the prime purpose of a college education as well as for the excellence of your classroom records. I hope you feel a real pride in this accomplishment and I trust that you are inspired with the determination to win new marks of distinction in whatever line of activity you may engage. I hope you have enjoyed the work in which you have been employed, that you have worked industriously in working hours, that you have played intently in hours of recreation, and that you have enjoyed the companionship of your associates in hours of relaxation. If this has been your record, you richly deserve the honor which is extended to you to-day. But however great our satisfaction for the good work of the past, I congratulate you more heartily for the opportunities which are opening before you. You are soon to become active factors in a world sick of war, worn by strife and perplexed by intricate political and economic problems. There is a great need for men and women who have been trained to think, to weigh, to decide and to act. Become an investigator of conditions as you find them and do your best to improve wherever you can. I congratulate you most heartily for the opportunity for hard work, intelligent accomplishment and useful service.

"So long as men shall be on earth
There will be tasks for them to do,
Some way for them to show their worth;
Each day shall bring its problems new.

And men shall dream of mightier deeds
Than ever have been done before:
There always shall be human needs
For men to work and struggle for."

B. S. HOPKINS

UNIVERSITY OF ILLINOIS

THE NEED FOR TRAINING TAXONOMIC BOTANISTS[1]

TAXONOMY is fundamental in its relation to other branches of botany in the sense that the correct identification of plants is the basis for all work which concerns the identity of species. Comparison of the results of investigations has value only in so far as there is certainty as to the plants compared. The cytologist compares the number of chromosomes in the allied species and their hybrids in a complex genus like Rubus or Rosa. The value of his conclusions depends on the accuracy with which his specimens have been identified. The pharmacist compares the oils derived from various species of oil grasses found in commerce. A taxonomist had to work over the group to which the oil grasses belong before the comparison was worthy of record. The proposition is so evident that further support would seem unnecessary.

[1] Read at the meeting of the Botanical Society of America, systematic section, held at Nashville, December 28, 1927.

I have shown in another place[2] that taxonomy was a dominant branch of botany during the early development of that science; that during the last half century taxonomy has lost that dominance; and that now, especially in this country, that branch of botany occupies a distinctly inferior position as compared to other branches. This unfortunate condition hampers the symmetrical development of botanical science as a whole. Taxonomy has its place as a primary coordinate branch of botany and its growth should be encouraged that it may keep pace with such other primary branches as physiology, morphology and genetics.

Within recent years the demand for exact information on the identity of species has become more insistent. This is noticeable in connection with the exploration and development of tropical regions. Those interested in the vegetable products coming from these regions wish to know the specific identity of the plants producing these. When chaulmoogra oil came into prominence in connection with leprosy it was found that the identity of the species producing it was uncertain. At once a taxonomic study of the group concerned was necessary. Information in such cases can be furnished only by the taxonomist. However, the number of taxonomists with sufficient training and experience is at present so limited that information can not be furnished as rapidly as wanted. In other words, the demand at present is far greater than the supply.

In another direction the demand exceeds the supply. It is now difficult to find trained young men or women to fill positions in taxonomy. At the present time there are positions awaiting properly qualified applicants, and there appear to be no such persons available.

The chief source of supply of people for positions requiring previous experience in taxonomy is the larger herbaria of the country of which there are few. The source of supply for these herbaria is the college graduates who have taken an interest in taxonomy and have specialized in that subject. In the main we must depend upon our colleges to equip students with sufficient training to fill positions requiring a fair knowledge of the principles of taxonomy. In my opinion the colleges are not doing this to the extent necessary. In fact I believe the colleges in the aggregate are not giving the attention to taxonomy indicated by its proportional importance as a primary coordinate branch of botany.

This condition appears to be due to two reasons, the lack of trained taxonomists in our colleges and the lack of interest in the subject itself. In the latter part

[2] "The Scope and Relations of Taxonomic Botany," SCIENCE, n.s., 43, pp. 331–342, 1916.

of the last century there was a gradual swinging away from taxonomy toward more recently developed branches such as morphology, ecology, cytology and genetics. The swing has been so great that few taxonomists were trained at the period when our present generation of teachers were in college. There are, therefore, few taxonomists of first rank in our colleges at present. This condition also accounts in part for the lack of interest in taxonomy among our undergraduate and postgraduate students. Consequently, taxonomy if taught as a distinct course is likely to be in the hands of a teacher whose primary interests are in some other branch of botany.

Assuming a desire to give the teaching of taxonomy a coordinate rank in the curriculums of our colleges, how can this be realized under the present conditions? I venture the following suggestions on what should be attempted as rapidly as practicable. It should be understood that taxonomy is now taught satisfactorily in a few of our educational institutions and there are a few taxonomists of high rank in charge of courses in taxonomy, but in the aggregate taxonomy is not receiving the attention that it should.

First, the larger universities should establish a division of taxonomy as a primary branch of the department of botany. The professor in charge of this division should be a taxonomist of first rank.

Second, the student should be given the same opportunity to specialize in taxonomy that is given in other branches of botany. This opportunity should include contact with the subject at the same time that he comes in contact with the other branches. It should include a sympathetic attitude toward taxonomy, that is, the student should be encouraged to specialize in taxonomy if he shows a liking for the subject.

It has been objected that the demand for professional taxonomists is so small that it is not worth while attempting to train them on the same scale as botanists in other lines are trained. This objection disappears when the subject is examined more closely.

In the first place I think it is not the function of undergraduate instruction in botany to train professionals. Even the instruction in postgraduate courses is scarcely of the nature to train professionals. Professional training with the taxonomist begins when he accepts a position in which taxonomy is the chief line of work. Such would be an assistantship in an herbarium or in state or federal government department. What our colleges should do is to give the student a training which will fit him for a position of this kind. It is true that professional positions in taxonomy are limited in number. It is also true that professional positions in other branches of botany are few. How many positions are there in which the occupant devotes himself to physiology, to genetics or to cytology? I am not here referring to teaching positions except as the teacher devotes himself entirely to one of these subjects. On the basis of specialization I think there is as much demand for taxonomists as for specialists in other lines.

Many of the botanists who take postgraduate work in our educational institutions become teachers of botany. If they are adapted to the prosecution of research they specialize in some branch in which they are interested. Much of the research in botany at present is carried on by teachers for whom the research is a side line. They are professional teachers rather than professional research workers. In this connection, then, my plea is that taxonomy be placed on an equality with other branches of botany in our colleges, then those who have taken special training in botany will have had an opportunity to equip themselves for research in taxonomy. Those who become teachers and have the opportunity and the inclination to carry on research in taxonomy can do this as a side line. In this way the amount of taxonomic research in America would be greatly increased.

It is true that comprehensive work in taxonomy can be pursued only in connection with a large herbarium and botanical library. But much can be done by the isolated worker if he confines himself to a definite group. He can accumulate specimens and books dealing with this group. He can supplement this by borrowing books and specimens. He can give the final touches to a piece of work by visiting a large taxonomic center.

Every institution teaching botany should have an herbarium, not a large one to compete with the great botanical centers, but a small well-selected collection of plants which can be used as a laboratory for teaching taxonomic botany.

However, the basis for the proper development of taxonomic botany is first a realization of its importance and, second, a sympathetic attitude toward this branch in our colleges.

A. S. HITCHCOCK
WASHINGTON, D. C.

THE FIFTH NEW YORK MEETING OF THE AMERICAN ASSOCIATION AND ASSOCIATED SOCIETIES[1]

PREPARATIONS for the fifth New York meeting of the American Association are much further advanced than is usual at this time. It is evident that this meeting will be larger and more important than any earlier

[1] This is the second announcement about the approaching New York meeting. The first announcement, by President Henry Fairfield Osborn, was published in SCIENCE for April 20.

meeting. Forty-one special scientific societies are planning to meet with the association on that occasion. A survey of available hotels and session rooms has already been made and the facilities have been shown to be ample for all needs.

Under the efficient and enthusiastic leadership of the president of the association, Professor Henry Fairfield Osborn, president of the American Museum of Natural History, several unusually attractive features are being planned for this meeting. It is hoped that those who come from away will arrive on Thursday, December 27, in time for the opening general session on Thursday evening and the general reception that is to follow it, and that they will remain throughout the period of the meeting, which will close with another general reception Wednesday evening, January 2. There is to be a general session of the association each evening at the American Museum. These general sessions on Friday, Saturday, Monday and Tuesday evenings are each to be devoted to a lecture by some eminent man of science, presenting interesting aspects of current progress in one of the larger science fields. These main public lectures are to be sufficiently non-technical to be useful to workers in other fields as well as to those in the respective fields of the lecturers themselves. Other general sessions for the same general purpose are being planned, and the fifth New York meeting will furnish exceptional opportunities for science workers in each field to become better acquainted with the recent accomplishments and aims of those in the other branches. This feature is being developed with the aim of counteracting to some extent the regrettable narrowing that inevitably results from modern specialization in science. While the special science societies and the sections of the association are devoted to the advancement of the several sciences, the American Association as a whole and the affiliated state academies of science need to give much attention to the broader aspects of science, the interlocking of all the many kinds of intellectual endeavor that together make up science in general. A social period is planned for each evening, following the general sessions, and those who attend are to have opportunity to examine the American Museum exhibits in the field of science to which the evening is specially devoted. These evening sessions will alone be well worth the trip to New York and the devoting of the entire week to science in the broader sense.

The retiring president of the association is this year Dr. Arthur A. Noyes, director of the Gates Chemical Laboratory of the California Institute of Technology. Dr. Noyes will deliver the retiring presidential address at the general session on Monday evening, December 31. The general session of Friday evening, December 28, is to be devoted to the annual Sigma Xi lecture, which is a regular feature of the annual meetings of the association. The lecturer will be chosen, as usual, by the Society of the Sigma Xi and his name will be announced in due time. A concert is being planned for Sunday afternoon and excursions to scientific institutions in and near New York are to be arranged for Sunday forenoon and for other times.

Reduced railway fares are being arranged for those who attend the New York meeting, which will amount to a fare and a half for the round trip. Plans are being made by which the validation of railway certificates may be accomplished with a minimum of trouble on the part of those who register. It is likely that there will be several registration offices, since scientific sessions will be held at several places.

The registration fee for the meeting is to be two dollars and each registrant is to receive the official badge, a copy of the "General Program," together with such program supplements as may be published, any other literature issued in connection with the meeting and an identification card entitling the recipient to all the privileges of the meeting, including the endorsement and validation of one railway certificate. But members of the American Association for the Advancement of Science who have been enrolled for the year 1928–29 may register by paying only one dollar. To secure the benefit of this lower registration fee one must be a life member of the association or an annual member whose current dues have been paid. Enrolment cards for 1928–29 will be issued from the Washington office to all life members on October 1, and to annual members upon receipt of dues for 1928–29, which are due October 1. These cards should be brought to the meeting and should be shown at the registration office in order to obtain the benefit of the lower registration fee.

Associates for the fifth New York meeting are to pay the regular associate fee of five dollars and are not to pay any registration fee. The associateship is provided for those who are willing to contribute to the meeting fund but who do not care to become members of the association. Associates do not receive the association journal, but they are to receive the special issues of SCIENCE that contain the reports of the meeting. They have all the privileges of the meeting except voting. All associate fees collected for this meeting, as well as registration fees and all entrance fees of new members who join at this meeting, are to go into the meeting fund, which is to be used for paying the extra expenses of the meeting.

A list of hotels and room prices will be published in SCIENCE as soon as assignments of hotel headquarters shall have been made by the local committee in charge of that feature of the preparations. It is hoped that reduced prices may be arranged for those from away who plan to stay in New York for Science Week. There are plenty of medium-priced hotels in the city and there will be no dearth of suitable rooms, but early reservation of rooms will be desirable. Reservations are to be sent directly to the hotels, after the appearance of the list showing the hotel headquarters of the several societies that are to meet with the association this year. The secretaries of these organizations will be promptly informed about hotel headquarters, prices, etc., so that they may transmit this information to their members.

The names of the forty-one organizations that have thus far intimated their intention to meet with the association in New York are as follows. Names of those that are officially affiliated with the American Association are indicated by one or two asterisks. One asterisk shows that the organization has one representative in the association council and two asterisks show that it has two representatives. Other officially associated societies are each indicated by a cross:

Organizations related to Section A (Mathematics)
**American Mathematical Society
**Mathematical Association of America

Organizations related to Section B (Physics)
**American Physical Society
*American Meteorological Society

Organizations related to Section D (Astronomy)
**American Astronomical Society

Organizations related to Section E (Geology and Geography)
**Geological Society of America
**Paleontological Society of America
*Mineralogical Society of America
**Association of American Geographers
†National Council of Geography Teachers

Organizations related to Section F (Zoological Sciences)
**American Society of Zoologists
**Entomological Society of America
**American Association of Economic Entomologists
*American Society of Parasitologists
Phi Sigma Biological Research Society

Organizations related to Section G (Botanical Sciences)
**Botanical Society of America
**American Phytopathological Society
**American Society of Plant Physiologists
†Sullivant Moss Society
†American Fern Society

Organizations related to both Sections F and G
**American Society of Naturalists
**Ecological Society of America
**American Microscopical Society
Genetics Section of American Society of Zoologists and Botanical Society of America
Geneticists Interested in Agriculture

Organizations related to Section H (Anthropology)
**American Anthropological Association
†American Folk-Lore Society

Organizations related to Section I (Psychology)
**American Psychological Association

Organizations related to Section K (Social and Economic Sciences)
†Metric Association

Organizations related to Section L (Historical and Philological Sciences)
*Linguistic Society of America
**History of Science Society

Organizations related to Section O (Agriculture)
**American Society of Agronomy
*Society of American Foresters
*American Society for Horticultural Science
†Potato Association of America
†Gamma Sigma Delta Honor Society of Agriculture

Organizations related to the American Association as a whole
**Society of the Sigma Xi
**American Association of University Professors
†Gamma Alpha Graduate Scientific Fraternity
*American Nature-Study Society
Sigma Delta Epsilon Graduate Women's Scientific Fraternity

As has been said, the fifth New York meeting will be unusually large, but it promises to be really less crowded than some of the smaller meetings have been. It is hoped that the society meetings may be distributed throughout the week so that the two halves of the meeting period (separated by Sunday) will not be very unequal in this respect. This meeting is to be specially interesting and unusually satisfactory on account of the inclusion of a Sunday in the period. This will offer exceptional opportunities for committee meetings, personal consultations, excursions to interesting points in the city, etc.

There will be no lack of suitable rooms to supply the needs of the numerous sections and societies. Some of these will meet in the American Museum and most of the remainder will meet at Columbia University, which cordially offers its very excellent facilities. Earlier New York meetings of the association and the associated societies have been held at the university, as those who have attended those meetings will remember with pleasure and satisfaction.

The great annual science exhibition, which has recently become a very important feature of the association meetings, will be especially large and valuable this year. A large number of firms that supply scientific apparatus for research and teaching and many publishers of scientific books are to take part. There will be an unusual number of exhibits by research workers and research institutions and laboratories.

Those who have new apparatus, methods or results that will be suitable and available for the New York exhibition should take up this question at an early date, by correspondence with the permanent secretary's office in Washington. Since many research workers are apt to be somewhat overmodest in bringing their work forward, those who know of apparatus and methods recently developed by others are asked to inform the permanent secretary, so that invitations may be sent out to secure as valuable and as representative scientific exhibits as may be had. Arrangements for this important feature of the exhibition should be taken up early, before October 1, for considerable correspondence will probably be necessary in each case and the press of other matters will be very great in the fall. The location of the general exhibition will be announced later. It will be convenient for those who attend the meeting and will be unusually valuable and attractive. The assignment of space for the commercial exhibits is in charge of Major H. S. Kimberly, manager of the exhibition.

An important feature of the New York meeting will be one or more sessions of the Secretaries' Conference, which has recently been organized under the special secretaryship of Dr. George T. Hargitt, Lyman Hall, Syracuse University. Another important feature will be a session and a complimentary dinner of the Academy Conference, also recently organized, the secretary of which is Dr. Howard E. Enders, Purdue University, Lafayette, Ind. The secretaries' complimentary dinner is planned for Sunday evening. That of the academy conference will probably occur Thursday evening. The first session of the executive committee of the association will be held at the general-headquarters hotel Thursday morning at 10 o'clock and the first council session will be held Thursday afternoon at 2 o'clock, after which will occur a session of the academy conference.

It is very desirable that as many as possible of the preliminary plans for the great New York convention in Science Week shall be completed before June. Little can be accomplished during the summer and both the local committees and the Washington office will be very busy after October 1. Correspondence about local arrangements should be addressed to Dr. Sam F. Trelease, American Association for the Advancement of Science, American Museum of Natural History, 77th St. and Central Park West, New York City. Carbon copies of all such communications should be sent, at the same time, to the permanent secretary's office, American Association for the Advancement of Science, Smithsonian Institution Building, Washington, D. C. Correspondence about space to be occupied by commercial exhibits in the general exhibition should be addressed to Major H. S. Kimberly, American Association for the Advancement of Science, Smithsonian Institution Building, Washington, D. C. Communications about scientific exhibits, by investigators and research workers, should be addressed to the permanent secretary.

Further notes concerning preparations for the fifth New York meeting will be published in SCIENCE as these become available and the "Preliminary Announcement" of the meeting will appear in the issue of SCIENCE for November 30.

BURTON E. LIVINGSTON,
Permanent Secretary

SCIENTIFIC EVENTS

THE INTERNATIONAL POPULATION UNION

AT the last session of the World Population Conference in Geneva, on September 3, 1927, there were passed the following resolutions:

The World Population Conference resolves that a permanent international organization be created for the object of studying population problems in a strictly scientific spirit.

A Provisional Committee is hereby authorized to prepare the constitution for this organization.

In accordance with these resolutions the following Provisional Committee for the organization of an International Union for the Scientific Investigation of Population Problems was then appointed, with power to coopt additional members until the total number of the committee was fifteen:

	Representing
Sir Bernard Mallet	United Kingdom of Great Britain
Professor F. A. E. Crew	
Professor E. M. East	United States of America
Professor Raymond Pearl	
Professor Leon Bernard	France
Professor Erwin Baur	Germany
Professor Corrado Gini	Italy
Professor W. Rappard	Switzerland
Professor A. Mahaim	Belgium

Under the power granted for cooptation the following persons have been added to complete the committee:

	Representing
Professor Severino Aznar	Spain
Professor Kiyo Sue Inui	Japan
Professor H. Lundborg	Scandinavia
Professor J. H. dePaula Souza	South America
Doctor Charles H. Wickens	British Dominions
Professor V. Bunak	Russia

The committee organized at Geneva and appointed Raymond Pearl, chairman, and Professor F. A. E. Crew, secretary.

Since last September this committee has been actively engaged in the preliminary work of the organization of the union, with the financial and moral aid and support of the National Research Council and the Social Science Research Council, acting in cooperation. A provisional draft of the statutes of the union is now in process of revision. The general plan of organization proposed is closely similar to that of other existing International Unions in the pure and applied sciences, with such differences only as are necessitated by the manifold and wide-ranging character of population problems. The basis of the union will lie in national committees in the various adhering countries, these underlying national organizations being composed of scientific men interested and active in research regarding various aspects of population. Such national committees have already been formed for Great Britain, France, Italy and the United States, and are in process of organization at the present time in a number of other countries. In the case of the United States committees on population have been appointed by the National Research Council and the Social Science Research Council, respectively, which bodies, acting conjointly, will be the official adherents to the union for this country.

The provisional committee will meet in Paris on July 2, 1928, for the purpose of finally completing the preliminary organization of the union, the first General Assembly of which will take place in Paris on July 4–6, 1928. According to the plan of organization provided for in the statutes, membership in the general assembly of the union will be restricted to delegates officially elected by the national committee of the adhering countries. In addition to the members a limited number of persons may be invited by the general assembly itself to attend its sessions.

The objects of the International Union will be purely scientific. Propaganda of any sort, for any purposes whatsoever, will have no place in its activities.

The purpose of the union will be to develop scientific studies pertaining to the problems of population, and particularly:

(a) To initiate and organize researches which depend upon international cooperation, and to provide for their scientific discussion and publication.

(b) To facilitate the establishment of common standards for the collection, tabulation and analysis of data regarding human populations, including economic, sociologic, demographic, agricultural and biologic data.

(c) To serve as a clearing house for the interchange and dissemination of information about population, especially for the purpose of facilitating research.

(d) To cooperate to the fullest extent with other scientific bodies having similar objects.

RAYMOND PEARL,
Chairman of the Provisional Committee

INTERNATIONAL CONFERENCES IN 1928

THE Institute of International Education of New York has issued a list of international conferences to be held during the present year. These include the following in the fields of science:

April 9–11, Fifth International Congress of Refrigeration, Rome.

May 26–29, Sixth International Congress of Doctors, Naturalists and Engineers, Prague.

June 3–9, One Hundredth Anniversary of Institution of Civil Engineers, London.

June 21–24, International Congress of Geologists, Copenhagen.

June 26–July 14, World's Dairy Congress, London. The program includes papers on all phases of milk industry.

July 5, Meeting of the International Astronomical Union, Leyden, representing twenty-three countries.

July 14–23, International Geographical Congress. Meets in London and Cambridge. In addition to the general meetings there will be meetings of six sections.

July 23–27, International Congress of Radiology, Stockholm.

July 23–28, Thirty-second session of the Congress of Alienists and Neurologists of the French-speaking world, Antwerp.

July,* International Convention on Cancer Research, London. Persons and organizations conducting research on cancer are invited to attend.

Summer,* International Health Congress, Havre and Paris. To consider the extermination of rats.

September 3–10, International Congress of Mathematicians, Bologna.

September 4–October 6, World's Power (Fuel) Congress, London. The technical program will be divided as follows: Composition and Classification of Fuels; Preparation of Fuels; Storage, Handling and Transmission of Fuels, and Utilization of Fuels.

September 10–14, International Psychotechnical Congress, Utrecht.

September 25–27, International Union against Tuberculosis, Rome.

September 28, International Congress on Iron and Steel, Bilbao.

September,* International Congress of Doctors, Budapest.

October 7–28, International Conference on Aerial Navigation, Berlin.

October,* International Technical Congress, Tokyo.

October,* International Congress of Microbiology, Paris.

November 19–24, Second International Conference on Bituminous Coal, Carnegie Institute of Technology, Pittsburgh.

November,* Second International Conference for the Protection of Plants, Rome.

November,* Ninth general meeting of the International Agricultural Institute, Rome.

December 15–22, International Congress of Tropical Medicine, Cairo.

FORESTRY ADVANCES IN THE UNITED STATES

THE official *Record* of the U. S. Department of Agriculture lists the more important advances in forest conservation which have been made in various states. Last year three states—Florida, South Carolina and Delaware—passed laws for the establishment of state forestry departments and the appointment of state foresters. Similar legislation was again proposed in Arkansas but failed. California created a department of natural resources under the general supervision of a director, with a division of forestry administered by the state forester and guided as to policies by a state board of forestry, the new department taking over all the powers and duties of the former state forester. Rhode Island made an important change in its forestry organization by putting it under the department of agriculture. North Carolina increased the membership of its state board of conservation and development. Louisiana provided for an additional member of its forestry board. Ohio passed legislation authorizing the board of control of the Ohio experiment station to acquire tracts suitable for research and demonstration in practical forestry. Maine provided for the establishment of town forests, and Wisconsin made similar provision for county forests. In Washington the State has been given authority to accept from counties tax lands suitable for State forests. Michigan provided for the retention of such lands by the state, and Minnesota set aside as state forests all state lands within the boundaries of the Minnesota National Forest. Pennsylvania appropriated $450,000 toward the acquisition of about 7,200 acres of private land in order to preserve some of the original forests of the state, and for other forests and tracts subject to the contribution of not less than $200,000 of private funds for the same purposes. Maryland authorized the formation of auxiliary state forests through agreement with private land-owners.

DR. B. L. HARTWELL AND THE RHODE ISLAND AGRICULTURAL EXPERIMENT STATION

THE New England section of the American Society of Agronomy has passed the following resolutions concerning Dr. B. L. Hartwell:

WHEREAS, Dr. B. L. Hartwell, during his many years of service at the Rhode Island Agricultural Experiment Station, has made many notable contributions to agricultural science, winning for himself and the Rhode Island station a national and international reputation; and

WHEREAS, The success of the investigations at the Rhode Island station in Dr. Hartwell's special field is largely the result of carefully planned and fostered cooperation of the station agronomists, chemists and plant physiologists; and

WHEREAS, The Rhode Island station experiments and researches respecting soil acidity, availability of phosphates, toxicity of aluminum, effect of one crop on another, crop response to fertilizer elements, manure substitutes for vegetable gardens, etc., have yielded results of incalculable value to agronomical science and practice; and

WHEREAS, Dr. Hartwell has taken an active part in the proceedings of the New England section of the American Society of Agronomy, working always for the best interest of New England agriculture through the promotion of agronomical science; has been known for his integrity, staunchness and untiring zeal; has been one whose counsel has been often sought and always esteemed by his fellow agronomists; and

WHEREAS, The New England agronomists feel that on account of Dr. Hartwell's long contact and detailed familiarity with the Rhode Island field experiments, into which he has put the best part of his life, his dismissal will cause agronomic science and New England agriculture to suffer a great loss and thereby affect the welfare of the people of New England; and

WHEREAS, The New England agronomists view with alarm any changes that would jeopardize the work, and with disfavor the summary dismissal of a scientist of Dr. Hartwell's record, character and ability, without a careful consideration of all the elements involved in the case; therefore, be it

Resolved, That the New England Section of the American Society of Agronomy earnestly requests a thorough investigation of the whole affair by some unprejudiced agency of Rhode Island, that the facts ascertained be made public, and that the board of managers of the experiment station keep an open mind for a reconsideration of its action in the light of the facts. Be it further

Resolved, That a copy of these resolutions be sent to Providence papers, the board of managers of the Rhode Island State College and to all other organizations or persons interested.

By A. B. BEAUMONT,
Chmn. New Eng. Sec. A. S. A.
FORD S. PRINCE,
Sec'y New Eng. Sec. A. S. A.

SCIENTIFIC NOTES AND NEWS

DR. WILLIAM H. WRIGHT, astronomer of the Lick Observatory, has been awarded the Henry Draper medal of the National Academy of Sciences.

* The information in the possession of the Institute does not give the exact date.

Dr. W. Nernst, professor of physical chemistry in the University of Berlin, has been awarded the Franklin medal of the Franklin Institute of Philadelphia.

The University of St. Andrews will confer the honorary degree of LL.D. upon Professor William Darrach, dean of the college of physicians and surgeons of Columbia University, and on Dr. E. P. Cathcart, Gardiner professor of physiological chemistry at the University of Glasgow.

The Bavarian Academy of Sciences has elected to its mathematics and natural history section as corresponding members the following: Dr. F. G. Hopkins, professor of biochemistry in the University of Cambridge; Dr. R. Robinson, professor of organic chemistry in the University of Manchester; Dr. S. Murbeck, professor of botany in the University of Lund; Dr. A. Angeli, professor of organic chemistry in the University of Florence; Dr. L. Dolle, professor of geography and paleontology in the University of Brussels.

Dr. A. W. Hill, director of the Royal Botanic Gardens, Kew, attended the annual meeting of the New Zealand Institute on January 26, when he was elected an honorary member. Sir John Russell, director of the Rothamsted Experimental Station, has also been elected an honorary member of the institute.

The Nichols Prize of the Royal Society of Medicine has been awarded to Dr. Peter L. McKinlay and Dr. Remington Hobbs, the prize being equally divided between them. This prize, of £250, under the will of the late Dr. R. T. Nichols, is offered every three years for the most valuable contribution by a British subject towards the discovery of the causes and the prevention of death in childbirth from septicemia.

Dr. Heinrich Kayser, who was for twenty-five years professor of physics in the University of Bonn, recently celebrated his seventy-fifth birthday.

A portrait of Dr. William H. Park, director of the laboratories of the New York City Department of Health, professor of bacteriology and hygiene in New York University and Bellevue Hospital Medical College and vice-president of the New York Academy of Medicine, was presented to the academy at a stated meeting on April 19.

At Tulane University, Dr. Erasmus Darwin Fenner has been appointed professor emeritus of orthopedics and surgical diseases of children and Dr. Rudolph Matas, professor emeritus of general and clinical surgery.

Dr. Frank C. Whitmore, chairman of the division of chemistry and chemical technology of the National Research Council and head of the department of chemistry at Northwestern University, has been elected a director of the American Chemical Society, to fill the vacancy created by the election to the presidency of S. W. Parr, of the University of Illinois.

Dr. John B. Whitehead, professor of electrical engineering and dean of the school of engineering of the Johns Hopkins University, has been engaged as a consultant for the engineering and research staffs of the General Cable Corporation. He is to act in an advisory capacity on wire and cable insulations.

Dr. Harry Everett Barnard, of Illinois, president of the American Institute of Baking in Chicago, has joined the scientific organization of the Royal Baking Powder Company as technical consultant, with headquarters in Indianapolis.

Dr. A. S. Patten, for the past twenty-two years chemist at the Michigan Agricultural Station, has resigned to take a position with the Huron Milling Company, Michigan.

C. E. Dobbin has been transferred from the fuel section of the geologic branch to the conservation branch of the U. S. Geological Survey, of which he is to be field representative of the mineral classification division, with an office in Denver, Colorado.

Dr. John Collinson, Jr., has been appointed head of the bureau of vital statistics of the Maryland Department of Health on a full-time basis to succeed Dr. Frederic V. Beitler, resigned.

Dr. Otto H. Schwarz has returned after about seventeen months abroad to become obstetrician-in-chief at the new maternity hospital and to head the department of obstetrics at the Washington University School of Medicine, St. Louis.

Commander Richard E. Byrd has made public the membership of his forthcoming Antarctic expedition, which includes the following scientific men: Dr. L. M. Gould, of the University of Michigan, will be geologist and geographer; William C. Haynes, of the U. S. Weather Bureau, meteorologist, and Dr. Francis D. Coman, of the Johns Hopkins Hospital, physician and surgeon.

Paul C. Standley returned to Washington on April 2, after spending four months in botanical field work in Honduras. Most of the time was devoted to a survey of the Lancetilla Valley, near Tela, but three weeks were passed in exploration of the pine forests of the interior of the Republic.

Dr. Graham Lusk, professor of physiology at the Cornell University Medical College, gave a series of three lectures under the Herter foundation of the University and Bellevue Hospital Medical College, New

York University, on April 23, 25 and 27. The subjects were, respectively, "Normal Metabolism," "Diabetes" and "Mechanical Work."

Dr. Robert A. Millikan, of the California Institute of Technology, will be the principal speaker at the dedication exercises on April 28 of the new science hall at Berea College and Allied Schools.

Dr. George E. Coghill, member of the Wistar Institute, will lecture on the subject of "Anatomy and the Problem of Behavior" at University College, London, on May 7, 8 and 10.

Dr. J. Frank, professor of experimental physics at the University of Göttingen, will lecture before the New York University Chapter of the Society of the Sigma Xi, May 2, on "Connections between Spectroscopy and Chemical Reactions."

Dr. Frank Schlesinger, director of the Yale Observatory, lectured before the Amateur Astronomers Association at the American Museum of Natural History on April 19.

Dr. S. Burt Wolbach, Shattuck professor of pathologic anatomy at the Harvard Medical School, delivered the annual lecture to the Philadelphia Pathological Society on April 19 on "The Pathology of Avitaminoses."

Dr. Charles H. Mayo, of the Mayo Clinic, delivered the Balfour lecture on Lister day, April 5, at the University of Toronto on "Focal Infection in Chronic and Recurring Diseases."

Dr. Aleš Hrdlička, of the Smithsonian Institution, gave three public lectures at the University of Wisconsin on March 26, 27 and 28 on "The Origin of the Living Races of Man, their Spread over the World and their Present Classification," "The Racial Composition of the Principal Now-existing Nations of the World" and "The American People."

Dr. F. E. Lloyd, MacDonald professor of botany in McGill University, gave two lectures at Purdue University, on April 16. In the afternoon he addressed the local biological society and the Purdue section of the plant physiologists on "Maturation and Conjugation in Spirogyra." In the evening he gave a popular lecture on "The Structure, Movements and Feeding Habits of Vampyrella Lateritia" at an open meeting under the auspices of the department of biology and the Purdue Chapter of Sigma Xi.

Dr. Julius Bauer, professor of medicine at the University of Vienna, gave a Mayo Foundation lecture on April 2, on "Individual Constitution in Clinical Pathology," at the Mayo Clinic. Dr. Bauer came from Vienna to deliver the oration at the recent meeting of the American College of Physicians in New Orleans.

Professor Bruno Bloch, director of the dermatological clinic of the University of Zurich at Strasbourg, will lecture at the Harvard Medical School on April 16, on "Formation of Pigment in the Skin."

Among the busts to be unveiled in the Hall of Fame at New York University on May 10 is that of Louis Agassiz. The bust is the work of Anna Vaughn Hyatt, the daughter of Alpheus Hyatt, who was a student of Agassiz.

A. Leroy Keyes, bacteriologist at the Rocky Mountain Spotted Fever Laboratory, of the U. S. Public Health Service, at Hamilton, Montana, recently died of the disease, which he had contracted in the laboratory.

Dr. Charles S. Boyer, of Philadelphia, known for his studies of Diatomaceae, recently died at the age of seventy-two years.

Professor Launcelot Harrison, Challis professor of zoology in the University of Sydney and president of the Linnean Society of New South Wales, died on February 20.

M. Félix Henneguy, professor of comparative embryology at the Collège de France, Paris, since 1900, and president for five years of the Société de Biologie, has died, aged seventy-seven years.

Professor Antonio Abetti, formerly director of the Institute of Astrophysics at Florence Arcetri, died on February 20 at the age of eighty-two years.

Professor Ritzema Bos, known for his work in connection with the diseases of plants, has died at Wageningen, Holland, at the age of seventy-eight years.

The Harvey Society of New York announces a celebration to commemorate the three hundredth anniversary of the publication of "Exercitationes de Motu Cordis et Sanguinis," by William Harvey, for the evening of Friday, May 11. The Harvey Society plans to celebrate the anniversary of this event in connection with the final lecture of the current year. The celebration is to consist of a dinner, in accordance with the ancient tradition established by Harvey at the Royal College of Physicians of London. After the dinner there will be an address, appropriate to the occasion, by Dr. Alfred E. Cohn, of the Rockefeller Institute. At the same time there will be on exhibition in the library of the Academy of Medicine a collection of Harveiana, arranged by Archibald Malloch, librarian of the academy.

THE Lehigh chapter of Sigma Xi was installed at Lehigh University on March 1, by Dr. G. B. Pegram, of Columbia University, the national treasurer of the society. There were thirty-nine charter members. The installation ceremony was followed by a banquet in the evening. The chapter elected the following officers: Dr. C. R. Richards, president of Lehigh University, *president;* Dr. B. L. Miller, *vice-president;* Dr. C. C. Bidwell, *treasurer,* and Dr. L. L. Smail, *secretary.*

THE annual meeting of the New Hampshire Academy of Science will take place at the Ashworth Hotel at Hampton Beach from June 1 to 3. Plans for the meeting include a general meeting addressed by an outside speaker, sessions for the reading of scientific papers and field trips.

THE fourth annual science dinner of the New York Association of Biology Teachers will be held on April 28 at the Hotel St. George, Brooklyn, N. Y. The program includes addresses by Dr. W. D. Bancroft, chairman of the department of chemistry at Cornell University; Dr. C. E. Baer, New York state supervisor of science, and Dr. F. C. Brown, director of the Museum of the Peaceful Arts.

GIFTS to the American Chemical Society aggregating $360,000, for "cooperative service in recording and indexing through the society's publications the chemical literature of the world," were announced at the society's closing session in St. Louis. The Chemical Foundation, Inc., of New York, of which Francis P. Garvan is president, gave $250,000. The remaining $110,000 came from the industries, among which a leading donor was the Allied Chemical and Dye Corporation, of which Dr. William H. Nichols, of New York, a charter member and a past president of the society, is chairman of the board.

THE Northeastern Section of the American Chemical Society has received a check for $1,000 from Mrs. Robert W. Neff as a contribution to the permanent trust fund of the section. Mr. Neff, who was a manufacturing chemist in Boston for thirty years, died a few weeks ago. He was a member of this section and was also treasurer of the board of trustees of this fund. He was deeply interested in the plans to provide a permanent source of income for the section and made provision in his will for this addition to the fund of which the income only can be spent for constructive work in chemistry by the Northeastern Section.

THE Academy of Natural Sciences of Philadelphia has received by bequest of the late Frank R. Mason, of Philadelphia, the important collection of Coleoptera accumulated by him over a period of nearly thirty years. The collection is especially rich in exotic species, and includes among other series the Cerambycidae of the famous Vanderpole collection and the Angell collection of Carabidae. The Mason collection contains representatives of 16,863 species and embraces about 76,650 specimens, contained in over 1,100 boxes housed in nine large steel cabinets. The collection of the family Carabidae alone contains about 10,200 specimens representing 2,338 species, while the series of Cerambycidae contains individuals of 4,660 species. The technique of the specimens in the collection is said to be exceptionally fine. By the terms of the bequest the collection is to be kept intact and to be known as the "Frank R. Mason Memorial Collection." It has been considered by competent students to be the best collection of the beetles of the world in America.

THE New York Botanical Garden has recently received from the American Museum of Natural History a collection of more than five hundred herbarium specimens from Mount Roraima, collected in 1927 by Mr. G. H. H. Tate, of the museum staff. Roraima stands at the boundary corner between Brazil, Venezuela and British Guiana, and rises to a height of more than 8,000 feet. Its flora is still imperfectly known, chiefly because of the difficulty involved in reaching it, but has long been noted for a large proportion of endemic species. Mr. Tate was able to spend two weeks on the actual summit of Roraima and collected specimens of every observed species, so that the gift is an important addition to the garden's South American material.

CONTRIBUTIONS toward the $1,000,000 sought by the Charles Sprague Sargent memorial fund for the Arnold Arboretum now total $906,551, according to an announcement made by Henry James, chairman of the New York committee for the fund. This amount includes a $50,000 gift which will be payable by Edward S. Harkness when the balance of the fund has been subscribed.

THE San Diego Society of Natural History has announced that in response to its appeal for a $250,000 building fund, pledges to the amount of $125,000 have been received. This building fund will make possible the erection of a new fireproof museum structure.

AT a recent meeting of the board of directors of the Desert Sanatorium of Southern Arizona, Tucson, $250,000 was voted to establish an institute of research to study the nature of solar radiations and their effects on living matter. The director will be Dr. Bernard L. Wyatt; the medical director, Dr. Roland A. Davison, and the research consultant, Dr. Daniel T. MacDougal.

THE *British Medical Journal* states that a national fund is being created in Sweden for presentation to King Gustaf V as a gift on his seventieth birthday in June this year. The King intends to expend the fund in promoting cancer research. A special institute may be established in Stockholm.

THE original thesis presented by David Starr Jordan for his master's degree at Cornell University has been given by Dr. Jordan to the university library. Dr. Jordan, a graduate of the class of 1872, prepared for his master's degree a manuscript on "The Wild Flora of Wyoming County, New York."

AN advisory commission of engineers has been organized to make a survey in Vermont with a view to preventing floods. J. W. Votey, dean of the University of Vermont College of Engineering, was named chairman of the commission and Professor H. K. Barrows, of Boston, consulting engineer. The commission plans to establish a number of stations along various streams to determine the flow of water at various times and under different conditions. From the data thus obtained, the locations of reservoirs to control the water flow will be determined.

CONTINUING its program of scientific research in cooperation with the United States Bureau of Mines and two advisory boards representing the mining and metallurgical industries, the Carnegie Institute of Technology in Pittsburgh will award ten fellowships in mining and metallurgical research during the coming year. Subjects to be studied by the fellows appointed for 1928–29 will be selected in the fields of origin and constitution of coal, coal mining, utilization of coal, mine safety and the physical chemistry of steel making.

ACCORDING to *Industrial and Engineering Chemistry* the Imperial Chemical Industries, Ltd., the British trust of which Sir Alfred Mond is chairman, has launched a move in England to promote chemical industrial research and stimulate interest in the chemical industry in general. To this end a research council composed of leading scientific men has been established. It is pointed out that coordinated industrial research in Great Britain has suffered in the past through lack of sufficient close associations with the academic and scientific world. The main functions of the council will be advisory, and it will act as a clearing house for ideas. The council will also provide close liaison between the industry and the universities, and will promote research along both industrial and purely academic lines. Sir Alfred Mond is chairman of the council. In further extension of this move the British chemical trust has also inaugurated a scheme to absorb research chemists and chemical engineer graduates from British educational institutions. The plan provides for selecting boys who indicate an aptitude along chemical lines and insuring them positions with initial salaries of $2,000 per year upon successful completion of their educational training in universities.

UNIVERSITY AND EDUCATIONAL NOTES

THE will of the late Chauncey M. Depew, of New York, includes an unrestricted bequest of $1,000,000 to Yale University.

ST. STEPHEN'S COLLEGE at Annandale-on-Hudson has been absorbed by Columbia University, according to an announcement by the officials of both institutions. Under the consolidation St. Stephen's becomes a unit of Columbia University on a parity with Columbia and Barnard Colleges.

THE *Journal* of the American Medical Association states that at a luncheon given by the University of Southern California in honor of Dr. Ray Lyman Wilbur, of Stanford University, and a group of sixty Los Angeles physicians on March 26, it was announced that the University of Southern California College of Medicine is to be reopened and that the trustees have agreed to set aside $500,000 as an endowment.

GROUND was broken with formal ceremonies at Lafayette College on April 26 for the John Markle mining building.

DR. CHARLES P. OLIVIER, of the University of Virginia, has been appointed professor of astronomy at the University of Pennsylvania and director of the Flower Observatory at Highland Park.

DR. RAOUL BLANCHARD, professor of geography at the University of Grenoble, has been appointed professor of geography at Harvard University.

DR. S. TIMOSHENKO, of the research department of the Westinghouse Company, has been appointed professor of applied mathematics at the University of Michigan. He is succeeded at the Westinghouse Company by Dr. A. Nádai, of Göttingen.

PROFESSOR F. C. KOCH has been made chairman of the department of physiological chemistry and pharmacology at the University of Chicago. Professor A. Baird Hastings has been transferred from the department of physical chemistry to be professor of biochemistry in the department of medicine.

AT Clark University, the following promotions from associate professorships have been made: Dr. W. Elmer Ekblaw, professor of agricultural geography; Dr. Clarence F. Jones, professor of economic geography; Dr. John P. Nafe, professor of experimental psychology. Oscar W. Richards has been appointed assistant professor of biology.

AT Rutgers University, Dr. Albert O. Hayes has been appointed full professor of geology and head of that department. He has served during the past two years as visiting professor of geology.

DR. CARL STEVENSON, of the University of Chicago, has been appointed acting professor of medical history at Cornell University, Ithaca, for the second term of the coming year, during the absence on leave of Professor Preserved Smith.

THE following promotions have been made in the department of chemistry at Princeton University: Assistant Professor Gregg Dougherty, to the rank of associate professor; instructors William T. Richards, Francis B. Stewart and Thomas J. Webb, to the rank of assistant professor.

DR. A. E. CAMERON, professor of zoology and entomology in the University of Saskatchewan, has been appointed lecturer in medical entomology in the department of zoology of the University of Edinburgh.

DR. JOHANNES WEIGELT, professor of geology in the University of Halle, has been appointed to the chair of geology in the University of Greifswald.

DR. HERMANN STEUDEL, of the department of physiology in the University of Berlin, has been made a full professor.

DISCUSSION AND CORRESPONDENCE

A NOTE ON THE FLUORESCENCE OF TEETH IN ULTRA-VIOLET RAYS

THAT teeth fluoresce under the excitation of ultraviolet rays has been known for some time. Hans Stubel[1] states that rabbit teeth fluoresce with a somewhat bluish intense white light. In human beings he finds the lens of the eye to be the strongest fluorescing organ, although the teeth are almost equally brilliant.

The following observations were made with a cored carbon arc and a Kromayer lamp, using as filters: (1) Corning purple-violet Ultra, (2) Corex G 986A, (3) Uviol cell with paranitrosodimethylaniline and a quartz cell of copper sulphate.

(1) The dentine fluoresces much more brilliantly than the enamel and seemingly with a bluer light.

(2) The white spot indicative of beginning dental caries does not fluroesce even though unpigmented. A similar effect is obtained by scratching through a paraffin coated tooth and placing in dilute acetic acid over night.

[1] *Arch. Ges. Physiol.*, 142, 1–14, 1911.

(3) Ashed enamel does not fluoresce, nor does dentine which has been boiled in 50 per cent. sodium hydroxide. On decalcifying dentine in dilute nitric acid the organic matrix retains its fluorescent power to an appreciable extent.

(4) Whereas serumal calculus fluoresces little if at all, salivary calculus fluoresces quite markedly with a reddish orange color (some old museum specimens emitted a white light).

These observations are significant in an investigation of the teeth as they may give a clue to the steps in the decalcification of enamel. From No. 3 the conclusion might be drawn that it was the organic matter which fluoresces. We have a means of determining on macroscopic pieces that we have enamel free from dentine. Further work is in progress.

H. C. BENEDICT

CHEMISTRY DEPARTMENT,
NORTHWESTERN UNIVERSITY DENTAL SCHOOL,
CHICAGO, ILL.

ON THE ANTIQUITY OF RELICS OF MAN AT FREDERICK, OKLAHOMA

IN the issue of SCIENCE for February 10, on pages 161 and 162, is an interesting contribution from Dr. Leslie Spier, of the University of Oklahoma, on the artifacts found recently at Frederick, Oklahoma. The present writer wishes to make some comments on this paper.

The most important statement made by Dr. Spier is that, according to the representations of Mr. Holloman, the owner of the pit, he picked up one arrow head from loose materials at the bottom of the front of the pit as it was being torn down by workmen. On the other hand, Mr. Holloman repeatedly told Director Figgins that he took it out of the hard conglomerate on the floor of the pit. Also the writer has Mr. Holloman's statement to the same effect in two or three letters. In one of these he informs me that he could not free the arrow-head himself, but had to call a workman to bring a tool. A pack knife was brought and with this the utensil was secured. Mr. Holloman further says that Dr. Spier misquotes him in saying that he picked the object from the loose materials. The writer can not for a moment doubt the veracity of either of these gentlemen. There must have been a misunderstanding of some remark made by Mr. Holloman.

In regard to the other flint object, probably a drill, Dr. Spier says that Mr. Holloman scratched it out of the face of the pit with his fingers. Now, if that object had fallen from the surface it would probably have become involved in the red clay which forms the uppermost stratum. In case it had fallen into the sand, this must have been sand which had been crushed, and it would have required no effort to pick up the little drill. Before the sand is disturbed it is compact enough to stand in a perpendicular face, and to release an instrument protruding from it would require some scratching with one's fingers.

Dr. Spier calls in question the genuineness of the metates. Before he cast this doubt on these utensils he ought to have requested Mr. Figgins to send him one or more of them for examination, and he doubtless would have received them.

Our writer thinks it possible that artifacts may yet be found on the surface of that ridge. I know of no reason why such things should not occur there, and if they are present and if the edge of the pit reaches them they will probably fall down; but this would not prove that those found by Mr. Holloman had fallen down and gotten into the compact sand and cemented conglomerate. And if arrow-heads and metates occur on the surface how is anybody to know whether they are recent productions or those of Aftonian time?

Our writer states certain other possibilities regarding the position of the artifacts. He tells us that we do not know the original position of the surface at this point with respect to the artifacts. He suggests that these lay on the surface of a depression and were subsequently covered by wash. It would be interesting to learn the probable history of a depression of this kind on that ridge. How did it begin, enlarge and finally disappear? It must have been from twenty to twenty-five feet deep in order to let the arrow head down to the conglomerate. There must, too, have been some way of escape for the water which first excavated and later refilled the depression. Mr. Holloman informs me that no ravine now comes within three hundred feet of the spot where the artifacts were discovered. The existing ravines at the foot of the ridge are cutting deeper instead of being refilled. Furthermore, the material filling such a hole or depression must have been mostly red clay; but Mr. Holloman did not observe any interruption of the strata furnishing the sand and gravel called for by his customers. He further says that there are now no depressions on the ridge where water stands after rains and no sink-holes.

Dr. Spier holds that there is an incongruity in the association of artifacts, as identified by our anthropologists, with fossil bones and teeth of animals of Aftonian age. There is an incongruity, but this is the creation of the anthropologists. They measure most things pertaining to human history in America by European standards. Because stone implements appear only late in Europe and are crude it is concluded that the art of working stone must have had a similar development in America. The writer believes that during the first interglacial stage men came from Asia and brought with them the art of skillfully chipping flint. Evidence of this has recently been furnished at Colorado, Texas; possibly, too, at Folsom, New Mexico.

Our anthropologists are forced to admit that the age of human bones and artifacts is to be determined by geology, but they insist on making their own geology. When the geology appears to be opposed to their view a variety of agencies are invoked to account for the apparent occurrences of Pleistocene man under the circumstances. It is rare that it can be established that the agency postulated has actually done the work. A long catalogue of these possible means might be compiled. The latest addition is the action of whirlwinds. This might well be called upon to explain the case at Frederick. What is more probable than that, while men slept, a mighty wind arose and, gathering up a cache of Comanchean implements of the wigwam and the chase, hurled them with violence against the face of that quarry and drove them into the hard sand and the conglomerate?

The writer has always admired the work done by Dr. Spier on the pebbles and artifacts systematically collected at Trenton, New Jersey. It had been declared that the deposit, a few feet thick only, had been so thoroughly disturbed by burrowing mammals, by the uprooting of trees, by the driving of palisades, and in other ways, that no conclusion could be reached as to the age of the artifacts embedded in it. Dr. Spier's work demonstrated that the pebbles and the artifacts had a definite arrangement in the stratum. There is general agreement that the deposit was laid down by Delaware River when the Wisconsin glacier had its front standing about sixty miles above Trenton. Dr. Spier's paper furnishes evidence hardly controvertible that the makers of the artifacts were in that region at the culmination of the Wisconsin glacial stage. The reader will enjoy a perusal of Dr. Clark Wissler's comments on the value of Dr. Spier's work.[1]

As is usual, our anthropological friends, on the announcement of the new discoveries of supposed Pleistocene man, sound the warning that we must proceed with caution. Do they exercise superior caution themselves? Was the anthropologist acting with due caution when he asserted, without the necessary investigation, that the deposit at Trenton had been thoroughly disturbed? Did another anthropologist display a cautious spirit when he insisted that masses of muck, sand and marl thrown back into a grave would soon rearrange themselves into their original relations and when he asserted he found muck, sand and marl undergoing restratification which had been

[1] *Scientific Monthly*, Vol. II, p. 234.

thrown on the dump by the dredge? Was even my friend Dr. Spier proceeding cautiously when he suggested a depression where the Frederick artifacts were discovered, apparently without inquiring of the owner of the pit and of the workmen whether they had observed anything of the kind?

Because certain existing tribes do not use metates Dr. Spier thinks it improbable that they were employed by people of early Pleistocene time. However, we do not yet know much about the climate of that period nor much about the resources and arts of the people.

OLIVER P. HAY

WASHINGTON, D. C.

ONE HUNDRED PER CENT. HATCH

ON October 31, 1927, the writer artificially impregnated 230 eggs taken from a small two-year-old hatchery reared brook trout, *Salvelinus fontinalis*. Two males were used to effect fertilization. Instead of following the accepted method of washing the eggs soon after insemination, the eggs were allowed to harden in the milt. After sixty-one days of incubation, 230 normal fry emerged tail first with elongated yolk-sacs which is an index of perfect fertilization.

In state, commercial and private hatcheries, the writer has met with wonderful success by holding the eggs in milt during the agglutination period.

These results indicate that the concentration of sperm suspensions may have a direct influence on the micropyle of the egg, which activates complete fertilization when agglutination takes place in the milt.

RALPH C. JACKSON

U. S. FISHERIES STATION,
NASHUA, N. H.

MORE DATA

IN spite of all the discussion on the subject that has been going on in SCIENCE, here is Mr. Sainton, of Cornell, saying (in the last number of the *Journal of The Optical Society of America*) "data is." It is known that Cornell is a special sinner in this respect.

As regards the two wrong pronunciations of *data* (lately discussed in SCIENCE), *dăta*, it may be pointed out, is far worse than *däta*, for the reason that those who adopt the thoroughgoing modern pronunciation of their Latin and Greek may feel obliged to apply it to *datum* too.

It is remarkable what a high literary standard the medical people have preserved in their scientific language. But they are wrong in sometimes saying "photo-sensitive." One can say "photo-esthetic" or "light-sensitive," but "photo-sensory" (or photo-sensitive) is a sad hybrid.

CHRISTINE LADD-FRANKLIN

COLUMBIA UNIVERSITY

SCIENTIFIC BOOKS

Romance of the Sun. By MARY PROCTOR, xii + 266 pages. Harper and Brothers, London and New York, 1927. $2.50.

MISS MARY PROCTOR'S book, "Romance of the Sun," contains many interesting pages for those who have little or no knowledge of astronomy, and who wish information about that part of this science which deals with the nearest star, our own sun. The book is written in popular language so that it can be read easily by any one. The sun is so important, not only to astronomers for their investigations, but also to every person and to everything living on this earth, that it is well to have books on this subject written for all types of readers.

After a brief description of the appearance of the sun's surface, four chapters are devoted to the problem of finding the distance from the earth to the sun. Accounts are given of the attempts made to find this distance accurately by observing the various transits of Venus across the sun's disc which occurred between 1629 and 1882. Horrock's observation of the transit of Venus in 1639 is well described, and made more vivid by quotations from the writings of that exceptional young minister who was such an enthusiastic astronomical observer. The chapter on Sir David Gill's observations of Mars in connection with this same problem is likewise made more interesting by several extracts from Lady Gill's book, "Six Months in Ascension." Just at the end of this chapter, on page 70, there is an important misprint. The sun's mass is given as 32,000 times that of the earth instead of 332,000 times the earth's mass.

The fifth and sixth chapters deal with the constitution of the sun and its atmosphere, the analysis of its light and the subject of solar energy, especially the fraction of that energy received by the earth. Several times in the descriptions of phenomena on the sun, phrases are used which might give to readers without astronomical knowledge the impression that the sun was at least in part liquid. The words "Vast oceans of molten metal," on page 71, form such a phrase which can hardly be considered appropriate when applied to a body like the sun, which is known to be purely gaseous.

Even in a popular book of this length, it would seem that a fuller treatment of the source of the sun's heat would have been of interest to any reader. No reference is made to the latest theory, now generally accepted by astronomers, that the sun's energy is due to the radiation of its mass. A more detailed description of the sun's surface would have increased the value of the book for the majority of readers. The subject of sun-spots is rather neglected. A brief and superficial description of sun-spots is given in the introduction. Nothing is said of the periodicity of these spots, or of the relation of the sun-spot curve to terrestrial phenomena and to the shape of the solar corona. Although hydrogen and calcium flocculi are referred to and also shown in two illustrations, no explanation of these terms is given.

Similarly there is a lack of explanation in the case of some of the instruments used in the study of the sun; especially in the case of the spectroheliograph and the spectrohelioscope, which are not so well known as the spectroscope. Brief descriptions of the main features of these instruments might have been given which would not have been at all technical but would have made much clearer the sections and quotations about observations with these instruments.

The remaining four chapters discuss the corona and its observation, and give descriptions of various eclipse experiences. It hardly seems worth while to give up twenty-five pages of one of these chapters to the unsuccessful attempts to photograph the corona without an eclipse, when in view of our present knowledge the reason for these failures is so obviously due to the feebleness of the light from the corona compared with the brilliant light of the sun itself.

In the description of the cause of a solar eclipse, no definition of a partial eclipse is given, though mention is made of a partial eclipse of the sun on January 24, 1925, in London. Those of us who remember this as the total eclipse seen under such favorable conditions by so many people in New York and Connecticut may be pardoned if we are a little disappointed to find no other reference in this book to this particular eclipse.

The quotations from the personal eclipse experiences of the writer and other observers can not fail to interest all readers, and to make those who have not seen a total eclipse eager to have that opportunity. After all, no description can do justice to the thrill of actually seeing this wonderful phenomenon. The description in the last chapter of the eclipse of June 29, 1927, visible in England and Norway, gives an excellent picture of the numerous activities connected with the observation of a total eclipse at the present time. The attempts to observe the eclipse from airplanes were only partially successful because of clouds, but gave to those who were in the airplanes experiences that would always be remembered.

Ida Barney

Yale University Observatory

SCIENTIFIC APPARATUS AND LABORATORY METHODS

MOUNTING CHICK EMBRYOS

In elementary courses in embryology sagittal sections often present considerable difficulty to the student. One reason for this is the practical impossibility of getting a truly sagittal section extending the

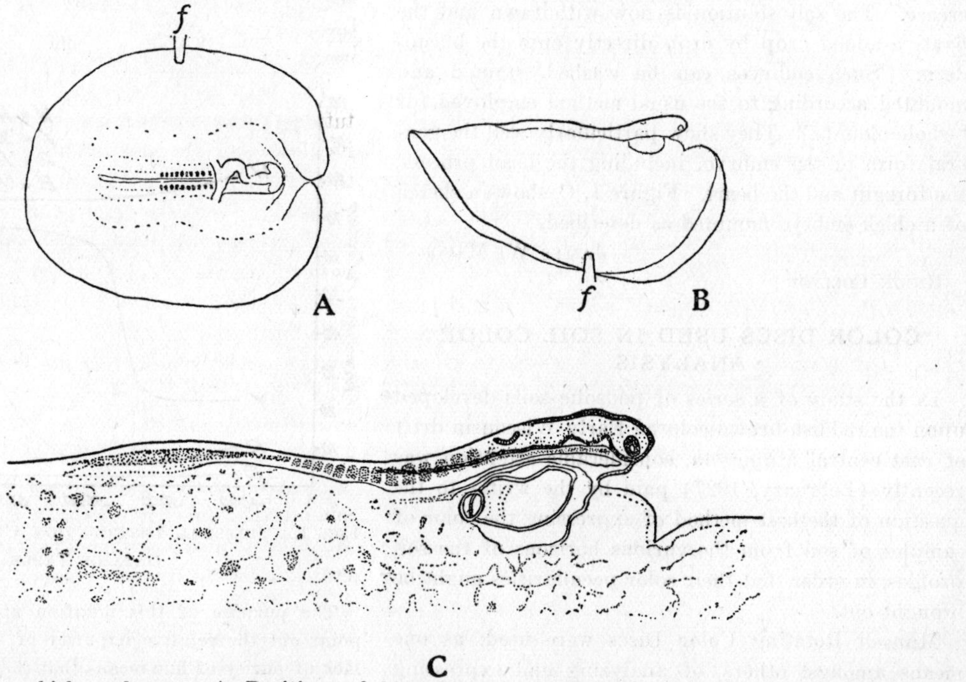

Fig. 1. Mounting chick embryos. A. Position of blastoderm in watch glass ventral side up, f, point at which forceps grasp edge of blastoderm. B. Folded blastoderm with right side folded over left side so that embryo lies along crease. C. Side view of embryo mounted as described.

whole length of the embryo; another is due to the fact that sagittal sections lack many of the structures which the student has come to regard as landmarks in his study of transverse sections. On the other hand, the preparation of sagittal sections presents difficulties for the technician.

The present writer has used for some years in his classes preparations which show the eight to fourteen somite (thirty to thirty-six hours incubation) chick in side view, in place of sagittal sections. Such preparations are scarcely more difficult to make than the usual whole mounts and help greatly the student in his attempt to visualize the structure of the embryo of this stage. The method has up to the present been used only on embryos before the beginning of torsion in the head region. It is possible, however, that it might be modified to apply to embryos of somewhat later stages.

The egg is opened in salt solution and the blastoderm cut from the yolk and floated into a watch glass in the usual way. It must then be turned over while still alive so that its dorsal surface is underneath (Figure 1, A). The lateral edge of the blastoderm directly opposite the middle of the embryo is then lifted with forceps and folded over so that the embryo appears along the folded edge and projects from it (Figure 1, B), while the half of the blastoderm which was lifted now lies over the other half which remained in position in the watch glass. The operation of folding the blastoderm can best be carried out under a binocular microscope. It is important to make the fold such that the entire length of the embryo lies along the crease. The salt solution is now withdrawn and the fixative added drop by drop directly onto the blastoderm. Such embryos can be washed, stained and mounted according to the usual method employed for "whole mounts." They show particularly well the general form of the embryo, including the head process, the foregut and the heart. Figure 1, C, shows a sketch of a chick embryo mounted as described.

JAMES W. MAVOR

UNION COLLEGE

COLOR DISCS USED IN SOIL COLOR ANALYSIS

IN the study of a series of podsolic soils developed upon the reddish-brown colored Early Wisconsin drift of east central Minnesota, considerable attention was recently (February, 1927) paid by the writer to the question of the best method of expressing the color of samples of soil from the various horizons of the soil profiles, in order that their color peculiarities might be brought out.

Munsell Rotating Color Discs were used, as one means amongst others, of analyzing and expressing the color of the disturbed soil samples. These discs are essentially Maxwell's discs, of stiff paper, colored "Red," "Yellow," "White" and Black." They are made to rotate upon a motor-driven shaft, and provide a means of matching a very great number of colors simply by altering the relative proportions of the different color discs exposed to the eye. Each one of the four almost new color discs was examined with a Keuffel and Esser Spectrophotometer, with the results given in Table I. Their spectral distribution curves are plotted in Figure 1. Each value for relative brightness represents the mean of five closely agreeing photometer readings. The standard white used in the machine was a freshly scraped surface of a block of magnesium carbonate.

TABLE I. ANALYSIS OF COLOR DISCS USED IN SOIL COLOR ANALYSIS

Wave length	Relative brightness expressed as percentage			
	"Red" Disc	"Yellow" Disc	"White" Disc	"Black" Disc
	Per cent.	Per cent.	Per cent.	Per cent.
7000 Å	60.2	70.8	75.6	3.4
6500	55.6	66.2	73.8	2.5
6000	22.5	66.8	74.0	2.3
5500	5.8	63.0	74.0	2.3
5000	6.0	22.0	76.2	2.2
4500	10.2	22.2	80.5	3.0
$\frac{I_{6500}}{I_{5000}}$	9.27	3.01	......	......
$\frac{I_{6500}}{I_{6000}}$	2.47	.99	......	......

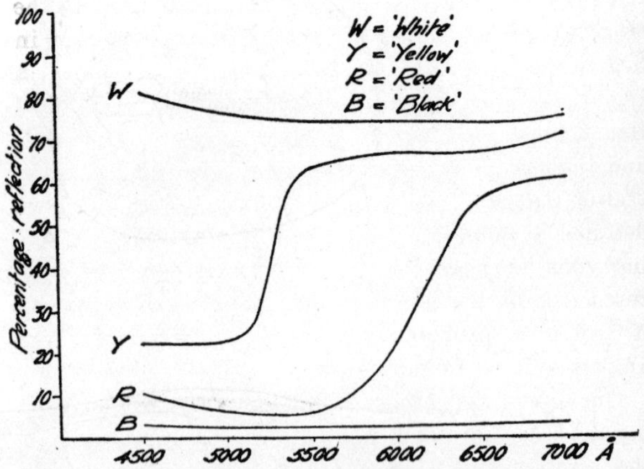

FIG. 1. SPECTRAL DISTRIBUTION CURVES PLOTTED FROM DATA OF TABLE I.

The purpose of this notation upon the subject is to point out the relative impurity of the color discs. This lack of purity of hue means that the percentages assigned to the various colors used on the disc are far from representing percentages of pure spectral hues. The actual percentage transmission of spectral red, for example, from the "Red" disc is lower than that from the "Yellow" disc. To the eye, of course, the differences in reflection of light of these wave lengths appears extreme in the opposite direction. By means of the ratio $\frac{I_{6500}}{I_{5000}}$ the different appearances to the eye of these two discs is more satisfactorily represented. Similarly the ratio $\frac{\text{"Red"}}{\text{"Yellow"}}$ as determined by color disc analysis is found to bring out better the apparent striking color differences of two soils.

G. B. BODMAN

DIVISION OF SOILS,
UNIVERSITY OF MINNESOTA

SPECIAL ARTICLES

LIVING CELLS TWO AND A HALF CENTURIES OLD

RESEARCHES dealing with the growth and hydrostatics of trees and other massive plants have led to a consideration of the activities of living cells in the interior of large stems. Rigidity and other mechanical features of tree-trunks are such that living cells in layers a year old can not grow or divide and hence the existence of a living cell in layers 50 or 100 years old may be taken as an example of a protoplast which has carried on an individual existence for that length of time. In many trees all living cells perish when the splint or sap wood of which they form a part is converted into heartwood. A notable case was recently described in SCIENCE in which medullary cells of the redwood remained alive in the heartwood attaining an age of over a century.[1]

Professor Faul has recently called attention to the work of J. H. White in which tyloses were seen in heartwood of beech, maple, oak and other trees in regions invaded by *Fomes applantus*. It is implied that these formations take place only in living cells and that their development was induced by the penetrating fungus. The case seems to call for a more detailed examination. Now that the existence of living cells in heartwood and in old wood has been rescued from the negations of widely used text-books it is highly probable that numerous additional examples will be found.[2]

Our quest for other examples of long-lived cells has had for its chief purpose the determination of the progressive changes in protoplasts which attain great age and to appraise the conditions endured. A desert tree *Parkinsonia microphylla*, which has been used for tests in conduction and growth has yielded results of interest in this matter.

This bean tree is a prominent member of the desert flora of the southwest and because of its smooth green bark is known as "Palo verde." Despite the fact that its growth in thickness is at an extremely low rate, 0.2 to 0.6 mm annually, the trunk is soft and brittle, losing 45 per cent. of its dry weight in two days in the drying oven at 100° C. Bark and wood are heavily loaded with crystals, mostly calcium carbonate. The ash constitutes as much as 3.4 per cent. of the dry weight.

Sections of stems 10 cm in diameter and over 75 years old, first examined, showed occasional living ray-cells near the center and also a number of tracheids in which the nucleus and cytoplasm were plainly in a normal and active condition.

An older excentric trunk which stood in a leaning position showed sound moist wood in the flank which was 9 cm in thickness. Several counts of layers by Dr. Forrest Shreve gave a basis for the estimate that the age of the trunk might be safely taken as between 275 to 300 years old. Living ray cells and tracheids could be seen in sections near the center without staining and with a dry objective. We have no hesitancy

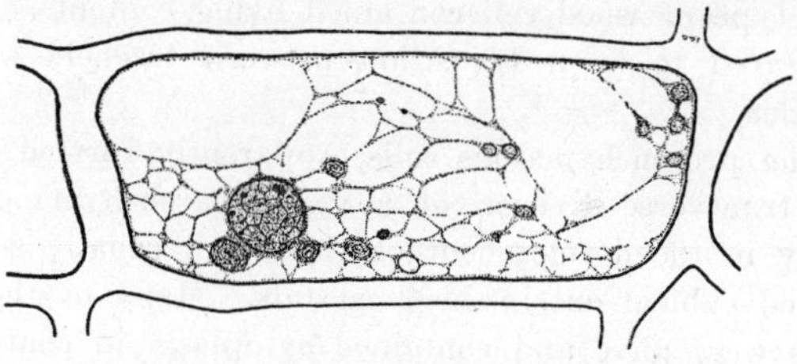

FIG. 1. Ray cell of Parkinsonia over 250 years old. Reticulum of nucleus and cytoplasm well defined.

in announcing that these elements may be safely considered as having an age of over 250 years.

Macroscopically the stele of *Parkinsonia microphylla* presented a nearly uniform light straw color sometimes with a small central core of heartwood (duramen). In other words, sapwood (alburnum) made up almost the entire mass of wood. Elements of the xylem consisted of tracheids typical in shape; coarsely pitted vessels; elongated thick-walled cells with blunt ends, and short prosenchymatous cells in vertical rows near the medullary rays.

The tracheids composed by far the greatest part of the xylem. They measured approximately 20 microns in length. Those laid down at the end of the growing season in the oldest wood near the central pith had walls averaging 4 microns when measured between lumina of two tracheids, while those formed in spring and summer and measured in the same way averaged 3 microns in thickness. Comparative measurements of tracheids in xylem formed in recent years was 3.2

[1] MacDougal, D. T., and G. M. Smith, SCIENCE 66, 456–457. 1927.

[2] Faul, J. H. "Living Cells in Heartwood," SCIENCE 67, 296. 1928.

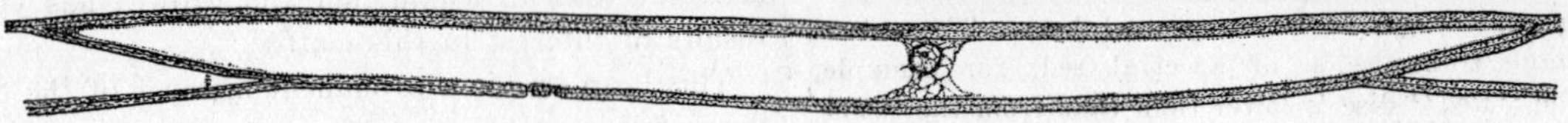

FIG. 2. Tracheid of Parkinsonia over 250 years old. Nucleus plump and normal.

microns for those laid down in the fall and 4.2 microns for those formed in spring and summer.

Living tracheids are numerous, even in the oldest part of the stem. Part of an annual ring in one bundle consisting of 120 tracheids showed nuclei and more or less cytoplasm in approximately 50 per cent. of the tracheids. Likewise many of the medullary ray cells were living. Nuclei in both tracheids and ray cells were large, well-rounded and clearly showed a reticulum. One to three nucleoli were present.

The vessels or tracheae were coarsely pitted and few in number. Some of them contained a substance which stained brown with Haidenhain's iron-alum haematoxylin. Otherwise they were not unlike those found in woody dicotyledonous plants.

Elongated cells with coarsely pitted end walls and abundant pits in lateral (radial) walls were found near the rays but extended vertically. Frequently this type of wood cell contained living contents. It appeared to be a transition between tracheid and trachea.

The prosenchymatous cells, apparently formed by the transverse division of a xylem parenchyma cell early in the development of the wood, usually contained cubical or six-sided crystals. Many of these cells were alive and contained cytoplasm in contact with crystals in various stages of development.

In previous discussions attention was called to the fact that cells attaining great age were of the thin-walled parenchymatous type. Later Dr. F. H. Long prepared a manuscript now ready for publication in which epidermal cells, including stomata of the tree-cactus of Arizona, are shown to attain an age of over a century.

The preceding paragraphs record the existence of ray cells of the thin-walled type in Parkinsonia and also of typical tracheids with heavy walls in parts of trunks formed over two and a half centuries ago. No observations have been made as to the length of the period of enlargement of these elements, but as the season's growth of this desert tree is completed within the brief period of the summer rains it may safely be taken to be something less than a week. Existence is continuous for 12 or 13 thousand weeks, thus setting a new high ratio between the developmental period and the period of mature existence.

Heartwood is not always formed in Parkinsonia, the vessels are large and the protoplasmic strands connecting neighboring cells are well defined and numerous. By this arrangement the innermost cells are much more closely connected with the surface layers of the trunk than in the redwood or the central parts of other trunks.

The cells capable of attaining great age appear to lose their embryonic character very early. At the same time surfaces of wounds of this tree dry out so quickly that rarely is any notable callus formation found. The living cells of the trunk endure a range of temperature higher than those to which trunks of mesophytic trees are subject. The actual range, however, may be not nearly so great as those attained by cells in flattened stems in cacti in which mid-day temperatures of over 50° C. are common.

The gases in the vessels and intercellular spaces of trunks of Parkinsonia are extractable at about the same rate as in Quercus. Samples taken from bores extending 10 to 12 cm or to the center of trunks at 0.3 to 0.4 atm showed never less than 1 per cent. carbon dioxide and the proportions in some cases were as high as 16 per cent.

The above notes are intended as an announcement of the discovery of living cells older than those noted in any record in which estimates of age have been included. Elements of Parkinsonia, including ray cells and tracheids, have been found near the center of a trunk nearly three centuries old. The appearance of the nuclei and cytoplasm is not widely away from that of young cells and it may be safely predicted that the examination of older trees would reveal living elements of even greater age.

The long-lived cells endure a wide range of temperatures and the gases in the vessels which are dissolved in their sap are very high in carbon dioxide. Mineral elements of which calcium is the chief component accumulate in the wood so that the ash constitutes 3.4 per cent. of the dry weight. The ash of beech wood forms but 0.355 per cent. of its dry weight. The caenocytic arrangement of the living cells is so marked as to suggest that the connections afforded by the heavy connecting protoplasmic threads may be important as conductive organs maintained between the deeply lying old protoplasts and the surface layers.

D. T. MACDOUGAL,
J. G. BROWN

LABORATORY FOR PLANT PHYSIOLOGY,
CARNEGIE INSTITUTION OF WASHINGTON
AND UNIVERSITY OF ARIZONA

SCIENCE

VOL. LXVII MAY 4, 1928 No. 1740

CONTENTS

The American Association for the Advancement of Science:

Malaria: DR. A. M. STIMSON 449

Parasitology in Relation to Medical Problems of the South: DR. C. C. BASS 454

Willem Einthoven: PROFESSOR H. B. WILLIAMS 456

Scientific Events:

Activities of the Rockefeller Foundation; The International Congress of Photography; The Selection of Chief of the U. S. Bureau of American Ethnology; Annual Meeting of the American Association of Museums; The National Academy of Sciences 458

Scientific Notes and News 460

University and Educational Notes 463

Discussion and Correspondence:

Deafness in Pre-Columbian Peru: DR. ROY L. MOODIE. *Production of Potato Tuber Necrosis:* PROFESSOR A. H. GILBERT. *"General Zoology":* PROFESSOR WILLIAM JOHN DAKIN. *The Pronunciation of Research:* DR. EDWIN E. SLOSSON, DR. PAUL NICHOLAS LEECH, PROFESSOR W. T. MAGRUDER 464

Quotations:

Popular Science 466

Scientific Books:

Carpenter on the Biology of Insects: DR. L. O. HOWARD. *Ramaley on Colorado Plant Life:* DR. JOHN W. HARSHBERGER 467

Special Articles:

Multiple Positively Charged Radioactive Ions: DR. LEONARD B. LOEB. *Crossing-over between Chromosomes of the Killifish:* DR. ALLAN C. FRASER and MYRON GORDON 468

Science News x

SCIENCE: A Weekly Journal devoted to the Advancement of Science, edited by J. McKeen Cattell and published every Friday by

THE SCIENCE PRESS

New York City: Grand Central Terminal.

Lancaster, Pa. Garrison, N. Y.

Annual Subscription, $6.00. Single Copies, 15 Cts.

SCIENCE is the official organ of the American Association for the Advancement of Science. Information regarding membership in the Association may be secured from the office of the permanent secretary, in the Smithsonian Institution Building, Washington, D. C.

MALARIA[1]

MALARIA is a subject of multifarious scientific interest. Its study leads us into many biological considerations involving an undetermined number of species representing at least three phyla of the animal kingdom: protozoa, articulata, chordata.

Considering only human malaria, the subject has important biological, medical, economic and cultural aspects. The topic could have been profitably discussed under the general heading of "Contributions of Science to Medicine," and it is equally adapted to consideration under the caption "Contributions of Medicine to Science," since it is a toss-up whether the scientists taught the doctors more than the latter repaid them. It was convenient when Dr. Laveran discovered the parasite to find that the systematists had a pigeonhole ready for it. It was of immense help when Dr. Ross demonstrated mosquito transmission to find that entomology could furnish many ready-made criteria for discriminating between various kinds of these insects, and many pertinent facts regarding their anatomy and physiology. It has been a pleasure to observe the repayment of these large debts in kind, in the numerous contributions which medical men have made to protozoology and entomology incidental to the study of malaria.

I am not competent to discuss malaria from the standpoint of the protozoologist, the entomologist, even the malariologist, or any other variety of scientist having an academically recognized standing. My contribution must emanate from the modest outlook of the student of public health. The only advantage to be claimed for this outlook is that while too shallow to claim authority in any one scientific specialty, it may be broad enough to appreciate the significance of scientific research in many apparently remote fields and to appropriate to the cause of human welfare scientific knowledge wherever found. I would not have you put a purely pragmatic interpretation on this attitude. Let me say in illustration that I think it is doubtful from which source the child who receives malaria lessons in school derives the greater benefit, from the purely informational source which tells him to swat the mosquito or he will become sick, or from

[1] Presented as part of a symposium on "The Medical Problems of the South" at a joint meeting of the American Association for the Advancement of Science and the American Public Health Association, Nashville, December 28, 1927.

the inspirational source which opens up to his vision a world in which knowledge for its own sake is something worth living for—and worth avoiding malaria for. Culture and malaria are directly opposed, and if we admit that malaria conquered the culture of Greece and of Rome, it was at that time a decadent culture, and we can reassure ourselves that the insurgent culture of America will conquer malaria. At the same time that we visualize a vicious circle in which malaria leads through disease to poverty and ignorance and back to malaria, we must not lose sight of that concentric circle in which education, improved living standards and even a little initial financial help tend to eliminate malaria and produce a higher culture and a greater human prosperity.

Malaria has been stated upon the eminent authority of Dr. Henry Carter to be the only disease of man which is able to render an area of the earth's surface uninhabitable. Such diseases as bubonic plague, Asiatic cholera, yellow fever and hookworm may take a terrible toll of a human population, but even at their worst they do leave a battered and ragged remnant to carry on. Malaria at its worst prevents people from living in the area where it prevails. Fortunately, we in America do not suffer from such intensities of prevalence or malignancy, but we still have areas, not large and not continuous, where more than half of the population may show evidences of past or present malarial infection. The actual death-rate is not considerable, and it is known to health officials not to be accurately measurable. Our malaria in general is of too mild a nature to permit of its measurement by the death-rate. Of far greater significance is the morbidity rate, for this gives us an index of the social importance of the disease. It is not the relatively few individuals who are killed outright whose removal importantly hampers the march of progress. It is the infinitely larger numbers of the maimed and stunted whose impaired product constitutes a cultural and economic loss.

In the United States malaria was formerly much more widely distributed geographically than it is at the present time. Even during the past generation it has become remarkably restricted. During my own memory it was fairly prevalent in one of the boroughs of New York City. At the present time we find it of considerable public health significance only in the south Atlantic coast, the Gulf coast and the lower Mississippi valley regions, with the exception of isolated areas, notably one in a Pacific coast state. And even in this distribution careful field surveys have shown the reassuring fact that the affected areas are not confluent, but spotted here and there, so that the problem of eradication has become less formidable with increasing knowledge. There is perhaps no hotbed of malaria, in the tropical sense, within our boundaries at the present time, but areas of serious prevalence do remain, chiefly in the so-called delta region of the Mississippi River valley. Moreover, in at least one area in the southwest, the disease is on the increase. It is, therefore, no time to stop control work, but rather time for redoubled effort with the positive assurance of ultimate success.

It has been claimed by some observers that the diminution of malaria in the United States has been due solely to the advance of civilization and culture. In some areas of low prevalence and intensities this has undoubtedly been true. Malaria has literally been built out in certain places incidentally to the concentration of populations, without intentional effort having been directed toward eradicating the disease. On the other hand, it has repeatedly been demonstrated that intentional effort on the part of health agencies has resulted in the virtual eradication of the disease from areas where previously no tendency toward diminution was observable. It may also be claimed with reasonable supporting evidence that in certain places of high incidence and intensity the intentional control of malaria must come before civilization and culture can gain a foothold.

It is, therefore, a matter of congratulation that at the present time in all the states in which malaria offers any considerable public health menace there is a definite established machinery in the state health department for the study and control of this disease. This provision has come about within less than a score of years, since at the time when the Public Health Service first undertook the intensive study of malaria not a single state had made this provision.

I have stated that malaria is a many-sided subject. According to the approach to this subject which our experience and training determine, we may entertain different views both as to the cause of malaria and as to the best methods of combating it. One may regard it merely as an instance of protozoan parasitism in man and advise concentration upon a program of medical treatment of individuals. Another with entomological leanings may think of it as a typical insect-borne disease and seek to get rid of it solely by exterminating the insect. Another with a historical background may see in malaria only a manifestation of crude unconquered nature which will succumb to the general improvements incidental to the growth of civilization—the so-called "bonification" of European writers. But we must let the sociologists and economists have their say, and they will put their fingers on the sore spot of social and economic maladjustment, and tell us, "Here is where your trouble lies, and this is the place to begin your curative operation."

I do not know how many more different kinds of specialists might wish to contribute their wisdom to this problem, but I do know that it seems to be clearly up to the health official to do something about it—and after all he is the logical man to do it. It is he and his research workers who must go into the swamps where the pestilence breeds, must go into the rickety homes of tenant farmers and learn to call the children by their first names and in other ways live with and learn at first hand the many aspects of this disease. Then in the laboratory they must examine blood smears, dissect mosquitoes, try out larvicides, and in the study they must read the world literature, for no hint is to be neglected.

And what does the student of public health make of all the various view-points and advice which the literature brings to his study. Perhaps I do not arrogate too much authority in saying that he feels very much with regard to malaria as a disease upon a population, as a competent physician does toward malaria as a disease of an individual patient, and that is that both as to cause and remedy one must discriminate, that there is no such thing as a stock diagnosis and that the treatment must be selected to fit local conditions and the individual. This parallel may be carried further. If a doctor visits a patient, makes a diagnosis of malaria, prescribes his routine treatment and goes on his way without having noticed that the patient is also suffering from a broken leg, we call him a charlatan and sue him for malpractice. So also we should discountenance the action of a health official, who having determined the existence of malaria in a community would immediately divert all its health resources toward the eradication of that one disease without first considering the other health needs.

If these premises be true, first that antimalaria measures must be selected with reference to local conditions, second that the emphasis on antimalarial work should be proportionate to the relative local importance of the disease, it must follow that effective work must be administered by some competent agency completely familiar with the local situation. This is essential not only to the work which a community may wish to do of its own initiative and at its own cost, but furnishes the only effective means through which outside agencies, be they governmental, benevolent or developmental, can effect the desired improvements.

This reasoning, applied not only to the malaria problem but to health problems in general, has actuated the program of the U. S. Public Health Service, which attempts to encourage the establishment throughout the country of effective official local health organizations or units. Since the rural areas suffer the greatest need, emphasis has been chiefly upon county or district organizations consisting of a health officer and such inspectors, visiting nurses and other personnel as he may require. While there is no panacea for malaria, there is one essential requirement for its eradication and that is a competent health authority on the spot.

Malaria, as it arises from what may for the time be called purely natural causes, presents problems enough, and it has only been after years of patient work that we are beginning to solve them, when to add to our troubles along comes man himself with a number of modern activities and artificially multiplies our difficulties. Curiously enough these activities are all intended to be beneficent, and would be so if their directors were properly concerned with health matters. High roads and railroads have been built through backward areas with the intent of developing them, of bringing in enlightenment and progress and taking out an increased product, but constructed in such a way as to bring this deadening disease malaria to the very populations which it was intended to benefit. This occurs, of course, through such bits of carelessness as blocking off loops of running streams and leaving undrained borrow pits which then become the breeding places of innumerable anopheline mosquitoes. Agricultural drainage, surely a beneficial undertaking in the abstract, has actually had the effect in some places of establishing permanent breeding places within a half mile of every inhabitant of the area treated. This is because the ditches become partly filled up at places and converted into a succession of small pools. Again, projects for the impounding of streams, intended to harness the force of gravity for the use of man, may succeed, so far as the health officer can see, only in greatly increasing the gravity of the local malaria problem. However, the correction of these errors is by fairly obvious means and probably offers no difficulties which may not be overcome within a few years.

Since we all have some personal bias, I may as well confess to mine with relation to malaria. To me it seems in final analysis, under our American conditions, to be chiefly an economic problem. Dr. Weir Mitchell once said that the majority of his patients could be cured merely by receiving a legacy of $25,-000. Undoubtedly health and happiness came cheaper in those days. Although malaria belongs to a far different category of diseases from that with which Dr. Mitchell dealt, it is nevertheless one of the diseases the immunity to which is purchasable. The proper approach, however, is not to solicit outside funds of charitable origin with which to bless the suffering for a brief period, afterwards forgetting about them, but to devise cheap enough methods of eradication so that those who really wish to get rid of malaria can afford to do so at their own expense and on a permanent basis. As regards thickly settled communities—cities, towns, villages—where the wealth, even though scanty, is relatively high per square foot of ground surface, this has already been fairly satisfactorily accomplished. It would indeed be a rather decrepit specimen of the American community which could not afford to rid itself of malaria by applying intelligently methods already at hand—or else one peculiarly unfortunately situated. But in rural areas where the population is sparsely scattered and money even scantier, and the surrounding breeding areas are vast, the problem is far more difficult. And here again we come upon those economic causes which are associated with faulty or questionable business methods. Tenant farming and single crops for example require for their successful management an intelligence and a humanity not always encountered, and one result of their failure is malaria. The program of education to correct these conditions must be a slow one. Perhaps it is too much to hope that farsighted statesmen will arise who will contribute to the solution of a part of the problem, or that inspired business organizations, alive to all the economies which arise from health protection, will see the gold mines which lie waiting to reward the application of higher intelligence.

Meanwhile, much has been done to help diminish malaria even under existing unfavorable economic conditions. We can now cheaply screen and otherwise mosquito proof almost the most disreputable tenant home which a negligent landlord will tolerate, and if the tenant will swat the few mosquitoes which succeed in getting in, and stay indoors at night during the breeding season he is much more likely to stay on his feet during the year than he is without these precautions, and his wife and children likewise. This means that the crops under his charge are much more likely to be planted, cultivated and gathered. In the aggregate this means much, but not the complete eradication of malaria.

Airplane dusting with Paris green will control the breeding of anopheles mosquitoes in almost any kind of tree or weed-grown swamp. The cost data are not completely worked out, but I will hazard the personal statement that it is within the means of, and would repay, any sufficiently large combination of owners of contiguous or nearby plantations where malaria is a serious matter. I can not at present see why this measure combined with medical treatment of those already infected should not completely control malaria during the seasons of its employment. This would liberate a considerable man power not only for the cultivation of existing farm land but for the reclamation to agriculture of swamp lands now worse than useless. This is one of the opportunities which big business may see.

We are accustomed to big things in America, and one big thing which I think many of us here present will live to see is the practical eradication of malaria. Such a hopeful prophecy, however, must be predicated upon the continued progressive acceptance of scientific findings and their intelligent application to this problem of human welfare.

I am quite aware of the fact that the Malaria Committee of the League of Nations, after able and prolonged study of conditions obtaining chiefly in Europe, advises a general policy of amelioration or palliation rather than one of thorough-going eradication, but this is apparently only because, as they state, their mandate confines them to measures which require little expenditure of money. They are thus led to ignore relatively such measures as the broad scale attack upon the breeding of mosquitoes, and to concentrate upon so-called direct methods which deal with the patient and his house, though advocating the general raising of the cultural and economic level. This is doubtless wise advice adapted to the areas concerned, and in some instances to conditions which may be found in America. However, places in the United States where conditions obtain which render such a restricted policy necessary do not represent the culture of America, which, as is well known, demands that every citizen may claim as a birthright a bathtub, a flivver, and a radio set, and if these, why not freedom from malaria which costs much less? Incidentally, we must ask the psychologists why it is possible for the knowledge of a popular subject like radio to become diffused throughout the land in a few months so that the majority of inhabitants over the age of fifteen are able to discuss ohms, wave-lengths, filaments and grids, interference, audio-frequency and a hundred other hitherto unfamiliar subjects, and to apply knowledge of them to getting results, when it takes years of teaching to spread the simple truth that malaria is conveyed by mosquitoes and that if you separate mosquitoes from man by whatever means, you prevent the spread of the disease.

Malaria is controllable in America at the present time if the public would be as lavish with money for that purpose as it is for radio. Since the public gives no indication of becoming lavish in this direction, it must be the work of science to cheapen the price until it becomes sufficiently attractive to make all classes willing to purchase freedom from this disease. At the same time we must work away at overcoming those psychological and social impediments which always stand in the way of innovations for the public good unless the latter have the happy appeal of radio—or chewing gum. These impediments are well known to consist of such factors as the inertia of habit, the conservatism of the self-interested, ignorance and the fear of loss in untried investments.

It would not be proper to complete this address without some reference to recent scientific research in the subject. The observations of what may be called experimental clinical malaria have been fruitful in correcting and making more precise our conception of the course of this disease. It is seldom that the physician is able to study a disease by direct inoculation of the human subject with the causative organism, and then by observing by all the means of measurement at his command the natural course of events. This was made possible in the case of malaria by the fact that inoculation with malaria organisms exerted a favorable and sometimes curative effect upon sufferers from general paresis and other forms of chronic and hitherto incurable diseases of the central nervous system. It became therefore not only legitimate but a duty to explore further this means of benefitting the suffering.

The cure of malaria itself by medication has been shown by investigations within the past few years not to be the simple matter which it was assumed to be only a generation ago. At that time quinine was considered a specific and when administered in time and properly an almost infallible remedy. We still find it invaluable for preventing the explosive manifestations of malaria and keeping our patients on their feet, but we have learned to our sorrow that there are grave limitations to its potency in completing the destruction of the parasite or "sterilizing" the patient with regard to it. The practical application of this fact to malaria control is obvious, since some other means is needed in order to render our patients incapable of infecting other persons through the mediation of the mosquito. New therapeutic preparations have been introduced which appear to be vastly superior to quinine in this respect, but which will require the test of large scale field application in order to determine their real and permanent value.

From the entomological standpoint much of interest is developing in this country. The extensive prevalence of an anopheles species hitherto regarded as a scientific curiosity has been determined for certain areas—I refer to *Anopheles atropos*. Its significance, real or potential, as regards malaria remains to be determined. That merely because it is an anopheles it is necessarily important to malaria of course does not follow, since it has been found, for example, that both *crucians* and *punctipennis* have very limited practical significance, although known to be capable of developing the parasite. Another species, *maculipennis,* distinguishable only with difficulty from the prevalent and destructive *quadrimaculatus,* but having different habits which would affect its control, is known to exist locally in this country and further study of its potentialities are demanded.

Despite the attitude of the Malaria Commission previously referred to, larvicides will continue to be useful in America, and their study is urgently demanded, not only from the standpoint of malaria control but from that of exterminating the salt marsh mosquito pests. Paris green has demonstrated its value, and we have Dr. Barber to thank for introducing its use as a larvicide, after painstaking tests. At first designed for the control of relatively small pools, by the simple process of dusting by hand, it has now been found absolutely effective in controlling anopheles breeding in large areas, even if they be overgrown with trees and other vegetation, when distributed by airplanes. An interesting feature of this latter mode of distribution is the almost incredible ability of the dust to penetrate the foliage of vegetation and become deposited on the underlying water which would seem to be protected by the trees and shrubs. This property appears to be associated with an electrical charge imparted to the dust by friction during its release. Studies of these electrical phenomena and the influence of materials and states of aggregation upon them are in progress. Paris green is cheap and efficient and may be the best larvicide which can be devised, but further studies are desirable to determine the exact limitations of this method and to devise refinements in the direction of economy.

RECAPITULATION

To recapitulate the factors concerning malaria which appear to me most important from the standpoint of the health official:

(1) Malaria in this country is in general a diminishing menace.

(2) Its continued diminution is dependent upon the persistence of those forces which have led to this diminution, the march of culture and active health work against the disease.

(3) In this country it is possible to look forward at no very distant date to the practical eradication of the disease, and the policy of mere amelioration should be only temporarily adopted in some local instances.

(4) Improved and more economical methods of eradication must be based upon rigid experimentation in many fields of inquiry.

(5) The means to be used in any given locality must be expertly selected after thorough knowledge of local conditions has been secured. There is no panacea.

(6) The first indispensable step toward undertak-

ing antimalaria measures is the establishment in the area concerned of an effective official health unit.

(7) Programs of malaria control should definitely aim at the eventual and even early taking over of activities by the local agencies and their support by local funds.

(8) Antimalaria programs should neither be allowed to take precedence over nor to be subordinated to other health activities in the area. After a careful study of local health needs they should be allotted their proportionate share in health activities.

(9) Malaria is as much due to social and economic causes as to the plasmodium or the mosquito. The problem as to just where to interrupt the vicious circle varies with locality and must be decided after local survey.

(10) Malaria in the United States could be not only controlled but virtually exterminated by methods already known and at not unreasonable cost.

(11) Impediments to malaria control and eradication arise from the well recognized psychological and social phenomena which always delay the adoption of useful innovations, unless the latter happen to come in peculiarly attractive form or are laden with considerable emotional appeal.

(12) It is essential that researches in malaria be continued. Not only are economic refinements of methods desirable, but from the standpoint of science a very productive field awaits further cultivation.

A. M. STIMSON
U. S. PUBLIC HEALTH SERVICE

PARASITOLOGY IN RELATION TO MEDICAL PROBLEMS OF THE SOUTH[1]

THE medical problems of the south include several diseases that are endemic in the region in addition to those that occur over the country as a whole. Some of the more important ones of these diseases are caused by large parasites like, for instance, the helminths, and intelligent dealing with them requires that advantage be taken of information to be derived from that division of parasitology which deals with this class of parasites—helminthology.

Other diseases endemic chiefly in the south are caused by microscopic parasites, the protozoa, and intelligent dealing with them requires practical application of information to be derived from the division of parasitology which deals with this class of parasites—protozoology.

The specific organism of some of the diseases of the south that are due to protozoa and some of those that are due to bacteria are transmitted from man to man, or in some instances from animal to man by insects, and these can be dealt with intelligently only by taking advantage of information to be gained from entomology, which we may include as another division of the general subject of parasitology. It often occurs that such a disease may be most successfully combatted by measures directed against the insect host of the specific organism or against the animal host of the insect host of the organism, as in bubonic plague.

The medical problems presented by a disease, parasitic or otherwise, are chiefly those of diagnosis, cure and prevention. Any and all of these are dependent more or less upon a knowledge of the life history of the specific organism or parasite, as in the case, for instance, of hookworm disease, or of both the specific organism and of the insect host as in malaria. Diagnosis is necessary for intelligent treatment of a parasitic disease, but both diagnosis and treatment may be applied only to the individual or either or both of them may be utilized in combatting or preventing the disease in the community. In other instances the cure of patients, as in the case of yellow fever or of plague, has little or no significance in dealing with the disease as a community problem.

Parasitology discovers the life history of the parasite and its environmental requirements for propagation and mischief. Unless we remind ourselves, we are likely not to fully realize how much the success we have had in dealing with several of the diseases that have been dealt with successfully during recent years was made possible by studies of the parasite or its insect host. During comparatively recent years yellow fever has been banished, never to return, thanks to the practical application of knowledge of the life history of the insect carrier; bubonic plague is under control and will never be a serious disease again, thanks to the practical application of knowledge of the life history of the rat-flea and its host; hookworm disease is no longer a serious disease in the south except in limited areas and in small numbers of people compared with twenty years ago, thanks to the practical application of knowledge of the life history of the parasite; malaria has been placed under control and practically eliminated from numerous demonstration communities, thanks to the practical application of knowledge of the life history of both the parasite and the insect host. Numerous other instances could be given in which the problem of endemic diseases has been solved to considerable extent at least through knowledge of the life history

[1] Presented as part of a symposium on "The Medical Problems of the South" at a joint meeting of the American Association for the Advancement of Science and the American Public Health Association, Nashville, December 28, 1927.

of the parasite or its host, provided largely through parasitology. Let us look more closely into the facts relating to some of these problems.

In 1901 Allen J. Smith (1) discovered hookworm ova in the feces of a number of students at Galveston, Texas, but it was the experienced zoologist, Charles Wardell Stiles (2), who fully recognized the significance of the observation. To him hookworm eggs in these students from different parts of the state could mean nothing less than wide distribution of this parasite. Examination of material from other parts of the south confirmed the opinion and showed that the parasite was widely distributed throughout the southern states.

It took months and, in fact, years for Stiles and others to thoroughly arouse the people of the south to a realization of the existence and importance of this great burden of hookworm disease and its effects upon the health and vitality of a large part of the inhabitants. For his pioneer work, which led to the creation of the Rockefeller Hookworm Commission and later the International Health Board, the country owes him an everlasting debt of gratitude that can never be repaid. Campaigns for the control of hookworm disease were conducted and extended from time to time until they have reached not only most of this country where the disease prevailed, but the four corners of the earth, resulting in untold benefit to many hundreds of thousands of people. These efforts to control the disease have been based largely on a knowledge of the life history of the parasite both outside of and within man that has been worked out by a great deal of scientific research by a host of workers.

Much valuable and indispensable information was supplied by the work of Loos (3) showing the mode of infection and the almost incredible route taken by the larvae in their passage through the skin, the blood vessels, heart and lungs to the intestine. These findings were soon confirmed and extended by Claude A. Smith (4) in this country. More recently most exhaustive studies have been made by a host of workers on the influence of different environmental factors on the hatching and survival of larvae, egg production and many other questions of the greatest practical interest. Great reduction has already been brought about in the prevalence of hookworm disease in the south, but it still remains one of the important medical problems to which parasitology is closely related.

A long warm season, abundant rainfall and a population that has not yet fully recovered from the consequences of a long exhausting war, all create favorable conditions for other intestinal parasites. A large part of the poorer people, especially the children who harbor hookworms and some who do not, also harbor other intestinal worms, ascaris, trichuris, oxyuris and strongyloides. While these probably do not constitute so great a menace to health they are still of great importance, and satisfactory methods of treatment and control, in some at least, await further knowledge of the life history of the parasites. Some of them may prove to have more significance than formerly believed as suggested by the more recent studies of Ransom, particularly on the course of ascaris larvae through the body. Cort and his co-workers are making an exhaustive study of ascariasis at the present time and their results are awaited with interest.

Intestinal protozoa, amoeba and flagellates are widely distributed throughout the south and amoebic dysentery is of frequent occurrence in most parts of the country. There is great need for improved methods of differentiating the pathogenic from the non-pathogenic species, and for improved methods of diagnosing the infection. The mode of transmission and the resistance or survival of the parasites outside of the body offer fields for research of the protozoologist.

The protozoa of the mouth, the tonsils, the vagina, require the most thorough study to determine whether they are pathogenic and the source of infection. Practically all people sooner or later lose their teeth from alveolodental pyorrhea if they are not lost from decay. Protozoa, especially amoeba, are found associated with the pyorrhea lesions. Are they pathogenic or not? Proven fact is what is wanted, not opinion.

Malaria constitutes one of the most important medical problems of the south. For many years it was far the largest cause of morbidity. At the time of the civil war malaria was the largest single cause of death. The prevalence and severity of the disease have gradually but surely declined during the past fifty to seventy-five years. Many years ago it was very prevalent not only in the south but also in large sections in New York, Pennsylvania, even Connecticut, and in Maryland, Ohio, Michigan, Illinois and Indiana. To-day there are only small endemic foci in some of these states and none in others. The area of endemic malaria in the United States has shrunk to not more than one third of its former extent. The rate of decline of the disease has been accelerated considerably during the past ten years, due to the greater activities of health agencies in combatting it in the light of the comparatively recent knowledge of its specific cause and mode of transmission and effective methods of dealing with them.

Prior to the discovery of the malaria parasite the only weapons against this disease, one of the greatest foes to civilization and colonization in warm countries, was quinine which was used extensively and deliberately and, in addition, clearing and drainage which were done chiefly for developmental purposes. The malaria parasite was discovered by Charles Louis Alphonse Laveran in 1880, and the mosquito was definitely incriminated as the transmitter of the parasite from man to man by Sir Ronald Ross in 1898. Knowing the cause of the disease and the transmitting insect it was desirable to learn all that could be known of the life history in nature of the parasite and of the insect mosquito host. Scientific workers throughout the world, entirely too numerous to name here, have added more and more to our knowledge, and further important studies are being made all the time. Present knowledge has shown where the most vulnerable points are in the life history of both the parasite and the mosquito. Attacks on them at these points have been successful in control of the disease in proportion to the thoroughness with which the measures could be applied.

In numerous instances practically 100 per cent. of control has been obtained in small areas. But the cost in effort and money has limited the control by intensive methods to these small areas as compared with the total area involved. Intensive work plus the more general application of measures directed against the parasite and against the mosquito have led to so great reduction until many are beginning to feel that malaria is no longer a serious problem in the south. Let us hope that there will be no disappointment in this regard. But let me point out the fact that while the decline in malaria prevalence and severity has been much greater during the past ten or twelve years than during any previous period of equal length, the year 1927 has brought a little discouraging news. Reports have been received that malaria incidence has increased noticeably in many localities (and, by the way, a good many of these are in the state of Tennessee). Whether this is only a temporary tendency or not remains for the future to determine.

There is great need for further knowledge about the influences that determine the life and survival of parasites in both the human and the insect host. Why does one man recover from the infection easily and another only with great difficulty? What causes the development of gametes? Why do they survive and infect mosquitoes sometimes and not others? What are the natural conditions, environmental, nutritional and otherwise, besides those already known, that influence mosquito breeding and transmission of malaria? These and many other questions of vital importance await further researches along parasitological lines.

Pellagra is one of the largest and most important medical problems of the south. The generally accepted theory that it is caused by faults in diet has only served to detract from interest in other lines of research as to the true cause of the disease. Until this is discovered we can only surmise as to the possible assistance parasitology may give in the solution of the problem of its control. Experimental transmission of the disease to monkeys by W. H. Harris (5), of New Orleans, in 1913, with material that had been passed through a Berkefeld filter, indicates that the infectious agent belongs to "the filterable viruses," but this does not lessen the probability of transmission of the specific virus by insects as in the case of other virus diseases carried by insects, like yellow fever, dengue, etc. In fact the long definite incubation period of experimental pellagra tends to encourage the thought of an insect host. The field is an inviting one, and as long as so little is known, it is reasonable to suppose that parasitology may help to solve problems of this disease that is killing hundreds in the south every year and from which thousands suffer.

These are only a few of the many medical problems of the south to which parasitology bears close relationship. Not only is research in parasitology to discover facts of practical application in medicine needed, but in my opinion there is great need for more parasitology, medical parasitology if you will, in the curriculum of the medical schools of the south. Medical students should be instructed in parasitology not merely from the standpoint of diagnosis and treatment but they should learn more of the life history of the parasites which cause the parasitic diseases they treat so they will be prepared to take the part they should as practicing physicians in prevention as well as cure.

C. C. Bass

School of Medicine,
Tulane University

WILLEM EINTHOVEN

Dr. Willem Einthoven, for forty-two years professor of physiology in the University of Leyden, died on September 28, 1927. He was born at Samarang, Java, and studied medicine at the University of Utrecht, receiving assistance from the Dutch government on condition that he would go back to the islands after graduation, to practice. Early in his student career he attracted favorable attention by an able investigation of the mechanism of the motions of pronation and supination of the forearm. While studying physiology under Donders, he developed an active interest in ophthalmology, the influence of which is reflected in several of his earlier researches and is to be perceived in much of his later work.

During Einthoven's last year as a student at Utrecht the chair of physiology at Leyden became vacant. Donders was asked by the government to nominate a new professor and finding no one of experience who could lecture in the vernacular, he urged that Einthoven be chosen on the basis of his great promise. The offer was made, carrying with it automatically a release from the obligation to return to the islands to practice medicine. The young medical student, not yet graduated, felt a natural hesitation about accepting so great a responsibility. It was largely due to the urging and encouragement of his fellow-student, Karl Koller, later to become well known as an ophthalmologist and the sponsor of cocaine anesthesia, that Einthoven finally accepted.

From the character of Einthoven's published work it might seem an easy inference that he had been especially interested in physics and mathematics as a student, or that he had fallen under the influence of some particularly inspiring teacher in these subjects, but this was not the fact. He realized, however, in taking over his academic responsibilities, that it would be necessary for him to know more about these subjects. In the course of a conversation regarding his days at Utrecht he recalled that one of his first acts after accepting the call to Leyden was to visit a bookshop and purchase a copy of a book on differential and integral calculus written by the late H. A. Lorentz, for many years his distinguished colleague at Leyden.

Einthoven is best known for his work on the electrical action currents of the heart. Following the discovery by Waller that these currents could be detected at the surface of the human body, he was quick to anticipate that their study might reveal important facts about the nature of the heart action in disease as well as in health. He commenced his studies in this field with the Lippmann capillary electrometer and an ingenious assemblage of accessory apparatus largely of his own devising. He was not long in discovering the limitations of the capillary electrometer, and independently of Burch, he discovered a method of correcting the readings of this instrument. Realizing that the time and labor required for a thorough study of the subject by this method would be almost prohibitive, he was led to consider other possible means of recording the rather feeble and somewhat rapid variations of electrical potential attending the heart-beat. As a result of his study he produced a new physical instrument, the string galvanometer, whose field of usefulness is by no means limited to the work of the physiologist. The original model of this instrument, after undergoing a few alterations suggested by experience with it, operated so well that it could hardly be improved except in the minor matter of mechanical simplification.

Within a few years after he described his string galvanometer, Einthoven began the publication of a series of papers dealing with studies made with its help in various fields of physiology. The earliest of these dealt with electrocardiography and covered the field so thoroughly that with the exception of the studies of auricular fibrillation and auricular flutter, which were made by others, little of major importance has been added which was not at least touched on in these first papers. Indeed, in his first long paper on electrocardiography there is to be found a record of a case of auricular fibrillation in man, though he was not aware of its significance.

Among his other published work the paper on the action currents of the vagus is a classic. His paper with Jolly on the action currents of the retina is also a remarkable piece of work. He wrote several papers dealing with the physical aspects of his galvanometer, which appeared in Drude's *Annalen,* and one on its construction, which was published in Pflueger's *Archiv.* The papers on graphic registration of heart sounds are also well known. In recent years he applied his knowledge of the production of extremely fine quartz fibers to the construction of a new instrument for direct registration of sound in which the quartz fiber is moved by the air molecules impinging immediately upon it. Among his recent papers also should be mentioned an important investigation of the relation between mechanical action of muscles and the accompanying action current.

In 1924 he visited the United States as the first lecturer under the Dunham Foundation at Harvard University. After delivering the Dunham lectures he lectured at a number of universities in the east and middle west, and while on this lecture tour he received the information that the Nobel prize in physiology had been awarded to him. In 1926 he was elected a foreign member of the Royal Society of London.

Cautious and painstaking in all his work, Einthoven was slow to publish and thought less of priority than of his duty to be correct. His sudden death has probably left numerous manuscripts unpublished, as it was his custom to keep them several years before publication. Charming in personality, his chief characteristic was modesty, though he could be very firm in defense of a thesis he believed to be well grounded. In his anxiety to avoid premature publication he possibly erred at times in withholding papers too long, but the young physiologist, who hastens to send off the paper written by him last night describing the results of a few experiments performed last week, will do well to consider the solidity of Einthoven's work and the confidence with which his successors have been able to build upon it.

H. B. Williams

Columbia University

SCIENTIFIC EVENTS

ACTIVITIES OF THE ROCKEFELLER FOUNDATION

A review of the activities of the Rockefeller Foundation in 1927, written by its president, George E. Vincent, will be issued in a few days.

The first instalment of the review summarizes the year's work in brief and discusses the ways in which the foundation seeks to promote the training of doctors and public health personnel for a new era in medicine, in which the emphasis is changing from cure to prevention.

During 1927 the Rockefeller Foundation, in disbursing from income and capital $11,223,124 (1) aided local health organization in eighty-five counties of six states in the Mississippi flood area; (2) operated an emergency field training station for health workers in this region besides contributing toward the support of nine other training centers elsewhere; (3) assisted nine schools or institutes of public health and three departments of hygiene in university medical schools; (4) gave aid to seventeen nurse training schools in nine countries; (5) furnished funds for land, buildings, operation or endowment to nineteen medical schools in fourteen countries; (6) supported the Peking Union Medical College; (7) paid two million dollars toward a new site for the University of London; (8) helped Brazil to maintain precautionary measures against yellow fever; (9) continued studies of that disease in West Africa on the Gold Coast and in Nigeria; (10) had a part in malaria control demonstrations or surveys in eight states of the Southern United States and in eleven foreign countries; (11) aided nineteen governments to bring hookworm disease under control; (12) contributed to the health budgets of 268 counties in twenty-three states of the American Commonwealth and of thirty-one similar governmental divisions in fourteen foreign countries; (13) helped to set up or maintain public health laboratory services or divisions of vital statistics, sanitary engineering, or epidemiology in the national health services of nineteen countries abroad and in the state health departments of sixteen American states; (14) made grants for mental hygiene work in the United States and Canada; (15) provided funds for biological research at the Johns Hopkins University and aided investigations in this field at Yale University, the State University of Iowa, the University of Hawaii, the Bernice P. Bishop Museum in Honolulu, and certain universities of Australia; (16) helped the League of Nations to conduct study tours or interchanges for 125 health officers from forty-four countries, to supply world-wide information about communicable diseases, to train government officials in vital statistics, and to establish a library of health documents; (17) provided, directly or indirectly, fellowships for 864 men and women from fifty-two different countries, and paid the traveling expenses of 115 officials or professors making study visits either individually or in commissions; (18) made minor appropriations for improving the teaching of the premedical sciences in China and Siam, for the operating expenses of hospitals in China, and for laboratory supplies, equipment and literature for European medical centers which have not yet recovered from the after-effects of the war; (19) lent staff members as consultants and gave small sums for various purposes to many governments and institutions; (20) made surveys of health conditions and of medical and nursing education in fourteen countries.

THE INTERNATIONAL CONGRESS OF PHOTOGRAPHY

In connection with the seventh International Congress of Photography to be held in London during the second week in July, 1928, it has been decided to hold exhibitions of an international character for each of the sections of the congress. These exhibitions will include pictorial exhibits and scientific apparatus, as well as matter illustrating new photographic processes and apparatus. There will also be a trade exhibition showing the recent trade developments in photographic goods.

The pictorial prints will be especially invited by the section of the congress dealing with pictorial photography, but all other material which American workers may desire to submit to the congress should be referred to Dr. C. E. K. Mees, Kodak Park Works, Rochester, N. Y., who is acting as secretary for the American division. As far as is known at present there will be no charge for space at the exhibition, although a small charge may be made later for inserting notices in the exhibition catalogues in order to cover the cost of printing the catalogues.

THE SELECTION OF CHIEF OF THE U. S. BUREAU OF AMERICAN ETHNOLOGY

The United States Civil Service Commission states that the position of chief of the Bureau of American Ethnology, Smithsonian Institution, is vacant, through the recent retirement of Dr. J. W. Fewkes, and that, in view of the importance of the position, and to insure the appointment of a thoroughly qualified man for the work, an unusual method of competition will be followed to fill the vacancy. Instead of the usual form of civil-service examination, the qualifications of candidates will be passed upon by a special board of examiners, composed of Dr. C. G. Abbot, secretary of the Smithsonian Institution; Dr. A. V. Kidder, ethnologist of the Carnegie Institution, and Mr. Frederick W. Brown, assistant chief of the examining division of the U. S. Civil Service Commission, who will act as chairman of the committee. For the purpose of this examination, all of these men will be examiners of the Civil Service Commission.

The examination will consist solely of the consideration of qualifications by the special board. The minimum qualifications for consideration are recognized eminence in American ethnological research, and experience of a length and character to demonstrate high ability in the direction and prosecution of ethnological research, administrative capacity of high order and thorough familiarity with the literature of American ethnology and archeology, and with the activities of scientific and professional organizations and institutions concerned with the subject. The applicant must possess the personality and demonstrated capacity for leadership, which will enable him successfully to lead and direct the personnel of research units and to enter into successful cooperative relations with other research and administrative agencies and the general public.

The entrance salary for this position is $5,200 a year. Applications must be on file with the U. S. Civil Service Commission at Washington not later than May 31.

ANNUAL MEETING OF THE AMERICAN ASSOCIATION OF MUSEUMS

THE twenty-third meeting of The American Association of Museums will be opened by the President of the United States, Calvin Coolidge, in Washington, D. C., on the morning of Wednesday, May 16. The occasion is to be a joint session held with The American Federation of Arts.

The meetings of both organizations will continue during three days, closing on the evening of Friday, May 18, with a joint annual dinner. On each of the days there will be sessions in the morning, afternoon and evening. This plan is an experiment and represents a reaction to recent meetings which have provided free afternoons for social functions and personal business of delegates.

The program is equally divided between the interests of those in each of the three major fields of museum work—art, science and history. A general session and a round table are scheduled for each group and in addition there will be sessions devoted to matters of concern to all. Several of the sessions will be held jointly with The American Federation of Arts.

The opening session—after the president's welcome and brief addresses—will be devoted to the vital problem of coordinating educational resources in the community. In the afternoon there will be a joint session on art museum problems. In the evening simultaneous round tables on special subjects will be held.

The second day will begin with a joint session on adult education. In the afternoon there will be a general session on science museum problems and in the evening one on history museum problems. The general topic in the afternoon will be trends in science museum exhibitions and in the evening the question of the historical museum in relation to the historical society. All of the sessions during the first two days are to be held at the Mayflower, which is hotel headquarters.

On the third day the scene will change to the Corcoran Gallery of Art. The morning and afternoon will be taken up with a symposium on educational problems and school people will join with museum workers in the program and the discussion. It is believed that the time allowed will enable the meeting to arrive at conclusions respecting many subjects which have been treated inadequately at former conferences for want of time.

On each of the first two days arrangements have been made for members of the federation and of the association to lunch at hotel headquarters and if circumstances are favorable impromptu programs of informal character will be arranged.

THE NATIONAL ACADEMY OF SCIENCES

AT the annual meeting of the National Academy of Sciences in Washington nine new members were elected as follows: Dr. John August Anderson, astronomer at the Mt. Wilson Observatory; Dr. William Mansfield Clark, professor of biochemistry at the Johns Hopkins Medical School; Dr. Arthur Keith, of the U. S. Geological Survey; Charles F. Kettering, head of the research laboratory of the General Motors Corporation; Dr. Alfred L. Kroeber, professor of anthropology at the University of California; Dr. Rudolph Ruedemann, state paleontologist for New York; Dr. Philip A. Shaffer, professor of biochemistry at the Washington University Medical School; Dr. George M. Stratton, professor of psychology at the University of California, and Dr. Lewis M. Terman, professor of psychology at Stanford University. Sir Robert A. Hadfield, British engineer, chemist and metallurgist, was elected a foreign associate. Dr. Joseph S. Ames, provost of the Johns Hopkins University, treasurer of the academy; Dr. W. B. Cannon, of the Harvard University Medical School, and Dr. Gano Dunn, New York engineer, were elected to serve three years on the council. Dr. George K. Burgess, director of the U. S. Bureau of Standards, was elected chairman of the National Research Council, succeeding Dr. Gano Dunn.

At the annual dinner of the academy on April 24 medals were awarded as follows:

Agassiz Medal for Oceanography—awarded to V. Walfrid Ekman, University, Lund, Sweden, in recognition of his outstanding work in physical oceanography. Dr. Ekman being unable to be in this country at the time of the meeting, the medal was received for him by Minister Bostrom, of Sweden, to be transmitted to Dr. Ekman through diplomatic channels.

Henry Draper Medal—awarded to William Hammond Wright, Lick Observatory, Mt. Hamilton, California, a member of the National Academy of Sciences, for his researches on nebulae, new stars and planetary atmospheres.

Public Welfare Medal (medal for eminence in the application of science to the public welfare)—awarded to Charles V. Chapin, Health Department, Providence, R. I., for his contributions to public health and his work in the administrative control of disease.

Mary Clark Thompson Medal and honorarium of $250.00—awarded to James Perrin Smith, Palo Alto, California, a member of the academy, in recognition of his accomplishment in paleontology of Triassic.

SCIENTIFIC NOTES AND NEWS

Elmer A. Sperry, inventor and engineer, has been awarded the Holley medal by the American Society of Mechanical Engineers for his achievements in the invention of the gyroscope. Presentation of the medal will be made on May 16 at a dinner which is to be held during the spring meeting of the American Society of Mechanical Engineers in Pittsburgh.

Dr. Charles-Edward A. Winslow, Anna M. R. Lauder professor of public health in the Yale University School of Medicine, has been awarded the Ling medal by the Ling Foundation of Los Angeles in recognition of his "work in behalf of the health progress of school children."

The Samuel Finley Breese Morse gold medal of the American Geographical Society has been voted to Captain George H. Wilkins by the board of directors of the society in recognition of his explorations in the Arctic, and particularly of his flight from Point Barrow to Spitzbergen. King George has approved the award of the Patrons royal medal of the Royal Geographical Society for this year to Captain Wilkins.

Dr. Jonathan A. W. Zenneck, professor of experimental physics at Munich, has been awarded the medal of honor of the Institute of Radio Engineers, for his "contributions to original research in radio and his scientific and educational contributions to the literature of the pioneer radio art." The medal will be presented to Dr. Zenneck's representative in this country on June 6 at a meeting in the Engineering Societies Building, New York.

The Plummer medal for 1927, granted by the Engineering Institute of Canada, has been awarded to Dr. J. W. Shipley and Charles F. Goodeve, of the department of chemistry of the University of Manitoba, for their work on alternating current electrolysis. This is the second time that Dr. Shipley has received this award, his work in conjunction with W. Nelson Smith on corrosion of metals earning the award in 1922.

The Faraday medal of the British Institution of Electrical Engineers was presented to Professor J. A. Fleming at the ordinary meeting of the institution held on April 19. The presentation preceded the nineteenth Kelvin lecture, by Sir Oliver Lodge, on "The Revolution in Physics."

The University of Liverpool will celebrate the twenty-fifth anniversary of its charter on May 10 and 11, when honorary degrees, including the following, will be conferred: D.Sc.: Professor J. E. Littlewood, Rouse Ball professor of mathematics in the University of Cambridge, for distinguished contributions to mathematical science; Professor Robert Robinson, professor of organic chemistry in the University of Manchester, for eminence as an organic chemist. LL.D.: Professor J. W. Gregory, professor of geology in the University of Glasgow, for distinguished services to geology, geography and exploration. D.Eng.: Professor J. A. Fleming, emeritus professor of electrical engineering at University College, London, for distinguished services in the advance and application of electrical science.

Dr. Emil Abderhalden, professor of physiology in the University of Halle, has been made an honorary member of the Chinese Physiological Society, Peking.

Dr. Hideyo Noguchi, of the Rockefeller Institute for Medical Research, has been elected a foreign member of the Società Medica Chirurgica di Bologna.

Professor Yukichi Osaka has retired from the chair of physical chemistry, which he has held for twenty-three years at the Kyoto Imperial University.

FOUR classes of the University and Bellevue Hospital Medical College (1928–1931) presented a bust of Dr. George David Stewart, who has been a member of the faculty for thirty years, to New York University at a ceremony on April 18.

A CAMPAIGN has been launched to raise $200,000 for the endowment of a chair of operative dentistry in honor of Dr. Edwin Tyler Darby, who recently celebrated the fiftieth anniversary of his appointment to the University of Pennsylvania School of Dentistry.

DR. RICHARD H. JAFFE, professor of pathology and bacteriology in the University of Illinois College of Medicine, has been named director of the new pathological and research laboratory of the Cook County Hospital.

PROFESSOR G. S. PARKS, of the department of chemistry at Stanford University, has been elected chairman of the California section of the American Chemical Society for 1928, in place of Professor W. H. Sloan, retiring chairman.

DR. LINSLY R. WILLIAMS, director of the New York Academy of Medicine and managing director, National Tuberculosis Association, has been appointed president of the New York Tuberculosis and Health Association, succeeding Dr. James A. Miller, who retired after nine years of service.

DR. REGINALD S. CLAY, principal of the Northern Polytechnic Institute, London, was elected president of the British Optical Society at the annual general meeting on March 8.

DR. ALBERT W. HERRE, chief of the division of fisheries in the Philippine Bureau of Science, has been appointed curator of the museum of zoology at Stanford University.

T. SWANN HARDING has been appointed editor of scientific publications, office of information, U. S. Department of Agriculture, vice C. M. Arthur, who recently resigned to accept a position as technical editor at the Forest Products Laboratory at Madison, Wisconsin. Mr. Harding has been engaged in research in the Department of Agriculture for many years, first in the Bureau of Chemistry and later in the Bureau of Dairy Industry.

DR. H. B. HUNGERFORD, of the University of Kansas, left on April 27 for eight months of research work in the museums of Europe. He will take with him specimens from the collections of the University of Kansas and the Smithsonian Institution, Washington, with which he is collaborating on the trip. Dr. Hungerford will spend most of the month of May in British museums, going later to Paris, Brussels, Amsterdam, Berlin, Halle, Copenhagen, Uppsala, Prague, Vienna and Budapest.

JOSEPH H. SINCLAIR, explorer and geologist, arrived in New York on April 24 after a five months' trip in Ecuador, which was made under the auspices of the American Geographical Society.

PROFESSOR FRED C. SEARS, head of the department of pomology at the Massachusetts Agricultural College, plans to go to Labrador and Newfoundland this summer to make a survey of the horticultural and agricultural possibilities of the region.

DR. HERMANN THOMS, professor of chemistry in the University of Berlin, has been invited to give a series of lectures in Buenos Aires.

DR. S. C. BROOKS, professor of zoology at the University of California, addressed a meeting of the University of California chapter of the Society of the Sigma Xi on April 11.

DR. J. H. MOORE, astronomer at Lick Observatory, will address the Astronomical Society of the Pacific in San Francisco on May 21.

AT the twentieth annual meeting of the Undergraduate Medical Association of the University of Pennsylvania on April 26, Dr. Anton J. Carlson, University of Chicago, spoke on "Recent Studies on the Thyroid Gland"; Dr. Allen O. Whipple, professor of surgery, Columbia University College of Physicians and Surgeons, New York, on "Bacteriologic Problems in their Relation to the Surgical Service," and Dr. Chevalier Jackson on "The Relation of the Bronchoscope to Research."

SIR ST. CLAIR THOMSON, London, past-president of the Royal Society of Medicine, gave the annual William Potter Memorial Lecture at Jefferson Medical College on April 25, on "The Strenuous Life of a London Physician in the Eighteenth Century." The *Journal* of the American Medical Association states that the board of trustees of Jefferson has founded these lectures as a memorial to the late William Potter, and has appointed for life Dr. Chevalier Jackson as the William Potter Memorial lecturer to deliver to the senior class each year a series of lectures on bronchoscopy, esophagoscopy and gastroscopy, and to arrange one additional lecture each year to be given by some eminent authority in any branch of science.

DR. VICTOR COFMAN, consultant to the research department of E. I. du Pont de Nemours and Company, lectured at Clemson College on "Colloids," on April 27 and 28.

RETIRING after two years as president of the Anthropological Society of Washington, Neil M. Judd, curator of American archeology in the U. S. National Museum, addressed the society at its annual meeting on April 17, on "The Present Status of Archeology in the United States."

Governor Fuller, of Massachusetts, observed Arbor Day by planting a white spruce tree on the state house grounds and dedicating it to the memory of the late Professor Charles Sprague Sargent, for fifty-four years director of the Arnold Arboretum.

The erection of memorials for Major-Generals Leonard Wood and George W. Goethals is called for in bills introduced by Representative Gifford, republican, of Massachusetts. The Wood memorial would be at Bourne, Massachusetts. That to General Goethals would be built at Tisbury, Massachusetts. Each of the measures would appropriate $100,000.

As already recorded in Science a bust of Louis Agassiz, among others, will be unveiled in the hall of fame at New York University on May 10. Funds for this bust were given by the American Association for the Advancement of Science and an admirer of Agassiz. The presentation will be made by J. Walter Fewkes, of the Smithsonian Institution, pupil of Agassiz, and the unveiling by Dr. Anna Agassiz Prince, great-granddaughter of Agassiz. The principal speaker will be Dr. Henry Fairfield Osborn, president of the American Museum of Natural History, and president of the association.

Elias E. Ries, of New York, known for his inventions in the field of electrical engineering, died on April 20, aged sixty five years.

G. Chisholm Williams, a distinguished pioneer in the medical use of X-rays, in England, died on April 10, aged sixty-three years.

Professor Wilhelm von Branca, emeritus professor of geology and paleontology in the University of Berlin, distinguished for his work on the evolutionary history of man and other animals, died on March 12, aged eighty-three years.

Dr. F. Ladislas Laskowski, formerly professor of human anatomy at Geneva University, died on April 16 at the age of eighty-seven years.

Professor Leon Guignard, director of the faculty of pharmacy in Paris, known for his work in microscopic botany, has died at the age of seventy-six years.

The one hundred and fifty-second regular meeting of the American Physical Society will be held at Pomona, California, on June 15, in affiliation with the Pacific division of the American Association for the Advancement of Science. The morning session will be a joint session with the Astronomical Society of the Pacific.

The annual meeting of the Wisconsin Academy of Sciences, Arts and Letters was held at Lawrence College, Appleton, on April 6 and 7. The Wisconsin Archeological Society and The Midwest Museums Conference joined with the academy in this meeting. President S. A. Barrett presided, and on Friday afternoon presented his lecture "Hawaii, the Paradise of the Pacific," which was illustrated with moving pictures. In all, thirty papers were presented at the sessions.

The New York State Geological Association will hold its next field meet at Cornell University, Ithaca, N. Y., on May 11 and 12.

The tenth biennial convention of Alpha Chi Sigma, national chemical fraternity, will be held at the University of North Carolina, Chapel Hill, North Carolina, from June 16 to 20. At this time the "History of Alpha Chi Sigma," by Dr. Harry A. Curtis, head of the department of chemistry at Yale University, will be officially introduced to the fraternity.

The ninety-sixth annual meeting of the British Medical Association will be held at Cardiff on July 20–28, under the presidency of Sir Ewen Maclean, who will deliver his address on the evening of July 24. According to *Nature,* the annual exhibition of surgical appliances, foods, drugs and books will be open from July 23 to 27. A pathological museum is also being arranged by Drs. J. B. Duguid and J. Mills, department of pathology and bacteriology, Welsh National School of Medicine. The following presidents of sections are announced in the provisional program: Sir Thomas Lewis (*medicine*), Professor A. W. Sheen (*surgery*), Dr. T. Watts Eden (*obstetrics and gynecology*), Professor E. H. Kettle (*pathology and bacteriology*), Dr. E. Goodall (*mental diseases and neurology*), Sir John Lynn-Thomas (*orthopedics*), Dr. A. Howell (*diseases of children*), F. P. S. Cresswell (*ophthalmology*), Dr. D. R. Paterson (*laryngology and otology*), Dr. H. M. Davies (*tuberculosis*), Dr. O. L. Rhys (*radiology and physio-therapeutics*), Dr. E. C. Williams (*preventive medicine*), R. M. F. Picken (*public health*), Dr. W. E. Thomas (*medical sociology*), Dr. Philip H. Manson-Bahr (*tropical medicine*), Walter G. Spencer (*history of medicine*), Dr. W. Langdon Brown (*therapeutics and pharmacology*), Sir Robert Bolam (*dermatology*).

Sigma Xi grants for research for 1928–29, available for workers in all fields of science, will be awarded by the middle of May. There are no restrictions as to the university or the country in which the holder is permitted to work. Applications should be made before May 10. Blanks may be obtained from Dean Edward Ellery, Union College, Schenectady, N. Y.

THE board of the University of Michigan Medical School has accepted two gifts of the fellowship corporation of Battle Creek, one of $20,000 to be paid in $1,500 instalments quarterly for studying problems of metabolism, the other of $2,500 for the investigation of bran as an article of diet. Dr. Louis H. Newburgh is to carry on the work in connection with these grants.

THE United States Shellac Importers' Association has founded a research fellowship in shellac, known as the shellac research bureau, at the Brooklyn Polytechnic Institute. The work will be done under the direction of J. C. Olsen and W. F. Whitmore.

ON the ten-acre plot of the Dominion Experimental Farm in Ottawa the government will erect the first unit of a national laboratory to be devoted to scientific and industrial research work and a central power plant. An appropriation of $750,000 has been made for the first year's work.

THE cornerstone of the new $150,000 testing laboratory of the American Gas Association, at Cleveland, Ohio, was laid on March 15. R. W. Gallagher, chairman of the managing committee of the laboratory, spoke on the steps taken to bring the laboratory to Cleveland and to make it a permanent institution. Since the temporary quarters were established in May, 1925, more than 7,300 appliances have been tested and approved for public use. The new building will make available about 30,000 square feet of space.

AT a meeting of the council of the American Chemical Society at the recent St. Louis meeting applications for granting charters for new sections with headquarters at Bozeman, Mont., Manhattan, Kans., and Pullman, Wash., were approved, all requirements having been met. Dr. Guy, of Atlanta, extended an invitation for the society to hold the spring meeting of 1930 in Atlanta, and the invitation was unanimously accepted. Reference was also made to an invitation from Omaha that the fall meeting of 1930 be held in that city. The invitation was placed on file for consideration at the appropriate time, together with one previously received from Cincinnati.

ACCORDING to *Industrial and Engineering Chemistry* some eight months ago, the British secretary of state for the colonies appointed a committee to investigate the question of the creation of a Colonial Agricultural Scientific and Research Service. This scheme aims at the establishment of a research department which will undertake work, the results of which will be available to the whole Colonial Empire, it being proposed to investigate such special problems as would be regularly submitted by any of the colonies. The committee has now reported and estimates the cost of an agricultural wing at $283,000, and a specialist wing at $171,000; in addition, $68,000 will be required for an advisory council and $98,000 for one central research station. The total estimated cost is thus $620,000. The fact is stressed by the committee that adequate salaries must be paid to the scientists to be employed by this scheme in order to attract distinguished men of proved ability. It is proposed to pay the chief adviser, who must have marked administrative and organizing ability, a salary of about $12,000 per annum. He would be provided with an assistant at about $9,800 per annum. The committee state definitely that, though the scales suggested might at first sight appear to be high, they are "convinced of the absolute necessity of framing them on bold, simple lines."

UNIVERSITY AND EDUCATIONAL NOTES

THE corner-stone of Du Pont hall at Hampton Institute was laid on April 26. The building is the gift of Senator T. Coleman du Pont, of Delaware, who gave $250,000 to the institute, with the provision that a hall of science should be erected with a part of the fund and other sums retained for the upkeep of the work.

THE new medical school building of Howard University was formally opened on April 9 and 10, when there were clinics and demonstrations and all laboratories were open for inspection.

DR. E. V. COWDRY, of the Rockefeller Institute for Medical Research, has been appointed professor of cytology in the department of anatomy of Washington University, St. Louis. The reorganized department includes all the anatomical sciences. Professor Robert J. Terry is chairman of the department and in charge of gross anatomy; Professor Cowdry will direct the microscopical work.

AT Columbia University the following have been promoted to full professorships: Dr. Robert H. Bowen in zoology, Dr. Clifford D. Carpenter and Dr. Arthur W. Thomas in chemistry, Dr. Colin G. Fink in chemical engineering, Dr. Selig Hecht in biochemistry, Dr. Harry L. Parr and Dr. Edward D. Thurston, Jr., in mechanical engineering and Dr. Albin H. Beyer in civil engineering.

AT Yale University, Dr. H. L. Seward and W. J. Wohlenberg have been promoted to be professors of mechanical engineering, and Dr. G. A. Baitsell to be professor of biology.

AT Vassar College, Associate Professor C. J. Beckwith has been promoted to professor of zoology and Ruth C. MacDuffie has been appointed instructor in zoology and anthropology. Assistant Professor H. M. Allyn has resigned to become academic dean of Mt. Holyoke College.

DR. JACOB C. GEIGER, executive secretary of the Chicago Health Department under the administration of Dr. Herman N. Bundesen, has accepted a position as professor of bacteriology at the George Hooper foundation of the University of California Medical School.

LARS G. ROMELL, of the Swedish Forestry Experiment Station at Stockholm, assumed his duties on April 1 at Cornell University as first incumbent of the Charles Lathrop Pack research professorship for the study of forest soils. Professor Romell will be associated with Professor T. L. Lyon, head of the department of agronomy and soils, and Professor Ralph Hosmer, of the forestry department. Professor Romell's appointment is for three years.

PROFESSOR J. J. R. MACLEOD, associate dean of the faculty of medicine at the University of Toronto, co-sharer of the Nobel prize in 1923 with Dr. F. G. Banting, the discoverer of insulin, will leave Canada in the autumn to become Regius professor of physiology at the University of Aberdeen, in succession to Professor J. A. MacWilliam, who recently resigned.

DISCUSSION AND CORRESPONDENCE

DEAFNESS IN PRE-COLUMBIAN PERU

THE determination of the causes of deafness in an ancient race of people, such as the pre-Columbian Peruvians, is well worth undertaking. The subject has already received some attention. Burton[1] has given an extremely useful survey of the nature of aural exostoses in general, with a brief account of otosclerosis.

The aural exostoses in the external auditory meatus in pre-Columbian crania from Peru are often definite osteomae with a typical ivory-like luster, and extremely hard and dense. These never grow very large, and I do not know that a single osteoma ever closes the auditory canal, but the presence of three tumors *does* close the canal completely, on one and on both sides. In addition to this the walls of the auditory canal itself often become swollen and sclerotic and close the canal, thus producing deafness.

The assignment of strain, brought on by the mastication of tough food, as a cause of the exostosial growths, and possibly the cause also of otosclerosis in general, requires an anthropological survey for confirmation. Infections played a part in deafness, for I have seen cases of pre-Columbian middle ear infections.

Aided by a grant of $300 from the Committee on Scientific Research, American Medical Association, a more exact investigation of the ancient conditions will be undertaken. Dr. L. C. Kinney, of San Diego, will do the roentgenological work on the pre-Columbian crania, and I have at my disposal scores of roentgenograms of unopened mummy-packs.

ROY L. MOODIE

SANTA MONICA, CALIFORNIA

[1] Burton, Frank A., 1927, "Some Considerations on Prehistoric Aural, Nasal, Sinus Pathology and Surgery." Santa Fe, N. M., pp. 1–38, Figures 1–17.

PRODUCTION OF POTATO TUBER NECROSIS

IN the course of investigations, chiefly histological and cytological, carried on during 1926–27 at the University of Wisconsin, but under the auspices of the Vermont Experiment Station, experiments were conducted by the writer to throw more light on the real relationship existing between leafroll and net necrosis of the Irish potato. Through the use of cages to exclude undesirable insects, potato plants were grown in the field both from healthy and from leafroll tubers and aphids of the species, *Myzus Persicae,* were colonized on leafroll vines under cage and transferred at intervals to the foliage of healthy vines also under cage. Some four or five such transfers were made, each transfer involving the introduction of 25–50 aphids into each of five cages where they were allowed to migrate from the detached leafroll leaves to the foliage of the enclosed healthy plants. Two cages of healthy plants from the same lot of tubers were kept as checks. One cage contained leafroll plants on which aphids were colonized for increase and distribution.

When the harvested tubers from these cages were first examined on October 25, very interesting results were found. Necrosis, of the phloem necrosis type, was found in abundance, even at this early date, in all the treated cages. In one of the five cages practically 100 per cent. of the tubers showed the characteristic discolorations. The necrosis was in early stages of development, that is, not extending far from the stem end of the tubers and not showing as extreme necrotic discolorations as are found in tubers later on in the storage period. Microscopic study of stained sections of these tubers showed the necrosis to be the characteristic phloem-necrosis which is being investigated. The tubers from the two check cages where the vines had been kept free from aphids and from all other insects showed no necrosis.

This is the first instance, so far as the writer is aware, of the production of net-necrosis under control conditions, and the first proof of what has been heretofore a hypothesis, though supported by considerable evidence, namely, a causal relationship between leafroll and net-necrosis.

The suggestion as to the above relationship is not new. Schultz and Folsom in Maine, showed in 1921 that net-necrosis occurred in varying percentages in hills adjacent to and in the near vicinity of leafroll plants. They further characterized the necrosis as a phloem necrosis rather than a necrosis of the xylem of the vascular tissues and suggested that it might be due to the same virus as that causing leafroll. The experiment here reported furnishes strong evidence that the above suggested explanation is a correct one.

The complete data connected with this investigation will be published in a forthcoming paper.

ALFRED H. GILBERT

VERMONT AGRICULTURAL EXPERIMENT STATION

"GENERAL ZOOLOGY"

I FEEL that I can not let Mr. H. L. Clark's review of my text-book of general zoology (SCIENCE, VOL. 67, No. 1726) pass without comment. Mr. Clark appears to have two main grievances which (with apologies) he airs at some length. They are (1) the choice of title and (2) the fact that I have omitted all mention of the Echinodermata! I omitted mention of many other groups of the animal kingdom, but I can quite understand that these omissions are nothing like so criminal to him. Mr. Clark is known to us as a very capable investigator of the Echinodermata. I am not sure what experience he has had of teaching work in the universities or higher schools of to-day. He starts off, however, by classifying teachers of zoology into three groups: (1) those stressing structure, (2) those emphasizing function and (3) those magnifying habits and life histories.

I venture to say that this classification is not only incomplete but unjust. There are many teachers of zoology to-day who realize the importance of a broad study of their subject and who endeavor to combine the studies of structure, function, life history and habits.

Now in England in the past it has been customary (and I think the arrangement may not have been different in the United States) to introduce the subject of zoology by a detailed course on the structure of a limited number of well-known types—amoeba, hydra, crayfish, dogfish, pigeon and rabbit. Many students who took this course never heard anything about the way the structures functioned, and it was very difficult for them to find anything in the literature about the physiology of these common types. This very one-sided study of zoology is now realized to be out of date. There is no need for me to discuss that here; it is universally recognized by the best teachers to-day.

Well, I was asked to write a text-book which would introduce the usual types, so that their structure could be studied in detail in the practical classes *together with a study of function.* The book was not to exceed five hundred pages—quite large enough for the purse of most first-year students in this country. If I had described the morphology of the types at length, I should have simply duplicated much that is found in many excellent text-books already in existence. I, therefore, expanded the functional side and introduced a very considerable amount of information not found in any elementary text-book of zoology or physiology with which I am acquainted. Structure was not neglected, but illustrations were used to save description and to aid the students in their dissections.

I do not apologize for the plan of the book. It is novel and that at least is something these days. To Mr. Clark's rebuke that I have omitted all mention of turtles, echinoderms and the songs of birds I retort that they do not come into our introductory text-books in this country. I still wonder whether he was serious when he wrote about the songs of birds.

My reply to his last sentence is that a student familiar with the contents of my book and with the laboratory training which accompanies it, will have a far better knowledge of animal life than one who has only studied the structure of representatives of a large number of animal groups and a far better training than one who has swallowed a superficial account of chatty nature study.

As to my choice of title "The Elements of General Zoology." Zoology to me is the study of animal life, and physiology is as important a part of it as morphology or taxonomy. I do not belittle either of the latter. The necessity of morphological work is clearly indicated.

WILLIAM JOHN DAKIN

DEPARTMENT OF ZOOLOGY,
UNIVERSITY OF LIVERPOOL

THE PRONUNCIATION OF RESEARCH

IN the issue of March 23, Nicholas Kopeloff expresses the opinion that "overwhelming usage seems to place the accent on the first syllable" of research. From such "datta" or "dayta" as I have collected on this question I am disposed to think that it is a drawn game at present. Last year, while I was sitting in at a conference of investigators from all parts of the United States held in the National Research Council, I kept tally of the rival pronunciations. Unfortunately I have mislaid my notes or laid them away carefully—which amounts to the same thing in my filing system—so I can not give the figures, but I remember positively that at the end of the afternoon the score stood exactly equal. In two cases I had to record a one half vote in each column because one man alternated in pronunciation and one woman always adopted the form used by the preceding speaker.

In case of transplantation to an exotic habitat about nine months is required for complete acclimatization to the alien accent. One June when a western professor came into my office to say good-bye at the expiration of his year on the National Research Council I expressed my regret that I had not seen as much of him as I had hoped to when he came in the fall but that the time of his stay seemed so short. "Yes," he responded, "The term of service on the Council is too short. No sooner does a man learn to say research′ instead of re′-search than he has to leave and another man takes his place to start at the same point."

Why not settle the question by dropping the first syllable? Does "research" have any advantages over "search," except in being longer and harder to pronounce?

Edwin E. Slosson
Science Service,
Washington, D. C.

In the issue of Science for March 23, 1928 (p. 319), Dr. Nicholas Kopeloff points out how annoying is the mispronunciation of the word, "research"; the common garden variety of usage places the accent on the first syllable, while the proper form is with the accent on the last syllable. Is this not as it should be? Are not about 90 per cent. of so-called original investigations "re′-search," whereas 10 per cent. may properly be dignified as "re-search′"?

Paul Nicholas Leech
Chicago, Illinois

Replying to the article by Dr. E. C. L. Miller on page 319 of Science for March 23, I would say that he has confounded the transitive verb "to believe" with the intransitive verb. The former is defined in the Century Dictionary as "to credit upon the ground of authority, testimony, argument or any other ground than complete demonstration." There is no reason why users of the English language should confine themselves to only one meaning or only one use of a given word, but as this troubles him, I would suggest that for believe, he should substitute "think," or "I am of the opinion," or "accept as true," or "to credibly state."

Answering Dr. Nicholas Kopeloff's article on "The Pronunciation of Research," I would say that even if the majority of people put the accent on the first syllable rather than on the second syllable of "research," it does not make it right, and that educated men, and especially scientists, should strive to overcome the mistakes and "foibles" of other people. The argument for re′-search is that the search is *again* made! There is some excuse for this pronunciation when this meaning is intended.

Wm. T. Magruder
Ohio State University

QUOTATIONS

POPULAR SCIENCE

The translation of scientific news—nowadays so enormous in its bulk—into suitable language, and its condensation to comparatively minute dimensions, are undertaken in a systematic manner in the United States of America by an organization known as Science Service, Inc., directed by Dr. E. E. Slosson, and functioning under the auspices of the National Academy of Sciences, the National Research Council and the American Association for the Advancement of Science. This organization publishes daily science news bulletins, and a weekly summary of current science entitled the *Science News-Letter*, in which current events, scientific discoveries, and résumés of progress, together with broadly-drawn reports of the proceedings of scientific conventions, are recorded in simple terms. In addition, there is compiled a weekly digest, intended to present the cream of the week's scientific news, which is regularly used by more than twenty broadcasting stations in the United States.

Fortunately, in Great Britain there is little fear that discoveries might be announced to the listening public in a manner savoring of sensationalism, or that accounts of scientific affairs might be so rendered as to appear ludicrous to the initiated, for the policy in this respect of the British Broadcasting Corporation and of its predecessor company has been exemplary. We are, however, familiar with the result of excursions by otherwise competent journalists into spheres with which they are not familiar; indeed, the distaste for publicity which is usually ascribed to undue modesty might, if the truth were known, quite possibly often be traced simply to a fear of misrepresentation. The American press is now able, however, to rely on telegraphic news "stories," prepared by the managing editor of Science Service, Mr. Watson Davis, and the members of his specialist staff, so that their reports of the proceedings of conferences and conventions shall be well-balanced and accurate, without losing their attractiveness as items of news.

In Great Britain there is, of course, fairly adequate publication and survey of the results of research, such publication being intended for the use of the scientific population itself, and being normally directed by members of that fraternity, but we seem to lack a widespread sense of the importance of an appeal to the non-specialist members of the community as part of their ordinary daily culture, an appeal which must, to be worth while, be sponsored by the most notable members of the professions, and to be effective by the more journalistically-minded among them. There is, after all, no valid reason why the dissemination of knowledge beyond the confines of schools and colleges, provided it is carried out with scrupulous honesty, dignity and restraint, should not be acknowledged to be as valuable a social service as the collection and arrangement of the knowledge itself. True, this view has been given practical effect in certain influential sections of the British lay press by acknowledged authorities in a number of the sciences, but apart from one or two publications of admitted standing, there is little organized continuous effort in this direction. An attempt was made a couple of years ago to secure the interest of scientific societies and institutions in Great Britain in the establishment of a science publicity service, but the response was so disappointing that the scheme was abandoned.

Dr. E. E. Slosson, in a recent address before the American Association for Adult Education, made the somewhat surprising statement that archeology and astronomy—essentially remote and unpractical—head the list of the sciences in order of popular interest, and that the essentially practical sciences are low in the list. He ascribes this, probably correctly, to the same cause as that operating in the selection of, say, "futuristic art" as a subject of study in a women's club rather than "domestic economy." He declares that scientific workers have been too humble and too modest in claiming credit for what they have done and what they can do in the control of human affairs, but have allowed statesmen, writers and financiers to take all the praise for the advance in civilization and the amelioration of living conditions that were really due to scientific research. If we look at the matter from the point of view of the wealth of nations, as Dr. G. E. Hale, the honorary chairman of the National Research Council, has recently done in *Harper's Magazine*, it is clear enough that the business of men of science is to help to guide mankind as well as to serve it. That is to say, if a scientific orientation can more universally be associated with moral and religious convictions in the equipment of the human mind, there will be less danger of the wicked and unscrupulous misuse of scientific power, less point in arguing the prohibition of poison gas, and an extension of that wider fraternal patriotism which distinguishes scientific international relations.—*Nature.*

SCIENTIFIC BOOKS

The Biology of Insects. BY GEORGE H. CARPENTER, D.Sc. 473 pp., 16 pls., 88 text figs. London: Sidgwick & Jackson, Ltd., 1928, 16 s.

WHEN Professor J. Arthur Thomson, in the series of biological handbooks which he is editing, came to the insects, he chose a very good man to prepare this volume. Dr. Carpenter had shown, in his "Insect Transformation" (1921), done while he was professor of zoology in the Royal College of Science in Dublin and at the same time secretary of the Royal Irish Academy, and by his "Insects: Their Structure and Life" (1924), published after he became keeper of the Manchester Museum, that he had a grasp of the subject and a power of presentation in a very thoughtful and most interesting way that made him the man to do the insect volume in the biology series as it should be done.

It is very obvious that Mr. Savory, for example, who wrote "The Biology of the Spiders" in this same series, had a much simpler task than Dr. Carpenter's; and in fact the author of the present volume must have been put to it to decide just what to use in a book of this restricted size. The overwhelming number of insects, their extraordinary diversity in form, habit and function, and the great mass of accumulated and published knowledge would seem to necessitate the publication of several volumes on their biology instead of one. Dr. Carpenter, in his preface, acknowledges himself chargeable with the offense of omitting many subjects which might be expected to appear in such a book.

But to the person who examines the book with its wealth of interesting facts and its profusion of illustrations, the omissions will scarcely be noticed. The main topics considered in the fourteen chapters are, Feeding and Breathing; Movement; Sensation and Reaction; Behavior, Instinctive and Intelligent; Reproduction and Heredity; Growth and Transformation; Family Life; Social Life; Adaptations to Haunts and Seasons; Classification; Evolution; Insects and Other Organisms; Insects and Mankind. In all these topics Dr. Carpenter shows an extraordinary knowledge of the work done in many countries by many competent workers. He has hit upon the significant things and has explained them in such a way that they are readily understood. And he has brought into logical form and in proper juxtaposition the work of isolated individuals so as to place before the busy worker in biology a comprehensive and readable whole.

Important papers on important biological investigations have a way of accumulating so rapidly that the average worker is confused or badly informed, until such a book as this appears in which a thoroughly competent man has digested them all into an understandable whole.

Thus, the topics just mentioned have been given a just and philosophical treatment, sufficiently condensed to be plain reading and yet sufficiently detailed to be convincing—a difficult task done in a masterly way. The fifty-page chapter on evolution, for example, will be a delight to many workers who have not followed the recent contributions of entomology to different aspects of this engrossing subject.

The plates are done from admirable photographs, and, like the text figures, are admirably chosen.

L. O. HOWARD

DEPARTMENT OF AGRICULTURE,
WASHINGTON, D. C.

Colorado Plant Life. By FRANCIS RAMALEY. Published by the University of Colorado, Boulder, Colorado, 1927.

THIS book of 299 octavo pages and illustrated with 133 figures and three colored plates of Colorado wild flowers has been issued as Volume II of the Semicentennial Publications of the University of Colorado. As the work is dedicated to the citizens of Colorado with presumably only a modicum of botanical knowledge, it is written in a simple style without sacrificing essential scientific accuracy. In this especially well-illustrated and printed book the author, who is professor of biology in the state university, describes in successive chapters plant sociology, life zones and altitude, the botany from a railway train or automobile, color in plants, plants of stream-sides and ditch-banks, mountain-parks, mountain-lakes, the life of a plant, the plains in springtime and autumn, mesas and foothills, plants of the true mountains, grasses and grass-like plants, forests and forest trees, the architecture of plants, flowers, fruits and seeds, and the flora of Colorado in which chapter the characteristics of the principal plant groups are emphasized. Keys are added, so that the trees of Colorado may be identified readily. A list of the early spring flowers of Boulder and vicinity, comprising 102 species, is given with a bibliography of publications dealing with Colorado vegetation. Appendix IV comprises a list of books on botany suitable for high-school and public libraries in Colorado. The author has included in the chapter dealing with the flora of Colorado a short history of the study of Colorado botany, which began with the collection of plants by Edwin James, who was historian and naturalist of Major Long's Expedition (1819–20). He has furnished a sample, which might be followed profitably by other states of the Union.

JOHN W. HARSHBERGER

UNIVERSITY OF PENNSYLVANIA

SPECIAL ARTICLES

MULTIPLE POSITIVELY CHARGED RADIO-ACTIVE IONS

IN a recent paper[1] the writer discusses the question of the existence of doubly charged positive ions in gases for intervals of time usually involved in gas ion mobility measurements. It is there shown that previous experiments supposed to be conclusive on this point are not so and that there is practically no evidence for the existence of such ions under the conditions above. There remains unexplained a very definite observation by Erikson[2] on the mobility of recoil atoms from active deposits of Ra, Th, and Act which if correct can not be passed over summarily. The results were not checked in recent experiments of Dee[3] in which however the data were too meager to constitute a real contradiction. Erikson observes positive ions of mobility 1.56 for these recoil atoms, which are doubtless the normal singly charged positive ions in air. He also observes in high fields with shorter time intervals simultaneously with the slower ions, ions of mobility of 4.35 cm/sec per volt cm. in each case. These apparently do not show the aging effects usually found for positive ions in other gases. This mobility is nearly three times the mobility of the normal ion. He ascribes it to a doubly charged[2] ion in air. This it can not possibly be, as doubling the charge can not more than double the mobility. Furthermore on the basis of ion theories it is doubtful if the mobility is directly proportional to the charge. It is probable that the mobility of a doubly charged ion would be between twice the mobility of a singly charged ion and the mobility of that ion. A mobility of 4.35 cm/sec might mean a triply charged positive ion. It is more likely that it would correspond to an ion with at least four positive charges. It is the purpose of this article to give reasons for believing that we may

[1] Loeb, L. B., Proc. Nat. Acad., SCI., 13, 703, 1927.

[2] Erikson, H. A., *Phys. Rev.*, 24, 622, 1924, and 26, 629, 1925.

[3] Dee, P. I., Proc. Roy. Soc., A 116, 664, 1927.

be dealing in this case with a multiply charged ion of charge at least three or greater.

Multiply charged positive ions are generated in certain cases of what one might term catastrophic ionization as directly observed by Auger[4] for photoelectric ionization of heavier atoms by high frequency X-rays using the C. T. R. Wilson cloud expansion method. In such an ionization the X-ray removes a high speed photoelectron from the K ring of a heavy atom. The L electron falls into the K ring and gives rise to K X-radiation of the atom in question. The atom in which such an X-ray pulse starts has a high absorption coefficient for its own radiation and this liberates from the atom an electron with the energy of the K radiation less the ionization energy of the emitted electron. An M electron then falls into the L ring and so on. Thus successively 1, 2, 3, 4 etc. electrons are ejected from the same atom. For heavier atoms therefore the primary photoelectron and three other secondary electrons were observed to be liberated. Now when a fast β-ray is shot from the nucleus, Ellis[5] and independently Meitner[6] have shown that similar effects probably occur in the nucleus, giving rise to the β-ray spectra. The softer of the X-rays must lead to the Auger effect. Again the α particle emission is accompanied by X-radiation of a soft sort and there seems no reason for believing that in the expulsion of an α particle internal rearrangements may not take place that lead to multiple ionization of the parent atom. Owing to the large recoil energy of these particles (at least 2×10^8 volts) and the high atomic number the recoil process with only a few collisions with gas molecules would also sometimes result in multiple ionization. Thus it seems reasonable to assume that multiply positively charged products of radioactive change must occur. Investigations which are not exhaustive and are very much complicated by impacts with gas molecules have shown that the recoil atoms are largely uncharged or singly positively charged.[7,8,9,10,11] It seems from the literature that no really careful investigations of the charge present have been made which are free from the effects of collisions with molecules and have sought for multiply charged recoil atoms.

[4] Auger, *Jour. de Physique*, 6, 205, 1925.

[5] Ellis, C. D., Proc. Roy. Soc., A 99, 261, A 101, 1, 1922, A 105, 165, 1924.

[6] Meitner, L., *Zeits. f. Phys.*, 9, 131, 1922, 11, 1, 1922, and 26, 169, 1924.

[7] Makower and Russ, *Phil. Mag.*, 20, 875, 1910.

[8] Wertenstein, L., Comptes. Rendus., 161, 696, 1915.

[9] Wellisch, E. M., *Phil. Mag.*, 28, 417, 1914.

[10] Henderson, G. H., Transact. Roy Soc. Canada, 10, 151, 1917.

[11] Briggs, G. H., *Phil. Mag.*, 41, 357, 1921.

Having now shown that such charges can occur in recoil atoms the question can be raised as to whether they can be detected as ions. The theory of Klein and Rosseland,[12] and the researches of Franck[13,14] and his pupils have led us to expect that an atom or molecule in an active state can in impact with a different inactive molecule or atom transfer its energy to that atom, causing it to be excited or ionized. This can hold as well for ionized molecules and atoms as for excited ones. The difference between the two energies in such impacts may go to other excited states, to the energy of the escaping electron, or to kinetic energies of the separating atoms or ions. The greater such energy differences are, the more involved are the relations and the less chance is there for a transfer of charge. In fact Franck assumes a parallel between probability of the ionization by a radiation and its energy content relative to the ionization energy of the ionized electron and the type of processes where transfer of energy occurs on impact as above. This has been well borne out by the experiments of Harnwell[15] on the transfer of charges from ionized atoms or molecules of higher ionization potentials to those of lower ones.

Therefore we may regard an ionized atom as a metastable state of the atom whose life is the longer the heavier the charge, but whose life is also conditioned by the ionization energies of the surrounding atoms or molecules. Thus as the ionization potential of a radioactive atom is very low for a single ionization, such ions will be stable in air and some other gases and will appear. The doubly charged ions will, however, be unstable in air, as may be the case for the triply charged ones. Those atoms with four charges with their high energies may, however, be relatively stable and should in short time intervals be detectable.

It is thus even to be expected that the chance in a gas like O_2 of some doubly charged ion losing its energy to an O_2 molecule to give a singly charged ion and O^+_2 with energy is comparatively slight. In the case of gas ion measurements at atmospheric pressure the impacts are so numerous, however, that the chance of detecting a doubly charged molecule in a few hundredths of a second is practically 0. With the energy, however, of a quadruply charged positive radioactive recoil atom the chance of loss of charge may become so small that in measurements such as Erikson's it

[12] Klein and Rosseland, *Zeits. f. Phys.*, 4, 46, 1921.

[13] Franck and Cario, *Zeits. f. Phys.*, 11, 3, 1922.

[14] Franck and Jordan, "Anregung von Quanten Sprüngen durch Stösse," Julius Springer, Berlin, 1926, p. 216 ff.

[15] Harnwell, G. P., *Phys. Rev.*, 29, 830, 1927.

could still be detected, though not under ordinary conditions. It is therefore not unreasonable to ascribe the results of Erikson to some such process.

The question is one of considerable interest and importance for the gas ion problem. It seems it should also be of some interest from the radioactive point of view. It could easily be verified by a positive ray investigation of recoil atoms of the active deposits and it is hoped some laboratory equipped to do this work will find it worth while to undertake the measurement.

LEONARD B. LOEB
PHYSICAL LABORATORY,
UNIVERSITY OF CALIFORNIA

CROSSING-OVER BETWEEN THE W AND Z CHROMOSOMES OF THE KILLIFISH PLATYPOECILUS

THROUGH the aid of a Heckscher Research Grant from the university, the writers have been conducting over the past three years a series of investigations on inheritance in certain of the Cyprinodont fishes. One of these studies has involved two sex-linked genes in the killifish *Platypoecilus maculatus:* a dominant gene for red body-color (R) and one for black spots (Sp). Bellamy[1] (22) showed that both of these characters are sex-linked and he concluded that they are members of the same allelomorphic series. He also showed that the mode of sex-determination in *Platypoecilus* is of the WZ type. Gordon[2] (27) confirmed the findings of Bellamy regarding the sex-linkage of red and spots, but believed them not to be allelomorphs since a normal red, spotted female will transmit both characters to her sons.

In the present work, crosses have been made between red, spotted fish and non-red, non-spotted (the *Gold* race of the fanciers). Two breaks have occurred in the linkage of these genes by crossing over between the W and Z chromosomes of the females. In at least one other case there is evidence that a crossover has taken place in such a way as to transfer both genes, *R* and *Sp,* from the *Z* to the *W* chromosome. The exceptional female resulting from this process was apparently of the constitution $Z_{r\ sp}\ W_{R\ Sp}$, where a normal red, spotted female is $Z_{R\ Sp}\ W_{r\ sp}$. Two different breeding tests of this exceptional female strongly support the belief that her genotype was $Z_{r\ sp}\ W_{R\ Sp}$. These tests show further that this type is best explained as the result of crossing over between the W and Z chromosomes in a female which was heterozygous for red and spots, and that such an individual can not be accounted for by non-disjunction or sex reversal. There is, of course, the very remote possibility that this fish arose by a coincidental mutation of two recessive genes to dominants. However, the fact that other crossovers have occurred between the W and Z chromosomes in the course of these studies renders the *mutation explanation* even more unlikely.

The exceptional red, spotted female was crossed to a male heterozygous for both red and spots ($Z_{R\ Sp}\ Z_{r\ sp}$). Two types of daughters were obtained from this cross: $Z_{R\ Sp}\ W_{R\ Sp}$ and $Z_{r\ sp}\ W_{R\ Sp}$. The first of these presents the unusual condition of homozygosity of sex-linked factors in the heterogametic sex. Aida[3] (21) had the same condition in the red males of *Aplocheilus latipes* ($X_R\ Y_R$). The further breeding of these homozygous females gives unusual results which might well prove confusing to one who was attempting for the first time to investigate the mode of sex determination in this fish. Crosses of such females with *Gold* (r, sp) males will give only males in the double recessive class in F_2. In this respect the cross is similar to that of a red-eyed female Drosophila with a white-eyed male, and it would suggest the XY type of sex determination. However, in the reciprocal cross of *Gold* female with red, spotted male ($Z_{r\ sp}\ W_{r\ sp} \times Z_{R\ Sp}\ Z_{R\ Sp}$), the W-Z type of sex determination is exhibited.

Another cross of the exceptional female with a Gold (non-red, non-spotted) male gave red, spotted daughters like the mother and non-red, non-spotted sons, like the father. Evidently this constitutes a case of "one-sided feminine inheritance" similar to the "one-sided masculine inheritance" observed by Schmidt[4] (20) in his studies of the *maculatus* spot in the fish *Lebistes reticulatus*. It is expected that further crosses of these red, spotted daughters with Gold males will give in turn, red, spotted female offspring, barring occasional crossovers.

Crossing over has been reported previously between the two Z chromosomes of the male fowl, and between the X and Y chromosomes of *Aplocheilus* (Aida '21) and the X and Y of the *Lebistes* (Winge[5] '23). The present work seems to involve the first case of crossing over between the sex chromosomes of an heterogametic female. A detailed report of these investigations will be published later.

ALLAN C. FRASER
MYRON GORDON
CORNELL UNIVERSITY

[1] Bellamy, A. W., *Anat. Rec.*, 24: 419–420, 1922.

[2] Gordon, M., *Genetics* 12: 253–283, 1927.

[3] Aida, T., *Genetics* 6: 554–573, 1921.

[4] Schmidt, J., *Comptes rendus des travaux du Lab. Carlsberg* 14, No. 8: 1–12, 1920.

[5] Winge, O., *Comptes rendus des travaux du Lab. Carlsberg* 14, No. 20: 1–19, 1923.

SCIENCE

Vol. LXVII MAY 11, 1928 No. 1741

CONTENTS

What Constitutes Publication? Dr. C. W. Stiles 471
The Seventh Cruise of the Non-magnetic Yacht "Carnegie": J. A. Fleming 478
Harris Hawthorne Wilder: Professor Henry S. Pratt 479
Scientific Events:
The Secretaries' Conference of the American Association and Affiliated Societies; Annual Meeting of Science Service; National Academy of Sciences; Appointments of the Carnegie Institution 481
Scientific Notes and News 483
University and Educational Notes 487
Discussion and Correspondence:
Does the Amount of Food Consumed Influence the Growth of an Animal: Professor Wm. C. Rose. *The Siberian Meteorite*: Dr. George P. Merrill. *A Rhizoctonia which forms Hymenial Cells and Basidiospores*: J. E. Kotila. *Modeling Clay as a Substitute for Colophonium Wax*: R. R. Durant. *A "Data" of Research*: Dr. F. L. Wells 488
Scientific Books:
Thomson's Brachiopod Morphology and Genera: Professor Charles Schuchert 491
Scientific Apparatus and Laboratory Methods:
The Use of Naphthalene in Narcotizing Earthworms: Dr. Elbert C. Cole 492
Special Articles:
The Effects of Selective Solar Radiations on Growth and Development: Dr. Charles Sheard and George M. Higgins. *Vitamin B—A Question of Nomenclature*: S. L. Smith 493
The Federation of American Societies of Experimental Biology: Dr. E. D. Brown 496
Science News x

SCIENCE: A Weekly Journal devoted to the Advancement of Science, edited by J. McKeen Cattell and published every Friday by

THE SCIENCE PRESS

New York City: Grand Central Terminal

Lancaster, Pa. Garrison, N. Y.

Annual Subscription, $6.00. Single Copies, 15 Cts.

SCIENCE is the official organ of the American Association for the Advancement of Science. Information regarding membership in the Association may be secured from the office of the permanent secretary, in the Smithsonian Institution Building, Washington, D. C.

WHAT CONSTITUTES PUBLICATION?[1]

Your secretary has assigned to me a Chinese puzzle. Kindly permit me, in accepting this assignment, to make one point unambiguous, namely, that in any views expressed to-day I am speaking only in my individual capacity, as a specimen of the genus *Homo* and not as secretary of the International Commission on Zoological Nomenclature. In fact, it is entirely conceivable that at some future time, as mouthpiece of the commission, I might express views at variance with the content of this paper.

A second point to be made clear is that no definition of zoological publication can be formulated which is not subject to debate, differences of opinion and criticism.

With this introduction I feel at liberty to discuss this very complicated theme.

"Publication" has numerous definitions, more or less subjective according to the particular field and goal under consideration. Our problem is "what constitutes zoological publication?"

Whatever subject we discuss, it is both interesting and instructive to consider the derivation of our terms in order to gain a starting point.

The English word "publication" comes from the Latin *publicatio*, which means "an adjudging to the public treasury, confiscation." Thus, when a zoological manuscript (legally the property of an individual) is published, its content becomes, by confiscation, the property of the *populus zoologicus*. *Ergo*, from the moment of publication the author has no more claim to the data or the ideas contained therein than has any other member of the zoological profession, except in so far as he may take out a copyright (which gives the exclusive right to multiply and to dispose of copies of an intellectual production—corresponding to a patent of an invention).

Consequently, the author has no more right to change a given published name than has any other zoologist—although the code of ethics provides that in case the author has inadvertently published a homonym, the colleague who notices this fact is to invite the attention of the author to it and, as an act of professional courtesy, to give him first opportunity to correct his error in technique.

The word *publicatio* is based on the Latin *publicare*, which means "to make public property, to seize and

[1] Address, by invitation, before American Ornithological Union, Nov. 15, 1927.

adjudge to public use, to confiscate; to show or tell to the public, to impart to the public, to make public; to publish, etc."

Publicare involves *publicus*,[2] a contraction of *populicus*, from *populus*, which from the root *ple*, of *pleo* (*cf. plenum*), means the people, multitude, host, crowd, throng, great number of persons, etc. *Pleo*, root *ple*,[3] brings us to rock foundation, and means "to fill, to fulfill."

The conclusion appears to be justified that the underlying basic idea in the English word "publication" involves the conception of reaching the *complete*, namely, *not abridged* public.

The completeness of a notice depends upon the audience it is intended to reach. A notice by the American Ornithological Union is complete and therefore published if it is intended only for the members of the American Ornithological Union and if it is addressed through regular channels to each and every member, namely, the *populus* of the American Ornithological Union.

Applying this idea to zoological publication, the conclusion appears justified, from the root *ple*, that a zoological document is published when it is addressed, through regular standard channels of communication, and therefore made potentially available, to the entire zoological public, *i.e.*, the zoologists of the world.

If this viewpoint, based on the conception *populus zoologicus*, be accepted, the corollary obtains that no document addressed to a "limited," "restricted," or "abridged" portion of the zoological public, is, theoretically, zoological publication—since it is not addressed to the entire profession. Thus, if a member of the American Ornithological Union communicates a thought, data regarding a new species, etc., to a colleague, or to all the members of the American Ornithological Union, and restricts or abridges its dissemination by any method which prevents it from reaching the entire zoological public, his act is not zoological publication.

On this principle, neither the date of manuscript nor the presentation of a paper before a restricted audience is accepted as zoological publication, but it becomes publication on the date when the document becomes potentially available to the entire zoological public. On this same principle, proof sheets sent to colleagues to obtain their criticisms have been declared (Opinion 87 of the International Commission) as not constituting zoological publication; and the same principle comes into consideration in connection with the much-discussed Huebner's Tentamen, which was by title addressed to experts, in this case specialists in *Lepidoptera* (see Opinion 97).

With this theoretically basic idea contained in the root *ple*, which thus represents the constitution of publication, so to speak, let us pass to the by-laws (or technique) by means of which the constitution is administered. Here we reach various *practical* aspects of the subject.

It is to be frankly accepted that the technique of publication varies according to the audience addressed, as, for instance, in the case of the board of health regulations of Washington, D. C., which do not involve the citizens of China or South Africa.

The practical problem is: What by-laws are necessary, reasonable and feasible in order that zoological publications may be potentially and reasonably available for use by the *populus zoologicus?* In this connection, it is well to consider—(1) Period of publication; (2) date of publication; (3) address of publisher; (4) language used; (5) status as record; (6) size of edition; (7) methods of manifolding manuscript; (8) sale; (9) daily newspapers; (10) separata; (11) sales-catalogues; (12) society programs.

(1) *Period of publication:* The *populus zoologicus* has varied at different times. In 1760, zoologists were located chiefly, but not exclusively, in Europe. To-day, they are widely distributed practically over the entire world.

The practical condition of making publications reasonably available to the zoological public in 1760 could be largely met by the system of distributing university theses, by exchange, to the leading university centers of Europe without placing the documents on sale. Thus, this system of university exchange could well be accepted in 1760 as largely meeting the necessities of the profession and thus it comes within the basic idea of publication.

To-day, however, the exchange system, not backed by public sale, is thoroughly inadequate to meet the reasonable requirements of the profession; hence this system, still in vogue to some extent, can no longer be reasonably accepted as zoological publication.

The moral is that the requirements as respects distribution vary according to the numbers and geographic distribution of the members of the profession; hence chronologically these requirements are a variable

[2] *Publicus* refers to a public officer; *publicum* to the public purse, also a public place; *publice* on account, at the cost, in behalf, or in charge of the state, also, before the people, openly, publicly.

[3] *Plenus*, from the same root (*cf.* Greek πλα; Latin *plerus, plebs, populus*, etc.), means full, filled; *plenum*, a space occupied by matter, full packed, laden, entire, complete, full, whole, at full length, not contracted, unabridged, abundant, plentiful, much, finished, ample. *Plene*, literally full, means fully, wholly, completely, thoroughly, largely, etc. The same root is found in *plerus* (very many), *plerusque* (a very great part), *pleraque* (all, everything, mostly, for the most part), *plerumque* (the greatest part, commonly).

factor, and what might be reasonably accepted as publication in 1760, 1800 or 1850 is not of necessity to be accepted as publication in 1927.

(2) *Date of publication:* As the law of priority is based upon chronological data, it is obvious that the date of publication is an essential factor in the by-laws of zoological publication.

In the vast majority of cases, the year date suffices; in a lesser number of cases, the month is necessary; in exceptional cases, the day of the month is imperative.

The general principle is universally recognized, so far as I recall, that the date borne by a publication is assumed to be correct unless and until proved to be incorrect.

In connection with the date, various complications—some theoretical, others practical—arise.

For instance, the point has been raised that it may still be November 15 in San Francisco at a moment when it is November 16 in London. Thus, two publications, differing in date by one day, might be issued at the same moment in London and in San Francisco. Which has priority? This same point has been raised in connection with the new wording of the law of priority, and the commission has settled it in advance by definitely stating in its report to the congress that the revised law of priority takes effect at Greenwich time midnight between December 31, 1930, and January 1, 1931. Accordingly, for the United States, the new wording actually becomes effective in the latter part of December 31, by our time.

In connection with the date of publication, serious printers' difficulties are often encountered which are beyond the control of either the author or the editor. Theoretically, it would be wise to print the year, month and day of the month on every zoological publication; but practically this is often impossible, for delays due to proofreading, breakdown of machinery, strikes, etc., etc., are always likely to occur and thereby invalidate the intended exact date of issue as set up in type. To prescribe these details is therefore not always practical, notwithstanding their desirability. But, as the saying goes, "there is more than one way to skin a cat": It is entirely feasible for a serial publication to print in its volume table of contents the exact dates of issue of the separate parts[4] or of each number in each succeeding number, or on the cover or last page of its final number, or in the first number of the next volume.

[4] As a side question in this connection, libraries should always bind in place the cover page of each number when they make up the volume. A failure to do this causes much extra labor for persons who use the serial.

But what is to be said of documents which bear no date at all? Theoretically, two possibilities come into consideration:

(a) Establish the date by evidence obtained elsewhere, as in the case of Huebner's (1806) Tentamen; and

(b) Reject the document on the ground that it lacks the evidence necessary for the application of the law of priority.

In principle, I favor the second alternative. In documents undated as to publication the publisher has not "played the game" with the profession; he has made a "foul play" and the "foul" should be ruled out. I should be inclined to support this as a thoroughly justified rule in connection with future publications. But ought it be made retroactive? Here certain practical considerations arise.

Some undated publications contain names which many authors have adopted. Should we not temper justice with mercy, as applied to some exceptional cases?

If one replies that a principle once adopted should be consistently carried out, and therefore be made retroactive, the answer can be made that we are often faced by choosing between two principles, one primary and more important, the other secondary and less important. As a matter of fact, does not everybody subordinate some secondary principle to some primary principle more or less frequently, possibly every day?

It would not hurt my conscience to vote to suspend the rules for Huebner's Tentamen, despite the fact that it was undated, provided entomologists prove that the rejection of this document will result in greater confusion than uniformity, although to my mind the Tentamen is not zoological publication, but essentially entomological correspondence addressed to a restricted audience.

In principle, I consider that undated documents do not correspond with the technique necessary to make them of reasonable use by the *populus zoologicus*, and, therefore, that they are not zoological publication. It seems eminently unfair to throw upon the reader the burden of proof as respects the date of a document; it causes extra and unreasonable work and easily leads to different conclusions, with later confusion in nomenclature.

For documents of indefinite year date (for instance, "Proceedings for the years 1891–95"), with no further clew as to date of issue, it would seem fair to consider December 31, 1895, as date of publication; and for documents issued with no more exact date than the year (example, "1927") it would appear fair to accept December 31 as date unless and until more definite date is proved.

(3) *Address of publisher:* The address of the publisher is scarcely a *sine qua non* of publication, for it is not zoologically essential to know whether or by whom a given document was printed in London, New York or elsewhere. But think of the unnecessary extra work caused our friends-in-need, the bookdealers and the librarians, when the address of the publisher is not stated. Some printed zoological documents have been distributed without any direct intimation as to whether they were printed in North America, England or Australia, and this point has been raised against one document which is supposed to have been printed at home by the author's son who is said not to be a trade printer.

Cases of this kind seem to have their origin in certain economic conditions which will be referred to later.

I would welcome a rule, effective (say) January 1, 1931, that no document be accepted as publication unless it bears the name of the publisher (or printer) with at least the name of the city in which his office is located. Before making such a rule retroactive, however, I would desire information as to its possible effect on nomenclature and further I would want the viewpoints of booksellers, librarians and publishers, with whom we should "play the game" fairly.

(4) *Language of publication:* Prior to 1800, the question of language of publication was relatively uncomplicated. Latin was read and written by most zoologists and thus formed an acceptable language for the *populus zoologicus.* Not unnaturally, however, even prior to 1800, some zoologists published in the modern languages—chiefly in those of western Europe, which also were understood more or less generally by the zoological public.

How much more complicated this problem is to-day! Professional zoologists are more widely distributed now as respects their mother tongue, some countries lay much less stress than formerly upon the ability to write in Latin, and the semi-professional and the amateur zoologists have increased tremendously in number and distribution.

Not only a theoretical question of national pride, but also practical questions of local economic conditions and other considerations now lead zoologists to publish in Hungarian, Japanese, Polish, Russian and other languages not ordinarily understood by the average zoologists, and the resulting international difficulties of potential availability of the contents of zoological literature are rapidly increasing. This represents a much more serious and more practical problem than is usually admitted and its solution is not so self-evident as I wish it were.

Many authors who write in languages not ordinarily studied clearly grasp the situation—as is evidenced by the fact that they append to their articles abstracts in one of the languages more commonly read than their own. Some of the publications in these exceptional languages are abstracted in journals published in the more international tongues.

That the profession will adopt either Latin or any one of the modern tongues as its official language is hardly to be expected and such a course would not solve the practical problem to-day. The most feasible solution appears to be a movement to urge all authors who publish in the exceptional languages to emulate the considerate example of so many of their colleagues by appending summaries in any one of several more or less generally studied languages. Whether it would be feasible to require this, as a premise to their admission under the law of priority, is a question upon which I scarcely feel in a position to make a pronouncement—for this requires an international consensus of opinion.

(5) *Status as records:* Manuscript can be manifolded for various purposes, for instance: Letters of inquiry, letters of instructions, duplicate proof sheets for criticism by colleagues, news letters regarding administrative or personnel items of an organization. These and some other documents are obviously of ephemeral nature and purpose, intended for the information of a restricted audience, and they do not serve the *populus zoologicus* as a permanent record—unless they are reprinted in a journal or definitely placed on sale through regular channels.

The intent of the document to serve as a permanent record of data would seem to be an exceedingly important, possibly a determining factor, in the pertinency of evidence as to zoological publication.

(6) *Size of edition:* We have seen that publication, through the root *ple,* involves the idea of general, unabridged or numerous. At first thought, one might be inclined to apply this concept in mathematical terms to the size of an edition (*i.e.,* the number of printed copies) as a practical standard to define publication. This, of course, would present difficulties, but it suggests certain general deductions.

An ornithological document issued specifically for the use of ornithologists is obviously not issued for the use of the general *populus zoologicus* but for only a fraction of the whole. Although that document may be of greater interest to this minority than it is to the majority, it can conceivably have a direct bearing on the work of the majority. If, however, by virtue of its being issued only to ornithologists it is limited to them, the conclusion seems justified that the edition is too small to be general, therefore it is not a zoological publication—no matter how universally it is distributed to ornithologists. In this hypothetical case, it is not really the *size* of the edition which comes into consideration, but the restriction of distribution.

Universities more or less generally require that graduates deposit a given number of copies (say twenty-five to forty, in cases personally known to me) of each thesis, and these copies are distributed, on an exchange system, to other universities. Does this represent zoological publication? My opinion is that *as of to-day* it can not be so accepted; this conclusion is based, however, not on the number of copies but on the method of distribution by exchange, a method which to-day does not make documents potentially and reasonably available to the *populus zoologicus*.

A state experiment station might issue a large edition, say five thousand copies, of a zoological bulletin for free and wide distribution *to the farmers of that state*. Here again it is not the size of the edition, but the audience to which it is addressed and distributed which is the more important factor. If that document is not available to the world-wide zoological public through regular channels, it is not theoretically published as a zoological record.

(7) *Method of manifolding manuscript:* The question as to the methods of manifolding manuscript (printing press, photograph, multigraph, stencil, photostat, etc.) is an important one. The printing press is (to a great extent) the standard method. But the multigraph is coming into widespread use in office work and has actually been used for at least one serial publication issued here in Washington by one of the government bureaus. Apparently stencil-made copies of an official serial were once issued by the German imperial government.

This question of method brings up the serious question of economics—and this latter problem carries us into more and more diverging necessities.

In view of the economic problems involved, I am not prepared to take a definite stand on the question of technique of manifolding manuscript as a condition precedent to recognizing publications.

(8) *Sale:* Reasonably to fulfill the requirements of the zoological profession, a document intended as a permanent record should be reasonably accessible to all zoologists.

The fulfillment of this requirement can be met theoretically in either of two ways, namely: (1) the publisher might distribute the document *gratis* to all public, university, college, laboratory and school libraries; or (2) the document might be placed on public sale through recognized trade channels, namely, dealers who are known to make a business of selling zoological publications.

Obviously, the first possibility, though theoretically conceivable, is impracticable for several reasons, *i.e.:* (1) it is economically too expensive; (2) it is inexcusably and economically wasteful; and (3) it is economically excluded from the standpoint of libraries, for public libraries in general have neither the space nor the personnel to take care of all documents. The deduction is, therefore, that free distribution is a most excellent policy—for this makes the document available to zoologists within practical range of the depository, but the conclusion can not be escaped that it does not make it reasonably accessible to the *populus zoologicus*. Accordingly, there is serious objection to making *gift* a determining factor in distribution.

The second possibility (*i.e., sale* through regular channels) makes the document potentially available to the entire zoological profession and therefore fulfills both theoretical and practical requirements.

Accordingly, the conclusion seems justified that as far as zoological documents of record are concerned, the offering for sale through regular zoological bookdealers at time of issue is theoretically a *sine qua non* of zoological publication.

(9) *Is a lay newspaper zoological publication?* Lay newspapers (daily, weekly, city, county, etc.) are on sale, are distributed through regular channels, are dated, their publishers are known, and they more than welcome additional subscribers. Thus they are undoubtedly generally and universally available, despite the fact that zoologists are only an infinitesimal fraction of the audience to which the newspaper is addressed. From this viewpoint, they are undoubtedly zoological publication.

But, are they reasonably available as professional documents of record? To be permanent records, they must be stored in zoological libraries. If the American Ornithological Union adopts the Washington *Post* as its regular medium of addressing the zoological public, each and every zoological society in the world would have the right to adopt the local newspaper of some other city, town or county for the same purpose.

We must pass from the theoretical to the practical. As a practical problem, would any zoological library in the world be in a position, either as respects space, finances or personnel, to keep these newspapers on file for our use? And since very few of them are indexed, could we use them if they were on file? This practical consideration places the daily press in the *reductio ad absurdum,* as respects zoological publication.

(10) *Are "preprints," "reprints," "separata," etc., zoological publication?* This much-discussed question can be approached from more than one angle:

(a) If a "preprint" is to be accepted as publication, then this is actually *the* publication of an article and the journal print is in reality a "reprint." Under this interpretation, how many editors would consent to furnish "preprints"?

(b) Some journals accept manuscript under the condition that the article is not to be published elsewhere. In this case, the author automatically agrees with the editor that neither reprint nor preprint is "publication."

(c) Assume that a manuscript contains "*Tweedledum* new genus" or "*Tweedledum tweedledee* new species": The publication of the new genus or new species represents its literary birth, so to speak. Can a genus or a species be born twice?

(d) Is the "separate" reasonably available to the zoological public through ordinary channels, *i.e.*, is it on sale? If it is, it is neither a "preprint" nor a "reprint" but a distinct publication.

(e) Separates (preprints, reprints, etc.) are essentially complimentary copies for the personal use of the author and his special mailing list, *i.e.*, a restricted distribution. Many of them bear the statement that they are not for sale, and this is *prima facie* evidence that these particular copies are not publication.

(f) To throw upon the reader the burden of proof whether an author uses his "separata" fairly or unfairly to the editor and publisher and has made his separates reasonably available to the zoological public, is not "playing the game" fairly with the reader.

The conclusion (from my viewpoint) is that, in general, evidence which proves that documents are separata (preprints or reprints), is *ipso facto* proof that they are not separate publication, but at best that they take the same date of publication as the journal article. Cases can, however, be imagined in which a so-called "separate" is actual publication and in which the journal article is the reprint. But the interpretation lies near, that republication in a journal is for the purpose of making the article reasonably available to the profession—and if this interpretation be correct, the conclusion seems justified that by republication the author automatically admits that his article was not reasonably available to the profession through his preprints, *ergo* that the preprints were not zoological publication.

It may be frankly admitted that there are viewpoints, *pro* and *con*, *ad infinitum*, other than those I have presented. For instance, if an author in Washington deposits a copy of a preprint in the Congressional Library, this document is available (after delay for cataloguing and other necessary "red tape") to all zoologists in and near Washington, and it is also available to any zoologist in South Africa who will buy a steamer ticket to an American port and a railroad ticket from there to Washington. But is this reasonable availability from the viewpoint of the zoological public? If this be acknowledged as "playing the game" fairly with the profession—a point I am so narrow-minded as not to support—then it is logical to accept as publication the deposit (in a public library) of a single copy of typewritten or photostatic manuscript, or of duplicate proof (either galley or page) as a preprint, months before the journal appears. This is surely a practical *reductio ad absurdum*, however theoretically correct it may be.

In connection with the general subject of "separata," may I invite attention to the enormous amount of waste to the profession, in time and energy, due to that invention (by some "printer's devil") known as "repaging" of reprints. Just why it is that publishers continue this vicious system which causes so much trouble and expense, I can not understand—but I am not a printer, therefore I do not look through the "book-maker's" spectacles. My view may be narrow and due to gross ignorance, but I labor under the impression that any factor (such as repaging, double-paging, etc.) which decreases the practical value of a document to the user can best be discontinued.

(11) *Are sales catalogues zoological publication?* Think of the amount of printer's ink used in discussing this subject! From my viewpoint (right or wrong as it may be considered), sales catalogues are of two distinct sorts:

(a) Most sales catalogues (example, the noted Brookes,[5] 1828, catalogue) are intended as ephemeral documents addressed to an exceedingly limited audience; they are not on sale; and they are not documents intended as permanent records; therefore they are not zoological publication.

(b) In very exceptional cases (example, the first edition, 1798, of the Museum boltenianum) the sales catalogue appears to be utilized for the issuance and recording of scientific data. If placed on sale, it can be reasonably interpreted as zoological publication; if distributed *gratis* during the period when the exchange distribution of university theses reasonably met the demands of the profession, it can be reasonably interpreted as publication. But assuredly, if the Museum boltenianum were issued in 1927 (instead of 1798) and not placed on sale, it would not come within my conception of publication—even if it were sent to every conchologist in the world. In other words, a document like the Museum boltenianum seems to me essentially on the same status as a university thesis—publication in the period prior to 1800, but not in 1927. No sharp line can be drawn at a given date between 1799 and 1927; some cases must of necessity be decided more or less arbitrarily by a specially appointed jury. Let the jury agree or differ with me, I am prepared to accept the jury verdict, for I am a

[5] Brookes, 1828, Cat. Anat. and Zool. Mus. of Joshua Brookes, London, ''a sales catalogue'' (''Eighth days sale, Wed., July 23, 1828, at twelve o'clock'').

firm believer in the legal maxim: *"Interest rei publicae ut sit finis litium"*—"it concerns the commonwealth (*publicus zoologicus*) that there be a limit to litigation [controversy]. Courts at law settle controversies about as frequently as they dispense justice, and some administrative decisions on cases of nomenclature and of publication are of necessity on this same general basis. Some court decisions are made on a very narrow margin which is subject to debate, and the same will always hold true in nomenclature and publication—but the important point is to obtain a decision and then accept it—in other words, "to play the game" with the profession.

(12) *Are society programs publication?* In answer to this question, I must use a witness's privilege in court, "Yes and no, and I will explain my answer."

The program of this meeting is free to everybody here, but it is not potentially and reasonably available to John Doe, protozoologist in Australia. Therefore, this sheet is not to be accepted as publication even were it to contain detailed abstracts of the papers presented.

But the moment this program is placed on permanent record in an annual volume offered for sale or in a journal, accepted as proper medium for publication, it becomes publication, and a new name thus printed would take date, *ceteris paribus,* as of the date of said journal—but not as of the date of this meeting.

Definition: On basis of the discussion thus far, but without expecting general agreement with me, I would define zoological publication theoretically as: *The manifolding of a dated zoological document which is intended as permanent record* and *which is made potentially and reasonably available to the populus zoologicus as of the decade of issue.*

The theoretical vs. the practical: While it is not difficult to point out certain theoretical factors in answer to the question assigned to me for discussion, the practical side of enforcing these factors is an entirely different question. Two very important principles in particular are to be considered, namely:

First: The basic question must always be considered, *"How much does it cost?* In other words, a practical application of theoretical ideals depends largely upon available funds. Economic conditions can not be escaped, and with the increased cost of printing the problem of finding prompt outlet for manuscript becomes increasingly more difficult. In absence of sufficient endowment and of adequate commercial returns to publishers, it is not unnatural that authors have followed directions of lesser resistance and have issued manuscripts under standards of manifolding which are not always ideal. If they did not know better, the fault is not theirs but that of their teachers; if they did know better, but did the best they could under the circumstances, should we not endeavor to improve the circumstances rather than blame the authors? *Why should not scientific journals be endowed, as well as university chairs, as permanent memorials to persons?* If any of you wish to establish a memorial of this kind to your parents or to a son or daughter, I feel quite confident that I can mention at least two worth-while serials which would welcome an endowment—and both of them need it very seriously.

Second: A rule, regulation or standard, voluntary as to adoption, is of practical value in so far as it has the approval of the *populus.* In this connection attention may be invited to the fact that the zoological profession is composed of specialists, therefore of individualists, who have an inherited idea that science must be free and untrammeled and who are occasionally somewhat inclined (I speak from personal experience in nomenclature) to resent decisions which are not in harmony with their own personal views. With all due respect I would good-naturedly invite attention to the fact that the words "freedom" and "disregard of propriety" are not synonyms.

The profession is not prepared to bow to the views of any one person, but I am persuaded that much good could be accomplished gradually if the International Zoological Congress would appoint a special "Commission on Principles and Practices of Publication" and assign to it the duty of studying this problem from the viewpoints of theory as well as from the practical economics existing in various countries, to determine in how far standards can be internationalized and in how far it would be feasible to reduce the present widespread waste (of publication space and subscription funds) by concentrating the present much-duplicated reviews into fewer journals, thereby releasing more much desired space for original contributions.

Such a commission could classify the current zoological publications in various groups, on a percentage basis or, let us say, as

Class A: Publications printed in or with summaries in certain languages, placed on sale, with a minimum edition of n copies, and with a free list of r copies at least x of which are sent abroad.

Class B: Publications placed on sale, printed in or with summaries in certain languages, with a minimum edition of n copies, but with no free list.

Class C: Publications printed in languages not ordinarily understood and with no summary in more generally understood languages.

Class D: Publications with editions composed of less than n copies.

Various combinations of important characters could be made and publishers would sooner or later endeavor to bring their works into the higher grades as defined by the commission, while two or more periodicals would probably unite, in many cases, in order to improve their standards, and some of the struggling serials would probably die a natural death more promptly than occurs at present.

Further, the commission could hand down opinions in respect to cases in doubt as to whether a given document is or is not to be accepted as published.

Self-understood, it would take time to obtain practical results. Civilization was not made in a day, and important reforms are developed by evolution rather than by revolution. A campaign of education by the commission would, however, work up a general sentiment in the profession in favor of the view that for the good of science publications should line up to certain prescribed standards of "playing the game" with the profession.

I have sufficient faith in the zoological profession to feel that a systematic campaign of education by an international commission, authorized by the congress and carefully selected as respects its personnel, would accomplish more good in standardizing the *sine qua non* of zoological publications than will any amount of individual essays or debate dealing with this subject which, year by year, is becoming a more complicated, more serious and more practical subject.

C. W. STILES

U. S. PUBLIC HEALTH SERVICE

THE SEVENTH CRUISE OF THE NON-MAGNETIC YACHT "CARNEGIE"

THE non-magnetic yacht *Carnegie,* of the Department of Terrestrial Magnetism of the Carnegie Institution of Washington, resumed on May 1, from Washington, D. C., the magnetic and electric survey of the oceans. Thus the plans visioned in 1904 under the enthusiastic and energetic directorship of Dr. Louis A. Bauer for the world-wide magnetic and electric survey will be further realized and the results already obtained will be greatly enhanced. This work was begun during 1905 to 1908 on the chartered brigantine *Galilee* in the then magnetically unexplored Pacific under the command, respectively, of J. P. Pratt for the first cruise and of W. J. Peters for the second and third cruises. With the completion of the specially designed yacht *Carnegie* in 1909 the survey was continued with greater efficiency, because of non-magnetic construction of the vessel and of the steady evolution of suitable instruments and observational methods, in all oceans during 1909 to 1921 under the command, respectively, of W. J. Peters for cruises I and II, of J. P. Ault for cruises III, IV and VI, and of H. M. W. Edmonds for cruise V.

Cruise VII of the *Carnegie,* to continue for three years during 1928 to 1931, will cover all oceans and will add 110,000 miles to the total of 290,000 miles already traversed by the vessel's first six cruises. Besides continued magnetic and atmospheric-electric investigations as heretofore with improved apparatus, determinations of natural marine electric-currents will be attempted as well as an extensive schedule in physical and biological oceanography.

The proposed increase in program is made possible through the addition of two to the scientific personnel which will total eight men. These and their special fields of activity are: Captain J. P. Ault, commander and chief of scientific staff; Wilfred C. Parkinson, senior scientific officer, atmospheric electricity and photography; Oscar W. Torreson, navigator and executive officer, magnetism, navigation and meteorology; F. M. Soule, observer and electrical expert, magnetism and physical oceanography; H. R. Seiwell, chemist and biologist, oceanography; J. H. Paul, surgeon and observer, medical work, meteorology and oceanography; W. E. Scott, observer, navigation and commissary; Lawrence A. Jones, radio operator and observer, radio investigation and communication. The sailing staff will consist of 17 men, making the total number of men on board 25; of the sailing staff, A. Erickson, first watch officer, C. E. Leyer, engineer and F. Lyngdorf, steward, occupied similar positions during the entire two years of the *Carnegie's* last cruise.

The necessary reconditioning of the vessel was completed last summer at Hoboken, New Jersey. The proposed program requires a great amount of instrumental equipment. Many improvements have been made by the department's shop in the magnetic and atmospheric-electric apparatus used on cruise VI; chief among these are the arrangements for electromagnetic determinations of magnetic inclination and intensity and for photographic registration of atmospheric potential-gradient. The oceanographic equipment includes an improved type of Wenner's electrical salinity apparatus made in the department's shop, Richter and Wiese thermometers and water-bottles, Nansen water-bottles, special non-magnetic winch with 6,000-foot and 20,000-foot aluminum-bronze cables for depth-work, sonic depth-finder loaned by the United States Navy Department, chemical and biological apparatus, silk meter and half-meter plankton-nets, various types of bottom-samplers and necessary appurtenances. The meteorological instruments are in general of the recording type and a special program of observation and control has been arranged. At Plymouth and at Hamburg additional recording wet- and dry-bulb thermograph and wet- and dry-bulb resistance-thermometer equipment with recording galvanometer for three stations at masthead, cross-tree and meteorological screen are to be installed.

The first leg of the cruise will be to Plymouth, England, where the vessel will arrive about the end of May. After a call at Hamburg the next ports of call will be at Iceland, at Barbados and at the Canal Zone (about the end of October, 1928). The balance of the cruise will cover the North Pacific, South Pacific, South Atlantic, Indian and North Atlantic oceans, and is planned to include ports of call at Easter Island, Callao, Papeete, Apia, Guam, Yokohama, San Francisco, Honolulu, Apia, Lyttelton, South Georgia, St. Helena, Cape Town, Colombo, St. Paul, Fremantle, Lyttelton, Rapa Island, Buenos Aires, St. Helena, Ponta Delgada, Madeira and Washington, D. C. (about September, 1931).

The preparations for this cruise have had generous cooperation and expert advice on all sides from interested governmental and private organizations and individuals both in America and Europe, who have also either loaned or presented much of the special oceanographic equipment and many books for the reference-library on board. Among these the Carnegie Institution of Washington is indebted to the following: United State Navy Department, including particularly its Hydrographic Office, Naval Research Laboratory, Signal Corps and Air Corps of the War Department, Coast Guard, National Museum, Bureau of Fisheries, Weather Bureau and Coast and Geodetic Survey; Scripps Institution of Oceanography of the University of California; Museum of Comparative Zoology of Harvard University; School of Geography of Clark University; American Radio Relay League; Geophysical Institute, Bergen, Norway; Marine Biological Association of the United Kingdom, Plymouth, England; German Atlantic Expedition of the *Meteor,* Institut für Meereskunde, Berlin, Germany; British Admiralty, London; Carlsberg Laboratorium, Bureau International pour l'exploration de la Mer, and Laboratoire Hydrographique, Copenhagen, Denmark, and many others. Dr. H. U. Sverdrup, of the Geophysical Institute at Bergen, Norway, research associate of the Carnegie Institution of Washington, is consulting oceanographer and physicist.

J. A. FLEMING

DEPARTMENT OF TERRESTRIAL MAGNETISM,
CARNEGIE INSTITUTION OF WASHINGTON

HARRIS HAWTHORNE WILDER

DR. H. H. WILDER, professor of zoology in Smith College since 1892, died suddenly in Northampton, Monday afternoon, February 27, 1928.

Dr. Wilder was born in Bangor, Maine, April 7, 1864, the son and only child of Solon Wilder, a musical director, and Sarah Smith Wilder, the daughter of a physician. In 1886 he graduated from Amherst College with the degree of A.B. He took the classical course in college, and the thorough grounding he received in Latin and Greek had an important influence upon his development as a scholar; the literary character of his scientific writings was throughout his life essentially scholarly. John M. Tyler was the professor of zoology at that time in Amherst, and his teaching and example were other powerful factors in the moulding of Wilder's tastes and habits of mind, in that they served to strengthen and develop a love for the natural sciences which had shown itself in him while still a young child and throughout his boyhood. After graduation he taught biology in one of the Chicago high schools for three years, and then, the impulse to make a special study of zoology and especially anatomy having become too strong to be longer resisted, he went abroad to pursue these subjects under Wiedersheim in the University of Freiburg. It was the beneficent influence of John Tyler, who had himself studied in Germany, which again became active in his interest and guided Wilder to Wiedersheim's laboratory.

His two-years' study-period with Wiedersheim and Weismann in Freiburg made a professional zoologist of Wilder, and gave him the technical and intellectual foundation and background of all his later work. He took the degree of Ph.D., *summa cum laude,* there in 1891. A mark of the breadth of his intellectual interests was the choice of medieval English as one of the minor subjects of his examination.

It was in Freiburg that Wilder's attention was first directed to anatomical studies in the Amphibia. This field of research was Wiedersheim's own special interest, in which he had first made his reputation as a comparative anatomist, and with his accustomed generosity towards his pupils he gave Wilder valuable material from his private collections for special study, while the latter was still a student under him.

The results of these researches were published in the *Zoologische Jahrbücher* in Wilder's first two papers, "Die Nasengegend von Menopoma," etc., and "A Contribution to the Anatomy of Siren lacertina." The skill with which he executed delicate dissections, his insight and often intuition in the interpretation of obscure anatomical structures, and the rare artistic talent shown in his drawings were all in evidence in these early productions. His interest in amphibian anatomy, thus auspiciously aroused, continued throughout his lifetime; his numerous contributions in this field of research and those of his colleagues and pupils have been of great importance and have made his laboratory in Smith College known throughout the world as one of the most important centers of amphibian studies.

On his return to America in 1891 Wilder taught again for a year in Chicago, and then, through the influence of John Tyler, was appointed professor of zoology in Smith College.

The following year, in 1893, Wilder caused a genuine sensation among zoologists by the publication in the *Anatomischer Anzeiger* of "Lunglose Salamandriden," in which he shows that in one family of common salamanders both lungs and gills are entirely wanting in the adult animal. This important and very surprising fact had not been observed or suspected up to that time, although these animals had been studied by numerous investigators both in America and Europe. The outstanding student of Amphibia in America at that time was the veteran comparative anatomist, Edward Drinker Cope, who, when shown Wilder's paper, scoffed at it, saying he had been dissecting salamanders most of his life and had always found lungs in them. He was mistaken, however, as to the large family of the Plethodontidae, which have none.

About 1897 Wilder began to interest himself in the epidermic markings on the palms and soles of primates and especially the friction ridges of the human hand and foot. This development was quite in line with his general interest in human anatomy, which had been active in him from a very early period. In fact, while still a high-school teacher in Chicago he had done human dissecting on the side, and during his first year in Freiburg he had joined the medical students in their anatomy courses and made a complete dissection of the human subject. His studies of palms and soles broadened and developed as time went on, and his numerous contributions to the subject, together with those of his colleagues and pupils, and especially his wife, have been of fundamental importance in this field of research.

The comparison of the palms and soles of the two members of pairs of human twins led Wilder into the field of teratology, and in 1904 and 1908, respectively, there appeared in the *Journal of Anatomy* his important papers, "Duplicate Twins and Double Monsters" and "The Morphology of Cosmobia." Similar studies, as well as his interest in human anatomy, also took him into the field of physical anthropology, which he cultivated during his latter years. In 1920 he published the first American text-book on the subject, "A Manual of Anthropology."

Wilder's grasp of the details of both human and comparative anatomy as well as of anthropology, the philosophic cast of his mind and the originality of his genius, and also the command of a facile English style have been productive of several treatises of importance: "The History of the Human Body," 1910 and 1923; "Personal Identification" (with B. Wentworth), 1918; "Man's Prehistoric Past," 1923; and "The Pedigree of the Human Race," 1926.

Of these books the first and last named are perhaps the most important. They are both outstanding works of pronounced originality, which will long be standard authorities on the matters of which they treat. The "History of the Human Body" is a comparative anatomy of man, written especially for medical students but also for an educated laity. It is a philosophy of human structure, and is distinguished in so eminent a degree by adequacy and breadth of treatment, by clearness of exposition and by facility of expression that it has become a classic in its field. And "The Pedigree of the Human Race" is probably a work of equal merit, although it is of too recent publication to have had its appeal to an interested public fully tested.

Wilder's publications comprise seven published books and some thirty-nine papers which have appeared in scientific journals. He was a member of the following scientific societies: American Society of Naturalists, American Society of Zoologists, Boston Society of Natural History, Association of American Anatomists, American Anthropological Association, International Association for Identification, American Academy of Arts and Sciences, Société des Sciences, Agriculture et Arts du Bas-Rhin, and the Galton Society.

On July 26, 1906, Wilder took the most important step in his career when he married Inez Whipple, who had been for several years an instructor in his department. The partnership thus formed was an ideal one from every point of view. Mrs. Wilder, who was also, and still is, a productive zoologist, had similar scientific proclivities to his own and carried on her researches in similar fields; consequently, although she and her husband conducted their scientific activities independently of each other and worked on different problems, they could give each other mutually the assistance and support which their closely related interests made possible.

In other and still more important ways also was Wilder's marriage fortunate; it ensured to him a congenial and happy home life, and enabled him to indulge his love of society and of familiar social intercourse with his friends and pupils. It also provided him with a companion for his travels. Both he and his wife were very fond of travel, and they made many trips together to distant countries. Less than a year ago they returned from a trip around the world which had occupied the greater part of a year. With Wilder, however, travel was not primarily a matter of sightseeing; he always felt that the most interesting and profitable aspect of it was the experience of meeting and knowing congenial people of other nationalities and races, and learning their point of view by actually living so far as possible, if only for a brief time, in their environment and manner. Thus he made numerous interesting contacts and warm friendships with scientific men and others in many parts of the world. As shown by the general tenor of the "Pedigree of the Human Race" he had developed a profound appreciation of the common humanity of all races and a belief in similar potentialities of all for intellectual and spiritual achievement.

The general public knows a scientific man by his published works and by his achievements in his chosen field of research, and H. H. Wilder will be long remembered. His family and friends, however, will think rather of other things when they look back on their association with him. They will remember the sweetness of his disposition, his modesty and gentleness, his gaiety and love of fun, the brightness of his wit and the brilliancy of his talk and his self-effacement when rewards and honors were being distributed. The many generations of Smith College students who sat under his teaching will recall the enthusiasm for his courses which he inspired in them, his vital concern for their welfare and progress and especially his hospitable home, where he loved to entertain and amuse them.

H. S. PRATT

HAVERFORD COLLEGE

SCIENTIFIC EVENTS

THE SECRETARIES' CONFERENCE OF THE AMERICAN ASSOCIATION AND AFFILIATED SOCIETIES

AT the second Toronto meeting of the American Association for the Advancement of Science, in December, 1921, was inaugurated a conference of the secretaries of sections and societies, together with members of the executive committee and some of the officers. A similar conference has been held in connection with each subsequent meeting of the association. Recently this conference has become organized as a standing committee of the association under the direction of the secretaries of sections and societies. Under the new plan the organization is permanent and is to be known as the Secretaries' Conference. It is planned that there shall be one or more sessions of the conference at each annual meeting and that the work of the conference will be carried on by correspondence in the interim.

The secretaries of the sections and societies are directly concerned with the details of arranging programs, rooms and the like, and they should be familiar with the needs of their own science groups. Efforts will be made by correspondence to determine some of the problems and questions which need study, and these will be made the topics for discussion at future sessions. It is expected that each secretary of a section or of a society will indicate modifications that seem desirable to make his sessions more successful, and that he will suggest possible changes that promise to lead to more satisfactory arrangements and procedure in general. There are numerous details which must be taken up anew each year by the local committees for the annual meeting and the combined experiences of the secretaries should be very valuable to the local committees as well as to the Washington office of the association. There might well be worked out by the secretaries' conference a series of directions to guide future committees in their work on arrangements for the meetings.

Some of the questions recently discussed in sessions of the secretaries' conference will give an idea of the problems which are still more or less unsolved. How may the scientific men themselves become better acquainted with the problems and work in other fields than their own? Will joint sessions or general papers on border-line questions be helpful? How may the interrelationships of different fields be presented to the general public so as to stimulate interest and support? How may room assignments be made to bring together related groups? How may the methods be improved for handling railway certificates, and facilitating the getting of return railway tickets and Pullman accommodations? What can be done to improve the procedure followed in making the award of the annual American Association prize? Can plans be worked out to develop the scientific side of the annual exhibition? Is there any way to reduce the great complexities that are more or less inherent in meetings of so many societies and groups?

It is hoped that some of these, or similar questions, may be arranged for study, report and discussion at the next session of the secretaries' conference in New York City next winter. The members of the conference will cooperate in this, and will welcome suggestions from others. The secretaries' conference might well become a sort of clearing-house for the consideration of the problems and questions arising in connection with the annual meetings of our scientific societies. Notes and suggestions may be addressed to the conference secretary.

GEORGE T. HARGITT,
Secretary of the Secretaries' Conference

LYMAN HALL, SYRACUSE UNIVERSITY,
SYRACUSE, NEW YORK

ANNUAL MEETING OF SCIENCE SERVICE

DR. WILLIAM E. RITTER was elected honorary president of Science Service at the annual meeting of the board of trustees of that organization held in Washington on April 26. This honor was conferred upon the occasion of Dr. Ritter's retirement this year as president and trustee of the organization for the formation of which he was largely responsible.

Science Service is the institution for the popularization of science organized under the auspices of the National Academy of Sciences, the National Research Council and the American Association for the Advancement of Science. The idea of the institution arose from the intellectual partnership of Dr. Ritter, formerly director of the Scripps Institution for Biological Research, with the late E. W. Scripps, newspaper proprietor, who furnished sufficient endowment to assure the institution's financial and intellectual freedom.

Dr. J. McKeen Cattell, editor of SCIENCE and psychologist, was elected president succeeding Dr. Ritter. Dr. Vernon Kellogg was reelected vice-president and chairman of the executive committee and H. L. Smithton, treasurer; Dr. David White and Marlen E. Pew, members of the executive committee, and Watson Davis, secretary.

Two new members of the board of trustees were elected at this meeting: H. L. Smithton, of Cincinnati, Ohio, as a representative of the E. W. Scripps estate, and Dr. Harrison E. Howe, editor of *Industrial and Engineering Chemistry,* Washington, D. C., as a representative of the National Research Council.

Annual reports presented by Dr. Edwin E. Slosson, director, and Watson Davis, managing editor, revealed that the past year has been one of progress for the institution. Its syndicate services are now used by some two hundred publications. The daily news report of Science Service reaches nearly a hundred daily newspapers and other publications. One fifth of the total daily circulation of the American press is reached by Science Service features. A substantial growth of the *Science News-Letter,* Science Service's weekly magazine, both in prestige and financially, was reported.

During the past year Science Service's service to newspapers has been extended to all of the twenty-six Scripps-Howard newspapers and arrangements have also been made to supply this important group of newspapers with a daily telegraphic news service. This service and other features have been extended to many other newspapers. Other activities of Science Service, such as the providing of magazines with periodical articles, the offering of lectures, the editing of books for prominent publishers and the establishment of collections of scientific photographs and information, have been extended in scope.

One of the matters given serious consideration at the annual meeting was cooperation with the Social Science Research Council in expanding the activities of the institution into the field of the social sciences. Plans and prospects for a Science Service Building are also receiving the attention of the trustees and officers of the institution.

The board of trustees as elected at the annual meeting is as follows: Representing the American Association for the Advancement of Science, J. McKeen Cattell (president) editor of SCIENCE, Garrison, N. Y.; D. T. MacDougal, director of the Desert Laboratory, Tucson, Ariz.; M. I. Pupin, professor of electromechanics in Columbia University, New York City. Representing the National Academy of Sciences, John C. Merriam, president of the Carnegie Institution of Washington; R. A. Millikan, director of the Norman Bridge laboratory of physics, California Institute of Technology; Dr. David White, senior geologist, U. S. Geological Survey. Representing National Research Council, Vernon Kellogg (vice-president and chairman of executive committee), permanent secretary, National Research Council, Washington, D. C.; C. G. Abbot, secretary of the Smithsonian Institution, Washington, D. C.; Harrison E. Howe, editor of *Industrial and Engineering Chemistry.* Representing journalistic profession, John H. Finley, associate editor, New York *Times;* Mark Sullivan, writer, Washington, D. C.; Marlen E. Pew, editor of *Editor and Publisher,* New York City. Representing E. W. Scripps estate, Harry L. Smithton (treasurer), Cincinnati, Ohio; Robert P. Scripps, Scripps-Howard newspapers, West Chester, Ohio; Thomas L. Sidlo, Cleveland, Ohio.

WATSON DAVIS,
Secretary

REPORT OF THE HENRY DRAPER COMMITTEE OF THE NATIONAL ACADEMY OF SCIENCES

THE Henry Draper Committee respectfully recommended to the council of the academy that the Draper Gold Medal for the year 1928 be awarded to William Hammond Wright, astronomer in the Lick Observatory, University of California, for the reasons here expressed:

Coming to the Lick Observatory in 1897, Mr. Wright at first participated in the program of radial velocity measurements which had been initiated by Dr. W. W. Campbell. To his ability as an engineer are due several improvements in the mounting and adjustment of the spectrograph that added greatly to its efficiency as a measuring instrument of precision. These features have been adopted in the design of practically all later spectrographs used in stellar radial velocity determinations.

Assigned to the duty of initiating the work of the Chile station of the Lick Observatory, he went to Santiago early in the year 1903 and within six months of the day of landing at Valparaiso, selected and secured the site for the observatory, erected the dome and telescope and began the actual work of securing spectrograms of the southern stars. He conducted the work of this station for nearly three years with distinguished success.

Returning to Mount Hamilton in 1906, he devoted the years to 1924 chiefly to spectrographic studies of the nebulae and of the novae. The former led, among other results, to the accurate measurement of the wave-lengths of the nebular lines, including some not previously reported; to the detection of the presence in the gaseous nebulae of the continuous emission of hydrogen, beginning abruptly at the end of the Balmer series, and extending into the ultra-violet; to the recognition of the remarkable variety of forms corresponding to the different nebular lines in the planetary nebulae; to the discovery that the nuclei of the planetary nebulae give a continuous spectrum strong in ultra-violet light, indicating that they are at a very high temperature, and to the conclusion that the nuclei of such nebulae are to be classed with the O-type stars. Some of these results were important factors in Bowen's recent brilliant work on the nature of nebulium.

Wright's studies of the novae can not be summarized briefly; it must suffice to say that they are more comprehensive and penetrating than those of any other investigator, covering in several cases the entire range of the spectrum and the entire known history of the star.

Since 1924 Mr. Wright has devoted his time largely to the photographic study of planetary detail, as revealed by plates sensitive to light of different colors, from the ultra-violet to the infra-red. This work is unquestionably the most significant and promising advance that has been made in the study of the planets in recent years, and has already resulted in important contributions to our knowledge of conditions on Mars and Jupiter.

Any one of these researches would in itself entitle Mr. Wright to recognition as one of the leading students of astrophysics; taken together they fully justify the award now made to him.

No grants of Draper funds in support of research in the field of astronomical physics have been made in the current year. The unexpended balance from the income of the Draper Foundation, available for this purpose, is $508.63.

Respectfully submitted,

W. W. CAMPBELL, *Chairman*

APRIL 3, 1928

APPOINTMENTS OF THE CARNEGIE INSTITUTION OF WASHINGTON

RECENT appointments of the Carnegie Institution of Washington include the following:

Dr. R. J. Havighurst, assistant professor of chemistry, Miami University, Oxford, Ohio, fellow of the Carnegie Institution of Washington in the history of science for the year beginning September 1, 1928, to enable Dr. Havighurst to undertake special studies in cooperation with Dr. George Sarton, associate in the history of science.

Dr. Wm. A. Heidel, Wesleyan University, research associate of the Carnegie Institution of Washington, for the period from July 1, 1928, to December 31, 1931, for the purpose of enabling Dr. Heidel to continue his studies on a comprehensive and critical history of early Greek thought, with special reference to its philosophical and scientific aspects.

Dr. Hubert L. Clark, Museum of Comparative Zoology of Harvard University, research associate of the Carnegie Institution of Washington, for the purpose of undertaking further studies of the echinoderm fauna of North Australia with a view particularly to interpretation of continental connections.

Dr. Henry E. Crampton, Columbia University, continuation of appointment as research associate of the Carnegie Institution of Washington, for the purpose of undertaking further studies of organic differentiation in nature as illustrated by land snails belonging to the genus Partula. Field studies will be undertaken especially in the Caroline and Pelew Islands, and it is hoped that further evidence may be obtained which may bear directly upon the problem of a pre-Pacific continent. Funds were provided for this study by Carnegie Corporation of New York.

Dr. Harald U. Sverdrup, Geophysical Institute, Bergen, Norway, research associate of the Carnegie Institution of Washington, for cooperation with the department of terrestrial magnetism of the institution in connection with development of a program for oceanographic studies during the forthcoming cruise of the non-magnetic yacht *Carnegie*.

SCIENTIFIC NOTES AND NEWS

DR. EDGAR F. SMITH, emeritus professor of chemistry at the University of Pennsylvania and formerly provost of the university, died on May 3 in the seventy-fourth year of his age.

PROFESSOR EDMUND BEECHER WILSON, of the department of zoology at Columbia University, has been awarded the gold medal of the Linnean Society of London. The presentation will be made in London on May 24 at the anniversary meeting of the society.

DR. LIBERTY H. BAILEY and Dr. W. R. Whitney were presented with the gold medals of the National Institute of Social Sciences on May 3. Dr. John Merle Coulter, adviser of the Boyce Thompson Institute for Plant Research, presented the medal to Dr. Bailey, who formerly was director of the State College of Agriculture at Cornell University. It was bestowed in recognition of "distinguished social service in the solution of human and scientific problems relating to rural life in America." The presentation to Dr. Whitney was made by General John J. Carty, vice-president of the American Telephone and Telegraph Company, in recognition of "distinguished service in promoting and leading electrical research, with its widespread favorable reaction upon human progress."

The gold medal for science of the Society of Arts and Sciences of New York has been awarded to Thomas A. Edison and will be presented at a dinner at the Hotel Astor, New York, on May 24. Mr. Walter Russell, president of the society, will preside and Dr. E. E. Slosson, of Science Service, will be toastmaster.

At the Washington meeting of the American Association of Physicians, presentation of the de Roaldes medal "for distinguished service to the science of medicine" to Dr. Chevalier Jackson, noted laryngologist of Philadelphia, was made on behalf of the Laryngological Society by Dr. Herbert S. Birkett, of Montreal. The association also conferred the George M. Kober medal on Dr. Victor C. Vaughan, of the University of Michigan.

P. H. Royster, associate chemical engineer, fertilizer and fixed nitrogen investigations, U. S. Department of Agriculture, has been given the 1928 Johnson award, made by the American Institute of Mining and Metallurgical Engineers to "some promising engineer, not over forty years of age, because of meritorious research, invention or contribution to the professional literature of iron and steel along the lines of blast-furnace process."

Dr. E. F. Armstrong, managing director of the British Dyestuffs Corporation, Ltd., has been elected a member of the Athenaeum Club for distinguished eminence in science.

At the annual dinner of the British Society of Dyers and Colorists, held in Manchester on March 23, the Perkin medal was presented to Dr. R. E. Schmidt, of Elberfeld, for "his remarkable work on anthraquinone and allied bodies, which has led to the discovery and commercial production of a whole series of fast dyestuffs."

Dr. Alexander Behm, professor of physics in the University of Kiel, has been awarded the gold medal by the Union pour la Sécurité en Aéroplane, Paris.

Dr. Konrad E. Birkhaug, assistant professor of bacteriology at the school of medicine in the University of Rochester, was recently elected to honorary membership in the Norwegian Royal Medical Society at Oslo.

At the meeting of the Royal College of Physicians of London, held on April 2, Sir John Rose Bradford, F.R.S., was reelected president.

L. H. Adams, of the Geophysical Laboratory of the Carnegie Institution, has been appointed secretary of the central petroleum committee of the National Research Council, which acts as adviser of the American Petroleum Institute in expending the funds for fundamental research on petroleum donated by John D. Rockefeller and the Universal Oil Products Company.

Dr. James J. Durrett, formerly professor of public health at the University of Tennessee, is to succeed Dr. George W. Hoover in charge of drug control in the food, drug and insecticide administration, U. S. Department of Agriculture.

Louis O. Sordahl, research assistant in physics at the University of Wisconsin, has been appointed field director of the Smithsonian Institution's station for the study of solar radiation at Mount Brukkaros, Africa.

The department of mathematics at the University of California will have as visitors on its faculty for the coming summer session Constantine Carathéodory, professor of mathematics at the University of Munich, Germany, and H. B. Phillips, professor of mathematics at the Massachusetts Institute of Technology.

Herbert W. Krieger, curator of ethnology in the U. S. National Museum, has returned from Santo Domingo, bringing many specimens from ancient village sites around Samana Bay.

Henry B. Collins, Jr., has left Washington for Alaska, where he will carry on archeological and ethnological explorations on St. Lawrence Island and the coast of Seward Peninsula under the auspices of the Smithsonian Institution.

Dr. Gerrit S. Miller, Jr., curator of the division of mammals in the U. S. National Museum, recently arrived in Sanchez, Dominican Republic, where he will spend the next few months investigating the caves of the region for bones of the extinct fauna of the island.

Dr. George T. Moore, director of the Missouri Botanical Garden, addressed the students of the American University in Cairo, Egypt, on April 3 on "Some of the Activities of the Missouri Botanical Garden."

On April 21, Dr. Davidson Black, professor of anatomy in the Peking Union Medical College, China, delivered an address to the Royal Canadian Institute on "Man's Origin from the Standpoint of Zoogeography."

A lecture before the science seminar of the Agricultural and Mechanical College of Texas, entitled "Measuring Distances of Stars," was given on April 30 by Dr. H. Y. Benedict, president of the University of Texas. On May 21 Dr. E. A. Lovett, president of Rice Institute, will address the science seminar on "Influence of Progress in Pure Science on Human Welfare."

Dr. Francis G. Benedict, director of the nutrition laboratory, lectured on "Basal Metabolism: The Modern Measure of Vital Activity" at the Carnegie Institution of Washington in Washington, D.C., on April 18, and at Teachers College, Columbia University, and at Wesleyan University, Middletown, Connecticut, on April 27.

Dr. Charles G. Rogers, professor of comparative physiology in Oberlin College, delivered a lecture before the biological students of DePauw University on April 5 on the subject "Physiological Evidences of Animal Relationships."

Dr. Michael F. Guyer, professor of zoology at the University of Wisconsin, addressed the regular monthly meeting of the University of Cincinnati section of the Society of the Sigma Xi on April 20, when he spoke on "Democracy as a Biological Problem."

On April 28, Dr. Chas. N. Gould, director of the Oklahoma Geological Survey, delivered an address before the North Texas Geological Society at Wichita Falls, Texas, on "Geology in Oil Finding."

Dr. Charles A. Shull, professor of plant physiology at the University of Chicago, is spending the spring quarter at West Virginia University. He is engaged in research and writing. On April 23 he addressed the botany seminar and on April 27 he delivered an address before the Society of Sigma Xi. He expects to make during the quarter trips to several neighboring institutions, one of these being Pennsylvania State College, where he will deliver an address entitled, "The Foundation of Experimental Plant Physiology: The Life and Work of Stephen Hales."

Dr. Haven Emerson, professor of public health administration at the College of Physicians and Surgeons, Columbia University, gave the Adolph Gehrmann lectures at the college of medicine of the University of Illinois on April 23, 24 and 25.

Dr. Irving Langmuir, assistant director of research of the General Electric Company, Schenectady, N. Y., gave a series of three public lectures on the evenings of April 30, May 1 and 2, under the auspices of the Carnegie Institute of Technology of Pittsburgh. His subject was "Electrical Discharges in Gases at Low Pressures." This series concluded the program of public lectures arranged by the Carnegie Institute of Technology for the benefit of residents of the district.

Dr. George Barger, professor of chemistry in relation to medicine in the University of Edinburgh, gave the fifth course of the Charles E. Dohme lectureship at the Johns Hopkins University on May 7, 8 and 9 on the general subject of ergot. On May 17 he will lecture on "The Chemistry of Hormones" and on May 18 on "The Chemistry of Thyroxine" at Buffalo, under the auspices of the Fenton Foundation and the Sigma Xi Club of the University of Buffalo.

The Cambridge University Press announces for early publication a volume of essays and addresses by the late William Bateson, F.R.S., edited, with a memoir, by Mrs. Bateson.

On February 14 the governor of the Falkland Islands unveiled the memorial over the grave of Sir Ernest Shackleton at Grytviken, South Georgia, which had been sent out in a whaling steamer by Lady Shackleton. It is a massive piece of sculpture in Scotch granite.

Memorial services for the late Dr. Thomas Forsyth Hunt, former dean of the College of Agriculture of the University of California, who died one year ago, were held on the university campus on April 22. Dean E. D. Merrill, of the college of agriculture, was chairman at the exercises and the speakers included Chester Rowell, representing the regents of the university; Vice-president R. G. Sproul, of the university, for the administration; Dr. H. J. Webber, director of the Citrus Experiment Station and former dean of the college of agriculture, representing the college, and R. E. Barrett, of Pasadena, senior student in agriculture, representing the students.

Dr. Cyrus C. Adams, of New York, geographer and formerly associate editor of the *Bulletin* of the American Geographical Society, has died in his seventy-ninth year.

Dr. John Smith Dexter, professor of zoology in the University of Porto Rico, died on April 19 at the age of forty-two years.

Professor Theodor Curtius, emeritus professor of chemistry in the University of Heidelberg, died at Heidelberg on February 9 in his seventy-first year.

The deaths are also announced of Dr. Bernhard Wanach, professor of astronomy at the Geodetic Institute in Potsdam, and of Dr. Theodore Zincke, professor of chemistry in the University of Marburg.

The alumni members of Sigma Xi at the University of Alabama met on April 24 and organized a Sigma Xi club. The club elected the following officers: Dr.

Emmett B. Carmichael, *president;* Dr. George I. Adams, *vice-president,* and Dr. W. P. Ott, *secretary and treasurer.*

The Society for Experimental Biology and Medicine, at its annual meeting on April 18, announced the election of the following general officers of the society: *President,* Stanley R. Benedict; *vice-president,* Peyton Rous; *secretary,* A. J. Goldforb; *council,* O. F. Avery, John Auer, W. R. Bloor, Robert Chambers, Alfred E. Cohn, Irving Hardesty, Alfred F. Hess, A. S. Loevenhart, A. B. Luckhardt, William Ophuls, W. W. Palmer, O. H. Plant, F. H. Scott, H. D. Senior and Hsien Wu.

At the annual meeting of the Boston Society of Natural History, held on May 4, the following officers were elected for 1928–29: *President,* Charles H. Taylor; *vice-presidents,* Nathaniel T. Kidder, Frederic T. Lewis, Glover M. Allen; *secretary,* Francis Harper; *treasurer,* Augustus P. Loring, Jr.; *trustees,* Thomas Barbour, Joseph A. Cushman, Laurence B. Fletcher, Frederic H. Kennard, W. Gordon Means and John C. Phillips. At the same meeting the annual Walker prizes in natural history, which were offered this year for the best papers submitted on any subjejct in the field of botany, were awarded as follows: a first prize of one hundred dollars to Chandrakant G. Kulkarni, of the University of Michigan, for a manuscript entitled "Meiosis in the Pollen Mother Cells of Some Strains of *Oenothera pratincola* Bartlett"; a second prize of fifty dollars to Miss Lydia B. Walsh, of Wellesley College, for a manuscript entitled, "Microsporogenesis in Petunia."

The committee on scientific research of the American Medical Association has recently made a grant of $2,000 to Professor A. S. Warthin, of the department of pathology, and Professor George R. La Rue, of the department of zoology, of the University of Michigan, to permit them to continue their studies on the broad tapeworm of man. A grant of $500 has been made to Dr. K. E. Birkhaug, assistant professor of bacteriology at the University of Rochester, for the study in European clinics of bacterial allergy in rheumatic fever patients.

The thirty-eighth annual meeting of the Nebraska Academy of Sciences was held on April 26, 27 and 28 at Midland College, Fremont, jointly with the Nebraska section of the Mathematics Association of America. Dr. W. D. Crouse, professor of physics at Midland College, is president of the academy. Chairmen for the sectional meetings were: biology, Professor C. J. Shirk, Nebraska Wesleyan; chemistry, Professor A. C. Rice, Grand Island; earth sciences, Professor E. F. Schramm, University of Nebraska; engineering, Professor Jiles W. Haney, University of Nebraska; mathematics, Professor W. C. Brenke, University of Nebraska; physics, Professor Chalmer N. Patterson, Hastings; social sciences, Professor C. K. Burkholder, Midland; high school teachers, Grant L. Stahly, Hastings High School.

The Utah Academy of Sciences held its twenty-first annual meeting at the Hotel Newhouse, Salt Lake City, on April 20 and 21, under the presidency of R. A. Hart, of the Western Clay Products Association. The program consisted of eight addresses. The following officers were elected: Dr. Joseph F. Merrill, Salt Lake City, *president;* Dr. Willard Gardner, Logan, Utah, *first vice-president;* Dr. Walter D. Bonner, Salt Lake City, *second vice-president;* Dr. Bert L. Richards, Logan, Utah, *councilman;* Dr. O. W. Israelson, Logan, *councilman;* Dr. S. Y. Cannon, Provo, *councilman;* Dr. Vasco M. Tanner, Provo, Utah, *secretary-treasurer.*

The Tennessee Academy of Science met at the University of Tennessee on April 20 for its twenty-second meeting. Dr. Walter S. Leathers, of Vanderbilt University, presided at the sessions on the first day, at which twelve scientific papers were read. A dinner was held in the evening at which W. F. Pond, state geologist, gave the principal address on "Contributions of Geological Surveys to State Development." The following two days were spent on a field trip to Mt. LeConte, Gatlinburg.

Universities in the middle west will be represented at the third annual meeting of the Midwestern Psychological Association at the University of Wisconsin on May 11 and 12 at which a series of symposiums, informal discussions and addresses will be on the program, according to an announcement by Professor C. L. Hull, in charge of local arrangements. Speakers and chairman of discussion groups include Professor M. F. Meyer, University of Missouri; Professor J. R. Kantor, University of Indiana; Professor Harvey A. Carr, University of Chicago; Professor A. R. Gilliland, Northwestern University, and Professor Hull.

A geological conference has been called to meet at Norman, Oklahoma, on May 19 by R. C. Moore, of Kansas, E. H. Sellards, of Texas, and Chas. N. Gould, of Oklahoma, to discuss the problem of the Pennsylvanian of the Great Plains. It is expected that the state geologists of Iowa, Nebraska, Kansas, Missouri, Arkansas, Texas and Oklahoma will be present and participate in the discussion, also a number of paleontologists residing in the region, as well as representatives of a number of geological societies.

DR. HOWARD A. KELLY, of Baltimore, has presented to the herbarium of the University of Michigan his mycological library to be called the "Louis C. C. Krieger Library and Collections." The library alone contains about 100,000 items and nearly all the older classical mycological literature, brought together during the last ten years. Included are 350 paintings by Krieger, many photographic prints, about 2,000 collections of fungi and a set of wax models. The collection will be housed in the herbarium quarter of the new museum building at Ann Arbor.

THE late Chandler Robbins, retired merchant and one of the founders of the American Geographical Society, has left $30,000 to the society.

GIFTS and pledges of $1,215,810 have been received towards the $2,000,000 fund which the Museum of the City of New York seeks to raise for building purposes by June 1, the date set to qualify for the offer of a city-owned plot at Fifth Avenue and 103d Street.

THE American Pharmaceutical Association has available a sum amounting to $550 which will be expended after October 1 for the encouragement of research. Investigators desiring financial aid in their work will communicate before July 1 with H. V. Arny, chairman, A. Ph. A. Research Committee, 115 West 68th Street, New York City, giving their past record and outlining the particular line of work for which the grant is desired.

PROFESSOR HENRY E. CRAMPTON, of Barnard College, Columbia University, associate of the Carnegie Institution of Washington, will leave New York on June 1 on an eight months' expedition to the islands of the western Pacific Ocean, under the auspices of the Carnegie Institution. During eight earlier field-journeys he has prosecuted studies on the variation, distribution and evolution of certain land organisms living in the islands of the South Pacific Ocean, from the Society and Cook Groups to Samoa and the Mariana Islands. It is now planned to extend these studies to the larger and higher members of the Caroline Islands, Palao Islands and Yap, in order to bring the western Pacific area into the entire scheme of the research. Professor Crampton will be assisted in the field-work by his son, Mr. Henry E. Crampton, Jr., and by Mr. Richard B. Goetze.

AN expedition of Italian scientific men to explore the upper reaches of the Amazon River is being organized at Padua, with the technical preparation of a large group of men. It is intended to study the flora and fauna and the lives of the natives. The expedition hopes to leave by the end of June. The venture is backed by the local press and popular subscription.

UNIVERSITY AND EDUCATIONAL NOTES

LAFAYETTE COLLEGE has received from Mr. Fred Morgan Kirby, of Wilkes-Barre, the gift of a building to house the department of civil rights which is expected to cost about $200,000.

DR. F. D. FROMME, professor of botany and plant pathology at the Virginia Polytechnic Institute and plant pathologist at the Virginia Agricultural Experiment Station, has been elected dean of the college of agriculture and director of the Agricultural Experiment Station of West Virginia University.

J. BURNS READ, assistant manager of the research department of the Metals Exploration Company, Golden, Colo., has been appointed professor of mining engineering at the Colorado School of Mines, in the place of Dean L. S. Grant, who recently resigned.

DR. ERNEST O. LAWRENCE, assistant professor of physics at Yale University, has been appointed as associate professor of physics at the University of California.

NEW appointments to professorships at Yale University include Dr. William Arthur LaField, who becomes clinical professor of radiology; Dr. Joseph Irving Linde, who is promoted from associate clinical professor to clinical professor of pediatrics, and Dr. Donald Wallace Porter, who is also promoted from associate clinical professor to clinical professor of pediatrics.

DR. RONALD MANSFIELD FERRY has been promoted to be assistant professor of biochemistry at the Harvard Medical School. Noel Ewart Odell, of the Mount Everest expedition, has been appointed lecturer on geology in the university.

DR. CHESTER K. WENTWORTH, formerly of the geology department of the University of Iowa, has been appointed associate professor of geology at Washington University, St. Louis.

DR. C. H. RICHARDSON, professor of mathematics at Georgetown College, Kentucky, has been appointed head of the department of mathematics at Bucknell University to take the chair formerly filled by Dr. W. C. Bartol, who retires after forty-seven years of teaching service.

PROFESSOR PASCAL, of the University of Lille, has been appointed professor of chemistry at the University of Paris to take the place of the late Professor Chabrié.

DR. FRIEDRICH ALVERDES, professor of zoology in the University of Halle, has been appointed to the chair of zoology in the University of Marburg.

Dr. Wilhelm Steinhausen, of the University of Frankfort, has been appointed to the chair of physiology at the University of Greifswald.

DISCUSSION AND CORRESPONDENCE

DOES THE AMOUNT OF FOOD CONSUMED INFLUENCE THE GROWTH OF AN ANIMAL?

Under the above title H. H. Mitchell[1] has recently published a general criticism of certain types of nutrition studies. In the course of his argument he refers to several papers from this laboratory (without specifically naming the authors) as illustrations of what he says appear "to represent an exaggeration of the importance of negative experimental results." In this category he places our findings that arginine and histidine are not interchangeable in metabolism.[2,3] His objection to our conclusions appears to be due to the fact that the animals which received arginine in the absence of histidine ingested less food than those which received histidine in the absence of arginine. We are convinced that the diminished food consumption of the arginine animals was *the result of the dietary inadequacy.* Such evidence as is available indicates the correctness of this conception. Sixteen years ago F. G. Hopkins[4] pointed out that when a deficiency occurs, the failure in appetite *follows* the failure in growth; which was interpreted by him as indicating that the latter is the *causal* factor, and the diminished food consumption merely the *result* of the inhibited synthetic processes. He says, "If then a factor or factors essential to growth be missing from, or deficient in, a dietary, the consequent arrest of, or diminution in, growth energy may diminish the instinctive consumption of food, while the supply of such factors may increase consumption as an indirect result of a direct effect upon growth." A similar conclusion was reached by Osborne and Mendel[5] in a study of the supplementing influence of yeast upon artificial diets. They state, "The food consumption of the rats on the smaller quantities of yeast was less than that of those on the larger quantities, because their growth was slower and consequently they needed less food; and the change from a small quantity of yeast to a larger one was followed by growth with a resultant increase in food intake."

The above quotations show clearly that the investigators in question regard the diminished food consumption of animals on inadequate diets as the *result* of the failure in growth. No one will deny that, within certain limits, an animal which ingests a liberal amount of an *adequate* food will increase in weight more rapidly than one which consumes a smaller quantity, but this fact is not incompatible with the mass of evidence which has been accumulated, indicating that the ability or inability of an animal to grow upon a given diet exerts a profound influence upon food consumption.[6] Indeed, so generally is this correlation observed that Osborne and Mendel[7] remarked several years ago, "It is a common experience that animals living on unsuitable diets tend to reduce their food intake." Evidently, therefore, the conclusions in our arginine-histidine experiments were arrived at by application of exactly the same principles employed by others in proving dietary deficiencies.

Acceptance of the doctrine that in a young animal growth is an indication of dietary adequacy, and failure of growth a characteristic having the converse significance, is regarded by Mitchell as evidence of amazing credulity since it involves, he says, belief in "the infallibility of the animal appetite." The writer doubts whether any one believes that appetite is infallible. The use by the human subject of various materials which do not contribute to nutritive well-being is quite sufficient to exclude such a view should one be disposed to adopt it. Appetite is a more or less imperfect (and therefore not infallible) response to a physiological need, but when an added dietary component leads to an appetite stimulation the explanation is to be found, we believe, in *the influence exerted by the substance upon the cells themselves.* In the words of Hopkins,[4] "any effect of the addendum upon appetite must have been secondary to a more direct effect upon growth processes." *Thus our view places the emphasis upon the cell processes* rather than upon the imperfect outward manifestations. It recognizes the fundamental and irrefutable fact that the animal organism is unerringly accurate in its syntheses. If a tissue is to be formed at all, every component required must be available or capable of being manufactured by the cells; otherwise the synthesis will not occur. If growth follows the

1 Mitchell, H. H., Science, 1927, lxvi (December 16), 596.

2 Rose, W. C., and Cox, G. J., *J. Biol. Chem.*, 1924, lxi, 747.

3 Rose, W. C., and Cox, G. J., *J. Biol. Chem.*, 1926, lxviii, 217.

4 Hopkins, F. G., *J. Physiol.*, 1912, xliv, 425.

5 Osborne, T. B., and Mendel, L. B., *J. Biol. Chem.*, 1917, xxxi, 149.

6 A few of the many contributions showing this fact, and involving both vitamine and amino acid deficiencies are, Osborne and Mendel, *J. Biol. Chem.*, 1915, xx, 351, and 1916, xxv, 1; Karr, *ibid.*, 1920, xliv, 255; Cowgill, *Am. J. Physiol.*, 1921, lvii, 420; and Jackson, *J. Biol. Chem.*, 1927, lxxiii, 523.

7 Osborne, T. B., and Mendel, L. B., *J. Biol. Chem.*, 1920–21, xlv, 277.

addition of an essential constituent to an inadequate diet, it does so because cell reactions which could not proceed in the absence of the added factor are now made possible. We believe that as the growth syntheses occur, the demand for raw materials is reflected in a stimulation of the appetite resulting in greater food consumption. It is difficult to see why such a view is unreasonable, or necessitates great gullibility for its acceptance. Furthermore, if food intake is not influenced by the adequacy of the ration it is a remarkable coincidence that of our histidine- and arginine-fed rats not a single one inadvertently made the mistake of eating more or less food than the other members of its group.

Mitchell also criticises in a similar fashion several papers dealing with the possibility of replacing essential amino acids (cystine and histidine) with synthetic compounds. It is scarcely necessary to defend these papers, inasmuch as no experimental data have been adduced indicating that our findings are incorrect. Suffice it to say that we are still of the opinion that taurine is "totally incapable" of replacing cystine in the diet for purposes of growth,[8] nor do we know of any reason for abandoning the conclusions expressed in the original publications regarding the availability of synthetic imidazoles.[9]

Mitchell cites the work of Lewis and Root[10] upon the replacement of lysine by nor-leucine as an example of a properly conducted experiment, in which the alterations in food consumption inherent in our investigations do not occur. If one calculates the average daily food consumption of Lewis and Root's rats, as may be done readily from the information supplied in the paper, it becomes evident immediately that *the foods were not consumed in equal amounts.* On the contrary, as would be expected, the change from an inadequate (gliadin) to an adequate (gliadin plus lysine) diet *was followed invariably by an increase in average daily food consumption. Supplementing gliadin with nor-leucine led to no appreciable change in food intake because both rations were equally inadequate for growth.* Furthermore, it must not be forgotten that gliadin contains some lysine. Were it completely devoid of this amino acid, the addition of the latter would lead to even greater alterations in food consumption than those observed. The experiments of Lewis and Root are comparable to our taurine investigations, in which the basal diet was not completely devoid of cystine. The magnitude of the changes in food consumption is of the same order in the two studies. There can be no reasonable doubt of the correctness of Lewis and Root's conclusions regarding the inability of nor-leucine to replace lysine, but the implication of Mitchell that there were no alterations in food consumption with the different types of diets is not in accord with the facts.

WM. C. ROSE
LABORATORY OF PHYSIOLOGICAL CHEMISTRY,
UNIVERSITY OF ILLINOIS

[8] Rose, W. C., and Huddlestun, B. T., *J. Biol. Chem.*, 1926, lxix, 599.

[9] Cox, G. J., and Rose, W. C., *J. Biol. Chem.*, 1926, lxviii, 781.

[10] Lewis, H. B., and Root, L. E., *J. Biol. Chem.*, 1920, xliii, 79.

THE SIBERIAN METEORITE

IN view of recent newspaper reports regarding a great meteorite supposed to have fallen in Siberia, I am sending you the following rather free translation of Mr. L. Kulik's story as it originally appeared in Russian.

From the two newspaper articles by Mr. L. Kulik, which you gave me, I have been able to obtain the following information concerning the so-called "Tungusk meteorite."

The appearance at 7 o'clock in the morning on June 30, 1908, of a "fiery body" of unusual brightness, rolling across the sky out of the north east and falling down in the "taiga" between the Yenissei and Lena Rivers, north of the Railroad line, was observed by a great number of people, mostly the native inhabitants, living in the basins of these rivers.

The fall of the meteorite was instantly followed by a column of fire rising skyward, by the formation of the heavy black clouds, and by a most deafening, resounding noise far surpassing in its magnitude, any thunderstorm, or artillery cannonade. This was heard for hundreds of kilometers within a radius of the cities of Yenisseisk, Krasnoyarsk, Kansk, Nijneudinsk, and Kirensk on Lena.

A terrific air-wave was formed which pushed ahead everything that it met in its way. The water in all rivers, lakes and streams was raised up; people and animals were lifted by it and carried along.

The vibrations produced by the fall of the meteorite were detected and registered by the seismographs of the Physical Observatory at Irkutsk, where Mr. A. V. Vesnesenski, who was in charge of the observatory, calculated the epicenter of the "earthquake" to be located in the upper part of the Podkamennaya Tunguska.

The phenomenon produced considerable panic, especially among the natives living in the basins of the Yenissei and all the various Tunguska Rivers, and adjacent part of the Lena River basin.

Several attempts, made in 1908, to find the body of the meteorite were fruitless, as for some reason all parties were searching near the city of Kansk, and not in the locality, determined by A. V. Vesnesenski, whose observations unfortunately remained unpublished. Gradually interest in the new meteorite died, and the whole matter was almost forgotten, except as a tale among the natives.

In 1927 Mr. L. Kulik attempted to find the exact location of the meteorite and led an expedition to the Tungusk region. Owing to the lack of funds and the extreme difficulties of transportation in the wilderness of taiga and tundra, the expedition was not altogether successful. However, Mr. Kulik was able to reach the area where the taiga bore distinct traces of the passage of the meteorite. An area struck by the meteorite is a water table between the upper part of the Podkamennaya Tunguska and its right tributary the River Chuni. The area is largely covered with tundra in the process of formation, intersected by hills, small lakes, swamps and typical tundra. The immediate area is surrounded by high naked hills, deforested by the falling meteorite. All trees are still on the ground, their tops are spread out in fan-like fashion away from the central zone of the fall. Exceptions are noted only in the ravines or in the gorges and deep perpendicular valleys and also in a zone which can be considered as the "interference" zone. And even in these places the trees, in most cases, are scorched and though still in upright position they are all leafless and dead.

The zone where the heat effect of the meteorite is evident is considered by L. Kulik to be 30 kilometers in diameter and the area of the air-wave breaking the trees is 50 kilometers in diameter.

The central part of the "fire zone" is covered by shallow "funnel" shaped craters, reaching in some instances many tens of meters in diameter and not greater than 4–5 meters in depth. The bottom of the craters is covered with swampy growth.

Unfortunately, Mr. Kulik was not able to find the body of the meteorite or determine the depth to which it had sunk.

He believes that the meteorite of 1908 was an aggregate (a swarm) of meteors, moving with a rate approaching 72 kilometers a minute. Some of the aggregates undoubtedly exceeded 130 tons in weight. Hot gases (above 1,000° C.) surrounded the meteorite and started fires before the meteorite had reached the ground and sunk into it, forming craters, uprooting the trees and burning everything that can burn in the center of its fall.

George P. Merrill
U. S. National Museum

CONCERNING A RHIZOCTONIA WHICH FORMS HYMENIAL CELLS AND BASIDIOSPORES IN CULTURE

While investigating root-rot diseases of alfalfa in October, 1924, a Rhizoctonia was isolated from a mass of hymenial cells and basidiospores which occurred on one of the diseased alfalfa plants. Several weeks later this Rhizoctonia was observed to have produced its perfect stage in pure culture and has continued to form hymenial cells and basidiospores up to the present time, when grown on certain artificial media and under proper external conditions.

Numerous single-spore isolations have been made from individual basidia of the spore-forming Rhizoctonia and with very few exceptions, all have formed spores. While under constant observation through a microscope, complete sets of spores have been picked from basidia by means of a Barber micromanipulator. All of the spores that germinated and continued to grow formed the perfect stage similar to the original isolation. This Rhizoctonia, therefore, is considered to be homothallic.

The hyaline mycelium formed by this Rhizoctonia can not be mistaken for that formed by *R. crocorum* (Pers.) D.C., which also occurs on alfalfa, and it is not believed that the two fungi are genetically connected. Cultures of Rhizoctonia were received from plant pathologists in various parts of the United States and amongst these one was found which is believed to be similar to the spore-forming Rhizoctonia isolated in Michigan. The former culture was isolated in Minnesota from an alfalfa root, which apparently was not affected with the violet root-rot disease. When grown under similar conditions the Minnesota Rhizoctonia was found to have spores and other characters identical with that of the Michigan strain.

The spore-forming fungus under consideration differs in many ways from *Rhizoctonia solani* Kühn (*Corticium vagum* B. & C.). The mycelium of the former is characteristically hyaline and lacks the brown color associated with *R. solani*. The sclerotia are smaller and less numerous. These differences are especially pronounced when the two fungi are grown on potato dextrose agar. Differences in sterigma length and in spore size distinguish the perfect stages of these two Rhizoctonias.

The perfect stage of the new spore-forming Rhizoctonia is apparently to be considered as a *Corticium* which is characterized, both on artificial media and upon inoculated alfalfa plants, by the unusual length of sterigmata.

J. E. Kotila
Michigan State College and
University of Michigan

MODELING CLAY AS A SUBSTITUTE FOR COLOPHONIUM WAX IN THE PHYSIOLOGICAL LABORATORY

In the experience of the writer and of several associates the colophonium wax which has such a general use in the physiological laboratory has proven unsatisfactory in several ways. Plasteline modeling-clay has been found a satisfactory substitute and free from some of the faults of the wax. This is due to its more stable consistency. It does not require warming before use. Low temperatures do not cause it to break loose, and warming, such as it may receive when used to attach writing points to signal magnets, does not cause it to melt.

R. R. DURANT

OHIO STATE UNIVERSITY,
COLUMBUS, OHIO

A "DATA" OF RESEARCH

WITH regard to the note on the pronunciation of "research" by Dr. Kopeloff in SCIENCE for March 23, 1928: To an ex-philologer the use of the singular verb with "data" is even more annoying than its mispronunciation (whatever the correct pronunciation may be). The next generation will very likely have forgotten that it ever had a plural verb. There has been suggested the ethical distinction that research denotes scientific investigation proper; while résearch denotes work of a compiling or reclassifying nature under direction.

From the point of view of linguistics we were taught that languages with stress-accents like the American-English tended to pull the accents towards the beginnings of words. Two examples of this process occur to me. As a boy I recall frequently having heard "advertisement" accented on the third syllable. One almost never hears this now and seldom on the second syllable, the dominant position of the accent being on the first. Within more recent years the word "automobile" has become generally accented on the first syllable, although in its early days it was frequently accented on the last and occasionally on the third syllable.

F. L. WELLS

BOSTON PSYCHOPATHIC HOSPITAL

SCIENTIFIC BOOKS

Brachiopod Morphology and Genera (*Recent and Tertiary.* By J. ALLAN THOMSON, director of the Dominion Museum, Wellington, New Zealand. Man. No. 7, N. Z. Board Sci. and Art, 1927. Obtainable from the Government Printer, Wellington, or the High Commissioner for New Zealand, London. Price, 17s. 6d.

STUDENTS of brachiopods, recent or fossil, will welcome this well-reasoned contribution to their literature, which is the culmination of a series of papers beginning in 1915. The book falls into three major divisions—morphology, classification and description of genera and species. As might be expected from the earlier papers, the section on brachiopod morphology (pp. 1–108) is particularly valuable, bringing together, as it does, all our present knowledge of the soft parts of these animals, the stages of development through which they pass, and the various shell parts, external and internal, with their growing terminology, treated in considerable detail and well illustrated.

In the section on classification, Dr. Thomson proposes two new major divisions, Gastrocaulia and Pygocaulia, which are practically coextensive with Huxley's Inarticulata and Articulata; in the new classification, however, the division is made on the mode of origin of the pedicle which in the Gastrocaulia develops "within the valves of the protegulum during the free-swimming stage from the ventral mantle-lobe and subsequently is protruded," whereas in the Pygocaulia it arises out of "the caudal segment of the embryo and is never enclosed within the shell." Well founded as these new divisions are, however, it will doubtless be difficult for them to displace the long-established Huxleyan terms. Within the Gastrocaulia he includes the orders Atremata and Neotremata of Beecher, with amended diagnoses, but within the Pygocaulia, in addition to Beecher's Protremata and Telotremata, he makes a new order, Paleotremata, to include the Rustellacea and Kutorginacea, *i.e.,* "primitive Pygocaulia without fully developed articulation or delthyria." The reviewer agrees that these two superfamilies should be removed from the Atremata, but would refer them to the Protremata rather than create a new order. Nor can he accept Thomson's reference of the Paterinidae (Paterinacea) to the Neotremata, since they show all the ordinal characters of the Atremata. The shell growth in typical *Paterina* is hemiperipheral, while in most of the Micromitras it is mixoperipheral; nevertheless, the pedicle issues from between the two valves instead of being restricted to the ventral valve as in Neotremata. The Acrotretacea of the Neotremata may, as Thomson thinks, have come out of the Paterinidae, but this remains to be demonstrated. His view that the most primitive Telotremata (Rhynchonellacea) arose in the Protremata is probably also correct, but here again we do not know the actual stock of origin.

The descriptive portion of the work (pp. 120–297) deals with sixty-nine genera, eight of which are new: *Hispanirhynchia, Abyssothyris, Japanithyris, Jaffaia, Pictothyris, Neobouchardia, Pirothyris, Malleia.* Each genus is classified, briefly diagnosed, its synonyms cited, and illustrated by a line drawing of (in the majority of instances) the genotype, making the book a dependable standard of reference. Two new subfamilies are proposed: Platidiinae, to include *Amphithyris* Thomson 1918 and *Platidia* Costa 1852; and Laqueinae, to include *Laqueus* Dall 1870 and *Pictothyris* n. gen.

The volume closes with a table showing the range in time and space of the Australian Tertiary brachiopods, a selected bibliography and a full index, thus rounding out an excellent little handbook, on the production of which both Dr. Thomson and the New Zealand Board of Science and Art are to be heartily congratulated.

CHARLES SCHUCHERT
YALE UNIVERSITY

SCIENTIFIC APPARATUS AND LABORATORY METHODS

THE USE OF NAPHTHALENE IN NARCOTIZING EARTHWORMS

THE preparation of earthworms for use in introductory courses in biology usually involves a more or less tiresome procedure of stupefying the animals with low grades of alcohol. In an effort to find some method which would shorten this procedure, experiments were made with a number of substances. Naphthalene in alcoholic solution gave excellent and uniform results.

A stock saturated solution of naphthalene in 95 per cent. alcohol was made up. Earthworms were gathered in the evening by the aid of a flashlight, during the months of May and June. Without preliminary washing the worms were placed in a dish of water, about one hundred specimens per liter. To each liter of water were added 40 cc of the stock naphthalene solution. Immediately the excess naphthalene was thrown out of solution as a curdy precipitate. This precipitate formed a stringy coagulum with the mucus secreted by the worms. In one hour or less the worms had become narcotized, so that pinching brought response only in an occasional worm. The animals were then washed entirely free of foreign matter. This process was not difficult, for the coagulum mentioned above did not adhere to the worms.

The specimens at this stage were found to be very flabby and wrinkled. They were laid, one by one, in fully extended condition, upon a dry paper towel in the bottom of a clean dish. All immature or injured individuals were discarded at this point. After some two or three hundred worms had been arranged on the towel, the latter was folded over and held in place, so that the position of each worm would not be disturbed while the following solution was poured on:

glacial acetic	10 cc
formalin	10 cc
copper sulphate	1 gm
water	1 liter

After a few hours in this solution the worms were found plump, fully expanded and well hardened. They were then transferred, without washing, to 95 per cent. alcohol for storage until needed.

Mixtures of alcohol and formalin may be used as storage solutions. In such solutions it is advisable to include a small quantity of copper sulphate. The bodies of worms as prepared for laboratory use contain a considerable amount of water, and this may dilute the alcohol to such a point that molds are likely to invade the solution and destroy the specimens. Molds which are able to live in fairly strong solutions of alcohol and formalin are unable to get a foothold in solution containing a very small quantity of copper sulphate. If this salt is present to the extent of one per cent., the tissues will be strongly colored. If this is deemed undesirable the amount may be greatly reduced without serious danger of invasion by molds.

It will be noted that acetic acid was a component of the hardening solution, but not of the storage solution. This reagent serves a valuable purpose in causing the worms to become plump and turgid before the formalin has had time to harden them. Long-continued treatment with solutions containing acetic acid has a tendency to make the body wall of the worm tender and therefore easily torn during dissection. Judging by the odor, it appears probable that the acetic acid carried over from the hardening solution to the storage solution combines with the alcohol of the latter to form ethyl acetate within a reasonably short time. This last compound does not appear to injure the tissues.

Comparative tests were made to determine the effects of naphthalene and of alcohol upon earthworms. Ten active worms were placed in a liter of water in each of two dishes. To dish A was added 40 cc of 95 per cent. alcohol; to dish B, 40 cc of saturated solution of naphthalene in 95 per cent. alcohol. At the end of three minutes the worms in dish A were active and writhing; in dish B they were performing peculiar movements as if tying themselves into knots. At the end of thirty minutes the worms in dish A were still active; those in dish B were quiet and moved only slightly after pinching. To test the depth of narcosis 5 cc of glacial acetic acid were added to each dish. The worms in dish A became very active immediately; those in dish B moved feebly. This experiment was repeatedly tried with uniform results. It appears clear that naphthalene has distinct powers as a narcotizing agent in the treatment of earthworms. Experiment demonstrated that worms showing slight movement after thirty minutes in the naphthalene solution, as used, could safely be placed in the hardening solution. The movements of the anterior ends were so feeble that in masses of closely compacted worms the anterior ends failed to get out of position to any serious extent.

This method has several attractive features. The naphthalene brings about narcosis in a relatively short time. Moreover, narcosis is accompanied by extreme relaxation both of the circular and of the longitudinal muscles of the worm. Full extension of the worm is therefore made possible. So great is the relaxation of the circular muscles that the body wall is thrown into a series of deep longitudinal wrinkles. These, however, entirely disappear during treatment in the hardening solution. The removal of mucus and foreign matter is easy, due to the fact that the strongly coherent coagulum does not adhere to the worms. If the worms are placed in running water the coagulum floats away as the mass is gently agitated. This method gives rapid narcosis, ease in freeing the specimens from foreign matter and mucus, and plump, well-hardened specimens.

ELBERT C. COLE

SPECIAL ARTICLES

THE EFFECTS OF SELECTIVE SOLAR RADIATIONS ON GROWTH AND DEVELOPMENT

TEN chicks (banded) were selected from each of the eight groups used by Higgins and Sheard in their investigations on the parathyroid glands as influenced by selective solar radiations. The filters used were: amber (Pittsburgh No. 48), blue (Pittsburgh No. 56), ordinary window-glass and vitaglass, each about 2 mm. in thickness. To the diet of half of the chicks, 2 per cent. (by weight) of cod-liver oil was added. The standard diet was the Wisconsin all-mash ration, consisting of eighty pounds yellow corn, twenty pounds shorts, five pounds bone-meal, five pounds limestone grits and one pound salt.

The growth of the chicks was estimated from the average weight of the same ten chicks from each of the eight compartments, respectively, the weights being taken biweekly. During the first eighty days it was found that the curves showing the relationship between average weight and age practically coincided when 2 per cent. cod-liver oil was added to the ration, and that similar curves of weight when the standard ration only was fed exhibited the greatest departure from normal (vitaglass or standard ration with cod-liver oil) in the case of the chicks under the amber filter, with blue-glass next. The influence of unfavorable weather conditions (heat and humidity) on the average weight was least marked under vitaglass and most noticeable under the blue and amber filters. The experiments over the eighty-day period indicate that cod-liver oil compensates, in a large part, for the absence of vitamin D, and that the presence of ultra-violet rays of short wave-length (300–330 millimicrons) is an added factor in overcoming various degenerative tendencies.

At the end of six months it was found that the average weight was practically the same (within 3 per cent.) under each of the filters if cod-liver oil was added to the diet. Without cod-liver oil, no departure in average weight was found under vitaglass, 10 per cent. under ordinary glass, 20 per cent. under blue-glass, and 30 per cent. under the amber filter. By reason of the percentages of transmission of solar energy through these filters, together with the fact that the blue-glass used transmits slightly lesser wave-lengths than does ordinary glass and a slightly greater percentage of ultra-violet light, we are forced to the conclusion that the presence of both the longer and shorter (ultra-violet) wave-lengths of sunlight is essential to normal growth.

These results also emphasize the rôle which the parathyroids play in the growth and development of chicks. Hyperplasia of these glands occurs under blue and amber filters in the absence of cod-liver oil. We may postulate that hyperplastic parathyroids develop in an attempted rectification of hypofunctioning through an increase in the size of the glands in order to produce as nearly normal metabolism and development as is possible. Initially, normal growth and development are accomplished through a multiplicity of the functional units. These ultimately break down, causing metabolic disturbances and deficiency diseases.

Our experiments, insofar as they parallel the investigations of others, are not in accord with conclusions commonly accepted. In the experiments of Bovie, young chicks were taken and variously grouped under an environment of sunlight and of light through a greenhouse roof. Their rations consisted of so-called regular feed, regular feed and green stuff, regular feed and cod-liver oil. At the end of the sixty-fifth day it was found that the total weight of the chickens receiving sunlight only through the greenhouse roof is about one-half of the total weight of all the chickens exposed to outdoor sunlight or to the light from the ordinary quartz lamp.

The difference in experimental data and conclusions may be due either to difference in quality of stock or the character of the ration or to both. Obviously, inferior stock will succumb to conditions which will have no effect on superior stock. The matter of ration is evidently important. Our ration was high in its content of minerals (calcium). Biweekly determinations showed that the calcium was about 12 mg for each 100 cc. of serum and the phosphorus about 6 mg. for each 100 cc. of serum during the first three months of observation, irrespective of the character of the light filter.

In conclusion, we have found from experimental data on the quality and quantity of energy in solar radiation transmitted by the various filters and calculations made therefrom, due regard being given to the experimental results on the influence of selective solar irradiation upon the parathyroids, that an energy-equivalent of the short or so-called vital rays (290 to 320 millimicrons) of 0.045 gram calorie per each square centimeter each minute is ample to produce normal development.

CHARLES SHEARD
GEORGE M. HIGGINS
MAYO CLINIC AND MAYO FOUNDATION

VITAMIN B—A QUESTION OF NOMENCLATURE

RECENT literature on the composite nature of vitamin B has been very confusing, partly through the failure of some investigators to accept, or at least make clear, the idea that neither of the two factors now believed to be contained in what was originally called water-soluble B and later vitamin B promotes growth in the absence of the other and partly through lack of conformity in naming the two factors.

The question of the identity of the antineuritic vitamin and vitamin B had always been a puzzling one, so closely did they resemble each other in many ways. In 1919 Mitchell[1] in a critical review of the literature on the subject called attention to certain discrepancies in solubility, stability and occurrence of the two vitamins which, in his opinion, cast considerable doubt on their identity and suggested the need of more quantitative experiments in which the same materials should be tested for the prevention of polyneuritis in pigeons and the promotion of growth in young rats—the criteria commonly employed for the study of the antineuritic vitamin and vitamin B, respectively.

Later work, chiefly along the lines suggested by Mitchell, including studies by Emmett and Luros,[2] Funk and Dubin,[3] Heaton,[4] Levene and Muhlfeld,[5] and Hauge and Carrick,[6] strengthened the growing belief in the non-identity of the two vitamins and threw some light on their relative distribution in nature. One or two of these papers contained suggestions to the effect that vitamin B might not be a single substance, but might include the antineuritic vitamin in its make-up, but these received little attention at the time on account of lack of evidence or emphasis on other points. In 1926, Smith and Hendrick[7] called attention to the supplementing action of autoclaved yeast for rolled oats as a source of vitamin B and a similar supplementing action of the autoclaved yeast for the Seidell antineuritic vitamin concentrate and suggested the possibility that a heat-stable vitamin was necessary in addition to vitamin B for the growth of rats. Their experimental work was confirmed by Seidell[8] and by Goldberger, Wheeler,

NOMENCLATURE OF THE HEAT-LABILE AND HEAT-STABLE FACTORS OF VITAMIN B

Author	Heat-labile factor	Heat-stable factor
Goldberger *et al.*	Vitamin B *sensu stricto*	P–P factor
Sherman	Vitamin F	Vitamin G
Randoin and Lecoq	Antineuritic factor	Maintenance or functioning factor
Salmon	Vitamin B–P	Vitamin P–P
Chick and Roscoe	Antineuritic vitamin	Vitamin B *sensu stricto*
Plimmer *et al.*	B_1	B_2
Plimmer *et al.*	Vitamin B	Vitamin P–P
Evans and Burr	Antineuritic vitamin B	Growth-promoting vitamin B
Williams and Waterman	Heat-labile factor	Heat-stable factor
Eddy	Antineuritic factor	Antipellagric factor

1 Mitchell, H. H., 1919: "On the Identity of the Water-soluble Growth-promoting Vitamin and the Antineuritic Vitamin." *J. Biol. Chem.*, 40, 399.

2 Emmett, A. D., and Luros, G. O., 1920: "Water-soluble Vitamins. I. Are the Antineuritic and the Growth-promoting Water-soluble B Vitamins the Same?" *J. Biol. Chem.*, 43, 265.

3 Funk, C., and Dubin, H. E., 1921: "The Vitamins of Yeast and Their Rôle in Animal Nutrition." Proc. Soc. Exptl. Biol. Med., 19, 15.

4 Heaton, T. B., 1922: "On the Vitamin D." *Biochem. J.*, 16, 800.

5 Levene, P. A., and Muhlfeld, M., 1923: "On the Identity or Non-identity of Antineuritic and Water-Soluble B Vitamins." *J. Biol. Chem.*, 57, 341.

6 Hauge, S. M., and Carrick, C. W., 1926: "A Differentiation between the Water-soluble Growth-promoting and Antineuritic Substances." *J. Biol. Chem.*, 69, 403.

7 Smith, M. I., and Hendrick, E. G., 1926: "Some Nutrition Experiments with Brewers' Yeast with Special Reference to its Value in Supplementing Certain Deficiencies in Experimental Rations." U. S. Pub. Health Rpts., 41, 201.

8 Seidell, A., 1926: "Comparison Between the Pigeon and the Rat Methods of Testing for Antineuritic Vitamin." Bul. soc. chim. biol., 8, 746.

Lillie, and Rogers,[9] but in interpreting their results Goldberger and his associates suggested what appeared to be the clue to the baffling problem of the relationship between the antineuritic vitamin and vitamin B—namely, that for the growth-promoting function of vitamin B two factors are necessary, (1) the antineuritic vitamin and (2) a heat-stable factor which they suggested might be identical with the factor which they believed to be responsible for the prevention and cure of pellagra.

Whether or not the heat-stable factor with which the antineuritic vitamin must be supplemented for the growth-promoting function of vitamin B is the vitamin responsible for the cure or prevention of pellagra has not been established with certainty, but the investigations of Salmon,[10] Chick and Roscoe,[11] Hassan and Drummond,[12] Sherman and Axtmayer[13] and Williams and Waterman[14] have furnished a convincing verification of the multiple nature of vitamin B and of the part played by the antineuritic vitamin and a heat-stable vitamin as components of the mixture. In fact, food materials are now being retested for vitamin B in terms of their relative content of the heat-labile antineuritic vitamin and the heat-stable vitamin and it is being demonstrated that certain foods previously considered to be deficient in vitamin B require supplementing only by very small amounts of preparations rich in one or the other of the two factors.

With the general acceptance of the belief that vitamin B is not a single substance, the present lack of uniformity in the use of the term vitamin B and in designating the factors of which it is composed is regrettable. A confusion of terms, necessitating in every paper dealing with vitamin B an explanation of the author's system of nomenclature for the two factors, tends to bewilder the reader who finds vitamin literature difficult to follow at best. Some of the terms which have been used in papers appearing within the past two years are given in the accompanying table.

In attempting to evaluate these terms, it should be kept in mind that the term vitamin B has always been used to denote the water-soluble, appetite-stimulating, growth-promoting vitamin originally named by McCollum water-soluble B and never the antineuritic vitamin, *except as the two were considered identical.* This being the case, the term vitamin B can not be used *sensu stricto* for either the antineuritic vitamin or the heat-stable vitamin, since neither of these fulfils the conception for which this term has always stood. It is the mixture of the two in suitable proportions rather than either one alone that is vitamin B *sensu stricto.* The same argument applies to the use of the term *growth-promoting* vitamin B for the heat-stable factor alone. The use of the terms B_1 and B_2 suggests that the two vitamins are not separate substances, but simply parts of a single substance, whereas even the proponents of this classification have stated in unqualified terms their belief in the separate existence of the two factors. Moreover, designations involving subscripts are awkward to handle and confusing to remember.

With the elimination, for the reasons stated, of the classifications in which the term vitamin B is used for either factor alone and the one retaining the letter B with subscripts, the remaining terms fall under three systems of nomenclature, (1) an entirely new system in which the first letter of the deficiency disease associated with absence of the vitamin in question is hyphenated with P for preventive, (2) the well-known system employing adjectives descriptive of the pathological symptoms induced by entire absence of the vitamin, and (3) the simple alphabetical system first suggested by McCollum in his "fat-soluble A and water-soluble B," simplified by Drummond to vitamin A and vitamin B, and followed consistently ever since of naming each vitamin in alphabetical sequence as soon as proof of its separate identity is established.

To accept the first of these systems of nomenclature involves an entire new series of terms. If vitamin B–P and P–P are to be used for the beriberi-preventive and pellagra-preventive vitamins, we should speak of vitamin O–P or X–P, vitamin Sc–P, etc. This would seem to be a sufficient argument against the adoption of B–P and P–P. The chief arguments against the second system are the unwieldiness of the terms for common usage and the undue emphasis which they place upon the outcome of complete absence of the vitamin, suggesting that the only func-

9 Goldberger, J., Wheeler, G. A., Lillie, R. D., and Rogers, L. M., 1926: "A Further Study of Butter, Fresh Beef and Yeast as Pellagra Preventives, with Consideration of the Relation of Factor P-P of Pellagra (and Black Tongue of Dogs) to Vitamin B." U. S. Pub. Health Rpts., 41, 297.

10 Salmon, W. D., 1927: "On the Existence of two Active Factors in the Vitamin B Complex." *J. Biol. Chem.*, 73, 483.

11 Chick, H., and Roscoe, M. H., 1927: "On the Composite Nature of the Water-soluble B Vitamin." *Biochem. J.*, 21, 698.

12 Hassan, A., and Drummond, J. C., 1927: "The Physiological Rôle of Vitamin B. Part IV. The Relation of Certain Dietary Factors in Yeast to Growth in Rats on Diets Rich in Proteins." *Biochem. J.*, 21, 653.

13 Sherman, H. C., and Axtmayer, J. H., 1927: "A Quantitative Study of the Problem of the Multiple Nature of Vitamin B." *J. Biol. Chem.*, 75, 207.

14 Williams, R. R., and Waterman, R. E., 1927: "The Composite Nature of Vitamin B." Proc. Soc. Exptl. Biol. Med., 25, 1.

tion of the vitamin is in the prevention of particular deficiency diseases.

If the third system is to be continued as the simplest and most usable, how can it best meet the peculiar difficulty of recognizing a subdivision of a previously named vitamin into two entirely separate substances, one of which is likewise a vitamin of long standing, but which hitherto has had only a descriptive name—antineuritic vitamin. As was stated earlier, vitamin B has always stood for a water-soluble, appetite-stimulating, growth-promoting substance. To shift the letter B to either the antineuritic vitamin or the heat-stable vitamin would mean an entire change in significance which, on historic grounds alone, would be unfortunate. To retain it in its original sense involves no real change in conception, even although we know that for the properties denoted in the descriptive adjectives associated with it at least two separate vitamins are involved, each with certain individual properties. These vitamins, to take their place in the vitamin alphabet, should automatically receive the letters F and G, F being assigned to the earlier known, heat-labile antineuritic vitamin and G to the heat-stable vitamin which possibly has antipellagric properties. To those who find it difficult to distinguish vitamins by letters, it is a happy coincidence that the letters are the initials of the two investigators, Funk and Goldberger, most closely associated with these vitamins.

S. L. SMITH

OFFICE OF EXPERIMENT STATIONS,
U. S. DEPARTMENT OF AGRICULTURE

THE FEDERATION OF AMERICAN SOCIETIES OF EXPERIMENTAL BIOLOGY

THE annual meeting of the Federation of American Societies for Experimental Biology was held at the University of Michigan, Ann Arbor, Mich., April 12, 13 and 14, 1928.

The first meeting, a joint session of the societies of which the federation is comprised, was held Thursday morning. The program consisted in the presentation of nine papers which had been selected as being of general interest to the members of all four societies. It would be impossible to select one or more of the papers as being of outstanding value without doing injustice to the authors of the others whose names appeared on the program. Suffice it to say, they were all meritorious, but differed in interest, depending upon the particular field in which the listener might be actively engaged.

The afternoon was devoted to the reading of papers by the constituent societies of the federation, namely, the Physiological Society, the Biochemical Society, the Pharmacological Society and the Pathological Society.

Owing to the large number of titles presented, the Physiological Society was obliged to hold a double session each day in order to allow for the presentation of all the papers.

The Biochemical Society likewise was obliged to hold a double session Friday morning.

Friday afternoon was devoted to joint demonstrations by all societies. Thirty-seven demonstrations were on the program, which was a marked increase above the number given at any previous meeting. They were in practically all instances most interesting and instructive.

The final meeting, a joint session, was held Saturday afternoon, when another group of papers of unusual interest was presented.

Regarding the meeting it may be stated that it was the largest in point of attendance of any held during the history of the federation. An unusually large number of titles was presented under the "introduced by" and "by invitation" list. The authors of these papers were, for the most part, of the younger generation, who in the majority of cases occupy minor teaching positions or are doing research work as undergraduates.

All the foregoing speaks favorably as regards the popularity of a spring meeting. This was the second meeting held at this time of the year, the first being one year ago when we met at Rochester, New York. The executive committee of the federation, recognizing the discomfort of traveling in the holiday season and the reluctance of some of the members in absenting themselves from their families during the Christmas holidays, recommended that the time of holding the annual meeting be changed. The proposition of making a change met with some opposition, but the experiment was made and has proved to be very successful.

It was voted that our next meeting be held at Boston, Mass., at the time of the meeting of the International Physiological Congress. The federation meeting will be merged with the meetings of the congress.

This report would be incomplete if the excellent services and the hospitality shown by the members of the University of Michigan were not mentioned. The local committee left nothing undone which could further add to our comfort and convenience.

The board of regents of the university kindly provided a complimentary dinner on Thursday evening, to which all in attendance were invited as their guests.

Everything considered, it was the most successful meeting ever held during the history of the federation.

E. D. BROWN, *Secretary*

SCIENCE

Vol. LXVII May 18, 1928 No. 1742

CONTENTS

The Berthelot Centenary and the Resulting International Efforts to Advance Chemistry: Dr. Atherton Seidell ... 497

Rainfall and Run-off: Professor Frank D. Adams 500

Edward Sandford Burgess: Professor W. K. Fisher ... 501

Scientific Events:
The Oxford Expedition to Greenland; The International Congress of Americanists; Building Plans of the American Museum of Natural History; New Building for Plant Industry at the University of Minnesota; Lectures under the Auspices of the Astronomical Society of the Pacific ... 502

Scientific Notes and News ... 505

University and Educational Notes ... 508

Discussion and Correspondence:
The Reapportionment Bill in Congress: Professor Edward V. Huntington. *Eye Soreness and Vitamin A Deficiency among the Nez Percés Indians:* Dr. C. A. Browne. *The Liter and Cubic Decimeter:* H. W. Bearce. *The Passing of the Circuit System of Collecting Weather Reports:* Alfred J. Henry. *The Abnormal Specific Heat of a Rarefied Gas at a Low Temperature, and the Cosmic Radiation:* Dr. R. D. Kleeman ... 509

Scientific Apparatus and Laboratory Methods:
Macroscopical Detection of the Medullated Wool Fiber: J. F. Wilson. *A Perfusion Fluid for Elasmobranchs:* Eleanor M. Kapp ... 512

Special Articles:
The Sexual Stage of Fungi Induced by Ultra-Violet Rays: Professor F. L. Stevens. *The Amide Nitrogen of Blood:* Dr. Sidney Bliss ... 514

The American Association for the Advancement of Science:
The Spring Meeting of the Executive Committee: Dr. Burton E. Livingston ... 516

Science News ... x

SCIENCE: A Weekly Journal devoted to the Advancement of Science, edited by J. McKeen Cattell and published every Friday by

THE SCIENCE PRESS

New York City: Grand Central Terminal

Lancaster, Pa. Garrison, N. Y.

Annual Subscription, $6.00. Single Copies, 15 Cts.

SCIENCE is the official organ of the American Association for the Advancement of Science. Information regarding membership in the Association may be secured from the office of the permanent secretary, in the Smithsonian Institution Building, Washington, D. C.

THE BERTHELOT CENTENARY AND THE RESULTING INTERNATIONAL EFFORTS TO ADVANCE CHEMISTRY[1]

In January last I had the pleasure of describing before the Chemical Society of Washington the celebration of the centenary of Marcelin Berthelot held in Paris from October 24 to 26 of last year. These remarks have been published in Science (Feb. 17, 1928) and possibly have been read by some of you.

Through the kindness of the French ambassador and M. Maurice Léon I am able to show you to-night a photographic record of the event, which will certainly give you a more vivid impression of it than I was able to convey by words alone to the chemists of Washington. Thanks to this pictorial presentation it will not be necessary for me to review again the details of the various ceremonies and more attention can be given to other aspects of the event.

Considering the celebration in its entirety there is no question but that it was the most magnificent tribute to chemistry but has ever been organized. More than fifty nations of the world sent distinguished chemists or governmental representatives. The president and entire government of France as well as the ministers and ambassadors of many other nations participated. Chemistry was extolled more highly than ever before. Judging by the space devoted to it by the newspapers the celebration attracted the attention of the general public to an extraordinary degree.

The gathering was noteworthy in being the first since the great war at which the chemists of the enemy nations have met together under such amicable circumstances. An especial effort was made to reestablish cordial relations between all, and the evidence of success in this direction was unmistakable.

The assemblage was unusual in that no other attraction than friendly regard drew the participants together. It is true that in the preceding week a program of chemical interest was provided by the Société de Chimie Industrielle, but at the Berthelot celebration nothing was presented other than discourses on Berthelot and the plan to perpetuate his ideals in regard to cooperation among scientists.

[1] Address delivered before the joint meeting of chemical societies at the Chemists' Club, New York, April 6, 1928.

As expressed by Berthelot science is a collective endeavor and owes its progress to the efforts of workers in all countries. It is truly international, and of all men scientists should be most interested in promoting friendly international relations. This was undoubtedly the keynote of the celebration and in emphasizing it French chemists demonstrated their outstanding interest in cooperative efforts to advance chemistry.

The desirability of intimate contact between those engaged in chemistry does not need to be emphasized. It is true that we may become acquainted with other chemists through their publications, and to many this is sufficient, but to others there is nothing so stimulating as personal intercourse with those interested in like problems. Any means which facilitates this contact may be expected to advance chemistry. This is believed by its sponsors to be one of the missions of La Maison de la Chimie.

The Chemists' Club of New York, although a local undertaking, has become a most powerful agency for the advancement of chemistry. It offers membership to chemists outside of New York and thus extends its field of usefulness. The Maison de la Chimie which will be erected in Paris will serve primarily those in its immediate vicinity, but it will also do for the chemists of the adjoining and other countries what the Chemists' Club of New York does for those of us who reside in other parts of the United States.

There is this difference between the two undertakings—whereas those who founded the Chemists' Club probably did not realize what an important factor for the advancement of chemistry they were inaugurating, the sponsors of La Maison de la Chimie are knowingly setting out to establish an international center for this purpose. Thus they have the advantage of a predetermined plan and a definite goal.

It can not be denied that such a center located in Paris will be of great service to the chemists of a large group of European countries. It is of course not so certain that many American chemists will be directly benefited by it. This, however, should not be a reason for the indifference with which the project has been received in our country. A more correct explanation of the attitude of American chemists is undoubtedly the great distance which separates us from Europe and the huge task in hand of developing chemistry in this country. We are captivated by our own affairs and will not allow our attention to be distracted by circumstances which we believe do not directly concern us.

There is, however, another reason which accounts for some of the criticism expressed by our society at Detroit. It was the solicitation by the French government of collaboration in the undertaking. We naturally question any governmental participation in scientific matters because we feel that anything having a political flavor can not be above suspicion. This, however, is an attitude which is peculiar to our country. In practically all others, it is the government which directly supports science. In France, for example, all the leading men of science in their capacity as professors in the universities or directors of institutions are government employees and every action they take in international affairs is with the financial and moral support of their government.

The movement for an international Maison de la Chimie was initiated by the chemists of France, but its realization would have been impossible without governmental aid. The reason it obtained such full support from the French government was that the prime minister and many of his associates are themselves scientists of the highest standing and have the very fullest appreciation of the benefits resulting from the progress of science. Berthelot was in his time minister of public instruction and Herriot, the present minister, occupied a prominent place in the ceremonies planned in honor of his predecessor in office. The close relation which exists between the governments and science in other countries was also shown by the number of ministers from other nations who participated in the Berthelot celebration. Finally, the small countries and colonies which contributed to the movement could have done so only through their governments. As with all other countries, the appeal to the United States to join in this movement was addressed to our government. It was the natural method, and if an exception had been made in our case and the request addressed directly to our society the action would have been considered, from their point of view, as one of disrespect to the United States government.

The fact that the leaders of our government are not men of science and that there is not a closer relation between science and government in the United States is regrettable. It is to be hoped that the organized effort to popularize science, being made by Science Service and the American Chemical Society (A. C. S.) News Service, may eventually arouse our government to greater interest in its benefits.

In another respect, however, we are particularly fortunate. It is that in the United States we have a single language and no political barriers between different sections of our great country. These handicaps exist in Europe, and the cooperation of the smaller groups of chemists in the various countries can be effected only by overcoming much greater resistance than oppose our efforts in America. It is this situation which makes desirable the concerted effort represented by La Maison de la Chimie. Aside from the countries in which the English and German languages are used there are many in which French is either the native or preferred language. These Latin countries are sorely in need of coordination of their efforts in respect to the dissemination of chemical literature. A central clearing house which can serve them in the way chemists are served by the organizations in Germany, England and America may be expected to facilitate greatly their contribution to the advancement of science. The International Office of Chemistry which will be given shelter in La Maison de la Chimie will undoubtedly perform an incalculable service to a large number of chemists in many different countries.

There is, however, a very difficult problem which confronts those interested in the establishment of this new project. Beginning now after such an extensive literature of chemistry has accumulated, the collection of a considerable part of it is a costly and laborious task. Even to establish a comprehensive French abstract journal for current contributions is a great undertaking, and with the present acceleration in the output of chemical publications necessarily becomes more and more difficult.

While talking to M. Gerard some months ago he told me of these problems and gave me a hint of a possible means to solve them. Although the solution he contemplated would necessarily be an experiment it would be one which the rapid increase in scientific literature is certain to make necessary sooner or later. Any improvement in the distribution of scientific literature is certainly desirable and the results of the experiment to be made by the International Office of Chemistry will be awaited with the greatest interest.

The plan contemplates the reproduction of printed chemical articles by a cinematographic process. The pages will be photographed upon a film and this sent to the user who will project it page by page before him on his desk and to such an enlargement as best suits his vision. The disadvantages to some resulting from the use of small type by certain journals will thus be avoided. Abstracts which attempt to give the substance of a paper will not be necessary, since the entire article may be sent out for a cost which it is expected will be no greater than that now required for preparing, editing, printing and distributing an abstract journal.

In order to acquaint chemists with the current articles as they appear a card catalogue system will be employed. The cards will be efficiently classified and describe only the scope of the paper. Each member will receive cards for the particular branches of chemistry in which he is interested and will select from these the papers of which he desires photographic copies.

This will be in effect a new kind of bibliographic service, and its success will of course depend upon the ingenuity displayed in perfecting the photographic apparatus required and the efficiency attained in the preparation and classification of the cards covering the current chemical literature.

The service which such a system will render to chemists of those countries in which the general distribution of chemical literature has not yet been developed may easily be imagined. The necessity for maintaining large libraries of chemical periodicals in each country will be greatly diminished and more money can be spent for compendia and text-books. The waste due to requiring those who subscribe to chemical journals to purchase a great quantity of material which they do not use and the necessity for condensing papers to an excessive degree will be largely eliminated. Each worker under the new plan will accumulate only that which directly concerns his own research activities.

This is the germ of an idea which will no doubt be considered by many to be fantastic, especially since it is contrary to the principle of mass production developed in our own society. Our three journals can be distributed to all our members cheaper than a smaller edition of each could be sent to those who would select only one of the three. What, then, would happen if eventually the edition of our publications should be reduced to the small number of copies required to supply libraries and distributing centers? It is difficult to predict, but it is easy to imagine that multigraphing processes will be so highly developed by that time that the printing of journals devoted solely to research will not be necessary.

The project of La Maison de la Chimie and of the International Office of Chemistry must be looked upon as an experiment in the cooperative advancement of world chemistry. The exact method by which this is to be accomplished can not be predicted, but that this is the sole aim of the sponsors of the movements no fair-minded person can doubt.

American good-will has made itself felt throughout the world. Our great philanthropists who have founded such international projects as those connected with the name of Rockefeller desire to improve conditions universally, both as regards health and learning. A larger portion of their funds are expended outside of this country than within it. Surely the chemists of the United States are not less magnanimous in regard to the advancement of our science and have nothing but good wishes for the earnest efforts of every one who desires to make chemistry a more powerful factor in world progress.

ATHERTON SEIDELL

HYGIENIC LABORATORY,
WASHINGTON, D. C.

RAINFALL AND RUN-OFF

IN a paper entitled "The Origin of Springs and Rivers—an Historical Review," presented by the writer at the annual meeting of the Geological Society of America held in Cleveland in December, 1927, it was shown that the statement of Aristotle to the effect that the rainfall on the earth's surface was quite insufficient to supply the amount of water carried off by the rivers and that some other contributory source of water must be found was accepted as correct by practically every writer on this subject down to the seventeenth century of the Christian era.

The first demonstration that this statement was not correct and that the rainfall is not only sufficient but much more than sufficient to supply the rivers with all their water is contained in a little book which was published in Paris in 1674 under the title "De L'origine des Fontaines." This work of duodecimo size and containing 353 pages appeared anonymously.

In the Philosophical Transactions of the Royal Society of London for A. D. 1674, p. 447, there appears (without signature) a short article which commences as follows: "A Particular Account given by an anonymous French Author in his book on the Origin of Fountains printed in Paris 1674 to show that the Rain and Snow waters are sufficient to make Fountains and Rivers run perpetually."

The early numbers of the Philosophical Transactions having run out of print, they were reprinted in an abbreviated form in 1731, the order for their publication being signed by Sir Isaac Newton as president of the society at that time.

A second abridged reprint of these early volumes was issued later, the first volume appearing in 1809. In both of these reprints the "Particular Account" above referred to reappeared, that in the latter being in a somewhat expanded form, and no mention of the name of the author of the book is made either in the original edition or in the first reprint of the Transactions. In the second reprint, however, the abstract is said to be that of *Papin's* book on the "Origin of Fountains" (Paris, 1674).

This statement was accepted as authoritative in fixing the authorship of this important little book and in his paper presented to the Geological Society of America the writer gave Papin the credit for having written it.

Papin as a matter of fact had, in a paper published in 1647, put forward the directly opposite opinion, but from the evidence referred to above it was supposed that in his latter years he had, after a detailed study of the subject, changed his views. The present writer had not been able anywhere to find a copy of the book in question before the presentation of his paper to the Geological Society of America, but since that time a copy has come into his hands through one of the dealers in old books in Europe.

An examination of the text of the book gives no clue to its authorship, but on the title page there has been written in ink by an unknown hand the words "par pierre Perrault."

On consulting the "Biographie Générale depuis les Temps les plus reculés jusqu'a nos Jours—Paris 1862" it was found that Pierre Perrault (whose name in the paper is mentioned as an associate of De la Hire and Mariotte), who was born about 1608 and died in 1680, is stated to have written a book having the title given above and which was published in Paris in 1674.

On comparing the abstracts in the Philosophical Transactions with the work itself it is clearly seen that this book which was attributed to Papin was really written by *Pierre Perrault,* to whom therefore belongs the honor of having discovered and established one of the fundamental facts of geology, namely, that the rivers of the earth derive their supplies of water from the rain which falls upon the earth's surface and not from the earth's interior or some other quaint source as held by earlier writers.

Pierre Perrault, who made this very important contribution to geological science, was not a member of the French Academy but a lawyer and man of affairs who took an interest in science, and who is therefore a member of that group of amateur workers who, like Clifton Sorby and others, have from time to time rendered such important services to science. It is a matter of regret that in certain other directions his activities were not viewed so favorably by his contemporaries, for it is recorded in the biographical sketch to which reference has been made that—"il fit ses études en droit et après avoir occupé quelques emplois secondaires dans l'administration acheta la charge du receveur général des finances de la généralité de Paris charge que Colbert, son ami cependant, le força de quitter pour avoir emprunté à sa caisse quelques sommes dont il avait besoin pour satisfaire d'avides creanciers."

Another point which may be worthy of mention in this connection is that in the abstract of Perrault's book which appears in the original edition of the Philosophical Transactions and which is reproduced without substantial change in both sets of the abstracts which appeared later, certain figures of rainfall and run-off in the district of the Upper Seine taken from Perrault are presented, upon which he based his conclusion that the rainfall of that district was six times as great as the run-off. These figures, however, do not bear out this result. This fact remained unnoticed until the publication of the second set of abstracts, when the editor remarked that some mistake must have been made in the numbers. On tracing this back to Perrault's book it is found that the abstracter for the original edition of the Philosophical Transactions, and whose abstract was copied by the others, confused the words "vingt quatre" (24) and "quatre vingt" (80), the amounts in the book being given in words and not in numerals. The amount of rainfall on the area selected for study is actually given by Perrault as 2*2*4,899,942 "muids"—and not "a little over 280 million" as stated by the abstracter. With this alteration the result given by Perrault—namely, that the run-off is one sixth of the rainfall—is seen to be correct.

In 1686 a book entitled "Traité du Mouvement des Eaux et des autres corps Fluides," by M. Mariotte, was published in Paris. This was twelve years after the appearance of Perrault's book. This work of Mariotte's was "mis en lumière" after the author's death by M. de la Hire, Professor of Mathematics, and, like Mariotte, a Member of the Royal Academy of Sciences of Paris. Mariotte was according to his biographer the first man in France to bring to the study of the science of Physics "un esprit d'observation et de doubt . . . si necessaire à ceux qui interrogent la nature."

In this book the question of the Origin of Springs is taken up in the Second Discourse. After referring to the "author of the book entitled on the Origin of Fountains" and his work, but without any mention of his name, Mariotte sets forth the results of certain measurements of the rainfall about Dijon which he had caused to be made, as well as measurements of the run-off of the Seine taken at the Pont Rouge in Paris. The annual rainfall according to these measurements was about seventeen inches. Taking it as fifteen inches, Mariotte calculated that the run-off was somewhat less than one sixth of the rainfall and that if taken as eighteen inches it would amount to one eighth of the rainfall.

In this way Perrault's work was confirmed by another of that brilliant group of men who were at work in Paris about this time.

The paper read before the Geological Society of America at the Cleveland meeting appears only in the form of an abstract in the Bulletin of the Society but will be printed *in extenso* in the Festband which is being issued by the University of Helsingfors in honor of Professor Sederholm and which is now in press. The present note will serve to correct the statement in both the abstract and in the extended paper which gives to Papin instead of to Perrault the credit for the important discovery made by the latter

FRANK D. ADAMS

MCGILL UNIVERSITY

EDWARD SANDFORD BURGESS

JANUARY 19, 1855—FEBRUARY 23, 1928

ALL too few are men of Louis Agassiz type, who combine a devotion to scholarly research with a marked gift for imparting to beginners their own zest for scientific pursuits. Such a teacher was Dr. Edward Sandford Burgess, for thirty years professor and head of the department of biological sciences (and for a time acting president) of Hunter College, New York City. A man of rare charm and unassuming manner, he chose always to elucidate, never to impress; gentle, selfless, kindly, he gave unstintingly of his time and energy to his students and to his chosen fields of work.

Dr. Burgess was not only a scientist; he had a wide and eager knowledge of many subjects and an especially deep appreciation of the finer things in the literature and art of many lands. His special spheres of labor were in botany and anthropology. He was a recognized authority on the genus Aster and on the history of botany, his major publications being a "History of Pre-Clusian Botany" (1902) and "Species and Variations of Biotian Asters" (1906). Among his other published works are: "The Chautauqua Flora" (1877); "Botanical Genera, Tribes and Families," in the Century dictionary, M to Z, 1891; "The Asters of the Northern United States" (with Dr. N. L. Britton, in Britton and Brown's "Illustrated Flora"), 1898; "The Asters of the Southern United States" (in Small's "Southeastern Flora"), 1903; "The Old South Road at Gay Head" (Duke's County, Mass., Historical Society Publications, Vol. 1, No. 4, 1926); a volume of poems.

During later years Dr. Burgess devoted much time to anthropology and taught this subject at Hunter College. Among his unpublished manuscripts are two extensive ones, entitled: "A Look at the Development of Man" and "A Series of Lectures on Anthropology." There are several genealogical and historical researches, especially on Indian lore of Martha's Vineyard.

Professor Burgess was a grandson of Dr. Jacob Burgess, who moved from Berkshire County, Massachusetts, to Silver Creek, New York, in 1811. His father, the Reverend Dr. Chalon Burgess, was long the pastor of the Presbyterian church of this place. His mother was Emma Johnston, daughter of the Reverend Charles Johnston, of Ovid, Seneca County, N. Y. Edward Burgess was born in Little Valley, Cattaraugus County, but his boyhood was spent in Panama, Chautauqua County. He was graduated from the state normal school of Fredonia, and, with distinction, from Hamilton College in 1879. For two years he held a graduate fellowship in Greek at Johns

Hopkins under the eminent Greek scholar, Dr. Gildersleeve. In 1899 he received from Columbia University the degree of doctor of philosophy, and in 1904 from Hamilton College that of doctor of science.

From 1882 to 1895 (when he became professor of natural science at Hunter College) Dr. Burgess taught botany in the Washington, D. C., high schools and from 1880 to 1895 at the Martha's Vineyard summer institute. He was instructor at Johns Hopkins in 1885. He was a member of the Phi Beta Kappa, the American Association for the Advancement of Science, the New York Academy of Sciences, the American Anthropological Association (a founder), the Society of American Folk-lore, the Century Club of New York, the Torrey Botanical Club, of which he was president, 1912–13, the New York Botanical Garden Corporation (a director, 1912–13).

Dr. Burgess's friends will cherish most the memory of him in his Yonkers home, Sweetbriarside. His marriage to Irene S. Hamilton, of Fredonia, N. Y., was one of rare companionship of spirit. Their garden, with its Shakespeare plot, its Wordsworth bed, its Keats corner, its Hellenica, its plants of western New York, its lily pool filled with native and exotic lilies, its dozen varieties of hybrid sweetbriars, its eighty or more different conifers, its wealth of tulips and roses, has been a delight to all flower lovers and is the expression of the lifelong devotion of the owners.

Dr. Burgess was modern in his conceptions of biology, yet from training and conviction he was deeply religious. Of the views of others, who differed, he was very tolerant: "Truth can not contradict itself," he was wont to say. His reverent attitude toward nature is reminiscent of two such different masters as Charles Darwin and Louis Agassiz. More accurately, Dr. Burgess recalls J. S. Henslow, of Cambridge, the wise professor of botany "who knew every branch of science," the beloved mentor with whom Darwin took long walks, until he became known as "the man who walks with Henslow."

A portion of Darwin's tribute to Henslow, as Romanes has pointed out, reflects the character of Darwin, but it is also an excellent likeness of Edward Burgess.

> Nothing could be more simple, cordial, and unpretending than the encouragement which he afforded to all young naturalists. I soon became intimate with him, for he had a remarkable power of making the young feel completely at ease with him; though we were all awe-struck with the amount of his knowledge. Before I saw him, I heard one young man sum up his attainments by simply saying that he knew everything. When I reflect how immediately we felt at perfect ease with a man older, and in every way so immensely our superior, I think it was as much owing to the transparent sincerity of his character as to his kindness of heart; and, perhaps, even still more, to a highly remarkable absence in him of all self-consciousness. One perceived at once that he never thought of his own varied knowledge or clear intellect, but solely on the subject in hand. Another charm, which must have struck every one, was that his manner to old and distinguished persons and to the youngest student was exactly the same: and to all he showed the same winning courtesy. In short, no man could be better informed to win the entire confidence of the young, and to encourage them in their pursuits. It always struck me that his mind could not be even touched by any paltry feeling of vanity, envy, or jealousy. With all this equability of temper and remarkable benevolence, there was no insipidity of character. A man must have been blind not to have perceived that beneath this placid exterior there was a vigorous and determined will. When principle came into play, no power on earth could have turned him one hair's breadth.[1]

Darwin adds, "I owe more than I can express to this excellent man."

In our strenuous era of high pressure research, when beginners emerge from courses in test-tube biology—*à la mode* and labeled "modern"—with a somewhat cynical and suspicious attitude toward Nature in her visible forms, it is perhaps permitted one to reflect upon the passing of the fine art of instilling an appreciation of natural history, and to wonder if youngsters of the future will experience the intellectual high adventure which has been the good fortune of those who have walked with Henslow, Agassiz, Jordan, Dudley, Burgess, Comstock and many another of the past or passing generation, too numerous to name.

Walter K. Fisher

Hopkins Marine Station

SCIENTIFIC EVENTS

THE OXFORD EXPEDITION TO GREENLAND

The Godthaab district of Greenland has been chosen as the scene of the Oxford University Greenland expedition of 1928, which has been initiated by the Oxford University Exploration Club, and has for its objects the continuation of the biological work begun in the Oxford Arctic expeditions of 1921, 1923 and 1924. A correspondent of the London *Times* writes that this area has been chosen as representing the region (to which the barren lands of Canada belong) where biological surveys have only just passed through their preliminary stages. Here a comparative survey of the wild life and the conditions con-

[1] "Life and Letters of Charles Darwin." Edited by Francis Darwin, Vol. 1, p. 186.

trolling it can be worked out by the ornithologist, the botanist and entomologist of the expedition, as a contribution towards researches in economic zoology and botany, which are necessary for the solution of important problems of human economy.

The study of malaria, of crop pests, of the means of developing and controlling the natural resources of countries, requires a clear understanding of the laws governing the interrelations of animals of all kinds and especially the regulation of their numbers. The data are not yet available for a complete understanding of these problems, but a preliminary contribution to them can be made through the working out of principles among a limited class of life in a place which the short northern season, the small number of species involved, and the absence of human interference make particularly favorable for the purpose.

Dr. T. G. Longstaff has consented to act as the leader of the party, which will consist of eight members. The expedition proceeds under the official authority of the university and with the official support of the Royal Geographical Society. It is assured not only of all facilities from the Danish government, but also of the benefit of the experience of the best Danish naturalists and explorers. The university has formally voted £50 towards the expenses of the expedition and the rest of the funds have been supplied by the members and their friends.

The personnel of the expedition will be as follows:

T. G. Longstaff, naturalist and topographer.
Major R. W. G. Hingston, entomologist.
E. M. Nicholson, ornithologist.
C. G. Trapnell, botanist.
W. G. H. D. Crouch, photographer and quartermaster.
B. D. Nicholson, ornithologist and assistant surveyor.
Sir John Hanham, assistant botanist.
H. P. Hanham, assistant ornithologist.

THE INTERNATIONAL CONGRESS OF AMERICANISTS

Arrangements are being made for the meetings of the twenty-third session of the International Congress of Americanists, to be held during the week beginning September 17 in New York. The invitations for the Americanists to meet in New York were extended at the twenty-second session, which was held in Rome in September, 1926, by the American Museum of Natural History, Columbia University, the Brooklyn Museum, the Museum of the American Indian, Heye Foundation, the American Geographical Society, the American Ethnological Society, the New York Academy of Sciences and the Archeological Institute of America.

The headquarters of the congress will be at the American Museum of Natural History, where the opening and closing meetings will be held. During the week there will also be meetings at Columbia University, the Museum of the American Indian, the Heye Foundation and the Brooklyn Museum. Prominent students of American Indian life and related topics will be in attendance from Europe and Latin America. The papers and discussions will deal with aboriginal inhabitants of the Americas, the origin and distribution of their cultures and matters of history, geology and geography bearing on the native populations.

Franz Boas,
Chairman of the Organization Committee
P. E. Goddard, *Secretary,*
American Museum of Natural History,
New York City

BUILDING PLANS OF THE AMERICAN MUSEUM OF NATURAL HISTORY

Plans for the construction of nine new sections to the American Museum of Natural History, to be completed by the seventieth anniversary of the institution in 1939, are contained in a report made to the trustees by President Henry Fairfield Osborn. In addition, a new building to be known as the Roosevelt Memorial, costing $3,250,000, is to be erected as a new entrance hall at the intersection of Seventy-ninth Street and Central Park West.

Two of the new wings, the African hall, costing $1,350,000, and the power and service section, costing $900,000, together with the Roosevelt Memorial are to be constructed in the immediate future. The other sections, the building of which will be spread out over the next eleven years, are to be the astronomic hall, to cost $1,689,525; Australian hall, $1,006,549; middle American hall, $2,306,592; south oceanic hall, $1,006,549; lecture amphitheater hall, $2,994,529; preparation and storage hall, $500,000. The complete cost of the new sections and the Roosevelt Memorial will be $15,004,744.

Dr. Osborn gave a *résumé* of the history of the museum since 1869, the year of its founding, and made note of the fact that only $8,390,599.68 had been spent on the institution since that time, and when added to the proposed expenditures will make a grand total of $23,394,343.68 for the nineteen section building as planned.

Dr. Osborn added that since 1902 more than $23,000,000 in gifts and bequests had been received by the museum. In this summary of the history of the institution, the president recalled that in 1869 New York had no museum of any kind, while such institutions flourished in Boston, Philadelphia, Chicago, Washington and in all the European capitals.

The father of President Roosevelt was one of the founders of the American Museum of Natural History, and in December, 1919, a movement was started to create a memorial to honor both father and son. In 1924 the State Legislature appropriated $250,000 to start the project.

NEW BUILDING FOR PLANT INDUSTRY AT THE UNIVERSITY OF MINNESOTA

DR. R. W. THATCHER, president of the Massachusetts Agricultural College, formerly dean of the department of agriculture of the University of Minnesota, has accepted an invitation to deliver the address at the dedicatory exercises of the new plant industry building for agricultural biochemistry at University Farm, St. Paul, on Thursday afternoon, June 7.

The building will be formally presented to the university by President F. B. Snyder, of the board of regents. The address of acceptance will be given by Dean W. C. Coffey. Greetings from the American Chemical Society will be extended by its president, Dr. S. W. Parr, professor emeritus of the University of Illinois. Greetings from the American Association of Cereal Chemists will be voiced by Leslie Olsen, its president and chief chemist of the International Milling Company of Minneapolis. As the association and also the northwest regional group of the American Chemical Society will meet in Minneapolis the same week, it is expected that a body of 400 to 500 chemists will attend the dedication exercises.

The new building, 152 feet in length and 70 feet deep at its maximum, cost with its equipment approximately $250,000. The construction material is cut limestone to the top of the basement, and brick the remainder of the exterior. Reinforced steel concrete was used throughout, with floors of concrete and terrazzo. The floor plans were designed with particular reference to research and teaching facilities.

The basement, which is largely above ground, combines a store room 24 by 42 feet and a laboratory of like proportions for semi-commercial scale experiments. The laboratory is provided with filter presses, vacuum pans and autoclaves. An optical room is used for physical-chemical research with the ultra-microscope and ultra-violet light. A large laboratory is used for cereal chemistry research. Constant temperature rooms are equipped and controlled for low temperature work.

The main floor is essentially a teaching floor, with the addition of offices and private laboratories for two members of the division staff. Two lecture rooms, capable of seating 70 students each, are on this floor. The second floor is a teaching and administration floor, with ample space for the division office and library, and for laboratories for assistants. The third floor contains large laboratories for graduate students who are working on thesis problems, a large room for office and study, offices of staff members and two animal nutrition laboratories.

A nutrition laboratory, 24 by 31 feet, on this floor is used by students working thesis on nutrition problems, where the use of small animals is required. The experiment station projects on vitamins are conducted on this floor.

LECTURES UNDER THE AUSPICES OF THE ASTRONOMICAL SOCIETY OF THE PACIFIC

TWELVE lectures were held during the past season in Southern California under the auspices of the Astronomical Society of the Pacific as follows:

At California Institute of Technology, Pasadena:

Sun Rays in the Service of Man
Dr. C. G. Abbot
Smithsonian Institution

The Exploration of Space
Dr. E. P. Hubble
Mt. Wilson Observatory

Sun-Spots
Dr. S. B. Nicholson
Mt. Wilson Observatory

Stars in Action
Professor A. H. Joy
Mt. Wilson Observatory

The Interior of a Star
Dr. W. S. Adams
Mt. Wilson Observatory

Our Planet Neighbors
Dr. R. G. Aitken
Lick Observatory

At Public Library, Los Angeles:

Beyond the Milky Way
Dr. E. P. Hubble
Mt. Wilson Observatory

The Great Meteor of Central Arizona
Dr. Mars Baumgardt
Southern California Academy of Science

Telescopes
Dr. F. G. Pease
Mt. Wilson Observatory

The Sun
Professor F. Ellerman
Mt. Wilson Observatory

The Solar System
Dr. R. G. Aitken
Lick Observatory

Giant and Dwarf Stars
Dr. F. C. Leonard
University of California at Los Angeles

SCIENTIFIC NOTES AND NEWS

DR. MAX MASON, president of the University of Chicago, previously professor of mathematical physics in the University of Wisconsin, has resigned to accept an appointment as director of the newly created division of Natural Sciences of the Rockefeller Foundation.

THE Rumford medal of the American Academy of Arts and Sciences has been awarded to Dr. Edward L. Nichols, emeritus professor of physics at Cornell University.

DR. JOHN C. MERRIAM, president of the Carnegie Institution of Washington, and Dr. Elihu Thomson, director of the Thomson Research Laboratories of the General Electric Company, will deliver the leading addresses at a banquet at the Hotel Astor, on the occasion of the conferring on May 24 of the gold medal for science of the Society of Arts and Sciences on Mr. Thomas Edison.

PRESENTATION of the seventeenth Willard Gibbs medal of the Chicago section of the American Chemical Society to Dr. W. D. Harkins, of the University of Chicago, will be made at a dinner to be held at Palmer House, Chicago, on May twenty-fifth.

PRESENTATION of a bust of Dr. John Dewey, professor of philosophy in Columbia University, was made to him at the Henry Street Settlement Building, New York, on May 16.

THE Vienna Society of Medicine, on March 23, elected as corresponding member Dr. Francis G. Benedict, director of the nutrition laboratory of the Carnegie Institution of Washington, Boston.

DR. ELVIN C. STAKMAN, professor of plant pathology at the University of Minnesota, has received the Emil Christion Hansen prize, consisting of a gold medal and 2,000 crowns, for his works on the diseases of plants. The prize was handed to the American chargé d'affaires at the legation at Stockholm on May 8 in the absence of Dr. Stakman.

PROFESSOR ALBERT EINSTEIN has been elected an honorary member of the British Physical Society.

THE council of the Royal Anthropological Institute has awarded the Huxley memorial medal for 1929 to Baron Erland Nordenskiöld, of Göteborg. He has also been invited to deliver the Huxley memorial lecture in November of that year.

THE John Hunter Medal in bronze, with the triennial prize of £50, has been awarded by the Royal College of Surgeons of England to Victor Ewings Negus, for his investigations into the comparative anatomy and physiology of the larynx and the anatomy of the bronchi in their relation to surgery.

DR. FRIEDRICH BECKE, professor of mineralogy at the University of Vienna, has been elected a foreign member of the Swedish Academy of Sciences.

DR. WILLIAM STERN, professor of psychology in the University of Hamburg, has been elected a corresponding member of the French Society of Psychology.

SIR WILFRED GRENFELL is to receive the honorary degree of doctor of laws from McGill University at the convocation, May 30. The degree is to be given in recognition of his service to humanity in establishing and maintaining a series of hospitals and nursing homes along the coast of Labrador.

THE awards of the medals of the Royal Geographical Society have been made as follows: The Founder's medal to Dr. T. G. Longstaff, for his discovery of the Siachen Glacier and long-continued geographical work in the Himalaya, and the Patron's medal to Captain G. H. Wilkins, for his many years' systematic work in Polar regions, culminating in his remarkable flight from Point Barrow to Spitsbergen. The Murchison grant to Captain C. J. Morris, for his recent journey in Hunza; the Back grant to Mr. George Binney, for his journey across North-East Land and his successful conduct of the Oxford Expeditions to Spitsbergen; the Cuthbert Peek grant to Mr. H. G. Watkins, in recognition of his leadership of the Cambridge Expedition to Edge Island and to assist him in his proposed expedition to Labrador, and the Gill Memorial to Mr. C. P. Skrine, for his exploration of the Qungur area and his work on Chinese Central Asia.

THE Association to Aid Scientific Research by Women awarded the Ellen Richards research prize of $2,000 at its annual meeting held on April 28 at the Massachusetts Institute of Technology. This prize, awarded for experimental research, was divided equally between Dr. Lisa Meitner, of the University of Berlin, and Madame Ramart-Lucas, of the University of Paris. Dr. Meitner's work has been in physics, especially radio-activity. Madame Ramart-Lucas's field is organic chemistry. Dr. Meitner was nominated by the German Federation of University Women and Madame Ramart-Lucas by the French Federation.

THE Italian correspondent of the *Journal* of the American Medical Association writes that special honors were conferred on Professor Benedetto Morpurgo, the incumbent of the chair of general pathology at the University of Turin, on the occasion of his completing thirty-five years of instruction. Two volumes containing scientific articles by eminent Italian and foreign scientific men were published to commemorate the event.

Sir Arthur Newsholme, fellow of the Royal College of Surgeons and formerly principal medical officer of England and Wales, who is visiting public-health institutions in this country, was the guest of honor at a dinner on May 10 given at the Hotel Roosevelt, New York.

The four hundredth meeting of the Washington Chemical Society took the form of a dinner in honor of Dr. F. W. Clarke, Dr. Harvey W. Wiley and Professor Charles E. Munroe, all of whom were early members of the Chemical Society of Washington, which later became the Washington section of the American Chemical Society. About one hundred and sixty members and guests were present.

At the annual meeting of the American Association of Anatomists, Dr. Charles R. Stockard, professor of anatomy in the Cornell University Medical College, New York, was elected president and Dr. Lewis H. Weed, the Johns Hopkins University School of Medicine, Baltimore, reelected secretary.

Paul J. Kruesi, of the Southern Ferro Alloys Company, Tennessee, has been elected president of the American Electrochemical Society, to succeed Professor S. C. Lind, of the University of Minnesota.

At the meeting of the American Laryngological Association, which met in Washington, D. C., from May 1 to 3, Dr. Charles W. Richardson, of Washington, D. C., was elected president.

On the occasion of the Linguistic Congress at the Hague in April an International Society of Experimental Phonetics was founded. The following elections took place: *President,* Professor E. W. Scripture, of Vienna; *vice-president,* Dr. E. A. Meyer, of Stockholm; *honorary members,* Professor A. Meillet, of Paris, and Professor L. Zwaardemaker, of Utrecht. The object of the society is the promotion of scientific research in experimental phonetics.

At the annual business meeting of the Central Ohio Physics Club held at the Ohio State University on May 5, the following officers were elected for the coming year: *President,* Professor E. H. Johnson, of Kenyon College, Gambier; *vice-president,* Professor C. W. Jarvis, of Ohio Wesleyan University, Delaware; *secretary-treasurer,* Professor J. H. McCloy, Otterbein College, Westerville.

Professor Thomas E. McKinney, of the department of mathematics and astronomy of the University of South Dakota, will retire from service at the end of the present academic year on account of blindness.

G. H. Collingwood, head of the office of cooperative forestry extension of the United States Department of Agriculture, has been named forester for the American Forestry Association, to succeed Shirley W. Allen, who recently resigned to join the staff in the forest school of the University of Michigan.

Dr. Blythe Eagles, holder of a Sterling research fellowship in Yale University, who has been working with Professor T. B. Johnson on the chemistry of sulphur in blood, has accepted a research fellowship given under the auspices of the British Medical Research Council and will begin his work in England in October.

Dr. J. J. Nassau, professor of astronomy and director of the Warner Swasey Observatory of the Case School of Applied Science, who is spending the present academic year at the University of Cambridge in the laboratory of Professor Eddington, recently read a paper before the Royal Astronomical Society. Dr. Nassau will return to Cleveland in September.

Dr. Charles F. Marvin, chief of the United States Weather Bureau, is on his way to Europe for conference with the directors of meteorological services. One of the subjects to be discussed is the collection and interchange of ship reports.

Dr. Ernest L. Walker, professor of tropical medicine, University of California Medical School, has returned from a fourteen months' stay in Honolulu, where he carried on investigations as to the cause of leprosy, at the invitation of the U. S. Public Health Service.

At the annual meeting of the division of chemistry and chemical technology of the National Research Council, the following chemists were appointed as members of the official American delegation to the meeting of the International Union of Pure and Applied Chemistry, which is to be held at The Hague on July 18 to 24: Ross A. Baker, Syracuse University; Wilder D. Bancroft, Cornell University; Edward Bartow, University of Iowa; John B. Ekeley, University of Colorado; W. H. Gesell, Lehn and Fink; F. G. Keyes, Massachusetts Institute of Technology; W. Lee Lewis, Institute of American Meat Packers; R. B. Moore, Purdue University; A. M. Patterson, Antioch College; C. L. Reese, E. I. du Pont de Nemours and Company; L. H. Ryerson, University of Minnesota; Atherton Seidell, U. S. Public Health Service; W. T. Taggart, University of Pennsylvania; C. P. Smyth, Princeton University, and R. E. Swain, Stanford University.

Dr. Fridtjof Nansen, professor of oceanography at the University of Oslo, gave a lecture before the

Washington Academy of Sciences on May 16 on "The Problems of Arctic Exploration."

DR. S. A. KINNIER WILSON, lecturer on diseases of the nervous system at King's College, London, lectured on May 11 on "The Nature of the Epilepsies" at Cornell University Medical College.

DR. RICHARD P. STRONG, professor of tropical medicine at the Harvard Medical School, lectured at the Johns Hopkins University School of Hygiene and Public Health, Baltimore, April 17, on "The Harvard-African Expedition of 1926–1927."

THE thirteenth Mellon lecture of the Society for Biological Research of the University of Pittsburgh School of Medicine was delivered on May 10 by Dr. Hans Zinsser, professor of bacteriology and immunology at the Harvard Medical School, on "The Present State of our Knowledge regarding Epidemic Encephalitis."

DR. T. WINGATE TODD, Hamann professor of anatomy of the Western Reserve University, delivered the annual public address of the James A. Gibson Anatomical Society of the University of Buffalo on May 8 on "The Anatomy of Digestion."

ON the evening of April 20 Dr. Barnum Brown, of the American Museum of Natural History, gave the annual public lecture before the Syracuse chapter of the Society of Sigma Xi at Syracuse University on "Prehistoric Man in America."

IN the presence of more than 10,000 employees, the board of directors and a few invited guests, a bronze tablet honoring the memory of Charles A. Coffin, founder of the General Electric Company, was unveiled on May 8 at the Schenectady plant of that company. Ceremonies included an address by E. W. Rice, Jr., honorary chairman of the General Electric board. The fund which made the tablet possible was established twenty-five years ago by General Electric employees.

SUBSCRIPTIONS to the Bayliss and Starling memorial fund (see SCIENCE, April 20, page 414) have, within three and a half weeks of being opened, attained the sum of £1,400.

THE Commitee on Foreign Relations of the U. S. Senate has ordered a favorable report on the bill authorizing an annual appropriation of $50,000 to be paid to the Gorgas Memorial Institute of Tropical and Preventive Medicine in Panama. The gift would be dependent upon the completion of the institute within five years.

THE three hundredth anniversary of the birth of Marcello Malpighi, the founder of histology, was celebrated at Bologna on March 10.

DR. JOSEPH NELSON ROSE, associate curator of botany in the U. S. National Museum, died on May 4, aged sixty-six years.

DR. BIRD T. BALDWIN, head of the Iowa Child Welfare Research Station at the University of Iowa, died on May 12, aged fifty-three years.

PROFESSOR V. L. OMELIANSKI, the Russian bacteriologist, member of the Russian Academy of Science, died on April 21. Professor Omelianski was one of the corresponding members of the Society of American Bacteriologists.

PROFESSOR S. NAZAWA, of the University of Hokkaido, at Sapporo, died on March 23, after a winter trip to Otaru. Dr. Nazawa was a well-known ichthyologist of northern Japan. He devoted himself largely to the development of the fishing industry.

THE bacteriologist who died on February 14 from Rocky Mountain spotted fever was A. LeRoy Kerlee, not A. LeRoy Keyes as incorrectly reported in SCIENCE and in publications from which the information was obtained.

THE twenty-seventh annual session of the North Carolina Academy of Science recently took place at the University of North Carolina, under the presidency of Dr. J. M. Bell, professor of chemistry in the university. The following new officers were elected: *President,* J. S. Holmes, of the state forestry commission; *vice-president,* Mary Petty, of the North Carolina College for Women; *secretary-treasurer,* H. R. Totten (reelected), of the University of North Carolina; new member to the *executive committee,* F. A. Wolfe.

THE Sigma Xi chapters of Union College and Rensselaer Polytechnic Institute held a joint annual dinner at the Rensselaer Polytechnic Institute on May 4. This is the second of such joint annual dinners held by the chapters of these two institutions. Dr. W. D. Coolidge, of the research laboratory of the General Electric Company, was initiated to membership in the Union chapter. The chemistry and the physics departments of Union College took this occasion to present Sigma Xi keys to Dr. W. R. Whitney, Dr. Irving Langmuir and Dr. W. D. Coolidge, for valuable assistance given to these departments during the past years. The Rensselaer chapter presented a Sigma Xi key to Mr. John Knickerbacker, of Troy, who was one of the founders of Sigma Xi when it was organized at Cornell University in 1886. The main speaker of the evening was Dr. W. F. Durand, of Stanford University, who gave an address on the Colorado River problem, devoting himself to the economic and physical aspects, rather than the political.

The Pasteur Society of Central California, recently organized under the tentative name of "Society of Bacteriologists," as recorded in Science (April 13), met in San Francisco on May 9. The new title was definitely voted upon as best representing the aims and ideals of the organization. The membership now numbers 125. Dr. J. C. Geiger, senior surgeon of the U. S. Public Health Service and associate professor of epidemiology of the University of California, addressed the meeting on "Scientific Aspects of Modern Health Department Organization," presenting the development of the Chicago department of health and its problems. The discussion was led by Dr. Charles F. Bacon, of Chicago.

The annual spring field meeting of the Oklahoma Academy of Science was held at Prices Falls, Arbuckle Mountains, on April 20 and 21. The attendance was about 140, representing faculty members and students from fifteen institutions in Oklahoma and neighboring states. The subject of geology was stressed, and geological excursions were conducted each day. Bird walks were held each day, also tree walks and flower walks. Lectures were delivered at night as follows: "Stratigraphy of the Arbuckle Mountains," O. F. Evans, University of Oklahoma; "Flowers," Paul B. Sears, University of Oklahoma; "Hawks," R. O. Whitenton, A. and M. College; "Oklahoma Forest Trees," George R. Phillips, state forester; "Structure of the Arbuckle Mountains," V. E. Monnett, University of Oklahoma; "Science and History," Jas. S. Buchanan, vice-president of the University of Oklahoma; "The Oklahoma Academy of Science," O. M. Smith, president of the academy, Oklahoma A. and M. College. Chas. N. Gould, director of the Oklahoma Geological Survey, was general chairman in charge of the meeting.

Announcement has been made of a gift of $750,000 for the development of the department of surgery of the Washington University in the Barnes Hospital. This sum will be expended for the construction of three additional floors on the surgical pavilion of the Barnes Hospital and for the surgical work in the hospital. Of the $750,000, $450,000 was contributed by the General Education Board and $150,000 each by Frank C. Rand, chairman of the board of trustees of Barnes Hospital and Jackson Johnson, a trustee of the Washington University. Construction of the new hospital wards will begin immediately.

The biological stations of the United States Bureau of Fisheries at Woods Hole, Mass., Beaufort, N. C., and Fairport, Iowa, will open for the summer's activities on June 20. Facilities for research work will be afforded at the various stations to independent investigators and dormitory facilities will be provided as far as possible. Applications for space may be made direct to the Commissioner of Fisheries, Washington, D. C. There will be accommodations for the usual number of workers at Woods Hole, but more space will be available at the other two stations, and workers who can not be accommodated at Woods Hole will be offered equally good laboratory facilities at either of the other stations.

Comparative Psychology Monographs have been taken over by the Johns Hopkins Press, and will be issued hereafter under the managing editorship of Knight Dunlap. The board of editors consists of J. E. Anderson, for child psychology; H. A. Carr, for the lower vertebrates; W. S. Hunter, for general human problems; A. V. Kidder, for racial studies; S. O. Mast, for invertebrates, and R. M. Yerkes, for the primates. Manuscripts offered will be referred to the appropriate editor immediately, and will be considered for publication only after being approved by him.

UNIVERSITY AND EDUCATIONAL NOTES

The reversionary bequest by Mr. E. J. Bles to the University of Cambridge of the residue of his estate (about £30,000) has been accepted and is to be used for founding a professorship of animal embryology or of biophysics in honor of Charles Darwin.

Dr. Francis Arthur Thomson, dean of the school of mines at the University of Idaho since 1917, has been called to the presidency of the Montana State School of Mines at Butte.

Dr. Herbert C. Sadler, head of the department of naval architecture and marine engineering, has been appointed dean of the colleges of engineering and architecture at the University of Michigan.

Dr. George R. Albertson, acting dean of the school of medicine of the University of South Dakota, has been appointed dean to succeed the late C. P. Lommen. Dr. Albertson was appointed to the chair of anatomy at the university in 1912.

Dr. Alfred C. Reed, a former member of the faculty of Stanford University School of Medicine, has been appointed professor of tropical medicine in the University of California Hooper Foundation for Medical Research and will take up his work in February, 1929. Dr. Reed is now studying at the London School of Tropical Medicine.

Howard F. Janda, head of the civil engineering department of the University of North Carolina, has been appointed professor of highway engineering and city planning at the University of Wisconsin.

DR. G. E. HILBERT has been appointed as research assistant to Professor Treat B. Johnson, Sterling professor of chemistry at Yale University for the academic year 1928–29.

ASSOCIATE PROFESSOR A. ELIZABETH ADAMS has been promoted to a professorship of zoology at Mount Holyoke College.

HARRY N. EATON has resigned the associate professorship of geology at Syracuse University.

DR. W. B. CROW, lecturer in botany at the University College, Cardiff, has been appointed head of the department of biology at the Technical College, Huddersfield, in succession to Dr. T. W. Woodhead, who will soon retire.

DR. ADOLF FRAENKEL, professor of mathematics at the University of Marburg, has been called to the University of Kiel.

DISCUSSION AND CORRESPONDENCE

THE REAPPORTIONMENT BILL IN CONGRESS

HOUSE RESOLUTION 11725, reported favorably by the House Committee on the Census on April 4, 1928, presents an interesting scientific situation.

This bill, which provides for an automatic apportionment of 435 representatives after each decennial census (unless Congress takes other action), specifies the method of major fractions as the method to be followed in the computation; and the report of the Committee (no. 1137) describes this method of major fractions as a "specific, concrete and exact scientific method." As a matter of fact, this method is an obsolete method which has failed to secure the approval of any scientific body.

The problem of selecting the best method of apportionment is a mathematical problem of quite unexpected complexity, on account of the necessity of obtaining a solution in whole numbers. The problem has been the occasion of bitter debates in Congress for over a hundred years. Several different methods have been used and later discarded. On one occasion, after a long speech by Daniel Webster, the Senate reversed the action of the House on purely mathematical grounds. Not until 1921 did a satisfactory solution of the problem become available. In that year, at the request of Senator Sutherland, the Joint Advisory Committee to the Director of the Census held extensive hearings on the subject and published a unanimous report in favor of a method, then new, known as the method of equal proportions—a method which in point of simplicity, directness and intelligibility leaves nothing to be desired. This method has since been endorsed by a general consensus of scientific opinion. It was adopted in the only bill which came up in the House in 1927, and at that time, according to Hasbrouck's "Party Government in the House of Representatives" (p. 126), the "method of equal proportions was pretty generally favored over the method of major fractions which had been the basis of the 1911 apportionment." All the bills introduced in the House in the early part of this winter, which specified any definite method, specified, as a matter of course, the method of equal proportions. Moreover, the question of the choice of method is vitally important at the present time, since, if the proposed legislation is carried, there are conceivable distributions of population for which the choice of a wrong method might affect the number of representatives in every state in the Union.

In spite of these facts, the present report from the House Committee on the Census makes no mention whatever of the method of equal proportions and totally ignores the scientific report of the Advisory Committee. Why this sudden change?

The change is attributable entirely to the efforts of one man, Professor W. F. Willcox, of Cornell, whose testimony before the House Committee, as printed in the hearings for February 21, contains an entirely false description of the method of equal proportions, by which, supported as it was by impressive charts and diagrams, the committee was completely misled.

In a carefully worded paragraph on page 61, repeated with emphasis on page 62, instead of presenting the simple definition of the method of equal proportions which is well known in the literature of the subject, he substitutes therefor a complicated definition which bears no resemblance to the standard method and leads to strikingly different results. For example, suppose 100 representatives are to be apportioned among the five states A, B, C, D, E, in the following table, according to the method of equal proportions. Column I shows the result under the true method of equal proportions; column II shows the result under Professor Willcox's erroneous idea of that method. The results are different for four of the five states.

State	Population	I	II
A	12,972,500	52	51
B	11,000,000	45	44
C	345,000	1	2
D	342,500	1	2
E	340,000	1	1
	25,000,000	100	100

Other parts of his testimony are equally erroneous and misleading, but no opportunity was afforded for rebuttal, and the committee had no reason to question the accuracy of the information offered it. Moreover, after a number of these errors were called to Professor Willcox's attention, he declined to take steps to correct them.

From the scientific point of view there is another feature of the situation which is even more unfortunate. After admitting (p. 88) that "a large majority of mathematicians and statisticians are on record in favor of the method of equal proportions," Professor Willcox secured and read into the hearings about a dozen statements from constitutional lawyers and professors of political economy in favor of his method of major fractions and thus persuaded the committee that there is a conflict of opinion among scholars on this subject. Inasmuch as these scattered statements were secured by means of the same unsuspected misinformation that had misled the committee, they can not be regarded as concerted or final judgments.

There is of course no conceivable conflict of interest between the mathematicians on the one hand and the political scientists on the other hand. On the mathematical side the problem is a highly technical one, requiring investigation of scores of different methods; the results of the mathematical analysis are indispensable to the statesmen who must make the final choice between the small number of methods that are found to be logically possible and workable. Among the logically possible methods, the method of equal proportions is the only method which has the approval of any organized body of scholars. If Professor Willcox has any serious objections to offer against this method, he owes it to mathematicians and economists alike to publish his views in some regular journal, so that they may be accessible to the scrutiny of all groups of scholars.

This is not the place to go into any detailed discussion of the problem. Full references may be found in a recent paper in the Transactions of the American Mathematical Society for January, 1928. The important thing in relation to Congress is to have scientific opinion united on a scientific question.

Professor Willcox has himself suggested that the American Political Science Association might well appoint a committee to investigate and report on this subject. This is a suggestion which should be welcomed by all those interested in the constitutional aspects of the problem. If it is generally accepted, as seems now to be the case, that the provisions of the constitution are not intended to favor systematically either the smaller or the larger states in any apportionment of representatives, then the question becomes a purely mathematical one. The mathematical evidence, which was seriously misrepresented in the recent hearings, clearly indicates that the method of equal proportions is the one method which has no bias in favor of either the smaller or the larger states. It would be most unfortunate to have any other method incorporated in permanent legislation.

Edward V. Huntington
Harvard University

A POSSIBLE CORRELATION OF EYE SORENESS WITH VITAMIN A DEFICIENCY AMONG THE NEZ PERCÉS INDIANS

The relation of vitamin A deficiency to a characteristic eye disease, known as xerophthalmia, keratomalacia, etc., was discovered by Osborne and Mendel in 1913 in their feeding experiments upon rats. Since the publication of their work various authorities have endeavored to determine whether a deficiency of vitamin A in the diet might not also be responsible for cases of eye trouble in man. The existing evidence upon this point by McCollum, Mori, Bloch and other observers has been summarized on pages 192 and 193 of Sherman and Smith's work upon "The Vitamins" of the American Chemical Society Monograph Series.

In the present note the writer wishes to call attention to what appears to be a much earlier recorded instance of eye soreness in man as a result of vitamin A deficiency. The references are contained in the journal of the expedition conducted by Lewis and Clarke to the northwestern territory of the United States in the years 1804–5–6, under the dates of May 10–12, 1806. The following extracts relate to observations made by the expedition during its stay with the Chopunnish or Nez Percés Indians within the present borders of Idaho. The page references are to Volume III of the "History of the Expedition under the Command of Captains Lewis and Clarke," published by the Allerton Book Co., New York, 1922.

> The chief spoke to the people, who immediately brought about two bushels of dried quamash roots, some cakes of the roots of cows (kouse), and a dried salmon trout: we thanked them for this supply, but observed that, not being accustomed to live on roots alone, we feared that such diet might make our men sick. (Page 102).

> Their chief subsistence is roots, and the noise made by the women in pounding them gives the hearer the idea of a nail factory. (Page 104.)

> We now resumed our medical labours, and had a number of patients afflicted with scrofula, rheumatism and sore eyes, to all which we administered very cheerfully as far as our skill and supplies of medicine would permit. We also visited a chief who has for three years past so completely lost the use of his limbs, that he lies like a perfect corpse in whatever position he is placed,

yet he eats heartily, digests his food very well, has a regular pulse, and retains his flesh; in short, were he not somewhat pale from lying so long out of the sun, he might be mistaken for a man in perfect health. This disease does not seem to be common; indeed, we have seen only three cases of it among the Chopunnish, who alone are afflicted with it. The scrofulous disorders we may readily conjecture to originate in the long confinement to vegetable diet; which may perhaps also increase the soreness of the eyes; but this strange disorder baffles at once our curiosity and our skill. Our assistance was again demanded early the next morning, Monday 12, by a crowd of Indians, to whom we gave eye-water. (Page 106.)

They then invited us into the tent, and told us that they now wished to answer what we had told them yesterday; but that many of their people were at that moment waiting in great pain for our medical assistance. It was therefore agreed that Captain Clarke, who is the favourite physician, should visit the sick, while Captain Lewis would hold the council. (Page 107.)[1]

Roots are all characterized by a very low vitamin A content and the absence of this important nutritional factor in the almost exclusively root diet of the Chopunnish Indians might very well give rise to eye soreness, a supposition which is hinted at with almost remarkable prescience in the report of the expedition. The cases of paralysis observed among the Chopunnish may also possibly have resulted from the lack of some necessary ingredient in the diet.

The observations of the Lewis and Clarke expedition upon the food and diseases of the various tribes of Indians which were visited are very complete but in no other case, besides the incident just cited, is the evidence so clearly marked of specific dietary deficiency on the one hand and of definite physical ailments on the other. With other tribes the use of roots was supplemented by the addition of cereals, vegetables, berries, nuts, fish and game. The general practice of the aboriginal Indians in eating the whole grain and in consuming all the organs of fish and game protected them no doubt from certain diseases which might have been incurred with the more civilized methods of preparing food.

C. A. BROWNE

BUREAU OF CHEMISTRY AND SOILS

THE LITER AND THE CUBIC DECIMETER

IN the original conception of the metric system of weights and measures all units of length, area, volume and mass were intended to be derived from the single basic unit of length, the meter, which was by definition equal to one ten millionth of the earth's quadrant from pole to equator. A cube having its edge equal to one tenth of the meter was provisionally adopted as the unit of volume, and was designated the cubic decimeter or the liter. The mass of this volume of water when at the temperature of its maximum density was provisionally adopted as the unit of mass, and was designated the kilogram.

It was found, however, that there were certain difficulties in the way of the practical realization of the original plan. For example, it was impracticable to determine accurately the length of the earth's quadrant and thus to fix the length of the meter on that basis. That difficulty was avoided by forsaking the original plan of deriving the meter from the figure of the earth and by defining the meter arbitrarily in terms of a specific material standard of length.

In attempting to establish the standard of mass in terms of the standard of length it was found that masses could be directly compared more accurately than they could be established through measurements of volume. It was, therefore, found advisable to depart again from the original plan and to define the kilogram arbitrarily in terms of a specific standard of mass without reference to the meter. Two arbitrary and independent standards were in that way established; the meter as the standard of length and the kilogram as the standard of mass.

As a result of the establishment of the kilogram independent of the meter there arose a need for a unit of volume which would also be independent of the meter. Such a unit was defined as the volume of a kilogram of water at the temperature of its maximum density. This new, or redefined, unit of volume was given the same name as that originally applied to the cube of one tenth of the meter; that is, it was still called the liter, although by the new definition it bears no direct relation to the cubic decimeter or to the meter. It is used in determinations of density and volume based on mass. That is, it is directly related to the kilogram.

We, therefore, now have two distinct units of volume in the metric system, the cubic decimeter derived from the unit of length and the liter derived from the unit of mass. These two units differ in volume by about twenty-seven parts in a million, the liter being the larger. The one thousandth part of the cubic decimeter is the cubic centimeter, and the one thousandth part of the liter is the milliliter. These units, of course, bear to each other the same relation as do the cubic decimeter and the liter, the

[1] The above references will also be found on pages 1002 to 1006 of Vol. III of the better known edition of the Lewis and Clarke expedition published by Elliott Coues in 1893.

milliliter being larger than the cubic centimeter by twenty-seven parts in a million.

It is a peculiar fact that although the one-thousandth part of the liter is the unit that is almost universally employed in measurements of volume and density of liquids, it is most often designated as the "cubic centimeter" or "cc" instead of by its correct designation "milliliter" or "ml." While the two units are so nearly equal as to be interchangeable for many purposes, yet the difference between them is sufficient to be very troublesome at times.

The only safe procedure is always to make sure which unit is being employed and then to designate it correctly. The preferable designation is "cm^3" for the cubic centimeter and "ml" (not "cc") for the milliliter.

It is unfortunate that the kilogram should not have been made a little lighter or the meter a little longer in order that the cubic decimeter and liter might have been equal and the original plan of interrelation of the units carried into effect.

H. W. Bearce
Bureau of Standards,
Washington, D. C.

THE PASSING OF THE CIRCUIT SYSTEM OF COLLECTING WEATHER REPORTS

On April 1, 1928, the Western Union Telegraph Company abandoned the circuit system, inaugurated in 1871 and used continuously since in collecting the twice-daily weather-reports from points in the United States and Canada.

A new and more flexible system was installed which obviated the necessity of withdrawing twice daily about 15,000 miles of wire from the usual commercial channels, for the exclusive use of the weather bureau. Two centers of collection and distribution, *viz.*, Chicago and New York, are a part of the new system. The largest factor in making the change was the very general use of automatic sending- and receiving-apparatus by the telegraph company in recent years whereby several channels of communication both ways are possible on a single wire.

The old system required hand operation, and traffic could flow but one way at a time.

Alfred J. Henry
Weather Bureau,
Washington, D. C.

THE ABNORMAL SPECIFIC HEAT OF A RAREFIED GAS AT A LOW TEMPERATURE, AND THE COSMIC RADIATION

In a paper that will appear in the May number of the *Journal of the Franklin Institute* it is shown thermodynamically that a gas at a very small molecular concentration, at which it is largely or altogether in the atomic state, near the absolute zero of temperature, has an abnormally large specific heat which may amount to thousands of calories per gram. This is due to three separate effects, each of which need not always occur. One of them is intimately connected with the remarkable result also obtained thermodynamically that the internal heat of evaporation of all substances is zero at the absolute zero of temperature. This result was obtained by means of the result deduced previously by the writer[1] that the adiabatic of zero entropy corresponds to zero absolute temperature. It was also obtained independently of considerations of the zero of entropy, thus incidentally furnishing welcome evidence from another direction of the truth of the foregoing result.

These abnormally large specific heats—they are likely to be specially large in the case of gaseous C, H_2, O_2 and N_2—are bound to be attended by great changes in the electronic configuration of the atoms with decrease of temperature, during which some of the electrons are likely to fall through very high potentials. This would give rise to an electro-magnetic radiation some of which might conceivably be of greater penetrating power than the γ radiation of radium. The cosmic radiation which appears to come from interstellar space might well be caused in this way. For no doubt this space contains various gases, especially the above, at an extremely low molecular concentration, whose temperature is near the absolute zero and still decreasing.

Since the air in the upper region of the atmosphere is at a low concentration and temperature, it is not improbable that a large part of the cosmic radiation proceeds from this region. If that is so the radiation arriving in a horizontal direction would be larger for a given solid angle than that in a vertical direction, a deduction which could be tested experimentally.

R. D. Kleeman
Schenectady, N. Y.

SCIENTIFIC APPARATUS AND LABORATORY METHODS

MACROSCOPICAL DETECTION OF THE MEDULLATED WOOL FIBER

The medullated wool fiber is considered a serious defect in the fleece. In the United States little if any attention has been given the problem of its elimination, possibly because most of the woven fabrics manufactured for clothing purposes in this country

[1] *J. Phys. Chem.*, 31, 940, 1927.

are made from the finer grades of wool, among which the medullated fiber does not so frequently occur. Among British wool manufacturers, however, the medullated fiber is looked upon as a menace to the prestige of British woven fabrics. It is thought to be responsible for harsh, wiry fleeces which do not work up well in the manufacturing processes. The medullated fiber is also criticised for lack of tensile strength and elasticity, and by some is accused of being responsible for uneven dyeing of certain goods.

Medullated fibers may be found among most of the improved breeds of sheep, including the Merino, but it is found in greatest quantity among the long-wool breeds, such as the Lincoln, Leicester, Cotswold and Romney. Sharp criticism of some New Zealand crossbred wools has recently been made by certain leading figures in the British textile trade, who point to the very great desirability of eliminating those "strong" or "hairy" fibers from the fleece. Obviously such elimination must be made by the breeder, if it is to be accomplished at all.

The presence of the medullated fiber can not be accurately detected by simple optical examination of the fleece, although the medulla is easily seen under the low power of the microscope when the fiber is prepared in a balsam mount. The literature on the subject contains no references to macroscopic detection.

A problem recently undertaken by the writer, involving the isolation of several thousand medullated fibers, led to the discovery of a method of detecting medullated wool fibers without the aid of a microscope. The method is simple and its use by breeders as well as by investigators seems warranted.

A rectangular piece of glass, of a size somewhat shorter in one dimension than the length of the fibers to be tested, is placed horizontally over a dull black or dark blue background. A small quantity of glycerin is then poured on the glass. The glycerin will have a tendency to spread over the glass and thus gradually become too shallow in depth to permit proper immersion of the fiber. This difficulty may be overcome by making on the glass a wall of paraffin in the shape of a parenthesis almost joined at the top and bottom. The fibers are cleaned in benzene to remove the excess of natural oil and dirt, and then are immersed one at a time in the shallow lake of glycerin. The ends of the fiber are held in the fingers and the two openings in the wall of paraffin permit the fiber to be held completely submerged and almost in contact with the glass.

The operation is carried on in natural light subdued to a point where reading would be difficult. The writer has found it convenient to work close to a window and to regulate the light by manipulation of a piece of very thick felt used in place of the ordinary window blind.

If the light has been properly regulated, a medullated fiber subjected to the treatment described can be seen as a faint white line across the glass, while non-medullated fibers can not be seen at all.

Tests of the efficacy of the method were carried out by examining under the microscope many fibers, both medullated and non-medullated, separated by use of the glycerin. These tests showed no errors in isolating medullated fibers, although a few which contained only traces of medullae were classed as non-medullated. The method is applicable to the examination of wool from any of the long-wool breeds, and with practice might be applied to finer fibers.

Tests with liquids other than glycerin, having a high refractive index, suggest that the index of refraction may be responsible for the phenomenon. Cottonseed oil, aniline, balsam, and other substances give fairly satisfactory results, while with water the detection is impossible.

J. F. WILSON

COLLEGE OF AGRICULTURE,
UNIVERSITY OF CALIFORNIA

A PERFUSION FLUID FOR ELASMOBRANCHS

THE use of diluted sea-water as a perfusion fluid for vertebrate tissues has been attended in the past with only partial success. Failure in the case of elasmobranch hearts, at least, was considered by Mines[1] to be due to the excessive magnesium content. The ratio of Mg to the other metals is about five times as great in sea-water as in elasmobranch serum, and about fifteen times as great as in the sera of land vertebrates.[2] Since the relative proportions of Na, K and Ca in sea-water are very similar to those found in vertebrate tissues generally, it seemed that the Mg might be the only disturbing factor.

It has been found possible to precipitate most of the Mg and relatively little of the Ca from sea-water by the addition of NaOH. To each liter of sea-water is added 12 cc of a 10 normal solution of NaOH, and the mixture is allowed to stand overnight in a stoppered flask. The flocculent precipitate settles in a compact mass at the bottom of the flask, and the supernatant liquid may be decanted easily through a filter. If the precipitate is not allowed to settle completely, filtration is unduly slow. The filtrate, after neutralization to pH 8 with a few drops of concen-

[1] Mines, G. R., "On the Relation to Electrolytes of the Hearts of Different Species of Animals," I—Elasmobranchs and Pecten, *Jour. Phys.*, 1912, 43, 467.

[2] Macallum, A. B., "The Paleochemistry of the Body Tissues and Fluids," *Phys. Rev.*, 1926, 6, 316.

trated HCl, may be used as the stock solution for a perfusion fluid which has proved highly satisfactory for dogfish and skate hearts. Preparatory to its actual use, this modified sea-water must be diluted as follows:

Modified sea-water	30 cc.
Urea, 20 per cent. sol.	10 cc.
Distilled water	60 cc.

The acidity will then need to be adjusted with dilute HCl to pH 7.4, to correspond with the pH of elasmobranch serum. The diluted mixture compares favorably in its physiological effects with Knowlton solution, the standard artificial salt-mixture for elasmobranch tissue; and it has the advantage of being much simpler and cheaper to make up.

Determinations of the Ca and Mg content of solutions prepared in this way yielded the following results. Unmodified sea-water similarly diluted and Knowlton solution are included in the table for comparison:

	Ca-Mols/liter	Mg-Mols/liter
Modified sea-water (a)	.0020	.0037
" " " (b)	.0019	.0046
" " " (c)	.0021	.0042
Plain sea-water	.0032	.0145
Knowlton solution	.0040	.0050

A detailed study of the precipitation of Ca and Mg from sea-water by NaOH[3] shows that the removal of more Mg entails the loss of so much Ca and the gain of so much Na that the physiological salt-balance is destroyed. It is therefore impossible to extend the foregoing technique to the preparation of a medium suitable for land-vertebrates.

Eleanor M. Kapp

Marine Biological Laboratory,
Woods Hole

SPECIAL ARTICLES

THE SEXUAL STAGE OF FUNGI INDUCED BY ULTRA-VIOLET RAYS

On January 29, 1928, while studying the effect of ultra-violet radiation of fungi in agar plate cultures radiated on January 25, it was noted that perithecia, the sexual stage of the fungus, had formed in great numbers on certain portions of the exposed plates.

The fungus under consideration was one, our laboratory number "G 10," of several strains of *Glomerella cingulata* that have been under close observation for some months. This culture was originally derived from apples affected with Bitter Rot and in October a single conidium was isolated in my laboratory. All cultures of "G 10" since that time have been from this monosporous strain. In no case were perithecia observed to develop on this monosporous strain.

This same essentially non-sexual strain in all agar cultures exposed to ultra-violet rays of certain intensity and for certain time develops perithecia literally by millions. Thus in the plate represented in the figure more than one hundred perithecia were visible in one focus of one low power field of the microscope or more than 1,500 on the exposed region of this small colony. It will be observed that no perithecia developed in the non-radiated part. Perhaps the most striking evidence that the radiation induces the perithecia was given by projecting the rays through a circular aperture of 0.5 mm. diameter upon a susceptible colony. The perithecia developed in great quantities in the small area radiated and

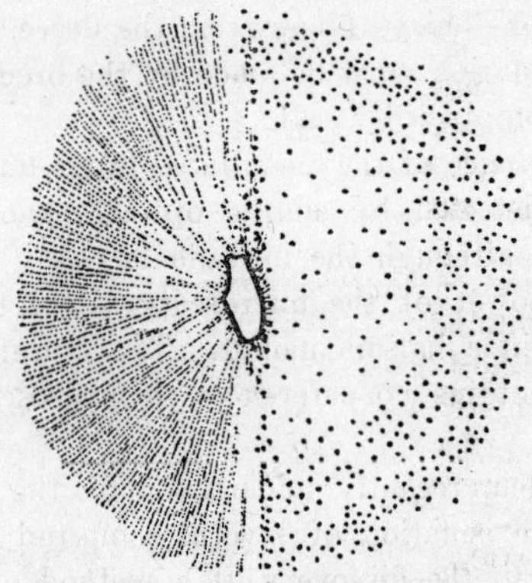

Fig. 1. Portion at right directly radiated; at left not so. Dotted region is perithecial; these on the right induced by direct radiation, the few at the left by indirect radiation.

only in that area. Their origins are visible two days after radiation as hyaline globose bodies and they can probably be traced to a much earlier time, since unusual branching is apparent within a few hours after radiation. In four days they appear as well-developed, spherical black bodies; asci and spores soon form. The perithecia differ from those naturally formed in that they are spherical and nonstromatic, but the asci and spores agree precisely with those found in nature.

All other strains of Glomerella that have been tested have given responses like those of "G 10." It appears certain that these ultra-violet rays or others near them have also a greatly accelerating effect on conidial production in this and other genera of fungi, for example, a Coniothyrium that normally produces pycnidia only at the end of several weeks and when the colony has completely occupied the petri dish, when radiated responds within a few days with numerous pycnidia.

[3] Kapp, E. M., Unpublished.

Exposure was to full radiation from a Cooper Hewitt quartz mercury arc, half of the colony shaded with cardboard to serve as a control. Two kinds of radiation resulted in perithecia: a, direct rays upon the exposed half of the colony, which resulted in perithecia deeply buried in the agar; b, indirect rays diffused to a few millimeters under the edge of the cardboard shield, which gave superficial perithecia.

The activating region of the spectrum has been determined by means of various screens as in the far ultra-violet, probably between the Ångstrom wave-lengths of 2760 and 3130.

That the effect is not the result of a chemical change produced in the medium by the radiation, but is a direct response by the mycelial cells to radiation, is rendered extremely probable by the results of several experiments directed to this special question.

Studies are now being made to determine the exact wave-lengths involved and the effect of these rays upon other species and genera of fungi both of the Ascomycetes and Fungi Imperfecti; the relation of the age of the mycelium to its susceptibility to stimulation; and the various steps in the development of the perithecium from the time of stimulation onward.

A presentation of this study was made at the meeting of the Illinois Academy of Science in April and a more complete account will be published soon in the *Botanical Gazette*.

F. L. Stevens

University of Illinois

THE AMIDE NITROGEN OF BLOOD

When it was established by Folin and Denis[1] that blood contains exceedingly small quantities of ammonia, it became necessary to consider whether or not such amounts were capable of furnishing the ammonia found in urine by simple excretion by the kidney.

Nash and Benedict[2] reasoned that the kidney must form the ammonia it excretes because they found no increases in blood ammonia with kidney ablation, and increases in urinary ammonia seemed to be unaccompanied by significant increases in the ammonia content of blood. Their belief in the special ammonia-forming function of the kidney was strengthened by their observation that the blood leaving the kidney is richer in ammonia than the blood that enters it.

The subsequent finding of Bliss[3] that other organs, notably the pancreas, show increases of ammonia in the blood leaving the organ suggested that ammonia formation, instead of being limited to the kidney, is a general tissue phenomenon.

He was not only able to demonstrate accumulations of ammonia in the blood of nephrectomized dogs, but found that such dogs only maintain low levels of blood ammonia concurrently with the elimination, by way of vomitus, of amounts of ammonia quantitatively comparable to their normal urinary excretion of ammonia.

While unsuccessful attempts have been made to demonstrate the existence of complex ammonia combinations in blood, this phase of the subject has now been studied with very favorable results. The demonstration of ammonia in a form not yielded by the ordinary methods, yet available within the body under the influence of enzyme action, would clear up a large body of facts already known about ammonia metabolism.

It seemed that the kidney might possess an enzyme that is capable of liberating ammonia from its combination in blood, and the search for such an enzyme revealed its presence.

The determination of ammonia that is obtained from blood by the use of this new kidney enzyme furnishes amounts of ammonia approximately a thousand times the old value—and for human blood the value is 115–125 mg instead of 0.05 to 0.10 mg nitrogen per 100 cc blood.

When purified casein was tried as a possible substrate for the enzyme, ammonia was liberated in appreciable amounts.

Using casein as a substrate, the new enzyme was compared with trypsin as to the rate of formation of amino-nitrogen and ammonia. Hunter and Smith[4] found that 37 per cent. of the casein nitrogen was in the form of amino-nitrogen after twenty-four hours' contact with trypsin, while the kidney enzyme liberated somewhat less than that amount in three days. A comparison of the formation of ammonia from casein by both enzymes shows that the kidney enzyme is much more specific for ammonia formation. Trypsin yielded 0.8 per cent. of the total casein nitrogen as ammonia in twenty-four hours, and 4.26 per cent. in eighty-eight days, while the kidney enzyme liberated more (5.1 per cent.) in four days than had trypsin in eighty-eight days (4.26 per cent.).

Hunter and Smith say:

> The absence of relation, in our experiments, between peptolysis and amidolysis is so conspicuous that these processes would really seem to have been catalyzed by two separate enzymes. We venture accordingly to suggest, as a working hypothesis, that the liberation of the

[1] Folin, O., and Denis, W., *J. Biol. Chem.*, xi, 161 (1912).

[2] Nash, T. P., Jr., and Benedict, S. R., *J. Biol. Chem.*, 1921, xlviii, 463.

[3] Bliss, Sidney, *J. Biol. Chem.*, 1926, lxvii, 109.

[4] Hunter, Andrew, and Smith, Ralph G., *J. Biol. Chem.*, 1924, lxii, 649.

amide-nitrogen of proteins is not, strictly understood, a function of trypsin at all, but is to be attributed to the action of a specific enzyme, possibly of tissue origin, by which trypsin as usually prepared is liable to be accompanied.

The discovery of the enzyme in kidney seems to justify the opinion quoted from Hunter and Smith—and this enzyme has been shown to be directly concerned with ammonia metabolism.

The action of the kidney enzyme suggested so strongly that it was amide-nitrogen that was being attacked that the more simple, direct and accurate method of acid hydrolysis was tried. This was particularly indicated by the fact that no ammonia was ever liberated by the new enzyme from the protein-free fraction of blood, so that it was possible to use the blood proteins only for the ammonia determination.

Acid hydrolysis was found to give results of the same magnitude as those obtained by the use of the new enzyme. The method that was developed is now in the course of publication elsewhere.

The amide-nitrogen of blood is to be carefully distinguished from the conception of an ammonia-precursor or ammonia "mother-substance." From the metabolic standpoint it has been shown by studying the changes in amide-nitrogen during changing conditions of acid-base balance in the body that the amide-nitrogen of blood comes from ammonia formed in the tissues.

Parnas[5] has measured the ammonia that develops when blood is allowed to stand, and his values, which are only 2 to 4 per cent. of the values hereby established, he has designated as representing an ammonia-precursor or "ammonia mother-substance." The work of Parnas has, therefore, no relation to the presence of amide-nitrogen. After considerable study by himself and collaborators, Parnas concludes that his "ammonia mother-substance" bears no relationship to the state of acid-base balance: "Es wird daraus geschlossen, dass die Ammoniakmuttersubstantz des Blutes eine andere physiologische Funktion hat als *Ammoniak* als solches zu bilden, und dass aus den abgespaltenen Aminogruppen in vivo andere Stickstoffverbindungen entstehen."

In the latest articles that have come to the attention of the writer, the "ammonia mother-substance" of Parnas has been abandoned and the attempt made to attach metabolic significance to the exceedingly low values for ammonia which must now be considered as accidental values developed during the course of the analysis.

SIDNEY BLISS

DEPARTMENT OF BIOCHEMISTRY,
MCGILL UNIVERSITY

[5] Parnas, J. K., and Heller, J., *Biochem. Ztschr.*, 1924, clii, 1.

AMERICAN ASSOCIATION FOR THE ADVANCEMENT OF SCIENCE

THE SPRING MEETING OF THE EXECUTIVE COMMITTEE

THE regular spring meeting of the executive committee of the council of the American Association was held at the Cosmos Club, in Washington, on Sunday, April 22, with the following members present: Cattell, Curtiss, Humphreys, Johnston, Kellogg, Livingston, Wilson. The absent members were: Moulton, Osborn, Pupin, Ward. The chairman, Dr. J. McKeen Cattell, presided. The following is a summary of the business transacted.

1. The minutes of the last meeting were reported as having been approved by mail.

2. The permanent secretary reported that, since last September 30, there had been a net increase in membership of 1,453. The number of members in good standing on April 21st was 15,074, with 1,241 additional names on the roll, but in arrearage for dues for one or two years. The total number of names on the roll was therefore 16,315. The number of those in arrears was proportionately somewhat less than for the same date last year. About next October 1 there will be sent out between 75,000 and 80,000 invitations asking non-members to join the association. Members are asked to continue to send to the Washington office names of persons who might be interested to join.

3. A letter was read from William L. Corbin, librarian of the Smithsonian Institution, who said, in part: "I am writing to thank you and, through you, the American Association for the Advancement of Science, for the very generous gift of miscellaneous publications that the association made not long ago to the Library of the Smithsonian Institution. We are deeply appreciative of this gift and most grateful for it. Already, in checking up these publications, we have discovered hundreds of complete volumes and parts of volumes needed in our standard sets. Not a few of these we had found it impossible before to get from any source. Other volumes and parts of great value to us are coming to light every day as the work of sorting the contents of the boxes goes on."

4. It was voted that the regular fall meeting of the executive committee will be held at the Cosmos Club, in Washington, on Sunday, October 21, 1928, the morning session to open at 11 o'clock.

5. A committee of three was named, to cooperate with the section committee of Section K (Social and Economic Sciences), to elect a section secretary and to arrange for the section at the approaching New York meeting. This committee consists of J. McK. Cattell, B. E. Livingston and Edwin B. Wilson, the last mentioned being chairman.

6. Dr. Wesley C. Mitchell, director of research,

National Bureau of Economic Research, was elected a member of the section committee of Section K for the term of office ending at the close of the annual meeting of December, 1931.

7. A special committee on linguistic sciences in the association was named, as follows: George M. Bolling, B. E. Livingston and Edward Sapir, the latter being chairman. This committee was requested to consider further the problems of Section L (Historical and Philological Sciences) with special reference to the needs of those interested in the linguistic sciences. It was also asked to name a chairman and a secretary for the section from the field of linguistics, to name an eminent scientist in this field to represent it by an address at the approaching New York meeting, and to arrange for a suitable program in linguistics for that meeting.

8. A petition from the Linguistic Society of America, for a special section on linguistic sciences in the association, brought up the general problem of section classification and subdivision, and it was the consensus of opinion of the executive committee that it would be well to consider in the near future the suggestion that a new arrangement of association sections be adopted, with perhaps just three sections or divisions (exact, natural and humanistic sciences, for example) instead of the present larger number. If such a plan were adopted there might be several subsection organizations in any section and the affiliated societies would function, in Association organization, as subsections. There would then be only three association vice-presidents and only three retiring vice-presidential addresses at an annual meeting. This suggestion should receive further attention.

9. Dr. R. G. Hoskins, of the Harvard Medical School, Boston, Mass., was elected to the secretaryship of Section N for the current year, his term to expire at the close of the fifth New York meeting.

10. In view of the present vacancies, caused by death and resignation, in the committee of one hundred on research and in its subcommittees, which will need to be filled in the near future, it was voted that the term of office of members of the committee and of its subcommittees shall extend from the time of their election to the close of the next following annual meeting of the association. It was also voted that the present members of the committee and of its subcommittees shall hold office till the end of the fifth New York meeting.

11. The executive committee expressed its great regret at the resignation of Dr. Maynard M. Metcalf, secretary of the subcommittee on research in educational institutions and chairman of the joint committee on research in colleges, and its appreciation of the work accomplished under Dr. Metcalf's leadership.

12. Dr. C. E. Seashore, dean of the Graduate School, University of Iowa, was named secretary of the subcommittee on research in educational institutions and the executive committee expressed its hearty approval of a continuation of the joint committee on research in colleges, if that seems desirable to the other organizations that have taken part in the work of the joint committee. These are as follows: National Research Council, American Council on Education, American Association of University Professors, American Council of Learned Societies, Social Science Research Council.

13. It was voted that matters coming before the executive committee of the association from the committee of one hundred on research or from its subcommittees shall be considered first by the executive committee of the committee of one hundred, which shall transmit them, with recommendations, to the executive committee of the association.

14. A report on the work and prospects of the committee of one hundred on research was presented, from Dr. Rodney H. True, secretary of the committee of one hundred, which was accepted and referred to the executive committee of the committee of one hundred, with power to arrange for carrying on the work of the committee until the end of the fifth New York meeting, including the use of treasury funds in that period to amount to not more than one thousand dollars.

15. The executive committee of the committee of one hundred on scientific research was asked to present to the executive committee of the association, for consideration at its next regular fall meeting, a plan for the future organization and work of the committee of one hundred.

16. It was voted that, for the four-year period beginning at the end of the fifth New York meeting, any member of any affiliated organization may join the American Association without paying the entrance fee.

17. It was voted that the price of the next volume of Summarized Proceedings and Directory of Members (which is to be published in the fall of 1929) shall be $2.50 (or $3.50 bound) to members who remit for it in advance of publication; $3.00 (or $4.00 bound) to members who remit for it after publication, and $4.00 (or $5.00 bound) to non-members.

18. The question of the desirability of altering the rules by which the annual American Association prize of $1,000 is awarded was considered, having been taken up previously by the permanent secretary in correspondence with the members of the executive committee, and it was voted to make no changes at this time. The permanent secretary was asked to arrange a committee of five to decide on the New York award of the prize, vice-presidents and retiring vice-presidents being considered especially suitable for appointment to this award committee.

19. The following resolution was adopted, recommending to the Congress of the United States the establishment of a National Institute of Health:

Resolved: That the Executive Committee of the American Association for the Advancement of Science, approving the action taken by the medical section of the association at Nashville, and representing the 16,000 members of the association, urges Congress to give special consideration to the desirability of providing means of maintaining human health in some such manner as is outlined in the Ransdell bill, S. 5835.

20. The academy conference was requested to consider the problem of providing increased facilities for the encouragement of junior scientific effort (reference being made to the article of Thomas Large, SCIENCE for March 9, 1928, page 272) and the conference was asked to make suggestions and recommendations on this subject for consideration by the executive committee at its next regular fall meeting on October 21. It was also requested that this subject be made a special order of business at the New York conference of academy representatives.

21. The following resolution was adopted concerning the provision of courses in elementary German and French in high schools:

Resolved: That it is highly desirable that all who are to undertake work in science should be familiar with German and French, and that a knowledge of these two languages should be acquired by students before they enter college.

22. Michael I. Pupin and J. McKeen Cattell were named as official delegates to represent the American Association at the conferring of a gold medal on Thomas A. Edison by the Society of Arts and Sciences on May 24, at the Astor Hotel in New York City.

23. A committee of three was named, to cooperate with the American committee on preparations for the World Engineering Congress to occur at Tokio in 1929. This committee consists of: E. Lester Jones (chairman), Robert L. Sackett (vice-president for Section M) and N. H. Heck (secretary of section M).

24. An appropriation of $50 from the permanent secretary's funds was made to aid the educational work of the American Institute of Sacred Literature.

25. In response to a request for a final subscription to aid the work of the National Conference on Outdoor Recreation, an appropriation of $50 was made for that purpose, from the permanent secretary's funds.

26. An appropriation of $100 from the permanent secretary's funds was made to aid the American Library Association's committee on work with the blind, to secure the printing of scientific books in Braille.

27. The American Library Association was officially affiliated with the American Association for the Advancement of Science. It is to have one representative in the association council.

28. The executive committee invited the Archaeological Institute of America to become affiliated with the American Association.

29. The College Art Teachers were invited to take part in the fifth New York meeting and to arrange a scientific program.

30. The American Philological Association was invited to have its New York program included in the General Program of the fifth New York meeting and to be otherwise the guest of the American Association as far as that may seem desirable to the Philological Association.

31. Sixty-nine members were elected to fellowship, distributed among the sections as follows: Section A, 1; Section B, 37; Section C, 2; Section E, 1; Section M, 21; Section N, 4; Section O, 1; Section Q, 2.

32. The permanent secretary was instructed to send, with the statement cards to be mailed next October 1, requests to all members asking for nominations for president of the association, as was done October 1, 1927.

33. A nominating committee was named for the fifth New York meeting, to present to the council nominations for general secretary, permanent secretary, treasurer, two executive committee members (to succeed Vernon Kellogg and Edwin B. Wilson), two council members (to succeed L. O. Howard and D. T. MacDougal), two members of the committee on grants for research (to succeed Joseph Erlanger and Nevin M. Fenneman), a member of the finance committee, and a representative of the association on the board of Science Service. The members named for the nominating committee are: Edwin G. Conklin (chairman), L. E. Dickson, Edward L. Thorndike, David White and Charles E. Mendenhall.

34. The permanent secretary was instructed to secure several nominations for secretary of each section and to present them to the executive committee at its fall meeting on October 21, elections to be by the council at the fifth New York meeting.

35. The permanent secretary reported that plans and arrangements for the approaching New York meeting were well advanced, that President Henry Fairfield Osborn is arranging a number of attractive special features, and that the local executive committee has held a number of meetings and has the various details of the preparations well in hand.

BURTON E. LIVINGSTON,
Permanent Secretary.

SCIENCE

Vol. LXVII — May 25, 1928 — No. 1743

CONTENTS

The Responsibility of the Agricultural Experiment Station in the Present Agricultural Situation: Professor C. G. Williams ... 519

Louis Agassiz and the Hall of Fame: President Henry Fairfield Osborn ... 523

Ernst J. Lesser: Dr. Carl F. Cori ... 523

Scientific Events:
The Second International Conference on Bituminous Coal; The Sixth National Colloid Symposium; A Bill to Promote Ethnological Research; The Award of Medals by the Franklin Institute ... 524

Scientific Notes and News ... 526

University and Educational Notes ... 530

Discussion and Correspondence:
The Little Circle of Reference: Professor Carl Barus. *Occurrence of a Mutant Meadow-Mouse:* Ruth D. Svihla and Arthur Svihla. *The Occurrence of Sarcocystis:* Dr. H. L. Osterud and Dr. K. F. Bascom. *Quails, Potato-Bugs and other Things:* N. L. Willet. *The Earliest Dynamo:* Dr. H. W. Wiley ... 530

Scientific Books:
Morrow's Biochemical Laboratory Methods: Professor William Seifriz ... 533

Scientific Apparatus and Laboratory Methods:
A Combined Fixative and Stain for Demonstrating Flagella and Cilia: Dr. Lowell E. Noland. *Reproducing Illustrations without a Camera:* Edgar P. Jones ... 535

Special Articles:
The Parathyroid Glands as Influenced by Solar Radiation: Dr. George M. Higgins and Dr. Charles Sheard. *A New Carbohydrate from Seaweed:* Dr. L. H. Cretcher and W. L. Nelson ... 536

Societies and Academies:
The Ohio Academy of Science: Wm. H. Alexander. *The Sigma Pi Sigma Convention* ... 538

Science News ... x

SCIENCE: A Weekly Journal devoted to the Advancement of Science, edited by J. McKeen Cattell and published every Friday by

THE SCIENCE PRESS

New York City: Grand Central Terminal

Lancaster, Pa. — Garrison, N. Y.

Annual Subscription, $6.00. — Single Copies, 15 Cts.

SCIENCE is the official organ of the American Association for the Advancement of Science. Information regarding membership in the Association may be secured from the office of the permanent secretary, in the Smithsonian Institution Building, Washington, D. C.

THE RESPONSIBILITY OF THE AGRICULTURAL EXPERIMENT STATION IN THE PRESENT AGRICULTURAL SITUATION[1]

Situations—good, bad or indifferent—are the common lot of man and of all groups and associations of men. Your program committee was therefore perfectly safe in assuming that there is an agricultural situation.

It was probably equally safe in assuming that the agricultural experiment stations of our country have some responsibility in connection therewith.

Some critics have gone so far as to hold the experiment stations responsible *for* the present situation, stating that were it not for the experiment station and the agricultural extension service there would be no agricultural situation, of the present sort at least. This is very likely true. Our agriculture might, however, be in the "fire" instead of the "frying pan."

I take it that the province of this discussion is to consider rather the responsibility of the agricultural experiment station *in* the existing situation.

Before the experiment station can get very far in the exercise of its responsibilities it will have to know very definitely what the agricultural situation is. As a "fact-finding" institution perhaps this is its first work, to find the facts as to the actual situation.

Having found these facts, it will be in order to determine the several causes which have resulted in the present situation; and, finally, to suggest courses of action, based upon researches, which give promise of remedying the situation.

We have quite a variety of opinions and pronouncements as to the agricultural situation—a situation which naturally changes very considerably month by month and year by year, as witness the change in the list of "basic" products in successive editions of the McNary-Haugen Bill. The price of eggs for several months past has indicated that the next edition of this bill would include eggs as one of the basic products, along with rice and tobacco!

The present agricultural situation has been described by some as "the farmer's failure to get his

[1] Address delivered at the forty-first annual convention of the Association of Land-Grant Colleges and Universities, Chicago, Illinois, November 15, 1927, by Director C. G. Williams, Ohio Agricultural Experiment Station.

share of the national income," and by others as his "inability to earn sufficient return upon his investment." Recently the agricultural committee of the International Economic Conference described the situation as "the disequilibrium which has arisen between the prices of agricultural products and manufactured products." This definition comes from an accredited source and is perhaps as satisfactory as any.

Now disequilibriums are usually brought about, the economists tell us, by maladjustments between the supply of and the demand for products. I take it, then, that the experiment station should make a thorough study of the production and consumption of the agricultural products in which its constituents are actively interested with a view of determining the actual situation.

Wheat Production and Consumption

Take the wheat crop, for instance. What has happened to it during the last forty years? Comparing the five-year period 1885–1889 with 1920–1924, it appears that our acreage per capita was 0.57 in the earlier period and 0.52 in the later, or a decline of 8.8 per cent. But, owing to increased yields per acre, our production per capita increased during this period from 6.77 bushels to 7.26, or 7.2 per cent. This increase in production would not seem to be a serious matter if the other factors bearing upon the wheat situation were unchanged. Unfortunately for the wheat farmer the factor of consumption has not remained the same. According to figures gathered by the U. S. Department of Agriculture the per capita consumption or "disappearance" of wheat has declined 1.1 bushels during the period in question. This, with the increased production of 0.49 bushel, makes an excess of 1.59 bushels per capita above the supply of thirty-five years ago.

How shall we account for this reduction in the consumption of wheat? Is it a permanent reduction, and is there a possibility of its increasing?

Wheat is one of our greatest energy-producing foods, and, in common with other foods of like character, is in less demand now than formerly because less hard physical labor is called for in the world's work. For one, and perhaps the most important thing, during the last forty years two hours have been clipped off the day's work of almost our entire population. While our farm population is not working an eight-hour day, it is probable that the farmer's working day has been shortened in proportion. Eight and ten hours of labor do not call for the amount of energy-producing foods that ten and twelve hours of labor require.

Then the tasks of the laborer, both in the manufacturing industry and on the farm, have been greatly lessened in so far as the physical energy called for is concerned by the marvelous line of machinery now in use.

Substituting One Food for Another

Partly as a result of these changed conditions and partly as a result of propaganda other foods, such as vegetables, fruits and milk, are being substituted for these energy-producing foods. Physicians, nutrition experts, and, sometimes it seems, the very "stars in their courses" are adjuring the public in their behalf. Still other foods have been called into increased use during recent years, notably poultry, eggs and sugar. All these changes mean a decreased demand for wheat and meats as a whole, though the consumption of pork shows an increase, but very likely a temporary one. Limits have been set to the capacity of the human stomach. More fruit, milk and eggs necessarily mean less bread and meat. And less hard labor means less energy-producing foods. So far as one can now see these conditions are here to stay and will result in a permanent, and possibly in a still further reduction in the demand for wheat as far as this country is concerned.

This study would have to take into consideration foreign production and consumption, for so long as we have to depend upon a foreign market for the utilization of a portion of our product so long will foreign conditions and tendencies be of concern to us.

Some such study as has been briefly and incompletely indicated for wheat would seem to be within the province of the experiment station for all the crops in which its constituency is interested. In so far as the present agricultural situation is due to production, consumption and consequent price relationships, such studies should prove of value. They should include investigations of the effect of temporary increases and decreases in production prices, concerning which our data are limited.

But there are doubtless many things which have had to do with the present agricultural depressions which need investigation.

Taxes

There is need for a thorough study of taxation as related to farm property. Our farmers are paying on the average 150 per cent. greater taxes now than in 1914. No other farm expense has increased in like ratio. A careful study should be made of rural as compared with urban taxation. Studies now under way in some sections are showing that while rural real estate is on the tax duplicate for 88.4 per cent.

of its sales value, urban property in the same county is assessed at 63.2 per cent. of its value. Reliable facts of this kind are being used very effectively in securing proper readjustments of the tax duplicate.

There are other tax burdens resting upon farm property that are in need of adjustment, which it would not be difficult to secure if all the needed facts were available. Fifteen years ago our cross-country roads were seldom used by traffic originating in the city. They were the farmer's own roads, and it was proper that he should make and maintain them. The situation is very different to-day and reliable facts on the existing situation would be very useful.

Our cities are not only interested in the country roads but in the youth of the country. These country boys and girls are educated at the expense of the rural community, but as soon as they arrive at a productive age many of them go to the city. Would it not be desirable to know all the facts involved in this transfer of rural wealth to the city? Is it not likely that such knowledge, if properly handled, would result in the shifting of a portion of this tax burden from the country to the city?

TARIFF

Does any responsibility rest upon the agricultural experiment station to make a study of the effect of the United States tariff on agriculture?

Of partisan opinions, both for and against the present tariff schedules, there are an abundance. While many investigations of a nation-wide bearing can very appropriately be undertaken by the United States Department of Agriculture it would hardly be possible for the department to conduct such an investigation because of its political connections. It would doubtless be difficult enough for a state experiment station to do so, but we surely need information as to the effect of the tariff on prices in this country. Such questions as:

Is the American price of protected articles always, usually, seldom or never equal to the foreign price plus freight and tariff?

To what extent are American products that are favored by a tariff sold abroad, and at what prices?

Are the products which are sent abroad sold at a loss or at a profit?

Is there any significance in the fact that many of the heavily protected articles, such as iron, steel, structural steel and chemicals, are selling nearer pre-war prices than grains, meats and dairy products?

How does the efficiency of the American laborer compare with that of the European laborer?

These questions may have some bearing upon the agricultural situation. The agricultural public would like information on them. Should not the experiment station help secure this information?

FARM LABOR

To what extent do the high wages of farm labor contribute to the agricultural situation?

In considering the principal items which make up the expenses of the farmer, including labor, machinery, feed, taxes, fertilizer, buildings, clothing, furniture, groceries, fuel and a group of miscellaneous items, farm labor is the second highest of the lot in comparison with pre-war prices, being exceeded by taxes only.

The wages of farm labor are influenced by the wages in manufacturing industries, though they have not increased in proportion to the latter.

It might contribute something to the mental condition of the farmer if he had some reliable data on the relative efficiency of farm labor now as compared with ten or twenty years ago. An investigation might show an increase of 30 to 60 per cent. in the productive efficiency of farm labor, as is believed by some people. Whatever the findings, it would seem that studies as to the efficiency of man power on the farm, the average working hours per day and working days per year would contribute information of considerable value in discovering what the agricultural situation is, and in adjusting ourselves to it.

In the time available it will not be possible to consider very many of the causes which may be contributing to the present situation. A few minutes should be given to lines of investigation tending to improve the situation.

ECONOMICAL PRODUCTION

Economical production is still the great question for a vast number of our farm people. A large proportion of the questions put up to the experiment stations to-day have to do with production. These questions have by no means been solved. When farm management studies conducted in one county of an important corn state show some corn growers investing in an acre of corn 260 per cent. more man hours and 177 per cent. more horse hours than other growers, and at the same time securing smaller yields per acre, there would seem to be room for improvement. There are individual variations of this sort in most neighborhoods, and frequently whole counties or sections of states show variations of moment which would be gradually corrected if attention were called to these differences by a comprehensive study of conditions. Such changes make for more profitable farming.

Most of our experiment stations have conducted, or are conducting, extensive soil surveys of their respective states. These soil surveys should be followed by equally thorough ecological surveys. Many of our farmers are attempting to grow alfalfa and sweet clover on land better adapted to alsike clover and timothy. Potatoes, tobacco, sugar beets and many other crops are often carried to soils and climates in which they are not at home and where they can not be grown economically. A better adjustment of crops to soil and climate will most certainly result in more economical production.

The Cereal-Legume Ratio

More investigations need to be conducted relative to the most desirable cereal-legume ratio. Grouping the non-legume potatoes and sugar beets with the cereals for the present purpose, it will be found that for the average of the years 1924–1926 the ratio of cereals to legumes seems to run from 2.7:1 in Michigan to 45:1 in North Dakota. And if cotton be included, Texas has a ratio of over 70:1, though possibly the legume figures as given in the Yearbook of the U. S. Department of Agriculture may not be complete for this state.

It is evident that if our leading corn belt states were to go from perhaps an average ratio of 8:1 to 3 or 4:1 our cereal surplus problem would be pretty well taken care of, even in a good season.

Our increased acreage of legumes would be used mainly for soil improvement, which would result in larger yields of non-legumes per acre, though in a smaller total production, and our production costs per unit would thus be reduced.

Adjusting Agricultural Production

It would seem that the time has arrived when our farm people must exercise a greater control over production. In so far as live stock is concerned this is comparatively easy, for we have matters largely in our own hands. If there is overproduction it is evident who is to blame. We are controlling production now, but not always in a wise and profitable way. Our hog men are simply a few months behind the game. Investigations like those reported in a recent bulletin from Illinois (Bulletin 293) on "Adjusting Hog Production to Market Demand" will have beneficial results.

In crop production matters can not be controlled as easily. A reduced acreage will, on the average, result in reduced production, but there will be exceptional seasons in which this will not hold good. If nature is especially kind one season we shall have to learn to limit our acreage the next season, or until the old surplus can be marketed satisfactorily. I fear that any plan to buy up surplus products and hold them until they can be marketed at a profit is doomed to fail unless some control over production is provided; but as yet no one seems to have suggested a workable control.

There is, however, no reason to believe that farmers can not learn to cooperate in these matters. The Canadian Wheat Pool, which controls 75 per cent. of the wheat acreage of Canada, is an encouraging sign of the times. Once we get over the notion that we are going to make Uncle Sam hold the bag and pay round prices for whatever we care to dump into it we may be able to engage in cooperative marketing as wisely and as satisfactorily as some other farm peoples have done. As a matter of fact the agricultural census of 1925 shows that the necessity for decreased production is being appreciated along many lines, and there is good reason to believe that the desired equilibrium between agricultural and other prices is gradually approaching.

America is anxious to maintain and increase its present high standard of living. This rests, in the main, upon the high-wage scale prevailing in this country. There would seem to be only two ways in which we can operate on a higher wage scale than Europe, and these are to produce more per man—*i.e.*, produce more economically—or confine our production to the needs of our own people. When we go into the markets of the world we shall have to accept world prices. Any attempt to give ourselves a bonus on exports will be almost certain to be met with a retaliatory tariff in every country except where it is desired to take advantage of cheap food, the better to compete with American manufacturers. And this would have to be offset here by a higher tariff, which means that we should soon get dizzy traveling around in a circle. Confirmation of this attitude on the part of foreign countries is to be had by the recent proposal of the National Farmers' Union of England that "counter-availing safeguards to home production, to meet bounty-fed competition from abroad be adopted."

There are two ways of attacking the problem presented by the present agricultural situation. One is agricultural research, followed by such economies and adjustments as may be indicated, together with commodity organization. The other is the Via Dolorosa of political nostrums. If the agricultural experiment stations rise to the occasion we may be saved from the latter.

C. G. Williams

Ohio Agricultural Experiment Station

LOUIS AGASSIZ AND THE HALL OF FAME[1]

NEARLY a century ago Louis Agassiz, following his friend Charpentier, boldly set before his confreres in the infant Academy of Neufchatel the novel and apparently revolutionary theory of a Glacial Age in which a mantle of ice covered the Alps and extended widely over Europe. This induction, conceived during his youthful encampment upon the Aar Glacier and his descent into its very heart, led step by step to our present knowledge of the repeated glaciations not only of the northern hemisphere but of the entire globe. The ten years between 1837 and 1847 Agassiz devoted to establishing this theory, and from the time of his arrival in Massachusetts in 1846 he was delighted to witness the vestiges of glaciation in North America, and before he passed away in 1873 he experienced the conversion of a startling and fantastic hypothesis into a well-established principle of the earth's history. This brilliant induction at the age of thirty yields the secret of Agassiz's great career, epitomized on the walls of his Penikese laboratory in four words: "Read Nature Not Books." For, next to his unrivaled inspiration as a teacher came his revolutionary insistence upon direct recourse to nature summed up in one of his most beautiful sentences, "If you study nature in books, when you go out-of-doors you can not find her." There never was a day in American educational history in which this observational method of Agassiz was more glaringly needed than the present day.

The little Swiss Canton of Neufchatel yielded not less than three great gifts of Switzerland to the United States—to Princeton University Arnold Guyot, comrade of Agassiz in glaciation; to our National Geological Survey Leo Lesquereux, classmate and comrade in botany; to all America Louis Agassiz, naturalist, geologist, zoologist. The French and Swiss social revolution of 1848, which hastened the departure to our shores of these three great men, inaugurated among us a scientific metempsychosis, the effects of which are quite beyond calculation. Into our practically virgin field of natural history, Agassiz brought the great traditions of his master, Cuvier, the brilliant founder of paleontology; of Humboldt, then the most influential scientist of Europe; of the British geologists, Buckland, Murchison, Sedgwick and Lyell. While never destined to be a disciple of Darwin, he paved the way for evolution through newer conceptions of creation in his titanic researches on living and fossil fishes, as well as through the vistas of geologic time in his glaciation theory and in his insistence upon the observation of nature.

Following to America the ardent French pioneers and explorers, Rafinesque, Bonaparte, Audubon and Lessen, Agassiz brought with him the great traditions and canons of the European school as well as the example of research and publication in all branches of natural history, especially the life of the sea. Our birds, mammals and reptiles had been discovered and described by early French, Spanish and English explorers; it remained for Agassiz to explore our beautiful seacoast and to show the romance in the life of the sea. Thus his third great contribution to America was his creation of a school of explorers of the world beneath the waters—a school which numbered among its pupils all the distinguished men of American biology enrolled in our National Academy of Sciences between the years 1846 and 1873, besides the hundreds and even thousands of laymen who were attracted by his contagious enthusiasm.

To his leadership, exerted to arouse public interest and attention, we owe directly our seashore laboratories and many of our museums. It was he who inspired young Albert Bickmore, the creator of the American Museum of Natural History, and his own son Alexander, the founder and benefactor of the Cambridge Museum of Comparative Zoology, in the days when the National Museum of the Smithsonian Institution and others were not yet dreamed of. Every American college and university of the fifties, sixties and seventies filled its chairs of zoology by a pupil of Agassiz. Thus his influence extended a thousandfold.

These are the four outstanding reasons why the bronze portrait of Louis Agassiz should be placed in this Hall of Fame to-day. Is it not a felicitous example of the power of heredity that Alpheus Hyatt, perhaps the most original and skilful disciple of Agassiz and a master of form in the science of paleontology, should be the father of Anna Vaughn Hyatt, the very gifted sculptress, who has to-day in this beautiful bronze perpetuated the name and fame of Louis Agassiz.

HENRY FAIRFIELD OSBORN

AMERICAN MUSEUM OF NATURAL HISTORY

[1] Address at the Hall of Fame of New York University, on Thursday, May 10, 1928, at the unveiling of a bust of Jean Louis Rudolphe Agassiz.

ERNST J. LESSER

THE sudden death of Dr. E. J. Lesser, biological chemist at the City Hospital in Mannheim, Germany, involves a very great loss to medical science. He possessed the qualities of the true research worker in a very exceptional degree. He had insight and enthusiasm;—and these were combined with exemplary patience, caution, self-criticism and a remarkable technical skill. Those who knew him were impressed by his gifted, generous and beautifully modest personality as well as by his deep understanding of other fields of knowledge. Dr. Lesser studied medicine in Freiburg and Munich. After taking his degree he worked in the physiological laboratories of Voit in Munich and Bernstein in Halle. In 1906 he was made "Privatdozent," submitting a thesis on the electromotoric force of the current of the frog skin. The following years mark the beginning of a series of investigations on life without oxygen, which led to the important observation that there occurs a restitution of glycogen when frogs are allowed to recover after a period of anoxibiosis. This phenomenon of oxidative recovery is now one of the basic laws of muscle physiology. In 1910 Dr. Lesser accepted the position in Mannheim, which he held until his death, with only a short interruption during the war, when he substituted as professor of biological chemistry at the University of Strasbourg. His work on the diastatic ferment of the liver led him into a broad investigation of carbohydrate metabolism which made him a recognized leader in this field. Here he succeeded in the preparation of an active extract of the pancreas, but before he was ready to publish his results, which he wanted to elaborate as far as possible, there appeared the first paper of Banting on insulin. Interested only in the progress of science and not in personal matters, he kept this fact secret—only his intimate associates knew of it—and never made any claims of priority. His series of papers on the nature of the action of insulin is a classic and his summarizing articles in text-books and reviews are proof of the clarity and penetration of his mind. Not surrounded by the glamor of an academic position, he did not receive the full recognition of the high qualities of his character and his work at the early age at which he died.

CARL F. CORI

STATE INSTITUTE FOR THE STUDY OF MALIGNANT DISEASE,
BUFFALO, N. Y.

SCIENTIFIC EVENTS

THE SECOND INTERNATIONAL CONFERENCE ON BITUMINOUS COAL

BETWEEN 60 and 70 scientists and fuel technologists in eleven different countries have tentatively accepted invitations to speak at the second International Conference on Bituminous Coal, which will be held at the Carnegie Institute of Technology in Pittsburgh, Pennsylvania, during the week of November 19. The list includes about forty Europeans whom Dr. Thomas S. Baker, president of the Carnegie Institute of Technology, personally invited while making his recent two months' visit in Europe in the interests of the conference.

It is announced that the purpose of the congress is similar to the one held in 1926 by the Carnegie Institute of Technology: to present the results of recent studies of coal that have to do with improved methods of utilization and combustion. The program will include the discussion of low temperature distillation, high temperature distillation, coal tar products, power, smokeless fuel, complete gasification of coal, hydrogenation, pulverized fuel and its new applications, fixation of nitrogen, coal beneficiation, etc.

Upon his return from Europe in April, President Baker expressed the opinion that the second conference will be much larger in scope and importance than the first, and that the number of delegates from foreign countries will be considerably in excess of that at the 1926 meeting, when thirteen different nations were represented.

Among the distinguished scientific men in Europe who have either definitely or tentatively accepted invitations to speak are the Right Honorable Sir Alfred Mead, Harald Nielsen, Dr. Cecil H. Lander and Dr. R. Lessing, of England; Donat Agache, president of the executive board of the Kuhlmann plants; André Kling, director of The Municipal Laboratories of Paris, and Henri Lafond, International Company for the Manufacture of Gasoline and Oils, France; Dr. Friedrich Bergius, inventor of the Bergius process for the production of oil from coal; Dr. Franz Fischer, director of the Kaiser Wilhelm Institute for Coal Research; Professor Fritz Hoffman, inventor of a process for manufacturing synthetic rubber from coal; Dr. Carl Krauch, director of the I. G. Dye Trust, and Rudolph Rawlikowski, of the Cosmos Machine Construction Institute, Germany, and many others.

Professor Sumner B. Ely, of the Carnegie Institute of Technology, is secretary of the conference. The advisory board includes John Hays Hammond, E. M. Herr, Samuel Insull, Frank B. Jewett, Otto H. Kahn, George E. Learnard, the Honorable A. W. Mellon, Auguste G. Pratt and Charles M. Schwab.

THE SIXTH NATIONAL COLLOID SYMPOSIUM

THE Sixth National Colloid Symposium will be held under the auspices of the Colloid Division of the American Chemical Society at Toronto, Canada, June 14, 15 and 16, 1928, with Sir William B. Hardy, of Cambridge, England, as the guest of honor. The following program of papers has been announced by the chairman, Professor Harry B. Weiser, The Rice Institute, Houston, Texas.

Sir William B. Hardy, Cambridge, England (title not yet available).

Dr. H. A. Abramson: Cataphoresis of blood cells and inert particles in sols and gels and its biological significance (with motion pictures).

Wilder D. Bancroft and C. E. Barnett, Cornell University: Adsorption of methylene blue by lead sulfate.

David R. Briggs, University of Minnesota: Surface conductance.

E. F. Burton and Beatrice Reid Deacon, University of Toronto: Influence of temperature on coagulation of colloidal solutions.

John R. Fanselow, University of Wisconsin: The influence of electrolytes and non-electrolytes upon the optical activity and relative resistance to shear of gelatin systems.

William D. Harkins, University of Chicago: Charges on colloidal particles, adsorption, and the spreading of liquids.

A. B. Hastings, University of Chicago: The rôle of hemoglobin in the blood.

Ernst Hauser, Frankfurt am Main, Germany: New microscopic methods in connection with the problem of vulcanization.

Emil Heuser, International Paper Company, Ontario: Problems of cellulose chemistry.

Harry N. Holmes and Robert C. Williams, Oberlin College: The uniform distribution of catalysts throughout porous solids.

F. B. Kenrick, University of Toronto: The effect of adsorbed water on electrical conductivity of powders.

John C. Krantz and Neil E. Gordon, University of Maryland: Hydrogen-ion concentration and stability of emulsions.

M. E. Laing, J. W. McBain and E. W. Harrison, Stanford University: Adsorption of sodium oleate at the air-water interface.

J. W. McBain, W. F. K. Wynne-Jones and F. H. Pollard, Stanford University: The activity and adsorption of p-toluidine in the surface of its aqueous solutions.

P. J. Moloney and Edith M. Taylor, Connaught Research Laboratories: Fractionation of diphtheria anti-toxic sera.

Stuart Mudd, Baludin Lucke, Morton McCutcheon and Max Strumia, University of Pennsylvania: Relation between surface properties and phagocytosis of bacteria.

H. A. Neville and H. C. Jones, Lehigh University: The study of hydration changes by a volume-change method.

J. B. Nichols, Dupont Company: The development of the ultra-centrifuge and its field of research.

Fred Olsen, Picatinny Arsenal: Influence of gel structure upon the technology of smokeless powder manufacture.

A. J. Phillips, Picatinny Arsenal: Structure of cellulose nitrate and cellulose nitrate gels.

W. L. Robinson, University of Toronto: The filtration of colloids by the spleen.

S. E. Sheppard and R. H. Lambert, Eastman Kodak Company: Grain growth in silver bromide precipitates.

A. J. Stamm, Forest Products Laboratories: The structure of soft-woods as revealed by dynamic physical methods.

H. L. Trumbull, B. F. Goodrich Company: The preparation and properties of rubber dispersions.

Hardolph Wasteneys and H. Borsook, University of Toronto: Emulsions and protein synthesis.

Harry B. Weiser and G. E. Cunningham, The Rice Institute: Adsorption of ions and the physical character of precipitates (with motion pictures).

G. S. Whitby, J. G. McNally and W. Gallay, McGill University: Studies of organophilic colloids.

A BILL TO PROMOTE ETHNOLOGICAL RESEARCH AMONG THE AMERICAN INDIANS

AN appropriation to provide for cooperation by the Smithsonian Institution with state, educational and scientific organizations in the United States for continuing ethnological researches among the American Indians, was approved by the Senate on May 8, when it passed the McKellar bill, which contains the following provisions:

Be it enacted by the Senate and House of Representatives of the United States of America in Congress assembled, That the secretary of the Smithsonian Institution is hereby authorized to cooperate with any state, educational institution, or scientific organization in the United States for continuing ethnological researches among the American Indians and the excavation and preservation of archeological remains.

Section 2. That there is hereby authorized to be appropriated, out of any money in the treasury not otherwise appropriated, the sum of $20,000, which shall be available until expended for the above purposes:

Provided, That at such time as the Smithsonian Institution is satisfied that any state, educational institution, or scientific organization in any of the United States is prepared to contribute to such investigation and when in its judgment such investigation shall appear meritorious, the secretary of the Smithsonian Institution may direct that an amount from this sum equal to that contributed by such state, educational institution, or scientific organization, not to exceed $2,000, to be expended from such sum in any one state during any calendar year, be made available for cooperative investigation:

Provided further, That all such cooperative work and division of the result thereof shall be under the direction of the secretary of the Smithsonian Institution.

THE AWARD OF MEDALS BY THE FRANKLIN INSTITUTE

THE annual meeting for the presentation of medals by the Franklin Institute took place in Philadelphia on May 16. Medals were presented to sixteen men for scientific achievement over a wide field. The Franklin medal, the highest award of the institute, was presented to Dr. Charles F. Brush, inventor of the arc light, and, through Baron F. von Prittz Witz-Gaffron, the German Ambassador, also to Professor Walther Nernst, of the University of Berlin. Dr. Brush read a paper on radioactive elements. Dr. Nernst's paper was read by Dr. Irving Langmuir, of the General Electric Company, one of his former pupils. Cresson medals were awarded to Henry Ford "in consideration of his rare inventive ability and power of organization"; to Charles L. Lawrance for his development of the air-cooled motor; Professor Vladimir Karapetoff, of Cornell University, for instruments for the mechanical calculation of magnetic and electrical constants of an electrical transmitting line, and Gustaf W. Elmen, of the Bell Telephone Laboratories, Inc., inventor of permalloy, a new alloy of nickel, 100 times more magnetic than iron.

The Henderson medal was awarded for the first time. It went to William F. Kiesel, in charge of the Altoona shop of the Pennsylvania Railroad, for improvement in locomotives and railroad equipment. Arthur Graham Glasgow, of London, received the Walton Clark medal for improvements in the manufacture of illuminating gas.

William E. Taylor, of Corning, N. Y., received for himself and his associate, Eugene C. Sullivan, the Potts medal for development of pyrex, a heat resisting glass. Oscar G. Thurlow, of the Alabama Power Company, also received the Potts medal for designs and inventions applied to hydroelectric plants.

Other awards were: Longstreth medals to Frank N. Speller, of the National Tube Company, for inventing scale-proof iron pipe, and to Warren P. Valentine, of New York, for improving the refractometer and other optical instruments; Wetherill medals to Albert S. Howell, of the Bell-Howell Company, for the development of movie cameras and projectors adaptable to the amateur, and to Frank E. Ross, of the Yerkes Observatory, for designing wide-angle photographic lenses which increase 100 times the astronomical area that can be photographed; and the Levy medal, to Vannevar Bush, of the Massachusetts Institute of Technology, for two papers on electrical power transmission contributed to the *Journal* of the Franklin Institute.

SCIENTIFIC NOTES AND NEWS

DR. HIDEYO NOGUCHI, member of the Rockefeller Institute for Medical Research, died on May 21 in Africa from yellow fever, which he contracted while working on the disease. Dr. Noguchi was fifty-one years of age.

DR. PERCY E. RAYMOND, associate professor of paleontology at Harvard University, has been awarded the Walker grand prize of $1,000, offered every five years by the Boston Society of Natural History. The prize, offered for outstanding discoveries or investigations in natural history, went to Professor Raymond for his work on the trilobites.

AS already recorded in SCIENCE, the Linnean gold medal for 1928 has been awarded by the Linnean Society to Dr. Edmund Beecher Wilson, Da Costa professor of zoology in Columbia University. In commenting on this award, *Nature* says: "Professor Wilson's early work dealt with descriptive embryology; in the 'nineties, he took a great part in founding the new science of experimental embryology, and many of his experiments, especially those on *Amphioxus, Nereis, Patella* and *Dentalium,* remain classical. He is known to a world-wide circle as the author of that admirable text-book, 'The Cell in Development and Heredity.' First published in 1896, a greatly enlarged third edition appeared in 1925. It is a model of what a text-book should be—encyclopedic, trustworthy and judicial—and shows the hand of a master."

AWARD of prizes for the best contributions to the arc-welding art were made at the opening session of the spring meeting of the American Society of Mechanical Engineers at Pittsburgh on May 14. These prizes were offered by the Lincoln Electric Company, of Cleveland, through its vice-president, James F. Lincoln, with the desire to promote the whole art and to reduce the cost of construction. The first prize, $10,000, was awarded to James W. Owens, of Newport News, Va., for a paper entitled "Arc Welding, its Fundamentals and Economics." Professor Henri Dustin, of the University of Brussels, Belgium, received the second prize of $5,000 for his paper on "Fundamental Principles of Arc Welding," while Commander H. E. Rossell, of the U. S. Naval Academy, took the third prize of $2,500 for his review of "Electric Welding of Ship's Bulkheads and Similar Structures."

SAMUEL REA, of Philadelphia, and Sir Ernest Rutherford, of the University of Cambridge, have, among others, been elected honorary members of the British Institute of Civil Engineers.

ON May 3, at the annual general meeting of the British Iron and Steel Institute, the Bessemer gold medal was presented to Mr. Charles M. Schwab, president of the American Iron and Steel Institute and the president of the Bethlehem Steel Corporation.

DR. DEAN LEWIS, surgeon-in-chief, the Johns Hopkins Hospital, has been made a foreign member of the Società Medico-Chirurgica of Bologna and an Ausserordentliches Mitglied der deutschen Gesellschaft für Chirurgie.

THE annual prize established in honor of Howard Taylor Ricketts, who at the time of his death in 1910 was assistant professor of pathology at the University of Chicago, has been divided between George W. Bachman, of Yochow City, Hunan, China, and James Roy Blayney, of Chicago.

THE council of the British Institution of Civil Engineers has made the following awards for papers read and discussed at the ordinary meetings during the session 1927–28: Telford gold medals to Dr. Oscar Faber, London, and G. L. Watson, Newark, New Jersey. Telford premiums to Professor John Goodman, Skipton; James Williamson, Wallington; R. M. Wynne-Edwards, Vancouver, and jointly to F. C. Vokes, Birmingham, and C. B. Townend, Birmingham.

AT the annual meeting of the Royal Institution on May 1, the Duke of Northumberland was elected *president,* Sir Arthur Keith, *treasurer,* and Sir Robert Robertson, *secretary.*

DR. CARLOS E. PORTER, of Santiago, Chile, editor of the *Revista Chilena di Historia Naturale,* has been elected president of the Entomological Society of Spain.

DR. W. R. BROWNE, assistant professor in the department of geology and physical geography of the University of Sydney, has been elected president of the Linnean Society of New South Wales.

DR. ELMER A. SPERRY, chairman of the board of directors of the Sperry Gyroscope Company, has been nominated for the presidency of the American Society of Mechanical Engineers.

PAUL JOHN KRUESI, president and general manager of the Southern Ferro Alloys Company, has been elected president of the American Electrochemical Society at the annual business meeting held in Bridgeport on April 26.

CARLETON W. STURTEVANT, civil engineer, of New York, has been appointed by President Coolidge to be the civil engineer member of the Mississippi Flood Control Commission, created by the flood control bill.

DR. JOHN P. BUWALDA, professor of geology at the California Institute of Technology, has been appointed a member of a committee of three advisers to assist in the solution of problems confronting the U. S. Department of the Interior in the managing of Yosemite Valley in California.

THE office of chairman of the National Council of Scientific Research for Canada has been accepted by Dr. Henry M. Tory, president of the University of Alberta.

DR. CHARLES BERRY WING, professor of structural engineering at Stanford University, has been appointed director of parks for the state of California.

JOHN P. WENTLING, formerly of the division of forestry in the University of Minnesota, has been appointed director of the research division of the Western Red Cedar Association, with headquarters at Minneapolis.

GEORGE LYNN, formerly physical chemist of the U. S. Bureau of Mines, Helium Division, Pittsburgh, Pennsylvania, has accepted the position of research chemist with the Pittsburgh Plate Glass Company, Barberton, Ohio.

S. C. LANGDON has dropped his teaching work at Northwestern University to take charge of chemical research for Curtis Lighting, Inc., Chicago.

Two members of the University of California College of Agriculture will be placed on the retired list next July: Dr. Elwood Mead, professor of rural institutions, becomes emeritus professor in that department, and Warren T. Clarke becomes emeritus professor of agricultural extension.

PROFESSOR JOHN W. HARSHBERGER, of the botanical department of the University of Pennsylvania, will visit Algeria, North Africa, this summer, crossing the Atlas Mountains to the northern part of the Sahara Desert to the oases of Biskra, Colomb Bechar and Touggourt. *En route,* he will visit the forests of Atlas cedar. Leaving North Africa, he will proceed *via* Naples, Rome and Leghorn to the Island of Corsica, to acquaint himself with its flora. Homeward-bound, he will cross the French Alps from Nice *en route* to Paris.

DR. A. G. MCCALL, director of soil investigation in the Maryland Agricultural Experiment Station, has arrived in England. He intends to visit the Rothamsted Station at Harpenden, afterward going to the Continent to confer with the chiefs of a number of European experimental stations on the subject of soil investigation.

DR. E. O. ULRICH, associate in stratigraphic paleontology at the U. S. National Museum, left on May 16 for six weeks' field work on the Cambrian and Ozarkian rocks of Oklahoma.

DR. NAGANICHI KURODA, the well-known Japanese ornithologist, visited the division of birds in the U. S. National Museum the last of April. Dr. Kuroda is on his way to Geneva to attend the International Congress for the Protection of Birds. Before his departure from Washington, he was given a dinner by the Baird Club.

Dr. E. Schratz, assistant in the Kaiser Wilhelm Institute für Biologie, Berlin, is the recipient of a fellowship from the International Education Board, under the terms of which he will carry on some studies of long-lived cells with Dr. D. T. MacDougal at the Desert Laboratory of the Carnegie Institution of Washington. Dr. Schratz will also be associated with Dr. Forrest Shreve in work on anatomy and distribution of desert plants with reference to lime formations.

Professor Friedrich Hund, of the University of Rostock, has been appointed lecturer in physics in Harvard University for the second half-year of 1928–1929. Professor Hund will lecture on "Molecular and Atomic Spectra."

The Massachusetts Institute of Technology announces a ten weeks' course of lectures and laboratory work in colloid chemistry, to be given the coming summer by Ernst A. Hauser, director of the Colloid Laboratory of the German Metallbank und Metallurgische Gesellschaft, Frankfurt.

Professor Ross G. Harrison, of Yale University, delivered a lecture on May 21 at University College, London, on "Modern Trends in the Study of Animal Development."

Dr. W. F. G. Swann, director of the Bartol Research Foundation of the Franklin Institute, addressed the Society of the Sigma Xi on May 4 at the Ohio State University on the subject "The Earth's Electric Charge." The following day he addressed the Central Ohio Physics Club in the Mendenhall Laboratory on "Some Recent Atomic Theories."

During a recent visit to the Pennsylvania State College, Dr. Charles A. Shull, professor of plant physiology at the University of Chicago, addressed the honorary agricultural society, Gamma Sigma Delta, on "The Relation of the Fundamental Sciences to the Agricultural Experiment Stations," and the Penn State Science Club on "The Life and Work of Stephen Hales."

Dr. W. J. Humphreys, of the U. S. Weather Bureau, gave an illustrated lecture on "Clouds and Cloud Splendors" before the New York Academy of Sciences on the evening of May 7.

Professor F. R. Watson, of the University of Illinois, gave an address on May 17 on "Ideal Auditorium Acoustics" at the annual convention of the American Institute of Architects.

On May 3, Dr. Maude Slye, of the University of Chicago, spoke at Iowa State College on her work concerning cancer and heredity.

Sir Frank Dyson, astronomer royal, delivered his presidential address to the British Institute of Physics on May 15, taking as his subject "Physics in Astronomy."

The Romanes lecture for 1928 was given in the Sheldonian Theater, London, on May 4 by Professor D. M. S. Watson, Jodrell professor of zoology and comparative anatomy in the University of London. Professor Watson took as his subject "The Paleontology and the Evolution of Man."

Dr. Charles H. Gilbert, professor of zoology at Stanford University, died on April 20, aged sixty-eight years.

Felix Deutsche, president of the Allgemeine Elektriziatets Gesellschaft and one of Germany's foremost industrialists, died on May 19, aged seventy years.

The Louisiana Academy of Sciences, which was organized at Centenary College on March 5, 1927, held its first annual meeting at Louisiana College, Pineville, Louisiana, on May 5, under the presidency of Professor I. Maizlish, of Centenary College. Dr. H. A. Wilson, professor of physics at the Rice Institute, gave the principal address. His subject was "Recent Theories of Atomic Structure." It was voted that the next annual meeting shall be held at the Southwestern Louisiana Institute, Lafayette, Louisiana.

The American Dairy Science Association will hold its annual meeting at the University of Wisconsin, from June 26 to 28 inclusive. The meeting will bring together research workers, agricultural extension agents, breeders and representatives of large milk plants, butter, cheese and ice cream manufacturers. Dairying in the broadest sense will be discussed from many different angles. Plans are being made for a number of demonstrations, inspection visits and conferences in some of the principal dairy centers of the state. It is expected that every agricultural experiment station and every agricultural school in the United States will be represented.

Two congresses of mathematicians have been held since the war; at Strasbourg in 1920, and at Toronto in 1924. It is proposed to hold a congress at Bologna in 1929, at which delegates from Central Europe will be present for the first time. M. Mussolini has agreed to act as honorary president and Professor Pasquale Sfameni as president. The executive committee is being organized by Professor Salvatore Pincherle, and the general secretariat by Professor Ettore Bartolotti. It is proposed to organize various sections, including pure mathematics, and mathematics applied to economic, scientific and technical problems. Members of the congress will be invited to make excursions to Florence and Ravenna.

IN celebration of the fiftieth anniversary of the foundation of the Folk-Lore Society, which was established in January, 1878, it has been decided to hold a Folk-Lore Congress in London from September 19 to 25. An advisory council is being formed to promote the congress, which is intended to be international in character. Many papers have already been promised, and it is proposed to include in the program exhibits and performances of folk-lore interest, visits to museums, etc. The subscription to the congress has been fixed at 10s. 6d. for members living in Great Britain, and at 7s. 6d. for those living abroad.

THE council of the Royal Geographical Society has received a radio message from Captain Wilkins thanking them for the award of the Patron's medal, and offering for the museum of the society the small British flag which he has carried through more than 15,000 miles of Arctic flying. The council accepted this gift, which will be placed beside the Union Jack flown by Sir Edward Parry on his sledge journey to latitude 82° 45′ North a century before. Captain Wilkins will be present to receive his medal at the anniversary meeting on June 18, and it is expected that both he and Lieutenant Eielson will be guests of the society at the anniversary dinner the same evening.

TWENTY-THREE honor graduates of British institutions of learning have received Commonwealth Fund Fellowships for study in the United States, including the following in the fields of science: Cyril D. Forde, University College, London; cultural history of North America from geographical and anthropological viewpoint, at the University of California. George A. Cumming, St. Andrews; geology, especially structure and stratigraphy, at the California Institute of Technology. Robert Spence, Armstrong College, Durham; physical chemistry, at Princeton University. Robert H. Angus, Sidney Sussex College, Cambridge; protection of high voltage and electric traction systems, at Stanford University. John M. Robertson, Glasgow; organic chemistry, at the University of Michigan. Norman Peter Inglis, Liverpool; strength of materials and fatigue of metals, at the University of Illinois. Catharine C. Steele, St. Andrews; organic chemistry with reference to optical activity, at the University of Illinois.

THE House on May 12 passed a bill designed to insure adequate supplies of timber by providing a 10-year program of reforestation. The bill sets up a series of authorizations covering the activities of the forest experiment stations. The House amended the Senate bill in passing it by providing for the establishment of additional forest experiment stations in Alaska and Hawaii and one additional station in a southern state. It is contemplated that appropriations under all the sections of the bill will approach the maximum authorizations under each section by approximately equal increases over the 10-year period until the maximum amount authorized, $3,575,000, is reached.

AT Ohio State University this spring a gold medal will be awarded for the first time from the Lamme Foundation, of which the late Benjamin Garver Lamme, who was chief engineer of the Westinghouse Electric and Manufacturing Company, is the donor. The medal, which contains $100 worth of gold, is to be awarded every five years to a graduate in any branch of engineering at Ohio State University.

COLONEL CHARLES LINDBERGH took his airplane, "Spirit of St. Louis," to Washington on April 30 for the purpose of turning it over to the Smithsonian Institution. The machine is to be exhibited in the Arts and Industries Building of the U. S. National Museum and plans have been made for suspending it just inside the main entrance. Approaches from galleries on either side will make it possible for visitors to see the interior of the cockpit at close range.

THE will of the late Harmon W. Hendricks, of New York, leaves $250,000 to the Museum of the American Indian, of which he was vice-president.

A TOTAL of $175,000 has been raised toward the building fund of the San Diego Natural History Museum. The total amount sought is $250,000.

ACCORDING to *Museum News*, the first arboretum in West Virginia will be established at Wheeling. It will cover an area of approximately 70 acres and will include several miles of trails, along which signs and labels will be placed to instruct visitors in natural history.

THE discovery of basket maker remains in cave shelters in southern New Mexico near Las Cruces, and in southwestern Texas in the vicinity of El Paso is the most important result of the Peabody Museum's Southwestern expedition of 1927 under direction of Mr. C. B. Cosgrove. Specimens recovered included the spear thrower or atlatl, long light darts with stone-tipped foreshafts, twined-woven bags, containers made from the skins of small mammals and other objects characteristic of the classic basket maker (Basket Maker II) culture, the earliest agricultural group in the Southwest. The find serves to extend southward by several hundred miles the known range of this very ancient people.

Two research fellowships in organic chemistry carrying a salary of $2,000 each a year have been organized for the coming year in the Sterling Chemistry Laboratory of Yale University. They will be known as the Milton Campbell research fellowships in organic chemistry and will be open only to men who have received their Ph.D. degree. Application for these fellowships with complete credentials should be directed to Professor Treat B. Johnson. A graduate fellowship in organic chemistry has been tendered to the Sterling Chemistry Laboratory by the Eli Lilly Laboratories for the year 1928–29. It has been awarded to Mr. Robert M. Herbst.

A census of the scientific workers of the Soviet Union has been taken by the Russian Academy of Sciences. There are altogether about 26,000 scientific workers active in the U. S. S. R., of which 12,000 are living in Leningrad and Moscow. A reference book on the scientific institutions of the U. S. S. R. is being issued by the academy.

Dr. J. McKeen Cattell, editor of Science, sails for Europe on May 26, returning on August 5. During this interval editorial communications should be addressed to Dr. McKeen Cattell, whose address is Garrison, N. Y.

UNIVERSITY AND EDUCATIONAL NOTES

Colton Laboratory, built and equipped to care for the departments of physics, chemistry and biology at Hiram College, was dedicated May 12. The building consists of three stories over a full basement and is constructed of concrete, brick and stone. It is named in honor of Professor George H. Colton, who was a teacher of the sciences at Hiram College from 1873 to 1926. Addresses were made by Dr. H. C. Cowles, Dr. Harry N. Holmes and Dr. H. B. Lemon, representing, respectively, botany, chemistry and physics.

The departments of mathematics and physics of Princeton University have announced the following special program of graduate courses and lectures during the coming academic year in the field of recent developments in mathematical physics: Professor H. Weyl will lecture on "Group Theory and Quantum Mechanics." He will be assisted by Dr. H. P. Robertson, visiting assistant professor from the California Institute of Technology. Professors Eisenhart and Robertson will offer a course in "The Mathematics of the Newer Quantum Theory." Professor E. U. Condon will give a course in "Wave Mechanics," with special emphasis on the physical concepts and applications.

Dr. James I. Scarborough has been appointed head of the department of surgery at the University of Arkansas, to assume his new duties on September 15.

Dr. Lee Wallace Dean, formerly of the University of Iowa, has been appointed full-time professor of oto-laryngology in the Washington University School of Medicine. Dr. Dean will assume his duties immediately.

The recent promotion of Dr. Selig Hecht to a full professorship of biophysics in Columbia University was incorrectly reported in Science as being in the department of biochemistry.

Dr. J. C. Geiger, for five years connected with the faculty of the University of Chicago, has arrived at the University of California to accept an appointment as associate professor of epidemiology in the medical school and Hooper Foundation for Medical Research.

Dr. M. T. Townsend, of St. John's College, Md., has been appointed associate professor of histology and embryology in the medical school at the University of Oklahoma.

Miss Hope Hibbard, fellow in the International Education Board, at present in Paris, has been appointed assistant professor of zoology at Oberlin College.

Dr. W. W. Jameson has been appointed to the chair of public health at the University of London, tenable at the London School of Hygiene and Tropical Medicine.

Dr. Hermann Sierp, professor of botany in the University of Munich, has been appointed to the chair of botany in the University of Köln.

DISCUSSION AND CORRESPONDENCE

THE LITTLE CIRCLE OF REFERENCE

One usually defines a simple harmonic motion as the motion of the projection of a uniformly circulating point on a fixed diameter. It may sometimes with advantage be defined as the motion of the projection of a fixed circumferential point on a uniformly circulating diameter, relatively to that diameter. In figure 1

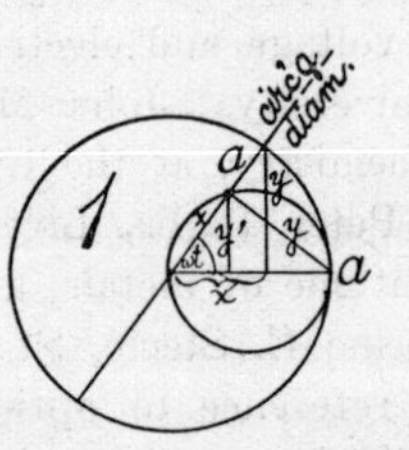

the two y's and the two x's are obviously the same, the angular displacement of the diameter at t seconds being ωt. The foot point from a lies on what may be called the little circle of reference; and since $x=$

cos ωt and $y' = x \sin \omega t = (a/2) \sin 2\omega t$, the new circulating point runs with twice the original angular speed, and half the amplitude. Now suppose the amplitudes a and b in figure 2 are at right angles, and

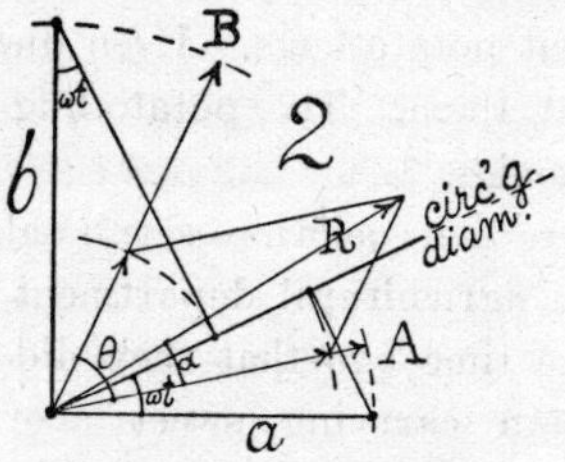

have a common circulating diameter. Their foot points from the ends of a and b will lie on little circles of reference with diameters a and b and at distances $a \cos \omega t$ and $b \sin \omega t$ from the center of the common circulating diameter.

Finally let A and B be any two given vectors of length a and b. Lay off the segments just obtained along the directions A and B, and let R be their sum. Then $R = A \cos \omega t + B \sin \omega t$ the familiar ellipse, selecting A and B as conjugate radii. The relation of the angles ωt and α which begin together, and the constant ϑ (see figure) though easily found, is naturally complicated; but it is usually of no interest.

CARL BARUS
BROWN UNIVERSITY

OCCURRENCE OF A MUTANT MEADOW-MOUSE

WHILE trapping for rodents along the roadside on the outskirts of Ann Arbor, Michigan, an adult female meadow-mouse, *Microtus pennsylvanicus pennsylvanicus,* with marked color differentiation, was captured alive on October 30, 1927. The roadside here slopes gradually to a natural depression, the sides of which are covered with uncut red clover and where Microtus runways are common. The mouse was captured not more than twenty feet from the concrete road. Compared with Ridgway's color chart, the color of the pelage is as follows: back and sides, drab-gray at the tips of the hairs and white at the bases; belly, pale smoke-gray; nose and extending up between and slightly above the eyes, drab; dorsal streak on tail, hair, brown. The eye-color was red. Unfortunately the mouse died on December 16, 1927, curtailing any chance of breeding. It is now preserved as a specimen in the mammalian collection of the University of Michigan.

The authors are indebted to Dr. H. W. Feldman for the following notes concerning the possible genetic constitution of this mutant:

The color-pattern is unmistakably agouti and compared with other mutant forms of murine rodents, the specimen bears a close similarity to the albino allelomorphs. It seems to indicate a condition midway between the ruby-eyed variety of the Norway rat, *Rattus norvegicus* (as described by Whiting and King[1]), and the extreme dilution of the house-mouse, *Mus musculus* (as found by Detlefsen[2]). If the differences in the normal intensity of the pelage coloration of the meadow-mouse are considered, this mutant represents a deviation as great for the former species as extreme dilution does for the latter. Since albino meadow-mice have been noted by Dunn,[3] the albino series in this form probably consists of at least three allelomorphs.

RUTH DOWELL SVIHLA
ARTHUR SVIHLA
MUSEUM OF ZOOLOGY,
UNIVERSITY OF MICHIGAN

NOTES ON THE OCCURRENCE OF SARCOCYSTIS

RECENTLY in the preparation of histological sections of muscle, we encountered two cases of parasitic infestation, which seem worth recording. The parasites appear to belong to the order Sarcosporidia, genus Sarcocystis. Wenyon[1] in his "Protozoology" discusses this order with other groups under the heading, "Parasites of Undetermined Position." The members of the genus Sarcocystis, as the name indicates, share the common characteristic of forming, in one stage of the life cycle, cysts within the fibers of skeletal and cardiac muscle. Within the typical cysts are found the characteristic "banana-shaped" spores. Considerable variation has been reported in the sizes of both the cysts and the spores.

In one of our cases cysts of this parasite occur in the heart-muscle of the ox. The preparations were made especially for the study of the Purkinje fibers, and the parasites are found within these as well as within the ordinary cardiac muscle-fibers. Large normal cardiac fibers measure 36 micra in diameter. The smallest cyst which we have observed in such fibers measures 36 micra. Another in oblique section measures 89 by 440 micra and the largest 105 micra in cross-section, in which latter case no definite remains of the muscle-fiber can be made out. Strands of the syncytium of Purkinje fibers measure from 36 to 240

[1] Whiting, P. W., and King, Helen Dean, 1918, "Ruby-eyed Dilution, a Third Allelomorph in the Albino Series of the Rat." *Jour. Exp. Zool.* 26: 55–64.

[2] Detlefsen, J. A., 1921. "A New Mutation in the House-mouse." *Amer. Nat.* 55: 469–473.

[3] Dunn, L. C., 1921. "Unit Character Variation in Rodents." *Jour. Mamm.*, vol. 2: no. 3: 125–140.

[1] Wenyon, C. M., 1926, "Protozoology," Vol. I, pp. 760–769.

micra in diameter. In a Purkinje fiber of the moderator band a cyst occurs which measures 170 micra. There are cysts in the fibers of the bundle of His ranging in diameter from 60 to 234 micra.

In the second case the cysts are found in the pectoralis major muscle of the turkey-buzzard. Fibers of this muscle measure 56 micra in diameter. Sections of three cysts measure, respectively, 52, 57 and 65 micra. Sections of the buzzard's heart were prepared and studied, but no cysts were found.

The spores within the cysts of the beef-heart measure 3 to 4 micra in diameter and 16 to 18 micra in length. Those in the buzzard measure 2 by 9 micra. In both the beef-heart and the buzzard-muscle the fibers adjacent to those containing cysts appear perfectly normal. Neither is there any connective-tissue-reaction to the presence of the cysts.

Although these parasites have been repeatedly described in the hearts of various species,[2] we have not found specific mention of their occurrence in the Purkinje fibers. Wenyon tabulates thirty-five species of Sarcocystis with four additional cases in which the species were not named. We have found no mention of these parasites occurring in the turkey-buzzard, either in the general literature or in Wenyon's book, although he lists nine other species of birds in which they have been found. The finding of these parasites in the buzzard is interesting in view of Crawley's statement[3] that "whereas the purely herbivorous cattle are practically invariably infected, records of the finding of sarcosporidian cysts in the muscles of carnivorous animals are very rare."

Alexeieff,[4] who studied these forms extensively, concluded that there is no means of telling what the species may be, and that, in spite of variations in size, all belong to the same species. Hence, we merely record that we found Sarcocystis sp. as described above in the Purkinje fibers of the beef-heart and in the skeletal muscle of the turkey-buzzard (*Carthartes aura septentrionalis*).

H. L. OSTERUD,
K. F. BASCOM

MEDICAL COLLEGE OF VIRGINIA,
RICHMOND, VA.

[2] Manifold, J. A., 1924–25, "A Case of Human Sarcosporidiosis." Trans. Roy. Soc. Trop. Med. & Hyg., London, xviii.

Hadwen, S., 1922, "Cyst-forming Protozoa in Reindeer and Caribou and a Sarcosporidian Parasite of the Seal (Phoca richardi)." *J. Am. Vet. M. Assn.*, Vol. lxi.

[3] Crawley, H., 1916, "The Zoological Position of the Sarcosporidia," Proc. Acad. Nat. Sc., Phila., Vol. lxviii.

[4] Alexeieff, A., 1913, "Recherches sur les Sarcospiridies." Arch. de Zool. exp. et gen., li, pp. 521–569.

QUAILS, POTATO-BUGS AND OTHER THINGS

HERE in Beaufort, S. C., there are many potato-bugs and quails. It may not be generally known that quails eat potato-bugs. Even ducks and guineas refuse to eat them. The potato-bug seems to have very few enemies.

Quails here eat acorns—scrub-oak and live-oak acorns. The agricultural department at Washington told me some time ago that they did not know of a live-oak strain carrying sweet acorns. There are three of these trees in Allen Park, Augusta, Ga., and I know one here on the Harvey place. The acorn is as sweet as the meat of a chinquapin, and by the way these chinquapin trees grow here thirty feet high an[d] have bushels of chinquapins on them.

Another interesting tree which grows wild her[e is] the Chinese tallow. Chickens fly up into the tree [to] eat these quite edible seeds. When the pods have burst and an oily seed is placed on a live coal it sends up a white flame six or eight inches high which burns steadily for three or four minutes.

In the up-country the *Magnolia grandiflora* is an ornamental lawn-tree. Down here it is a regular forest-tree only, with diameter of three or four feet and grows along with slash pine and live-oak in the forest.

N. L. WILLET

BEAUFORT, S. C.

THE EARLIEST DYNAMO

I NOTE in your issue of April 13 a notice of the approaching fiftieth anniversary of the invention of the dynamo. I desire to call your attention to the fact that in the Centennial Exposition of 1876 there were two dynamos on exhibition known as the Gramme Dynamo. These machines were made in Paris. At the close of the exposition, Professor Barker, of the University of Pennsylvania, bought the larger of these machines and I bought the smaller one for the young institution of learning, Purdue University. Following the close of the exposition my Gramme machine was sent to Lafayette and installed in the chemical laboratory. I also built a lamp which was very successful, mounted it in the cupola of the university and illuminated the city of Lafayette late in November with the first electric light ever shown west of the Alleghenies and generated by a dynamo. This machine remained in use in the physical and chemical laboratory of Purdue University up to a recent date, and is still in an excellent condition. It has now been installed in the museum of Purdue, properly labeled with the data which I have just described. Evidently the celebration of the fiftieth anniversary of the dynamo should have been held about two years ago.

H. W. WILEY

SCIENTIFIC BOOKS

Biochemical Laboratory Methods for Students of the Biological Sciences. By CLARENCE AUSTIN MORROW, PH.D., John Wiley and Sons, New York, 1927.

THIS book by the late Clarence Austin Morrow, until his death in 1926 professor of biochemistry at the University of Minnesota, is a volume which will be welcomed by all teachers and students in biochemistry, botany, general physiology, pathology, agronomy and bacteriology. It was written by a man who had had extensive teaching experience in biochemical laboratory methods. Each of the experiments given in the book, and there are two hundred and thirty-three, has been thoroughly tested out in the student laboratory by college classes.

The general field of physical and chemical biology is greatly in need of texts. This volume by Dr. Morrow fulfills one of these needs. As one reads the interesting experiments outlined, one wishes again and again that the author had wandered astray to discuss the theory of the behavior of nitrogen-containing compounds. It is hoped, therefore, that this laboratory manual of biochemistry will soon have a companion volume, by some equally capable teacher and writer, dealing with the theory of biochemical behavior.

Too often in laboratory manuals are the time-honored and time-worn methods given so that the student comes to think that this is the only way and these the only materials, but in Dr. Morrow's book this is not the case. The experiments are well chosen and depart in the main from stereotyped forms.

The first chapter is on the "Colloidal State" and covers the subject briefly but well. The only adverse criticism which I can make of Dr. Morrow's book has to do with subject-matter handled in this first chapter. The faults are not serious, and I call attention to them more because they happen to touch upon two subjects in which I, for some time, have had a personal interest. Morrow helps to perpetuate the now antiquated term "emulsoid." This expression has become so firmly established in physical and chemical biology that it seems difficult to eradicate it even though it has long since been discarded by most chemists and never was accepted by such colloidists as Zsigmondy and Donnan. There is not sufficient reason to believe, nor do many workers in the field now believe, that hydrophilic colloids of the gelatin type are fine emulsions. We can, however, partially forgive Dr. Morrow for continuing the use of this expression, a relic from the early days of colloidal chemistry, since he has done the very correct thing of putting the emulsions in a class by themselves, where they, as liquid suspensions, belong.

The second adverse criticism has to do with the support which is given to the attempt of others to draw a distinction between viscous and plastic flow; but here Dr. Morrow has numerous capable investigators on his side. The conception that plastic flow is fundamentally different from viscous flow is a sound one and is based on the fact that viscous substances flow no matter how low the rate of shear, provided the shearing force acts over a sufficient interval of time, while plastic substances do not flow until a certain definite shearing force has been exceeded. Plasticity is made up of two fundamental properties, yield value and mobility. The former is dependent upon the shearing stress required to start deformation, while the latter is proportional to the rate of deformation after the yield value has been exceeded. These properties and the distinction they emphasize between viscous and plastic flow are generally recognized and hold for such a substance as lead which does not exhibit viscous flow until a maximum stress is applied. The fact that lead will flow, as when forced through small holes under pressure, does not interfere with our conception of lead as a solid; but with colloidal jellies the case is different.

To call a thin solution of gelatin or soap a solid, because it possesses such solid properties as elasticity and rigidity, even though its viscosity may be but twice that of water, is as misleading and as meaningless as it would be to call metallic lead a liquid. The distinction between liquid and solid becomes purely arbitrary when applied to colloidal substances of the gelatin type.

But a more serious objection to the point of view that elastic colloidal solutions exhibit plastic flow is that plasticity already has a definite meaning in physics and refers to that property which permits a substance to be deformed and yet show no tendency to return to the original shape. This is not true of elastic colloidal substances such as gelatin, rubber, protoplasm or any jelly.

The whole difficulty in this matter seems to me to lie in the failure to realize that in solutions of gelatin and the like we are dealing with two properties, viscosity and elasticity, and the type of flow is determined by the presence of these two properties. Gelatin is not plastic. No elastic substance can be if we stand by our old and recognized definitions. Gelatin does not at first show true viscous flow because of the interference of elasticity, or, if we get back to the cause of elasticity in jellies, because of the presence of a structural framework. When this structure is broken down, *i.e.*, when the elastic property is completely overcome, as is true at maximum stress, then true viscous flow results. This is seen in determinations by Freundlich of viscosity coefficients of elastic solutions by the capillary (Hess viscometer) method. The measured viscosity value rapidly falls with increase in pressure until a maximum stress (of 60 mm. Hg) is reached when the curve becomes a straight line. At this point of maximum pressure elasticity no longer interferes with capillary flow. The structure of the liquid elastic jelly is broken down and true viscous flow, with constant viscosity values, results. This, then, is the explanation of the deviation from Poiseuille's formula of elastic colloidal solutions.

The preceding criticisms are directed not against Morrow's excellent volume but against two viewpoints which, in the first case, has long persisted in biology, and, in the second case, is a new conception for which there does not appear to be sufficient justification.

The second chapter of Biochemical Laboratory Methods has to do with the Physical Chemical Constants of Plant Saps. Here Morrow gives methods for determining osmotic pressure, molecular weight, water binding power, and electric conductivity, using in every case plant sap as experimental material, thus pointing out that what sometimes appears to be a course in physical-chemistry is really the application of physical-chemical methods to biology.

Chapter three, on H-ion Concentration, illustrates again the excellent method of presentation followed in the book. In this chapter Morrow has given the biological student all he needs to know of H-ion concentration in order to do good work and to understand the subject without losing himself in a maze of theory and mathematics.

Chapter four is on the Proteins, their tests, and their preparation. It is this phase of the subject with which Dr. Morrow was especially well acquainted, and it is also that field of experimental endeavor which has made the Division of Agricultural Biochemistry of the University of Minnesota so well known. The chapter, therefore, becomes a valuable contribution to our knowledge of the isolation of natural plant proteins. Some of the experiments have to do with animal material, as cystine from hair, tryptophane from casein, etc.

Perhaps the most encouraging thing which the teacher of biochemistry will find in the fourth chapter of this book is the realization that it is possible to prepare in the student laboratory reasonably pure plant proteins. The preparations are not easy, but they can be done by the student and have, in addition, the pedagogical value of teaching the student that pure proteins are things to be worked with under carefully controlled conditions. By the time the student has isolated globulin from the peanut, or gliadin from wheat flour, or prepared some of the amino acids such as tryptophane from casein, as described by Morrow, he will have a wholesome respect for the value of his preparations, and yet have the satisfaction of knowing that he can do the work and do it well. The classical work of eminent investigators on plant proteins is likely to discourage not only the student but the teacher from attempting to duplicate even the simplest of these experiments in class laboratories. When confronted with such difficulties it has always been my policy to go ahead and do the best that I can. If the answer to the question of whether or not an experiment is to be attempted is to rest on the degree of precision or purity of the results, then many a biological problem will remain untouched. Who, after all, knows what a pure protein is? The same difficulty confronts every worker on living matter. One of the most impressive features of Morrow's book is the realization that precise physical-chemical methods are brought to bear on biological problems and that biology is gradually becoming an exact science, an encouraging thing when one realizes the many almost insurmountable difficulties involved in experimental work on living matter.

I recall with amusement the irritable attitude of a physicist who objected to my crude method of determining the viscosity of protoplasm. He said it would be so simple a matter to make precise observations by merely running the protoplasm through a capillary viscometer! I remember, too, the similar state of mind of a chemist who was annoyed at my speculating on the structure of protoplasm when he did not yet know the structure of such relatively simple non-living substances as gelatin. It is a joy, therefore, as one reads Morrow's book to appreciate the extent to which chemistry has brought accuracy into biology, just as physics brought accuracy into chemistry, and as mathematics has brought accuracy to all.

Chapter five deals with the Carbohydrates. Methods of extraction and identification of the saccharides are given. A considerable variety of plant material is selected as a source for extracting sugars.

Chapter six on the Glucosides, and seven on the Fats. Animal material is again resorted to, as a source for cholesterol and lecithin.

Chapter eight has to do with Enzymes and chapter nine with Plant Pigments.

These last chapters of the book are much more complete than this brief review indicates, for they represent, as I have said, that field of biochemistry to which Morrow devoted his life. The value of these chapters is greatly added to by the giving of methods which have not before appeared in print, methods developed not only by Morrow himself but by his colleagues.

Dr. Morrow's book on biochemical laboratory methods is one which should be in the hands of every teacher and student in biochemistry, biophysics and physiology.

WILLIAM SEIFRIZ

SCIENTIFIC APPARATUS AND LABORATORY METHODS

A COMBINED FIXATIVE AND STAIN FOR DEMONSTRATING FLAGELLA AND CILIA IN TEMPORARY MOUNTS

BELOW is given a new fixative-stain combination, which has proved to be especially suitable for the rapid preparation of temporary mounts to show flagella and cilia. The reagent contains:

80 cc	saturated solution of phenol in water
20 cc	40 per cent. solution of formaldehyde in water
4 cc	glycerine
20 mgms	gentian violet

It is advisable, in order to facilitate the dissolving of the dye, to moisten it thoroughly with a cubic centimeter of water before adding the other ingredients.

Mix a drop of the reagent with a drop of the culture or infusion containing the organisms to be studied. The flagella and cilia stain clearly, while the cell body remains quite natural in shape and sufficiently transparent to observe the nucleus and the other cytoplasmic structures, such as granules, pharyngeal rods, chloroplasts, pyrenoids, paramylum bodies and the like. The background remains practically colorless, the dye concentrating itself in the organisms. The depth of the stain can be regulated by varying the proportions of reagent to infusion.

The reagent promises to be extremely useful in demonstrating flagella to elementary classes and in identifying the minute flagellates in protozoology courses. It has been used with surprising success on Oicomonas, Tetramitus, Menoidium, Peranema, Euglena, Astasia, Chilomonas, Polytoma, Naegleria and others. It will undoubtedly prove useful as a quick method for studying the flagellated stages of algae, fungi and myxomycetes.

The cilia, cirri, membranelles and undulating membranes of the ciliates are stained by it in approximately natural form, permitting an accurate determination of the number of the ciliary rows, and the arrangement and number of the cirri, membranelles and membranes. To any one who has tried to work out the exact arrangement of the locomotor organelles of a small hypotrich the advantage of such a reagent is obvious.

For staining internal protozoan parasites it is advisable to use more glycerine and dye (approximately 8 cc glycerine and 25 mgms gentian violet have given good results). The presence of mucus interferes with the staining process. It is consequently advisable to mix the material to be examined with three or four times its volume of normal salt solution before using the reagent. With these precautions the method has been used with success on Trichomonas, Chilomastix and Balantidium. With further work along this line it might be possible to develop a method that would materially facilitate the diagnosis of intestinal and other parastic protozoa.

Unfortunately the reagent does not work well with Paramecium, since the discharge of the trichocysts tends to tear away the cilia, but satisfactory preparations have in some cases been obtained in spite of this difficulty. With smaller ciliates, such as Cyclidium, Colpidium, Urotricha, Colpoda and Aspidisca, the method works beautifully; and in larger forms without a heavy trichocyst layer very satisfactory results have been obtained, for example with Stylonchia, Ophryoglena and Chilodon. The cilia stand out as clear blue, individual threads.

Bacteria stain clearly and stand out distinctly against the colorless background. It is possible in the filamentous types to observe the gelatinous sheath in which the rods are imbedded. However, the flagella of the motile forms, such as the larger spirilla and bacilli commonly found in laboratory infusions, do not take the stain.

LOWELL E. NOLAND
UNIVERSITY OF WISCONSIN

REPRODUCING ILLUSTRATIONS WITHOUT A CAMERA

EXACT copies of drawings or photographs are reproduced cheaply and effectively by the following method:

(1) Make the drawing transparent. Saturate the drawing with oil of cedar, oil of cloves or "Three-in-one" oil. Remove the excess of clearing-oil from the surface by blotting the print between sheets of any absorbent paper.

(2) Make a negative. Use an ordinary photographic printing-frame. Print through the transparent original onto glossy paper. The ink of the

original must bear against the emulsion of the paper. Expose approximately the same length of time as a normal negative. Develop and dry the paper.

(3) Make the negative transparent. Repeat processes outlined in (1).

(4) Make any number of the desired prints. Print the transparent negative as in (2). The prints are made on any desired surface of paper. Greatest definition is secured by the use of glossy paper. A good glossy print is as detailed as was the original.

(5) Recover the original drawing. Wash the original print or drawing in xylol, and dry. It returns to its original opaque condition and is none the worse for the processes through which it has passed.

This method is used for reproducing drawings made on stock of as great thickness as an ordinary index-card.

For many kinds of scientific work, the negative secured in (2) is more effective than is the positive secured in (4), due to the reversal of the colors.

EDGAR P. JONES

ZOOLOGY DEPARTMENT,
UNIVERSITY OF PITTSBURGH

SPECIAL ARTICLES

THE PARATHYROID GLANDS AS INFLUENCED BY SELECTIVE SOLAR RADIATON

SINCE hyperplasia of the parathyroid glands occurs in animals kept upon a diet deficient in calcium, and since calcium metabolism is dependent upon vitamin D, present either in the diet or in the lesser wave-lengths of sunlight, an experiment was tried to determine the effect of selective solar radiation upon the parathyroid glands of chicks maintained upon diets in which the content of calcium was adequate.

Four convenient pens were constructed and screened upon their southern exposure by amber, blue, ordinary and vitaglass filters, transmitting variable portions of the sun's spectrum. Each of these four pens was divided by a median partition, so that four pairs of compartments, each pair illumined through a single filter, were thus arranged. The basic diet employed throughout the experiment was the Wisconsin ration, Bulletin 371, Agr. Exp. Station, Madison, Wis. This ration, without the cod-liver oil, was provided the chicks in one compartment of each filter; while the cod-liver oil was added to the diet in the other compartment of each filter. The chicks were placed in he filters on April 22, 1927, and the experiment was discontinued October 25, six months later. Certain chicks in each pen were killed after two, three, four, eight and twelve weeks of experimental observation. The thyroids and parathyroids were fixed in Bouin's fluid, sectioned and stained for histological study. Differential blood counts, serum calcium and phosphorus were determined at frequent intervals throughout the study.

The normal parathyroid tissue in the chick is massed into a pair of small glands which lie at the caudal angle of each thyroid lobe. Each gland is an epithelial structure, surrounded by a thin capsule which continues within the gland as the stroma. The cells comprising the gland are arranged into irregular groups or cords, sometimes alveolar or tubular in organization. The cells are usually large and contain elliptical nuclei with numerous nucleoli. Mitotic figures are frequently seen.

After three weeks of observation a differential growth in these glands under the various filters is manifest. Hyperplasia is more apparent in the glands of those chicks grown under the blue and amber filters on a diet devoid of cod-liver oil. In the chicks kept under these filters and fed the cod-liver oil the glands are smaller than those without the oil, but are larger than the parathyroids of chickens grown in the compartments having vitaglass or ordinary window-glass. Vitamin D, present in the cod-liver oil, appears to compensate partially for the absence of direct sunlight, at least in so far as the size of the parathyroids is concerned.

In the absence of the optimal wave-lengths of sunlight the chicks immediately evidence an increase in the number of parathyroid cells, apparently normal and of entirely functional significance. Chickens taken from compartments with blue or amber filters and maintained upon a diet without the cod-liver oil have parathyroids at the end of one month nine times the size of the gland in a chick grown under the vitaglass filter on the same diet.

Progressive changes within the hyperplastic glands become manifest about the end of the first month. Such regression is first manifest by an increase in the extent of the connective tissue stroma followed by a destruction of the normal cords and columns of cells. Hyperemia is also characteristic of such regression. Two distinct types of cystic degeneration occur within these hyperplastic glands. These cysts appear to be composed of extensive mucoid deposits walled off, in one case, by a high columnar epithelium and in the other case by a series of pavement cells concentrically arranged. The columnar cells of the first type appear to be formed by parathyroid cells of the normal columns, which break away to wall off the developing cyst from the adjacent parathyroid tissue. The origin of the concentric pavement cells is not clear, although those cells appear to arise in connection with the hyperplasia of the connective tissue stroma. Giant cells are frequently found associated with these cysts.

Light of certain wave-lengths appears to bear a definite relationship to the physiology of the parathyroid glands. In the absence of the optimal light factors, an attempt is made by the organism to compensate for this loss by an increase in the total functional activity of the gland. Hyperplasia ensues in the absence of the lesser wave-lengths of sunlight but such hyperplasia is partially obviated by the addition to the diet of a small portion of cod-liver oil. These experiments indicate that normal development of the parathyroids will best maintain in the presence of both the lesser and the greater wave-lengths of sunlight.

GEORGE M. HIGGINS
CHARLES SHEARD
MAYO CLINIC AND MAYO FOUNDATION

A NEW TYPE OF ACID CARBOHYDRATE FROM SEAWEED

NATURALLY occurring acidic materials, essentially carbohydrate in nature, have been known for many years, though they have been investigated comparatively little from the standpoint of structural chemistry. We know little more about the chemistry of gums than was known by the chemists of thirty years ago. Many gums occur in nature as inorganic salts of complex organic acids, which on hydrolysis break down to mixtures of both pentoses and hexoses, and form also acidic products of unknown composition. That these acidic substances are *uronic* acids or polymers or derivatives of such acids is indicated by the fact that they liberate CO_2 when boiled with 12 per cent. HCl and that they give the naphtho-resorcin test.[1] That conjugated *uronic* acids are constituents of many polysaccharides found in plants is indicated by the work of various investigators, among them Nanji and others,[2] Erich Schmidt and coworkers,[3] Schwalbe and Feldtman,[4] and also by unpublished observations of the present writers.

Of late certain substances of this general class, namely, the pectins and the soluble specific substances produced by various types of pneumococcus have been submitted to careful study with interesting results. Ehrlich[5] and his coworkers have found that digalacturonic acid is formed by hydrolysis of pectin, along with sugars—mainly arabinose and galactose—and that this acid or polymers of it constitute a considerable proportion of the pectin molecule. Very recent work by Heidelberger and Goebel[6] shows an aldobionic acid—glucoso-glucuronic—to be the fundamental building stone of the polysaccharide derived from Type III pneumococcus and to be an important constituent in that from Friedlander's bacillus.

We are now able to report, in a preliminary way, a new type of carbohydrate material which apparently is made up completely of *polyuronic* acid. Quantitatively, at least, this material bears the same relation to *uronic* acid that starch does to glucose.

A sample of seaweed, gathered at Woods Hole, Massachusetts, in April and classified as *laminaria agardhii,* was extracted with cold dilute Na_2CO_3. After filtering, the so-called alginic acid was precipitated by addition of HCl and freed from salt by washing and dialysis. It was dried over P_2O_5 to constant weight and analyzed. The results of analysis indicate the formula $(C_6H_8O_6)n$, which is also closely checked by titration with standard alkali. The compound loses 24.5 per cent. of its weight as CO_2 on boiling with dilute HCl. This indicates that the molecule is at least 98 per cent. *uronic* anhydride, probably even more, as the loss of CO_2 from a *uronic* acid is said to be not quite quantitative.[7]

We have also isolated alginic acid from *macrocystis pyrifera*—the giant kelp of the Pacific coast. Our work to date indicates that this material is also a polyuronic anhydride to the extent of at least 98.6 per cent.

But little study, beyond the determination of the analytical data, has been made of the alginic acid from *laminaria agardhii.* Enough work has been done, however, with that from the *macrocystis pyrifera* to indicate that it is a very interesting substance, worthy of careful investigation. The pure acid does not reduce Fehling's solution, but becomes reducing if dried at 100° or if boiled with distilled water for a short time. By the action of heat in the presence of water, the substance loses CO_2. Because of these facts, it is our opinion that the analytical data and physical constants, obtained by previous investigators[8] working with this material, may be inaccurate. Changes were undoubtedly brought about in the substance, before it was analyzed, on drying at 100°.

Schmidt and Vocke[9] have recently isolated what they considered to be a mixture of polyglucuronic acids from *fucus serratus.* These acids, as they found them in the plant, were bound with varying amounts of other carbohydrates. They obtained, on hydrolysis of this material, an acid whose cinchonine salt

[1] Tollens, *Ber.,* 41, 1788, 1908.
[2] *J. Soc. Chem. Ind.,* 44, 253T, 1925.
[3] *Ber.,* 58, 1394, 1925.
[4] *Ber.,* 58, 1534, 1925.
[5] *Biochem. Z.,* 168, 263, 1926; *ibid.,* 169, 13, 1926.
[6] *J. Biol. Chem.,* 74, 613, 1927; *ibid.,* 74, 619.
[7] Nanji, Paton and Ling, *loc. cit.*
[8] Hoagland and Lieb, *J. Biol. Chem.,* 23, 287, 1915.
[9] *Ber.,* 59, 1585, 1926.

melted at 204°, the melting-point of the cinchonine salt of glucuronic acid as reported by Neuberg.[10]

We have hydrolyzed the alginic acid from *macrocystis,* following exactly the method of Schmidt and Vocke, and have obtained a substance having the properties of a hexonic aldehyde acid. Its cinchonine salt melts at 152°. The acid is, therefore, not glucuronic. That this is the case is also indicated by the fact that on oxidation with bromine or nitric acid no saccharic acid was obtained.

The absence of mucic acid in the oxidation products also excludes galacturonic acid as the structural unit of the original material.

Glucuronic and galacturonic acids are the only aldehyde sugar acids hitherto found in nature.

We are continuing work on the chemistry of plant gums and the acidic portions of the algae, and will report more fully in a short time.

LEONARD H. CRETCHER,
WILLIAM L. NELSON
MELLON INSTITUTE OF INDUSTRIAL RESEARCH,
UNIVERSITY OF PITTSBURGH

[10] *Ber.*, 33, 3317, 1900.

SOCIETIES AND ACADEMIES

THE THIRTY-EIGHTH ANNUAL MEETING OF THE OHIO ACADEMY OF SCIENCE

THE thirty-eighth annual meeting of the Ohio Academy of Science was held at the University of Cincinnati, Cincinnati, O., on Friday and Saturday, April 6 and 7, 1928, under the presidency of Dr. Harris M. Benedict, of the University of Cincinnati. The attendance was good, the atmosphere notably congenial, the programs well balanced, the public lectures and sectional papers highly satisfying, and the hospitality of the City of Cincinnati generous and winning. The central theme of the meeting was the relation between physics and biology, as emphasized by the presence and notable lecture of Dr. William T. Bovie, of the Medical College, Northwestern University, on "The Relation of Physics to Biology," the lecture by President Schneider on results from the Basic Laboratory of the University of Cincinnati, the lecture by Dr. S. J. M. Allen on the use of the X-ray as a means of investigating the structure of protoplasm, the lecture by Dr. Albert P. Mathews on some aspects of the problem of coagulation of the blood, and the lecture by J. B. Kelly, of the Bell Telephone Laboratories of New York, on "Recent Researches in Audition." In addition, there were some 85 or 90 papers read before sectional meetings.

The officers elected for the coming year were: *President,* James S. Hine, Ohio State University; *vice-presidents,* zoology, Annette Braun; botany, E. Lucy Braun; geology, Charles H. Behre, Jr.; medical sciences, Albert P. Mathews; psychology, Samuel Renshaw; physical sciences, E. H. Johnson; *secretary,* William H. Alexander; *treasurer,* A. E. Waller; *elective members of the executive committee,* R. C. Osburn and Stephen R. Williams; *trustee research fund,* George D. Hubbard.

Fellowship was bestowed upon the following members: Chas. H. Behre, Jr., Fred A. Hitchcock, Robt. A. Moore, Katharine Dooris Sharp, John P. Visscher and Frank J. Wright, and some 60 or more new members were elected.

The academy went on record as unanimously in favor of H. R. 6091, Seventieth Congress, first session, by Mr. John McSweeney, M. C.

WM. H. ALEXANDER,
Secretary.

SIGMA PI SIGMA CONVENTION

SIGMA PI SIGMA, national honorary physics fraternity, held its convention at Davidson College, Davidson, N. C., April 10 and 11. The reports of the national officers and the delegates from the various chapters showed growth in the strength of the fraternity and an increasing interest in its work. Chapter representatives were present from Davidson College, Duke University, the Pennsylvania State College, Furman University, Centenary College and the College of William and Mary. All the officers and members of the Executive Council were present, as follows: *President,* R. W. Graves; *vice-president,* Marsh W. White; *secretary-treasurer,* H. E. Fulcher; *councilors,* J. M. Douglas, W. N. Mebane and C. C. Hatley.

At the conclusion of the business session on the afternoon of April 10 Professor R. C. Young, of the College of William and Mary, presented a paper on "The Use of the Vacuum Tube Oscillator in Making Laboratory Measurements."

At an open meeting at 7:30 P. M. Professor J. M. Douglas gave a short talk on "The Aims and Ideals of Sigma Pi Sigma." Professor McConnel, of Davidson College, welcomed the fraternity upon behalf of the faculty and the administration of the college. The principal address of the evening was given by Dr. Marsh W. White, of the Pennsylvania State College, upon the subject: "The Energy Relations in X-ray Tubes."

Officers were elected at the business sessions on April 11 as follows: *President,* Professor C. C. Hatley, of Duke University; *vice-president,* Professor R. C. Young, of the College of William and Mary; *secretary-treasurer,* Professor Marsh W. White, of the Pennsylvania State College; *councilors,* Professors J. M. Douglas and W. N. Mebane, of Davidson College.

SCIENCE

VOL. LXVII JUNE 1, 1928 No. 1744

CONTENTS

The Place of Research in the College: PROFESSOR HARRY N. HOLMES ... 539
Early Psychological Laboratories: DR. J. MCKEEN CATTELL ... 543
William Barnum: IRVING M. GREY ... 548
Scientific Events:
The Enlarged Program of Forest Research; The Lasker Foundation for Medical Research; Standard Mathematical Symbols; The Week on Agriculture at the Institute of Chemistry; Award of the Willard Gibbs Medal to Professor W. D. Harkins ... 548
Scientific Notes and News ... 550
University and Educational Notes ... 554
Discussion and Correspondence:
Archimedes and Trigonometry: PROFESSOR G. A. MILLER. *Reproduction Rate in Wild Rats:* PAUL EATON and C. S. STIRRETT. *Vitamin B:* DR. CHAS. H. HUNT. *What is Osmosis?* ORTON K. STARK. *The Preparation of Biological Specimens by Filtration of Paraffin:* DR. OLIVER P. HAY ... 555
Scientific Books:
Pearl's Alcohol and Longevity: DR. W. R. MILES 557
Reports:
The Western Cooperative Oil-Spray Project: E. J. NEWCOMER ... 560
Scientific Apparatus and Laboratory Methods:
A Method for Cutting Glass Tubing: DR. J. L. ST. JOHN. *An Ineffectual Attempt to Demonstrate the Vacuome of Certain Plant Cells:* BERNICE B. RICE ... 561
Special Articles:
The Effect of X-Rays in Producing Return Gene Mutations: PROFESSOR FRANK BLAIR HANSON. *A Spontaneous Modification of the Viscosity of Fresh Blood Serum:* DR. LECOMTE DU NOÜY ... 562
Science News ... x

SCIENCE: A Weekly Journal devoted to the Advancement of Science, edited by J. McKeen Cattell and published every Friday by

THE SCIENCE PRESS

New York City: Grand Central Terminal

Lancaster, Pa. Garrison, N. Y.

Annual Subscription, $6.00. Single Copies, 15 Cts.

SCIENCE is the official organ of the American Association for the Advancement of Science. Information regarding membership in the Association may be secured from the office of the permanent secretary, in the Smithsonian Institution Building, Washington, D. C.

THE PLACE OF RESEARCH IN THE COLLEGE[1]

IT is a common idea, all too common, that research should be left to the universities, research institutes and the great corporations.

"The primary function of the college is to teach!" is a statement often made with misleading emphasis. All good educators agree on the dominant position of teaching in the college, but many know that teaching attains its highest degree of efficiency only when the research attitude of mind is developed in the student and a research atmosphere fostered in the institution. I know teachers whose scholarship and teaching have been vitalized by enthusiasm over their own research problems. The limited time spent on these problems paid rich dividends not measured in dollars alone.

The general misunderstanding of the true nature and the methods of research is appalling. The typical research professor is not, as so many fear, a retiring and very peculiar genius irritated by teaching duties and interested only in his own selfish problems. Instead of neglecting teaching the ideal teacher brings to his lectures the freshness of originality and gives to his words the ring of authority. There are, of course, brilliant men who have no place on a college faculty, but there are also many, ever so many, priding themselves on their exclusive attention to teaching, whose words are as dry dust in the mouth.

Pure research is sometimes damned with the triumphant question, "Of what use is it?" Let J. J. Carty, of the American Telephone and Telegraph Company, give answer. "The pure scientist is the advance guard of civilization." Herbert Hoover adds, "Our whole banking community does not do the public service in a day that Faraday's discoveries do us daily." In speaking of the chemical research on coal-tar that has given the world a thousand beautiful dyes such as were never known before, indispensable medicines, liquid fuels, wood preservatives, high explosives and many other remarkable products, H. H. Gray pays a merited tribute to originality. "After all, only mind can transform the pence of coal-tar into the sovereigns of fine chemicals. Capital can draw the dividends and labor can plume itself on its indispensability, but it is mind which performs the miracle."

[1] Address given at Wittenberg College on the occasion of the dedication of the Laboratory for Chemistry.

It is idle and unfair to quote a few examples of silly and futile research as proof that the whole business would be a waste of college time and money. Sane supervision will protect it from abuse.

There is far too much stress on the informational side of college teaching. We boast that we train the student to think and indignantly deny that we are fact-stuffers, yet most college faculties withhold from the student the most effective method of thought ever developed, the scientific method, the research method. The worst of it is that some of our leaders pride themselves on thus cheating the undergraduate out of his intellectual rights and privileges. The faulty habits of thought that should be trained out of college students are summarized in a forceful way by Fairchild (pamphlet issued by the Character Education Institution of Washington).

INTELLECTUAL IMMORALITIES

(1) Carelessness in observations.

(2) Inaccuracy in determining units to be counted in statistical research.

(3) Slovenliness in logic, fantastic explanations.

(4) Generalizing beyond one's data.

(5) Confusing opinions with knowledge.

(6) Contentment with "discussion."

(7) Egoism allowed to crowd one to the invention of "new" theories for personal distinction.

(8) Inventing interesting theories for the sake of selling them in books, articles, lectures and conversation.

(9) Formulating an hypothesis on weak bases of facts, and then becoming blind to facts in opposition.

(10) Emotionalism during research, "I believe" instead of "I have proved."

(11) Opposition to a theory merely because of ignorance and stupidity, "I can not see how."

(12) Rushing into print with a report of research work that justifies no conclusions.

(13) Cowardice in supporting a verified generalization because it is unpopular and conflicts with selfish interests.

(14) Impatience, unwillingness to proceed step by step through a research.

(15) Indulgence in dense verbiage for the sake of appearing superlearned.

(16) Poularizing tentative generalization for the sake of personal publicity.

(17) Resort to the authorities, or to sarcasm and ridicule, against data, arguments and verifications.

"Verification" seems to have been too little appreciated in college circles as a factor essential to all research supposed to be on the scientific level. We must do more than indulge in "views, theories and endless discussions."

An indignant believer in the scientific method of thinking writes me, "My cousin is the wife of a great scientist, but she has lost her senses over the modern fake imitations of psychology and writes articles without any conscience as to verification of her generalizations; the spirit of the fantastic thinker is in her rather than that of the scientist."

Ira Remsen believed in the ethical virtues of research. The essential honesty of a scientist with his problem appealed to Remsen as making for superior character. The late Charles D. Walcott, former secretary of the Smithsonian Institution, went further and insisted that a good research man ought to make a good Christian and a good Christian ought to make a good research man because both are in search of truth.

Herbert Hoover well says, "If we would command the advance of our material, and to a considerable degree, of our spiritual life, we must maintain the earnest and organized search for truth. We could well put such an appeal wholly upon moral and spiritual grounds; the unfolding of beauty, the aspiration to knowledge, the ever-widening penetration into the unknown, the discovery of truth, and finally, as Huxley says, 'the inculcation of veracity of thought.'"

If we hope to inspire the college youth we must make him feel that he is drinking from a fresh spring of knowledge rather than from a stagnant pool. As one keen student remarked, "I notice that the teaching is better when there is some research going on around the corner."

Oberlin's great librarian, Azariah Root, in the last year of a scholarly life, announced to a college committee, "What Oberlin must do is to spend more money on research and to encourage it in every way in order to keep our faculty from growing stale." Oberlin is probably doing as much in research as any pure college, but there is much more to do. An inspired faculty develops an inspired student body.

"Research by stealth" is an unpleasant phrase used to describe the situation in some colleges where the professor is expected to spend his entire time in routine teaching. A recent questionnaire disclosed the fact that only a very limited number of college presidents are willing to encourage research by financial aid for productive work. Some others are willing to have national honor brought to the college by research publications of its faculty if no expense is involved. This short-sighted policy cheats the students by driving away the ambitious, productive scholars of the faculty.

Without a staff of productive men how shall the college meet the challenge of the gifted students? Informational teaching is not adequate, but sound instruction in the research method of approach to all problems will stimulate the gifted student to his best. Even a freshman will ignite from the right sort of spark, although he will not actually engage in research. Instead of describing achievements to him in the final form the instructor can lead him in fancy, step by step, through all the difficulties preliminary to great discoveries, disclose the original plans and hopes, and arrive at the climax of successful achievement with dramatic force. It is more than the historical method, it is the living, breathing, thrilling method of teaching.

In actual practice undergraduates respond eagerly when asked to walk occasionally in the footsteps of the great masters of the past. Many of them get from the experience "a sense of unlimited possibilities, of adventure and of exultant hope." They can be thrilled with the conception of research as service to humanity in conquering yellow fever, in making the surgeon's work safe with antiseptics and merciful with anesthetics, in averting a predicted world wheat famine, in making every man your neighbor by marvelous improvements in communication and transportation, and by reducing the working day of fifteen hours, common a century ago, to the modern day of eight hours with its increased possibilities for health, comfort, culture and the pursuit of happiness. To prove to the youthful mind that the pure research of Faraday, Henry and others made possible the electrical industry which in the United States now multiplies the man-power of our population is to give a vivid impression of service. Slaves rushing along a wire at the touch of a button to run our errands, lift us to the lofty floors of our office buildings, run our washing machines, sweep our floors and save us from drudgery even as a thousand captives once slaved for a petty king of the long ago!

Beyond the question of inspiring the undergraduate and training his mind in the mastery of the varied problems of life is the moral obligation on the college to acknowledge its debt to the past by adding something new to the sum total of knowledge. Is it right for a great institution of learning to hand out facts other faculties have gathered without sharing in production? Carlyle exclaimed, "Produce, if it be but the pitifullest infinitesimal fraction of a product, in God's name produce."

The sciences, it must be admitted, have done more than the non-sciences in recognizing this obligation. Professor John R. Commons, of the University of Wisconsin, has extended this statement to include the universities, "To acquire knowledge—the existing knowledge—is the retail store method, the hand-me-down method. The research method is just opposite; it is the discovery method. We do not acquire knowledge, we discover knowledge, using the dig-it-up method. In economics, in sociology, in philosophy, in all those sciences which have to do with the great laboratory of human life throughout the community, we have not yet learned the laboratory method, the dig-it-up method."

The American Historical Association, in a recent report, admits that fewer than one fourth of the holders of the Ph.D. degree in history are productive scholars. A quotation from this report follows: "Presidents, especially of the smaller colleges, insist on having Ph.D.'s on their faculties, not because they expect or wish them to be productive scholars, but largely for advertising purposes. The large universities are thus crowded with mediocre graduate students, many of whom can not be taught the technic of research except with great difficulty. It is still more difficult, and often impossible, to inspire them with a passion for research. One important reason for lack of production is a widespread belief that research does not pay. It is alleged that many who are productive fail to gain the reward they might reasonably expect; that presidents of colleges and universities give lip-service to research, but do not take it into consideration to any great extent in making promotions or increases in salary; that, therefore, Ph.D.'s seek to advance by teaching, wire-pulling and 'social stunts.'"

Bertrand Russell and the Bishop of Ripon are suggesting that if scientists desist from discovery for ten years the rest of the world might catch up and adjust itself to a condition of tranquility. This is an admission of weakness, not an acceptance of a challenge. Evidently the eight hundred thousand college students of this country need an insight into the scientific method of collecting facts by many accurate, unbiased observations, of classifying and comparing facts, of explaining the facts with a theory or generalization, of rigidly and honestly testing the theory and of using the tested theory to predict future behavior.

There are, of course, difficulties in making research an integral part of college teaching. Many men now on college faculties, though trained to research, in the struggle for the Ph.D. degree have allowed this acquired talent to atrophy. Now they shrink from any belated demand for productivity. It is difficult to blame them. Rather let us blame the college for overloading such men with mere routine teaching and for a general failure to recognize, encourage and reward a proper amount of productivity. The cost is a veritable lion in the path, but must it forever stand in the path to the highest excellence?

Adequate reward for research will doubtless bring on its attendant evils. Publications of an inferior order will be cited for promotion, but it is easy to get the judgment of leaders in a given field as to the quality of original work. Time will, in a few instances, be frittered away on silly struggles to be original, but why not, in the future, deny to such men the opportunities to continue this waste? "To him that hath (the Divine spark) shall be given, and to him that hath not shall be taken away."

The Division of Educational Relations of the National Research Council suggests:

WAYS TO AID RESEARCH IN COLLEGES

Give research a place in faculty meetings on a parity with teaching problems.

Give research, as a matter of course, recognition in the budget of each department of study; grants for apparatus, literature, research assistants, etc.

Have special research fund for special grants, this to be administered by the research committee. Emphasize dignity and importance of this committee.

Give stenographic and clerical assistance to faculty members to conserve their time and energy for teaching and research.

Cut down hours of teaching.

Large faculties, small classes.

Leaves of absence, on salary, for intensive study.

Consultation trips by college men to the research centers for advice and conference and reading.

Exchange of teachers between universities and colleges (and perhaps exchange of research men between industry and the colleges).

Assistance toward expense of attending professional society meetings.

Research as well as teaching success recognized as a basis for promotion.

Special professorships for those markedly successful in both research and teaching, with added time and assistance for research, and additional salary.

Appointment of occasional research associates giving full time to research.

Encouragement of research for the M.A. degree; also special stipends for M.A. students who shall assist professors in their research.

Research scholarships for outgoing seniors and for recent graduates to study in research institutions.

Develop the library for assistance to research as well as to teaching.

The appointment or election of a standing research committee on the college faculty is vitally important.

FUNCTIONS OF A COLLEGE RESEARCH COMMITTEE

Promote appreciation of importance of research on the part of all members of the college community, including trustees, administrative officers, faculty students and donors.

Survey and list the researches in progress in the institution.

List the more important researches published in the past from the college.

Gather and classify information in regard to the entrance of graduates upon research, and list the ablest men among the graduates of the college.

Learn, classify and list the assistance needed for: (a) researches in progress, (b) researches it is desired to undertake. Assist in plans for securing such aid.

Publish these items for circulation in the college community.

Publish an annual report for circulation in the college.

Assist in securing cooperation between faculty members in research.

Study and suggest possible correlations between researches under way in the college.

Consider publication of research results—perhaps advisable, especially for studies of local environment. Publication assistance is especially needed in the so-called ''humanities.'' Avoid encouraging publication of unworthy papers.

Secure a liberal research fund, grants from which shall be administered by the research committee.

Exchange with local committees in other colleges information as to methods and success in promotion of research.

Arrange for presentation to the students, by men from the several departments and from outside the college, of the life devoted to research, in the several major fields. This is important in securing recruits for the life of research.

Encourage departmental clubs which shall report and discuss research and newer phases of progress in knowledge, discussing also the men through whose research mankind have made great advance.

Encourage work by semi-research methods in the curriculum, putting some of this work as early as the sophomore year.

Encourage establishment of societies and fraternities which reward research ability.

Present research to community by lectures and exhibits.

Urge value of administrative assistants to relieve faculty members of detailed committee work.

Ten years ago Oberlin College, at the request of the National Research Council, elected a science research committee and made it a standing committee of the faculty with all the privileges thus implied. The small original committee set a high standard of election. Every man on a science faculty was asked to submit a list of his research publications exclusive of his doctor's thesis. If his independent work published in journals of good standing measured up in quality and quantity he was recommended for election, which always followed as a faculty endorsement. It is now considered an honor to be a member of this committee. At occasional dinners the members discuss the situation and plan for the future.

In addition to this group of scientists a "Committee on Productive Scholarship" is now being formed in somewhat similar fashion. However, the qualifications include authorship of books (other than mere compilations) and musical compositions of merit as well as scientific research. Obviously productive work in the entire faculty will be encouraged and made prominent.

All this is eminently worth while if we agree with President Angell, of Yale, who urges that "Individual initiative, resourcefulness, ingenuity, imagination, vision, must be kept at a high pitch all along the line."

HARRY N. HOLMES

OBERLIN COLLEGE

EARLY PSYCHOLOGICAL LABORATORIES[1]

LABORATORIES for research and teaching in the sciences are of comparatively recent origin. They may be regarded as part of the industrial revolution, for there is a close parallel in causes and effects between the development of the factory system and of scientific laboratories. The industrial revolution began with the exploitation by machinery of coal and iron in England; it may perhaps be dated from the use of the steam engine of Watts in the coal mines of Cornwall about a hundred and fifty years ago.

The laboratory had its origin fifty years later in Germany as part of the scientific renaissance following the Napoleonic wars. The University of Berlin was founded by Wilhelm von Humboldt and Frederick William III in 1810. The first laboratory of chemistry was opened by Justus von Liebig at Giessen in 1824. This was followed by similar laboratories at Göttingen under Wöhler in 1836, at Marburg under Bunsen in 1840, and at Leipzig under Erdmann in 1843. The first English laboratory was the College of Chemistry, now part of the Imperial College of Science and Technology of the University of London, which was opened in 1845 by von Hoffmann, brought from Germany by Prince Albert. Benjamin Silliman founded at Yale University the first American laboratory for the teaching of chemistry.

Prior to the industrial revolution the artisan worked at home, sometimes with 'prentices, who were often his children. The factories, the mines and the systems of transportation, with their machinery, their skilled overseers and division of labor, their owners and entrepreneurs, their exchange of commodities and ideas, created a remarkable economy in production, so that now each individual may perhaps work half as long and consume twice as much wealth as formerly. But there are serious drawbacks in the lack of freedom and initiative of the workman, in the loss of joy in creative work. The situation in the laboratory is similar. A professor may have many associates, assistants and students; expensive apparatus and extensive libraries may be installed; division of labor in each laboratory and among laboratories can be planned; there may be exchange of ideas and of information on the progress of research; students are taught in large groups. Production is greatly increased, perhaps quadrupled, as in the industrial system. But the scientific man is subject to administrative controls; he is no longer free; he must compromise with others and teach all sorts of students. The system is useful for the production of a large mass of routine work; it may not be favorable to creative genius.

Anatomy has been called the mother of the sciences; dissecting rooms go back to the medieval universities of Italy. Observatories, museums, botanical gardens, academies of science and university schools, where research was undertaken and in which students and assistants were taught and trained, preceded organized laboratories. Chemistry is the gold transmuted through alchemy; we have all seen on the stage the laboratory of Faust. Christian fathers say that when "the sons of God saw the daughters of men, that they were fair and they took them wives," as told in the sixth chapter of Genesis, these fallen angels taught the fair daughters of men the arts of astrology and alchemy. Scientific men who do not care for special creations may assume that there has been a gradual development from the time of the first experiment by an anthropoid ape, or it may be by a paramecium or an electron. If, however, we want an official beginning for the first scientific laboratory, it will be the laboratory of chemistry at Giessen, the hundredth anniversary of whose foundation was celebrated three years ago.

Chemical laboratories were followed by laboratories of physics and biology. I worked in the first American biological laboratory in its early days. It was established at the Johns Hopkins University by Newell Martin, a student of Huxley, who at the Royal College of Science had founded the first laboratory of biology. From the laboratories of Martin and Brooks at the Johns Hopkins have proceeded many of our most eminent biological workers. The Johns Hopkins also led in the establishment under Welch, Mall, Abel and Howell of laboratories in the medical sciences. But there is obviously no sharp line of demarcation between the modern laboratory and earlier groups of workers, such as the great school of zoology conducted by Agassiz at Harvard.

The first laboratory of psychology was established by Wilhelm Wundt. In an article on the Leipzig laboratory, published in *Mind* in 1888 and submitted to Professor Wundt, I give the date as 1879. The fiftieth anniversary of the founding of the labora-

[1] Address on the occasion of the inauguration of the Psychological Laboratory of Wittenberg College, Springfield, Ohio, October 21, 1927.

tory was, however, celebrated at Leipzig in 1926. Wundt published his "Grundzüge der physiologischen Psychologie" in 1874 and was called from Zürich to a chair of philosophy at Leipzig in 1875. The *Psychologische Institut* there was a gradual development. Wundt writes in his autobiography "Erlebtes und Erkanntes," published in 1920, that Kraepelin, Lehmann and I were his three earliest "Arbeitsgenossen" who remained faithful to psychology and that we worked with him at a time when the institute was his private undertaking and lacked official recognition on the part of the university. The first research published from the Leipzig laboratory was apparently a doctor's dissertation by Dr. Max Friedrich carried out during the winter semester of 1879–80.

Wundt writes in the preface to the "Physiologische Psychologie" that it undertakes "ein neues Gebiet der Wissenschaft abzugrenzen," but he was partly anticipated by Hermann Lotze, whose "Medizinische Psychologie" was published in 1852. Both Lotze and Wundt had a medical education and were professors of philosophy. Their books are landmarks in the history of our science. It was my privilege to hear the last course of lectures on psychology by Lotze given at Göttingen in the winter semester of 1880–81. In accordance with the custom of that university Lotze dictated summaries which could be written down verbatim even by one who had small psychology and less German. The "Dictata" of that year were published and have been translated into English. In the spring of 1881 Lotze, then 74 years of age, migrated to Berlin and died, according to Göttingen opinion, of homesickness.

Herbart, whom Lotze succeeded at Göttingen, had tried to give a mathematical formulation to psychology as Spinoza had to philosophy. He published the first edition of his "Einleitung in die Philosophie" in 1813. There followed Drobitsch, Lindner, Benecke, Volkmar and other German psychologists. In England we have the notable development of association and analytic psychology from Locke through Berkeley, Hume, the Mills and Bain to Ward. The first edition of Carpenter's "Mental Physiology," to-day a useful and readable book, was published in 1874, the same year as Wundt's "Grundzüge." In England and in France there were numerous workers in the fields of physiological and pathological psychology.

The most important developments for laboratory psychology were through the great German physiologists and physicists, most of all Helmholtz, who passed from physiology to physics. His "Physiologische Optik," recently translated under the editorship of Professor Southall and published as an act of piety by the Optical Society, and his "Tonempfindingen," of which there is an earlier translation, are classics in the history of science. E. H. Weber became professor of anatomy at Leipzig in 1818 at the age of twenty-three, being later transferred to physiology. The law that bears his name was stated in his "Annotationes," published from 1834 to 1851. Fechner was appointed professor of physics at the same university in 1834; his "Zendavesta" was published in 1851, his "Elemente der Psychophysik" in 1860. When I was a student at Leipzig he was over eighty-five years old and blind from experiments on vision, a charming man, intensely interested in his psychophysical experiments, though chiefly in philosophical interpretations.

The middle fifty years of the last century were the golden age of the German university and of science, its *Wunderkind.* It is marvelous what was accomplished then and there. Thus in the little corner of the field of science concerned with the psychology of the sense of vision there worked, in addition to Helmholtz and Fechner, a notable company, including Aubert, Brücke, du Bois-Reymond, Donders (in Holland), Exner, Fraunhofer, Fick, von Graefe (who examined my eyes when I was a child of eight), Hering, Hermann, von Kries, Listing, Johann Mueller, Nagel, Purkinje, Vierordt, the Webers and many more. There is no such group in the world to-day working on vision or in any other part of experimental psychology. At that time the investigation of the other senses, of movement, of the time of reaction and much else was pursued probably to greater effect than in all the innumerable laboratories of to-day.

The fields so fertile in the nineteenth century were of course cleared at an earlier time. Experiments on vision go back to Kepler, Huygens and Newton. Weber's law was anticipated by Bouguer and Lambert; Fechner's law by Bernouilli and Laplace; the personal equation by the astronomers. Observations on after-images were made not only by Goethe, the elder Darwin, Buffon and Newton among others, but also by Augustine and Aristotle. Very curiously the problems of psychological measurement were clearly stated by the poet Shelley, who more than a hundred years ago wrote: "A scale might be formed, graduated according to the degrees of a combined scale of intensity, duration, connexion, periods of recurrence, and utility, which would be the standard, according to which all ideas might be measured."

When I came across this passage in Shelley it seemed almost incredible that he of all men should have written it, as indeed it is that the most unearthly of poets should have been the son of a country squire. But England has always given birth to great men in families and as sports. It has been said that Graham Bell—he too was British—could not have invented the telephone if he had been a physicist, for he would have known that it was impossible; so it may be said that Francis Galton could not have accomplished his great work toward founding modern psychology if he had been a psychologist, for he would have known that it was not psychology. Galton, like Darwin, his cousin, had no university position and no laboratory. He published his "Hereditary Genius" in 1869, his "Inquiries into Human Faculty" in 1883.

With intermissions I was a student at Leipzig under Wundt from 1881 to 1886, serving during the last year as laboratory assistant in psychology, the first to be appointed there or anywhere. Wundt had a higher opinion, doubtless with good reason, of American enterprise than of American scholarship. In his reminiscences he writes that with "bekannter Amerikanischer Entschlossenheit" I approached him and declared: "Herr Professor, you need an assistant and I shall be your assistant." He was the most kindly of men and was much worried lest I should not pass my doctorate examination in physics under Hankel and in zoology under Leuckhart, but these distinguished professors also fortunately made due allowance for a child of the wilderness. Wundt's combined courtesy and remoteness from the modern world may be illustrated by an incident. At that time women were seldom admitted to university lectures, but at my request he gave permission to an American of fine intelligence to attend his course on psychology, which was frequented by two or three hundred students, among them the most stupid in the university, for all theological students were required to attend. One day he said: "I am sorry that I let Miss X attend my lectures; it embarrasses me; I feel that I ought to speak in a way that a woman can understand."

When I showed Wundt an outline of the work that I proposed for a doctor's thesis on the reaction-time, including complicated responses and a study of individual differences his comment was: "ganz Amerikanisch." As a matter of fact I did the work in my own rooms and with my own apparatus. At that time students were expected to work in the laboratory on a subject assigned by the professor, during certain definite hours in the afternoon and with the apparatus supplied, which had to be put away neatly in the cases after a two-hour period. We used two batteries of Daniel cells and when these were set up and got into running order it was nearly time to take them apart, wash the zincs and coppers and put the fluids into bottles. As in this process we were likely to splash sulphuric acid on our clothes we kept handy a bottle of ammonia, which was very promptly applied to the stains. At that time I anticipated Dr. Watson in an observation on the conditioned reflex, for when the German student who worked with me drew a mouthful of dilute sulphuric acid through the syphon that we used, he immediately reached for the ammonia bottle and took a mouthful of that.

In the early eighties Wundt's laboratory was housed on the top floor of the *Convict* building, where indigent students had their meals. He used to walk through the laboratory after his lecture, always courteous and ready to answer questions, but, as I remember it, usually limiting his visit to five or ten minutes. He was interested in the laboratory as a system and as a method of introspection, but he was not himself a laboratory worker. His interests were very broad. His "Logik," published from 1880 to 1883, contains in the second edition 1,995 pages; his "Ethik," also published while I was at Leipzig, contains in its third edition 933 pages. The "System der Philosophie," published in 1889, contains in its third edition 738 pages. The last edition of the "Physiologische Psychologie" contains 2,317 pages, the "Völkerpsychologie," 3,161 pages. And they are very large pages.

These books and others Wundt composed on a typewriter that I gave him, one of the first in Germany. Avenarius once remarked that I had by this gift done a serious disservice to philosophy, for it had enabled Wundt to write twice as many books as would otherwise have been possible. At that time the relations of German professors were curious from an American point of view. Wundt was not in friendly relations with Helmholtz, Stumpf, Müller and others. Stumpf, next to Wundt the most distinguished of German psychologists, was professor at Halle, only three quarters of an hour by train from Leipzig, and Wundt was asked for an introduction. He said that he was sorry that he could not give it, as he did not know Professor Stumpf personally; it was better so, for they could then write more freely when there was a difference of opinion—and they did a couple of years later.

At the beginning of the semester students who wanted to undertake experimental work stood before Wundt in a row and from a slip of paper that he held in his hand he assigned topics in order. The year that I appeared there were six or seven of us, representing nearly as many nationalities. I was given the problem of reacting to colored lights; first when the light was seen, and second when the color was distinguished, and by subtracting one time from the other of obtaining what Wundt called the "Apperceptionszeit." This I could not do, but the problem was most useful to me, for it led me to realize the limitations of introspection and to base my work on objective measurements of behavior. Wundt's refusal to admit any subject to the laboratory except a psychologist who could use the results introspectively was also useful, for it led me to transfer the work to my rooms and make there the first psychological measurements of individual differences and to attempt to develop the useful applications of psychology—with both of which efforts Wundt had no sympathy.

Wundt rejected as a doctorate dissertation Münsterberg's very able monograph on "Die Willenshandlungen" because it did not coincide with his own theories. He calls Stanley Hall's excellent sketch of his life and work an "erdichtete Biographie die von Anfang bis zu Ende erfunden ist." But such things were only the righteous indignation of the Hebrew prophet denouncing the enemies of the Lord. The academic life in Germany in those days was exalted. The nation, the university, the professor, were sacrosanct. It was a fine experience to be admitted to the outer court of the temple before the money changers had entered. Wundt himself was the ideal German professor, with boundless learning shading toward the pedantic, fully conscious of his plenary inspiration, yet withal most modest, shy and kindly; a seer before his students, a child at home, a truly great man.

Wundt's laboratory of psychology was international in its reputation and influence, attracting students from all parts of the world, Americans and Russians predominating. In 1892 it received larger quarters and in 1897 was removed to one of the buildings vacated by the Medical School, where fourteen rooms were remodeled for its purposes. In the late eighties there were beginnings of laboratories under Ebbinghaus at Berlin, under Müller at Göttingen, and under students of Wundt who were my contemporaries and friends, Münsterberg at Freiburg, Martius at Bonn, and Lehmann at Copenhagen.

The second laboratory of psychology was organized by G. Stanley Hall at the Johns Hopkins University early in the year 1883. I was there before Hall, holding a fellowship in philosophy, this award for a thesis on Lotze having been made by the professor of Latin, who knew even less about philosophy than I did, or the fellowship would have been given to John Dewey. He was there as a student, as were also Joseph Jastrow and H. H. Donaldson. We helped Hall set up a modest laboratory in a private house adjacent to the center of ugly little brick buildings and great men that formed the university. The small group of professors working there included Remsen, Rowland, Sylvester, Gildersleeve, Haupt, Adams, Brooks and Martin.

It is a curious fact that neither of the founders of our first two psychological laboratories was a laboratory worker. Hall's chair, like Wundt's, was not limited to psychology; he lectured on philosophy and he also conducted courses in pedagogy. The range of his interests was large, but it was the human aspects of life that he cared for rather than abstract quantitative measurements. Like James he was a man of literary genius swayed by the emotions, which are such a large part of life and as yet such a small part of our science. Minot, the distinguished Harvard embryologist, once said that he envied my occupation with a science concerned with human interests. My reply was that my experiments had as little to do with such things as his had with love and children. Hall wrote about children, adolescence and senescence, religion and sex, the drama of life. He and James were giants in the land, overtowering their descendants of a work-a-day world.

As Wundt established the *Philosophische Studien* to publish the work from his laboratory and his own articles on psychology and philosophy, so Hall established the *American Journal of Psychology*. The early volumes give a survey of the work done in Baltimore, which was largely physiological and psychiatrical. Hall was much interested in insanity and other pathological aspects of psychology and we used to go regularly to the Bayview Hospital for the Insane. These interests were maintained and in the last conversation that I had with him in his lonely house at Worcester he wanted especially to know why orthodox American psychologists cared so little for Freud and psychoanalysis. He showed me a mass of publications and notes that he had collected on the subject.

Hall was called upon to organize Clark University in 1888 and gathered there a group of outstanding scientific men, including Michelson, Webster, Bolza, Neff, Whitman, Mall, Donaldson, Lombard, McMurrich and Boas. The financial support of the university by Mr. Clark was less liberal than had been anticipated and Dr. Harper took over in a body a large part of these men for the faculty of the new University of Chicago. In his "Life and Confessions" Hall remarks: "I felt his act comparable to that of a housekeeper who would steal in at the back door to engage servants at a higher price." Sanford went with Hall from the Johns Hopkins to Clark and became director of the laboratory of psychology which was opened in 1889. The Johns Hopkins laboratory was closed and the apparatus dispersed until it was reestablished by Professor Baldwin and Professor Stratton. Hall and Clark University long maintained a dominant position in psychology and the psychological side of education. In his death there ends the romantic and heroic era of our science.

The laboratory of psychology at the University of Pennsylvania was founded by me in 1887, though it was only in January, 1889, that a special laboratory with adequate equipment of apparatus was opened. The laboratories at Leipzig and the Johns Hopkins were for research, and psychology was only part of the field covered by the professor. At the University of Pennsylvania a professorship of psychology was for the first time established and laboratory courses for students were for the first time given. It might consequently be argued by a partial advocate that this was the first laboratory of psychology in the sense that Liebig's chemical laboratory at Giessen was the first scientific laboratory. More significant is the circumstance that in this laboratory the research work and the courses for students were based on objective measurements of responses to the environment with special reference to individual and group differences and to the useful applications of psychology, thus leading to the development of modern educational, clinical and industrial psychology.

In 1888 I was also lecturer at Bryn Mawr College and at the University of Cambridge, conducting in both institutions laboratory courses for students. At Cambridge the work was in conjunction with the lectures of Professor James Ward and in the Cavendish laboratory of which the present Sir Joseph Thomson was the director, having just before, at the age of twenty-six, succeeded Maxwell and Rayleigh in the professorship of physics. In the Cavendish laboratory was also set up apparatus for research and this was the beginning of the first British laboratory of psychology. At that time I had the privilege of assisting Galton in the arrangement of the Anthropometric Laboratory in the South Kensington Museum and we began in cooperation the preparation of a book of instructions for a laboratory course in psychology.

The five-year period from 1887 to 1892 is distinguished for the development of laboratories of psychology in the United States. For earlier work tribute should in passing be paid to James McCosh, Presbyterian clergyman from Scotland and president of a Presbyterian college, who at Princeton promoted the study of organic evolution and physiological psychology. George Trumbull Ladd, also a clergyman, was called to Yale as professor of philosophy in 1881 and developed there courses in physiological psychology, leading to the publication in 1887 of his "Outlines of Physiological Psychology." With James and Hall he shares the honor of leading in the development of psychology in America. The laboratory at Yale was organized by Professor Ladd in 1892 with Dr. E. W. Scripture as instructor.

Work in experimental psychology leading to the establishment of a laboratory was begun by Professor Joseph Jastrow at Wisconsin in 1888. His service as professor of psychology is the longest in the history of our science. A year or two later laboratories were established at Indiana University by President W. L. Bryan, at the University of Nebraska by Professor H. K. Wolfe, at Brown University by Professor E. B. Delabarre and at Stanford University by Professor Frank Angell. Professor J. Mark Baldwin was called to Toronto in 1890 and established there a psychological laboratory, as he did at Princeton when he returned to that university in 1893. In 1895 we together founded the *Psychological Review*, which, with its children, *The Psychological Monographs*, *The Psychological Index*, *The Psychological Bulletin*, the *Journal of Experimental Psychology*, and the newly established *Psychological Abstracts*, have now, through the generous cooperation of Professor Warren, been acquired and are being conducted by the American Psychological Association.

The professorship of psychology and the laboratory of psychology at Columbia University date from 1891. There worked Professor Thorndike, Professor Woodworth and many others who have led in the development of modern psychology. The following year is notable for the establishment of the psychological laboratories at Harvard and Cornell and the calling to America of Hugo Münsterberg and E. B. Titchener. At Cornell the traditions of the Leipzig laboratory have been best maintained. Titchener brought to us the scholarship of the Oxford don and the research ideals of the German professor. Now he has followed James, Hall and Münsterberg, leaving the world more drab and empty.

Where were James, Royce and Münsterberg was the center of psychology. James was appointed professor of psychology at Harvard in 1889, having been from 1872 to 1880 instructor and assistant professor of comparative anatomy and physiology, after 1880 assistant professor of philosophy, becoming again professor of philosophy in 1897. His great work, "The Principles of Psychology," was published in 1890. In a letter addressed to me as editor of SCIENCE in 1895 James thus tells of the development of work in experimental psychology at Harvard: "I, myself, 'founded' the instruction in experimental psychology at Harvard in 1874–5, or 1876, I forget which. For a long series of years the laboratory was in two rooms of the Scientific School building, which at last became choked with apparatus, so that a change was necessary. I then, in 1890, resolved on an altogether new departure, raised several thousand dollars, fitted up Dane Hall, and introduced laboratory exercises as a regular part of the undergraduate psychology-course. Dr. Herbert Nichols, then at Clark, was appointed in 1891 assistant in this part of the work; and Professor Münsterberg was made director of the laboratory in 1892."

With the publication of James's "Principles of Psychology" in 1890, the opening of the laboratories at Harvard, Yale and Cornell in 1892, and the establishment of the American Psychological Association in the same year, the earlier period of psychology in America may be closed. The few survivors may look back upon it as the golden age of our science, but that is doubtless due only to the presbyopia that obscures the vision of objects near at hand. In the thirty-five years that have since passed the number of our workers in psychology has increased to an extent perhaps without parallel in any other country or in any other science. We welcome the opening at Wittenberg College of a new laboratory which, under the direction of Professor Reymert, will become a new center for psychological teaching and research.

J. McKEEN CATTELL

WILLIAM BARNUM

THE Carnegie Institution has recently lost two of its most illustrious friends—Charles D. Walcott and William Barnum. By a strange coincidence both of these men came from Utica, New York, both were pillars in the formative period of the Carnegie Institution of Washington, and they died within a few months of each other. Dr. Walcott was a trustee of the institution since its founding and Mr. Barnum its editor since 1903.

It was in June, 1904, the school holidays, that the writer was given a little note in pencil written by Dr. Walcott and addressed to Mr. Barnum. The gist of the note was "and here is the red-headed boy of whom I spoke this morning." That summer holiday job stretched itself through the years to the present time.

To have worked beside such a man as William Barnum in these past years was an education in itself; to have felt the inspiration that seemed to generate from a noble soul was a blessing indeed; but to have known what this man meant to hundreds of others, to all who came in intimate contact with him, was to know a man the like of which one sees none too often.

Withal, William Barnum was a practical man. Assistance he would render to any one—provided it was an intelligent request. He despised the bluff or insincere. As editor, he would take a fifty-page pamphlet and perhaps reduce it to ten pages. Fine phrases in science writings do not necessarily bring out new information, and Mr. Barnum was an expert in aiding the author to express his thoughts. So too would he turn tables in such a fashion that the author thought the editor knew more about the subject than he did. The late Dr. Alfred G. Mayor, a prolific writer and a most sincere scientific writer, too, relied wholly on Mr. Barnum's judgment in his institutional writings.

The three presidents of the Carnegie Institution of Washington, Dr. Daniel C. Gilman, Dr. Robert S. Woodward and Dr. John C. Merriam, valued and depended upon the great abilities of Mr. Barnum. Dr. John C. Merriam has recently extolled his ability.

As editor of the publications of the institution for nearly a quarter of a century, William Barnum's monument is a library of over five hundred volumes on nearly every scientific subject, the author of each book a debtor to the editor.

The writer would pay a tribute to his friend if he knew how. Perhaps the memory of him in years to come will compensate for my lack of ability to do him justice.

IRVING M. GREY

SCIENTIFIC EVENTS

THE ENLARGED PROGRAM OF FOREST RESEARCH

THE McSweeney-McNary bill, which became a law with the approval of the president on May 22, represents the most important piece of fundamental forestry legislation enacted since the Clarke-McNary law of 1924, according to a statement by Secretary of Agriculture Jardine, who also said:

> Forest research has hitherto failed to keep pace with many other forestry activities, notwithstanding the fact that research is the foundation upon which forestry development should be built. A greatly enlarged research program is called for by this situation, and the comprehensive policy of forestry research provided in the new bill will enable the department to cooperate with other agencies in a definite and far-reaching program of investigations which will form the basis for a permanent system of forest production and utilization for the entire nation.

The new bill establishes and outlines a ten-year program for forest research. A little more than $1,000,000 is now being expended by the federal government each year for this purpose. Under the terms of the McSweeney-McNary bill this amount may be increased each year by about $250,000 until the maximum annual expenditure of $3,500,000 is reached. All classes of forest research are contemplated by the bill, including investigations in growing, managing and utilizing timber, forage and other forest products, watershed protection, fire prevention, insects and disease. The various lines of research contemplated will be conducted by several bureaus of the department, including the Forest Service, the Bureau of Plant Industry, the Bureau of Entomology, the Biological Survey, the Weather Bureau, the Bureau of Chemistry and Soils and the Bureau of Agricultural Economics.

The McSweeney-McNary bill was backed by a widespread, aggressive public interest from all parts of the United States and representing widely diversified groups, including many Chambers of Commerce and development associations, the lumber and wood-using industries, nature, outdoor and recreation groups and women's clubs.

THE LASKER FOUNDATION FOR MEDICAL RESEARCH

AT the meeting of the board of trustees of the University of Chicago held January 12, a communication from Mr. and Mrs. Albert D. Lasker was presented, in which are set forth the particulars by which is created the Lasker Foundation for Medical Research. The fund thus contributed to the university adds another large endowment for research in medicine, an endowment which provides the means for investigation of notable significance.

Added to the resources of the Douglas Smith foundation, of the Mr. and Mrs. Frank G. Logan fellowships, of the Seymour Coman fellowships (all of which funds are designed to encourage research in various branches of medical science and in the prevention, cause and cure of disease), the new foundation greatly increases facilities and opportunities for medical research.

The Lasker Foundation (established by Albert D. and Flora W. Lasker) consists of $1,000,000, "the net income of which shall be used for the promotion of medical education and research at the University of Chicago." Already a liberal portion of the founding fund has been transferred to the university and the remainder will be paid with interest during the next three years. The offer to pay interest during the period of deferred payment enables the university to begin at once with the full amount of income from the fund the beneficent inquiries and to seek the hoped-for results which are contemplated by the creators of the foundation.

The donors' letter says in part:

> We express the desire that the income from this fund be used in the first place to support research into the causes, nature, prevention and cure of degenerative diseases. In the event, however, that in the opinion of the advisory board—which we shall subsequently mention—and the board of trustees of the university, the income of this fund can be used most effectively for medical education and research in other and further directions, the university shall be authorized to make such changes in the use and purposes of the income derived from said foundation. The general direction of the income shall be determined by an advisory committee, to be appointed by the trustees of the university. It is understood as part of this offer and agreement, and any agreement based thereon, that the publication of researches conducted wholly or partially through the support of this foundation shall, if possible, in the title recite the fact that said research has been supported by the Lasker foundation for medical research.

STANDARD MATHEMATICAL SYMBOLS

APPROVAL of mathematical symbols as American standards has completed the first step in a program of unification of the scientific and engineering symbols and abbreviations used in engineering and industry, under the auspices of the American Engineering Standards Committee. The confusion resulting from variations in symbols used in different publications, reports and tables, led to the initiation of a project of unification by the standards committee early in 1923. The work has been progressing since that time, with 14 national organizations participating.

The approved mathematical symbols include those for arithmetic and algebra, elementary geometry, analytic geometry, trigonometric and hyperbolic functions, calculus, special functions and vector analysis. The effort was made to select from symbols already in use those which are most clearly understood and least likely to lead to confusion with other symbols.

Professor E. V. Huntington, of Harvard University, representing the American Mathematical Society, was chairman of the mathematical symbols subcommittee. This subcommittee is part of the sectional committee on scientific and engineering symbols and abbreviations, of which Dr. J. Franklin Meyer, of the U. S. Bureau of Standards, is chairman. The sectional committee includes other subcommittees on symbols for hydraulics, symbols for heat and thermodynamics, symbols for aeronautics, navigation and topographical symbols, electrotechnical symbols (including radio), symbols for photometry and illumination and symbols for mechanics, structural engineering and testing materials.

THE WEEK ON AGRICULTURE AT THE INSTITUTE OF CHEMISTRY

THE week of July 23, 1928, at the American Chemical Society Institute in Evanston will be devoted to a discussion of the ways chemistry can help agriculture by developing markets for its products other than for food and clothing. To date the twelve speakers listed below have accepted the invitation of the society to take part in the institute sessions during the week of July 23.

W. E. EMLEY: Bureau of Standards, Washington, D. C. He has charge of the work supported by the Department of Commerce on the industrial utilization of farm wastes. He has made a careful and extensive survey of this entire field as to the past and the future.

G. J. ESSELEN, JR.: Skinner, Sherman and Esselen, Boston, Mass. An expert on cellulose. He will discuss cellulose in modern industry and the influence of cellulose on civilization.

H. T. HERRICKS: Color and Farm Waste Division, Department of Agriculture, Washington, D. C. He will discuss the processes by which moulds are being used to convert corn sugar into valuable materials such as citric acid. It will perhaps soon be possible to go from corn to glucose and then to citric acid more readily than to go from cull lemons to citric acid according to present practice.

H. G. KNIGHT: The new chief of the Bureau of Chemistry and Soils of the Department of Agriculture, Washington. He will take a leading part throughout the week. He will pay special attention to future possible developments of agricultural chemistry along new lines.

C. S. MINER: Miner Laboratories, Chicago. Under his direction furfural has been changed from a chemical curiosity found only in museums to an important industrial chemical sold in tank cars for a few cents a pound. Its largest use is in artificial resins. He will tell how this development took place, but more especially how other similar advances may be made.

A. S. RICHARDSON: Procter and Gamble, Ivorydale, Ohio. His subject will be hydrogenation, the process by which an oil like cotton seed oil is made to unite with hydrogen gas to form a solid fat suitable for cooking.

G. A. RICHTER: Brown Company, Berlin, N. H. On the preparation of pure cellulose from wood. This material can be used in place of cotton cellulose for almost all purposes.

G. M. ROMMEL: New York. An expert agricultural economist, retained by the Department of Agriculture for special studies on farm wastes with special reference to the preparation of cellulose from them.

H. J. SCONCE: Cornstalks Products Co., 42 Broadway, New York, and Danville. The preparation of useful products from farm wastes.

O. R. SWEENEY: Iowa State College. An authority on the preparation of hundreds of useful products from corn stalks and cobs. He is also working with the Department of Commerce on this problem.

A. W. SCHORGER: Burgess Laboratories, Madison, Wis. A leading authority on the chemistry and utilization of cellulose.

R. W. THATCHER: President, Massachusetts Agricultural College. Formerly dean of department of agriculture, University of Minnesota; formerly director of New York Experiment Station. He will present the broader aspects of the subject with special reference to future possibilities.

CHARLES D. HURD,
Executive Secretary.

AWARD OF THE WILLARD GIBBS MEDAL TO PROFESSOR W. D. HARKINS

PROFESSOR WILLIAM D. HARKINS, of the University of Chicago, received on May 25 the Willard Gibbs gold medal, awarded annually by the Chicago section of the American Chemical Society to a chemist whose work in either pure or applied chemistry has received international recognition. The ceremony took place at a national dinner gathering of scientists at the Palmer House.

Professor Harkins delivered an address on "Surface Structure and Atom Building." Professor S. C. Lind, director of the school of chemistry of the University of Minnesota, made the presentation address, discussing "Harkins the Scientist." Professor G. L. Clark, of the University of Illinois, a former student of Professor Harkins, spoke on "Harkins the Teacher and the Man." S. L. Redman, chairman of the Chicago section, discussed "The Willard Gibbs Medal."

Other speakers were: Professor Arthur H. Compton, of the University of Chicago; Dr. Leo Hendrik Baekeland, honorary professor of chemical engineering in Columbia University and former president of the American Chemical Society, New York; Dr. Harrison E. Howe, of the National Research Council, editor of *Industrial and Engineering Chemistry,* Washington; President Max Mason, president of the University of Chicago, and Professor S. W. Parr, of the University of Illinois, president of the American Chemical Society.

Previous Willard Gibbs medallists have been: Svante Arrhenius, T. W. Richards, L. H. Baekeland, Ira Remsen, Arthur A. Noyes, Willis R. Whitney, E. W. Morley, W. A. Noyes, W. M. Burton, F. G. Cottrell, Madame Curie, J. Stieglitz, G. N. Lewis, M. Gomberg, Sir James Irvine and J. J. Abel.

The 1928 jury which made the award was composed of: Dr. A. D. Little, Boston; Professor F. C. Whitmore, director of the institute of chemistry of the American Chemical Society; Professor J. F. Norris, Massachusetts Institute of Technology; L. M. Tolman, Hammond, Ind.; E. W. Washburn, U. S. Bureau of Standards, Washington; Professor Edward Bartow, University of Iowa; W. Lee Lewis, Chicago; Professor William McPherson, Ohio State University; Professor Julius Stieglitz, University of Chicago; Professor Roger Adams and Professor S. W. Parr, University of Illinois, and Professor Moses Gomberg, University of Michigan.

SCIENTIFIC NOTES AND NEWS

AT a dinner on May 23 the Holley medal of the American Society of Mechanical Engineers was presented to Dr. Elmer A. Sperry for his invention of the gyroscope compass.

ORVILLE WRIGHT, pioneer aviator, would be awarded the distinguished flying cross, the highest award for American aeronautical achievement, under a bill introduced in congress by Representative James, of Michigan.

FOR outstanding service to his profession, Dr. Charles H. LaWall, dean of the Philadelphia College of Pharmacy and Science, was awarded the Remington medal, at a dinner given in his honor at the Hotel Pennsylvania, New York, on May 14.

THE American Academy of Arts and Sciences has announced the election of new foreign honorary members including Friedrich Paschen and Wolfgang Kohler, of Berlin; Soren Peter Lauritz Sorensen and Carl Hansen Ostenfelt, of Copenhagen; Guglielmo Marconi, of Bologna; Francis Arthur Bather, Alfred Barton Rendle, Charles Tate Regan, Karl Pearson and Richard Burden Haldane, of London; Louis Dollo, of Brussels; D'Arcy Wentworth Thompson, of St. Andrews; Mikinosuke Miyajima, of Tokio; Henri Louis Bergson, of Paris; Benedetto Croce, of Naples; Edmund Husserl, of Freiburg; Hans Oertel, of Munich, and Arthur Cecil Pigou, of Cambridge.

IN connection with the celebrations commemorating the twenty-fifth anniversary of the foundation of the University of Liverpool honorary degrees have been conferred, among others, upon Dr. J. A. Fleming, emeritus professor of electrical engineering, University College, London; J. E. Littlewood, lecturer in mathematics, Cambridge University, and on Dr. Robert Robinson, professor of organic chemistry, Manchester University.

HONORARY degrees are to be conferred by Cambridge University upon Professor A. Einstein, Professor Cumont, Professor W. A. Craigie, Lord Lugard, Lord Justice Scrutton, Sir Cecil Hurst and Sir D. Y. Cameron.

PROFESSOR A. G. TANSLEY, Sherardian professor of botany in the University of Oxford, has been elected a member of the Athenaeum Club for distinguished eminence in science.

M. JOSEPH AUCLAIR was recently elected a correspondent of the Paris Academy of Sciences in the section of mechanics.

DR. WALTHER HORN, director of the department of entomology in the Kaiser Wilhelm Institute, Berlin, has been made a corresponding member of the Hungarian Entomological Society, Budapest.

THE eightieth birthday of Professor A. P. Karpinsky, the well-known Russian geologist, president of the Academy of Science, was recently celebrated in Leningrad.

AFTER ten years' service as dean of Cornell University Medical College, Dr. Walter L. Niles, about to retire, was presented with a bronze plaque by the College Alumni Association at its annual dinner in the Hotel Commodore on May 10. On May 23 Dr. Niles was tendered a dinner at the Waldorf Hotel by the faculty of the college.

PROFESSOR HENRY H. WING, professor of animal husbandry in the college of agriculture at Cornell University, will retire in June after forty years on the faculty.

DR. R. E. SCHUH, professor of geology in Howard University, is resigning after twenty-one years of service.

THE following officers have been elected for the American Section of the Society of Chemical Industry: *Chairman,* Charles Lunn; *secretary,* Foster Dee Snell; *treasurer,* F. C. R. Hemingway; *new members of the executive committee,* Samuel Cabot, Moritz Dittmar, L. V. Redman, R. T. Baldwin and Stephen P. Burke.

THE Southern Appalachian section of the Society of American Foresters recently elected the following officers: *Chairman,* Dr. C. F. Korstian, silviculturist, Appalachian Forest Experiment Station; *vice-chairman,* M. A. Mattoon, supervisor, Pisgah National Forest; *secretary,* F. W. Haasis, assistant silviculturist, Appalachian Forest Experiment Station.

AT the recent convention of Sigma Pi Sigma, national honorary physics fraternity, the following officers were elected: *President,* Professor C. C. Hatley, of Duke University; *vice-president,* Professor R. C. Young, of the College of William and Mary; *secretary-treasurer,* Professor Marsh W. White, of The Pennsylvania State College; *councilors,* Professors J. M. Douglas and W. N. Mebane, Jr., of Davidson College.

PROFESSOR OLLIE E. REED, head of the dairy husbandry division of the Michigan State College of Agriculture, has been appointed chief of the Bureau of Dairy Industry of the U. S. Department of Agriculture. He will take up his duties in Washington about September 1. The position has been vacant since the first of the year, when Dr. C. W. Larson resigned to become director of the National Dairy Council.

DR. OSCAR C. WILLHITE has been appointed chief of the neuropsychiatric division of the United States Veterans Bureau at Washington, D. C., to succeed Dr. L. M. Wilbor.

GEORGE N. SCHRAMM, assistant physicist in the electrochemical section of the U. S. Bureau of Standards, has taken a position as research chemist in the Vandergrift, Pa., laboratory of the American Sheet and Tin Plate Company, and will conduct research on the corrosion of iron and steel.

H. W. HOOTS recently resigned as a geologist in the U. S. Geological Survey to engage in commercial geology.

Louis O. Sordahl, research assistant in physics at the University of Wisconsin, has been appointed field assistant of the Smithsonian Institution's station for the study of solar radiation at Mount Brukkaros, Africa, and not director as was incorrectly reported in Science and other publications.

Professor Harlan T. Stetson, of the Harvard Astronomical Laboratory, has been appointed exchange professor from Harvard University to Carleton, Grinnell and Pomona Colleges for the second half of the next academic year.

According to the *Journal* of the Washington Academy of Sciences, Dr. E. G. Zies, of the geophysical laboratory, Carnegie Institution, will spend several months in the Dutch East Indies, in a study of the gases and other volatile products of the volcanoes of that region. Messrs. E. T. Allen and C. N. Fenner will spend the summer in a chemical and geological study of the geysers and hot springs of the Yellowstone National Park.

Members of the third University of Michigan Greenland Expedition are sailing on the *Stavangerfjord* on June 5. Dr. William H. Hobbs, director of the expedition, has already left the United States and will join the other members in Copenhagen and sail on the *Disko* about June 15 for their base at Holstensborg, Greenland.

Australian newspapers note that Dr. Frank Blanchard and his wife, Dr. Frieda Cobb Blanchard, both of the University of Michigan, are spending 1927–28 studying the fauna and flora of Australasia, particularly the mountainous temperate portions of New Zealand, Tasmania and Australia. They also intend spending some time on the Great Barrier Reef, Queensland. Dr. Blanchard is studying particularly the herpetology of Australasia, and Mrs. Blanchard the flora of the cooler portions, with a view to securing plants suitable to the conditions of the botanical gardens of the University of Michigan, of which she is assistant director.

C. W. Gilmore, curator of vertebrate paleontology in the U. S. National Museum, left on May 12 to take charge of an expedition in the Two Medicine Formation of Montana, in search of dinosaur and other vertebrate remains, which will be in the field for two and a half months.

Dr. C. Poulsen, of the Mineralogical Museum, Copenhagen, spent April and May at the U. S. National Museum in connection with his study of the Silurian fossils collected in North Greenland by Dr. Lauge Koch.

Dr. Russell L. Cecil, assistant professor of clinical medicine at the Cornell University Medical College, delivered the commencement address at the Medical College of Virginia, Richmond, on May 29. On this occasion the honorary degree of doctor of science was conferred upon him.

H. E. Howe, editor of *Industrial and Engineering Chemistry,* Washington, D. C., during the months of April and May has made a number of addresses before groups of engineers, college students and luncheon clubs in Oklahoma, Missouri, Minnesota, Illinois and Pennsylvania, emphasizing various applications of scientific research to industrial achievement.

Dr. Jerome Alexander addressed the New England Association of Chemistry Teachers at their 109th meeting at Wesleyan University, Middletown, Conn., April 19, on "Colloid Chemistry and its Applications." Films were shown which were loaned by Dr. Alexis Carrel and Mr. Heinz Rosenberger, of the Rockefeller Institute for Medical Research.

Dr. R. W. Boyle, dean of faculty of applied science in the University of Alberta, addressed the Philosophical Society of Washington on "Ultrasonics," on May 26.

Dr. E. S. London, professor of physiology in the University of Leningrad, gave two illustrated lectures under the joint auspices of the Institute of Medicine of Chicago and the University of Illinois College of Medicine on May 3 and 4, on "Experimental Fistulas of Blood Vessels" and "Enzymes, Hormones and Vitamins."

Sir Jagadis Bose lectured at University College, London, on "The Motor Mechanism of Plants," on May 8 and demonstrated by new types of sensitive recorders the contractility and rhythmic pulsations of plants.

At the last meeting of the University of Pennsylvania chapter of the Society of the Sigma Xi, on May 9, the following minute was unanimously adopted: "This chapter of the society of the Sigma Xi sincerely mourns the passing of Edgar Fahs Smith, former provost of the University of Pennsylvania, for many years a most highly valued member of this society. In his going, science loses one of its most distinguished servants, and the many who enjoyed his friendship lose a rare blessing."

A Copenhagen message reports the death of Dr. C. G. Johannes Petersen, for 40 years director of the Danish Biological Station. Dr. Petersen had been associated with Danish fishery research work since 1883, and was known for his investigations of the life history of various food-fishes.

The eighty-fourth annual meeting of the American Psychiatric Association will be held at the Hotel

Radisson, in Minneapolis, on June 5, 6, 7 and 8, under the presidency of Dr. Adolf Meyer, of Baltimore, Md. The program will cover such subjects as administration, mental hygiene, pathology, clinical psychiatry, phylogenetics, psychoanalysis and psychopathology, with round-table discussions in addition to the regular meetings. A feature of the meeting will be the annual address by Professor Roscoe Pound, dean of the Harvard Law School.

THE Chemistry Research Club met on May 17 in the Natural History Museum, New York City. It was voted to make application to become an affiliated society in the New York Academy of Sciences. Professor Arthur E. Hill, of New York University, read a paper on "The Alkali Periodides." Dr. K. G. Falk, of the Harriman Research Laboratories, read a paper on "Lipase Actions in Normal Tissues and Tumors," in which he summarized the research which he has carried on in the past ten years.

THE third symposium on general organic chemistry will meet at Princeton University late in December, 1929, under the auspices of the division of organic chemistry of the American Chemical Society. The executive committee of the division consists of William Lloyd Evans, Frank C. Whitmore, F. B. Dains, E. Emmet Reid and James B. Conant.

THE annual meeting of the Chicago Neurological Society was held at the Billings Memorial Hospital on May 17. Among others, Drs. Anton J. Carlson, Arno B. Luckhardt, Dallas B. Phemister, John Favill and Roy R. Grinker spoke. The president of the society invited the members to be his guests at dinner at the Shoreland Hotel.

A GEOLOGICAL field conference was held in northwestern Arkansas on May 12 and 13, under the auspices of the department of geology of the University of Arkansas. About 50 geologists were present, representing Arkansas, Oklahoma, Kansas, Missouri and Nebraska. Formations of late Mississippian and early Pennsylvanian age were studied.

THE Alpha Gamma chapter of Phi Sigma was installed at the University of South Dakota on May 15 by Professor Don B. Whelan, of the department of entomology of the University of Nebraska.

ON May 11, a public address was given under the auspices of the Maryland chapter of the Society of Sigma Xi by Dr. F. C. Whitmore, chairman of the division of chemistry of the National Research Council. His subject was "The Habits of the Atoms." On May 18, the first annual initiation and banquet was held. Twenty-four active and associate members were initiated. Dr. William Crocker, director of the Boyce-Thompson Institute for Plant Research, delivered the address of the evening. His subject was "The Work of the Boyce-Thompson Institute."

PLANS for participation of the United States in the World Engineering Congress in Tokio next year were formulated at a meeting of the American committee at the Carlton Hotel, New York, on March 22, following a dinner tendered to the committee by the Japanese Ambassador, T. Matsudaira. Officers elected by the committee follow: *Honorary chairman,* Herbert Hoover; *chairman,* Elmer A. Sperry, New York; *vice-chairman* and *chairman of the executive committee,* John W. Lieb, New York; *vice-chairman,* C. E. Grunsky (Pacific Coast), San Francisco; C. E. Kettering (Middle West), Detroit; *executive secretary,* Maurice Holland; *executive committee,* Gano Dunn, New York; George W. Fuller, New York; Maurice Holland, New York; Dugald C. Jackson, Cambridge, Mass.; Frank B. Jewett, New York; John W. Lieb, New York; J. H. McGraw, New York; O. C. Merrill, Washington D. C.; Calvin W. Rice, New York; Charles F. Scott, New Haven; Dr. Sperry, Brooklyn; W. E. Wickenden, New York; *finance committee,* John W. Lieb; *technical program committee,* D. C. Jackson; *transportation committee,* F. B. Jewett; *entertainment committee,* O. C. Merrill; *publicity,* J. H. McGraw; *promotion and attendance,* George W. Fuller; *nominating committee,* Gano Dunn.

JAMES L. CLARK, of the Carlisle-Clark African expedition of the American Museum of Natural History, sailed from New York on May 9 to get material for the Akeley African Hall of the museum. They will proceed to Nairobi, British East Africa, the expedition's headquarters, where they will meet G. Lister Carlisle, Jr., who left New York with Mrs. Carlisle on April 1. W. R. Leigh, an artist who accompanied the late Carl Akeley to Africa, and C. C. Raddatz, of the department of preparation, will also be members of the expedition. Leaving Nairobi the expedition will spend at least four months in the field, then go out through Uganda and the Sudan to Khartum and across the desert to Wadi Halfa on the second cataract of the Nile, and from there travel down the river to Cairo.

PHYSIOLOGICAL optics as a study for scientific study and instruction has received important recognition at the Wilmer Ophthalmological Institute, the Johns Hopkins University School of Medicine. On October 1, 1928, carrying out the provisions of a special gift, a research laboratory will be opened, designed and equipped for the study and investigation of all phases of pure and applied physiological optics. The work of this laboratory will be conducted by Dr. C. E. Ferree, professor of experimental psychology and director of the psychological laboratory at Bryn Mawr

College, who has been appointed resident lecturer in ophthalmology and director of the research laboratory of physiological optics; and by Dr. Gertrude Rand, of Bryn Mawr College, who has been appointed associate professor of research ophthalmology.

The Fleischmann mammal wing of the Santa Barbara Museum of Natural History was opened on April 3. This new portion of the building is the gift of Major Max Fleischmann, who recently returned from a hunting expedition to French Indo-China. Four large habitat groups were completed in time for the initial opening of the wing and others are now in progress.

Studies of landslides in unconsolidated materials are being begun at the University of Cincinnati, with the intention of determining causes and of considering such factors as angle of slope, soil saturation and mode of movement. Dr. James K. Rogers, of the department of geology, would like to hear from readers of Science who know of the location of landslides in unconsolidated material in the states east of the Mississippi.

A trust fund for the maintenance of neurological research at the Wistar Institute of Anatomy, Philadelphia, has been established by Mrs. Carlos F. MacDonald, widow of the New York psychiatrist, who died on May 29, 1926. The amount of the fund was not made public, but it is to be increased to several hundred thousand dollars.

A collection of medical books containing many of the earliest printed works on the subject, brought together by Dr. E. C. Streeter, of Boston, over a period of twenty years, has been purchased by the New York Academy of Medicine. The purchase price was $185,000, of which $85,000 was contributed by the Rockefeller Foundation. Fellows of the academy contributed an additional $10,000 and other large contributors included Edward S. Harkness, $25,000; Carl Tucker, $10,000; Mrs. Walter S. Ladd, $10,000; Felix Warburg, V. Everit Macy and Harry P. Whitney, $5,000 each; Clarence A. Mackay, $2,000, and Dunlevy Milbank, Jeremiah Milbank and Harry H. Flagler, $1,000 each.

Delivery of the William Libbey geographical library to the Clark University library has been completed. The Libbey library was presented to the university as a memorial to Dr. William Libbey, late professor at Princeton, by his widow, Mrs. William Libbey. Before his death, Dr. Libbey left instructions that his collection of geographical material be placed in an institution promoting geographical research. Mrs. Libbey decided in favor of Clark University. The library of Dr. Libbey contains about 8,000 volumes, including leading geographical publications of Germany, France, Great Britain and the United States. The gift to the university library also includes the Libbey card catalogue of all the important articles in geography that have been published. The collection also includes 14,000 lantern slides with views from all parts of the world, accompanied by a full index to the slides.

UNIVERSITY AND EDUCATIONAL NOTES

Frank G. Tallman, vice-president of the E. I. du Pont de Nemours Company, has made a gift of $100,000 to Bowdoin College, to establish the Tallman lecture fund as a memorial to the Bowdoin members of his family. The income is to be used to provide visiting professors and lecturers.

Ground-breaking ceremonies for the George Herbert Jones chemical laboratories, at the University of Chicago, were held on May 29. Mr. George Herbert Jones, director of the Inland Steel Company, whose gift of $665,000 made the chemistry laboratory possible, was one of the speakers at the ceremony. President Max Mason and Professor Julius Stieglitz, head of the department of chemistry, also gave addresses.

Albany Medical College, Albany, N. Y., has announced plans to raise a $2,000,000 endowment fund.

Dr. Kenyon S. Butterfield, president of Michigan State College, has resigned and Dr. R. Shaw, dean of agriculture in the college, has been appointed his successor.

Earl D. Hay, head of the department of mechanical and industrial engineering at the University of Wyoming, has been appointed to a similar position at the University of Kansas.

Dr. Carey Croneis, instructor in geology at Harvard University, has been appointed assistant professor of paleontological geology at the University of Chicago, where he will have charge of the work in invertebrate paleontology, succeeding in that field the late Professor Stuart Weller. Dr. Croneis will conduct the field courses in geology in Missouri this summer and begin his full-time work in Chicago in October.

At Yale University, the following have been promoted from the rank of instructor to assistant professorships: Dr. Harold Kirby, Jr., biology; Francis Thomas McNamara, electrical engineering, and Frederic William Keator, mechanical engineering.

Dr. A. Schmincke, of Tübingen, has been appointed professor of pathology at Heidelberg.

DISCUSSION AND CORRESPONDENCE

ARCHIMEDES AND TRIGONOMETRY

ARCHIMEDES (287–212 B. C.) is commonly regarded as the greatest mathematician of antiquity, but it is only recently that he has been credited by modern writers on the history of mathematics with fundamental developments in trigonometry. Our text-books on this subject usually refer to the Greek astronomer, Hipparchus, who lived about a century later than Archimedes, as the founder of trigonometry. It should therefore be of wide interest to note here that recent discoveries relating to the works of Archimedes, especially to one devoted to the heptagon, seem to establish the fact that we now have more substantial reasons for regarding Archimedes as the founder of trigonometry than we have for giving this credit to Hipparchus. In particular, Archimedes seems to have known rules which are equivalent to our common formulas for the sine and the cosine of the sum and the difference of two angles.

In a recent number of the *Archiv für Geschichte der Mathematik, der Naturwissenschaften und der Technik,* Volume 10, page 432, the well-known German writer on the history of elementary mathematics, Johannes Tropfke, discusses at considerable length some of the necessary modifications relating to the history of trigonometry which result from the recent discoveries as regards the work of Archimedes. He points out, in particular, that Archimedes knew the rule which is now commonly expressed by the following formula:

$$\sin\frac{A}{2} = \sqrt{\frac{1-\cos A}{2}}$$

The ancient Hindu and Arabian writers regarded this rule as one of the most important ones of trigonometry, and it has been assumed heretofore that it was probably due to Ptolemy, who used it without referring to its earlier use by others. It is very interesting to note therefore that it now seems to be due to Archimedes, who lived about four hundred years earlier than Ptolemy. The recent discoveries to which we have referred tend also to give additional support to the view that the so-called Heron formula for the area of a plane triangle in terms of its sides is due to Archimedes, and this constitutes another substantial reason for regarding him as the founder of trigonometry.

It should be added that these discoveries relate to Arabian translations and to references found in Arabian works, and it is well known that many such references are unreliable. In the present instance there are, however, many indirect evidences which tend to support these references. At any rate it is interesting to know that discoveries which promise so much for the history of trigonometry have recently been made, especially since the work of writers who preceded Archimedes seems to show clearly that the fundamental rules to which we referred above could not have been known in their times, and hence it does not seem likely that they could have been known long before the times of Archimedes. Such discoveries also tend to emphasize the important fact that the rapid advances which are being made in the history of science are apt to affect our views as regards some of the oldest and most fundamental developments.

G. A. MILLER

UNIVERSITY OF ILLINOIS

REPRODUCTION RATE IN WILD RATS

As a contribution to the subject dealt with by Dr. Donaldson in SCIENCE for March 20, 1925, "Control of Rat Population," we submit the following:

In 1922 the board of health of New Bedford, Mass., at the suggestion of the U. S. Public Health Service, undertook a rodent survey of the town which was carried on for a period of about two years. Two trappers were employed to trap rats in the business portion of the city and along the water front. The rats were brought to the laboratory of the board of health and examined for lesions of plague by one of us (C. S. S.). Since the whole number examined was small (about 6,000) it was possible to extend the examination beyond the mere search for plague. Careful observations of pregnancy in the female and of the number of fetuses were recorded. Of the total number of female rats examined, seven per cent. were found to be pregnant. This percentage varied little from season to season.

The female rat becomes sexually mature at about three months of age and remains fertile until about twenty months of age. The average life-span of the rat is about three years. Thus the period of fertility is approximately one half of the whole life-span. If the rats which were trapped were equally distributed as to age, approximately one half of the females brought to the laboratory would be fertile. The period of gestation in the rat is about twenty-one days. Pregnancy is grossly visible in the exposed uterus for about sixteen days. If the female rats which were trapped were all reproducing at the rate of one litter per year and there was a purely random distribution as above-mentioned, there would be about one chance in forty-five ($16/365 \times \frac{1}{2}$) of finding pregnancy in any female, that is, about 2 per cent. of the females would be pregnant. The fact that 7 per cent. of the rats were found to be pregnant seems to indicate that rats under the conditions obtaining in New Bedford were bearing at the rate of from three to four litters per year.

Limitation of numbers in nature is thus seen to be accomplished by a restriction of the reproduction rate as well as through the action of natural enemies. In other words, a physiological limit is imposed probably through the influence of nutrition. Trapping or poisoning merely serves to increase the available food supply for survivors.

PAUL EATON,
C. S. STIRRETT

AUGUSTA, GEORGIA
NEW BEDFORD, MASS.

VITAMIN B

Now that the vitamin originally known as "Vitamin B" has been definitely shown to be made up of at least two other vitamins, this laboratory has devised a method of separating these vitamins from each other and thus leaving them in a liquid form which can be easily used.

When these two fractions are fed alone and separately from the basal diet there is only a slight stimulation of growth for two or three weeks and then a gradual decline, but when the two are fed together there is a moderate rate of growth. This rate of growth, however, is not what one expects from the amount used (equivalent to 1.0 gm of original yeast daily) nor is the rate of growth comparable to that produced by the original yeast. In looking about for an explanation it was thought that possibly the yeast-residue contained the missing factor. A check lot of rats was given this yeast-residue, but instead of a good growth there was slight growth for about two weeks and then a decline and death. However, when these two other vitamins were added to the yeast-residue and the same fed to rats, excellent growth resulted. This new substance found in the yeast-residue after the two other vitamins have been removed meets all the definitions of a vitamin. It appears to be thermostable, and insoluble in water. It activates the two other vitamins of the vitamin-B complex and causes a greater growth than the two alone.

CHAS. H. HUNT

OHIO AGR. EXP. STATION,
WOOSTER, OHIO

WHAT IS OSMOSIS?

THE recent edition of the text-book of General Botany by Holman and Robbins states:

> The word osmosis has been given such a variety of meanings by those who have used it that it has lost any precise meaning whatever. As far as possible we shall avoid its use.

That it has been badly used, or rather misused, is evident, but should it be abandoned for this reason? The word is applied to a very definite physical phenomenon and has an exact meaning regardless of whether it has been misused or not.

Examination of standard text-books of botany reveals the source of the present status of the term. A single illustration will suffice. One widely used text states:

> Diffusion through a membrane is osmosis. When two fluids (liquids or gases) of different densities are separated by a porous membrane, diffusion through the membrane will take place until equilibrium results. The diffusion will be more rapid from the less dense to the more dense fluid.

The use of the term *dense* in this connection is meaningless. Students usually interpret it in terms of viscosity, a condition unrelated to osmosis. If it be considered to mean specific gravity then again the definition will not account for the direction of movements of all materials, for the dissolved salts of an egg, to use the illustration given in connection with this definition, will diffuse out into the water in which the egg is immersed at the same time water diffuses in. In this case, however, the movement is from the egg or "denser" medium, to the water or "less dense" medium. Therefore, the "law" is not applicable and consistent for the relatively simple example used to illustrate the process.

Any discussion introducing such terms as "dense solution," "less dense solution," "weaker solution," "stronger solution," and similar descriptions of the concentration of materials in a solution is entirely misleading and can but cause confusion.

A clear statement of the principles involved should remove all possibility of misunderstanding and restore to usage a term too important to be discarded.

In the first place osmosis follows the simple law of diffusion in that the direction of major movement of any material is determined by the concentration, *i.e.*, the number of molecules or ions of that material. The general direction of movement is always from a region where the diffusing material is higher in concentration of particles. The particles of the diffusing material are moving in *both* directions through the membrane, but more are moving away from the position in which most are found than are returning.

Materials move independently of each other, no matter how heterogeneous the solution in contact with the membrane may be. In no case are the diffusing particles dependent on the movement of water or any other material for their own movement.

Osmosis, then, can be defined briefly and accurately as diffusion through a membrane, the direction of major movement being from a region of high concentration to a region of low concentration of the thing diffusing.

Such a definition will apply to all cases of the phenomenon, no matter how complicated. It is easily applied and avoids the misconceptions introduced by the use of inexact terms.

ORTON K. STARK

UNIVERSITY OF WYOMING

A NOTE ON THE PREPARATION OF BIOLOGICAL SPECIMENS BY FILTRATION OF PARAFFIN

IT is only recently that the writer has seen and read No. 233 of the *American Museum Novitates*. This contains an article written by Dr. G. K. Noble and M. E. Jaeckle and entitled "Mounting by Paraffin Infiltration." Naturally I am interested in learning how these authors received the first suggestions of the possibilities of the method and how they have, with diligence and ingenuity, brought it to a high stage of efficiency.

A special reason for my interest in the matter arises from the fact that I may regard myself as the original inventor of the process. In Volume XIX of the *American Naturalist,* issued May, 1885, on page 526, I detailed the manner in which I filled all the tissues of various small animals with paraffin. Among these were small turtles, fishes, lizards, salamanders, mussels and earthworms. Noble and Jaeckle employ some media which were not at my command, but the result to be attained is the same. I congratulate them on their success.

It appears to the writer that economy of time might be effected, especially in the case of the larger specimens, by more use of injections of the hardening and clearing fluids into the body cavities, perhaps also into the alimentary tract, that seat of rapid putrefaction, and even into the blood-vessels. Certainly freshly-killed animals of moderate or large size will in warm weather begin to decay and become bloated by gases before the preserving formalin or alcohol can penetrate the skin and muscles.

OLIVER P. HAY

U. S. NATIONAL MUSEUM,
WASHINGTON, D. C.

SCIENTIFIC BOOKS

Alcohol and Longevity. BY RAYMOND PEARL. Knopf, New York, 1926, pp. xii + 273.

NOT only Professor Pearl's "Friends of the Saturday Night Club" to whom he dedicates this work, but his other friends and indeed the whole alcohol-interested public will find matter of great importance in this volume. It records a unique investigation in human life statistics and makes the results clear, even for the non-scientific reader. Doubtless many careful readers, who are students of the problem, will be surprised at Professor Pearl's finding on page 226:

> "In a fairly large and homogeneous sample of the working population of Baltimore the moderate drinking of alcoholic beverages did not shorten life. On the contrary moderate steady drinkers exhibited somewhat lower rates of mortality, and greater expectation of life than did abstainers."

The problem of the effect of alcohol on the duration of human life is inherently such that we must turn to large groups for our observations and "to the mathematics of large numbers, to the theory of mass phenomena, to interpret safely our observations." Few if any scientific workers to-day doubt the metabolism results of Atwater and Benedict in reference to the utilization of alcohol in the human body. These results have recently been further extended by Carpenter[1] at the Nutrition Laboratory, who has administered alcohol in the form of rectal enemata and finds the same promptness of oxidation as his predecessors. In the well-known study by Dodge and Benedict on the psychological effects of single doses of alcohol it is pointed out that taken the world over there are very many people who "regularly obtain a somewhat larger proportion of their total energy requirement (calories) from alcohol than from protein." Moreover, it is generally agreed now that alcohol is not a stimulant but a depressant. The results of many studies, including those by Dodge and Benedict and more recent ones by the reviewer, have shown that even small or moderate single ingestions of dilute alcoholic beverages tend to slow up and disarrange reflex and voluntary functions particularly at the time when the alcohol in the blood is on the increase. From these results it appears that we have in alcohol an environmental factor which the body can handle at least in moderate quantities, a contribution to nutrition that needs no digestion, that can to some extent replace other food, but that has a characteristic effect on the central nervous system. As a rule, people take alcohol not so much for its calories as for its colorful relaxing influence on mental life. But it is recognized as

[1] Carpenter, Thorne M., "Human Metabolism with Enemata of Alcohol, Dextrose, and Levulose." Carnegie Institution of Washington, Washington, 1925, Pub. No. 369.

an unsuitable potion for a tight rope artist, an aeroplane pilot, or even for that mundane creature the bank cashier. Subjectively time drags less after alcohol; the individual is not so hard to satisfy, his attentional field becomes somewhat narrowed and he experiences an added increment of interest in his own mental states. Will he pay a penalty of shortened life span for this, shall we say, semi-dreamy and often altogether pleasing existence? These are not the words and this is not exactly the line of argument used by Professor Pearl. He does not say that since alcohol exercises a depressant action (has been used for ages as a "night-cap") it might perhaps reasonably be expected to conserve the quota of human energy and spread it out over a somewhat longer time axis, as increasing the average number of hours of sleep might possibly do. The question of voluntary alcohol indulgence and life span is his problem in the present volume.

Professor Pearl states that his interest in alcohol as an environmental agent began about 1916 when he tried experimentally to modify the germ cells of domestic fowl by this agent. The alcohol was given by the inhalation method. The birds were placed in metal chambers which contained alcohol vapor at about the point of saturation. One hour's occupancy of such a chamber was enough nearly to intoxicate the usual bird. Daily treatment with alcohol was continued for two and one half years. The control birds were of course placed in a similar chamber, but without the alcohol vapor. The results were surprising in that the alcohol-treated birds lived longer than the controls, had progeny that showed considerably less prenatal and postnatal mortality, and as treated organisms demonstrated less incidence of such diseases as roup. The autopsy records are reported as showing no clear indications of the ravages of alcohol. Stockard has used precisely the same inhalation method over a long period with guinea-pigs and has obtained results which very closely parallel those of Pearl with domestic fowl. Professor Pearl in commenting on the striking results in reference to roup says, "A possible explanation is that the daily inhalation treatment acts as a disinfectant of the air passages, and the treated birds do not take the disease because its germs are killed or greatly weakened before they have an opportunity to get an effective foothold." The reviewer can see no reason why this same possibility can not be extended to include the treated organism's entire body surface. Aside from this disinfectant action on the skin and feathers, when the bird is first removed from the chamber the rapid evaporation of the alcohol from the body surface can not but exercise through cooling the usual stimulating effect on the skin. The experimental routine of Pearl and Stockard does not eliminate these external factors which can not be appraised without further data. Nevertheless the results on the fowl were surprising and served as a natural starting point in the study of alcohol and longevity in man.

In approaching the human problem one recognizes instantly that it is impossible to prescribe the hour's daily bath in alcohol vapor and most of the other conditions that can in general be so neatly controlled in animal experimentation. It might be supposed that the essential data were reposing in the record books of insurance companies quietly awaiting the coming of the man with the statistical mill. Professor Pearl largely explodes this idea, making clear that such companies in general are not geared to the research drive. They have not the machinery and as a rule have no interest in prying into the daily or occasional practices of their policy-holders after once they have been accepted. Census reports are of course of even less value in the study of this problem. His material has resulted from family history records obtained by trained field workers under his personal direction. At the request of the National Tuberculosis Association he began about 1920 a comprehensive study of factors concerned in the incidence of tuberculosis, "with special reference to genetic elements." The individuals selected for study were very carefully questioned in reference to the use of alcohol and tobacco because of the possible bearing of these habits on tuberculosis. The field workers stated their problem directly to each examinee and it is believed in this way got the most trustworthy frank statements that can be had. Starting with an individual known to be a case of tuberculosis the field worker traced the family history both backward to ancestry and collaterals and forward to descendants and their collaterals. Numerous environmental factors were taken account of. In exactly the same manner individuals known not to be tuberculosis cases were studied. All the material (both groups) "was taken from one socially and economically homogeneous group of the population of the city of Baltimore and Maryland; namely, what might inclusively be called workingmen's families." An item to be included in a history had to be corroborated by the independent testimony of at least two persons acquainted with the individual in question. For each individual studied there is a record for the kind and amount of alcoholic beverages used, the frequency or regularity of use and such habits at different periods throughout life. The field workers had no hint that these data would be used for a study of alcohol and life duration. These items "sharply differentiate the present material from anything available for the study of this problem in the records of insurance companies, or indeed anywhere else, so far as is known to the writer."

When it comes to the matter of classifying the material in reference to amount of alcohol used numerous difficulties are encountered. The first classification into (1) total abstainers, (2) moderate and occasional drinkers, and (3) heavy or steady drinkers, which was used when this material was presented as an appendix in Starling's "The Action of Alcohol on Man," was criticized as too rough a grouping. Hence eight groups are made for the present treatment: abstainers, three moderate drinker classes and four heavy drinker groups. In all these the question has been *the amount* and the degree of *occasional* to *steady* use. Supposedly the question of dilution has figured somewhat in placing a particular person. Another very important factor, which is in effect a matter of dilution, is whether the alcohol is characteristically, for the given individual, taken with or after food or between meals on an empty stomach. Most assuredly it is not just the total of alcohol dumped into the stomach that is worthy of chief note. The conditions that modify the rate of its getting into the blood and so of its gaining access to the various tissues including the central nervous system are highly important here. Together with the amount and rate of ingestion they define the dosage. A good deal of the so-called idiosyncrasy to alcohol probably consists in these varying conditions which modify absorption. If we take the famous hard drinker, Dr. George Fordyce, for whom Dr. Pearl expresses such unrestrained admiration (p. 68), it will be noted that this one-meal-a-day man did not begin on his alcohol until after he had started to eat. And considering the amount that he ate he could (the size of his stomach permitting) drink a great deal without having the gradient of alcohol concentration in his blood reach a toxic value.

Results are analyzed for 2,164 females and 3,084 males. These populations are classified under sixteen racial groups. In general the females distribute themselves 3.1, 29.8 and 67.1 per cents. for heavy, moderate and abstainer classes. For the three classes in the same order males show 27.4, 42.6 and 30.0 per cents. Scandinavian women showed the largest per cent., 17.6, in the heavy class, while Hebrew, Scotch and Welsh and Old American show 0 here. The Hebrew men give the lowest, 8.3, "heavy" value. Between the three general groups there was not much difference in weekly income. Divided into the eight groups we find that the "moderate in amount, unspecified as to frequency" is 86 per cent. men and 14 per cent. women, which indicates that women gave a more accurate account of their habits. In all forms of the "heavy" classes men constitute more than 90 per cent. of these groups.

The data for the 5,248 individuals studied are presented in numerous tables and graphs where various comparisons between different subgroups and against other data are made. Individuals who changed their group status are discussed. Those who decreased drinking show death-rates below the general population, while those who increased are as decidedly above, but this subgroup whose habits changed during life have not been included in the general actuarial calculations. Numerous questions of an actuarial nature are asked and answered and the author defends as justifiable the calculation of life tables from the material under review. In the case of Dr. Pearl's data a person drops out of "the exposed to risk" group only because of death, never because of a "lapsed policy." The material as a whole without distinction as to the several classes of alcohol users and in respect to both sexes shows a higher expectation of life at all ages than does the general white population of Baltimore, which naturally also includes alcohol users. Although the more refined division into eight groups is proposed there is a tendency throughout the discussion to lump all the "moderates" together for comparison against the abstainers. All the tables and curves show them to compare rather closely and in some the "moderates" make a slightly better showing in life expectancy. So it is possible for Professor Pearl to draw the following conclusion which he places in italics: "In the males the death rates for moderate drinkers are slightly higher than those for abstainers from age 30 to age 55 inclusive, but, in my opinion, there is no statistically significant difference in the specific death rates, in the range of age from 30 to about 70, between abstainers and moderate drinkers, in this experience. In the same range of age the heavy drinking group exhibits a markedly higher rate of mortality than either of the other two groups." A particularly interesting comparison is between 94 male abstainers. and 113 moderate drinking brothers of the abstainers. The death-rates are a little higher for the moderate drinkers up to the age of thirty-five, while after that they are a little lower.

The earlier evidence on alcohol and mortality is reviewed and there is an extensive chapter on racial effect of alcohol. There is a bibliography of 269 titles a large single fraction of which (Nos. 158–197) relates to alcohol and cirrhosis of the liver as a disputed question. The book is well gotten up and satisfactorily indexed as to subject and author.

Dr. Pearl feels constrained to disclaim more than once "any responsibility for the application of the results of this investigation to the business of individual living." Notwithstanding this no small amount of space is devoted to straightforward arguing for the "moderate use" and in the face of the disclaimer the author has certainly not been fortunate in his selection of a final quotation to end his treatise. Dr. Pearl states it as his firm conviction that carefully conducted research with animals will in the long run produce more reliable and trustworthy evidence as to the effect of alcohol, as such, upon duration of life as such, including human life, than will any human data.

W. R. MILES

STANFORD UNIVERSITY

REPORTS

THE WESTERN COOPERATIVE OIL-SPRAY PROJECT

THE use of oil as an insecticide has increased rapidly during the last few years. Much experimental work has been done by various agencies, but most of this work has not been coordinated in such a way that comparisons could be made. In order partially to overcome this difficulty, a conference of entomologists and chemists was held at Tacoma, Washington, June 30, 1926, chiefly at the instance of J. R. Parker, associate entomologist at the Montana Agricultural Experiment Station. At this meeting, the Western Cooperative Oil-Spray Project was formed. The participants in this project included the Canadian department of agriculture, the agricultural experiment stations of Washington, Oregon, California, Idaho and Montana and the United States department of agriculture. Mr. Parker was named chairman of the organization. As practically nothing has been published regarding the intentions or results of the project, this brief report is presented at this time.

A further conference was held in Spokane, December 5, 1926, which plant physiologists and horticulturists were invited to attend. The oil-spray problem is not merely entomological in scope. The physiological effects of oils on plants must be considered, as well as the chemical aspects of oil-sprays. It was decided to limit the project to work of a fundamental nature, that is, primarily to investigate the effect of various types of oils on insects and plants and to ascertain the best methods of emulsifying the oils. It is believed that work of this nature will be more valuable than work with oil emulsions that may be on the market. In order to coordinate the work, a definite plan was formulated and the investigators were supplied with uniform materials. This has made the work of the various investigators much more comparable than has been the case heretofore. And to quote from the memorandum of understanding between the various agencies, one result of the project has been "to broaden the knowledge of the individual worker by the exchange of ideas and brief annual reports on work accomplished and to establish mutual confidence and to avoid trespass in matters of credit."

One year's work has been completed, and the results have been discussed and further plans made at a meeting held in Spokane, December 17 and 18, 1927. As the agencies involved are chiefly interested in horticultural work, the investigations so far have been limited to fruit trees. Possibly the most striking feature of this work has been the need of careful observations on the part of plant physiologists and horticulturists as to the effect of oil-sprays on trees and their products. This has been more or less overlooked in the past by entomologists, possibly because of their inability to measure carefully such effects.

The project feels that the use of dormant oils is fairly well standardized, and recommendations can be made and have been made regarding their use for the control of the fruit-tree leaf-roller, scale-insects, aphids and red spider eggs. However, there is still much to be learned as to the best time for application and the effect of low temperatures following application, and this portion of the investigation is to be continued.

The use of oil for summer spraying is not well standardized. On account of this, manufacturers are continually changing their products. Good results have been obtained in the control of red spiders and the codling moth, but the application of a number of summer sprays of oil has often resulted in injury, in one form or another, to the trees. For example, the fruit of yellow apples is particularly susceptible to oil injury; and trees in poor physical condition may be more severely injured than those in good condition. Moreover, the use of oil with lead-arsenate may complicate the subsequent removal of the spray residue. For these reasons, aside from the use of a single application of oil of sufficient strength to kill red spiders, no recommendations for using summer oils can be made by the members of this project until further investigations have been carried out.

The members of the project engaged in the 1927 investigations were as follows:

Dominion of Canada, Department of Agriculture:
- E. P. Venables, (Entomology), Vernon, B. C.

Washington Experiment Station:
- Dr. R. L. Webster, (Entomology), Pullman
- E. L. Green, (Chemistry), Pullman
- Anthony Spuler, (Entomology), Wenatchee
- F. L. Overley, (Horticulture), Wenatchee
- W. A. Luce, (Horticulture), Wenatchee

Oregon Experiment Station:
- D. C. Mote, (Entomology), Corvallis
- B. G. Thompson, (Entomology), Corvallis
- R. H. Robinson, (Chemistry), Corvallis
- Leroy Childs, (Entomology), Hood River
- R. K. Norris, (Entomology), Talent

California Experiment Station:
E. R. deOng, (Entomology), Berkeley
A. D. Borden, (Entomology), Sebastopol
Idaho Experiment Station:
Claude Wakeland, (Entomology), Parma
Montana Experiment Station:
J. R. Parker, (Entomology), Bozeman
Dr. W. C. Cook, (Entomology), Bozeman
H. E. Morris, (Plant Physiology), Bozeman
B. L. Herrington, (Chemistry), Bozeman
United States Department of Agriculture:
D. F. Fisher, (Plant Physiology), Wenatchee, Wash.
H. C. Diehl, (Plant Physiology), Wenatchee, Wash.
C. P. Harley, (Plant Physiology), Wenatchee, Wash.
L. E. Reeves, (Plant Physiology), Wenatchee, Wash.
L. A. Fletcher, (Plant Physiology), Wenatchee, Wash.
E. J. Newcomer, (Entomology), Yakima, Wash.
M. A. Yothers, (Entomology), Yakima, Wash.

At the present time E. J. Newcomer is chairman of the project and Anthony Spuler is secretary.

D. F. FISHER,
E. L. GREEN,
E. J. NEWCOMER, *Chairman*

SCIENTIFIC APPARATUS AND LABORATORY METHODS

A METHOD FOR CUTTING GLASS TUBING

A THIRD method for cutting heavy glass tubing may be added to those described by Seemann, SCIENCE, No. 1726, and Tolmachoff, SCIENCE, No. 1733.

A piece of stout string about two feet long is wound once and a half around the tube. The two ends are allowed to hang down on opposite sides of the tube. The tube is held in a wooden vise, clamped on a desk with a wooden clamp, or held by a fellow worker, so that the edge of the desk acts as a guide for the string at the point where the tube is to be cut. The two ends of the string are grasped firmly, one end in each hand. The hands are pumped rapidly up and down, keeping the string tightly pulled around the tube. This is continued a short time until the tube and string are hot enough so that the string begins to smoke. Cold water from a beaker is quickly poured on the hot tube causing a clean break. The entire process may be completed in two or three minutes.

J. L. ST. JOHN
DIVISION OF CHEMISTRY,
AGRICULTURAL EXPERIMENT STATION,
STATE COLLEGE OF WASHINGTON

AN INEFFECTUAL ATTEMPT TO DEMONSTRATE THE VACUOME OF CERTAIN PLANT CELLS

IN an investigation concerning the nature of the plant-vacuole the writer had occasion to attempt a silver impregnation of the vacuome of various kinds of cells. The Golgi method of Da Fano was used because it is recommended by Guilliermond. This method involves the following steps:

(1) Fixation of the tissues in Da Fano fluid, a solution of cobalt nitrate in dilute neutral formalin. This fluid has a pH of 6.7.

(2) Impregnation of the tissues with a silver salt solution, silver nitrate.

(3) Reduction of the pieces of tissue thus treated by means of a modified photographic developer, Cajal solution.

(4) The customary procedure of dehydration, infiltration with paraffin, embedding, sectioning, mounting and counterstaining the tissues.

Root-tips of four-day-old wheat, barley and pea seedlings were used. Guilliermond recommends the use of root-tips of barley and pea seedlings.

By means of the Da Fano method, using the concentrations of Da Fano, Cajal and silver nitrate solutions recommended by Da Fano, the writer attempted to demonstrate the vacuome of the cells of the above tissues. In four of the experiments, the concentration of the solutions used was increased and the time of exposure of the tissues to the solutions was increased. Material on 153 slides, each containing from eight to ten sections, was subjected to the Da Fano procedure and examined carefully. In all cases examination of the sections failed to reveal the existence of a silver impregnated vacuome described and sketched by Guilliermond. In a few sections of wheat-root-tips examined, round black granules appeared in the vacuoles of 80 per cent. of the cells of the meristem. These granules resembled very closely in general appearance, distribution and occurrence the granules described by Guilliermond.

Changes in hydrogen-ion concentration of the fixative used, cobalt nitrate in dilute formalin, were tried. This modification has not been recorded by Guilliermond. The solution was brought to pH 2.4, 3.0, 4.6, 7.0 and 8.0 by the use of potassium acid phthalate and potassium dihydrogen phosphate buffer mixtures. The root-tips fixed in these solutions were then submitted to the remaining steps in the Da Fano procedure. Examination of sixty-two slides, twenty-three of barley containing the sections of ten root-tips and twenty-seven of wheat, containing sections of eight root-tips, revealed empty vacuolar spaces. Nuclei of cells of material fixed in solutions of pH 7.0 and 8.0 contained more granules of reduced silver than did those of material fixed in more acid solutions. The cytoplasm of the former cells also contained a much heavier deposit of silver than did that of the latter cells.

The results herein recorded indicate the extreme capriciousness of the method recommended by Guilliermond. The success of the method seems to be a matter largely of chance or depends upon factors which are as yet unknown.

BERNICE BURKHARDT RICE

UNIVERSITY OF MISSOURI

SPECIAL ARTICLES

THE EFFECT OF X-RAYS IN PRODUCING RETURN GENE MUTATIONS[1]

MOST of the natural mutations known in Drosophila are to the recessive condition. With the exceptions of the reversions from bar eye to full eye and possible return mutations at the white-eye locus there is but scant evidence that this is a reversible reaction.

Muller found that gene mutations produced by X-rays are, in general, in the same direction and of the same nature as those occurring spontaneously in the fruit fly. In the numerous mutations arising in his recent experiments as a result of irradiation Muller has only two cases of return mutations—both involving the same factor locus, *scute*. This raises the problem of why it is more difficult to find mutations in one direction than in another.

Mutations by X-rays are also fortuitous or chance occurrences at the present time. The operator may be likened to a hunter shooting birdshot into a flock of ducks. As the hunter "accepts with natural piety" what comes down, so the investigator shooting X-rays into a flock of genes accepts what is given. For it is impossible to aim at any particular gene at the present time.

However, in spite of the infrequency of return mutations to the normal condition and the impossibility of controlling results, it appeared to the writer that an experiment carried out on sufficiently large scale might give the mutation rate of mutant genes to normal and the relative frequency with which certain specific genes are hit.

The problem then was: Return mutations at specific loci due to the action of X-rays.

The males used in the experiment carried five mutant genes in their X or sex chromosome; those for yellow body, white eye, forked bristles, bar eye and Beadex wings. The first three of these are recessive to normal, the other two are dominants. Part of these males were exposed to X-rays, using a dosage of 50 K. V.; 5 M. A. M.; 15 cm from the target and forty-eight minutes' exposure (known in Muller's Lab. as the T-4 treatment). The remainder were treated for twice this length of time (T-8). During treatment the flies were placed in gelatin capsules punctured by a fine needle to admit air.

Immediately following treatment these males were mated to virgin double-X yellow females. These females are peculiar in that the two sex chromosomes are attached at the right hand end and go together into the same gamete, which is equivalent to 100 per cent. non-disjunction. The double-X yellow females also carry a male Y-chromosome. In such a cross the sons get their X-chromosome from their fathers and their Y-chromosome from their mothers, a reversal of the usual procedure in this species. There are several advantages in using a stock made up in this way. Practically all mutations occurring in the sex chromosome of the treated fathers show up in the first generation of sons, whether recessive or dominant, as they are not covered by normal allelomorphs in the Y-chromosome.

One thousand such virgins were mated to irradiated males, two pairs to a bottle. This gave five hundred bottles and after seven days the parents were transferred to new bottles and remained there for seven days more. This gave one thousand bottles of offspring among which to look for changes in the five specific loci described above. Such heavy dosages of X-rays as were used in this experiment decrease productivity to a marked extent. The writer has shown elsewhere that following dosages of the magnitude used here only 12 per cent. of the eggs laid complete their life history.

The following table gives the count of the young hatching in the one thousand mating bottles. The average young per bottle was only 10.7 per cent. Many bottles contained no offspring at all.

	Males	Females	
T–4	3,796	4,811	
T–8	866	1,243	
	4,662	6,054	10,716

Gene mutations apparently are produced by a dosage which is just under that rendering complete sterility.

While an experiment involving one thousand mating bottles is not exactly small in scale the poor viability of rayed males reduces the offspring to a point where extensive results could hardly be expected. This defect is being remedied by a repetition of the work on an even larger scale. However, the results secured at the bar gene locus throw considerable light on a mooted question and seem worthy of record at the present time.

[1] This work was done in the Zoological Laboratory of the University of Texas during a recent sabbatical leave of absence from Washington University. My appreciation for the many courtesies received is hereby expressed to Professor J. T. Patterson and Professor H. J. Muller.

There were no return mutations at the yellow, white or forked loci. Considering the small number of offspring examined and the rarity of return mutations this is not a matter for surprise. There were eight cases of normal wings instead of the expected Beadex wings. These were either extreme overlaps of the beaded characters or somatic mutations. They did not breed true when mated to double-X yellow virgins, but gave again the beaded wings. There were four cases of reversion to full eye, and these bred true to full. Two were in the T-4 group and two in the T-8 group. This is a ratio of one reversion in 433 males in the T-8; one in 1,898 in the T-4. These are the results of the observations upon the five definite loci studied in the X-chromosome of the male offspring.

In addition, approximately one hundred other mutations, mosaics and abnormalities of various sorts were observed. These occurred in both males and females and affected all parts of the body. The strong temptation to preserve and breed everything that turned up was resisted and the original plan of rigidly concentrating on the five loci described above will be adhered to in further work now under way.

The four reversions to full eye at the bar locus are of considerable importance. Zeleny[2] has studied the bar-eye gene very extensively. He found that bar eye reverts to round eye about once in 1,600 times; and also discovered an allelomorph of bar, called ultra-bar, whose reversion rate is approximately the same. Zeleny considered the bar-eye character to be due to a gene mutation not different from other gene mutations in Drosophila. Upon evidence based on the sex ratio Zeleny concluded that mutations to full eye may occur in the male germ tract as well as in the female.

Sturtevant[3] assumes that Zeleny's data indicate that reversion occurs only in the female and reports extensive experiments which seem to show that reversions at the bar locus are due, not to gene changes at all, but rather to unequal crossing-over between the two X-chromosomes of the female. Hence no reversion in the male is possible, since no crossing-over occurs.

According to Sturtevant crossing-over in the bar region occurs in such a way that the respective points of interchange lie to the left of the bar locus in one chromosome, but to the right of it in the other one. Sturtevant made many crosses and all his data, compiled in nineteen tables, indicated that both reversion to round and to ultra-bar eye (called by him double-bar) was due to unequal crossing-over. He also made a count of 10,179 males derived from a cross with double-X yellow females, in which all males got their X-chromosome from the father, and in these males no rounds or double-bars were observed.

Furthermore, Muller and Dippel[4] counted 35,000 sons that had derived their X-chromosome from a bar-eyed father, and in this large number not a single case of reversion to full eye occurred. These results of Sturtevant and Muller and Dippel seemed to warrant the conclusion that mutations to round eye occurred exclusively in the female. And Sturtevant's experiments indicated that reversion to round eye was due to unequal crossing-over in the female and not to a gene mutation such as is responsible for character changes at other loci.

However, that reversions to round eye *are* possible without crossing-over seems proved by the work with X-rays. Muller (unpublished data) got two reversions to round eye in females in cases where there was no crossing-over near the bar locus (between forked and Beadex), one in control material and the other from lightly X-rayed flies. My results (described above) give one reversion to round in 433 males from heavily treated fathers and one in 1,898 males from fathers less heavily treated. These reversions were obtained under conditions which clearly rule out Sturtevant's theory of unequal crossing-over.

It is of interest that a mutation rate of one in 433 males is probably the highest rate of gene change yet reported in *Drosophila melanogaster*.

FRANK BLAIR HANSON

DEPARTMENT OF ZOOLOGY,
WASHINGTON UNIVERSITY

[2] Zeleny, Charles, 1921. "The Direction and Frequency of Mutation in the Bar-eye Series of Multiple Allelomorphs of *Drosophila*," *Jour. Exp. Zool.*, 34: 203–233.

[3] Sturtevant, A. H., 1925. "The Effects of Unequal Crossing-over at the Bar Locus in *Drosophila*," *Genetics*, 10: 117–147.

[4] Muller, H. J., and Dippel, A. L., 1926. "Chromosome Breakage by X-rays and the Production of Eggs from Genetically Male Tissue in *Drosophila*," *British Jour. Exp. Biol.*, 3: 85–122.

A SPONTANEOUS MODIFICATION OF THE VISCOSITY OF FRESH BLOOD SERUM

IN order to study such unstable solutions as blood serum, it is important to dispose of methods which enable us to follow continuously the evolution of a phenomenon, as a function of time, or temperature, for example, without introducing uncontrollable or disturbing factors. The viscometer described in 1923 (based on the principle of coaxial cylinders) was devised in order to fulfil these requirements, and was used recently to determine the viscosity of fresh normal horse serum, as a function of time. It was found that such a serum, centrifuged immediately after separation from the clot and placed in the viscometer, behaved in the following way: At first, its viscosity, which is rather high (relative viscosity $\frac{\eta}{\eta_0}$ *i.e.*, ratio of the absolute viscosity, of the solution, to that of the solvent, of the order of 3) generally increases for a short time—say ten minutes—then decreases rapidly, almost proportionally to the time, and finally reaches a stable value, considerably lower than the original one (order of magnitude $\frac{\eta}{\eta_0} = 1, 8$). Towards the end, the curve is logarithmic. The total phenomenon requires from one to two hours, as a rule, this time depending mainly, as far as we can see at present, on the amount of handling to which the serum has been submitted.

TABLE I

SPONTANEOUS DECREASE OF THE VISCOSITY OF FRESH BLOOD SERUM (HORSE)

(Exp. N° 10 Ser. N° 3) (Relative viscosity, η)

Time minutes	η
0	2.640
5	2.730
7	2.640
10	2.580
15	2.440
20	2.140
26	1.905
30	1.870
35	1.845
40	1.835
45	1.830
60	1.824
70	1.824

Important fluctuations are sometimes observed at the beginning of the experiment. The spot moves jerkily, as if the bob (inside suspended cylinder of the viscometer) were attached to the outside moving cup and suddenly released.

When the spot is allowed to come back to the zero, that is, when the constant speed motor is stopped, during the first minutes of an experiment, it does *not* come back all the way to the zero, but stops at a certain distance—say thirty or fifty divisions of the scale. As the experiment progresses, however, the distance becomes shorter and shorter, and when the stable value of the viscosity is attained, the zero checks perfectly.

It seems to us that the aforesaid facts can readily be accounted for in the following way: the chemical evolution of the serum begins the minute it is separated from the fibrinogen. It has lost its power of coagulating rapidly, but the splitting, if we may be allowed to say so, of the "plasma molecule" leaves a "serum molecule," which does not immediately reach a stable state. The amputation of the fibrinogen exposes certain unstable chemical groups, which rearrange themselves in time by shifting or otherwise. While they are exposed, however, they still retain to a small extent the power of adhering to one another and to form reticular structures in the solution. These structures are invisible even under the ultra-microscope. But they are strong enough to apparently increase the viscosity of the serum, and, when the rotation of the cup is stopped, to prevent the spot from returning to the zero. As time elapses, the number of molecules capable of adhering to one another decreases, and when the transformation is complete, the zero checks, and the *true* viscosity is measured. Before that, what was measured was really viscosity *plus* a kind of plasticity, and the curves obtained express the progressive passage from one state to the other.

This hypothesis seems to account for the observed phenomena. The increase which takes place at the beginning may be due to the fact that handling of the serum (aspirated and poured into the cup by means of a pipette) breaks down the existing structures, which tend to rebuild themselves up as soon as the serum is in the cup; this would also account for the fluctuations described at the beginning of this paper.

This phenomenon is not without precedent in the colloidal world. Certain iron sols will coagulate, and become fluid again on mere shaking. It is known that the so-called "stabchen-sole" studied by Siedentopf, Szegvari and Zocher show the tendency to form structures by sticking to one another. This phenomenon is different from adsorption, as only certain parts of the particle seem capable of sticking, usually the extremities: Orientation of colloidal molecules or particles is one phase of this phenomenon.

We may now understand why, when studying living cells with dark-field illumination, certain particles can be seen in what seems to be a perfectly structureless protoplasm, obviously agitated with brownian movement, but apparently limited in all direction, as a bird in a cage. The bars of the cage are not visible: yet they are there; this explains how difficult it is to measure the "viscosity" of protoplasm, and also why the protoplasm does not flow out of fibroblasts which usually show at the end of one of their arms an "opening" which is not limited by any visible line. The protoplasm is not coagulated, yet it is maintained, not by surface tension, but by these reticular structures.

In finishing this preliminary note, I wish to express many thanks to Dr. Simon Flexner, director of the Rockefeller Institute, for having allowed me to take over the instruments and apparatus which made this work possible.

LECOMTE DU NOÜY

INSTITUT PASTEUR, PARIS

SCIENCE

VOL. LXVII JUNE 8, 1928 No. 1745

CONTENTS

The Theory of Chemical Action in Electrical Discharge: PROFESSOR S. C. LIND 565
The Plateau Habitat of the Pro-Dawn Man: PROFESSOR HENRY FAIRFIELD OSBORN 570
The Use of Charts in the Natural Sciences: PROFESSOR A. C. NOÉ 571
Scientific Events:
An International Committee for Research on Infantile Paralysis; Dedication of the Santa Catalina Natural Area; Researches and Publications of the Princeton University Expeditions to Patagonia; Reorganization of the Department of Zoology at Columbia University 574
Scientific Notes and News 577
University and Educational Notes 580
Discussion and Correspondence:
The Apportionment of Representatives: PROFESSOR WALTER F. WILLCOX. *Transplantation of the European Oyster:* DR. J. H. ORTON. *The Boiling-Point and the Latent Heat of Vaporization of Water:* DR. J. B. NATHANSON. *Coryneum Canker of Cypress:* WILLIS W. WAGENER. *More Research:* PROFESSOR JAMES S. STEVENS, W. H. KUN, E. H. MCCLELLAND. *Corrections to the Biographical Directory of American Men of Science:* DR. J. MCKEEN CATTELL 581
Reports:
Work Accomplished by the Field Museum Paleontological Expeditions to South America: ELMER S. RIGGS 585
Scientific Apparatus and Laboratory Methods:
Making a Correct Mechanical Analysis of Soils in Fifteen Minutes: PROFESSOR GEORGE J. BOUYOUCOS. *A Simple Method of Picking up Correlations:* DR. CECIL D. MURRAY 587
Special Articles:
A Bioelectric Potential: DR. SAMUEL GELFAN. *Studies on the Physiology of Ascaris Lumbricoides:* JUSTUS F. MUELLER 589
Science News x

SCIENCE: A Weekly Journal devoted to the Advancement of Science, edited by J. McKeen Cattell and published every Friday by

THE SCIENCE PRESS

New York City: Grand Central Terminal

Lancaster, Pa. Garrison, N. Y.

Annual Subscription, $6.00. Single Copies, 15 Cts.

SCIENCE is the official organ of the American Association for the Advancement of Science. Information regarding membership in the Association may be secured from the office of the permanent secretary, in the Smithsonian Institution Building, Washington, D. C.

THE THEORY OF CHEMICAL ACTION IN ELECTRICAL DISCHARGE[1]

THAT slow chemical action accompanies various types of electrical discharge in many gases has been long known. Berthelot[2] summarized and reviewed the earlier as well as his own work, in which the arc, spark or silent discharges were applied to a large number of gases or gaseous mixtures. At that time little or no attempt was made to find a general mechanism or theory. This is not surprising if we remember that almost nothing of our present ideas of discharge in gases was then known. While some of the early results have not been confirmed by later work, most of them have been, and many of the unusual products have also been found in other ways, for example, under *alpha* radiation, proving that the early work of Berthelot, Thenard, Brodie and their contemporaries offers many valuable leads and forms a basis for further progress.

Naturally the first attempts to find a theory for the electrochemical effects in gases were directed toward a correlation between the current flowing and the amount of action produced according to Faraday's law. The disagreement found in the exhaustive researches of Warburg and of others, while unexpected, was so unmistakable that these efforts had to be abandoned.

The theories advanced since then attribute the effects to one of the following agencies: (1) Photochemical; (2) Static ions; (3) Critical activation by kinetic ions. Upon failing to find a relation between current and chemical effect, Warburg quite early adopted the idea that ozone formation, for example, might be due to the ultra-violet light accompanying the discharge. In his review[3] of the subject in 1925 he still adhered to this hypothesis.

The equality of ozonization and ionization of oxygen by means of Tesla discharge convinced Krüger in 1912 of a static-ion theory of ozone formation. Simultaneously a study of ozonization under α radiation led me to the same conclusion, and to a generalization of this theory (as also Krüger) to explain all

[1] The presidential address, presented at the fifty-third general meeting of the American Electrochemical Society at Bridgeport, Conn., April 26, 1928. Colin G. Fink in the chair.

[2] M. Berthelot, "Essai de Mécanique Chimique," Vol. II, Chap. 11 (Dunod, Paris, 1879).

[3] *Zeit. f. techn. Physik.*, 1925, p. 625.

cases of excess of chemical action over current prediction in gaseous discharge, which excess Warburg had shown might readily reach 1,000 fold.

The central hypothesis of the static-ion theory is that the chemical action is the direct result of recombination of positive and negative ions in the bosom of the gas, which never reach the electrodes and hence can have no relation to the current. In fact this represents in some respects a complete antithesis to the conditions of electrolytic reaction. In electrolysis it is the ions which conduct that react chemically, while in gaseous discharge it is the ions that recombine without conducting that react chemically; possibly the ions which conduct also react chemically at the electrodes, but their proportion is a negligibly small part of the total ionization under usual conditions of chemical action in gaseous discharge. In other words, an intensity of ionization that corresponds to measurable chemical action on a basis of equivalence is far outside the range in which saturation current can be produced or even approached. Any attempt to attain saturation by applying more voltage simply produces more ionization by electronic collision, and defeats its purpose by a yet wider margin.

Not only is it impossible to measure the total ionization accompanying electrical discharge through gases, but the theory of the discharge is so imperfectly understood that we are not able to calculate any comparison of the chemical yield with ionization in gaseous discharge.

The question must arise then: Is it important to establish this yield factor? The answer must be affirmative from several standpoints. The information gained about the chemical yield per ion in other types of ionization, especially by *alpha* radiation, has indicated that it is a fundamental constant for a given reaction. We also have much evidence, which is rapidly being strengthened, that the nature of the reaction and of the products is the same for different types of ionizing agencies. This is just what we should expect if the reactions are due to ionization, that the means of producing the ions ought to make no difference, or at least only secondary differences in the character of the reaction.

If this principle can be thoroughly established, then we can reverse the process and use a reaction of known chemical yield per ion to determine the ionization in electrical discharge. This suggestion applies equally well to the high-speed electrons from a Coolidge tube, or to any other ionizing agencies that produce chemical effects, excepting, of course, those types such as arc or spark discharge when temperature effects intervene. If the chemical yield per ion-pair remains constant for a given reaction, whether this ionizing agent be α rays, β rays, X-rays or heavy recoil atoms, there is no reason to foresee that it will not also be true in ionization by electronic discharge.

It has been quite certain for some time that chemical action produced by α rays is not only proportional to, but strictly equivalent to, the ionization. This equivalent is not equal to the Faraday equivalent, but greater within restricted limits. Since for nearly all α ray reactions the value of M/N[4] exceeds unity, usually having values between 2 and 20, we must assume some kind of multiplying process which acts either collectively or successively. The former seems more likely as a working hypothesis, so that we may assume ion clusters, for the existence of which there is also some physical evidence.

Unfortunately, the positive ray method, which gives us the most definite information about gas ions, is not applicable to the study of ion clusters, because it can be operated only at very low pressures, where the collisions necessary for clustering can not occur, and where the clusters if once formed would probably dissociate. Another general method, that of studying ions by means of their velocity of migration in a field, has not proved satisfactory in obtaining the mass of ions. Therefore the chemical method once firmly established may prove to be the best method of studying clustering.

The clustering hypothesis of mechanism of chemical action produced by gas ions may be briefly stated as follows: When a gas molecule is ionized by having one of its electrons removed, a minimum amount of work is required, which regarded thermally is very large, 10 to 20 electron-volts (or 230,000 to 460,000 calories per mole.) for different gases. This leaves a positive ion possessing a large amount of latent energy, and which owing to its charge will exert an induced attraction on neutral molecules that approach or collide with it, thus forming an ion cluster while still retaining its positive charge.

We do not know precisely the size of these clusters nor the efficiency of collision in clustering, but the chemical M/N ratios give a minimum—probably a critical—value for the portion which we may call the *chemical cluster;* while the physical cluster may be larger, and possibly is in dynamic (not kinetic) equilibrium with the colliding neutral molecules and is hence variable rather than critical in size. When the free electron or, in case a gas with electron affinity is present, the negative ion or cluster again unites with the positive cluster, the high energy of ionization is set free, and the cluster either dissociates to the original components (the energy being kinetically degraded to heat) or it may dissociate partly or wholly into the

[4] M/N is the chemical yield per ion-pair, M being the number of molecules reacting for N ion-pairs produced.

elements or into new products of higher heat content, or may be largely stabilized to a product of high molecular weight. The heat of ion-recombination is either radiated[5] away or carried off by some of the molecules from the cluster.

The following empirical rules have been found for the size of that part of the cluster which reacts chemically, that is, for the M/N ratio. (1) In gaseous systems of one component with no affinity for free electrons, $M/N = 2$ (approximately), which means first a positive cluster of about two molecules, which reacts chemically upon being restored to electrical neutrality by the free electron. (2) In gaseous systems of two components one of which is oxygen and the other an oxidizable substance, $M/N = 2 \times$ (simplest stoichiometric reaction formula), one cluster belonging to the positive ion and the other to the negative (oxygen) ion. (3) In unsaturated compounds M/N is usually greater, lying in the region 5 to 20 molecules per ion-pair, the direct products being liquid or solid, confirming a high degree of clustering.

Recent work[6] on the effect of different kinds of electrical discharge, on ethane and on propane gases, has shown that the products both gaseous and liquid are quite similar to those obtained from the same gases by α radiation. Lower hydrocarbons are condensed to higher ones by the elimination of hydrogen or methane, with the formation of some liquid hydrocarbons. In the action on ethane in a Siemens tube, the ratio of methane to hydrogen liberated was quite close to that found for the condensation of ethane, propane, or butane under α radiation.

This makes it evident that the reaction has the same character and general mechanism in both cases, and if due to ionization, as is very probable for the α ray cases, then ionization must also be the primary step in chemical action under electrical discharge. Further we may predict that the character of the reaction should be more or less independent of the type of discharge, which we have found to be the case. Some secondary differences are found. For example, the more disruptive the type of discharge the more tendency there is for liberation of free carbon, and for the formation of insoluble solid hydrocarbons.

All of the predictions made from the α ray results, however, have been so thoroughly supported by the subsequent experiments in electrical discharge, that it seems safe to assume the same general kind of mechanism in both cases.

The acceptance of the static-ion mechanism of reaction in discharge has, however, not been general, perhaps mainly due to the lack of a knowledge of the ionization in order to evaluate the equivalence (M/N ratio). The conditions in electrical discharge are much more complicated than in ionization by radon, and suffer from the great disadvantage that the generation of ions is dependent on the field, and at any pressure above a few millimeters varies with it in a very complicated way.

Even in the α ray work some authorities have felt that it ought to be possible to demonstrate directly the chemical effect of ionization by diminishing or increasing in some independent way the number of ions, and correspondingly the number of molecules made to react. This is however quite impossible, because we have no means of adding more ions, from an independent quantitative source, to the intense ionization already necessary to produce a measurable rate of chemical action. Nor is it possible, as we have seen, to withdraw any considerable fraction of the ions, since such high fields must be applied that a larger but unknown quantity of new ions is at once produced.

The recent success of applying the quantum theory in various directions, especially to photochemistry, has frequently led to the belief that although the reactions under discussion are accompanied by and are proportional to ionization, they must, however, be directly caused by *excited* rather than by ionized molecules. It is sometimes lost sight of that ionization itself represents a wholly quantized as well as a highly energized state, and that there is every theoretical reason to believe that ions are equally if not more reactive chemically than excited molecules, because on account of the high electrical field of ions they exert a larger sphere of influence. We have then just as good reason to expect that the quantum law should apply to ionic-chemical as to photochemical reactions and, as a matter of fact, we have been successful in demonstrating its application in many cases, and without the prevalence of the marked exceptions which characterize the experimental tests of the Einstein Law.

The principle of a third theory, recently proposed from Prof. Donnan's laboratory by Elliott, Joshi and Lunt,[7] might be identified with excitation, though apparently it originated from analogy with a yet less energetic type of activation. They postulate that the concept of "critical activation" may be applied to chemical action in electrical discharge. They assume, as in the collision theory of chemical activation, that the reaction rate is a function of the kinetic energy of the constituent particles, and that it is im-

[5] F. L. Mohler, *Phys. Rev.*, 31, 187 (1928).

[6] Lind and Glockler, *Trans. Am. Electrochem. Soc.*, 52, 37 (1927).

[7] G. A. Elliott, S. S. Joshi, and R. W. Lunt, Trans. Faraday Soc., 23, 57–60 (1927).

material whether the kinetic energy be of thermal or of electrical origin. According to this idea the activating energy might be the sum of kinetic energies of thermal and electrical origin. It would therefore be interesting to see whether reaction in electrical discharge has a positive temperature coefficient, as would be predicted by the theory. Many of the reactions under α radiation do not have, thus supporting a static rather than a kinetic-ion theory.

Based on the hypothesis of the kinetic action of ions, Elliott, Joshi and Lunt developed an equation which it seems would apply equally well for activation by either ions, excited molecules or kinetically activated molecules. Two kinds of experimentation might give a decision in the case of electrical discharge: evaluation of the proportionality factor, as in the determination of M/N or $M/h\nu$ values, or else by increasing the speed of homogeneous electrons until reaction begins. The difficulty of the former has been discussed. Work of the latter kind[8] on the reduction of CuO by H_2 gave no indication of reaction until the excitation potential of H_2 (11.4 volts) was reached, while Storch and Olson[9] and Andersen[10] found no synthesis of ammonia in low voltage arc until the ionization potential of nitrogen (17 volts) was reached.[11] Neither of these results supports the view that electrons produce chemical activation at low speed corresponding to critical activation potential—about 2 volts or 45,000 cal.

Hutchinson and Hinshelwood[11] have also recently investigated in a different way the possibility of a parallelism between electrical and thermal reaction mechanisms. They determine the relative decomposition of N_2O and NH_3 gases in two similar discharge tubes, connected either in series or in parallel. Their results were hardly those to be expected from kinetic activation nor from thermodynamics, but appear to be capable through the following analysis of affording strong support of the ion-cluster hypothesis. They find under parallel conditions that about 4.8 to 7.6 times as many molecules of N_2O are decomposed as of NH_3. The electrode material made little difference, and the rates were first order with respect to pressure, both of which indicate reaction in the gas phase.

While we have rather meager information about the relative chances for different molecules to be ionized in a stream of electrons under potential fall much greater than the ionization potential, it seems probable that the relative ionization of two gases might be about the same as for ionization by α particles. Therefore we may expect at the same pressure in equal electron streams (approximately the same current) that N_2O would be ionized $1.53/0.81 = 1.9$ times more than NH_3.

Furthermore, if the ions produced are of the same character as those from α particles, we may assume that the chemical yield per ion pair will be equal for each reaction to the ion yield in α radiation, which from Wourtzel's[12] results at 18° is 0.8 for NH_3 and 1.74 for N_2O or a ratio $1.74/0.8 = 2.2$. Both of these factors operate in the same direction, to make the decomposition of N_2O $1.9 \times 2.2 = 4.2$ times that of NH_3, which approximates the factor found experimentally by Hutchinson and Hinshelwood.

It should be emphasized that the relative ionization of two gases is not directly related to their ionization potentials, but is as shown by Glasson, proportional to $Z^{2/3}$ (Z = atomic number), or to the cross-sectional density of orbital electrons in the molecules through which a stream of α particles (presumably also a stream of electrons) is passing. For example, the ionization potential of NH_3 is 11.1 volts, while that of N_2O (hitherto not determined) should according to Eve's rule be about the same as that of CO_2, or about 14 volts, which in itself would give no grounds to expect that N_2O would be more readily decomposed than NH_3. Nor could we expect that N_2O on account of a higher ionization potential would be less frequently ionized than NH_3, because the electrons in Hutchinson and Hinshelwood's experiments are produced by an induction coil, and hence move under voltages far above the ionization potentials.

Claims that reaction in electrical discharge may be attributed to excitation rather than ionization have also been made. On a reexamination of the yield of O_3 per ion-pair, Krüger and Utesch[13] estimate from new experiments a yield of 30 to 40 O_3 molecules per ion-pair which they attribute to excitation. Owing, however, to later confirmation[14] of the ion yield in ozone formation under α radiation as $M_{O_3}/N = \mathit{1\ to\ 2}$ and to the uncertainty of the measurement or calculation of ionization in electrical discharge, we are not prepared to accept the high yield as definite.

8 Geo. Glockler, W. P. Baxter, and R. H. Dalton, *J. Am. Chem. Soc.*, 49, 58 (1927).

9 H. H. Storch and A. R. Olson, *J. Am. Chem. Soc.*, 45, 1605 (1923).

10 E. B. Andersen, *Z. Phys.*, 10, 54 (1922).

11 W. K. Hutchinson and C. N. Hinshelwood, Proc. Roy. Soc., 117A, 131–6 (1927).

12 E. Wourtzel, *Jour. de Phys. Rad.*, 11, 341, 345 (1919).

13 F. Krüger and O. Utesch, *Ann. d. Physik.* (4), 78, 113–56 (1925).

14 J. D'Olieslager, *Acad. Roy. Belg.*, 1925, 711; Mund and D'Olieslager, *ibid.*, 1926, 309; *Bull. Soc. Chim. Belg.*, 36, 399 (1927); Lind and Bardwell, "Chemical Effect of Alpha Particles," 2d Ed., p. 92. Chem. Catalog Co., N. Y., 1928.

Finally, I should like to discuss briefly the mechanism of condensing lighter to heavier (condensed or polymerized) molecules either thermally, catalytically, photochemically or electrically. It appears that all of these methods have something in common, though the mechanisms that have been proposed may be differentiated into two quite distinct classes. (1) Primary reaction consisting of clustering followed by splitting (when it takes place) or (2) Primary reaction consisting in first splitting followed by a reassembling of the elements or radicals.

Of these two processes the former has appeared more plausible in conceiving mechanisms for the ionic reactions, and it has recently been suggested[15] that it may also be plausible in some photochemical processes. The hydrocarbon gases, for example, which were formerly thought to be quite difficult to change one into another, have only recently been shown to have great facility, for such changes. H. A. Wilson[16] has proposed, and thermodynamically supported, thermal equilibria of the type

$$2C_nH_{2n+2} \leftrightarrows C_{n+1} + H_{(n+1)2+2} + C_{n-1}\ H_{(n-1)2+2}$$

according to which, ascension in the hydrocarbon scale can be accomplished only by production of an equal number of molecules of lower molecular weight.

It is possible that this type of condensation may occur also in electrical discharge, but apparently more pronounced types predominate, which consist in doubling or multiplying through the elimination of one product of very low molecular weight (H_2 or CH_4) which evidently allows the other product to be correspondingly higher. To illustrate: thermally, according to Wilson, $2C_4H_{10} \leftrightarrows C_3H_8 + C_5H_{12}$; while ionically, according to Lind and Bardwell,[17] $C_4H_{10}^+ + C_4H_{10} = C_8H_{18} + H_2$ or also

$$C_4H_{10}^+ + C_4H_{10} = :C_8H_{16} + 2H_2$$

and

$$x :C_8H_{16} = (C_8H_{16})_x \text{ (liquid)}.$$

Evidently the ionic processes arrive more directly at the product of higher molecular weight, but with a much higher energy expense.

A mechanism by which building up of large molecules is effected by clustering, followed by partial splitting, seems more plausible than to assume that the splitting occurs first and building up subsequently. This may apply to some photochemical as well as to ionic syntheses.

Referring to the statement of Elliott, Joshi and Lunt (*loc. cit.*) that, "Despite the numerous investigations that have been made on chemical changes produced by an electric discharge through a gas, no satisfactory general hypothesis has yet been suggested to describe the mechanisms of such changes," I should say that the fault lies rather with the inadequacy of the theory of electrical discharge in gases than with the hypothesis of the nature of the chemical changes produced. As long as we can neither measure nor calculate the ionization, any theory based on ionization must lack quantitative support and depend on indirect evidence, although it may later prove to be a correct theory. Proof that the velocity of reaction (K) is related to the pressure (p) at constant current by a linear relation of p to log K/p would be equally true for the static-ion theory, since p must have a double function in determining the energy received from the electron stream (by any mode whatsoever—ionization, excitation or critical activation) and again in determining collisions between energized and ordinary molecules in the completion of the chemical reaction.

To review the two theories more generally, it would appear that if enough energy has already been expended to produce ions, a very large amount of latent energy is possessed by the ions, so that they need no additional kinetic energy to make them reactive toward other molecules. The only way to disprove this by energy considerations would seem to be by showing that a larger amount of action is accomplished than can be accounted for on the cluster theory. This involves evaluation of the proportionality factor which for electrical discharge has not yet been done and, as we have seen, can not be accomplished until the ionization can be determined. But if we may reason by analogy from the α ray results, static ions without any kinetic energy (resulting from a field) are quite sufficient, and the yields found do not exceed the possibilities of clustering. That the α ray results for the hydrocarbon gases may be applied by analogy to the chemical action of *electrical discharge* in the same gases has already been discussed.

Continuation of the work reported at the last meeting of the Society has yielded further confirmation of the ion cluster theory. By controlling the conditions of condensation[18] the average molecular weight of the liquid product from ethane has been lowered from 467 to 120.

S. C. LIND

SCHOOL OF CHEMISTRY,
UNIVERSITY OF MINNESOTA

[15] Lind, *J. Phys. Chem.*, 32, 575 (1928).

[16] H. A. Wilson, Proc. Roy. Soc., 116A, 501–15 (1927).

[17] *J. Am. Chem. Soc.*, 48, 2346 (1926).

[18] Lind and Glockler, *J. Am. Chem. Soc.*, 50, June (1928).

THE PLATEAU HABITAT OF THE PRO-DAWN MAN

GROUNDS for the pro-Dawn Man theory[1] are directly derived in part from existing embryological, anatomical and zoological evidence, in part from certain principles of animal descent or phylogeny which were entirely unknown in the period when Charles Darwin published his classic work, "The Descent of Man" (1871), and the shortly succeeding period when Huxley wrote his famous essay, "Man's Place in Nature." Although following Lamarck, who early in the nineteenth century sketched the apes as human ancestors, Charles Darwin required great courage to draw in 1871 the following picture of our ancestors:

> The early progenitors of man must have been once covered with hair, both sexes having beards; their ears were probably pointed, and capable of movement; and their bodies were provided with a tail, having the proper muscles. Their limbs and bodies were also acted on by many muscles which now only occasionally reappear, but are normally present in the Quadrumana. At this or some earlier period, the great artery and nerve of the humerus ran through a supra-condyloid foramen. The intestines gave forth a much larger diverticulum or caecum than that now existing. The foot was then prehensile, judging from the condition of the great toe in the foetus; and *our progenitors, no doubt, were arboreal in their habits, and frequented some warm, forest-clad land.*

I take the liberty of italicizing the two most salient lines in this oft-quoted passage because they give the key to the thought of Darwin and of subsequent advocates of the ape-man theory down to the present time. Over against such a habitat which has framed the structure of all anthropoid apes may be placed the conclusion theoretically reached by the brilliant geologist, Joseph Barrell, in 1917, and independently reached by myself by direct observation during my journey of 1923 into the heart of the desert of Gobi. To my knowledge Barrell was the first to formulate what may be called a semi-arid plateau theory of the origin of man, as recently quoted by Charles Berkey in "Geology of Mongolia":[2]

> . . . Among the many suggestive thoughts offered by Joseph Barrell (1917) as guiding hypotheses for our explorations in central Asia, his idea about primitive man is especially ingenious. Man's strong padded foot, his relatively long leg and his erect posture, are all distinct departures from an adaptation to life in the trees, and tend, instead, to fit him for running and for tramping long distances; in short, for life on open plains where trees grow in patches along the stream courses, rather than for life in a dense forest. Granting that the more distant ancestors of men lived in trees and in jungles, it seems probable that they would have remained arboreal in an environment of jungle and forest. But in a region where forests were thinning, where open, treeless plains were beginning to appear, and where the climate was changing toward cooler and more arid conditions, it seems probable that arboreal types must adapt themselves to the plains, or become extinct.

I am not conscious of having seen or heard of Barrell's generalization prior to my own discovery of the same principle, which I enunciated before a gathering of geologists and natural philosophers in Peking:[3]

> Mongolia was probably not a densely forested country—this is indicated by the animal remains found there in the earlier deposits. An alert race can not develop in a forest—a forested country can never be a center of radiation for man. Nor can the higher type of man develop in a lowland river-bottom country with plentiful food and luxuriant vegetation. It is upon the plateaus and relatively level uplands that life is most exacting and response to stimulus most beneficial. Mongolia always has been an upland country, through the Age of Mammals and before. It was probably a region forested only in part, mainly open, with exhilarating climate and with conditions sufficiently difficult to require healthy exertion in obtaining food supply. . .
>
> In the uplands of Mongolia conditions of life were apparently ideal for the development of early man, and since all the evidence points to Asia as the place of origin of man, and to Mongolia and Tibet, the top of the world, as the most favorable geographic center in Asia for such an event, we may have hopes of finding the remote ancestors of man in this section of the country. However, this Mongolian idea must be treated only as an opinion; it is not yet a theory, but the opinion is sufficiently sound to warrant further extended investigation.

No pro-human habitat could present a wider contrast than does the central Asiatic plateau to Darwin's "warm, forest-clad land." All recent ethnologic and physiographic evidence points in the same way, namely, that intelligent progressive and self-adaptive types of mankind arise in elevated upland or semi-arid environments where the struggle for food is intense and where reliance is made on the invention and development of implements as well as

[1] Before the American Philosophical Society, April 20, 1928, the author renewed his attack upon the ape-man theory of human ancestry which he began at the bicentenary meeting of the society in April, 1927.

[2] Charles P. Berkey, Frederick K. Morris: "Geology of Mongolia. Natural History of Central Asia," Vol. 11. Published by the American Museum of Natural History, New York, 1927.

[3] H. F. Osborn: "Why Mongolia may be the Home of Primitive Man." *The Peking Leader*, October 10, 1923.

weapons. On the contrary, there is no premium on invention, intelligence, or self-adaptation in mammals of any kind living in warm forests.

Granting all the very strong *circumstantial* evidence in favor of the ape-man theory, which has been piled mountain high by investigators since the time of Darwin and has been recently revived and stimulated to new force by the attacks of the fundamentalists on the whole evolution theory, we must look for the direct evidence which can come only from geology and palæontology. The final solution of this problem of problems therefore rests with the fossil hunter and explorer, whose task is an extremely difficult one because fossil remains of Primates, always scarce, are becoming increasingly scarce as the Primates rise in the scale of intelligence. I do not know the exact figures, but I think it is safe to say that 50,000 to 1 is about the ratio of probability of discovery of fossil remains of lower orders to fossil remains of Primates in Tertiary time.

Meanwhile, the circumstantial evidence of geology and of geography is all in favor of the theory that the pro-man stock was well established in Oligocene time, now conservatively estimated at sixteen million years ago. At this time occurred the first *modernization* of the entire mammalian kingdom. So far as we can observe geologically, this modernization was due to the first great wave of aridity concurrent with the complete elevation of great continental plateaus, especially in central Asia and in the western region of North America.

This wave of aridity and of elevation caused a profound cleavage in the mammalian world, the first great natural divorce between the warm forest-loving types developed during the preceding Eocene period and the temperate plains and plateau-loving types which apparently invaded the great Oligocene belt of the 40th parallel from the north. This cleavage profoundly affected the whole mammalian world of this region; not only the horses, rhinoceroses, tapirs, and even-toed animals like the progenitors of the deer, the cattle, and the camel families had to make their choice between forest regions and the plains, but the carnivorous enemies—wolves and foxes and the progenitors of the greater carnivores in the cat family—were compelled to go forest-ward or plains-ward. It is not at all probable that the Primates—lemurs, North and South American monkeys and the hypothetic division of pro-man—were exempt from this compelling and fateful decision. Why was it postponed by the progressive progenitors of man when adopted by all the progressive elements in the remaining mammalian world? Why theoretically postpone this fateful decision on the part of our primate ancestors to Miocene or Pliocene time, as is still done by many conservative writers who continue to adhere to the abandoned conceptions of the period of Charles Darwin's speculation partly because of loyalty to him and reverence for his classic contribution to anthropology?

This concludes the seventh address which I have devoted to this absorbing subject. In the succeeding or eighth address I shall continue the attack and try to demonstrate that while the anatomical and embryological evidence for the *kinship* of the apes to man is overwhelming, the same evidence, when closely analyzed and subjected to conditions of modern principles of phylogeny discovered since Darwin's time, compels us to replace the ape-man hypothesis by the new pro-Dawn Man theory.

HENRY FAIRFIELD OSBORN

THE USE OF CHARTS IN THE NATURAL SCIENCES

OLD teachers of natural science subjects will remember the time when charts were used extensively in classroom and laboratory instruction. That was before the general introduction and universal use of the lantern, now the principal means of classroom demonstration. The lantern slide has almost completely driven out the chart, and many university departments of zoology, anatomy, physiology, bacteriology and botany have practically no charts at all, or whatever they have is antiquated material or home-made, crude and unattractive.

A recent inspection of new German charts suggested the question whether we have not gone too far in our abandonment of the use of the chart and have deprived ourselves of a help, which the lantern-slide can not and will not render. In Germany it was undoubtedly the reason of economy which prompted the continuous use of charts instead of slides. Under present circumstances no German university institute could afford to equip each classroom with a lantern or to have enough portable lanterns on hand to put one at the disposal of each lecturer or laboratory instructor. Of course there are some lanterns in German universities, but they are few and far between. The same is true to a still higher degree of French educational institutions. Also, the high perfection in graphic arts in Germany and the comparatively low cost of publishing charts of a high artistic value have contributed in a large degree to the universal demand for charts in German classrooms.

Sometimes the lantern-slide is superior to the chart. It allows a much greater variety of illustrations. It is handy to use and every biological laboratory has the equipment to make lantern-slides from micro-photographs, from field-photographs, from book illustrations and drawings. The costs are comparatively low, and it is easy to build up a collection of thousands of slides in the course of years. When the classroom is darkened and the lantern in operation, it is easy to run through a series of sixty to seventy-five slides during a classroom period of one hour. But there is one great disadvantage connected with this form of instruction. It invites haste and superficiality and the attention of the student is purely voluntary and frequently very inadequate. He looks upon the lantern-slide demonstration as an entertainment which he may follow or not. Since he can not take any notes in the dark classroom and can make no drawings from lantern-slides, he has no record and he knows that he can not be examined about the material shown in this way. He is also deprived of a chance to review these pictures at his convenience after class. Also the lantern-slide can never be used for laboratory purposes, since a continuous comparison between object and picture is impossible. In spite of these drawbacks the lantern-slide will undoubtedly continue to hold its place as a means of convenient and rapid demonstration.

Where the lantern-slide fails, the chart can take its place to greater advantage. If charts are used in a class, the student can make notes of the lecture and if he has enough time he can accompany these notes by drawings. If the charts are left in the room, the student may use them for additional notes, drawings and reviews after recitation. Charts can be exhibited in a laboratory and left there during the entire laboratory period and the student can constantly compare what he sees in the microscope or what he has on his dissecting table with the information supplied by the chart. Good charts will emphasize certain features of an object and omit details which make a photographic picture frequently less lucid. Also, the charts can picture objects of which photographs are hard or impossible to obtain and maybe the results of a teaching experience which is not available for many instructors. These are sufficient reasons to suggest a revision of our present abandonment of charts and to consider seriously whether departments of zoology, botany, physiology, anatomy, general biology, not to mention geography and geology, should not give very serious attention to charts, as means of rounding out their equipment for illustrative material.

Of the many new charts which have recently been published, mostly in Germany, a few of the outstanding sets will be discussed in the following.

In the field of general biology should be noted Haecker's Wandtafeln zur allgemeinen Biologie. Among other subjects they illustrate Mendel's law, the De Vries' theory of mutation, also the protective coloring of insects and the influence of temperature on insect colors. Matzdorf's Lebensbeziehungen und Gewohnheiten der Tiere shows the effects of mimicry in animals and their different habitats. The life of protozoa is illustrated in Täuber's Mikroskopische Wandtafeln.

In zoology the front rank is still held by Leuckart and Nitsche's Zoologische Wandtafeln. This large series has one hundred sixteen large-sized charts and covers the whole ground which may be taken up by any general zoology course dealing with invertebrates. These charts are masterpieces of accuracy and scientific detail and supply inexhaustible material for laboratory study.

Among the other charts in general zoology two main groups may be observed, one in which the animals are pictured detached and without reference to biological features, like habitats or ecologic relation to man, and the other where the animal is considered as part of its natural surroundings. The first group is represented by such collections as Jung, Koch and Quentel's Neue Wandtafeln für den Unterricht in der Naturgeschichte, Schroeder and Kull's Biologische Wandtafeln zur Tierkunde, Pfurtscheller's Zoologische Wandtafeln, or Engleder's Wandtafeln für den naturkundlichen Unterricht (Tierkunde). There is another group as mentioned above which pictures the animals with their natural background. These charts are mostly of high artistic value, having been executed by painters of ability following the advice of scientists. Many of these charts are so beautiful that they could be used for decorative purposes and might find permanent places in museum rooms, classrooms and corridors. Here should be mentioned Täuber's Zoologische Wandbilder, Schmeil's Zoologische Wandtafeln, and Lehmann-Leutemann's Zoologischer Atlas. For instruction in animal anatomy should be mentioned Brass-Lehmann's Zootomische Wandtafeln and Täuber's Zootomische Wandtafeln.

A very attractive series of instruction in embryology and histology is represented by Smalian's Histologische embryologische Tafeln.

Among various entomological charts may be mentioned Schlüter's Schädlingstafeln der Deutschen Gesellschaft für Angewandte Entomologie. On fourteen charts the most important harmful insects are given in relation to their human and plant hosts. Another interesting set describing entomological objects are Meinhold-Pascal's Biologische Charakterbilder der Niederen Tiere. This set of seventeen charts deals with representative types without reference to harmfulness and shows them in their natural surroundings and activities.

For bacteriology two sets of charts have been published by F. Lucksch. Series I shows the general forms, structure, sheaths and cilia of bacteria. Series II deals with pathogenic bacteria.

The best set of charts ever produced on human anatomy are unquestionably the American Frohse Life-Size Anatomical Charts. These eight charts are the most valuable means of instruction in human anatomy and are known to all medical men. A smaller set along the same lines is formed by Zschommler's Buntfärbige Röntgenbilder, in which the human body is pictured as if seen transparent. In this way the bones and softer organs can be seen in their natural relation to each other. The set consists only of two charts and gives the front and rear view of the body. Other sets of charts dealing with human anatomy are Fiedler and Hoelemann's Anatomische Wandtafeln and K. G. Lutz's Anatomische Wandtafeln. There is also a French series of charts, the Deyrolle, on human anatomy, but it does not compare in any way with the American or German publications.

It is especially the science of botany where the German charts excel, although a slight disadvantage is the difference in species which characterizes the North American and the German floras. This difference is not large enough to form a serious handicap for the use of the foreign charts, since a great many species are common or internationally known.

The most important series in general botany are L. Kny's Botanische Wandtafeln. The former is a set of 120 charts and represents an extensive botany course in itself. Its complete study would take at least a year for any beginning class in botany, but many of these charts could also be used in various advanced courses dealing with anatomy or morphology of plants. The manual which is published with these charts covers 563 octavo pages of German text. Other large sets illustrating botany are Balslev-Warming's Botanische Wandtafeln and Engleder's Wandtafeln für den naturkundlichen Unterricht, Pflanzenkunde. The two last-mentioned sets do not deal with general botany but are more or less useful for courses in local floras and in plant taxonomy. A very beautiful set of charts illustrating the principal tree types are Hartinger's Wandtafeln: Bäume. The set pictures on twenty-five charts the most important tree types of the temperate zones. The execution of the charts is so beautiful that every one of them could be used for exhibition. They give the local background and natural setting of the trees.

The modern botanical subject of plant ecology is well represented in Potonié-Gotham's Vegetationsbilder der Jetzt- und Vorzeit. Six of these charts deal with the different ecologic types of modern vegetation as climax forest, swamp vegetation, mural flora, alpine flora, prairie vegetation and high moor flora. Two other charts are reconstructions of ancient floras and are unique in their way, being devised by men who were thoroughly familiar with plant paleontology and executed by prominent artists. One of these two charts represents a late Paleozoic swamp forest from the coal age while the other chart pictures a Mesozoic forest probably from the Jurassic period. The Potonié-Gotham charts are 50 x 38 inches and their size makes them highly acceptable for decorative purposes in classrooms and museums. A number of sets are devoted exclusively to the subject of plant anatomy. Among these is most complete the collection of Frank and Tschirch's Wandtafeln für den Unterricht in der Pflanzenphysiologie. This set pays special attention to plant anatomy from the viewpoint of physiology. A much smaller series containing only eight charts brings out some of the most important data of plant anatomy as different types of cells and tissues.

There are two well-known sets dealing with the subject of plant pathology, one in French and one in German. The first one is Fron's Maladies des Plantes Cultivées et leur Traitement. It contains only a limited number of charts dealing with important diseases of agricultural plants. A much more complete treatment of the same subject is found in Appel-Riehm's Atlas der Krankheiten der Landwirtschaftlichen Kulturpflanzen. This collection of rather small charts ($11\frac{1}{2}$ x $17\frac{1}{2}$) commends itself not only for classroom purposes but also as a laboratory text-book and field guide. The illustrations are excellent and picture the different diseases of cereals, vegetables, fruit and seed plants.

There are several sets of charts dealing with foreign useful plants, mostly tropical. Since the charts are published in Germany, the American cotton and tobacco figure amongst the foreign plants. One series of charts along these lines is Zippel's Ausländische Kulturpflanzen. There are sixty-seven charts divided into three series in the set, and the plants are shown on black background with analytic drawings of various organs as insets. Another series on the same subject is Goehring-Schmidt's Die wichtigsten ausländischen Kulturpflanzen. The charts of this series show the plants in their natural setting and with their human relations and therefore are also valuable for geographic instruction. The coloring and design are very beautiful. Apparently the

Goehring-Schmidt charts have been drawn from first-hand information because all details with regard to plantations, to natives and to the preparation of plant products are true to nature and not made from imagination. The entire series is one of the most attractive sets of charts that has ever been produced.

Recently a number of geological and paleontological charts have come to the writer's attention. Very useful for the teaching of historical geology are Lindner's Wandtafel zur Erdgeschichte. The chart summarizes the principal facts of earth history and can be used not only for an introductory lecture but would also be valuable for permanent use during such courses in zoology and botany where constant reference to geologic epochs must be made. It is a chart which the students should carefully study provided that they know enough German to understand a limited number of geologic terms. The chart is divided in columns which deal with the different epochs and their subdivisions, with the distribution of sedimentary and igneous rocks in geologic time, with the history of structural changes, climates and organic developments, and with the varying distributions of land and water during the earth's history.

An attractive set of charts on paleontology is Fraas' Die Entwicklung der Erde und ihrer Bewohner, in seven colored charts, representing the most important epochs in the history of the earth. Each chart contains in its upper part a reconstruction of the principal animal and plant types arranged in an ideal landscape picture, with a legend in the left-hand upper corner, while the lower half of the chart shows the geologic profile of the rock formation on the right side, and a plate with index fossils of the respective period on the left side. The ideal landscape represents merely life at a given moment during the formation in question, but the profile generalizes the geologic sections through all important horizons of the entire period. Therefore the profiles of the different charts, taken together, give a continuous sequence of the geologic deposits through the earth's crust. It is obvious that this series would prove not only useful in introductory courses in the earth's history but would be very profitable for a short series of historical lectures connected with courses in evolution.

Physiography is a subject which leads from geology into geography. It is well represented in a series of charts by Fraas, Die Naturerscheinungen der Erde. The charts deal with the phenomena and the effects of volcanic action, the mechanical forces of water and air, the rôle which ice is playing to-day on the surface of the earth and with such physiographic character types as the prairie, the coral reef, and the desert.

There are numerous charts devoted to the teaching of geography, especially human ecology. Let us select as a representative series for this discussion Wünsche's Land und Leben. In forty beautifully executed pictures, scenes from cities, harbors, rivers, primitive forests, jungles, prairies, all over the world are shown, with groups of people in their peculiar activities. There is an immense geographic information accumulated in these pictures which seem to have all been prepared by artists on the basis of first hand knowledge. They all look so real and are in no way a product of imagination or second-hand information.

With the exception of one set which is American, and two sets which are French, the charts mentioned in this article are all "made in Germany." They are well executed in colors, in high type of German graphic workmanship. Each set is accompanied by a manual written in Germany and only in very few instances this manual contains an English and French translation. The fact that the manual is written in a foreign language is unquestionably a disadvantage, but it also reminds the American scientist that he can get only the full benefit of the world's treasure of information if he is able to read German with sufficient fluency. There seems to be no escape from this fact in spite of the idea which sprang up during the Great War that the German language can be counted out of the necessary equipment of a scientist. At least it won't be true as long as the Germans continue to publish information of general usefulness.

A. C. NOÉ
UNIVERSITY OF CHICAGO

SCIENTIFIC EVENTS

AN INTERNATIONAL COMMITTEE FOR RESEARCH ON INFANTILE PARALYSIS

AN international committee for the study of infantile paralysis has recently been formed under the chairmanship of Dr. W. H. Park, director of the bureau of laboratories of the New York City Health Department. Arrangements have been made for a concerted three-year attack on the difficult problems of prevention and therapy presented by this formidable and crippling disease. To enable research to be conducted at a number of centers in the United States and in Europe, a sum of $250,000 has been contributed by Mr. Jeremiah Milbank, a New York financier, who takes an active personal interest in hospitals and charities. The following centers have been chosen for the proposed researches: Bureau of Laboratories, New York City Health Department; the pathological laboratories of Columbia, Harvard and Chicago Universities; the Pasteur Institute, Brussels, and the Lister

Institute, London. These various institutes are represented on the international committee by their respective heads. The personnel of the committee is as follows: *Chairman*, Dr. W. H. Park; *vice-chairman*, Dr. Joseph A. Blake, of Tarrytown, N. Y.; Drs. E. O. Jordan and Ludvig Hektoen, of the University of Chicago; Drs. F. P. Gay and Frederick Tilney, of the College of Physicians and Surgeons, Columbia University; Drs. Milton J. Rosenau and Hans Zinsser, of Harvard University; Dr. Lee K. Frankel, of the Metropolitan Life Insurance Company; Sir Charles J. Martin, of the Lister Institute, London, and Dr. Jules Bordet, of the Pasteur Institute, Brussels. Mr. Samuel M. Greer and Dr. Josephine N. Neal will act, respectively, as treasurer and secretary, and the committee's headquarters will be Dr. Park's office at the Bureau of Laboratories, East 16th Street, New York, N. Y. Directors of research at each selected center will be free to initiate such investigations as seem to them desirable and within the compass of their respective institutions. The results of such researches will, however, be studied and coordinated by the international committee, and will thus constitute a joint piece of work. At the Lister Institute special arrangements are being made for research on poliomyelitis under the direction of Professor J. C. G. Ledingham.

DEDICATION OF THE SANTA CATALINA NATURAL AREA

ON May 12, 1928, the Santa Catalina Natural Area, near Summerhaven in the Santa Catalina Mountains of southern Arizona, was dedicated by the Tucson Natural History Society and representatives of the United States Department of Agriculture.

The area lies at an elevation range of from 4,800 to 9,150 feet and includes 4,464 acres. It embraces the summit of Mount Lemmon, Marshall Gulch (where the Desert Laboratory of the Carnegie Institution of Washington has several experimental plots), the Wilderness of Rocks and a considerable part of the headwaters of Lemmon Creek. It contains samples of nearly all the ecologic communities represented in the higher parts of the mountains.

The dedication is the result of a movement initiated several years ago by the Tucson Natural History Society. After a period of investigation by the society's committee on preservation of natural areas and by officials of the Forest Service, the matter was taken up with the forester and the Secretary of Agriculture in Washington. On March 3, 1927, favorable decision was made by the secretary.

Administration and management of the area is to be by the Forest Service. Regulations applying to the tract have been worked up jointly by the society and the service.

The dedicatory program was opened by Dr. Chas. T. Vorhies, of the University of Arizona. Assistant District Forester John D. Jones, of Albuquerque, New Mexico, explained the Forest Service policy, adopted by the forester on December 30, 1926, providing for five categories of tracts: (1) Wilderness areas, more than 500,000 acres; (2) semi-wilderness areas, 25,000 to 250,000 or 300,000 acres; (3) natural areas, 320 to 4,000 or 5,000 acres; (4) scenic areas, of varying size; (5) scenic strips, along selected highways. These areas are planned to care for different phases of the scientific and recreational needs of the people.

Other speakers on the program included G. A. Pearson, director of the Southwestern Forest Experiment Station, Flagstaff, Arizona, and Dr. Walter P. Taylor, of the U. S. Biological Survey.

The dedicatory program was concluded by the exhibition, in the lobby of La Mariposa Hotel, Summerhaven, of five reels of motion pictures, through the courtesy of the Forest Service and Mr. J. D. Jones. These were "Forest and Waters," "Horses and Men" and "Trees of Righteousness."

The committee in charge of the dedication was A. A. Nichol, secretary of the Tucson Natural History Society, *chairman;* Chas. T. Vorhies, of the University of Arizona, and Fred Winn, supervisor, Coronado National Forest.

RESEARCHES AND PUBLICATIONS OF THE PRINCETON UNIVERSITY EXPEDITIONS TO PATAGONIA—1896–1899

AT the recent meeting of the American Philosophical Society, Professor William Berryman Scott reported on the imminent completion of a very great scientific undertaking begun in 1896. The publication of reports of Professor Scott's work in Patagonia between the years 1896 and 1899 was originally rendered possible through the interest and generous donations of the late J. Pierpont Morgan, supplemented by gifts from the Carnegie Institution and Princeton University. In recognition of the high scientific value of this work, Professor Scott has been awarded the Wollaston medal by the Geological Society of London. Professor Scott's informal statement of the progress of work is as follows (*H. F. O.*):

Like everything else in connection with the Princeton Patagonian expeditions, the plan of the series of reports was due to Mr. J. B. Hatcher, the leader of the explorations. So great were the collections in all departments of natural history, that he felt it would be a great misfortune to have the results scattered through many publications—journals and transactions and proceedings of learned societies; and he therefore proposed to me that I should endeavor to finance the independent publication of these remarkable results. The late Mr. J. Pierpont Morgan gave me $24,000 for the work; and, so far as could be foreseen at that time (1900), this sum should have been sufficient, as the plan called for only eight quarto volumes. Unfortunately, however, every contributor far exceeded his estimates as to the amount of text and the number of plates which he would require, and the nominal eight volumes have expanded to fourteen. The additional sums necessary for the publication have been obtained partly from the Carnegie Institution of Washington ($1,500) and Princeton University ($6,000), and from sales of the work to subscribers.

Volume I contains the narrative of the expeditions and the geography of Patagonia by Mr. J. B. Hatcher, whose untimely death prevented his taking any further part in preparing the Reports.

Volume II (Ornithology) was mostly written by the late Messrs. W. E. D. Scott, of Princeton, and R. B. Sharp, of the British Museum, both of whom died in 1910, leaving that volume unfinished. Their remaining manuscript was taken by Dr. Witmer Stone, of the Philadelphia Academy of Natural Sciences, and the final part was entirely written by him.

Volume III (Zoology) is due to a number of hands. The late Dr. J. A. Allen, of the American Museum of Natural History in New York, wrote the chapters on the Mammals; Dr. L. Stejneger, of the U. S. National Museum, prepared those on the Reptiles and Amphibia; the late Dean Eigenmann, of the University of Indiana, wrote the report on Fishes; the late Dr. A. E. Ortmann, formerly of Princeton and then of the Carnegie Museum in Pittsburgh, reported on the Crustacea; Professor Calvert, of the University of Pennsylvania, wrote that part on the Leeches, and Professor Moore, of the same institution, was also a contributor.

Volumes IV to VII, inclusive, were devoted to paleontology. Volume IV contains the reports of Dr. T. W. Stanton, of the U. S. National Museum, on the Cretaceous Invertebrates, by Dr. Ortmann on the Tertiary Invertebrates, and finally the report by Dr. W. J. Sinclair, of Princeton, on the Marsupials of the Santa Cruz formation. Volume V was entirely written by myself, and contains the descriptions of the Edentata and Glires (Rodentia) of the Santa Cruz. Volume VI has Dr. Sinclair's chapters on the Santa Cruz Typotheria, and mine on the Toxodontia and Entelonychia. The remaining part of this volume, my report on the Astrapotheria and the monkeys in the Santa Cruz, is now in the printer's hands, and will, I trust, appear in a few weeks. Volume VII contains my chapters on the Litopterna. Dr. M. S. Farr, of Princeton, is preparing the report on the fossil birds of Patagonia, and that will go to the printer as soon as the Astrapotheria are completed. And, finally, is a brief summing up of the Santa Cruz fauna and the Patagonian geology by myself. This will contain nine plates in heliotype reproduction of Mr. Charles Knight's restorations of Santa Cruz mammals, plates which are now being made in Boston by the firm of E. O. Cockayne. I am particularly glad to publish these restorations, because of the great interest which Mr. Morgan took in them. One of the first things he said, on agreeing to furnish the funds, was that we should immediately turn to Knight for a series of restorations.

Volume VIII, and a supplementary volume, are devoted to botany. The great bulk of this Flora Patagonica was prepared by the late Professor George Macloskie, of Princeton, with the most valuable criticism and assistance of the eminent Swedish botanist, Per Dusen, who also wrote the chapters on the Patagonian mosses. The report on the Hepaticae was written by Professor Evans, of Yale University.

I can already give a very close approximation to the number of pages of text and of plates which the finished work will contain, as all the plates are either finished, or in the hands of the engravers. The great majority of the plates are lithographs, which were made by the firm of Werner and Winter, of Frankfurt, in Germany; but some photographic processes were made in this country, partly in New York, and partly in Boston. The water color drawings for the modern birds were done by Mr. Keulemans, who was so long associated with Dr. Sharp in the work of the British Museum. The botanical plates were mostly prepared in London, as Dr. Macloskie, through his connections there, was able to exercise a closer supervision than he could have done in Frankfurt. The total number of pages of text is approximately 4,880, of a preliminary text cvii, and of plates 421, of which latter 37 are colored. Much of the value of the work is derived from its admirable plates and for these the original drawings were principally made by the late M. von Itenson and Bruce Horsfall. The work of Messrs. Knight and Keulemans has already been mentioned.

In this country there are about 100 subscribers, and in addition there are a number of free and exchange copies. I have, as yet, had no report from the European publishers at Stuttgart.

The long delay in the completion of the work has been due partly to the war, and partly to the period of extravagant prices which followed. This inflation affected especially everything connected with the making of books, having more than doubled the cost per unit of the parts which remained to be issued after the war. The end is now in sight; and I can not but esteem myself fortunate in having been able to see the great work thus far on its way.

REORGANIZATION OF THE DEPARTMENT OF ZOOLOGY AT COLUMBIA UNIVERSITY

Columbia University has announced plans to develop the department of zoology. These include the appointment of Dr. Leslie Clarence Dunn, of the Agricultural Experiment Station at Storrs, Conn., and James Gray, of the University of Cambridge, England, to carry on the experimental work in genetics. This program of expansion also embraces broadening of research, creation of a new professorship and a new lectureship, reorganization of courses, enlargement of equipment and, ultimately, the construction of laboratories for the biological sciences rivaling those recently provided for physics and chemistry.

Dr. Edmund B. Wilson, Da Costa professor of zoology and executive officer of the department, who has been at Columbia for thirty-seven years, will retire from active service on July 1 with the rank of professor emeritus in residence. With President Henry Fairfield Osborn, of the American Museum of Natural History, he organized the department of zoology at Columbia in 1891. Professor Wilson will continue to conduct research at the university, and will be available for consultation and advice by advanced students. He will not, however, offer any stated instruction leading to a degree. As previously announced, Professor T. H. Morgan will leave the university in July for the California Institute of Technology, at Pasadena, Calif., where he will be the head of the division of biological sciences.

Dr. Gary N. Calkins, who holds the professorship of protozoology, will succeed Dr. Wilson as executive head of the department.

Dr. Dunn, who will occupy the new professorship of zoology, was born in Buffalo, N. Y., in 1893, and was graduated from Dartmouth College in 1915. He pursued advanced studies at Harvard University, taking the degree of doctor of science in 1920. For four years he was assistant in zoology at Harvard.

Mr. Gray, the new lecturer in zoology, is now lecturer in zoology at King's College, Cambridge. He is well known in the younger British group in zoology. He is thirty-eight years of age and was trained at Cambridge, where he received the degree of A.B. in 1912 and A.M. in 1916. Mr. Gray will lecture on experimental zoology and embryology. His researches have been in the field of experimental embryology and cytology, including researches on artificial parthenogenesis, cell division and the development of the lower animals.

SCIENTIFIC NOTES AND NEWS

BOTH branches of Congress have adopted a resolution providing for the striking of a gold medal commemorative of the achievements of Thomas A. Edison and the presentation of the medal to Mr. Edison by congress. Duplicate medals in bronze are to be made and sold at cost.

GOLD medals will soon be presented, under authority of an act of Congress just approved by President Coolidge, to Lincoln Ellsworth, Umberto Nobile and Roald Amundsen in recognition of their joint transpolar flight in the dirigible *Norge*.

CAPTAIN WILKINS, who with Lieutenant Eielson recently flew from Alaska to Spitzbergen, was awarded the Carl Ritter medal by the centenary session of the Geographical Society on May 24.

THE Imperial Order of the Second Class of the Rising Sun has been conferred by the Emperor of Japan upon Dr. Hideyo Noguchi, the discoverer of the yellow fever germ, who died May 21 while conducting investigations for the Rockefeller Institute on the Gold Coast of Africa.

IN recognition of his work in the study of nephritis, Dr. Thomas Addis, of the Stanford Medical School, has been awarded the Gibbs memorial prize of $1,000. He will devote it to the Wellington Gregg fund of the school, through which research work in this disease is being financed.

DR. DAVID RIESMAN, professor of clinical medicine at the University of Pennsylvania School of Medicine, was recently made a Knight of the Order of the Crown of Italy.

FREDERICK E. BRASCH, of the Library of Congress (Smithsonian division), has been awarded a grant for research from the American Council of Learned Societies to complete his studies upon the history of astronomy during the Colonial period in the United States.

THE research prize awarded by the Scientific Club of Winnipeg for the best research work done in the University of Manitoba during a period of three years by a recent graduate has been divided between Leonard B. Clark and Charles F. Goodeve, whose work was carried on in the departments of zoology and chemistry, respectively.

DR. W. REID BLAIR, director of the New York Zoological Park, has had conferred upon him on May 28 by McGill University the honorary degree of doctor of laws.

DR. ABRAHAM FLEXNER has resigned as director of Studies and Medical Education of the General Education Board.

PROFESSOR ARTHUR E. SEAMAN, head of the department of geology in the Michigan College of Mining and Technology, is retiring after forty years of service. Dr. C. O. Swanson, of the Michigan Geological Survey, will succeed Professor Seaman.

DR. T. T. QUIRKE, chairman of the department of geology at the University of Illinois, has been relieved of his administrative duties and will continue his work at the University of Illinois as professor of geology. During the summer he will continue his field researches which he has been carrying on for several years in the Precambrian complex north of Lake

Huron. Professor W. S. Bayley has been made head of the department at the university.

Dr. Lynn Thorndike, professor of history at Columbia University, was elected president of the History of Science Society by the council, to fill the unexpired term of Dr. Edgar Fahs Smith, who died on May 3.

Professor H. B. Dwight, of the Massachusetts Institute of Technology, was elected chairman of the Boston section of the American Institute of Electrical Engineers at the annual meeting.

Dr. W. H. Eccles, F.R.S., has been elected president of the British Physical Society.

Clark C. Heritage, of the Paper Board Corporation, has been appointed to the position of senior chemical engineer in charge of the section of pulp and paper of the Forest Products Laboratory at Madison, Wisconsin, succeeding John D. Rue, who recently resigned.

Dr. J. A. LeClerc, grain specialist in the foodstuffs division of the U. S. Department of Commerce, has accepted appointment in the food research division of the chemical and technological research unit of the Bureau of Chemistry and Soils.

H. S. Bean, chief of the gas measuring instrument section of the Bureau of Standards, will take charge of the cooperative investigation in Buffalo, of the Bureau of Standards, the Bureau of Mines and the Natural Gas Department of the American Gas Association, on methods for measuring large volumes of gas.

Dr. Claude Fuller, formerly chief entomologist of the Union of South Africa, has left Pretoria for Lourenco Marques, where he will assume the duties of chief entomologist to the government of Mozambique.

Under the direction of Dr. Johannes Schmidt, of Copenhagen, a scientific expedition, chiefly financed by the Carlsberg fund, is leaving Denmark at the beginning of June on a journey around the world. The object of the expedition is to carry out oceanographic and zoological investigations, more especially regarding the species of eel in the Pacific and it is expected to take two years.

Dr. Elias Melin, soil botanist of the Swedish College of Forestry, Stockholm, has spent the last year visiting and studying at various agricultural experiment stations in the United States.

Dr. J. C. Th. Uphof, head of the department of botany at Rollins College, will be connected during the coming summer with the Tropical Plant Research Foundation in Washington, D. C., to prepare reports on sugar cane growing and sugar technique of the Dutch East Indies.

Professor Kirtley F. Mather, head of the department of geology at Harvard University, will lead a party of geological students into the Swiss Alps this summer. On reaching Switzerland the group will combine with a party headed by Dr. L. W. Collet, professor of geology in the University of Geneva.

Samuel J. Record, professor of forest products in the school of forestry of Yale University, sailed for Europe on June 2 to enlist the cooperation of scientists there in a comprehensive investigation of the forest resources of the tropics, and particularly of western Africa. The trip is sponsored by Mr. Harvey Firestone, president of the Firestone Rubber Company, Akron, Ohio.

Dr. A. S. Hitchcock, custodian of grasses in the U. S. National Museum, will leave for Newfoundland about July 1 to collect grasses.

Dr. W. F. Book, chairman of the department of psychology and philosophy in Indiana University, returns on June 10 from a tour around the world. He will resume his work at Indiana in September. Dr. Geo. S. Snoddy was acting chairman of the department in Dr. Book's absence.

James L. Peters, research associate in ornithology in the Museum of Comparative Zoology at Harvard University, and Edward Bangs recently returned from a collecting trip in Central America. In all, some six hundred birds were added to the collection in the museum.

Dr. William S. Thayer, of the Johns Hopkins University, president-elect of the American Medical Association was a delegate to the Harvey Tercentenary celebration in London in May.

Dr. R. J. Tillyard, commonwealth entomologist of Australia, and Mr. J. W. Evans, one of his assistants, visited the Kansas State Agricultural College on May 19 to 22. On May 20, a special field meeting of the Kansas Entomological Society occurred at the fossil beds at Elmo, Kansas. On May 21, Dr. Tillyard addressed the zoological and entomological seminar on the subject of "The Relation of the Study of Fossil Insects upon Insect Evolution."

Professor C. U. Ariens Kappers, director of the Central Institute of Brain Research, Amsterdam, is giving a series of six lectures in the neurological department of Columbia University at the new medical center from June 4 to 9 at 4:00 P. M.

Dr. F. d'Herelle, of Alexandria, Egypt, who is to give the Lane lectures at Stanford University during the week beginning October 22, will address a joint meeting of the Chicago Society of Internal Medicine and the Institute of Medicine of Chicago in October.

DR. GEORGE BARGER, professor of medical chemistry at the University of Edinburgh, now lecturing at Cornell University, addressed a meeting of the New York section of the American Chemical Society, the American Electrochemical Society, the Society of Chemical Industry and the Société de Chimie Industrielle on June 1, when he spoke on "Thyroxine and the Thyroid Gland."

DR. RAYMOND PEARL, director of the institute for biological research of the Johns Hopkins University, lectured at Cornell University on May 9, on the Schiff Foundation, on "Experiments on Longevity," and on May 10 and 11 he delivered the eleventh series of Harrington lectures at the University of Buffalo Medical School, the subjects being, "Alcohol and Life Duration" and "Cancer from the Viewpoint of the Human Biologist."

DR. DONALD C. BARTON, of Houston, Tex., consulting geologist and geophysicist, recently gave a series of lectures on certain phases of oil geology and geophysics at the University of Chicago, at the Massachusetts Institute of Technology and at Harvard University.

THE Hermann M. Biggs Memorial Fund has given more than $55,000 to New York University to establish a professorship in preventive medicine in Dr. Biggs's name in the medical college.

THE Louis Agassiz Fuertes memorial room in Ithaca was opened May 28 to the public. The room contains a collection of memorabilia of Dr. Fuertes, including three thousand five hundred birds which he used for his working models in his illustrations and paintings.

THE display of works, illustrations and other data, marking the tercentenary of Harvey's discovery of the circulation, is now open to visitors at the New York Academy of Medicine. The collection of loan specimens occupies eleven cases in the main reading hall.

AT the thirty-seventh annual general meeting of the British Institution of Mining and Metallurgy in London, Mr. Peter Larkin, High Commissioner for Canada, presented to the institution a portrait of the late Dr. Willet G. Miller, provincial geologist of Ontario. The portrait, which is a replica of the original now hanging in the Ontario Legislative Buildings, is the gift of Canadian friends and admirers of the late Dr. Miller.

WILLIAM H. NICHOLS, JR., vice-president of the Allied Chemical and Dye Corporation, known for his work on the metallurgy of copper, died on May 28, aged seventy-six years.

DR. W. M. L. COPLIN, emeritus professor of pathology and bacteriology in the Jefferson Medical College, died on May 29, aged sixty-three years.

PRESS dispatches announce the death from yellow fever of Dr. William Alexander Young, director of medical research at Accra, on the African Gold Coast. Dr. Young was working with the late Dr. Hideyo Noguchi on yellow fever.

DR. JOHN HORN, the well-known geologist of Scotland, has died at the age of eighty years.

DR. H. F. GADOW, Strickland curator and reader in morphology of vertebrates in the University of Cambridge since 1884, died on May 16, at the age of seventy-three years.

DR. ARTHUR HERBERT LEAHY, emeritus professor of mathematics at the University of Sheffield, died on May 16, aged seventy years.

DR. EMIL FROMME, professor of chemistry at the University of Vienna, died on May 29, at the age of sixty-three years.

THE thirteenth International Physiological Congress will be held from August 19 to 23, 1929, at the Harvard Medical School, Boston. This congress meets for the first time in the United States, and is to be under the auspices of the Federation of American Societies for Experimental Biology.

FORTY-FIVE geologists from Iowa, Nebraska, Missouri, Kansas, Arkansas, Oklahoma and Texas met in conference at the offices of the Oklahoma Geological Survey at Norman on May 19 for a discussion of the problem of the Pennsylvanian of the western interior region. Dr. Raymond C. Moore was elected chairman of the conference. After much profitable discussion, it was decided that a general committee be appointed to outline methods for the solution of the Pennsylvanian problem. It was voted to work in conjunction with the American Association of Economic Paleontologists and Mineralogists.

LEADERS in the field of oil engine power, manufacturing, operation and research will convene at the Pennsylvania State College on June 14, 15 and 16 for the first national meeting of the oil and gas power division of the American Society of Mechanical Engineers and the second annual oil power conference arranged by the Pennsylvania State College. Developments in the Diesel engine in all parts of the world will feature the discussions. Among the speakers who will discuss technical phases of the industry are Charles M. Schwab, former president of the society, and George Heath, of the Carels corporation of London, England. The Atlantic division of the American

Relay League will hold its third annual convention on the same dates.

Free public lectures will be given at the New York Botanical Garden on Saturdays during June and July at 4:00 P. M. as follows: June 2, "Japanese and Siberian Irises," Dr. George M. Reed; June 9, "A Naturalist in India, Kashmir and Burma," Mrs. Barnum Brown; June 16, "Life Zones of the Rocky Mountains," Dr. P. A. Rydberg; June 23, "Roses," Mr. F. L. Atkins; June 30, "Botanical Rambles in Panama," Dr. Marshall A. Howe; July 7, "The Story of the Redwoods," Dr. Arthur Hollick; July 14, "Wild Flowers," Mrs. N. L. Britton; July 21, "Selecting a National Flower," Dr. Edgar T. Wherry; July 28, "Fungous Diseases of Plants," Dr. B. O. Dodge.

The U. S. Civil Service Commission announces an open competitive examination for assistant chemical engineer, applications for which must be on file not later than July 5. The examination is to fill vacancies in the federal classified service, for duty in Washington, D. C., or in the field, at an entrance salary of $2,400 a year.

Announcement is made by Dean Franklin Moon, of the New York State College of Forestry, Syracuse University, that twenty-eight members of this year's senior class received instruction at the Pack demonstration forest from April 28 to June 2, situated near Lake George in the heart of the finest pine region of the state. This forest was given to the college about two years ago by the Charles Lathrop Pack Forestry Trust for the purpose of serving as a demonstration forest and research area combined. Being located on the main highway from Albany to Montreal the roadside demonstrations in field reforestation and underplanting, thinnings to accelerate growth, pruning of young pines to improve the quality of the timber, can be observed by the thousands of tourists who pass this forest each year. In addition to the regular staff of instructors, foresters from Denmark and Switzerland conducted research and assisted in instruction during the period.

Dr. George Grant MacCurdy announces the completion of plans for the eighth summer session of the American School of Prehistoric Research, of which he is director. The term will open in London on July 2 and will close on the continent the middle of September. Among the special invitations received by the director is one from Professors Depéret and Mayet, of the University of Lyon, which will give the students of the school an opportunity to take part in the excavations at the celebrated station of Solutré. Beginning in October, representatives of the school will cooperate with representatives from Oxford University on a joint exploring expedition in Irak. Dr. and Mrs. MacCurdy will sail for London on June 15 on the *Tuscania*.

Early human remains will be sought in Southwest Africa by the Cameron-Cadle Kalahari Desert expedition, which sailed from New York on June 1. Ethnological, geological, medical and photographic experts make up the expedition, which has booked passage from Southampton to Cape Town on the steamer *Kenilworth Castle,* sailing on June 15. The expedition's financial backer is Will J. Cameron, of Cameron's Surgical Specialty Company, of Chicago. Mr. Cameron will undertake to find a specimen of the web-footed lizard to bring back for the Field Museum of Chicago, also other specimens which that museum wishes to add to its collections. Dr. C. Ernest Cadle will represent the Colorado Museum of Natural History. Another member of the expedition is Professor R. L. Mannen, of San Antonio, who will represent the University of Texas and the Willie Museum of San Antonio. Fred Parrish and Hank Hoder, of Colorado Springs, will make motion and still pictures for the expedition.

The Russian Academy of Sciences, jointly with German scientific institutions, is organizing a scientific expedition to the Pamir for the exploration of the Altai mountain range. Part will be taken in the expedition by Professor Stcherbakov, Professor Belayev, Professor Korzhinevsky, of Tashkent University; Professor Sicker, of the Geological Institute of Berlin; the German geologist Ritmer, and others.

A sum of $25,000 has been placed at the disposal of the Royal Society of Canada as a nucleus for an endowment fund by the Carnegie Corporation of New York, according to an announcement by Sir Robert Falconer, president of Toronto University.

UNIVERSITY AND EDUCATIONAL NOTES

Gifts to Columbia University amounting to $241,159 have been announced by President Butler. F. W. Vanderbilt was the largest contributor, giving $116,666.66 toward a pledge of $350,000 to enable the university to install the Vanderbilt Clinic in the new medical center. Harold S. Vanderbilt, who has pledged $150,000, gave $50,000 to the clinic.

Dr. Allen W. Rowe, director of research at the Evans Memorial Hospital, Boston, has been elected president of the Boston School of Physical Education.

Dr. Gerald Wendt, who was recently appointed director of the new Battelle Memorial Institute for scientific and industrial research at Columbus, Ohio, has resigned from that position after completing the plans for the laboratory and the award of the contracts and has been appointed assistant to the president of the Pennsylvania State College, where he has for four years been dean of the school of chemistry and physics. He will continue as acting dean for a year but will devote himself primarily to research administration and the development of the large research program of the college.

DR. JACQUES BRONFENBRENNER, of The Rockefeller Institute for Medical Research, has been appointed professor and head of the department of bacteriology and immunology at Washington University Medical School, St. Louis.

DR. OSCAR V. BATSON, professor of anatomy at the University of Cincinnati College of Medicine, has been called to the chair of anatomy in the graduate medical school of the University of Pennsylvania, where he will take up his duties in the fall.

IN the department of anatomy in Columbia University, Dr. Dudley J. Morton, assistant professor of surgery at Yale University, has been appointed associate professor, and Dr. W. M. Copenhaver, instructor in anatomy at the University of Rochester, assistant professor.

PROFESSOR L. W. CURRIER, associate professor of mineralogy at the Missouri School of Mines, has been appointed associate professor of engineering geology at Purdue University.

DR. J. E. WELSTER, Ph.D. (Ohio State, '28), formerly of the Boyce Thompson Institute, Yonkers, has been appointed assistant professor of agricultural chemistry at the Oklahoma Agricultural and Mechanical College.

DR. DEA B. CALVIN, now holder of a Porter fellowship of the American Physiological Society at Yale University, has been appointed instructor in physiological chemistry at the University of Missouri.

DR. HUBERT ERHARD, professor of zoology at the University of Giessen, has accepted the chair of zoology at Freiburg.

DISCUSSION AND CORRESPONDENCE

THE APPORTIONMENT OF REPRESENTATIVES

PROFESSOR HUNTINGTON'S criticism in SCIENCE for May 18 (p. 509) of my action regarding apportionment invites me to discuss in your columns a question of much public importance.

A census of the United States was taken in 1920, but no apportionment law redistributing members of the House among the several states has since been passed and it seems practically certain that none will be passed until the next census is taken. This is the first time in 130 years that Congress has neglected its duty to apportion representatives. The primary reason for the failure is the sharp difference of opinion between two groups of representatives nearly equal in size, one wishing to apportion but unwilling to increase the present size of the House, the other unwilling to apportion unless that size should be increased by the same act, perhaps to the point at which no state would receive less than its present number of members. The second group has been successful in each apportionment since 1880 and the size of the House increased thereby from 332 to 435 members. Owing to this clash of opinion Congress has been deadlocked for seven years. After the next census shall have measured the population changes between 1910 and 1930 it will probably appear that if the House is not increased in size about seventeen states would each lose one or more representatives and that if each state is to retain or increase its present membership it would be necessary to increase the House by about 100 members, nearly one fourth of the present number. Under those conditions the difficulty in securing the passage of an apportionment law will be greater and the precedent for inaction set in the decade now ending seems likely to be followed.

To diminish this danger I revived a suggestion which I had made in 1915 that Congress should revert to the precedent set in 1850 and make the decennial apportionment a ministerial act. For that purpose it would need to pass a law authorizing the President or the Secretary of Commerce, in whose department the bureau of the census lies, to apportion the present number of representatives, 435 (or any other number that might be preferred) by the method last used by Congress (or any other method that might be preferred) as soon as the figures of each successive census were announced and report the results to Congress. This would not, of course, tie the hands of any future Congress but it would secure an automatic readjustment of the number of members last approved to the changes of population in each decade in case Congress by its inaction failed to express any other preference in the matter. The committee welcomed the suggestion and amended the original draft to give Congress one session after the census figures were reported in which to agree upon a bill. If it did not so agree the apportionment was to be made by the executive acting under these instructions.

This proposal raised the question: What method should be prescribed in such a bill? My own view was and is that the method as well as the number of representatives last approved by Congress should be prescribed and that view was adopted by the committee.

It is this decision which is distasteful to Professor Huntington. After the census of 1910 improved methods of dealing with the apportionment problem were laid before the committee on the census by Dr. J. A. Hill and by me. The committee approved my proposal and based the apportionment law of 1911 upon it. In 1921 Professor Huntington improved upon Dr. Hill's method and urged this method of equal proportions, as it was then called, upon Congress. It was considered and approved by the advisory committee to the director of the census but neither Congress nor a committee of Congress has endorsed it. In 1927 and 1928, when the committee on the census held hearings on the bill for ministerial apportionment, each method was advocated and the committee decided to follow congressional precedents in the matter. In my opinion the prescription of a novel method would have increased the obstacles to the bill, obstacles which I regret to say have proved insurmountable, the bill having been defeated in the House May 18th by a vote of 164 in favor and 186 opposed.

Perhaps the main difference between Professor Huntington and me is over the nature of the problem. He treats it as a statistical or "purely mathematical" question which mathematicians and statisticians are to solve, while Congress should accept their solution. I regard it as a political problem in which the scholar should attempt first to find what end the constitution or Congress aims at and then devise or improve a method by which Congress may accomplish that end. The function of mathematicians in the problem is not to choose among ends but merely to determine how some primary end of apportionment can best be secured.

Upon this main difference another depends. Professor Huntington thinks I owe it to the world of scholars to defend my heterodox opinions by publishing them "in some regular journal." My main purpose, however, has been to help Congress out of a dilemma and I am not interested in justifying my course in so doing to my academic colleagues. If any reader wishes to obtain the material for an independent judgment about my position and arguments and the validity of Professor Huntington's criticisms of both he can best do so by asking the Chairman of the House Committee on the Census, Honorable E. Hart Fenn, for a copy of the Committee Hearings of February, 1927, and February, 1928.

One of the main objections to the method of equal proportions is that to the non-mathematician in Congress or out it is almost unintelligible. The comments upon that method made by two scholars who at my request read the hearings before the census committee, including testimony and memoranda by Dr. J. A. Hill, Professor A. A. Young and Professor E. V. Huntington, may be cited in support of this claim. The late James Parker Hall, dean of the University of Chicago Law School, wrote about the method of major fractions: "It is much easier to explain (to any one but a society of mathematicians)." A distinguished teacher of political science in one of our leading universities wrote: "I read very carefully Professor Huntington's explanation of the method of equal proportions contained in the hearings. I confess my inability to comprehend it." In the congressional debate on the bill just defeated the leader of the opposition to it and the senior Democratic member on the Census Committee said: "I presume the mathematicians know what they are talking about. Nobody on the committee knew whether they were right or not."

WALTER F. WILLCOX

CORNELL UNIVERSITY

TRANSPLANTATION OF THE EUROPEAN OYSTER

IT is well known that the accidental introduction of the Portuguese oyster (*O. angulata*) into Arcachon Bay in France has led to the establishment there of a great breeding-ground and immense production of this oyster on beds which were formerly occupied only by the European oyster (*O. edulis*).[1] Portuguese oysters, which do not occur naturally on English oyster-beds, are also grown and well fattened on these beds on a commercial scale after transplantation of the young from Portugal or France. There is, therefore, evidence that this kind of oyster will live and thrive in situations other than those in which it occurs naturally, and there is every reason to believe that other kinds of oysters can be transplanted—with circumspection—to obtain similar results. The European oyster is generally regarded as a superior article of food to the American oyster, and for that reason should be of greater commercial value. There are indeed physiological reasons for believing that *O. edulis* fattened on the West Atlantic Coast would compare favorably with the best American shell-fish. The object of this note is to suggest that the European oyster especially may be expected to breed and flourish in the beds in the northern states and in Canada on the Atlantic coast and that the transplantation of this species should not be a difficult matter.

[1] M. Dantan, *Comptes Rendus Acad. des Sci.*, Feb. 2, 1914, Paris.

In reviewing the characters of the dominant species of oysters throughout the world it has been shown that two distinct types may be recognized. Type I consists at present of *O. virginica-elongata,* the American and Canadian oyster; *O. angulata,* the Portuguese oyster; *O. cucullata,* an oyster of world-wide distribution in tropical and subtropical regions.

Type II consists at present of *O. edulis,* the European oyster; *O. lurida,* the British Columbian oyster; *O. angasi,* the south Australian mud-oyster.

The oysters of Type I flourish in tropical or subtropical regions; have small eggs, which are thrown directly into the water, and are either male or female.

The oysters of Type II, on the other hand, flourish in temperate regions; have large eggs, which are incubated inside the shell until developed into a free-swimming larva, and the individuals are hermaphrodite.

Now the oysters of Type II occur, in the northern hemisphere, on the west coast of Europe and the west coast of North America, but not on the Atlantic coast of North America. In the southern hemisphere this type occurs in the south of Australia and the south of New Zealand. Why, then, is a dominant member of this type absent from the Atlantic coast of America?[2] It seems highly improbable that there can be any other answer to this question than could be supplied by geological changes, if sufficient knowledge were available. There is every reason to believe that the biological conditions in the estuaries in the middle part of the Atlantic coast of North America would be eminently favorable to the European oyster. The reverse of this has been proved[3] in the case of the American slipper-limpet, which was introduced on American oysters into the Thames estuary in England and has flourished there exceedingly well. It is equally probable that both the European and British Columbian oysters would also thrive on the Atlantic coast, and quite probably increase at a great rate on the warmer beds.

In these days of rapid transport it should be possible to relay oysters from Europe or British Columbia to the American or Canadian Atlantic beds within a few days and with no greater mortality than occurs on relaying from one European bed to another. Any scheme of transplanting, however, ought to be well thought out and should aim at relaying a maximum number of individuals in a small area in secluded estuaries where there is a minimum tidal current.

J. H. ORTON

MARINE BIOLOGICAL LABORATORY,
THE HOE, PLYMOUTH

[2] J. S. Gutsell in SCIENCE, LXIV, No. 1662, 1926, describes a small species of this type from Beaufort, N. C.

[3] J. H. Orton, *Proc. Roy. Soc.*, B, Vol. 81, 1909.

THE BOILING-POINT AND THE LATENT HEAT OF VAPORIZATION OF WATER

THE teaching of loose concepts in physics in the high schools and colleges may lead to the acquisition of incorrect habits of thinking. Many text-books of physics leave the student with the impression that the boiling-point and latent heat of vaporization of water are immutable constants. The concept of the boiling-point of water being 100° C. is drilled so deeply in the mind of the student that it becomes exceedingly difficult later to uproot this idea. Invariably, when the boiling-point of water is mentioned, the student thinks of 100° C. or 212° F. and a latent heat of 540 calories per gram; that water exists as such only below 100° C., and only as steam above this temperature. Neither is it sufficiently impressed on the student that the latent heat of vaporization is not a constant, but a variable which is a function of the vaporization temperature.

Illustrative of the looseness found in the statement of calorimetric problems is the following one taken from a standard text-book. "How much steam at 150° C. must be added to 1 kg of ice at −10° C. to give nothing but water at 0° C.?" Since no pressure is stated, presumably the student is to assume a boiling-point of 100° C.

Another well-known text-book makes the following statement in explaining the determination of the latent heat of vaporization of water: "In condensing, its latent heat of vaporization is given up and the condensed water is cooled from 100° to the final temperature of the calorimeter." Apparently the figures 100 represent a sacred number.

In a third text-book it is stated that "brine must be raised above 100° C. to boil." As if pure water can not be made to boil above 100° C. or that it must boil at 100° C.! What must the student think of his physics text-book when he observes water above 100° C. being fed to the boiler of a power-plant?

In a fourth text the author after carefully showing that the boiling-point and latent heat of vaporization are variables rather than constants, then proceeds to give an illustrative problem of an experimental determination of the latent heat of vaporization, and without stating any pressure, tacitly assumes that the boiling-point is 212° F.

In a fifth text the following usual problem is given: "How much heat would be required to change 10 grams of ice at −10° C. to steam at 110°? Assume a specific heat of steam at constant pressure equal to 0.5." To solve this problem the student takes for granted that the boiling-point is 100° C., and that the steam has been heated from 100 to 110. Soon he arrives at such a habit of thinking that no problem in saturated or superheated steam can be solved unless that mystic number 100 is introduced into the problem. It would be very desirable if authors of general physics text-books could be induced to exercise greater care in the treatment and statement of problems in calorimetry.

J. B. Nathanson
Carnegie Institute of Technology

CORYNEUM CANKER OF CYPRESS

The Monterey cypress (*Cupressus macrocarpa*) is widely planted in the warmer temperate parts of Europe, South America, Australia and New Zealand. It has long been a favorite for hedges, windbreaks and for park purposes in the coastal region of its native California, occurring so generally that, like eucalyptus, it has become a characteristic of the landscape. The early California plantings enjoyed comparative freedom from pests and diseases. Then insects gained a foothold, becoming particularly active in trees on unfavorable sites and in the warm, dry interior valleys. Nearer the coast the cypress fared better and, while a gradual increase in damage from insects and root troubles has been noted, the loss among trees under proper care has not been large until the last two or three years, when dying back of specimens of all ages became general around the south half of San Francisco Bay. The injury was first attributed to the attack of bark-beetles, as these insects were commonly present in the dead trees. Mr. J. M. Miller, entomologist, United States Department of Agriculture, in the spring of 1927, reported to this office that he was unable to trace the dying back in certain trees at Palo Alto and Stanford University, California, to insects. From the appearance of the affected parts he was led to believe that a fungous disease might be responsible. The same trouble has since been found to be general in the portions of Alameda, Santa Clara and San Mateo Counties adjacent to San Francisco Bay. It has also been reported from Sacramento County, but is not yet definitely known to occur elsewhere.

Affected trees become conspicuous through the dying of individual parts of the crown, either branches or portions of the top. This continues until finally the entire tree is either killed or is rendered so unsightly that its removal becomes necessary. An inspection shows the dying to be due to the girdling action of bark cankers caused by a fungus. The affected bark first swells and soon begins to die in the central portion of the canker. The dying is accompanied by heavy resin flow, which furnishes one of the most characteristic indications for the presence of the canker. Ordinarily branch cankers are less than a foot in length, but on the main stem they may be longer. A pitch moth commonly works among the resinous material on the diseased bark, giving the appearance at first glance of being connected with the injury. The causal fungus is an apparently undescribed species of Coryneum, the blackish pustules of which usually appear irregularly scattered over the surface of the discolored, dead bark of the cankers. Inoculations on young Monterey cypress with spores of the fungus resulted in positive infections, both on wounded and unwounded young bark and on unwounded foliage. Typical acervuli of the Coryneum developed from a number of the infections. The common avenues of infection in the open have not yet been definitely determined. As control measures the removal of sources of further infection by the cutting-out and destruction of all cankers followed by applications of a standard fungicidal spray are indicated. So far the disease is confined mainly to Monterey cypress, but the well-known Italian cypress (*C. sempervirens*) is also severely attacked and it is not unlikely that other cypress species may be found susceptible.

No clue as to the origin of the disease has been found. To all appearances it has been present in certain of the localities where it is now serious for perhaps four or five years, but beyond that nothing is known. There is no record of any disease resembling it on the native cypresses of the state. Irrespective of its origin the canker has sufficiently demonstrated its destructive possibilities to warrant efforts for the prevention of its spread to localities where it is not now present. Further studies of the disease are under way.

Willis W. Wagener
Office of Forest Pathology,
Bureau of Plant Industry,
San Francisco, California

MORE RESEARCH

Speaking of *research:* Ré-search is bad enough, but how about ré-zearch? One hears this occasionally from doctors of philosophy in various sciences. I once knew a minister who used frequently to pray for ré-zawrse, thus perpetrating three distinct errors in one comparatively short word.

James S. Stevens
Orono, Maine

In reference to the letters as to "The Pronunciation of Research," in Science for May 4, I think there will be universal agreement that the Oxford Dictionary is the final court of appeal as to spelling and pronunciation of English. That gives the accent on the second syllable of "research" used both as a noun and a verb, and also places the accent on the second syllable in "researcher."

W. H. Kun

IF there were any valid argument for accenting "research" on the first syllable, it would equally well apply to a great number of other words beginning with "re-," in which the force of the prefix is exactly the same (for those who advocate accenting the penult, "reinter" is a good one for practice!).

The solution of this problem (and of all others of similar character) is clearly and definitely indicated in an admirable little book by Martin C. Flaherty, entitled "How to Use the Dictionary" (Ronald Press Co. 1923). It can be read in a few hours and will richly repay the effort.

E. H. MCCLELLAND

CARNEGIE LIBRARY OF PITTSBURGH

CORRECTIONS TO THE BIOGRAPHICAL DIRECTORY OF AMERICAN MEN OF SCIENCE

IN the fourth edition stars should be attached to the subjects of research of Dr. Atherton Seidell, chemist in the hygienic laboratory of the U. S. Public Health Service, and of Dr. T. Wingate Todd, professor of anatomy in Western Reserve University. The copy was correct, but unfortunately the errors were passed by the proofreaders.

In the table (page 1128) showing the strength of institutions in the different sciences, Harvard University should be given a rating of 4.6 in anthropology, one man who was called to Harvard before the date of reference not having been so recorded. This places Harvard first among universities in anthropology and further emphasizes its dominant position. Changes in position are frequent, the situation having altered in a number of institutions between the date to which the table refers and the time of its publication.

Several less serious errors have been discovered, as also the omission of names that should be included. The latter situation, however, is inevitable, partly owing to the large number of individuals concerned and partly because some scientific men will not reply to requests for information.

J. MCKEEN CATTELL

REPORTS

WORK ACCOMPLISHED BY THE FIELD MUSEUM PALEONTOLOGICAL EXPEDITIONS TO SOUTH AMERICA

THE work undertaken by the Field Museum paleontological expeditions to Argentina and Bolivia has been finished. The party composing the second expedition returned to Chicago in November, 1927. Collections brought together by these expeditions from many localities have now been received at the museum.

These expeditions, made possible by the generous support of Captain Marshall Field, were active from 1922 to 1927. The work has been carried on by two successive expeditions under the leadership of the present writer. The object was to make collections of fossil mammals from as many as possible of the known fossil-bearing horizons of South America. A similar undertaking had not been made by a North American institution since the Princeton University expeditions to Patagonia of 1896–99.

The first expedition, consisting of E. S. Riggs, G. F. Sternberg and J. B. Abbott, set out from Chicago early in November, 1922, and proceeded to the Santa Cruzean formations of southernmost Argentina. Near the Port of Rio Gallegos the first working base was established. Collecting was carried on in the province of Santa Cruz until the end of the following May, when the approach of southern winter made a movement northward advisable. Collections amounting to 282 specimens of fossil mammals, together with a few specimens of fossil birds, were made from the Santa Cruzean formation. This number included 177 skulls, with a few skeletons more or less entire. According to field determinations, this collection included thirty-two genera of fossil mammals, and a considerably larger number of species.

With the approach of winter the party moved northward to the vicinity of Commodoro Rivadavia. There the months of July and August were passed in collecting recent mammals and birds when weather conditions permitted.

The second working season, from September to May, 1923–4, was devoted to collecting fossil mammals from the earlier fresh-water formations, designated by North American geologists as the Deseado Series, and referred by them to the Oligocene period. Collections of fossil shells to the number of three hundred, and a few specimens of cetaceans, were also made from the Patagonian Beds. Some collections of Cretaceous dinosaurs were made from the San Jorg formation. A fossil forest of *Araucaria* was discovered near Cerro Madra y Higa of the province of Santa Cruz, and a collection of 250 specimens of cones, twigs and branches made from it. Unrecorded occurrences of Deseado mammals were examined near this point and at another locality in the vicinity of Pico Truncado.

Of the Eocene mammals, only a limited collection was made from the "Nothostylops Beds" of Ameghino. A larger collection, comprising 256 specimens, was collected from the upper fossil-bearing horizons of the Deseado formation, including the "Astraponotus Beds" and the "Pyrotherium Beds" of Ameghino. No less than eight widely separated fossil-bearing localities were examined, and a reconnaissance was made through the northern part of the province of

Santa Cruz and the southern part of the province of Chubut.

In May of 1924 the party again moved northward to escape the severe weather of winter. The two collectors then returned to the museum. The leader with one assistant visited the Pliocene (Araucanian) exposures along the River Parana without discovering any promising collecting grounds. A collection of 110 Pliocene invertebrates was there made. The party then proceeded northward to Bolivia. The succeeding winter was devoted to collecting in the Pleistocene formation about Tarija. Local men were employed as collectors and work was carried on there from July to December. This resulted in a collection of 126 specimens of Pleistocene mammals of both indigenous and immigrant stocks. Among this number are three large skeletons and a number of skulls.

Returning to Buenos Aires in December the party disbanded. Plans were then laid for the work of a second expedition. Reconnaissance was made by the leader through the Pampean formations and westward along the Rio Negro as far as Neoquen. The dinosaur-bearing localities of the Roca formation were there examined. The leader of the expedition then returned to the museum to recuperate and to organize a second expedition.

The personnel of the second expedition included, under the same leader, Mr. R. C. Thorne, of Chicago, and Dr. Rudolf Stahlecker, of the University of Tübingen, as collectors. Camp men and other helpers were employed as occasion arose. The party set out from Chicago in April, 1926, proceeding to Buenos Aires and thence to the northern provinces of Argentina.

The first task of this expedition was to find a productive locality and to make collections of Pliocene mammals. The Araucanian formations of the River Parana and of the southern coast of the Province of Buenos Aires had long been exploited by Argentine collectors and did not at this time offer promise of good collections. Attention was therefore directed toward the Catamarcan formation of the northern provinces. The known locality of the Valley of Santa Maria in the Province of Catamarca was first visited. Local help was employed, pack-animals and mounts were secured, camp established and collecting begun about the twentieth of May.

The massive sandstone and indurated clays exposed in abrupt cliffs at the base of the Aconquija Mountains yielded important returns. This locality was small and soon exhausted. The Santa Maria valley was then explored northward into the provinces of Tucuman and Salta. Finding less promising fields in that direction, the base camp was moved to Puerta Corral Quemada in the Department of Belen. A new field was there developed which proved most productive. The Catamarcan formation, composed of sandstones and clays similar to that of the Valley of Santa Maria, was found to reach a thickness of more than six thousand feet. This series was exposed in mountain ridges, with included valleys, everywhere highly inclined and folded, and evidently of pre-Andean age. The fauna contained in this formation proved to be essentially the same as that of the type locality near Santa Maria. The lowermost measures of reddish sandstones yielded a scant fauna of toxodonts and glyptodonts. The middle measures yielded a typical Araucanian fauna similar to that of Entre Rios, the type-locality in the Valley of Santa Maria. The upper measures revealed a more varied, and somewhat later, fauna, which appeared to be forerunners of well-known Pleistocene animals.

Collecting was carried on along the River Corrall Quemada until the beginning of the rainy season in November. The entire collections were then gathered at Andalgala for shipment by railway and the party moved southward for the ensuing summer. The collections made from the Catamarcan formation included glyptodonts of five or more genera, gravigrade sloths of two genera, armadillos in considerable variety, two or more forms of toxodonts, four forms of typotheres, one of macrauchenids, a procyonid, one or two marsupials and a profusion of rodents of indigenous forms. There were also found some variety of large birds, a single species of great tortoise and a few small batrachians. The collection from the Catamarcan formation numbers 181 specimens of fossil vertebrates. Invertebrates were found in the lower horizon only. The entire fauna is so different from that of the Santa Cruzean beds as to indicate a prolonged interval of time between the close of the Santa Cruzean period and the beginning of the Catamarcan.

The expedition had by this time secured representative collections from the Deseado series, the Santa Cruz formation, and from the Catamarcan formation, which, following North American geologists, may be designated as of Oligocene, Early Miocene and Pliocene age, with a moderate representation of early Pliocene mammals from the Tarijan formation. Attention was now fixed upon the great indigenous mammals of the South American Pleistocene. From the discoveries made by South American paleontologists during the past seventy-five years, this fauna appears to have found its best expression in the Pampean formations of central Argentina. In this populous region the Pampean fossils had been correspondingly exploited by local and visiting collectors. The task of making collections from this formation was therefore entered upon with some doubt as to success. On the other hand, specimens of the great ground sloths and of glyptodonts were especially desired because of their immense size and their unique characteristics, which render them of especial value as museum exhibits.

Localities along the southern coast of the Province of Buenos Aires were selected as offering the best prospect of securing good specimens of the great Pampean mammals. The motor equipment, which had been stored since the first expedition, was again brought into use. The coastwise exposures from Bahia Blanca to Miramar were gone over. Some collecting was done on the beaches as exposed at low tide, along the low sea-cliffs and among sand dunes near the shore, where small areas had been denuded by wind erosion. More favorable collecting grounds were found along the banks of certain rivers, whose channels have, in their lower courses, cut through the entire Pampean formation. These steep banks, swept clear of débris by floods in every period of high waters, offered the most favorable opportunity for discovering specimens.

From these localities a collection of sixty-two specimens was secured. Among the number is more than half of an articulated skeleton, including head, of the greatest of the ground sloths, *Megatherium americanum.* Excellent articulated skeletons of the intermediate-sized sloths, *Scelidotherium* and *Glossotherium,* good specimens of the great saber-tooth tiger and of the Argentine mastodon, and various specimens of fossil horses, llamas and rodents were also secured.

This work held the expedition in the south until the close of the southern summer. In May the party again moved northward to continue collecting in the Pleistocene valley-deposits of Bolivia. Dr. Stahlecker, who found it necessary to return to Germany at this time, was replaced by Sr. Jose Strucco. A new force of camp men and helpers also was employed.

As soon as preliminaries had been arranged, the party pushed on from Tarija into the small, isolated valley of Patcaya. There a formation of valley sediments similar to that of Tarija was found. Quarters were established for the winter and collecting was begun among the arroyos and thornbushes of this mountain district. The prize specimen here secured was an articulated skeleton, almost entire, of the mountain species of the great sloth, *Megatherium tarijensis.* Specimens of the equally large sloth, *Lestodon,* rewarded prolonged excavations in an old stream-channel. Two articulated skeletons of *Glossotherium* compensated for months of patient search through bush-lands. Various specimens of the Andean horse and of camels and llamas added to the sum total of the winter's collection.

By the end of September, 1927, collecting by the second expedition was terminated. Shipments were made during the succeeding month. The party then returned to Chicago by way of Peru and the western coast.

The results of the two expeditions may be summed up as follows: Representative collections of fossil mammals were made from the Eocene, Oligocene, Early Miocene, Pliocene and the Earlier and Later Pleistocene of Argentina and Bolivia. During this work the Field Museum parties examined most of the formations of Argentina and Bolivia which have yielded fossil mammals. Collections were made from no less than twenty-two different localities, several of which were first made known by the labors of these expeditions. Fossil invertebrates were collected from Cambrian, from Miocene and from Pliocene formations. A rare collection of fossil cones, twigs and branches of the genus *Araucaria* was made from fossil trees found *in situ* near Cerro Madre y Higa, of the province of Santa Cruz. Small collections of recent mammals, birds and reptiles were made; also collections of flowering plants from the provinces of Chubut and Catamarca. Studies of stratigraphy in the several fossil-bearing localities were carried on and a number of geological sections were prepared. A series of some twelve hundred photographs were made for the purpose of recording the work of the expedition, as well as to illustrate subjects of more general interest.

Through the courtesy of the Argentine and the Bolivian governments, all these collections, excepting a certain number of duplicated specimens, were permitted to be exported to the United States. The various shipments, totaling nearly three thousand specimens of fossil mammals, birds, reptiles, mollusks and plants, have safely arrived at the Field Museum. The preparation and the study of these collections will require a period of years. A number of specialists in various lines have been invited to assist in this task.

ELMER S. RIGGS
FIELD MUSEUM OF NATURAL HISTORY

SCIENTIFIC APPARATUS AND LABORATORY METHODS

MAKING A CORRECT MECHANICAL ANALYSIS OF SOILS IN FIFTEEN MINUTES

IN previous communications the use of the hydrometer method has been proposed as a rapid and simple method for the study of soils.[1] A very comprehensive study has been made to ascertain if the method could be used for making a mechanical analysis of soils. It has been discovered that if the soil particles are grouped into three main groups—sand, silt and clay or colloids—these three groups can be determined by

[1] *Soil Science,* No. 5, 1927; No. 4, 1927; SCIENCE, July, 1927.

the hydrometer method rather remarkably correct in only fifteen minutes by making only two readings, one at the end of one minute and the other at the end of fifteen minutes. In making these studies about thirty different soils were obtained from the United States Bureau of Soils whose complete mechanical analysis was known. It was found that the percentage of material that settles out at the end of one minute in the regular hydrometer method is almost exactly the same as the percentage of all the combined sands obtained by the mechanical analysis method. If the percentage of material that settles out at the end of fifteen minutes minus the sand which settles out at the end of one minute is considered to be silt, and if the material that still stays in suspension at the end of fifteen minutes is considered to be clay or colloids, it was found that the mechanical analysis and hydrometer methods agreed quite closely in the soils whose silt content was composed mostly of the coarser size—in the neighborhood of .05 mm and disagreed rather widely in the soils whose silt content was composed of the finest size —in the neighborhood of .005 mm. This is as should be expected because recent studies go to show that the finer silt has practically the same characteristics as the clay and should be classed, therefore, with the clay, while the coarser silt does not possess the same characteristics. The hydrometer method, therefore, includes in its clay or colloidal determination the finer silt but not the coarser silt, consequently the hydrometer method would agree with the mechanical-analysis method in soils with the coarse silt content but not with the finer silt content. In other words, the hydrometer and mechanical-analysis methods agree almost perfectly in the determination of the combined sands, coarser silt and clay. Where they do disagree is in the finer silt. The mechanical analysis classes this fine silt with the coarse silt, where the hydrometer method classes this fine silt with the clay, because it has more of the characteristics of clay. Hence there is no serious and radical disagreement between the two methods.

If it is desired to determine only the total sand and the total silt and clay, these determinations can be made by the hydrometer method in only one minute and will be very correct.

With the aid of Stokes's law, the hydrometer method can also be used to make a very detailed mechanical analysis of soils.

Although the method may appear too ideal to be true, yet all facts point such to be the case. Indeed, the method appears to be a rather remarkable and unique means of studying soils quickly, simply and accurately. For all general and practical purposes this method gives nearly all the information that is necessary and essential regarding the physical composition of soils. And in many cases such information seems to be more true than that of the mechanical-analysis method.

Finally, it must be stated that the criticisms which Joseph and Keen have made in *Soil Science* regarding the hydrometer method are not justified and do not apply to the method as is shown elsewhere.

GEORGE JOHN BOUYOUCOS
MICHIGAN AGRICULTURAL EXPERIMENT STATION

A SIMPLE METHOD OF PICKING UP CORRELATIONS[1]

IN dealing with a long series of systematic observations on individuals, as in the routine work of the Constitution Clinic in the Presbyterian Hospital—besides the opportunity of working out the type characteristics of any group under investigation—there is the possibility of finding a large number of correlations. If there are n observations on each subject or patient, there are $n\,(n-1)/2$ correlations of the first order. A fair estimate of the significant correlations can be obtained by means of the home-made sorting machine to be described.

The observations on one individual are recorded on a long card about 5 cm. high in vertically ruled spaces

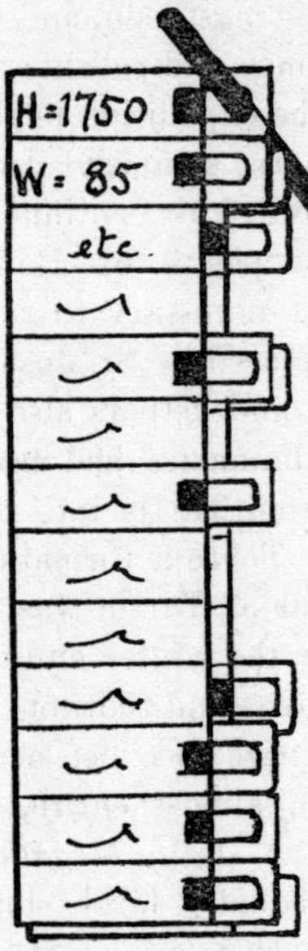

1 cm. wide. Each observation is then compared with some given criterion and classified as plus or minus, yes or no. If the observation is plus, a clip is attached in the appropriate position along the top of the

[1] From the department of medicine of the College of Physicians and Surgeons of Columbia University and the Presbyterian Hospital, New York.

card. When all the cards are filed together, the spaces in which a certain observation has been recorded lie one behind the other; and the clips protrude above the level of the file in their respective rows. Each clip has a hole in it so that a rod may be passed through all the clips in any particular row.

Supposing that there are forty-eight cards in the group, and that for each character the median value has been selected as the criterion. If then it is desired to find the association between one character (*e.g.*, height) and any other character (*e.g.*, weight), the cards for the twenty-four tallest individuals are raised by passing a rod through the clips in the height row. If there were no association between height and weight, there would be, on the average, twelve out of the twenty-four heavy individuals among the twenty-four tall ones—less than twelve if the association is negative, more than twelve if the association is positive. The actual number can easily be determined by counting the clips (or the empty spaces) in the weight row which appear among the cards which have been lifted. In fact, the single operation of raising the cards belonging to the tall subjects reveals at a glance any significant association between height and any other character observed. A second rod enables one to examine "second-order" associations, *i.e.*, to raise the cards belonging to the individuals who are both tall *and* heavy.

For the mathematical treatment of data obtainable by the above procedures, for calculating correlation coefficients, and for some of the pitfalls of interpretation, reference may be made to Yule's book[2] especially chapters V and XI.

Arrangements are being made for the manufacture of the sorting-clips. It is thought that these clips will also be useful in the analysis of questionnaires and in the investigation of sociological problems.

CECIL D. MURRAY

PRESBYTERIAN HOSPITAL,
NEW YORK CITY

SPECIAL ARTICLES

A BIOELECTRIC POTENTIAL

BY means of a pair of non-polarizable micro-electrodes that can be inserted into a single living cell,[1] a difference of electrical potential between two points in the protoplasmic stream of the plant cell *Nitella* was detected and measured. The electrodes are operated by means of a Taylor micro-manipulator, and the electromotive force measured by means of a galvanometer (sensitivity 29,200 megohms), and a potentiometer. The two electrodes are both in the protoplasmic stream, usually about 125 μ to 150 μ apart. The difference of the electrical potential ranges from .002 to .004 volts. The E. M. F. drops to zero when the streaming is caused to stop, but will approach the initial magnitude if streaming is resumed. The direction of the current generated with respect to the direction of the protoplasmic streaming is always the same.

Ettisch and Péterfi,[2] using a binant electrometer and micro-electrodes, were unable to detect any potential difference between two points in the interior of the small *Amoeba terricola*. They consequently concluded that no ionic equilibrium that can be measured existed in the protoplasm of this form. In *Nitella* the conditions are somewhat different because of the continual and rapid streaming of the protoplasm. The observed potential difference not only is directly associated with the streaming of the protoplasm, but the two phenomena seem to be dependent upon each other. This is indicated by the fact that the E. M. F. drops to zero when the streaming is caused to stop by a slight mechanical stimulus with one of the electrodes.

In the electrical theories of protoplasmic streaming[3] the view is held that electrical currents are in part concerned in the production of these streaming movements. There is, however, the difficulty in explaining the origin of the E. M. F. The cessation of streaming upon stimulation makes it equally difficult to explain the disappearance of the E. M. F.

The observed potential difference might on the other hand be considered as being produced by the streaming of the protoplasm. We would have, then, in this case, an electrokinetic phenomenon, an E. M. F. that is set up by the impressed motion. This type of an electrokinetic phenomenon is the *streaming potential* and is the reverse of *electrosmosis*.[4] The stationary wall and ectoplasm of *Nitella* are analogous to the solid walls of the capillary tube, and the streaming protoplasm is the moving liquid layer. In *Nitella* the system is a closed one, and the diameter of the cells used ranged from .2 to .4 mm. The conditions for the production of a Helmholtz electric double layer, which is the basis of the explanation of

[2] G. U. Yule, "An Introduction to the Theory of Statistics," London, 1924.

[1] Gelfan, S., Univ. Cal. Publ. Zool., 29, no. 17, 453, 1927.

[2] Ettisch, G., and Péterfi, T., *Plüg. Arch. Phys.*, 208, 3./4. Heft, 1925.

[3] For a discussion of the theories of protoplasmic streaming see Ewart, A. S., "Protoplasmic Streaming in Plants," 1903.

[4] Freundlich, H., "Kapillarchemie," 3rd ed., p. 335.

all capillary electrical phenomena, seem to be present in *Nitella*.

The difficulty encountered in this explanation is the relatively high conductivity of the protoplasm. The E. M. F. of the streaming current is inversely proportional to the conductivity of the liquid. In *Nitella* the conductivity of the protoplasm is equivalent to a .04N KCl solution.[5] According to Kruyt,[6] in a 10^{-3}N KCL solution, the stream potential is equal to four millivolts. In higher concentrations no measurable potentials were observed.

The production of the observed E. M. F. would, therefore, only be possible if the ζ, or electric double layer potential, to which it is directly proportional, were relatively great. This factor, however, is not known for the ecto-endoplasmic surface. A test might be made were it possible to apply the formula for the stream potential, but very little or nothing is known, for protoplasm, of some of the physical constants which are factors in the formula.

Samuel Gelfan

Zoological Laboratory,
University of California

STUDIES ON THE PHYSIOLOGY OF ASCARIS LUMBRICOIDES

For three years past the writer has been engaged in work on the physiology of *Ascaris lumbricoides*, part of which, because of its practical significance, may well be announced at this time, although the complete report of these investigations will be brought out within the near future. Much of the older work in the form under consideration has been critically repeated, with a resulting revision of accepted views.

Comparative studies on the so-called excretory system have shown that in the forms of the subfamily Anisakinae the supposed excretory system is probably a salivary gland for the secretion of an anticoagulin, and this fact has been reinforced by the demonstration of fragments of the tissues of the host, together with large quantities of blood-corpuscles in the intestine of worms previously not known to have blood-sucking habits. On the other hand, in members of the genus Ascaris, evidence has been adduced to show that the so-called excretory system probably serves some as yet unsuggested function. It can not have any important part in the excretory processes, however. In the first place, it would not be expected that the same fundamental structure would in different closely-related worms have such diverse functions as salivary secretion in one case, and the excretion of waste products in the other. In the second place, conclusive experiments prove that the cuticula, which throughout the literature of helminthology seems to be regarded as a very impermeable membrane, is permeable to excretory products and is the channel through which the end-products of metabolism are carried to the exterior. Thus the nematodes have a cutaneous type of excretion.

Experiments also show that substances may pass in through the cuticula. Sugar in high concentration passes in appreciable quantities through the body wall. Chloroform, in water-solution or suspension, passes into the worm directly through the cuticula and the same is true of carbon tetrachloride. Not only is the rate of ingestion on the part of the worm too slow to account for the rapid toxic effect of these substances, but experimental evidence shows that under unfavorable conditions the movement of the alimentary tract ceases altogether.

Observations with the polarizing microscope demonstrate the sparsity of lipoid in the tissues of the worm and show that the aggregates of fatty globules immediately surrounding the nuclei of the muscle cells are true lipin, and not lipoid, as was thought by von Kemnitz. The presence of large quantities of fat in the subcuticula and the occurrence of clusters immediately surrounding the nuclei of the worm are sufficient to account for and enhance greatly the effect of anthelmintics, the most effective of which are usually either fatty in character, or fat soluble.

In contradiction of Weinland's conclusions and confirming those of Slater, it is certain that these worms can and do live aerobically. On the assumption of anaerobic life, fat-storage and oxidation can not be regarded as economical processes, and previous workers have regarded fat oxidation as impossible in the worm, and its storage as a mystery. Part of the past misunderstanding on this point has been due to the difficulty of keeping these worms alive under culture conditions long enough to make any careful experiments. I have succeeded in demonstrating by tissue-culture methods that stored fat is burned by the tissues in the usual manner.

Detailed work has been done in connection with the cytological background of the above-mentioned facts, and some further investigations have been made into the tissue chemistry of the worm. The complete evidence for these findings will be discussed at length in my later paper.

Justus F. Mueller

Zoological Laboratory,
University of Illinois

5 Paper giving these results in press.

6 Kruyt, H. R., *Kolloidzeitschr.*, 22, 81, 1918.

SCIENCE

VOL. LXVII JUNE 15, 1928 No. 1746

CONTENTS

The Pathology of Certain Virus Diseases: PROFESSOR ERNEST W. GOODPASTURE 591
Analogies between Physiological Rhythms and the Rhythmical Reactions in Inorganic Systems: PROFESSOR RALPH S. LILLIE 593
Joseph Nelson Rose: PROFESSOR WM. TRELEASE 598
Scientific Events:
The Glasgow Meeting of the British Association; Centenary of the London Zoological Society; Exhibit of Optical Instruments and Products; The Place of Science in Education 599
Scientific Notes and News 601
University and Educational Notes 605
Discussion and Correspondence:
Ovarian Secretion and Tumor Incidence: PROFESSOR LEO LOEB. *The Ring Method in Changing Surface Tension:* DR. LECOMTE DU NOÜY. *"Nutrilites":* DR. ROGER J. WILLIAMS. *An Ancient Walrus Skull:* BIRGER R. HEADSTROM. *The Royal Photographic Society:* A. J. NEWTON. *Low Humidity and High Taciturnity:* PROFESSOR ERNEST A. VUILLEUMIER 605
Reports:
Horizontal versus Vertical Forces in Crustal Movements of the Earth: DR. JOSEPH L. GILLSON 608
Scientific Apparatus and Laboratory Methods:
The Use of the X-Ray in Biological Investigations: DR. VICTOR PIETSCHMANN. *A Convenient Method of Determining the Rate of Cleavage:* DR. E. ALFRED WOLF 610
Special Articles:
The Effect of a Secondary Sound upon Hearing: E. G. WEVER. *Remarkable Musical Technique of the Larger Angular-Winged Katydid:* H. A. ALLARD 612
Societies and Academies:
The Kentucky Academy of Science: A. M. PETER. *The North Dakota Academy of Science* 614
Science News x

SCIENCE: A Weekly Journal devoted to the Advancement of Science, edited by J. McKeen Cattell and published every Friday by

THE SCIENCE PRESS

New York City: Grand Central Terminal.

Lancaster, Pa. Garrison, N. Y.

Annual Subscription, $6.00. Single Copies, 15 Cts.

SCIENCE is the official organ of the American Association for the Advancement of Science. Information regarding membership in the Association may be secured from the office of the permanent secretary, in the Smithsonian Institution Building, Washington, D. C.

THE PATHOLOGY OF CERTAIN VIRUS DISEASES[1]

THE term "virus diseases," as used in this title, has reference to that group of acute infectious diseases whose etiological agents have not yet been cultivated with certainty on artificial media but have the common property of filterability through earthenware or porcelain filters.

Notwithstanding the fact that a very great number of infectious agents, both bacterial and protozoan, have been demonstrated and cultivated during the past fifty years, there remains a surprisingly large residuum of infections which may be included under the term "virus diseases."

There is a very wide distribution of the virus infections both within the animal and plant kingdoms. For example, among the diseases of man belonging to this group are such important examples as smallpox, poliomyelitis and rabies. The group may be represented among the lower animals by such instances as foot and mouth disease, rinderpest and hog cholera. In plants there is the mosaic disease of tobacco and numerous others. It is probable also that the bacteriophage of D'Herelle belongs in the same category. The biological importance of the filterable viruses may be further illustrated by the fact that certain tumor-like diseases are known to be caused by these agents, namely, Rous's chicken sarcoma and fowl leukemia.

It is of particular interest from the standpoint of pathological and cytological studies that the lesions of many virus diseases are associated with specific cellular inclusions, the nature of which has not as yet been determined with certainty. The inclusions may be situated either within the cytoplasm of the cells involved, within the nucleus or within both. As examples of intra-cytoplasmic inclusions may be mentioned those of rabies, smallpox, vaccinia, trachoma and molluscum contagiosum of man. In the fowl characteristic inclusions occur in epithelioma contagiosum. Inclusions confined within the nucleus have been demonstrated in herpes simplex, herpes zoster and varicella in man, and in the nuclei of cells of the central nervous system in the encephalitis of horses, known as Borna's disease.

These inclusions from time to time have been considered to be protozoan parasites, or the products of

[1] Read before Section N (Medical Sciences) American Association for the Advancement of Science, Nashville, Tennessee, December 28, 1927.

cellular degeneration or reaction products incorporating the virus. The last hypothesis was formulated several years ago by von Prowazek; and he designated the viruses inciting the specific cellular reactions Chlamydozoa. Lipschutz, a little later, included under the term Strongyloplasms the minute, uniform, granular components of inclusions which could be demonstrated in fresh preparations and in smears. He regarded these minute bodies as the visible form of the infectious agent. In this group he included the viruses of fowl-pox, molluscum contagiosum of man, sheep-pox, variola and vaccinia. These minute structures were demonstrated in smears from the lesions of fowl-pox and sheep-pox first by Borrel in 1904, in smears of molluscum contagiosum by Lipschutz in 1906, and about the same time in the lesions of variola and vaccinia by Paschen.

In the present study which I will report, our interest has been directed toward an investigation of the nature of the inclusions, particularly in the lesions of fowl-pox and molluscum contagiosum.

Fowl-pox is a contagious, eruptive disease which occurs often in epidemic form in chickens, pigeons, turkeys, geese, pheasants and other species of fowl. The lesions consist of a nodular exanthem which appears particularly on the unfeathered parts of the body, especially about the head. They represent essentially an epithelial hyperplasia. Only surfaces lined by squamous epithelium are affected, the lesions being strictly confined to the epidermis and to the mucosa of the mouth, nasal pharynx, the esophagus, crop and occasionally the cloaca. During the eruptive stage of the disease the virus is present in the blood and probably in all the organs of the body, although there are no demonstrable lesions in the internal organs. Within the eruptive lesions the virus is present in a very high concentration, and the disease may be induced by inoculating a susceptible fowl at any point on the skin, where epithelial cells have been injured by scarification or by plucking feathers. In early stages of the disease, while the virus is circulating in the blood, local lesions may be induced by simple scarification or the removal of feathers at any point. Notwithstanding its wide dissemination in the body it appears that this virus proliferates for the most part, if not entirely, within the eruptive lesions.

On microscopic examination the nodular lesions are found to be due essentially to an epithelial hyperplasia. Practically every epithelial cell of the lesion contains within its cytoplasm a large, discrete, compact body which possesses an eosinophilic staining reaction and has a hyalin appearance. These inclusions are larger and more numerous as the surface is approached. They may be absent in the cells of the Malpighian layer. It has been demonstrated that their formation begins near the basal layer by the condensation of an apparently amorphous material about one or more intracytoplasmic globules, or as they appear in fixed preparations, clear vacuoles. This material increases in abundance until it entirely covers or replaces the vacuole. Cells containing these inclusions are larger than normal, the mitochondria are intact, the nucleus shows no evidence of disintegration, and there is no indication that the cell thus altered is degenerating. Not infrequently one may find particles within the cytoplasm which appear to have been extruded from the nucleus. These particles do not take part in the formation of the specific inclusions. From a study of the cells in which the inclusions are developing we are convinced that the latter are not derived from preexisting material within the cell through degeneration nor through the formation of any constituent which the cell may produce during its differentiation. On the contrary, the inclusion appears to be constituted of a new and foreign material which accumulates in abundance within a vitally active cell.

In fresh preparations it is easily possible to tease out from fragments of a nodule numerous inclusion bodies, so that they are free from the cell. Such liberated bodies suspended in physiologic saline solution have the appearance of round, elliptical or lobulated, refractive, homogeneous, hyaline masses which are plastic and can be pressed or squeezed easily into various forms. When these masses are suspended in distilled water they swell rapidly, increasing greatly in size within a period of one half to one hour. As they imbibe water they assume a grossly granular appearance, later becoming transformed into a mulberry-like mass of globules suspended within a hyalin matrix. When the globules have reached a considerable size it can be seen by ordinary illumination under high magnification that they contain innumerable minute particles exhibiting an extremely rapid molecular motion. Sometimes the rapidly moving particles will stick to the periphery of a globule so that they may be photographed. The inclusions do not swell to the point of rupture, but remain definitely circumscribed. By compression, however, the minute bodies may be liberated and can be seen with ordinary illumination or in a dark-field preparation, as minute, spherical bodies having a diameter of about .25 micron. If physiological saline be added to the distilled water preparation the unruptured bodies will rapidly contract through the loss of water, becoming hyaline, wrinkled and apparently homogeneous.

By compressing an inclusion and staining it by a suitable method in a dry preparation it can be seen that it is composed essentially of two constituents; the one consisting of great numbers of minute, spherical bodies uniform in size and staining reaction, the other a homogeneous, faintly staining, amorphous material in which the minute bodies are suspended. The staining method which we have devised for this purpose is as follows:

A smear preparation dried over a flame is mordanted one minute with a .25 per cent. aqueous solution of potassium permanganate. It is then rinsed in running water and stained one minute with a few drops of the following solution: Alcohol (30 per cent.), 100 cc.; basic fuchsin, 1 gram; phenol (crystals), 1 cc.; anilin oil, 1 cc.

The stain is washed off in running water, and the preparation, blotted and dried, is ready for examination. This method of staining is not attended by the formation of any precipitate and stains the minute bodies quite sharply.

Thus from a morphological standpoint it is possible to demonstrate that the specific inclusions of fowl-pox are formed within the cells by the accumulation of a foreign material within the cytoplasm unattended by evidences of degeneration, and that these specific inclusions are constituted of minute, uniform bodies in great numbers, suspended and surrounded by a hyaline matrix. Morphologically, therefore, it is possible to demonstrate structures which resemble a minute micro-organism as the important constituent of the inclusion. These minute structures are in numbers sufficient to account for an infectiousness of material from the lesion in high dilutions. The minute bodies are small enough apparently to pass through the pores of a Berkefeld filter. It would appear from the fact that minute bodies are surrounded by a homogeneous matrix that filtration experiments might be attended with difficulties, and this experimentally is found to be the case. The incorporation of the minute structures within a hyaline matrix, which seems to be of a semipermeable nature, and appears to have a lipoid and proteid structure, might protect an enclosed micro-organism against such physical changes as dehydration by drying or glycerination.

We have demonstrated that the minute bodies are preserved in dried or glycerinated preparations after periods of many months (six) by soaking such material for twenty-four hours in distilled water, making smears and staining as above indicated. This material was infectious.

It has further been possible to show, we believe, that active virus is associated with the inclusions. By bacterial putrefaction it has been possible to soften and disintegrate the epithelial cells of lesions, leaving the inclusions apparently intact. By repeated washings and centrifuging at low speed the inclusions have been freed in large part from adherent cellular material and bacteria. A suspension of these inclusions was centrifuged at high speed. The supernatant fluid inoculated upon the skin of a susceptible fowl proved to be non-infectious, while the sediment, consisting of inclusions, proved to be highly infectious when similarly inoculated upon the skin.

From these observations we are convinced that in fowl-pox we have to do with a specific infectious disease due to a living microorganism which is visible under the microscope. This microorganism, we believe, invades the epithelial cells of the lesion; and the daughter cells, resulting from the division of an infected cell, will carry the virus by direct transmission. The microorganism proliferates within the cytoplasm of infected cells resulting in the formation of minute colonies suspended in a hyaline lipo-protein material which constitutes the specific inclusion.

The epithelial inclusions of molluscum contagiosum of man are composed essentially of the same type of minute bodies which can be demonstrated in suitably stained smear preparations and in fresh preparations with ordinary illumination. In fresh preparations the minute bodies can be seen in rapid molecular motion in every way similar to that exhibited by the bodies within the globules of swollen fowl-pox inclusions. In molluscum, however, there is not so dense a matrix; consequently, the inclusions are more diffuse and, because of their corpuscular content, appear finely granular in stained sections of the lesion. In molluscum contagiosum it is believed that we have to do with an acute infectious disease similar to fowl-pox, and caused by a visible microorganism which penetrates and proliferates within the affected cells of the lesion. This conception has been advanced by Lipschutz and by da Rocha-Lima.

Through the studies of Borrel, Paschen and others it seems possible that a similar microorganism may be the etiological factor in the diseases sheep-pox, variola and vaccinia.

This group of virus diseases then offers, we believe, a particularly favorable material for further etiological investigations.

ERNEST W. GOODPASTURE
DEPARTMENT OF PATHOLOGY,
VANDERBILT MEDICAL SCHOOL

ANALOGIES BETWEEN PHYSIOLOGICAL RHYTHMS AND THE RHYTHMICAL REACTIONS IN INORGANIC SYSTEMS

THE periodic or rhythmical reactions of inorganic chemistry are surface reactions, characteristic of polyphasic systems of a somewhat special type.[1] Typically they occur at the boundary between certain metals (iron, chromium, nickel and others) and electrolyte solutions, usually acids, and are always associated with variations in the electrical potential of the metallic surface. In some cases the metal shows a spontaneous rhythmical reaction with the solution (*e.g.*, iron in nitric acid, mercury in hydrogen peroxide); in others the rhythm occurs only during electrolysis, usually with the metal as anode (*e.g.*, periodic sulphide or iodide electrode reactions). A constant feature of each single reaction in the rhythmical sequence is the formation of an insoluble reaction-product which is strongly adsorbed by the metallic surface, forming over the latter a thin impermeable coating or film. This film limits or prevents the reaction between the phases and at the same time alters the interfacial potential; the reaction then ceases (or its velocity is greatly reduced) until it is renewed by some secondary reaction which removes or alters the film. In the spontaneous rhythms, *e.g.*, of iron or mercury just cited, the removal or dissolution of the film occurs rapidly as the result of a local electrochemical reaction which is propagated over the whole surface; the film is then reformed and the cycle is repeated. Under uniform conditions the succession of reactions exhibits a rhythm of remarkable regularity. From the standpoint of the physiological comparison it is of special interest to note that the formation of interfacial films and their dissolution under a transmitted electrochemical influence are the essential factors governing the peculiar behavior of such systems.

The parallels with the rhythmical reactions of living tissues (of the heart, nerve centers, cilia) have long attracted attention; and some years ago Bredig and his students,[2] in a series of studies on the rhythmical catalysis of hydrogen peroxide by mercury, pointed out various features of special physiological interest, such as the synchronism between the rhythms of reaction velocity and electromotor change, the dependence of the rhythm on the alternate formation and dissolution of an interfacial film, the high temperature coefficient, the sensitivity of the rhythm to H-ion concentration and the presence of foreign substances, and the part played by local circuits in electrolyzing and removing the film. Such striking resemblances point to some fundamental identity in the general conditions controlling the reaction velocities in both types of system.

The rhythmical reaction of pure iron wire in HNO_3 exhibits under certain conditions even more detailed analogies with the physiological rhythms. The tendency of iron to react rhythmically with nitric acid and the similar behavior of iron anodes in sulphuric acid have long been known; the precise conditions of the rhythm have, however, not been clearly analyzed; in particular its relation to the varying properties of the surface-film has been insufficiently considered. This relation is important because the whole resemblance to the physiological rhythm depends on the control of the reaction cycle by periodic variations in this film. It is now widely recognized that variations in the semipermeable protoplasmic membranes or surface-films underlie the response of irritable tissues to stimulation. The primary reactions in stimulation are surface reactions, as is shown clearly by their sensitivity to changes of electrical polarization and to the presence of surface-active compounds. The bioelectric variations of stimulation are also evidence of the part played by surface processes; these variations are now very generally referred to changes in the polarization of the protoplasmic membranes (membrane theories), and there is independent evidence of parallel variations in permeability. The well-known dependence of electrical stimulation on the polarizing action of the current (shown by Nernst and others), and such general physiological facts as chronaxie, polar stimulation and inhibition, together with the temporary existence of a non-reactive or refractory period following excitation, are other features of agreement between the living system and the inorganic model.

The rhythmical reaction of iron in nitric acid consists essentially in an alternation of active and passive periods, the latter corresponding to the film-covered condition. Not all specimens of iron show a regular rhythm in nitric acid; an irregular or local rhythm is common, but a rhythm in which all parts of an extensive surface—*e.g.*, of a long wire—are simultaneously active is found only in iron having special properties, the chief of which are a rapid and complete transmission of the active state over the whole surface when the metal is locally activated (as by scratching or touching with zinc) and a rapid return of transmissivity after activation. Such properties are shown most completely in soft iron of low carbon content; pure iron wire prepared by electrolysis[3] and the pure commercial wire known as Armco[4] exhibit an especially beautiful and regular rhythm under the conditions described below. In hard steel wire (piano

[1] A comprehensive account of these reactions is given in the monograph by R. Kremann, "Die periodischen Erscheinungen in der Chemie," Ahrens Sammlung chemischer und chemisch-technischer Vorträge, 1913, Bd. 19, p. 289.

[2] *Cf.* Bredig and Wilke: *Biochem. Zeitschr.*, 1908, Vol. 11, p. 67; Antropoff: *Zeitschr. f. physik. Chem.*, 1907, Vol. 62, p. 513.

[3] Kindly supplied by the U. S. Bureau of Standards, Washington.

[4] American Rolling Mill Co. The carbon content is *ca.* 0.1 per cent., according to analyses furnished by the Company.

wire), on the other hand, the tendency to rhythm is almost entirely absent. In this case the non-transmissive period ("refractory period") following activation lasts for several minutes (in 70 v. per cent. HNO_3 at 20°), indicating the presence of a relatively thick or resistant passivating film; while in Armco wire under the same conditions complete transmission is again possible within less than one second after the passage of an activation wave. The remarkable rhythmic properties shown by this wire are closely connected with its power of rapid recovery, the rate of rhythm being directly determined by the duration of the brief non-transmissive period following each activation. Armco wire was used in the following experiments.

When short pieces of iron wire (1 to 2 mm thick, 1 to several cm long), previously passivated, are placed in a flat-bottomed vessel containing nitric acid of 60 to 75 v. per cent. concentration[5] and activated by a single brief contact with zinc, usually a rhythmical reaction begins at once. At regular intervals (of one half to one second) the dark effervescent surface of the metal becomes momentarily bright and inactive, indicating the passive state; in 70 v. per cent. HNO_3 the passive period is brief as compared with the active period; as the strength of acid is increased up to 80 per cent. its relative duration becomes longer.[5a] If the acid is well stirred during the reaction the rhythm continues uniformly until the metal is largely dissolved away; if stirring is omitted the reaction soon becomes irregular and passes into a continuous effervescence.

Further study of this phenomenon soon showed that the essential condition determining the persistent rhythm is the presence of some local area or areas in which the reaction of the metal with the acid is continuous. From such an area waves of activation travel at intervals over the whole wire. Such an active region is formed wherever a sufficient surface of the metal is in contact with the glass or is otherwise protected against free renewal of the acid; the latter is there depleted by the reaction and soon becomes too weak to repassivate the iron. When the wire is suspended freely in the acid (by thin glass threads) no rhythm is shown; a touch with zinc then elicits a single reaction which is transmitted rapidly over the whole wire; the latter then immediately becomes again passive and remains so until again activated. The interval between such successive activations may be less than one second; at every touch the wire gives a single reaction and reverts automatically to the passive state. Such experiments illustrate the brevity of the period of recovery in this wire; they also show that the passive state is the state of equilibrium in acid of more than a certain critical concentration. In acid of less than this concentration (*ca.* 55 v. per cent.) automatic repassivation does not occur; the wire when activated continues to react until it is completely dissolved. This is the condition in the local protected area of the rhythmical wire. Such a continually active region may be compared with the nodal or pace-making region of the heart, or with the basal body (or "blepharoplast") of a cilium; it exerts a constant activating influence to which the external passive part of the wire responds as soon as it is sufficiently recovered. The rate of the rhythm is thus dependent on the duration of the temporary non-transmissive period, which is comparable with the refractory period of the living irritable tissue.

The chief conditions for the maintenance of a regular rhythm may be defined as follows: (1) acid of uniform concentration sufficient to reform the passivating film promptly after each activation (60 to 80 v. per cent.); (2) rapid recovery of transmissivity by the wire; and (3) presence of a local continuously reacting region sufficiently large and active to exert a constant activating influence[6] on the adjoining passive regions. These conditions were satisfactorily met by the following simple arrangement. The wire was supported horizontally, about 0.5 cm from the bottom, in a crystallization dish 10 cm wide, furnished with an outflow tube inserted into its side *ca.* 1.5 cm above the bottom. The support was furnished in some experiments by two thin glass threads suspended between the two limbs of a U-shaped glass rod lying on the bottom; in other experiments a bent wire was used, one end of which was attached to a key for making electrical connections; in this case a straight length of wire, 4 to 6 cm long, was exposed to the acid, while the bend (where the wire passed into the air) was coated with paraffin to prevent irregular action. Acid was led into the dish by a siphon connected with a large supply bottle; the slow flow of acid provided the necessary stirring.

[5] Volumes of HNO_3 (C. P., sp. gr. 1.42) in 100 volumes of solution.

[5a] This variation in the relative durations of active and passive periods is clearly shown in photographic records of the electromotor variation, taken with the string galvanometer. The current was led to the string from the sliding contact and terminal of a low resistance tube rheostat connected with the pulsating wire and an indifferent platinum electrode immersed in the acid.

[6] *I.e.*, An influence similar to that which the continual contact of zinc would have. In fact, contact with zinc will maintain a rhythm in an iron wire suspended in 70 per cent. HNO_3, but it is impossible to keep the conditions constant in such an experiment and the rhythm is irregular.

Opposite the free end of the wire was placed a short glass tube of caliber slightly wider than the wire. When the wire is inserted into this tube for a short distance (2 to 4 mm) and activated by touching with zinc a continuous reaction is readily started in the enclosed region, which is protected from free renewal of acid. The area of this active region can be adjusted by inserting the wire more or less deeply into the tube. From this region waves of activation pass in regular succession over the whole wire. The rhythm shown under these conditions is remarkably regular and continues indefinitely, *i.e.*, until the enclosed end of the wire is dissolved away. At any time the reaction may be brought to a stop by removing the tube from the wire; the latter then immediately becomes passive.

Since complete transmission and rapid recovery are necessary conditions for the rhythm, their general conditions should first be considered. The transmission itself, as is well known, is an effect of the local circuit formed between the active and the passive areas, the latter being cathodal; the film is there broken down by electrolytic reduction and the process of disruption spreads automatically, since it is repeated wherever anodal and cathodal areas adjoin each other. The process may be regarded as in the nature of a two-dimensional explosion, *i.e.*, an explosive reaction confined to the thin layer (probably monomolecular) of reactive material at the phase boundary. According to the usual conception of explosions, a reaction becomes explosive when heat is produced locally more rapidly than it is conveyed away. The film-conditioned type of chemical transmission differs, however, from the three-dimensional explosion in that the essential factor determining the spread of reaction is not a certain critical local heat-production, but a certain critical intensity of electric current between the reacting area of the surface and the passive region adjoining. If the current intensity (or density) is insufficient, the reaction fails to spread; in other words, a certain threshold must be overpassed. When the current intensity exceeds the critical level required, there is an automatic spread of the reaction to an indefinite distance, *i.e.*, over the entire area of the film—assuming the latter to have uniform properties throughout.

In another respect this type of explosive process differs from that in three-dimensional masses of material, such as explosive gas mixtures or compounds: *i.e.*, materials are at hand, in the direction of the third dimension, for replacing the film, so that a second reaction may become immediately possible. A certain interval is required, but this may be brief; in pure iron wires in 70 v. per cent. HNO_3 it is about one half second at 20°; in living systems, such as nerve, it may be much less; the system can then react as before. The interval represents a temporary non-transmissive or "refractory" period, during which the reactive molecules are to be regarded as assembling at the surface, and presumably there undergoing orientation or other change favorable to reaction. The refractory period thus corresponds to the interval required for the formation of an adsorption film having definite characteristics. In general it should be noted that such surface reactions, since they depend on the conditions present in thin layers—where distances are small and the time required for access of material from either adjoining phase is correspondingly brief—are subject to rapid fluctuations of velocity. The quick initiations and arrests shown in the stimulation processes of living organisms—as well as their electrically conditioned character—are in themselves evidence that the controlling chemical reactions are surface reactions. Similar considerations apply to the physiological rhythms, which represent automatic and regularly repeated stimulations.

Conditions Determining the Rate of Rhythm

Extent of pace-making area: In general any increase in the area of the continuously active or controlling region is found to accelerate the rhythm, while any decrease retards it. The rate can thus be regulated by inserting the wire for a greater or less distance inside the tube. If the active region be decreased beyond a certain length (of 1 or 2 mm) it becomes suddenly passive, by spread of the external passive area, and the rhythm ceases. There is thus for each concentration of acid a certain minimal area of the controlling region, corresponding to the slowest rhythm which is stable under the conditions. The rhythm can readily be doubled by inserting the wire for 4 to 5 mm into the tube; this increases the anodal area of the local circuit, and hence also the intensity and reducing effectiveness of the current at the adjoining passive area. A dependence of the rhythm in the rate of the local cathodal reduction is thus shown. This effect is readily understood when we consider that the film at its first deposition is refractory to reduction and attains its final state of maximum reactivity by a progressive process.[7] Hence at a given interval a stronger local current may cause activation while a weaker one is ineffective.

Concentration of Acid: Within the range of concentration in which a regular rhythm is shown (60 to 80 v. per cent.) the rate increases with concentration, in a manner approximately linear. With the controlling region kept at its minimal area, as above de-

[7] Following a curve of the type $R_t = R_o (1 - e^{-kt})$, as indicated by my earlier results on steel wires (*Journ. Gen. Physiol.*, 1925, vol. 7, p. 493).

scribed, the following rhythms were found characteristic (at 22–23°).

Concentration (v.per cent. HNO_3)	Rate per minute
60	34–36
65	50–56
70	62–70
75	80–90
80	> 100 (becomes irregular)

In 80 v. per cent. acid a regular reaction is difficult to maintain, probably because of too great heat-production at the site of the controlling reaction.

Temperature: The temperature of the acid was controlled by a water bath surrounding the supply bottle. The following rates are typical for 65 v. per cent. acid at temperatures between 10° and 30°. Below 10° the rhythm is uncertain and above 30° it tends to accelerate and become irregular. As before, the wire was adjusted to give the slowest rhythm that was stable under the conditions.

Temperature	Rate per minute
10°	14– 16
15°	28– 32
20°	46– 50
25°	84– 88
30°	122–128

The range of temperature within which the rhythm is stable is not large and is similar to the physiological range, although the precise significance of this correspondence is not clear. It may be that the film is not sufficiently stable at higher temperatures, while at lower temperatures the reaction is too slow for effective reduction.

The correspondence of the temperature coefficient with that of the physiological rhythms is striking; the Q_{10} value is 2½ to 3, equivalent to a value of 17,000 to 22,000 for μ in Arrhenius' exponential formula, $\frac{k_2}{k_1} = e^{\frac{\mu}{2}\left(\frac{1}{T_1} - \frac{1}{T_2}\right)}$ where k_1 and k_2 are the velocity constants at the absolute temperatures T_1 and T_2. As already pointed out, the interval between successive reactions represents the time required for the surface-film to attain a certain degree of reactivity, *i.e.*, of reducibility by the local active-passive current. In the case of steel wires the rate of change in the film at different temperatures has been determined, using the recovery of transmissivity as criterion; the temperature coefficient of this recovery process is the same as that of the rhythm.[8] This correspondence is further evidence that the chemical change in the film determining the recovery of transmissivity is also the condition determining the rate of rhythm. This is apparently also the case in the cardiac rhythm, where the temperature coefficients of refractory period and of rhythm are closely similar or identical.

Other factors influencing the rhythm: As in the case of the heart beat, the rhythm of passive iron is affected by electrical polarization. When the pulsating wire is connected through a rheostat to an external source of current, making the wire anode has a retarding or inhibiting effect, while making it cathode causes acceleration. These effects vary characteristically with the intensity of the polarizing current; sufficient anodal polarization stops the reaction, while sufficient cathodal polarization renders it continuous. Polar effects of an analogous kind are well known in living tissues. A more detailed description of these and other parallels will be given elsewhere.

There is also a remarkable relation between the rate of rhythm in a pulsating wire and the total length of the wire, the rate decreasing at first rapidly, then slowly, with increase in the length. The following rates were found characteristic for different lengths of regularly pulsating wires, at one end of which a pace-making region was established by encircling the wire by a glass ring 3 mm long. The same ring was used in all experiments; the concentration of acid was 70 v. per cent. and the temperature 20°–21°.

Length of wire (cm)	Rate per minute
30 and 18	40– 46
12	42– 46
8	46– 50
6	48– 54
4	60– 64
3.5	64– 68
3	66– 72
2.5	68– 74
2.0	82– 92
1.5	84– 96
1.0	100–108
0.75	> 120 (less regular)

This phenomenon appears to be an expression of the mutual influence which the active and passive areas of the same wire exert upon one another.[9] The presence of a passive region has a restraining or inhibiting effect upon activation in other regions of the wire; reactivation at the region adjoining the pace-making area is thus delayed until the activation wave has extended over the whole length of the wire. There are biological analogies here also; in general it is observed that the frequency of ciliary beats or heart beats decreases as the linear dimensions of the tissue increase. In such cases it seems clear that a dis-

[8] *Journ. Gen. Physiol., loc. cit.*, p. 500.

[9] This influence was early noted by Schönbein, *Philos. Mag.*, 1836, Vol. 9.

tance action, possibly of the same kind as that observed in the experiment just described, plays a controlling part in the determination of rhythm: *i.e.*, the latter depends on a coordinating influence, in the general nature of a removal of restraint, transmitted at a finite velocity from the pace-making region. Correspondingly, we find that when transmission is locally impaired in the heart, fibrillation often occurs, at a rhythm typically faster than the main rhythm. In such cases local pace-making regions are to be assumed, each controlling the rhythm over a relatively small area.

Ralph S. Lillie

University of Chicago

JOSEPH NELSON ROSE

1862–1928

On the afternoon of May fourth an assembly-room in the United States National Museum was filled to overflowing in response to a call issued that morning by the secretary of the Smithsonian Institution. The gathering was called as a means of showing and recording his late associates' appreciation of Dr. Rose, who had left his desk in order late the preceding afternoon—never to return to it.

The meeting was impressive. To those of us who listened, as speakers rose here and there in the room, the kindly personality of a friend and the talented devotion of an able man to earnest work unfolded. To those of us who spoke, the sadness of the occasion was blended with a consolation born of the knowledge that a well-rounded-out life had come to ripe fruition.

I recalled that last winter Dr. Rose had reminded me of the fact that over forty years ago he had asked to do the work for his doctorate with me, but had been prevented by circumstances from doing so; and I thought of the original and thorough-going study of a difficult group of plants—the Umbelliferae—that came out of his candidacy under Professor Coulter. I remembered that when a preliminary dip into the Crassulaceae, which are ill-preserved in herbaria, had convinced me that they were beyond my own understanding, he disentangled them with masterly skill. There came to my memory a long day's tramp with him down a lava-covered mountainside bordering the valley in which the City of Mexico lies, and the keen, detailed and comprehensive way in which he examined the many agaves that we found—in which at that time he was more interested than I. Even a few days before his death he had shown me a collection of specimens and full-sized photographs of what passes for *Acacia Farnesiana,* and which for years he has known to comprise more than one species.

Interwoven with these memories were many others, like them indicative of a close observer, an energetic worker, a deliberate thinker and a friendly man even when critical.

Except for two years before attaining the doctorate, Rose was not a teacher—unquestionably to the loss of young men in whom his deliberate weighing of questions and facts would have conduced to the early formation of a judicial habit.

For forty years his connection has been with the government botanical service—first in the Department of Agriculture and later, when the present national herbarium was established under the National Museum, in this institution. To his efficiency in building up and using this great collection his associates all bear witness, and the collection itself and the long series of published "Contributions" are in evidence to the same effect; but of recent years the brunt of this responsibility has been borne by his coadjutor, Mr. Maxon.

Custodianship of a large herbarium, with an impulse to investigation, not only offers great possibilities to one who knows how to use them, but almost of necessity drives one afield. With familiarity with the contents of the larger European collections Dr. Rose also came to know many of the objects of his study in their haunts—Central and South America; and his work, especially on succulent plants, never could have acquired its lasting value in any other way. The necessary routine handling of the accessions in such an establishment as the National Herbarium affords in itself the basis of a liberal education to one keen on floristic and taxonomic studies. New material comes in from unfamiliar regions and the specimens must be named.

Among Dr. Rose's earlier tasks was naming several west-Mexican collections made by Edward Palmer, a pioneer in that field, and enumerations of such collections are among his earlier publications. It probably was in doing this work that he formed a habit of which he once spoke to me—that of synoptically bringing under his eye the characters of all the known species of a group, preliminary to naming adequately those before him; and this was a most valuable habit in his later and more difficult studies.

Though his most monumental work was on the Cactaceae, Crassulaceae, Umbelliferae and Amaryllidaceae, his interests were broadly distributed over the flowering plants. This is not the place for an enumeration of his publications, but they covered the North American representatives of Burseraceae, a considerable series of "Studies of Mexican and Central American plants," often from an economic standpoint, and a carefully executed study of the anatomical characters of certain pines applicable to their classification—for which Engelmann had marked the way. Occasionally, as of Canby in 1904 and Greene in 1916, he wrote appreciative sketches of botanists whom he had known.

It is chiefly through his comprehensive handling of the difficult succulents, tuberose-like Amaryllids and Umbelliferae that his memory will be kept fresh in science; but those who knew him well will remember him also as a devoted public servant and a sympathetic and helpful friend, whom the last call found still active at the end of a long and successful professional career.

WM. TRELEASE

SCIENTIFIC EVENTS

THE GLASGOW MEETING OF THE BRITISH ASSOCIATION

THE British Association for the Advancement of Science has issued the preliminary program of its meeting to be held in Glasgow from September 5 to 12, under the presidency of Sir William Bragg, who in his address will deal with modern developments of the physical sciences and their relation to national problems. The subjects of the presidential addresses and discussions in the various sections include the reflection of electrons by matter, the photography and measurement of radiation, ancient geography in modern education (by Professor J. L. Myres), the nature of skill (by Professor T. H. Pear), the influence of engineering on civilization (by Sir William Ellis), the archeology of Scotland (by Sir George Macdonald) and increasing returns and economic progress (by Professor Allyn Young). Dr. Cyril Norwood will give the presidential address in the education section, which also will hold a discussion on broadcasting in the service of education, opened by Sir John Reith.

One of the customary evening discourses will be given by Professor E. A. Westermarck, on the study of popular sayings; this will be the Frazer lecture in social anthropology, which is due for delivery in Glasgow, and to which members of the association will, by the courtesy of the university authorities, be admitted. The other evening discourse will be given by Professor F. G. Donnan under the title of "The Mystery of Life," the subject being considered from the viewpoint of physical chemistry. The delegates of corresponding societies, under the presidency of Dr. Vaughan Cornish, will discuss the preservation of scenic beauty in town and country. All the meetings, except those in the evening, will be held in the university, an unusually convenient arrangement. The Lord Provost and Corporation of Glasgow will give a reception and dance in the city chambers, and the local committee a reception in Kelvingrove Art Galleries.

Ample opportunity will be provided for visits to places of scientific interest in the country around Glasgow, and for studying the manifold economic interests of the city and the Clyde area, with their many outstanding examples of the value of applied science in industry and social conditions. Saturday, September 8, is, as usual, devoted entirely to excursions, but in addition there will be numerous half-day and afternoon excursions during the week. Many of these will be of special sectional interest, or will be devoted to visits to particular works and industrial centers. The Port of Glasgow, with its quays and docks and shipyards, will be of special interest to many visitors, and to facilitate its inspection the Clyde trustees are proposing to place their steamer *Comet* at the service of members of the association.

CENTENARY OF THE LONDON ZOOLOGICAL SOCIETY

THE Zoological Society of London will celebrate the completion of its hundredth year of work next year, as it received its royal charter in 1829. The London *Times* gives the following details of the early history of the society:

As is often the case with an institution which came into existence by stages, there are several dates on which a centenary celebration might have been justified, but, as the council has announced in its annual reports for some years, 1929 was selected as the most appropriate.

The first possible date was 1822, for in November of that year some fellows of the Linnean Society, meeting at the house of William Kirby, the entomologist, gratified their discontent with the disproportionately small attention given to zoology by the Linnean Society by deciding to form a Zoological Club. They were still tied by loyalty to their parent society, and when they drafted the rules of the new body they limited membership to fellows of the Linnean Society, and arranged that their scientific work should be published by that society. The work they contemplated and for some time carried out did not include the maintenance of a living collection. There is still uncertainty over the transition from the Zoological Club of the Linnean Society to a Zoological Society with the chief object of establishing a zoological garden, and there is reason to believe that the latter had an independent origin, largely at the instigation of Sir Stamford Raffles, who, although a fellow of the Linnean Society, does not appear to have been a member of the Zoological Club.

The first known prospectus of the Zoological Society was issued in 1825 and announced as its object the formation of a society that should have the same relations to zoology and animal life that the Horticultural Society bore to botany and the vegetable kingdom. There were 77 original subscribers, among whom may be mentioned Sir Stamford Raffles, Sir Humphry Davy, president of the Royal Society, the Duke of Bedford, the Marquis of Lansdowne, Robert Peel and Alexander Baring, M.P. In this prospectus there was no suggestion of the existence of the Zoological Club of the Linnean Society, or of limitation of the members of the new society to fellows of the Linnean Society. But there was overlapping of interest, and Mr. Vigors, who was the first secretary and last chairman of the Zoological Club, was the first secretary of the Zoological Society. The club was dissolved, apparently, in 1829, by which time most of its members had joined the new society.

A house was obtained in Bruton-street for the new society, where meetings were held, a museum established, and a certain number of living birds and mammals kept. In the course of 1826 negotiations with the Crown were successfully conducted for the use of part of Regent's Park, and the latter part of 1826 and 1827 were occupied with the laying-out of the new Zoological Gardens. Early in 1828 there were a few pinioned wild duck on a lake, an emu, an otter, some silver-haired rabbits and several birds of prey. It is reported that on February 25, 1828, there were four visitors to the gardens, but under what conditions they were admitted is not known. On April 27, 1828, a superintendent was appointed, and it was decided that visitors should be admitted on the presentation of a voucher from a fellow and the payment of 1s. Considerable progress was made during the remainder of 1828 in stocking and laying out the gardens. The first report of the council appeared in 1829, when the society received its Royal Charter, and the oldest voucher for admittance that has been traced was signed by a fellow who did not join the society until 1829.

EXHIBIT OF OPTICAL INSTRUMENTS AND PRODUCTS

UNDER the joint auspices of the Optical Society of America and the Bureau of Standards there will be an exhibit of optical instruments and optical products in the buildings of the bureau at Washington, D. C. This exhibition will be open from 9:00 to 4:30, October 31, November 1, 2 and 3 and for one evening session to be designated later by the Optical Society.

It is the desire of the committee to include in this exhibit all the newer instruments which have been developed by scientific investigators and our commercial firms. Research workers are particularly invited to contribute exhibits designed to illustrate the progress of their work and their attention is called to the fact that such an exhibit is often more useful than the presentation of a formal paper for emphasizing the significance and importance of an investigation. All American made instruments or products in which the application of optical principles is an important part in design, construction or use are eligible for exhibition. The following lists will serve to partially indicate the contemplated scope of the exhibit: optical and colored glasses, fused silica, optical components, spectacle lenses, ophthalmic instruments, binoculars, microscopes, photographic apparatus, colored photographic processes, motion-picture apparatus, astronomical instruments, interferometers, spectral apparatus, metrological instruments, surveying and nautical instruments, search lights, telescopic gunsights, photometric apparatus, optical pyrometers, colorimetric instruments, vacuum discharge tubes, special systems of illumination, etc.

I. C. GARDNER, *Chairman,*
Committee on Optical Instruments Exhibit
BUREAU OF STANDARDS

THE PLACE OF SCIENCE IN EDUCATION

THERE has just been published a report of the committee of the American Association for the Advancement of Science on "The Place of Science in Education."

This report is organized under seven headings as follows and the summarizing sentence is given for some of them:

I. The Committee's Understanding of its Functions.

II. The Search for Enduring Facts and the Growth of Confidence in the Guidance of Scientific Truth. Science instruction both in school and out needs better organization, more effective cooperation to make even the health knowledge now available function more completely in the lives of people generally.

III. Obligations of Science Knowledge. Science, not to be discredited, must devise effective ways and means of developing, in its devotees first and in the whole people ultimately, a sense of moral obligation that will prevent the newly acquired knowledge and method of science serving base ends.

IV. The Science Subjects in Educational Programs. The hopeful element is that the stereotyped science courses of the college are being replaced in the earlier years at least by new types, tentative at present but frankly experimental, looking toward a more satisfactory college science sequence. The whole problem needs careful study.

V. Summaries of Types of Specific Studies Relating to the Educational Uses of Science. The above represent but a beginning in the application of the objective scientific method to the problems of science teaching. Such investigations must be multiplied and verified by those truly interested in the scientific solution of such questions.

VI. Those who Teach Science. A more thoroughgoing preparation in the fundamentals of science is needed by all who aspire to teach it.

VII. Those who have Developed Science. Science as method is quite as important as science subject-matter and should receive much attention in science instruction.

The committee offers the following recommendations:

(a) That some organization of national scope such as the United States Bureau of Education, or the Research Division of the National Education Association, be asked by this committee to undertake a comprehensive and intensive study of the situations, tendencies and needs of science instruction in educational systems.

(b) That the services of a field secretary be secured, to work with existing agencies, to distribute information on research in science education, to stimulate further research, to operate as a sort of clearing-house agent and to continue the organizing of new groups of science teachers, writers for popularization of science, etc. This field secretary should work under the guidance of the Committee on the Place of Science in Education, or under the guidance of a national council of science teachers as soon as such a council is formed.

(c) That a national council of science teachers be organized to advance science teaching, to increase public appreciation of science and to secure for science teachers increased facilities and a wider usefulness. The services of a field secretary would be very useful in the organization of such a council.

A copy of the full report will be mailed on request sent to Elliott R. Downing, School of Education, University of Chicago, Chicago, Illinois.

SCIENTIFIC NOTES AND NEWS

DR. WILLIAM WALLACE CAMPBELL, director of the Lick Observatory and president of the University of California, received the honorary degree of doctor of science from Columbia University on June 5.

AMONG the honors listed on the occasion of the birthday of the King of England is a knighthood conferred on Captain George Hubert Wilkins, who with Lieutenant Carl B. Eielson recently flew from Alaska to Spitzbergen.

DR. G. H. HARDY, professor of geometry in the University of Oxford, and Dr. F. G. Hopkins, professor of biochemistry in the University of Cambridge, have been made foreign members of the Society of Sciences of Göttingen.

THE first award of the Dalby memorial prize, for the best original work in otology during the previous five years, has been made to Dr. Otto Mayer, of Vienna. The award is in the hands of the council of the Royal Society of Medicine, acting on the recommendation of the president and vice-president of the section of otology.

PROFESSOR LIONEL WILLIAM LYDE, professor of geography in the University of London, has been appointed a foreign member of the Hungarian Academy of Science.

DR. MAX PLANCK, professor of physics in the University of Berlin, celebrated his seventieth birthday on April 23. To commemorate this occasion his friends and colleagues have founded a gold medal to be awarded for distinguished work in theoretical physics.

PROFESSOR KARL VON NORDEN, professor of medicine at the University of Frankfort, and Professor Friedrich Müller, professor of medicine at the University of Munich, will celebrate their seventieth anniversaries in September.

EMILE PICARD, professor of mathematics in the University of Paris, celebrated in May the fiftieth anniversary of his scientific career.

PROFESSOR HERMANN T. VULTÉ, who retires in June as professor of household chemistry in Teachers College, Columbia University, was tendered a farewell luncheon by his colleagues at the Columbia faculty house, on which occasion a gold-banded ebony cane, suitably inscribed, was presented to him. By action of the trustees Professor Vulté will continue to occupy his research laboratory.

PROFESSOR EVAN THOMAS, one of the oldest professors at the University of Vermont, retires this June under the provisions of a Carnegie pension, having completed over a quarter of a century of service at the university.

AT the annual meeting of the American Society for Clinical Investigation, held in Washington, D. C., on April 30, Dr. Jonathan C. Meakins, Montreal, was elected *president;* Dr. James L. Gamble, Boston, *vice-president;* Dr. George A. Harrop, Jr., Baltimore, *treasurer,* and Dr. Joseph T. Wearn, Boston, reelected *secretary.*

AT the anniversary meeting of the Linnean Society of London on May 24 the following were elected officers for 1928–29: *President,* Sir Sidney Harmer; *vice-presidents,* Dr. W. T. Calman, H. N. Dixon, H. W. Monckton and Dr. E. J. Salisbury; *treasurer,* H. W. Monckton; *secretaries,* Dr. G. P. Bidder (zoology) and J. Ramsbottom (botany).

PROFESSOR LEO EDWARD MELCHERS, head of the department of botany and plant pathology, Kansas State Agricultural College, who is on leave in Egypt, was recently made chief mycologist in charge of the section of mycology in the Ministry of Agriculture. During his stay in Egypt he is undertaking the reorganization of the mycological work for the Egyptian government. He was recently made chairman of a committee on plant quarantine and inspection work in Egypt, the plan being to improve the present service and facilities for conducting the work.

DR. B. T. DICKSON, until recently professor of plant pathology of McGill University, Canada, has been appointed chief of the division of economic botany of the Commonwealth Council for Scientific and Industrial Research of Australia, which division he is now in process of organizing. Dr. Dickson originally went to Australia to take charge of the plant pathological work of the council and this is now being absorbed in the larger division.

PAUL C. STANDLEY, formerly of the U. S. National Museum, has been appointed associate curator of the herbarium in the Field Museum of Natural History, Chicago. He began work in his new position on June 1.

CLIFFORD S. LEONARD, assistant professor in the department of pharmacology and toxicology at Yale University, has joined the staff of the chemical research laboratories of Burroughs Wellcome and Company, Inc., in New York.

JAMES GIRVIN PETERS has been appointed chief of the branch of public relations in the United States Forest Service. Mr. Peters succeeds Major R. Y. Stuart, who on May 1 took over his duties as chief forester.

THE U. S. Coast and Geodetic Survey announced on June 1 the appointment of Leo O. Colbert as director of coast surveys of the Philippine Islands, to succeed R. B. Derickson, who will be assigned to other duty.

DR. S. HERBERT ANDERSON, associate professor of physics at the University of Washington, has been granted a year's leave of absence to engage in research work for the Guggenheim Foundation of New York. His studies will concern the field of sound as related to aeronautics to develop instruments for landing in fog and other safety devices. He will report at Wright Field, Dayton, the army engineering headquarters, on July 1.

AUGUST F. FOERSTE, of Dayton, who was granted an award from the Marsh fund by the National Academy of Science, sailed on June 8 to spend the summer visiting collections and field localities in northern Europe.

FRANCIS J. PETTIJOHN, on leave for study from the department of geology, Oberlin College, will spend the summer studying the ancient crystallines near Sioux Lookout, Ontario. He will be accompanied by Mr. Walter Chappel, a recent Oberlin graduate in geology. The work will consist of a reconnaissance survey, followed by an intensive study of the critical areas.

HUGO WINKENWERDER, dean of the college of forestry at the University of Washington, left on May 26 for Europe, where during the summer he will make a study of botanical gardens and ancient forests.

THE department of vertebrate paleontology of the American Museum of Natural History is sending out three men, Peter Kaisen, Ernest Kaisen and Glen Streeter, to cooperate with the Colorado Museum of Natural History in completing the Folsom, New Mexico, bison excavations, noted because of the association of human artifacts with an extinct species of bison.

DR. ALBERT ERNEST JENKS, professor of anthropology in the University of Minnesota, will head an expedition which was to leave about June 10 by motor and railroad to dig for six weeks in the Mimbres Valley, New Mexico, where they expect to find traces of prehistoric culture.

PLANS for an expedition this summer to study marine sedimentation and its influence on ocean life at the West Indies, with Dr. William Beebe, of the New York Zoological Society, and Dr. Charles Fish, director of the Buffalo Society of Natural Sciences, among its members, have been announced by Professor Richard M. Field, of the department of geology at Princeton University.

DR. HENRY J. COX, of the United States Weather Bureau, has been appointed a delegate of the Geographic Society of Chicago to the International Geographical Congress, which meets in London and Cambridge, England, from July 13 to 26. He has also been named as a delegate to the same congress by the National Academy of Sciences and National Research Council in Washington.

PROFESSOR CHARLES P. BERKEY, professor of geology in Columbia University, has been invited to take part in an arranged discussion on the geology of Central Asia at the meetings of the British Association for the Advancement of Science, which will be held in Glasgow next September. Professor Berkey will attend the convention as an official delegate of the American Museum of Natural History and of Columbia University.

DR. G. STRUVE, director of the Berlin University Observatory at Neu-Babelsberg, Germany, arrived in the United States on June 4. Dr. Struve came at the invitation of the University of Chicago and of Yerkes Observatory, of which he was recently nominated honorary research associate professor. He will also visit the Lick Observatory.

DR. HANS WILDBOLZ, professor of surgical and diagnostic urology in the University of Berne, gave a Mayo foundation lecture on June 7, at the Mayo Clinic, Rochester.

PROFESSOR G. W. RITCHEY, of the Solar Observatory, Pasadena, delivered an address on May 11 before the Royal Astronomical Society, in which he explained the method of the construction of "cellular" mirrors carried on at the Paris Observatory. On May 16, Professor Ritchey spoke on "The Modern Reflecting Telescope," before the Optical Society in the Imperial College, South Kensington.

DR. GEORGE C. SHATTUCK, assistant professor of tropical medicine at the Harvard Medical School, gave a lecture in London, on May 21, on his recent expedition to Liberia and the Congo, before the Royal Geographic Society.

PROFESSOR W. F. G. SWANN, of the Bartol Research Foundation, addressed the colloquium at the Bell Telephone Laboratories, New York City, May 28, on "Possible Modifications in Electrodynamics and Their Consequences."

ARTHUR E. MORGAN, president of Antioch College, formerly chief engineer of the Miami Conservancy District, addressed a meeting of the geology section of the Ohio Academy of Science, June 2, on the subject of the problems connected with flood prevention in the Dayton area.

THE surgical papers of Dr. William Stewart Halsted, who died in 1922 and who was for thirty-two years surgeon-in-chief of the Johns Hopkins Hospital, have been published in two volumes as a tribute to his memory.

A MEMORIAL volume, containing more than 200 pages with photographs, prepared by employees of the Panama Canal to commemorate the life and works of the late Major-General George W. Goethals, has been sent to his widow.

THE one hundred and twenty-fifth anniversary of the birth of the chemist Justus Liebig, who was born at Darmstadt, is to be celebrated by rebuilding with the original material the house in which he was born, and the addition to it of a museum.

DR. HOWARD A. LOTHROP, professor of surgery at the Harvard Medical School, died on June 4, at the age of sixty-four years.

WILLIAM EDWARD PLUMMER, director of the Liverpool Observatory, died on May 22, aged seventy-nine years.

DR. F. M. PERKIN, of England, one of the founders of the Faraday Society, died on May 24.

THE deaths have been announced of the following German scientific men: Dr. Otto Staude, professor of mathematics at the University of Rostock; Dr. Gustav Schultz, professor of chemical technology and metallurgy in the University of Munich; Dr. Johannes Gadamer, professor of pharmaceutical chemistry in the University of Marburg, and Dr. Julius Hirschwald, professor of mineralogy and geology in the University of Berlin.

PROFESSOR OTTO NORDEÑSKJOELD, well-known Swedish Arctic and Antarctic explorer and professor at the University of Gothenberg, died on June 2, at the age of fifty-nine years.

THE Pacific section of the American Association for the Advancement of Science is meeting at Pomona College from June 13 to 16. Various affiliated societies are holding their meetings in conjunction with it, including the Astronomical Society of the Pacific, the American Meteorological Society, the American Physical Society, the Pacific sections of the American Chemical Society, the American Association of Economic Entomologists, the Botanical Society of America, the Western Society of Naturalists, the Society for Experimental Biology and Medicine and others. The meeting is presided over by the president of the section, Dr. Charles A. Kofoid, professor of zoology at the University of California. On Wednesday evening, June 13, he delivered an address on "The Luminescence of the Sea." Other general lectures are to be given by Dr. F. H. Seares, assistant director of the Mt. Wilson Observatory, on "Counting the Stars," and by Dr. Charles K. Edmunds, president of Pomona College, on "Some Physical Features of China."

PROBLEMS confronting federal, state and local health authorities, including prevalence of leprosy in the United States, the present status of trachoma and its treatment, the relation of iodine to goiter, and other public health matters of mutual concern, were considered by the joint sessions of the annual Conference of State and Provincial Health Authorities of North America, meeting in Minneapolis, June 8 and 9, under the auspices of the United States Public Health Service.

THE fourth Pacific Science Congress will be held at Batavia, Buitenzorg and Bandoeng, Java, during May and June, 1929, under the auspices of the Pacific Science Association. The general president of the congress and chairman of the Netherlands Indies Pacific Research Committee is Dr. A. A. L. Rutgers.

AT a general meeting of members of the British Institute of Metals on May 8, an invitation was presented on behalf of the American Institute of Mining and Metallurgical Engineers for the Institute of Metals to visit America and meet with the American body in 1932. According to the *Electrical Review* the president of the institute, Dr. W. Rosenhain, F.R.S., suitably acknowledged the receipt of the invitation, and indicated that it would be gladly accepted by the institute.

PLANS for the twenty-third International Congress of Americanists, to be held in New York the week of September 17, have been announced. The congress, which holds biennial sessions, is devoted to the study of the peoples of pre-Columbian America, both ethnically and from the point of view of environmental factors. Sessions of the congress will be held at the Natural History Museum, at the Museum of the American Indian, at Columbia University, and at the Brooklyn Museum. The program includes general and sectional meetings and various entertainments. Henry Fairfield Osborn is chairman of the honorary committee and Franz Boas of the organizing committee. Other members of the latter committee include George G. Heye, Stewart Culin, A. V. Kidder and P. E. Goddard. Two previous meetings of the congress have been held in this country: the thirteenth in New York in 1902 and the nineteenth in Washington in 1915.

FOLLOWING the action taken by the executive board of the National Research Council on April 24, that the National Research Council adhere through its division of geology and geography to the International Geographical Union, the following seven delegates have been named to the International Geographical Congress to be held in London and Cambridge from July 14 to 25: Dr. Wallace W. Atwood, president and professor of physical geography, Clark University; Colonel C. H. Birdseye, chief topographic engineer, U. S. Geological Survey; Dr. Isaiah Bowman, director of the American Geographical Society, New York City; Dr. Albert P. Brigham, professor of geology in Colgate University; Dr. Henry J. Cox, senior meteorologist, U. S. Weather Bureau, Chicago, Ill.; Dr. Douglas Johnson, professor of physiography, Columbia University, and Colonel E. Lester Jones, director of the U. S. Coast and Geodetic Survey.

THE United States Civil Service Commission announces an open competitive examination for senior physicist, applications for which must be on file with the commission at Washington not later than July 5. The examination is to fill a vacancy at the Signal Corps Laboratory, Monmouth, N. J., and vacancies occurring throughout the United States in positions requiring similar qualifications. The entrance salary for this position in the departmental service in Washington, D. C., and of the present vacancy in the Signal Corps Laboratory at Monmouth, N. J., is $5,200 a year. Competitors will not be required to report for examination at any place, but will be rated on their education and experience, and writings to be filed with the application.

ACCORDING to the annual report of the Rockefeller Foundation, the following medical schools were assisted during 1927: State University of Iowa, University of Montreal, National School of Medicine and Pharmacy, Haiti; Faculty of Medicine, São Paulo, Brazil; University College, London; London Hospital Medical School, University of Cambridge, University of Edinburgh, University of Lyon, Free University of Brussels, University of Strasbourg, twenty departments in twelve French and Italian medical schools, Institute of Psychiatric Research, Munich; University of Zagreb, American University in Beirut, Chulalongkorn University, Bangkok; Shantung Christian University, Tsinan; Shanghai Union Medical School, Hsiangya Medical College, Changsha; Keio University, Tokyo.

Two prizes are offered by the Eugenics Research Association for the best essays written by an American author and two prizes for essays written by European authors on the topic: "A comparison of both the crude birth-rate, the birth-rate per 1,000 females 15 to 45 years of age, and the 'vital index' (or 100 births/deaths ratio) of the Nordic peoples and non-Nordic peoples in the Americas." Data are to be considered in different periods from 1850 to the present time, or that of the last available census or registration. Nordic peoples in the Americas are considered to be those whose ancestors came mainly from Nordic countries. For the purposes of this investigation Nordic countries are defined as including the Scandinavian countries south of about 63° N. lat., the Netherlands, England, Scotland, North Ireland and the German States of Schleswig-Holstein, Mecklenburg, Hannover and Westphalia. Any other section of Europe, any part of Asia and Africa north of the Zambezi, may be regarded, for the purposes of this study, as "non-Nordic." The prizes offered in each of the two groups are: $1,000 for the best essay and $200 for the second best. The essay is to be typewritten and mailed in time to reach Cold Spring Harbor by February 1, 1929. Further details may be obtained by addressing the Eugenics Research Association, Cold Spring Harbor, Long Island, New York.

THE sea life along the Great Barrier Reef will be studied by a British expedition that sailed for Australia on May 26. Naturalists of the expedition staff will investigate the composition and formation of the enormous coral reef and feeding habits of the sea animals. They also hope to study the commercial possibilities of the region, including oyster, pearl, turtle and trochus shell resources. The expedition, which will be in the field for one or two years, is headed by Dr. C. M. Yonge, naturalist, who has been on the staff of the Marine Biological Association. The project of studying the coral reef was promoted by the British Association for the Advancement of Science, and a number of scientific organizations have subscribed to it.

UNIVERSITY AND EDUCATIONAL NOTES

A GIFT of $100,000 has been made by Mr. and Mrs. R. T. Crane, Jr., Ipswich, Mass., toward the endowment of the department of therapeutics of New York University and Bellevue Hospital Medical College.

THE University of Southern California plans to ask the medical profession of Southern California to raise $500,000 for the endowment of the new medical school which will open in September. An entire new faculty is to be appointed in the reopening of the medical school. The appointment of the full-time professors for the preclinical work will be made in the next few months.

THE corporation of Yale University has increased by $500 the salaries in each grade of the assistant professorships and associate professorships and has raised the minimum salary for full professors from $5,000 to $6,000.

CAPTAIN EDWARD STEIDLE, of the Carnegie Institute of Technology, has been appointed dean of the school of mines and metallurgy at the Pennsylvania State College.

DR. JOHN FRAZER, professor of chemistry and for the past sixteen years dean of the Towne Scientific School of the University of Pennsylvania, has resigned as dean in order to continue his teaching and to devote himself to research in chemistry. He has been granted a leave of absence for the coming year.

DR. ROBERT CHAMBERS, JR., professor of microscopic anatomy in the Cornell University Medical College, has been appointed by New York University to be chairman of the department of biology and research professor of biology at its Washington Square College.

DR. SYDNEY W. BRITTON, associate in physiology at the Johns Hopkins University, will leave at the end of the scholastic year to become professor of physiology at the University of Virginia Department of Medicine, Charlottesville.

DR. SHERMAN C. BISHOP, zoologist in the New York State museum since 1916, has been appointed professor of zoology in the department of biology at the University of Rochester.

DR. JOHN G. SINCLAIR, of the department of anatomy at the University of Wisconsin, will go to the University of Texas as associate professor of embryology and histology in the medical school at Galveston, Texas.

PROFESSOR J. M. BRYANT, of the University of Texas, has been appointed professor of electrical engineering and head of the department at the University of Minnesota. Professor I. M. Kolthoff, of the University of Utrecht, Holland, has been appointed professor of analytical chemistry and chief of the division.

DR. ARTHUR T. EVANS, for the past five years head of the department of botany and plant pathology at South Dakota State College, has resigned to become head of the department of botany at Miami University, Oxford, Ohio.

AT the University of London the following appointments have been made: Dr. Percival Hartley, of the National Institute of Medical Research, has been appointed to the university chair of biochemistry tenable at the London School of Hygiene and Tropical Medicine. Dr. C. B. Fawcett, reader in geography in the University of Leeds, has been appointed to the university chair of economic geography tenable at University College. Dr. Geoffrey Hadfield has been appointed to the university chair of pathology tenable at the London School of Medicine for Women.

DISCUSSION AND CORRESPONDENCE

OVARIAN SECRETION AND TUMOR INCIDENCE

IN SCIENCE for April 13, 1928, Dr. W. S. Murray[1] has published, in reply to my note in SCIENCE of January 27, 1928,[2] a second article on the relation between the internal secretion of the ovary and the origin of tumors of the mammary gland in mice. Inasmuch as the statements of this author as to the facts, on which the proof of the significance of internal secretions of the ovary for the development of mammary cancer in mice is based, are incorrect, and in particular as his statements as to my work concerning this problem are incorrect, I feel constrained to state briefly what I believe to be the correct interpretation of the facts in this case.

(1) According to Dr. Murray, in my series of experiments (published twelve and nine years ago),[3] my own figures prove that the reduction of tumor rate through castration on the one hand, and through prevention of breeding on the other hand, are of approximately the same order. This conclusion is made possible only by adding together all my castration experiments, irrespective of the time at which the castrations were carried out. This is a procedure which is misleading, the inadvisability of which I have emphasized in my paper published nine years ago. There I pointed out that mice castrated at the age of three to four months remain practically free from tumors. There was one doubtful case among fifty-four castrated animals between the age of three and six months

[1] Murray, W. S., SCIENCE, 66, 600, 1927, and 67, 396, 1928.

[2] Loeb, Leo, SCIENCE, 67, 104, 1928.

[3] Loeb, Leo, *Am. Journ. Cancer Research*, 1, 1, 1916, and *Journal of Medical Research*, 40, 477, 1919.

in which a tumor arose, and, as I then stated, there was some reason for believing that in this instance we had to deal with an animal which was older than four months. But even conceding that there developed one tumor among fifty-four castrated mice, we would have accomplished through castration in mice, at an early stage of sexual maturity, a reduction in the tumor rate from 68 per cent. to 1.8 per cent. These results, and similar ones obtained by Cori,[4] whose mice were castrated at a still earlier period of life and remained entirely free from tumors, show that castration carried out in early life, by removing the cyclic stimuli exerted on the mammary gland through internal secretions given off by the ovary, prevents the development of mammary cancer in mice, which otherwise were destined hereditarily to have a higher tumor rate.

There was in addition one group of seventeen mice castrated between the age of four to six months, among which there were therefore no mice younger than four months; in this group there appeared four tumors. If we include this group among the animals castrated between the age of three to six months we obtain five mice with tumors among seventy-two castrated mice; this corresponds to 7 per cent. It is only if we castrate mice fully six months old or older that the incidence of cancer becomes higher.

(2) This is a result totally different from the effect produced through prevention of breeding. Through the latter procedure it was possible, in these investigations carried out by Miss Lathrop and myself, to effect in some strains a reduction of 30 per cent. or slightly more; but in other strains the reduction was much smaller. In one strain of non-bred mice there was even an increase in the tumor rate, partly owing to the increase of length of life due to non-breeding. On the average the tumor rate of the mice belonging to families with a high tumor rate fell to about 30 per cent. and in one case to about 23 per cent., while in other cases it remained considerably higher. In general, in non-breeding mice the tumor appeared later in life than in mice which were bred. Different strains varied as to the effect of prevention of breeding on the cancer rate, but we did not obtain by these means a diminution of the tumor rate below 20 per cent. In the strain used by Dr. Cori the non-breeding caused only a slight reduction in the tumor rate.

The fact, shown in my previous experiments, that prevention of breeding, in general, reduces the tumor rate, although to a less extent than early castration, proves that, in addition to the cyclic stimuli exerted by other ovarian structures, also the stimuli given off by the internal secretion of the corpus luteum and the stimuli associated with the abrupt cessation of the action of the corpus luteum following the preceding growth period, may play a rôle in the development of mammary carcinoma in mice.

(3) As I pointed out in my previous note, I attempted to confirm the results thus obtained through transplantation of ovaries into castrated male mice belonging to strains with a high incidence of cancer. Owing to conditions over which I had no control, the number of experiments had to be limited and I obtained therefore negative results. Murray, in operating upon a much larger number of male mice, succeeded in obtaining positive results in a small minority of his animals. I consider his results as a valuable contribution to this problem; however, as far as the main point at issue is concerned, the importance of the internal secretion of the ovary in the production of mammary tumors in mice and of the quantitative interaction of these substances with hereditary factors, this had been demonstrated conclusively through our earlier experiments and it has been confirmed by the work of Cori.

(4) As far as the stock of mice is concerned which served for these experiments and which is referred to by Dr. Murray, I may state that I observed personally not only the mice castrated by myself previously, but also certain control mice which developed tumors under conditions under which the mice castrated, at an early period, remained free from tumors.

I may further state that the investigations on heredity of mammary cancer in mice, on which the experiments concerning the action of internal secretions were based, were jointly carried out by Miss Lathrop and myself. While the mice used for breeding were almost exclusively attended to personally by Miss Lathrop, I visited the breeding establishment from time to time, and had occasion to convince myself of the untiring energy, care and trustworthiness with which Miss Lathrop carried out the breeding experiments which I had suggested and in which she was deeply interested. In many cases, I controlled the results as to the development of tumors through autopsies performed on this stock, and if a mistake did happen Miss Lathrop made it a point to inform me of such an occurrence. I have no doubt that the care which Miss Lathrop gave to the actual breeding of the mice was vastly superior to the attention which an ordinary attendant in laboratories is accustomed to give to such work; and it is on the cooperation of others that investigators have to rely in breeding experiments which are carried out on a large scale. Furthermore, in its important aspects the results which we have obtained as to the hereditary transmission of tumor rate in distinct strains of mice have been confirmed by subsequent investigators, a fact which may be considered as a proof that the breeding

[4] Cori, C. F., *Journ. Exper. Med.*, 45, 983, 1927.

experiments had been carried out with the necessary care.

(5) In these investigations we considered it sufficient to divide the mice to be used in the castration experiments into age groups covering in some cases two, in other cases three months periods. For statistical purposes, I combined these mice into one class, including the mice between three and six months of age. However, Miss Lathrop kept a record of the time of birth of each litter used in our work on the heredity of cancer in mice, and there is no justification for the conclusion on the part of Murray that such records were not kept. As to the mice which were castrated at this age (between three and six months), they had been prevented from breeding previous to the operation; but if, contrary to our plans and knowledge, they should have bred, the result of castration in preventing the development of mammary cancers in these mice would have been the more striking.

(6) In conclusion I may state again that the investigations, on which Murray reports, without exception represent the type of experiments which I had carried out previously and that through this earlier work the significance of the various internal secretions, given off by the ovary, for the development of mammary cancer in mice had been proven.

LEO LOEB

DEPARTMENT OF PATHOLOGY,
WASHINGTON UNIVERSITY
SCHOOL OF MEDICINE

THE RING METHOD IN CHANGING SURFACE TENSION

I HAVE just seen a very excellent paper by S. L. Bigelow and E. R. Washburn, published in the *Journal of Physical Chemistry*, on "Variations in the Surface Tension of Solutions."

It is a great pleasure indeed to read such a reliable and conscientious piece of work. I hope the authors will find it natural that I should explain a statement which I made somewhere and which they quote as "remarkable," not in the complimentary sense of the word, I am afraid. The sentence read: "It is only through the ring method that it is possible to observe and study this phenomenon (changing surface tension) as it is the only procedure which permits the measurement of surface tension of the same layer of liquid at very short intervals." This statement is not accepted by the authors of the paper, who decide that it is 'manifestly in error," and they are quite surprised that I should have found anything by this method.

In the first place, they are right, as it is obviously not the "only" method whereby such changes can be observed, but I maintain that it is the only one which, as I said, makes readings possible at "very short intervals." Of course we may not call "very short intervals" the same thing. What I meant were intervals of the order of one second and less. I have published in my book experiments where eight measurements were taken in the first minute. The technique is described in the same volume. That, I still believe, is impossible with the capillary method. Furthermore, if Messrs. Bigelow and Washburn had read the aforesaid book carefully, they might have understood how it was I managed to observe phenomena which they confirmed: "Pulling off a ring, they say, and replacing it must seriously upset any molecular arrangement in the surface . . ." Well, it does, but I did not always pull it off and replace it. I used a different sample of the same solution for every measurement. The ring was pulled off only once.

However, I must add that, even when such precautions are not taken, the phenomenon of time-drop can be followed, but not as accurately, of course.

LECOMTE DU NOÜY

INSTITUT PASTEUR, PARIS

"NUTRILITES"

THE term "vitamine" was introduced by Funk to designate those unknown factors in nutrition which were thought to prevent various diseases. This term with a modified spelling has become widely adopted in spite of its obvious defects. The term has been applied in some cases to unknown substances which in small amounts are effective in the nutrition of fungi (including yeast), bacteria and other organisms. At present, however, the tendency is to restrict the use of the word "vitamin" entirely to substances concerned in *animal* nutrition.

The word "bios" was introduced by Wildiers to designate an unknown substance which in small amounts stimulates yeast growth. The word "auximones" was likewise introduced by Bottomley to designate substances of a similar nature which were thought to be effective in the nutrition of certain green plants. It is increasingly apparent that there are unknown factors which function in the nutrition of many types of organisms. It is also obvious that there is need for a general term to designate these factors. Otherwise it will be necessary to invent new names for substances found to be effective in the nutrition of bacteria, molds and other forms of life. None of the terms in use at present applies.

It is suggested that the word "nutrilite" be used to designate all those vitamin-like substances which in small amounts function in the nutrition of organisms in general. The term has the advantage that it indicates that the substances function in nutrition, but does not indicate in advance of our knowledge *how* they function. The term makes no extravagant claim as to the indispensability of the substance or to any peculiar relationship to life, as unfortunately the terms "vitamin" and "bios" do. In form the new word is similar to the word "metabolite." There is a closely related word already in the dictionary, "nutrility," which pertains to nutrition, but is rarely used.

We may then define a nutrilite as a substance, other than the well-recognized nutrients, which functions in small amounts in the nutrition of organisms. It is to be expected that borderline cases will appear in which it will be difficult to decide whether or not the material in question should be regarded as a nutrilite. This will not seriously impair the usefulness of the term, however, since a similar situation exists in the case of many words such as, for example, "carbohydrate" and "alkaloid."

ROGER J. WILLIAMS

UNIVERSITY OF OREGON

AN ANCIENT WALRUS SKULL

A RATHER interesting find, in the nature of an ancient walrus skull, recently made on Georges Bank off Cape Cod, has been presented to the Boston Society of Natural History. The skull, consisting of the fore part with tusks, which are twelve and fourteen inches long, and most of the flat-crowned crushing teeth of the upper jaw still in place, belongs to an animal now unknown as far south as the New England coast.

It has not been determined how this skull came to be on the bank, nor is it known how long it may have lain on the sea bottom, but it is probable that it came there two hundred and twenty or three hundred years ago. The walrus occurred, during the Ice Age, as far south as Virginia and the Carolinas, where fossil remains have been reported; in the seventeenth century it was found on Sable Island, off the coast of Nova Scotia, while during the last century it was quite common in the Gulf of St. Lawrence and on the shores of Labrador. It is quite possible at that time some of them may have visited the waters of the Gulf of Maine, or even strayed as far south as the Georges Bank, and that the specimen recently found belongs to one of these.

BIRGER R. HEADSTROM

MEDFORD HILLSIDE,
MASSACHUSETTS

THE ROYAL PHOTOGRAPHIC SOCIETY

The Royal Photographic Society of Great Britain is holding its seventy-third annual exhibition in September and October of this year. It is hoped that the American representation in the scientific section will be such as to demonstrate the place held by this country in applied photography. I am collecting and forwarding American work for the scientific section again this year. Exhibits should consist of prints showing the use of photography for scientific purposes and its application to spectroscopy, astronomy, radiography, biology, etc. Photographs should reach me not later than June 8, and should be mounted but not framed. There are no fees.

A. J. NEWTON

EASTMAN KODAK CO.,
ROCHESTER, N. Y.

LOW HUMIDITY AND HIGH TACITURNITY

ARIZONA is perhaps best known in the demi-lands of letters as the abode of strong, silent men. So steeped in sentimentality is the lore of their laconism that a pragmatic interpretation has become imperative.

The low humidity of Arizona is almost as proverbial as the silence of her strong men. This is no mere fortuitousness. For low humidity begets parched throats, and it is axiomatic that a desiccated larynx and a vociferous tongue are incompatible.

A practical application suggests itself. Repression of verbosity has been, at times, a problem of national concern, actually jeopardizing the Senate rules. The atmosphere of the district is notoriously humid, and in such an environment loquacity thrives. But to euthenics there is available an effective antidote, a local anesthetic of uncanny selectivity. Even the most garrulous of filibusters could be silenced quickly by the aid of a potent air-dehumidizer.

E. A. VUILLEUMIER

DICKINSON COLLEGE

REPORTS

HORIZONTAL VERSUS VERTICAL FORCES IN CRUSTAL MOVEMENTS OF THE EARTH

PROFESSOR BAILEY WILLIS, of Leland Stanford University, and now president of the Geological Society of America, addressed the Boston Geological Society on January 11, 1928, on "Horizontalist or Verticalist?"

The doctrine of the direction of forces causing diastrophism is a question of faith. Willis states that he was brought up a horizontalist, and in 187[illegible] G. K. Gilbert had told him to study Appalachian structure, and he was carried far in seeing the effect of horizontal thrusting. On later expeditions into the Alps, the Andes and into Patagonia Willis found his faith in horizontalism supported. Later he went to California, where Gilbert had studied the structure of the Basin Ranges and had concluded that there the forces had acted upward from below. Willis first accepted the fact that the Sierra Nevada had been tilted but not deformed.

Louderback had described normal faults, arranged as step faults, dipping east, along the eastern front of the Sierra Nevada, and which there bound the range. Willis considered these as superficial slides into the eastern basin, and that the tilting of the mountain had been accomplished by rotation of the mountain block on a rounded base by a horizontal force from the west.

Two recent field seasons in Owens Valley and Mona Lake country along the east base of the Sierra Nevada showed Willis that the normal step faults are but minor slips, and the crest of the range is not the top of the fault scarp, but the top of an arched surface. The arch ends at an elevation of nine thousand feet on the east side, and from there the blocks on the east dip into the valley. The main fault is curved back toward the west beneath the range. The westward back slope of the main range instead of being merely tilted is curved, or domed, and is intersected by faults with throws as great as a thousand feet.

Willis coupled these observations with studies made in tunnels and drifts in the serpentine of the New Almaden mine where the rocks display an extreme squeezing beneath the Sierra Nevada. He thus conceived that the main force was horizontal, and was a tremendous deep-seated thrusting from the west against a stable block on the east. The rocks were squeezed as in a vise. A component of the pressure was necessarily upward, doming the Sierra Nevada upland, and lifting the blocks along faults, which instead of being normal faults are reversed upthrust faults.

This conception took Willis back to his experiments of wax and turpentine made in 1887 and 1888, in which he reproduced the folding of the Appalachian type. The lower surfaces of the material yielded by shear, and shearing planes developed at 45 degrees to the shearing force and caused displacements on a relatively large scale.

If the upswelling is due to a movement in a deeper zone, it must have been due to the conversion of a deep-seated crystalline rock into a gneiss, with vertical schistosity. In order to test this theory, Willis kept the problem in mind on a recent trip around the world. He had become a horizontal verticalist, because he saw how vertical movements of the earth's crust could result from horizontal compression.

During his visit to Japan, he examined the ranges of Hokkaido, the northern island of Japan. The central range, about seven thousand feet in height, is deeply dissected and rugged, revealing complexly folded Paleozoic sediments injected by tongues of granite. The block as a whole has an arched appearance. West of the range, Cretaceous beds are folded and overthrust westward toward Asia. They abut on the west against folds of early and mid-Tertiary strata, which have a more simple structure, but are also overturned toward the continent. Still farther west on the same island the folded Tertiary zone is succeeded by a platform of uplifted, but nearly horizontal Pliocene beds, from which one descends to the coast.

A Paleozoic geosyncline, folded and intruded by granite, must have been peneplaned during the Mesozoic time. Then a new Cretaceous geosyncline formed west of it, and received its fill of sediments, and was in turn folded, by pressures which arched up the Paleozoic mass on the east. The cause of this swelling was the shearing and the development of schistosity in deep-seated crystalline rocks. The active force had come from the Pacific. A third geosyncline formed during the Tertiary time and west of the Cretaceous folds; and having received in turn its load of sediments, was folded before Pliocene time. The fourth, or Pliocene trough, has not yet been folded.

The presence of folds en echelon, especially in the newer Japanese arcs, points to their lying in the shear zone between two rounded disc-like blocks—the one under the Pacific and east of northern Japan, the other under the Asiatic continent. The rotation of both blocks in a clock-wise direction has developed the shearing and folding en echelon between them. The location of granite intrusions in northern Japan was determined by tension.

In the southern island of New Zealand, Willis made a section westward from Dunedin. On the eastern half of the island there is an elevated plateau separated by a deep valley from the Southern Alps to the west. The plateau is broken in an irregular fashion by rift valleys described by Cotton. The plateau is underlain by mica gneisses, as Willis termed them—rocks with horizontal banding but in which the sedimentary structures are preserved. The Southern Alps he found to be a tightly compressed isoclinal fold, which must have been an old fold. On the west side of the range there is a shear-zone recorded by networks of quartz veins, while shatter-zones reveal the modern revival of shearing. The region is probably underlain by a batholith of late Paleozoic age. Willis pictures the movements as being mainly a horizontal thrust from the east, along the curving thrust-plane which dips from the western side of the range and eastward under the range. As a component of this thrusting there was a vertical uplift of the plateau, due mainly to shearing in the mechanical zone.

The island of Cyprus, in the eastern Mediterranean, Willis found to be of especial interest to him who seeks horizontal forces. Three main structural elements are found in the island; in the north an east-west range of mountains; in the south a higher and broader range, and between them a central plain or lowland. The northern range includes Cretaceous Oligocene sediments, folded and faulted. The central lowland is of tilted and beveled Miocene shales and limestones, overlain unconformably by the horizontal Pliocene. In the Miocene sediments at the foot of the northern range, there is a marvelous exhibition of crushing. The southern massif is the famous Mt. Troodos, the old Olympus of Greek mythology. It is a mass of hornblendic igneous rock, an old plutonic mass, now gneissic.

There has been a thrusting from the north, so that the northern mass has been moved southward. There are no faults in the Miocene central plain except normal faults due to tension. The Miocene dips northward off the northern flank of Mt. Troodos at about 15 degrees, and the rocks have been stretched. The upland of Mt. Troodos is a smoothly rolling mature-land, and on it the ancient Miocene shoreland is approximately indicated by a longitudinal valley, high up on the flank of the mountain, where, banked in by the former cuesta front of the Miocene, a subsequent river has cut a trench into the crystallines of the Troodos massif.

This old shore-line indicates that there was a vertical movement of Mt. Troodos, probably as much as four thousand feet, while twenty miles to the north there is a great overthrust. Here, therefore, is another example of vertical movement in connection with great horizontal compression. The great movement came from the north and was deep-seated (the overthrusting of the northern range is only a shallow expression of it) and as a result of the development of gneissic structure in the Troodos mass in response to the horizontal compression, the southern part of the island was considerably uplifted.

In response to questions on the Cyprus mass, Willis said that he thought that the movements were still going on in Cyprus, of which the recent destructive earthquake of Salamis is testimony. This raised the question of the cause of destructive earthquakes. Willis stated that in his opinion such earthquakes are not the result of slight movements on normal faults, but rather the elastic spring of rocks, from the energy stored up in them through years of compression.

Willis stated that he thought the thrusting upward of a piston of crystalline rock, like that at Mt. Troodos, with a drag along the side of the piston, and consequent removal of material from beneath the contingent areas of the lee side, away from the side of active horizontal pressure, is the cause of subsidence, and the formation of geosynclines.

A lively discussion by Professors Lane, Daly, Terzaghi, Collet, Morris and Dr. Boydell followed Professor Willis's address.

Joseph L. Gillson

Boston Geological Society

SCIENTIFIC APPARATUS AND LABORATORY METHODS

THE USE OF THE X-RAY IN BIOLOGICAL INVESTIGATIONS

Though X-ray pictures have been generally adopted by the medical sciences, they have been little used in the descriptive natural sciences where I believe they would greatly facilitate studies. A picture may save months of painstaking technical work. For students it would save the laborious work of microtomy and the subsequent reconstruction of organs from sections.

By using this method many a valuable organism can be kept intact that otherwise would have to be sacrificed for the purpose of study.

As far as I know, X-ray pictures have been used in zoology and botany only by a few workers and by them in only a small way. Probably the first to use them was Dr. David Starr Jordan, who reproduced X-ray photographs of fishes, but confined himself in the main to showing the pictures without giving a detailed description of the objects represented.

One of the main reasons why this method has been so little employed by biologists is the fact that its use necessitates expensive apparatus and that the pictures have to be made by carefully trained experts, who are thoroughly familiar with all the details of the process. In addition to that, the pictures themselves are quite expensive, and as a consequence only institutions with large available funds are able to undertake the work.

Because of the splendid cooperation between the Queen's Hospital and Bernice P. Bishop Museum of Honolulu, I have been able to realize my ambition to study by means of X-rays the majority of the representatives of the ichthyological fauna of a relatively large area and also to make observations and experiments regarding the adaptability of this method to biological studies as a whole.

An undeniable advantage of the Roentgen method, as compared with all others, is that every bone, even the finest, may be seen in its natural position. Even the intermuscular ossifications not connected with the skeleton can be clearly observed; whereas by any other known method their accurate position in relation to the rest of the body can be determined only with the greatest difficulty. Even while dissecting in the most careful and exact manner, one can not avoid cutting off some very fine points of the ribs or projections from some other bones. An X-ray picture makes this unnecessary.

The X-ray picture would be especially valuable for studying fossils; above all for the study of fossil fishes. An X-ray picture resembles such a fossil much more than a skeleton without any of the soft parts could possibly do. While these parts are rather dim on the negative, they are sharply circumscribed and remind one of the shape of the fossilized animal, whose outlines and soft parts of the body can only be distinguished by a discoloration of the stone.

In differentiating a number of closely related species of the same genus, whose only differences consist in colors and small dissimilarities of the body, the paleontologist is faced with an extremely difficult problem. It might be said that, in the meaning applied to living species, such a procedure is futile. By means of X-ray pictures *real* species distinguish themselves through constant differences between each other (small differences of the skeleton, in the air-bladder, etc.). These differences, however, in many species are so inconsiderable that we can hardly use them as a basis for distinguishing paleontological species, if we consider that the fossil print incorporates a number of changes and disturbances of the several parts of a body.

In studying the skeleton, the possibilities of biological investigation are by no means exhausted. Even the usual X-ray picture shows that the soft parts of the body appear on the negative in varying degrees of intensity. On fishes, for instance, the air-bladder will appear very clear and sharply outlined, especially if the picture has been taken immediately after the death of the animal. A procedure, so generally adopted in medical practice, to inject certain solutions or emulsions into cavities on account of their relative impermeability to X-rays in order to make them visible on the negative, points a way to a method which has been hardly used at all.

I injected barium sulfate solutions into the heart and the larger vessels of fishes and obtained pictures which are clear to the most minute detail; many show even the last capillary vessels absolutely plain. That in such pictures each vessel will be shown in its true position and relation to the rest of the body goes without saying. Here again the advantage of saving a great amount of time and work is apparent. Biologists are well aware that investigations involving the smaller vessels demand preparations which involve months of painstaking technical work.

I know of a distinguished scientist whose studies of the position and relations of the smaller vessels of the human heart demanded years of his time. An X-ray picture of a properly injected organ might have shortened that time to a few hours. It is possible to make just as easily studies of the vessels of invertebrate animals. As a matter of fact, these promise even more success, because there are no skeletons to disturb the picture. The practice of using certain selective staining methods for representing certain elements of the body—for instance, the nervous system—seems to me to be altogether within the limits of adaptation.

In the same manner as vessels, other cavities can be shown by means of injections. Here is the main field for roentgenographical work in botany. Also the entomologist, who studies plants that have been attacked by insects, will surely find in X-ray pictures a valuable help.

Naturally each field of investigation and its peculiar technic must be studied in all its particulars. The representation of the blood vessels, too, necessitates certain preliminary conditions and a certain practice which can be acquired only through experience.

In a forthcoming paper I am discussing the methods and advantages of X-ray pictures as applied to zoological and botanical materials. The use of this method is fully demonstrated in a monograph on Hawaiian fishes, now in preparation.

VICTOR PIETSCHMANN
MUSEUM OF NATURAL HISTORY
OF VIENNA

A CONVENIENT METHOD OF DETERMINING THE RATE OF CLEAVAGE

FOR the study of factors influencing the rate of cleavage of developing eggs, it is essential to determine that rate for a large number of eggs. Since the individual differences in the time of cleavage usually extend over a period of only a few minutes, the counting has to be done quickly. The inexperienced worker will have to spend some time in acquiring the necessary skill for obtaining reliable data.

The following convenient and accurate method is suggested. The camera lucida is used. Note the time of the appearance of the first cleavage of the eggs in the microscopical field, and from now on mark on the drawing paper, with the aid of the camera lucida, all those eggs that divide within the first two minutes with No. 1 written across the image of the egg. Eggs dividing within the next two-minute period, mark with No. 2, and so on until the whole field has divided. A record is left on the paper. Now count from this record the number of eggs marked with 1, 2, 3, etc. You thus obtain the data for a regular distribution curve from which you read off the average time at which cleavage of a large number of eggs occurred.

The advantages of this method are: a permanent record is left on paper; the counting is done with ease after the process has passed; each egg is counted only once, the mark across the image of the egg on the paper indicating the eggs already counted in the preceding period.

E. ALFRED WOLF

DEPARTMENT OF ZOOLOGY,
UNIVERSITY OF PITTSBURGH

SPECIAL ARTICLES

THE EFFECT OF A SECONDARY SOUND UPON HEARING

THE problem of hearing in the presence of a secondary sound has of late received considerable attention from correspondents of this journal. The ancient belief that certain persons suffering from paracusia, in the form of a partial deafness of the conduction-type, are able to hear more acutely in noisy surroundings than under conditions of quiet has been brought to question and debated on various sides.[1]

The matter seems at last to be decided by the excellent experiments of Knudsen and Jones, reported recently.[2] The threshold of hearing was ascertained for speech-sounds and for a faint tone both in silence and with a constant noise, and it was shown that for all subjects, normals and defectives alike, acuity is reduced in the presence of a noise. This finding is not incompatible, it must be noted, with the well-attested fact that under particular conditions the paracusic can carry on conversation more easily in the presence of a secondary sound. The phenomenon is a consequence not of an increased sensitivity of the acoustic mechanism, but rather of a relative advantage which the situation affords the paracusic over his normal companion.

The explanation is plain. The commonest auditory defects involve a considerably greater reduction of low tones than of high tones, and since most extraneous noises are made up predominantly of low-pitched tones, it follows that the person of impaired hearing is deaf to the secondary sound relatively more than he is to the essential tones of speech (which are of higher pitch) and thus in conversation is disturbed by the sound relatively less than is a person of normal hearing. Now since the loudness of one's voice is adjusted by reference to the background as he hears it, the normal person, being greatly disturbed by a sound, speaks much louder than usual, but the defective, selectively deaf to the sound, raises his voice but little. The net result of the background, in this situation, is a favoring of the person of impaired hearing, though actually the acuity of both persons is reduced as compared with silence. This explanation is supported by the fact that the illusion of improved hearing in the presence of a noise occurs only in conversation between a normal and a defective, and never between two normals or two defectives.[3]

All this seems clean-cut enough. The writer has merely to add some remarks upon an experiment which in a measure confirms, and further extends, the findings of Knudsen and Jones and which brings forth an additional problem for settlement. The experiment, conducted at the University of California last year in collaboration with Mr. Stanley R. Truman, was concerned with the effect of a background of tone upon the acuity of the normal ear.[4] Various frequencies and intensities of tone were used for the background and for the testing-tone, and we found, as Knudsen and Jones did, that at the introduction of a tonal background hearing is always reduced.

However, we came upon the further discovery that the threshold does not remain constant under such conditions. At the entrance of the secondary tone the acuity is considerably diminished, but recovery of sensitivity begins immediately and proceeds at a rapid rate until, under a given set of conditions, it may become three or four times as great as it was at first. Sensitivity does not, however, reach the level shown under conditions of silence; after about two minutes it has attained its highest extent and from then on we found no indication of further significant change.

Just what is the cause of this change in threshold-sensitivity we are thus far unable to state with conviction, but experiments are in progress which it is hoped will afford a clue. It would be interesting as well as significant in this relation to know whether paracusics would show the same type of curve of threshold-recovery as do normal persons under the conditions stated, and whether with prolonged stimulation by a secondary tone the relative advantage which, as has been pointed out, circumstances may afford the paracusic would continue to be maintained. Unfortunately, Knudsen and Jones do not tell us the temporal conditions of their tests, and the presumption is that they took no pains to control them—though it is plain on the basis of our results that the temporal factor is of first importance. It is to be hoped that some investigator with the necessary clinical facilities will extend the work of Knudsen and

[1] See, *e.g.*, 60 (1924), 360; 61 (1925), 260 ff.; 62 (1925), 109–111 and 182; and esp. Kranz, 60 (1924), 549.

[2] V. O. Knudsen and I. H. Jones, *Laryngoscope*, 36 (1926), 623–663.

[3] See Knudsen and Jones, *ibid.*, and *cf.* H. Fletcher, *Volta Rev.*, 26 (1924), 443 f., 447 f.

[4] See *J. Exper. Psychol.*, 11, 1928, 98–112.

Jones, and trace the sensitivity of the paracusic ear in the presence of a tonal background throughout its course of change; the result might lead us to a better understanding of this phenomenon not only in paracusia but in normal hearing as well.

E. G. WEVER
PRINCETON PSYCHOLOGICAL LABORATORY,
PRINCETON, N. J.

REMARKABLE MUSICAL TECHNIQUE OF THE LARGER ANGULAR-WINGED KATYDID

IT is evident that there has been marvelous specialization in the vocal music of the birds, the flute-toned thrushes, including the marvelous hermit, probably leading them all with their tonal embellishments. There has been a parallel specialization among the musical insects of the world. The insects have turned especially to instrumental music, adopting microscopic teeth to be operated upon by a scraping edge as the more common type for their frictional music, in the majority of instances. A mere file-vein and scraper or plectrum to rasp across its teeth seem simple enough as a musical instrument, but even this primitive chitin xylophone offers many possibilities of specialization. It may have teeth of different sizes and spacing, to produce different notes as in the case of certain sound-making ants and beetles, or more than one file-vein may be present on an insect. For the present these specializations of the physical structures of the instrument itself need not be considered. There is a further possibility, and that concerns the technique, the manner of handling the instrument to produce the greatest variety of tones and notes. In the music of man, technique has become the big factor, and marvelous progress has been made in this direction alone by the modern masters over the ancients. In spite of the fact that the crickets have somehow hit upon tonality in their music, and the katydids have not, the latter have nevertheless shown a marvelous specialization in the direction of technique far excelling the crickets. The larger angular-winged katydid has proven himself a master-artist with his xylophone. He has specialized in a manner that makes him a pioneer in his art, at least in our own country. Unfortunately we know too little of the musical behavior of insects elsewhere in the world. This fine katydid, as veritably leaf-adorned as the trees themselves, has somehow learned of the full potentialities of his microscopic file-vein and is making good use of his acquirement. The file-vein is a mere thickened ridge or vein bearing parallel chitin bars or teeth, like the teeth of a comb, these being set practically at right angles to the vein and perpendicular to the surface from which they arise. An almost universal technique among the crickets and katydids is to draw the scraper entirely across this music-file one or more times to produce a note. In the single chirp of a cricket or the intermittent rasp of many katydids, an extremely rapid back-and-forth movement several times delivered produces the sound. The quaver of the cricket-chirp is due to these alternate wing-strokes. In this manipulation all the teeth of the file-vein are used practically simultaneously. The larger angular-winged katydid has somehow gone far beyond this and has learned to produce a long, slow crepitation of thirty to forty or more clicks, making use of the individual teeth, or perhaps sometimes slipping over two or more teeth. The wing-covers along their upper edge are opened nearly three sixteenths of an inch, and set at an angle that will bring the file-vein of the under side of the upper tegmen against the scraper of the upper side of the under tegmen. The scraper is now slowly moved with nice adjustment and precision over the individual teeth, in a gradual closing movement of the wings to produce the long series of individual clicks characteristic of the more typical "song" of this species.

A count of the teeth of the file-vein, including poorly-developed ones at each end of the file, reveals only from fifty-five to sixty teeth, in a length of about three mm. It is probable that not many more than forty to fifty well-developed teeth are present on this file, which would allow not more than an average of one tooth per click in a series of thirty to forty clicks. This is a remarkable specialization in technique and shows the nice control of the katydid in this behavior. It would appear that no other katydid or cricket in our own country has progressed this far in the matter of technique, and we know as yet too little to speak with any authority covering the technique of any foreign species. This katydid not only makes use of this specialized technique, but it has in addition an intermittent zip, produced by striking all the teeth with one quick draw of the scraper across the teeth.

One wonders how this fine katydid sensed this new technique of tapping the chitin-bars of its dorsal, organic xylophone very slowly, to make each tooth emit a note or tone. The most marvelous thing about life, however, is the way it always seems to sense possibilities in every detail of form and function. Once the chitinous xylophone came into being on its wing-covers, once the scraper began to touch the bars to produce a rasp, potentialities were ahead. In the case of the intermittent rasp or zip of this katydid, one quick closing draw produced the note. Slowing down this closing draw of the scraper upon the file-vein was the next step, and some weird prescience of life has in some manner taught the katydid to do just this.

While the crickets have evolved tone in their musical expressions, the matter of technique such as the katydids have specialized upon, seems quite beyond their moods at present. Yet if any of our crickets could strike pure musical tones upon the individual chitin-bars, as the larger angular-winged katydid is attempting to do with its sounds, their tinkling chimes would mark a new era in the spontaneous expressions of insects. A number of the katydids have evolved complicated little instrumental "songs," involving wide departures in time-relations and variety of phrases, from the simple repetitive rhythms of the more primitive type. All this marks some unconscious specialization, it would seem, toward a fuller self-expression with the potentialities of sound.

It is hard to see just how an uncouth and prehistoric scaled-reptilian type should evolve into a beautiful bird, feathered, songful or finally into an inimitable hermit thrush with a soul sensitized for music or pleasurable sounds and whispered tonal harmonies. Yet the lowly insects with their primitive musical instruments, a simple file-vein and scraper, are following the same trend, it would seem. Tonality they have, in the case of the crickets; highly specialized technique and variety they have in the case of the katydids; rhythm and even an ear for synchronous rhythm is evident in both great groups. Is it something unconscious, external and cosmic operating upon life, or is there a subconscious urge, which sooner or later becomes translated into the conscious experience of life? Surely, now are the crickets and katydids conscious of their sound-experiences, but the methods, the genesis of it all constitute a mystery as deep as life itself. The individual seems to have as little to do with it all as the individual cells of our bodies have to do with our own running, our talking, seeing or what-not in body-behavior as a whole. The organic unfolding of the phylum at times seems to be the unit, with the individual functioning as a mere cell in its continuity, but this savors too much of the ultimate meaning of life of which we can have no adequate concept.

H. A. ALLARD

U. S. DEPARTMENT OF AGRICULTURE,
WASHINGTON, D. C.

SOCIETIES AND ACADEMIES

THE KENTUCKY ACADEMY OF SCIENCE

THE Kentucky Academy of Science held its fifteenth annual meeting at the University of Kentucky May 12, President Valleau presiding at the general sessions, at one of which Dr. E. C. Stakman, of Minnesota, representative of the American Association for the Advancement of Science to the academy, delivered a very interesting lecture on biologic specialization.

The three divisions, biological sciences, physical sciences and philosophy and psychology, had full programs of papers.

Officers elected were:

G. Davis Buckner, University of Kentucky, *president.*
George D. Smith, Eastern State Normal School, Richmond, *vice-president.*
A. M. Peter, University of Kentucky, *secretary.*
W. S. Anderson, University of Kentucky, *treasurer.*
A. R. Middleton, University of Louisville, *representative* in the council of the A. A. A. S.
Division of Physical Sciences—W. R. Jillson, *chairman;* C. S. Crouse, secretary.
Division of Biological Sciences—G. D. Buckner, *chairman;* E. N. Fergus, *secretary.*
Division of Philosophy and Psychology—R. M. Bear, Centre College, Danville, *chairman and secretary.*

A. M. PETER,
Secretary.

THE NORTH DAKOTA ACADEMY OF SCIENCE

THE twentieth annual meeting of the North Dakota Academy of Science was held at the North Dakota Agricultural College on May 4 and 5. Dr. H. L. Walster, dean of the School of Agriculture of the North Dakota Agricultural College, presented the president's address on the theme "The Pursuit of Science in North Dakota." A notable feature of the program was the showing by Mr. Russell Reid, of the North Dakota State Historical Society, of a series of fifty colored lantern slides showing the beauty spots in western North Dakota and illustrating the characteristics and nesting habits of many North Dakota birds.

In his invitation address on "The Biological Value of Practical Agricultural Experimentation," Dr. J. Arthur Harris, head of the department of botany of the University of Minnesota, urged the point of view that much of the material results from agricultural experimentation could, through careful biometrical analysis and similar studies, be made to yield much material of great value in pure science.

The following officers were elected for the ensuing year:

President—Dr. G. A. Talbert, professor of physiology, University of North Dakota.

Vice-president—Dean R. M. Dolve, school of mechanic arts, North Dakota Agricultural College.

Secretary-Treasurer—Dr. G. A. Abbott, professor of chemistry, University of North Dakota.

Additional members of Executive Committee: Professor J. H. Seymour, Valley City State Teachers' College; Professor C. H. McLees, School of Forestry, Bottineau.

Representative of the North Dakota Academy of Science on the council of the American Association for the Advancement of Science—Dr. H. L. Walster, dean, School of Agriculture, North Dakota Agricultural College.

SCIENCE

VOL. LXVII JUNE 22, 1928 No. 1747

CONTENTS

The Differentiation of Species: PROFESSOR HENRY E. CRAMPTON ... 615
Research and the Training of the Researcher: T. H. EATON ... 619
The Promotion of Knowledge of Precambrian Life: DR. DAVID WHITE ... 620
Scientific Events:
The Award of Prizes and Grants by the Belgian Academy of Sciences; Exhibit of the Bingham Oceanographic Collection at Yale University; Oklahoma Geological Survey Field Parties; Appointments and Promotions at Harvard University 622
Scientific Notes and News ... 624
University and Educational Notes ... 627
Discussion and Correspondence:
Research Plus News-Gathering: DR. EDWIN E. SLOSSON and WATSON DAVIS. *Agronomic Jabberwocky:* J. H. KEMPTON. *Note on the Inertia Dyadic:* I. F. MORRISON. *A New Amphibian Record from Kansas:* CHARLES E. BURT. *Geologic Age by Lead Uranium Ratios:* ALFRED C. LANE. *Datum, Data:* F. E. ... 628
Scientific Books:
Shaw's Manual of Meteorology: DR. ALEXANDER MCADIE ... 632
Reports:
Intellectual Cooperation and Biology: DR. J. E. DE VOS VAN STEENWIJK ... 633
Special Articles:
Variation in Solar Radiation: DR. C. G. ABBOT ... 634
Societies and Academies:
The North Carolina Academy of Science: DR. H. R. TOTTEN. *The Kansas Academy of Science:* DR. GEORGE E. JOHNSON. *The Indiana Academy of Science:* HARRY F. DIETZ ... 635
Science News ... x

SCIENCE: A Weekly Journal devoted to the Advancement of Science, edited by J. McKeen Cattell and published every Friday by

THE SCIENCE PRESS

New York City: Grand Central Terminal.

Lancaster, Pa. Garrison, N. Y.

Annual Subscription, $6.00. Single Copies, 15 Cts.

SCIENCE is the official organ of the American Association for the Advancement of Science. Information regarding membership in the Association may be secured from the office of the permanent secretary, in the Smithsonian Institution Building, Washington, D. C.

THE DIFFERENTIATION OF SPECIES[1]

WITH the lapse of another year, it is again my privilege and my obligation to present what is technically known as a "presidential address." This occasion is one of particular personal interest, for it marks the close of continuous active service to the academy throughout a period of more than three decades, during which it has been my privilege to serve in almost every designated capacity. And with the close of this evening, I shall pass to the long and venerable list of ex-presidents, however unworthy that association may be with the notable men of science of our community who have directed the life and work of our institution.

A choice of subjects is inevitably controlled by circumstances; the topic must be general in scope, it must be of timely interest, and it ought to be one with which the speaker is familiar, at least to some extent. I have chosen to discuss briefly some aspects of evolution. No other is more comprehensive or more fundamental. Each of the natural sciences, with its own materials and by its own methods, has demonstrated the reality of incessant change, in the heavenly bodies, in mountains and seas and continents, and in the wide array of plants and animals that constitute the organic world.

The further circumstance determining this choice is the fact that for more than twenty odd years I have been engaged in the study of a definite group of animal organisms in an effort to understand the processes by which evolution comes about in wild nature. The natural history of animals is like that of plants, and hence this topic is directly related to botanical generalization. It is of real concern to the geologist also, who, as paleontologist, must deal with the bygone organisms that have lived and have passed away. It is axiomatic, of course, that the student of fossil species can not observe directly the dynamics of specific evolution; what he may know about the actual processes of transmutation can be learned only by the study of existing organisms and their changes, which he then projects into the past—precisely as the geologist can not see his age-old strata in process of

[1] Address of the retiring president, delivered at the annual meeting of the New York Academy of Sciences, December 19, 1927. Photographic illustrations of topographic features, specimens and tabulated statistics, which were employed at the time, are necessarily omitted here.

actual formation, although he can understand their origins from what he now observes in the way of erosion, deposition, solidification and uplift.

The material with which I shall deal specifically consists of certain land-snails that dwell in the larger and higher islands of the western and southern Pacific Ocean. They belong to various and varied species of the single genus Partula. In the course of the past twenty years more than 150,000 individuals have been secured in several groups of islands. As the adult animals are viviparous, the young dissected from the brood-chambers of their parents afford valuable data for heredity. The young number about 250,000. Hence the material comprises an ample array of over 400,000 individuals for the study of distribution, variation, heredity and organic differentiation—which last phrase means evolution.

Last year I presented a general description of these animals and their local distribution, showing how each group of islands bears its own characteristic species, and how each island of a single group is inhabited by forms that occur nowhere else. Indeed, in some instances a given species is confined to a single mountain peak or to a restricted area not more than a hundred yards in any diameter. From such facts of distribution, and from the correlation between geographical proximity and specific similarity, it is possible to decode the history of organic differentiation by which the present situation has come about. And incidentally it was shown also how the zoogeographical data are valuable for the purely geological problem of a pre-Pacific continent.

On this occasion, employing the identical facts of Partula nature and distribution, I purpose to discuss some other aspects of the problem of organic differentiation, and to express some of the convictions that have gained form and definition in the course of the detailed studies of an unusual wealth of material. No claim is made that my conclusions are original or novel, for their like are to be found in commentary and controversial literature. But even at this date in the discussion of evolutionary dynamics, conflicting views are presented to us, more often on theoretical grounds than on the basis of an analysis of organic variation in nature. The Partula work is concrete and circumstantial, and its results make it possible to present definite statements regarding many of the controverted questions of evolutionary procedure.

In particular, the topics are, first and principally, the concept of species, and the change in focus that I believe to be essential if progress is to be made in the analysis of the origin of species in nature; the second is the Darwinian formula of natural selection, and the precise form of its statement that holds for the history of Partula evolution, particularly as regards the problems of utility and the survival value of small congenital variations. The third topic, to be dealt with very briefly, is the opposition of fortuity and orthogenesis. A final profession of evolutionary faith will conclude the discussion.

Our present concept of a species is a heritage from the eighteenth century. It has been useful, and indeed indispensable for the organization of biological information, but at the same time in some ways it has deterred progress in analyzing and understanding the modes by which diverse organic types have come into existence. In medieval times the concept did not exist as such, until with the era of Suarez the evolutionary views of earlier centuries, sanctioned and expounded by the orthodox fathers of the church like St. Augustine and St. Thomas Aquinas, were cast aside in favor of the dogma of supernatural creation, according to which, once for all time, all kinds of living creatures came into being in the Garden of Eden, unchanged and unchangeable. Yet the special creationists themselves were by no means in agreement as to the natures and numbers of organisms thus first constituted. According to some, like Bory de Saint Vincent and Gmelin, the original kinds were what would be called to-day the generic types—Felis, Canis, Homo. As time passed, by natural resolution, each of these was supposed to be divided up into lesser components, such as the species, *Felis leo, Felis tigris,* etc. Others, like Ray and Linnaeus, held that the latter were the primary types; and while at first Linnaeus contended that these had undergone no organic diversification since their creation, later he espoused the belief that transmutation within species had produced different varieties or sub-species. Again, Jordan held that these lesser units—the varieties—were the original things and that a species was an arbitrary aggregate, precisely as a Linnaean genus was a convenient collection of essentially similar types, assembled by convention.

During this period, when the idea of supernatural creation held sway, there was no problem of the *origin* of species, for the various kinds were postulated *ab initio,* just as in embryology the false preformationist views of Bonnet and Haller excluded the problem of embryological differentiation. Such a concept could not have other than a baneful effect upon investigation, for whatever allowance was made for transmutation within genera or within species, this was regarded as quite subordinate to the supernatural fixation of the first-formed kinds, and a general program of organic evolution was impossible.

With Darwin and his work, the whole matter entered its modern phase, when universal organic transmutation came to be fully established, and when the species came to be understood as an artificial concept, like the concept of genus, of order, of family and of class. It is true that the Linnean form of the idea still controlled taxonomy among the major divisions of biology, and it still rules evolutionary discussion to an extent which many, myself included, hold to be unjustifiable and harmful. It is impossible to outline the true conception of species more clearly than in the words of Darwin himself, and while the correct idea is now axiomatic, we must not forget that this was by no means the case when Darwin wrote. He says:

Certainly no clear line of demarcation has as yet been drawn between species and sub-species—that is, the forms which in the opinion of some naturalists come very near to, but do not quite arrive at, the rank of species: or, again, between sub-species and well-marked varieties, or between lesser varieties and individual differences. These differences blend into each other by an insensible series; and a series that impresses the mind with the idea of an actual passage.

Hence I look at individual differences, though of small interest to the systematist, as of the highest importance for us, as being the first steps towards such slight varieties as are barely thought worth recording in works on natural history. And I look at varieties which are in any degree more distinct and permanent, as steps towards more strongly-marked and permanent varieties; and at the latter as leading to sub-species, and then to species . . . A well-marked variety may therefore be called an incipient species . . .

Here we have a definite statement that a species is only one term in an array of assemblages of lesser or greater comprehensiveness and scope. To focus attention on just that degree of difference which by convention is taken to be specific in degree is no more helpful than to concentrate on the greater degree of difference between two genera or two families. In fact, it diverts attention from the point where the enquiry into the origin of diverse organic types must begin, namely, the production of the individual variant itself, and the passage from parent to offspring. For here, and here only, can the dynamics of organic differentiation come under direct observation. Anything else is deduced. It is admitted, of course, that comparative morphology, crystallized into taxonomy, must take some conventional degree of difference from which to work, and on account of the historical strength of the species idea, it starts with what *on detailed analysis* proves to be a relatively large and a derived degree of difference. From this, it works mainly upwards to genera and to larger groups. But when it proceeds downwards from the same point, namely, to varieties, subvarieties and ultimately to individual variants, it is working in the direction opposite to that of natural organic differentiation.

For purely descriptive purposes, in my own work, it has been necessary to start with the individual variants, and to establish groupings below variety which have the same relation to subspecies as that of subspecies to species, species to genera and so on. All individuals that are alike in at least one distinguishable quality, however they may differ in others, constitute what I call a *gens*—a name that is closely similar to the word gene of the geneticists, and the similarity in name correctly implies that the identical manifest qualities are due to similar genetic factors. Aggregates of *gentes* form a *cohort*—a more inclusive grouping with greater intrinsic diversity than the *gens*. *Cohorts* constitute a *socius*—that is, a geographically outlined assemblage built up of the lesser components. Several *socii,* or indeed a single *socius,* may present a complexion that is collectively distinctive, and hence, they, or it, will form a *variety,* or better a *primary variety,* still more comprehensive and with a still greater diversity among its members. Such *varieties* constitute the *species,* and the rest follows according to convention.

It may sound paradoxical, but it has become increasingly evident to me in prosecuting my own work, that little if any understanding of the *origin* of diverse organic types can be gained through the study of genera, species or even varieties, *after* they have arisen. We can gain knowledge of their evolutionary connections, it is true, on the principle that the degree of likeness is an index of the degree of genetic relationship, for there is no known reason for organic similarity other than common ancestry. But the factors that have made varieties dissimilar, species more unlike, and genera still more so, are not there to be discovered. Let me repeat that we must concentrate on the initial episode when individual offspring present themselves as something different from their parents. What happens when gentes come to differ within their cohort, cohorts within their socii, varieties within the species and species within their genera, is universally the same, and it is nothing but the initial episode repeated again and again.

The conclusion at which we arrive therefore is in effect that the geneticists and they alone are working on the fundamental dynamics of organic differentiation. With the conjunction of Weismannian cytology and Mendelian experimentation a new era was begun, and its accomplishments in the brief period of twenty-five years are known to all. Now, I believe, we require the same kind of combination of effort, on the part of geneticists who work in the experimental garden and laboratory with complete control of conditions, and of what might be called the analytical taxonomists, who deal with organisms in open nature. Having the assured principles of genetics, the field-worker is justified in postulating an internal genetic control of his minor variations exactly like that which manifests itself in the succession of changing laboratory generations, just as a pair of qualities that are newly found to Mendelize may confidently be referred to chromosomal direction, even though the cytological demonstration in question may not have been made.

So far as the material of Partula is concerned, the elementary episodes of organic differentiation that have been demonstrated, and the long history of evolution rewritten by deduction, reveal no primary or originative factors at work other than those of congenital nature and location. Thus the results are in full accord with those of laboratory genetics, which allow for external control of the behavior of qualities, it is true, but find no evidence that external conditions actually originate new qualities as such. Despite the fundamental importance of this subject, this brief statement is all that can be given in the present connection.

And now a few words regarding mutation and the supposed conflict between the doctrine of mutation and Darwin's views. The antithesis in question, for which De Vries is largely responsible, has long since disappeared from the only writings that deal directly with the facts, namely, those in the field of genetics. Nowadays the word mutation is used to apply to any congenital departure or variation, whatever it may be in degree. Its real antithesis is a change due to the operation of an external influence, or a somatic modification, sometimes named a fluctuation. Numerous instances of true mutations have been discovered in Partula and in numerous species. Sometimes the new type is rare, like the sinistral mutants in *P. taeniata,* where they number only four out of sixty thousand individuals. Sometimes the novel condition is more frequent, as in many of the color-varieties, or cohorts. These instances prove to be true mutations, for some among the embryonic offspring repeat the new parental character and thus carry it over to posterity.

We come now to the second topic, natural selection, and the way natural selection enters into the evolutionary history of the Partula material. To forestall any possible misapprehension later, let me state at once that I hold myself to be a true believer in orthodox natural selection. Darwin clearly separates this from congenital variation and takes the latter as given, so to speak. Others of the neo-Darwinian school attempted to expand natural selection so as to make it originative in effect as well as discriminatory, notably those who propounded the theory of germinal selection. As to the truth of the elements of natural selection, there can be no two opinions. Given the fact that congenital variations do arise universally, it is found that in general organisms multiply at an excessive rate, and they are thus plunged into some sort of struggle for existence; the unadapted perish, and thus the only ones to carry on are those which are predestined to succeed by their congenital make-up. The crucial point in the whole formula is the matter of the survival value of small differences. Darwin himself did not insist on the positive utility of such individual differences, for he discusses at length a whole series of what he calls "indifferent characters." But Wallace took the extreme position and argued that whether the observer can or can not discern just how a small difference may have been useful, yet it must have been so, else the possessor could not survive. This really begs the whole question. Of course the literature is full of citations of directly useless and eliminative characters that are congenital in origin as mutations, such as the lethal factors in Drosophila and the uni-sexual organization of some of De Vries' primroses. But an unprejudiced review of the many individual differences displayed by the Partulae, whether they be small or large in degree, finds no reason to believe that they are of direct benefit to their possessors, or otherwise. The statement that congenital variation *must not be inutile* or detrimental has really the correct form, as I believe; and I do not regard it as any less Darwinian than any other element of the doctrine of natural selection.

The third topic—fortuity *vs.* orthogenesis—must be dismissed with very brief consideration. There is no evidence that the variations in the Partula material have proceeded along orthogenetic lines, while all the evidence is to the contrary effect. It is not possible here and now to present the detailed facts which warrant the foregoing general conclusion and the following brief statement. The qualities of the gentes which compose a cohort differ fortuitously in such a way as to form a continuous polygon of frequency. The cohorts, when treated statistically, also disclose a continuous relationship. When the socii themselves are assembled, they vary about an average condition in the same way that individual variants group themselves about a median condition. Let me recall the primary contention that it is here in the earlier stages of organic differentiation that we must look for the true facts. If orthogenesis is real, it will be found here. But the evidence is all to the contrary. I am well aware that this may seem to be a very cavalier treatment of a large subject, but it is my purpose only to present the conclusions which are authorized and justified by the results of the present investigation. And this summary statement must suffice.

And now, by way of conclusion, I may outline what I believe to be the full and correct statement regarding the history of organic differentiation among the Partulae, as it has gone forward in the past and as it is proceeding to-day. The efficient causes of evolution are congenital, and their work is manifested by the continuance of some among the parental qualities; but these are never repeated faithfully, for the hereditary chromosomal machinery is such that exact similarity is impossible. The individual differences may be small or larger, but the degree is unimportant—it is congenital causation that is the essential element. The variants then exercise their hereditary endowments as they may, with success or failure as the outcome of their accord with the whole complex of surrounding circumstances. They must not be unadapted—this is the true biological categorical imperative. Nature makes a wide allowance in the matter of actual utilitarian values.

Variation and heredity, then, are the two aspects of the workings of the internal factorial machinery; natural selection, with which I include spatial and physiological isolation, does the rest. The whole complex of external conditions, whatever these may chance to be, does nothing in the way of originating variations; its effects are limited to an acceptance, a tolerance or a rejection of the varied aspirants for the career of a complete organic life.

HENRY E. CRAMPTON

BARNARD COLLEGE,
COLUMBIA UNIVERSITY

RESEARCH AND THE TRAINING OF THE RESEARCHER

I

RESEARCH is systematic and critical investigation into the sources of truth; it is a characteristic and proudly accepted function of the university. In the eyes of the world the university degree, the doctor's degree, stands for competency in scholarly pursuit of truth. In granting the degree the university acknowledges, tacitly at least, responsibility for *training in research* of potential researchers. Are the functions desirably to be differentiated?

(1) One policy, not uncommon, admits the candidate for the doctor's degree to a professorial undertaking in research. He may, at the discretion of the professor, take such part in the investigation as appears compatible with its validity and profit therefrom in "training" as he can. Responsibility, however, lies with the professor; the investigation is his investigation. Thus, properly, the candidate is follower and not director of inquiry; he pursues a technique chosen and directed by another; he is executor of a plan not his own. If he plays his part of technical assistant to the satisfaction of the professor, thereby, so far as research enters, he qualifies for the doctor's degree.

(2) A second policy does not admit the candidate to staff research; it assigns him to independent research. The candidate is not an assistant whom the professor may use at his discretion for the forwarding of his own researches; he is, rather, an initiate in self-directed inquiry, for whom the professor is a resource of advice and criticism. His independent research is both a medium for the development of research ability, and a test of that ability. By it he is judged to be competent or not competent in research.

(3) A third policy is intermediate. The policy admits the candidate to a part in execution of more than one professional inquiry, each designed, directed and controlled throughout by the responsible staff member. When the candidate by repeated practice under direction appears to have mastered the essentials of a variously flexible technique, he is released from his auxiliary status and assigned to independent research. Again by his independent work as researcher he manifests his competency or incompetency.

II

Now the end of research is truth discovered. To that end error, so far as is humanly possible, must be kept out of investigations. The obligation of the university in its research function is to maintain the highest quality of truth-seeking that the capacities of its membership and the extent of its material resources permit. Hence research must be directed and controlled by the select and the proven in research—namely, the experienced and competent staff membership.

(1) In the first policy described above, that principle is clearly accepted. There is no research other than staff research. The policy permits, if it does not ensure, the highest attainable quality in all research for which the university stands sponsor.

(2) The second policy segregates staff research from the research of candidates. The staff is in no wise hindered in the most effective use of its resources

for discovery of truth. But the policy does admit a second level of research. For it is neither assumed nor to be assumed that the norm of acceptability in student research shall equal the norm of staff production in research. The standard is, rather, the minimal level of acceptable staff research. Hence, if student research be placed in the same category with staff research, the level of quality in the total research product of the university is lower than it is under the first policy of strict staff responsibility.

(3) The third, or intermediate, policy protects staff research exactly as does the first policy. But, like the second policy, it admits a second level of research. The level of student product, however, is likely to be raised. For the policy involves training in the essentials of technical procedure preliminary to the undertaking of independent research. Hence, the level of total research under university auspices will, in quality, lie between the extremes.

III

The end of the training function is the competent researcher—a man able to locate and define a problem for investigation; able to plan and carry through a technique of inquiry appropriate to the solution of his problem; able to organize and interpret, in their immediate bearings at least, the findings to which his inquiry leads.

(1) The first policy, well designed to the maintenance of quality in research, is deficient as a means to the qualification of the researcher. The candidate is not the original and responsible agent in location and definition of the problem for investigation; nor is he selecter and organizer of the method of attack; nor, again, is he organizer and interpreter of findings. In all those phases of the investigation he is but observer, or, at best, "vicarious participant." He is responsibly active only in execution of technique. That is, his "training" is alongside of research rather than in it. If the candidate has originality he has not demonstrated it. He is trained only as a technical assistant, not as a researcher.

(2) Under the second policy the candidate is placed in the position of the researcher. He must find and define his problem, plan and execute his technique of inquiry, organize and interpret his findings. His participation in research is genuine and not vicarious. He is trained in research by performance of "a complete act" of research.

(3) The third policy, by keeping the candidate in contact with "a complete act" of a competent researcher, provides for him a pattern of research. By repeated practice in certain essentials of technique it trains him in elements of habit usable in research. By assignment to independent research it educates him in "a complete act" of research. The candidate learns both by imitation of research and by genuine research of his own.

IV

It appears, then, that an organization of university function to the end of highest quality in research is not an organization best adapted to the production of the competent researcher. On the other hand, an organization to the end of competency in the researcher is not best adapted to the highest product in research. The functions of research and of training in research are coordinate, but they are not coincident.

Can not the university best serve both ends by a frank recognition of distinction in functions? Let us have in one category research of the highest quality, performed by the experts in research—what I should like to call university research. In another let us have research of high quality, performed by initiates in research, undertaken by the university not for the sake of its value in contributing to the sum of known truth, but undertaken as a means to the development of competency in prospective researchers. This I have, without license, already called student research.

T. H. EATON

CORNELL UNIVERSITY

THE PROMOTION OF KNOWLEDGE OF PRECAMBRIAN LIFE

THE promotion of the knowledge of Precambrian life is the object of an award and medal founded by Mrs. Mary Vaux Walcott, in memory of her late husband, Dr. Charles Doolittle Walcott, internationally distinguished for his investigations of Cambrian life and preeminent in his explorations of Precambrian life. A trust fund providing for an honorarium and inexpensive medal has been established under the auspices of the National Academy of Sciences in accordance with Mrs. Walcott's letter as follows:

> I inclose herewith the outline for a medal and honorarium, to be awarded every five years by the National Academy in memory of the work of my husband, Charles Doolittle Walcott. I hope this trust will be acceptable to the Academy and serve to stimulate investigation along the scientific lines which were of such great interest to Doctor Walcott.

The essential provisions governing the award are:

> (1) The fund ($5,000) is to be known as the Charles Doolittle Walcott Fund.

(2) The income shall be used for the award of medals and honoraria to persons between the ages of 21 and 48 years, the results of whose published researches, explorations, and discoveries in pre-Cambrian history shall be judged by the Trust Fund Board to be most meritorious. The award shall be made without respect to nation, race, sex, or academic degree.

(3) A medal to be known as the Charles Doolittle Walcott Medal, for the promotion of knowledge of pre-Cambrian life, is to be awarded every 5 years, beginning with 1932, unless in the judgment of the Board no candidate worthy of the award is in view at the end of the period. The medal is to be cast in bronze or some other inexpensive metal and the accrued income in highest even hundreds of dollars is to accompany the medal as an honorarium. The same person shall not receive the medal and prize on two successive periods.

(4) The selection of the recipients is in the hands of the Fund Trustees, whose recommendations are submitted to the Council of the National Academy for approval. The Trustees, 5 in number, are to include the Secretary of the Smithsonian Institution in Washington, *ex officio*, a member to be proposed by and represent the Institut de France, a member similarly representing the Royal Society of London, and two members of the National Academy of Sciences distinguished in Paleozoic paleontology, to be appointed by the President and Council of the Academy.

(5) The awards will be bestowed at annual meetings of the Academy.

An interesting and notable feature of the terms of the gift is the stipulation that it is awarded only to young men and women who have not yet passed the age of forty-eight.

The announcement of the gift of the fund by Mrs. Walcott and of its acceptance by the council of the Academy was made in the session of the Academy on April 23. The formal acknowledgment by the president of the Academy follows:

Permit me, on behalf of the council of the Academy, to express the satisfaction felt by it that you are commemorating the life and work of Dr. Charles Doolittle Walcott by establishing a medal and honorarium bearing his name for the promotion of knowledge of Precambrian life, and also to thank you for your confidence in placing in trust of the Academy this memorial to a distinguished member, who did much to advance its welfare.

The history of Precambrian life runs from the origin of the first living organism to the high development of the lower orders of life found in the early Cambrian, in the study of which Dr. Walcott was for many years preeminent. The period covered by this history, during which terrestrial conditions, including seas, lands, sunlight, rains, winds and currents appear to have been favorable for life on earth, may well have been as long or even longer than all time that has elapsed since the first Cambrian sediments were laid down. The story of the sequence of plants and animals during Precambrian time to be told by the actual fossil remains is as yet almost wholly unknown. Most of its pages have been torn away or effaced by mountain building and erosion, or blotted and disfigured beyond hope of discernment by the forces which have produced metamorphism or even complete destruction. Some doubtless now lie buried deeply from sight beneath the strata of later ages, to be revealed, perhaps, by erosion following new revolutions in the course of hundreds of millions of years to come. Only in comparatively few areas, where the sediments, after having first escaped obliterating metamorphism have fortunately escaped erosion or deep burial, can we expect to find surviving fragments of the record which future students may laboriously piece together. In some cases, the records, though offering indisputable proof of life, do not permit the revelation of the structure of the organism and its meaning, just as an old letter, faded and torn, is unquestionably in writing, though it can not now be read. In other cases the student may not for a time understand the language, many of whose characters are nevertheless distinct. Eventually, however, large portions of the history of Precambrian life will be built up, piece by piece, and with it the larger understanding of the conditions, the processes and the contemporaneous products of the evolution of life on earth.

For over thirty years Dr. Walcott was deeply interested in the search in Precambrian formations for the remains of life antecedent to that in the earliest Cambrian with which he was so familiar. His early discoveries in the Appalachian and the southwestern regions paved the way for his later discoveries of the highly varied and impressive organic formations in the Belt series and associated terranes of the Northern Rocky Mountains, which form the nucleus of our greatest contribution to Precambrian life, especially as it is revealed in deposits laid down through the vital activity of different types of plant life. Not only was Dr. Walcott deeply interested in Precambrian life; to his zeal and persistent faith we owe the greater part of our knowledge of it.

It is appropriate that through these awards you seek to stimulate the interest and zeal of young men and women in this field so long cherished by Dr. Walcott, while perpetuating the association of his name with the advancement of knowledge of Precambrian life.

The Academy accepts your trust in this spirit and in homage to your late husband.

As is well known, Dr. Walcott was for many years an active and productive member of the Academy, which through different periods he served as treasurer, councillor, and, not long before his death, as president. He took a leading part in the acquisition of the lands and in securing the funds necessary for the erection of the magnificent home of the Academy and the National Research Council in Washington.

DAVID WHITE

SCIENTIFIC EVENTS

THE AWARD OF PRIZES AND GRANTS BY THE BELGIAN ACADEMY OF SCIENCES

ACCORDING to *Nature,* the following prize awards have recently been announced by the Belgian Royal Academy of Sciences: Maurice Nuyens (1,500 francs), for his memoir on the resolution of problems with axial symmetry in general relativity; A. Monoyer (1,500 francs), for anatomical and ethological researches on one or more plant species interesting through their mode of life; Théophile Gluge prize (1,300 francs), to L. Dautrebande for his work on the study of gaseous metabolism in man in health and disease; P. J. and Ed. van Bereden prize (3,400 francs), to Hans de Winiwarter for his work published during 1924–26; Adjutant H. Lefévre prize (1,500 francs), to Hélène Massart for her researches on the phenomena of secretion in plants; Ad. Wetrems prize (7,500 francs), to Louis Verlaine for his studies on instinct and intelligence in Hymenoptera Agathon de Potter Foundation. The following grants have been made: W. Conrad (2,000 francs), for the continuation of his researches on the lower organisms, particularly on the Belgian fresh-water flagellates; J. Pasteels (500 francs), to continue at Wimereux his researches on the cyto-physiological action of the dilution of sea-water on the eggs of lamellibranchs; the Jean Mascart experimental garden (5,000 francs), to continue a series of experiments on plant physiology commenced by the late Jean Mascart; E. Zunz (6,000 francs), for the purchase of instruments necessary to the continuation of his researches on glycaemia; Th. De Donder (7,500 francs), for the publication of his "Théorie des invariants intégraux"; Gilta (1,000 francs), for the publication of plates of chemical crystallography; E. De Wildemann (3,000 francs), for assisting the publication of parts of volume 4 of "Plantæ Bequærtianæ"; Comité national de Géodésie (5,000 francs), to enable it to print the reports of 1920–25 and 1926, on the geodesic work done by the Institute cartographique militaire since the war; Beeli (500 francs), for the execution of plates relating to the mycological flora of the Congo. Jean Servais Stas Prizes to Lucie De Brouckère, Léon Navez, Louis Henry; the Decennial prize of the mineralogical sciences to Armand Renier.

EXHIBIT OF THE BINGHAM OCEANOGRAPHIC COLLECTION AT YALE UNIVERSITY

THE Bingham oceanographic collection, which consists of over 3,000 items, and which was collected by Harry Payne Bingham, of New York City, has been placed in the Peabody Museum of Natural History at Yale University, and was exhibited in connection with the university's 227th commencement activities. This collection of marine animals, containing over one hundred new species, is so arranged that it may be of utmost benefit to students and the public.

Three oceanographic expeditions by Mr. Bingham and a group of scientists were required to bring together this material. The first expedition visited West Indian waters and the coast of the British Honduras. Efforts were chiefly directed toward making a collection of the less common fishes and other animals in the shallower waters, and of the various organisms which inhabit the sea-bottom to a depth of about three thousand feet. As a result of this expedition, twenty new species of shallow water fishes and seventeen new species of crustaceans from various depths have already been described. The second expedition went to Perlas Islands in the Bay of Panama and the Gulf of California, the latter a comparatively little explored faunistic region. Many valuable items were found there, of which already fifteen species have proved to be new.

The third expedition conducted by Mr. Bingham, considered the most successful of the three, visited the waters about the Bahama and Bermuda Islands. As a result of this expedition, thirty new species have already been described, and it is expected that many more will be found.

About one hundred and twenty fishes representative of the regions visited by Mr. Bingham during his expeditions have been mounted by Francis West, who accompanied him on these expeditions, and whose work is well known in American museums. Wilfred S. Bronson, also a member of the expeditions, has made over fifty oil and water paintings in color of the fishes and other animals as they were taken fresh from the water. In his paintings Mr. Bronson has worked on the relationships of the fishes to each other and to their surroundings, with the result that each picture serves almost as a habitat group. Over one hundred species of fishes are represented in these paintings.

In order that his collection could be studied and the results published, Mr. Bingham has placed in charge of his collections Alfred E. Parr, a Norwegian oceanographer and ichthyologist, who has been appointed to the staff of Peabody Museum as assistant curator of zoology in charge of the Bingham Oceanographic Collection. It is planned not only to continue the taxonomic work but to take up investigations in other important biologic aspects of oceanography.

OKLAHOMA GEOLOGICAL SURVEY FIELD PARTIES

DURING the present summer eight geological field parties will be working in Oklahoma under the direction of the Oklahoma Geological Survey, according to Chas. N. Gould, director.

Professor Charles E. Decker and C. A. Merritt, of the University of Oklahoma, will continue their studies begun last year in the Arbuckle Mountains in southern Oklahoma. A paper recently published by these investigators states that the thickness of the Arbuckle limestone is approximately 8,000 feet. Dr. E. O. Ulrich, of the U. S. Geological Survey, was with this group the first two weeks of June collecting fossils from the Arbuckle limestone.

Professor F. A. Melton, of the University of Oklahoma, will spend two months in the Arbuckle and Ouachita Mountains measuring the tension joints in the formations, and applying the Cloos methods of investigation, in the endeavor to ascertain the relative ages of these two mountain uplifts. Professor W. T. Thom, of Princeton University, assisted by C. W. Miller, will spend three months in the coal fields of eastern Oklahoma tracing coal outcrops of the segregated coal lands of the Choctaw nation.

Professor Joe E. Moose, of the University of Oklahoma, will collect samples of Oklahoma coals and make B. T. U. thermal tests of the same. Paul E. Shelly, of the department of petroleum engineering of the University of Oklahoma, will collect asphalt samples in southern Oklahoma and conduct weathering tests on Oklahoma asphalts. A. J. Freie, of the University of Iowa, will continue his sedimentation studies on the Anadarko basin. G. G. Suffel, of Stanford University, will spend two months in western Oklahoma studying field exposures of the dolomite formations of the Permian red beds preparatory to a report on Oklahoma dolomites. John A. McCutchin is undertaking the work of ascertaining deep well temperatures in Oklahoma, this being part of Research Project No. 25, sponsored by the American Petroleum Institute under the direction of the petroleum committee of the National Research Council.

The results of the various investigations will be embodied in reports to be published by the Oklahoma Geological Survey.

APPOINTMENTS AND PROMOTIONS AT HARVARD UNIVERSITY

AMONG the promotions and new appointments recently announced by Harvard University are the following:

William H. Weston, Jr., professor of cryptogamic botany. Professor Weston has served as a pathologist in the Bureau of Plant Industry, U. S. Department of Agriculture, and during the past year has been associate professor of botany in the university.

Leon W. Collet, professor of geology. Professor Collet was in the geology department of the University of Edinburgh, and later professor of geology at the University of Geneva, before becoming a visiting lecturer at the university in 1927.

Joseph H. Faull, professor of forest pathology. Professor Faull comes from the Department of Botany in University of Toronto.

Joseph C. Aub, associate professor of medicine and physician at the Collis P. Huntington Memorial Hospital. He has been a member of the Medical School faculty since 1920.

Charles H. Berry, professor of mechanical engineering. Since 1925 he has been an associate editor of the magazine *Power* and an assistant professor at Cornell University.

Edwin J. Cohn, associate professor of physical chemistry. Since 1925 he has been an assistant professor in the department.

William L. Aycock, assistant professor of preventive medicine and hygiene. In 1916 he served as diagnostician with the New York State Department of Health, and later as director of the research laboratory of the Vermont Board of Health and instructor in preventive medicine in the university.

Chester M. Jones, assistant professor of preventive medicine and hygiene. Since 1925 he has held the Henry Pickering Walcott fellowship in clinical medicine.

Monroe A. McIver, assistant professor of surgery. In 1921 he was national research fellow in physiology and has been an instructor in surgery in the university since 1924.

John Homans, assistant professor of surgery. Since 1916 he has been an instructor in surgery in the university.

Richard H. Miller, assistant professor of surgery. Since 1919 he has held the position of instructor in surgery.

Robert C. Cochrane, assistant professor of surgery. He has been an instructor in urinary surgery in the university since 1924.

Merrill C. Sosman, assistant professor of roentgenology. He has served as instructor in the Medical School, consulting physician in the Collis P. Huntington Memorial Hospital since 1924.

Clifford L. Derick, assistant professor of medicine. Was recently connected with the Peter Bent Brigham and since 1924 with the Rockefeller Hospital in New York City.

Hermann L. Bhemgart, assistant professor of medicine. He has been connected with the Medical School since 1923 as instructor in medicine.

Derwent Stainthorpe Whittlesey, assistant professor of geography, now associate professor of geography at the University of Chicago.

Harold Coe Stuart, assistant professor of child hygiene. Dr. Stuart has been a member of the department since 1922.

SCIENTIFIC NOTES AND NEWS

Dr. M. L. Harris, professor of surgery at the Chicago Polyclinic Hospital, was elected president of the American Medical Association at the Minneapolis meeting to succeed Dr. W. S. Thayer, of Baltimore. It was decided to hold the next meeting at Portland, Oregon.

Yale University has conferred the honorary degree of doctor of science on Dr. C. U. Ariëns Kappers, director of the Central Institute of Brain Research, Amsterdam, Holland, and on Dr. H. E. Ives, physicist of the Bell Telephone Laboratories. The degree of master of science was conferred on Dr. Evarts Ambrose Graham, professor of surgery at Washington University, St. Louis.

Dr. Barton W. Evermann, director of the museum of the California Academy of Science; Professor Aldred Scott Warthin, head of the department of pathology of the University of Michigan, and Dr. John A. Miller, astronomer, and vice-president of Swarthmore College, all graduates of the University of Indiana, were among those receiving honorary degrees at the ninety-ninth annual commencement exercises at the university on June 11.

The honorary degree of doctor of laws was conferred upon Dr. Henry Fairfield Osborn, president of the American Museum of Natural History, at the annual commencement exercises of Union College, on which occasion Dr. Osborn gave the principal address.

Professor Albert R. Mann, dean of the college of agriculture at Ithaca, and Professor Samuel T. Dana, dean of the College of Forestry at the University of Michigan, received honorary doctorates of science at the fifty-seventh annual commencement exercises of Syracuse University.

The honorary degree of doctor of science was conferred on Chas. N. Gould, director of the Oklahoma Geological Survey, by the University of Nebraska at the commencement on June 2.

The president of the French Republic has conferred the cross of officier de la Légion d'Honneur on Dr. George H. F. Nuttall, Quick professor of biology in the University of Cambridge.

Among those honored on the occasion of the birthday of the King of England are Professor J. H. Jeans, secretary of the Royal Society, who has been knighted, and Professor J. S. Haldane, honorary professor of mining at the University of Birmingham, who has been appointed to the order of the companions of honor.

At the anniversary meeting of the Royal Society of South Africa on March 31, Dr. W. A. Jolly, professor of physiology in the University of Cape Town, was elected president. Dr. A. Ogg, professor of physics in the University of Cape Town and retiring president of the society, was elected honorary general secretary, and Dr. L. Crawford, professor of pure mathematics in the University of Cape Town, honorary treasurer.

At the annual meeting of the Harvey Society held on May 16 the following members were elected to serve as officers for the coming year, 1928–1929: *President,* Dr. Peyton Rous, of the Rockefeller Institute; *vice-president,* Dr. Horatio B. Williams, Dalton professor of physiology, Columbia University; *members of the council,* Dr. Robert Chambers, professor of microscopic anatomy, Cornell University Medical School; Dr. Harold D. Senior, professor of anatomy, New York University and Bellevue Hospital College; Dr. Alfred F. Hess, clinical professor of pediatrics, New York University and Bellevue Hospital College; *secretary,* Dr. Philip D. McMaster, Rockefeller Institute.

At the meeting of the American Association of Pathologists and Bacteriologists held at Washington, D. C., on May 1, the following officers were elected for the ensuing year: *President,* E. B. Krumbhaar; *vice-president,* George H. Whipple; *secretary,* Howard T. Karsner; *treasurer,* F. B. Mallory, and incoming *member of council,* Ward J. MacNeal. The next meeting of the association will be held in Chicago on March 28 and 29, 1929.

The American Society of Experimental Pathology has elected the following officers for the ensuing year: *President,* E. B. Krumbhaar; *vice-president,* W. F. Peterson; *secretary-treasurer,* C. V. Weller. The next meeting will be held in conjunction with the International Congress of Physiology in Boston in August, 1929.

Dr. Forman T. McLean has resigned from the staff of the Experimental Station of Rhode Island State College, to accept the position of superintendent of public education at the New York Botanical Garden.

Lloyd S. Tenny, chief of the bureau of agricultural economics of the U. S. Department of Agriculture, has resigned to take a position with the Associated California Fruit Industries.

William Newton has been appointed plant pathologist for the Dominion Department of Agriculture in British Columbia.

Dr. Harlan T. Stetson, assistant professor of astronomy at Harvard University, has been appointed exchange professor to western universities for the second half of the next academic year.

Dr. W. F. Meggers, chief of the spectroscopy section of the U. S. Bureau of Standards, has left for

Europe, where he will represent the bureau at the meetings of the International Astronomical Union in Leyden, Holland.

DR. EMANUEL G. ZIES, of the geophysical laboratory of the Carnegie Institution, is proceeding to Java to engage in research in connection with volcanic activity.

DR. ROBERT L. PENDLETON, soil technologist in Los Banos College, Philippines, has recently been granted three months leave in order to visit various colleges and experiment stations in the Orient. After two weeks in Tokyo he went north to Morioka and Sapporo, then down the west coast and to Kyoto, Nagoya and Fukuoka. On the homeward trip he expects to stop in Formosa and at Canton Christian College.

DR. PAUL BARTSCH, curator of mollusks of the U. S. National Museum and holder of the Walter Rathbone Bacon research scholarship, will spend the next four months in Cuba, where he will be joined by Dr. Carlos de la Torre, president emeritus of the University of Havana, on a search for salt and fresh-water mollusks.

DR. E. O. ULRICH, paleontologist of the United States Geological Survey, is spending a month in Missouri, Arkansas and Oklahoma collecting fossils from the lower Paleozoic formations in these states. The information obtained will be embodied in a report which Dr. Ulrich is now writing on the Paleozoic formations of the Arbuckle Mountains of Oklahoma.

DR. IRVINE H. PAGE will sail in August for Munich, Germany, where he will be a guest research worker and physician to the Kaiser Wilhelm Anstalt Forschung under the directorship of Professors Willstätter and Plaut.

WILLIAM BEEBE, of the New York Zoological Society, has returned from a month's visit to England, where he went to study the deep-sea fish in the British Museum and to complete certain portions of his ichthyological library. He gave several addresses on his diving work on the coral reefs of Haiti, including one before the Zoological Society of London.

PAUL S. MARTIN, curator of archeology and ethnology at the museum of the Colorado State Historical Society, has returned from his second season in Yucatan as assistant archeologist for the Carnegie Institution of Washington. While in Yucatan he excavated and completely restored a Mayan temple. He is planning to do some excavating for the State Historical Society in the southwestern part of Colorado during July and August.

FREDERICK G. CLAPP has completed a reconnaissance in southern and western Persia and eastern Iraq and has returned to Teheran.

DR. W. M. DAVIS, emeritus professor of geology at Harvard University, lectured on "The Coral Reef Problem" before the Sigma Xi of the University of Arizona at Tucson on May 26, and on May 30 delivered the commencement address on "The Value of Useless Knowledge" at the same university, where he has been lecturing on physiography through the spring term. On June 3 he conducted a field meeting of the Rift Club of Southern California at the base of the dissected fault-scarp which limits the San Gabriel mountains on the south near Pasadena.

DR. R. J. GARBER, head of the department of agronomy and genetics at West Virginia University, gave two lectures at the eighth annual convention of the Canadian Society of Technical Agriculturists, which was held in Quebec, June 11 to 14, inclusive. The subjects of the lectures were "Breeding for Disease Resistance with Particular Reference to the Smut of Oats" and "The Nature and Significance of Mutations in Present-day Breeding Methods."

DR. R. W. THATCHER, president of the Massachusetts Agricultural College, will give an evening lecture at the Institute of Chemistry of the American Chemical Society, July 27, on "The Development of Agricultural Research."

THE following lectures have recently been given at the physical laboratory of the University of Minnesota: Professor Léon Brillouin, of the University of Paris, lectured on May 14 on "Quantum Statistics" and "Recent Developments in Quantum Theory." On May 16, Dr. G. Cario spoke on "Recent Work on Collisions of the Second Kind." On May 25 and 26 Professor Kramers, of the University of Utrecht, gave lectures on "The Uncertainty Principle in Quantum Theory," "The Anomalous Refraction of X-rays," and "The Quantum Theory of the Electron."

AT the annual graduation exercises at Clark University a scholarship as a memorial to the late Dr. Edmund C. Sanford, psychologist, former president of the university, was presented by the alumni, and a portrait of the late Professor William Libbey, of Princeton University, was presented by Dr. W. Elmer Ekblaw, representing Mrs. Libbey.

A MARBLE bust of the late John Collins Warren, done by J. F. Paramino, will soon be placed in the Warren anatomical museum at the Harvard Medical School.

SAMUEL B. PARISH, honorary curator in the herbarium of the University of California and lecturer in Stanford University, died on June 5, aged ninety years.

THE *Experiment Station Record* notes the death on March 7 of Dr. Hjalmar von Feilitzen, one of the leaders in agriculture and agricultural research in Sweden.

DR. CHARLES PLATT, emeritus professor of biological chemistry in the Hahnemann Medical College, Philadelphia, has died at the age of fifty-nine years.

THE Northern Arizona Society of Science and Art has been founded to increase and diffuse both the knowledge and appreciation of science and art, to protect historic and prehistoric sites, to protect scenic places, and conserve vanishing wild life. The society will maintain in the city of Flagstaff a museum where the archeological and ethnological treasures of Northern Arizona can be displayed and where the geological wonders of the plateau can be interpreted. Dr. Harold S. Colton is the director of the museum. A board of fifteen trustees has been appointed.

THE twentieth annual meeting of Poultry Science Association will be held from August 21 to 24, at Purdue University, Lafayette, Indiana. The annual meetings are largely attended by extension, teaching and research workers, who devote most of their time to poultry science, of various state universities, experiment stations and state departments.

THE executive committee of the International Geodetic and Geophysical Union has voted to hold the next meeting of the union at Stockholm, Sweden, between the dates, August 18–25, 1930.

AN Empire Forestry Conference will open in Perth about the first week in September, and delegates will spend six weeks in Australia, the last week being occupied in Canberra. They will spend three days in each state inspecting forestry activities.

THE Institution of Civil Engineers began on June 4 the meetings associated with the celebration of the centenary of its incorporation by royal charter. The inaugural ceremony took place in the hall of the institution, Great George Street, Westminster, when the president, Mr. E. F. C. Trench, welcomed delegates from various parts of the world, many of whom presented addresses of congratulation. In addition to engineering, scientific and professional societies and universities in the British Isles, there were representatives present of kindred institutions in Canada, South Africa, Australia, New Zealand, India, Austria, Chile, Czechoslovakia, Denmark, France, Germany, Holland, Italy, Japan, Norway, Portugal, Sweden, Switzerland and the United States.

WE learn from *Nature* that by the will of Lieutenant-Colonel A. J. C. Cunningham, who died on February 8, the London Mathematical Society will receive £1,000 for the improvement of the method of factorization of large numbers, and £2,000 for the publication of Colonel Cunningham's unpublished printed mathematical works and the completion and publication of his mathematical manuscripts, and also his library of mathematical books. The residue of his estate is to be divided as to one twelfth to the London Mathematical Society, and one twelfth to the British Association, mathematical subsection, for preparing new mathematical tables in the theory of numbers.

THE Chilean Nitrate of Soda Educational Bureau has offered an annual award of $5,000 to research workers in North America for outstanding research that will contribute to the fund of knowledge regarding nitrogen in crop production. The award is sponsored by the American Society of Agronomy, of which P. E. Brown, Iowa State College, Ames, Iowa, is secretary-treasurer.

THE board of regents of the University of Wisconsin have accepted a fund of $15,000 by a Wisconsin group of foundries for metallurgical research in the college of engineering. The fund provides $5,000 a year for three years for equipment to carry on the experiments.

THE Johns Hopkins University has received $500,000 from an anonymous donor to complete the endowment of the Welch Medical Library. An anonymous donor also gave $100,000 to the Wilmer Clinic, subject to an annuity.

Two donations of $200,000 each by John D. Rockefeller, Jr., and James Speyer have sent the building fund of the Museum of the City of New York over the $2,000,000 mark. This assures the museum the city-owned plot of land at 103rd St. and 5th Ave.

THE formal opening of the new museum building at the University of Michigan took place on June 14.

THE important collection of diatoms assembled by the late Charles S. Boyer has been presented by Mrs. Boyer to the Leidy Microscopical Club of the Academy of Natural Sciences of Philadelphia, together with Mr. Boyer's complete library covering the literature of the Diatomaceae. The collection contains over six thousand slides with a card catalogue, includes many types, and embraces practically all the material studied by Mr. Boyer in preparing his "Synopsis of the Diatomaceae of North America," recently published by the Academy of Natural Sciences of Philadelphia.

THE University of Virginia has announced a gift from the General Education Board of $175,000, to be expended within a period of seven years in support of research in biology, chemistry and physics. Research fellowships, open to properly qualified graduate students, have been established in each of these subjects. A number of fellowships at $1,000 each are still available for 1928–29 in the schools of biology and chemistry. Applications should be addressed to the secretary of the appropriate department.

THE new Daniel Guggenheim aeronautical laboratory at the Massachusetts Institute of Technology was formally dedicated and opened for use on June 4.

THE three-story science building of St. Leo's College in Florida was destroyed by fire on June 1, the damage being estimated at $35,000.

AGASSIZ MUSEUM, the Harvard University museum of comparative zoology, was opened again to the public, beginning June 19, following the first extensive remodeling it has had in fifty years. The museum has been closed for about six months while repairs were being made. During the past six months the whole museum has been redecorated and repainted; the building has been entirely renovated. Several old collections which were deemed unsuitable for further exhibition have been discarded and all the exhibits have been rearranged. Several exhibits, new to the university, have been prepared, one being a hall of oceanic mammals, another one of domesticated animals and others designed to show heredity and the variation of animals under domestication.

PRESIDENT COOLIDGE has by executive order reestablished for the protection of native birds the Pathfinder Bird Refuge, embracing 22,700 acres on the North Platte River in central Wyoming, according to an announcement by the U. S. Department of Agriculture. The area is set aside as one of the numerous refuges administered by the Bureau of Biological Survey.

To exchange ideas with the leaders of forestry and outdoor life in Europe and to study the problems of European forests, a group of members of the American Forestry Association, Washington, and others vitally interested in forests, parks and wild life sailed from New York on June 30. The tour will include France, Germany, Switzerland, Finland and Sweden.

UNIVERSITY AND EDUCATIONAL NOTES

ESTABLISHMENT of a trust fund of between $5,000,000 and $6,000,000 for the University of Virginia has been announced by President Edwin A. Alderman. The money was given by an anonymous donor. Half of the income from this fund is to be used for the establishment of scholarships and fellowships, and the remainder for the general educational purposes of the university.

BOWDOIN COLLEGE received over $1,000,000 in gifts during the last year. This includes a $250,000 bequest from F. A. Munsey; $150,000 from the estate of Thomas Upham Coe, of Bangor, Me., and $50,000 from David Pingree, of Salem, Mass.

THROUGH the generosity of an anonymous donor interested in the subject of chemical education a professorial chair in this field has been endowed for the immediate future in the Johns Hopkins University, and Dr. Neil E. Gordon has been elected to the position. Dr. Gordon is at the present time head of the department of chemistry at the University of Maryland and state chemist.

DR. CHARLES F. HOTTES, professor of plant physiology at the University of Illinois, has been appointed professor of botany and head of the department to succeed Dr. H. L. Shantz, who becomes president of the University of Arizona.

DR. F. D'HERELLE, director of the bacteriological laboratory at Alexandria, Egypt, has been appointed professor of bacteriology at Yale University. Dr. d'Herelle was born in Montreal and still retains his Canadian citizenship. He will arrive in the United States about September 1.

PROMOTIONS and appointments on the faculty of the Massachusetts Institute of Technology have been announced. Those promoted from the grade of associate professor to full professorships include: John B. Babcock, professor of railway engineering; J. W. M. Bunker, professor of biochemistry and physiology; H. H. W. Keith and George Owen, professors of naval architecture; Charles Terzaghi, professor of foundations, and Clair E. Turner, professor of biology and public health.

DEAN EDWARD H. ROCKWELL, of the College of Engineering, Rutgers University, has been appointed professor of civil engineering in Lafayette College.

ROBERT L. SPENCER, chief engineer of the McAleenan Corporation of Pittsburgh, has been elected dean of the department of engineering of the University of Delaware, to succeed the late Professor V. G. Smith.

DR. E. D. RIES, director of the division of industrial research in the school of chemistry and physics at the Pennsylvania State College, has resigned to give all his attention to his duties as head of the chemical engineering department, he having filled both positions for the past year. Dr. William J. Sweeney, formerly of the chemistry faculty and for the past two and a half years at the Massachusetts Institute of Technology, has been appointed assistant professor of research and director of the division.

At the University of Edinburgh, Dr. F. A. E. Crew has been appointed professor of animal genetics and director of the university department of research in animal breeding. The chair, which is to be known as the Buchanan chair of animal genetics, was founded by a donation from Lord Woolavington, supplemented by a grant from the International Education Board.

DISCUSSION AND CORRESPONDENCE

RESEARCH PLUS NEWS-GATHERING

Although not primarily a research institution, Science Service is now contributing in a small measure to the advancement of science.

In some instances it is possible to combine a certain degree of research with the news-gathering activities of the Service. The most successful instance to date is the earthquake reporting service that Science Service organized and conducts with the cooperation of the leading seismological observatories, the U. S. Coast and Geodetic Survey and the Jesuit Seismological Association. This system serves the needs of seismologists as well as newspapers. During the year ending March 31, 1928, twenty-seven earthquakes were located and reported through this service. As many as eighteen seismological observatories, some as far away as Alaska and the Philippines, have cooperated. Whereas before the inauguration of this service scientists and the public were often in ignorance for weeks as to the location of many earthquake epicenters, now practically every shock of any importance is located within six to twenty-four hours. We often locate disastrous earthquakes, and predict loss of life that occurred, days and weeks before the news reaches the world through the routine news channels. When the Bulgarian city of Philippopolis was destroyed on April 18, Science Service reported the earthquake early the next day, stating the probability of disaster, while the cables did not carry the news until April 21. On April 10 our instrumental data located a severe earthquake in eastern Peru; a week later on April 17 the news came from the region itself. On May 23, 1927, a severe earthquake in Kansu Province, China, was recorded, and Science Service announced its exact location and predicted heavy loss of life. Not until the latter part of July, two months later, did the confirmation of this great disaster filter out from the interior of the yellow continent.

This combination of research and news activity is now being extended to the fields of anthropology and archeology.

It is very important to be able to send to the spot of the alleged archeological find a competent investigator. Prompt action is necessary from the point of view of anthropology because of the liability that evidence as to the character of the discovery of its geological position or the indications of the age of the deposits may be forever destroyed by careless excavators or faked relics; and from the point of view of Science Service because it is our job to see that exaggerated and misleading reports do not get the start of authentic news. To meet such emergencies we proposed to cooperate with the department of psychology and anthropology of the National Research Council by offering to provide funds sufficient for the preliminary inspection of the find if we were supplied with a list of authorized "scientific minute men" located at strategic points all over the country to whom we should be at liberty to wire for advice in cases of disputed questions. If plans for action are made in advance they might, without delaying to consult us, take train or automobile at once to the place where a prehistoric inscription or the bones of an antediluvian giant has been reported.

The division of anthropology and psychology of the National Research Council has authorized cooperation with Science Service in this undertaking and will arrange with us in preparing such a list of anthropologists and other specialists who will wire us at our expense directly from the field. This obviously requires cooperation with geologists, paleontologists, archeologists and ethnologists. By taking measures for the prompt preliminary investigations we may forestall such squabbles as those of the French savants over the alleged Glozel finds.

The volcanoes of the world will be watched as carefully and thoroughly as the earthquakes, if our plans for cooperation between Science Service and the section of volcanology of the American Geophysical Union materialize.

A committee of the section of volcanology was authorized at the recent meeting of the American Geophysical Union to work out methods of cooperation.

The volcano observatories in this country and abroad, scientists who have paid particular attention to volcanoes and who live in their vicinity and others will be invited to participate in a volcano reporting organization by means of which accurate and prompt information on volcanic activities will be obtained by wire and cable, supplemented by mail reports. It is also planned to bring together historical data upon known active volcanoes which will be of service to both newspapers and scientists. Volcanologists have expressed themselves as feeling that this service will aid their science as effectively as the earthquake reporting service of Science Service has aided the science of seismology.

Science Service desires to extend in the future such combined news-gathering and research activities, and we should like to receive from scientists and scientific bodies suggestions for other such cooperative investigations.

EDWIN E. SLOSSON
WATSON DAVIS
SCIENCE SERVICE,
WASHINGTON, D. C.

AGRONOMIC JABBERWOCKY

WHO among us has not thrilled to Lewis Carroll's sonorous and gruesome lines:

> Twas brillig and the slithy toves
> Did gyre and gimble in the wabe
> All mimsy were the borogoves
> And the mome raths outgabe.

Now after these many years the jabberwock has been aroused again and with eyes of flame is whiffling through the tulgey wood and burbling as he comes:

> The rugaplanes in thickth midlux
> Midodored in the coolth
> But straighth and plumpth the illth umblux
> Midceptisist in fulth.

The new ululations of this fearsome beast are not neglected *Dodgsoniana* resurrected by the antiquarians. They are the grotesque inventions of three moderns who, if not so mellifluous as Dr. Dodgson, are almost as whimsical.[1]

Incomprehensible though it may be, these present fantasies of sounds are not intended as poetic amusement for adolescents. They are offered in all seriousness as aids to American agronomists who, it appears, are struggling perspiringly to be articulate in the refractory English language. That these etymological freaks are welcome is evidenced by the approval with which they were accepted at the Chicago meeting of the agronomists. Presumably hereafter these scientists are to seek lucidity in a ludicrous lexicon of such words as midceptimmune, thickth, plumpth, straighth, midgoodth and rugaplane.

There may be those who will espy the Machiavellian hand of "Big Bill" in this attempt to besmirch the King's English, but that the act took place in Chicago is believed to be the purely fortuitous result of more deep-seated genetic causes.

Proceeding apparently on the theory that the case of the agronomists required heroic treatment the committee on terminology made a herculean effort. The energetic chairman distinguished himself in linguistic prestidigitation, pulling monster after monster out of his hat to be added to a language already reputed to contain 50,000 (or is it 500,000?) words. Whichever the correct number, there surely are enough to meet all the rhetorical requirements of the agronomists, once they have been thoroughly mastered.

It is true that agronomic literature like that of most sciences is open to criticism, but the defect is to be found in the lack of a facile command of the language rather than in a shortage of suitable words. Since "the ultimate aim of research is publication,"[2] inability to express one's thoughts fluently is a fault worthy of most serious study. Any sensible effort to discover a corrective should be welcomed, but an effective cathartic for costive minds hardly is to be obtained by compounding new words, however bizarre. The hapless agronomists have fallen upon evil times and are not likely to find an alleviating diagrydium in the upas shadow of Dr. Ball's Carrollian pastiche.

One can not but be astonished at the egotistic effrontery of a group of men who, after a few weeks' consideration, attempt to improve a language which has met the test of world-wide use for so many centuries. English speech lacks median terms? Forsooth they shall be supplied and presto with a flourish of the pen these diaskeuasts create a veritable Walpurgis of words.

Their words tell us precisely nothing. Objects may be large, small or middle-sized, like the three bears in the nursery tale, but these terms are recognized as being purely relative. They have no meaning in the discrete units of quantity nor should they have. As with general size so with other qualities; things may be tall or short, stout or slender, broad or narrow, deep or shallow, dark or light, straight or crooked, just as committeemen may be wise or foolish, profound or superficial, inferior or superior, grave or comical, sharp or dull, sensible or silly, brilliant or stupid. In fact, there is an almost interminable number of words designating opposite extremes of variable scales. For the positions between the extremes there is an appropriate series of qualifying words such as intermediate, middle, normal, medium, moderate, partial, semi, ordinary, etc. These terms are useful in describing general conditions but are always relative to each other and require definition anew with each discussion where some specific limit is intended.

Not satisfied with having words for the extremes and middle, Dr. Ball's committee is now urging a whole series of new words to mark the quarter positions! These new words, formed by combining adjectives and nouns, are required, presumably, for ac-

[1] Ball, C. R., Shantz, H. L., and Shaw, C. F. "Median Terms in Adjectives of Comparison." *Jour. Amer. Soc. Agronomy*, Vol. 20, No. 2, pp. 182–191. February, 1928.

[2] Allen, E. W. "The Publication of Research." Lecture before the class in "The Nature and Method of Research." Graduate School, Department of Agriculture. Published in mimeograph form for the information of the staff of the Department of Agriculture, February 11, 1925.

curacy of expression, but are likely to create more mental obfuscation than they dispel.

Perhaps the agronomists need a few distinctive terms to add dignity to their science, but the chairman of their committee is not content to restrict his changelings to agricultural science.[3] He seems to feel that his "words" deserve a more widespread popularity and will fill a need in the language at large. The ignominious fate of simplified spelling has been forgotten; a reform justified by sound logic and sponsored by the indefatigable Roosevelt with the full weight of his dynamic personality.

Apparently the agronomists are no longer content to permit the cultured to determine good usage in American speech. Hereafter these matters are to be more democratically decided. The ignorant minority must prevail in language as in politics, and illiteracy is to displace culture. This is an innovation and if we accept agronomic canons of good taste there is no logical reason for rejecting pathological or genetic canons, or for that matter amalgamated truck-drivers' canons. If the agronomists are successful in having their orthographic solecisms incorporated in the respectable dictionaries we may expect similar minority domination from all quarters and our language will become the plaything of irresponsible committeemen.

Nothing could be more absurd than such an arbitrary method of adapting a language to changing conditions. Culture ever has been identified with intellect and never will be achieved by means of the ballot despite the cajoleries of these modern Malaprops with their complacently acquiescent organizations.

All work and no play is detrimental even in matters scientific, but the agronomists, having had their little excursion behind the looking-glass, should now take their vorpal swords in hand and slay the jabberwock. They can then return contentedly to a consideration of their researches, secure in the knowledge that the elegance of their published reports will not be marred with pleonasms imposed by philological mountebanks.

J. H. KEMPTON

BUREAU OF PLANT INDUSTRY,
WASHINGTON, D. C.

NOTE ON THE INERTIA DYADIC

FOR the dynamics of a rigid body it has been shown that the moment of momentum may be expressed as the scalar product of a dyadic—called the inertia dyadic—and the angular velocity. The inertia dyadic is defined by the relation

$$\Phi = \Sigma m(\mathbf{r} \cdot \mathbf{r}\mathbf{I} - \mathbf{r}\mathbf{r})$$

[3] According to the *Jour. of the Amer. Soc. of Agronomy,* for December, 1927, the case for general adoption of these new words is to be presented in "American Speech."

Thus, it plays the same rôle for rotational motion as the mass for translational motion. There is an important difference, however. Whereas the mass is assumed constant, the dyadic is not constant and as a consequence it becomes necessary to obtain its time-derivative.

Starting with the expression given above it can be shown that

$$\dot{\Phi} = \mathbf{p} \times \Phi - \Phi \times \mathbf{p}$$

in which $\mathbf{p}$ is the angular velocity. This shows, as was to be expected, that the time-rate of change of the dyadic is due only to the angular velocity. The form, however, is not so simple as in the case of vectors and I am not aware that any one has ever taken the trouble to express the derivative in this way. The expression is useful as a step in the development of rotational dynamics, for when taken in conjunction with the fundamental principle

$$\frac{d(\Phi \cdot \mathbf{p})}{dt} = \mathbf{L}$$

Euler's equations for rotational motion are obtained immediately.

I. F. MORRISON

UNIVERSITY OF ALBERTA

A NEW AMPHIBIAN RECORD FROM KANSAS, HYLA PHAEROCRYPTA (COPE)[1]

IN the spring of 1925 a specimen of tree-frog was collected near Wildcat Creek, west of the Kansas State Agricultural College at Manhattan, Riley County, Kansas. It differed from any that had been taken in the region and in life somewhat resembled *Hyla crucifer* because its irregular and asymmetrical dorsal markings tended to form a cruciform pattern.

Later the specimen was sent to the U. S. National Museum for identification and was kindly identified as *Hyla phaerocrypta.* Because of the close resemblance of this species to other members of its genus I did not include this report in my list of the amphibians and reptiles of Riley County (1927),[2] but held it for further study. The specimen was consequently sent to Dr. G. K. Noble, who independently agreed with the previous identification.

Hyla phaerocrypta is an amphibian of unusual interest. It was described by Cope (1889)[3] from a

[1] Contributions from the zoological laboratory of the University of Michigan.

[2] Burt, Charles E., 1927, "An Annotated List of the Amphibians and Reptiles of Riley County, Kansas," Occas. Pap. Mus. Zool. Univ. Mich., 189: 1–9.

[3] Cope, E. D., 1889, "The Batrachia of North America," Bull. U. S. Nat. Mus., 34: 1–515.

single specimen from Mount Carmel, southeastern Illinois, as a subspecies of *H. versicolor*. Mount Carmel still remains as a northern record for the form. Viosca (1923)[4] has reported it from Mandeville, southeastern Louisiana, and has removed its subspecific classification. He has found that the size averages about one and a quarter inches and that the body is generally smaller than that of *H. versicolor*. Both Viosca and Ridgway (1924)[5] have called attention to the bird-like notes of *H. phaerocrypta* and its great difference from the croak of *H. versicolor*. An eastern point in the distribution of *H. phaerocrypta*, namely, Nashville, central Tennessee, has been given by Dunn (1927),[6] and I believe that this present paper sets a western record.

For the purpose of comparison the Kansas specimen (Univ. Mich. No. 65029) and an adult *H. versicolor versicolor* (Univ. Mich. No. 65018) from Cheboygan County, Michigan, have given data for the table below.

Measurement	*H. phaerocrypta*	*H. v. versicolor*
Width of head	11 mm	17 mm
Length of body	35 mm	48 mm
Length of arm	17 mm	23 mm
Length of foot	49 mm	65 mm

The dimensions given above not only illustrate the size-difference of the two forms, but also show the close similarity in their bodily proportions.

CHARLES E. BURT
UNIVERSITY OF MICHIGAN

GEOLOGIC AGE BY LEAD URANIUM RATIOS

DR. KIRSCH has kindly called my attention to a slip I made with regard to the atomic weight of the lead determined by Richards and Hall from the Etta Mine at the Black Hills, South Dakota.

The result was 206.07, and I suggested that to get the atomic weight of uranium lead .05 should be subtracted, whereas, allowing for the slower decay of thorium, it should be .02, making the atomic weight of uranium lead 206.05, practically the same as had been found before.

May I take the occasion to say that at the recent meeting of the committee on the estimation of geologic age by atomic disintegration Dr. Fenner reported some analyses of Brazilian minerals from the same pegmatite which checked remarkably well as to age, one contained mainly thorium and the other mainly uranium. Also Dr. R. C. Wells had obtained from the Upper Cambrian Swedish Kolm the lead: uranium ratio .056, which perhaps means that the upper Cambrian is twice as old as the lower Permian, though final results can not be obtained until the atomic weight of the lead upon which Bliss is working in Professor Baxter's laboratory is determined.

ALFRED C. LANE

DATUM, DATA

DOWN in sunny Buenos Aires,
  They call a vamp *patata,*
They speak *la lengua español,*
  And insist upon *la data.*

But up in bleak New England,
  Not quite so cold as Etah,
They follow Webster's unabridged,
  And intonate it *dayta.*

Barbarians out in Arkansaw
  Care not to whom they cater,
Any old parlance goes with them,
  They call it simply *dayter.*

Some reckless folks in other climes,
  Disgracing Alma Mater,
When questioned on their own research'
  Reply, "I'm accumulating *dater."*

Then, there's the chap, who should be shot,
  (His ré-search doesn't matter)
Who every time he opes his mouth,
  Talks about his *dătta.*

And last we treat the hopeless guy,
  If he doesn't know better he oughta,
Who in spite of profs and courses and books
  Still pronounces it *daughta.*

So with *dayter, dayta, dătta,*
  And with *data, daughta, dater,*
No matter where the mean may lie,
  Statistically, there's too much scatter.

I don't know what in h—l to do
  In this seeming simple matter;
But so long as God will grant me breath
  I'll never call it *dătta.*

F. E.

[4] Viosca, Percy, 1923, "Notes on the Status of *Hyla phaerocrypta* Cope," *Copeia*, 122: 96–99.

[5] Ridgway, Robert, 1924, "Additional Notes on *Hyla phaerocrypta* (?)," *Copeia*, 128: 39.

[6] Dunn, E. R., 1927, "*Hyla phaerocrypta* in Tennessee," *Copeia*, 162: 19.

SCIENTIFIC BOOKS

Comparative Meteorology, Manual of Meteorology, Vol. II. By Sir Napier Shaw, with the assistance of Elaine Austin. Royal 8vo, 225 illustrations. pp. xl + 446. Price $10.00. Cambridge University Press. Macmillan, Agents in United States.

When Sir Napier Shaw retired from the directorship of the Meteorological Office he set himself the task of preparing four volumes covering the general field of what we now call *Airgraphics*. This volume, although numbered as the second, is the third to appear; and, good as the others were, we are inclined to think this much better. Encyclopedic is the proper term to describe it. There is to begin with a dictionary of technical terms from "absolute" and "adiabatic" to "vortex" and "waves"; and those of us who teach thank him for such an aid to memory. Under "Lest We Forget" are definitions of symbols; and Heaven be praised a given letter stands for one and the same quantity throughout.

Furthermore, conversion tables are given in convenient places, for example, in entablatures with the maps. The result is that a student clearly visualizes the layout; and then, with systematic units, can proceed to tackle his problem without cluttering his desk with an armful of reference books. Will not future text-book writers take the hint? Before one undertakes to prepare a text-book, he should have a clean-cut conception of the physical quantities and processes that are operative. An indiscriminate use of symbols not only baffles the student, but may often trap a tired teacher. The detail of the auxiliary conversion tables deserves much credit. For example, if one wants to know the equivalent in a twenty-eight-, twenty-nine-, thirty-, thirty-one-day month of an annual rainfall of 70 mm., it is given to the third decimal place. Or if one wants at a glance the swing of the pressure over the northern hemisphere, the fine-print heading the chapter on pressure and wind explains a graphic integration of monthly charts of normal pressure; and one easily grasps the situation as a sine curve which follows the curve of total power of solar radiation over the hemisphere with a lag of twenty-seven days. Thus a generalized representation of what otherwise would require a treatise is given in a few lines. Subject to a correction of not more than five per cent. for air displacel by mountains, the mass of air on the Northern Hemisphere varies from its mean value by

Oct.	Nov.	Dec.	Jan.	Feb.	Mar.	Apr.	metric ton × 10^{12}
+ 0.1	1.7	4.2	5.1	4.4	1.7	0.3	
May	Jun.	Jul.	Aug.	Sept.			
− 1.6	4.2	5.1	4.1	2.5			

This is just one of many such treatments. The book is full of condensed data, the meat of each nut without much shell. Because of this new volume, reference books on a five-foot shelf within reach will no longer be consulted by this reviewer, as of yore. In his opinion it enables one who lacks easy access to a large library to meet on equal terms those who are thus fortunate. It may or may not have occurred to Sir Napier and to those who helped him (it was of course impossible for any one man to compile, assemble and analyze all the data which of necessity had to be licked into shape; and Sir Napier fully acknowledges the services of many coworkers, especially Austin, Harding, C. E. P. Brooks, Captain Brunt, Commander Garbett and the staffs of various official organizations) that they have laid the corner-stone of a coming all-important applied science. It is a strange thing that college presidents, with few exceptions, have been sound asleep concerning the need and value of instruction in *airgraphics,* heretofore rather disjointedly called meteorology, climatology, aerology, or physics of the air. Surely no college graduate can regard himself as an intelligent member of society, if he does not know something of the major circulations of the atmosphere and a little about minor circulations and the physical processes involved in the "endless making and unmaking of weather," to borrow from Professor James. Our college presidents concern themselves greatly with modern methods in education and talk at much length of this, that and the other need; but it seems never to have occurred to them that a chair of *airgraphics* is now much more needed than any existent chair. To say nothing of constant application to all phases of human industry, such a course of study would offer the student a tremendous intellectual stimulus. For the field is developing at an astonishing rate. To-day "the air's the thing!" and man is mastering his environment. He realizes at last that while he walks on the ground and sails the seas, he *lives in the air.* Here is high adventure for both brain and hand. So, then, every instructor in any of the sciences dealing with man in relation to his environment, must, if he would keep abreast of the times, read and profit by the information contained in this manual.

Needless to say, the University Press at Cambridge has done its best on this volume. The type work, the legends, the distribution of matter on the page, are all such as might be expected from master craftsmen. Doubtless the text came to them in excellent shape; but it lost nothing at the hands of those who gave it permanent form and dress.

Sir Napier Shaw must feel a large measure of satisfaction as he nears the completion of a work that is truly monumental. What younger man of our generation could have carried on so valiantly?

Alexander McAdie

Blue Hill Observatory,
Readville, Mass.

REPORTS

INTELLECTUAL COOPERATION AND BIOLOGY

SINCE its early days, the League of Nations has devoted attention to problems concerning the organization of intellectual life, apart from the political activity with which it is more commonly associated in the mind of the general public.

In 1922 an International Committee on Intellectual Cooperation was especially established for this purpose, composed of well-known men and women from the world of science, art and literature, and of which the late Professor Lorentz, the world-famous Dutch physicist, was chairman.

The position of this committee was considerably strengthened by the foundation in 1925 of the International Institute of Intellectual Cooperation in Paris, which provided a permanent international body recruited from specialists in the various branches of art and science for carrying out the resolutions of the committee and preparing the ground for future action.

Problems of scientific bibliography were among the first to engage the attention of the international committee and continue to occupy an important place in
The inquiry was first directed to the analytic bibliography of current literature in the case of the differ-
the activity of the scientific section.
ent sciences with a view to obtaining better results from the general bibliographical work which has been hitherto carried out in a disorderly and uncoordinate fashion in the different countries.

Having dealt with the physical and economic sciences, the question of biological bibliography was placed on the agenda of the international committee.

It should be pointed out that the technical difficulties encountered in the different sciences are practically the same and therefore the methods previously adopted for the other sciences have been applied in the case of biology.

The first step was to convene a meeting of experts, composed of editors of reviews especially devoted to the biological sciences. This meeting was held at the International Institute of Intellectual Cooperation on April 7 and 8, 1927.

The following were present:

Miss Bonnevie, professor of zoology at the University of Oslo, member of the International Committee on Intellectual Cooperation.

M. Apstein, *Zoologischer Bericht.*

M. Baur, *Zeitschrift für induktive Abstammungs- u. Vererbungslehre.*

M. Fedde, *Botanischer Jahresbericht.*

M. Kerkhof, Reichszentrale für Wissenschaftliche Berichterstattung.

Mr. Hutchinson, *Biological Abstracts.*

M. Fauré-Fremiet, *Année Biologique.*

M. Mesnil, Institut Pasteur.

Mr. Chalmers-Mitchell, *Zoological Record.*

M. Kooiman, *Resumptio Genetica.*

M. Racovitza, professor at the University of Cluj, correspondent of the International Committee on Intellectual Cooperation.

M. Strohl, *Concilium Bibliographicum.*

The above committee considered the actual problems of biological bibliography from many different aspects and passed the following resolutions concerning the methods to be employed in attempting a practical solution:

I. The committee of experts recognize that to obtain access to the literature is one of the greatest difficulties in the way of biological bibliography.

They are of the opinion that a great step in intellectual cooperation would be the reception, by those responsible for the preparation of abstracting and indexing publications, of separata (with the original pagination) of each memoir in scientific publications.

They recommend that steps should be taken, under the authority of the league, to induce the editors of journals publishing original work in biology to provide a limited number of separata of each paper sufficient to supply a copy to each bibliographical authority agreed upon by the conference, or its successors, as of international value.

They further recommend that an international organization (working through national bureaus if found more practical) be founded to receive the separata and distribute them to the appropriate bibliographical authorities.

II. The conference of experts are of the opinion that it would materially assist abstracting publications if an author's abstract were printed with every published paper.

They have been informed that the editors of some journals will not accept papers unless the authors have provided such an abstract, and they recommend that all editors should be invited to conform to this practice; such abstracts should average three to five per cent. of the original paper.

III. The committee of experts has considered a set of periodicals dealing with biological bibliography and has made a preliminary classification of them into groups, with the object of examining the possibility of cooperation and mutual help.

The classification is as follows: General biology; zoology; botany; systematics—zoology; systematics—botany; genetics; anatomy and embryology; microbiology and parasitology.

The following methods of cooperation are contemplated for each of these groups:

(1) Exchange of final proof-sheets (printed if possible on one side of the paper only), or of the publications themselves with rights of reproduction and translation, under conditions which might vary in the different cases.

(2) Separate sale of the bibliographical parts

(printed if possible on one side of the paper only) of those periodicals which also contain original matter.

IV. The committee of experts has charged certain of its members with the duty of getting into touch each in his own country with those most competent to prepare the details of cooperation.

The results of these negotiations shall be communicated to the institute, which shall make use of them in summoning first those interested in each separate group, and afterwards for the reunion of the full conference, which will be necessary before the attempt to bring into operation the proposed cooperative arrangements.

V. The conference of experts consider that a universally adopted system of abbreviations of the titles of periodicals would be an advantage which would outweigh the temporary inconvenience of changing the many existing systems.

They have been informed that bibliographical experts belonging to the British Museum have considered current systems and have devised a system which they have applied to the titles of 24,000 periodicals and that this list of abbreviations has been printed in Volume 2 of the World List of Scientific Periodicals.

They recommend that at their next meeting the possibility of the universal adoption of this system should be taken into favorable consideration.

These resolutions were approved by the international committee in July and by the Plenary Assembly of the league of Nations last September, and the institute was instructed to take the necessary action in order to put them into force.

It now remains to be seen whether biologists in general and in particular the editors of biological journals are sufficiently interested in this undertaking to make it a success.

As appears from the resolutions, the experts were of opinion that the different subdivisions of biology should be treated separately and the question now is to decide which of these subdivisions can most easily be made the subject of a common agreement, so as to concentrate on it in the first place.

Another aspect of the problem, which could not be dealt with at the time of the experts' meeting, is the extent to which our scheme should be altered in view of the publication of the *Biological Abstracts* in the United States, because before the meeting of the committee only one number had appeared.

The International Institute will welcome suggestions from the editors of biological reviews concerning the biological problems referred to in the experts' resolutions and will be glad to avail itself of their recommendations and collaboration in pursuing this work.

J. E. de Vos van Steenwijk

Section for Exact and Natural Sciences at the Institute of Intellectual Cooperation

SPECIAL ARTICLES

VARIATION IN SOLAR RADIATION

The Lick Observatory Bulletin No. 401 carries a series of measurements of the brightness of the planet Uranus and of the satellites of Jupiter by Stebbins and Jacobson. Similar measurements were made by Stebbins in the year 1926, also at the Lick Observatory. They employ a potassium cell, most sensitive in the blue, at approximately 4,600 Ångstroms.

Measurements were made on about twenty nights of August and September, 1926, and on about fifty nights in July, August and September, 1927. During these intervals the Smithsonian Institution maintained daily observations of the solar constant of radiation at its station on Mount Montezuma, in Chile. It is interesting to compare the two series (omitting dates not common), to see what they may indicate as to the variation of the sun during these intervals.

In making such a comparison, one might proceed with the theory that the sun is equally bright at all parts of its surface, and, if it varies, it varies as a whole in brightness. But many indications lead us to the other view that although, associated with the march of solar activity revealed in sun-spots, there are changes of the general brightness of the whole solar surface, yet, just as the solar corona and the solar surface present much detail to the telescope, so the sun as a source of radiation presents inequalities of surface brightness turned toward the dfferent directions in space. Accordingly, it seems best to take into account the heliographic longitude of the satellites and the planet observed by Stebbins, and also to consider the time occupied by light in traveling from

Observations of 1926

Dates: Montezuma	Dates: Lick	Departures: Tenths per cent. Montezuma	Departures: Tenths per cent. Lick	Difference—Montezuma from Satellites
August				
24	24	−1	+1	2
25	25	−1	+1	2
27	27	+4	−5	9
28	28	−1	−2	1
30	29	+2	−10	12
32	31	−2	+1	3
Sept.				
2	1	+1	−2	3
3	2	−2	−2	0
4	3	−1	0	1
5	4	+2	−4	6
6	5	+2	+5	3
7	6	+4	+2	2
8	7	−1	−1	0
9	8	−2	+7	9
	Means:	2	3	4

the sun to these distant mirrors and thence to the earth, and to correct the dates of the observations of Stebbins and his colleague to correspond with the dates of observation of the solar constant, by allowing for the time intervals required for the sun to rotate from the direction of the satellites and the planet to the direction of the earth.

The Lick observations are published as departures in stellar magnitudes from the mean brightness of the objects during the whole interval of observation. The

OBSERVATIONS OF 1927

Dates Montezuma	Dates Lick Satellites	Dates Lick Uranus	Departures: Tenths per cent. Montezuma	Departures: Lick Satellites	Departures: Lick Uranus	Differences—Montezuma from Satellites	Differences—Montezuma from Uranus
July	July						
27	24	23	+2	−4	−1	6	3
28	25	24	+1	−24	−2	25	3
29	26	25	−3	−8	−2	5	1
30	27	26	+1	−10	−4	11	5
31	28	27	0	......	−1	3	1
32	29	28	−1	−4	−1	3	0
33	30	29	+1	−2	−1	1	2
34	31	30	−1	−2	0	3	1
35	32	31	−1	+2	0	......	1
August	August						
5	2	1	0	+6	−2	6	2
6	3	2	0	−6	−2	6	2
7	4	3	+1	......	−2	......	3
9	6	5	−2	−13	−2	11	0
10	7	6, 7	−1	−1	−1	0	0
11	9	8	−5	+4	0	9	5
14	12	11	−2	......	+4	......	6
17	15	14	0	+4	+10	4	10
18	16	15	+2	−1	+11	3	9
19	17	16	−5	+6	−3	11	2
20	18	17	−1	+11	−9	12	8
21	19	18, 19	−6	+10	+4	16	10
22	21	20	−4	−1	+9	3	13
23	22	21	−5	+2	−6	7	1
24	23	22	−4	−4	+1	0	5
26	25	24	−2	......	+11	......	13
28	27	26	−2	......	−2	......	0
31	30	29	+5	......	+6	......	1
Sept.	Sept.						
3	3	2	0	......	+6	......	6
6	6	5	0	−20	−4	20	4
19	19	19	0	0	+4	0	4
20	20	20	+1	......	−3	......	4
21	21	21	+5	−2	−2	7	7
22	22	22	0	......	−6	......	6
23	23	23	+3	−2	−4	5	7
24	24	24	+2	0	+5	2	3
29	29	29	−1	−2	−2	1	1
Means:			2	6	4	7	4

solar constant measures at Mount Montezuma are given in calories per square centimeter per minute. I have reduced all these results from both stations to the corresponding condition of percentage departures from the mean values prevailing during the periods of observation. To avoid repetition of useless figures, I express these departures in tenths of a per cent.

It will be noted that the range of departures for the solar constant scarcely exceeds 1 per cent., while the range of the photoelectric measurements is somewhat greater. Stebbins and Jacobson decided that the measurements on Uranus in 1927 have greater weight than those on the satellites, as is indeed indicated by their smaller range.

The solar constant values as here employed are all reduced by the definitive method in which every known source of error has been eliminated, including systematic errors requiring several years of observation for their determination. They are as accurate, we think, as can ever be obtained.

On the whole, there is agreement on both sides that the short-interval solar variations during these periods were very minute. As the photoelectric measurements are not quite equal in accuracy to the solar constant measurements, it is not possible to be sure whether they really support one another in singling out any of the apparent minute solar variations as real. The agreement between Montezuma and Uranus from July 27 to August 10, 1927, is very close, but reveals no considerable solar changes. During the interval from August 19 to August 31, when Montezuma seems to indicate a range of 1 per cent. very consistently, the agreement, otherwise close, is marred by four considerable departures.

C. G. ABBOT

SMITHSONIAN INSTITUTION

SOCIETIES AND ACADEMIES

THE NORTH CAROLINA ACADEMY OF SCIENCE

THE twenty-seventh annual meeting of the North Carolina Academy of Science was held at the University of North Carolina, Chapel Hill, N. C., on April 27 and 28, 1928. Papers were presented before the general section of the academy on Friday morning and afternoon. Friday evening the retiring president, Dr. J. M. Bell, gave his presidential address on "Some Approaches to Fundamental Theory of the Physical Sciences." Saturday morning the academy met in the following sections: General section, chemical section, mathematics section and physics section. Seventy-nine papers and five exhibits were on the program (abstracts of most of these papers and complete papers of several will appear in an early number of the *Journal of the Elisha Mitchell Scientific Society*).

The executive committee reported the election of fifty-seven new members during the year and the reinstatement of eight former members. One hundred and sixty-five were present for the meeting.

Mr. H. E. Biggs, Jr., a student in the Greensboro high school, was declared the winner of the high school science prize, a silver loving cup, for the best essay submitted by a high-school student. (Essays for 1928 were confined to the fields of chemistry and physics).

The officers elected for the year 1929 were:

GENERAL ACADEMY

President, J. S. Holmes, state forester.

Vice President, Miss Mary Petty, North Carolina Woman's College.

Secretary and treasurer, H. R. Totten, University of North Carolina.

Executive committee, The above officers and J. W. Nowell, Wake Forest College; A. H. Patterson, University of North Carolina; and F. A. Wolf, Duke University.

Representative to the A. A. A. S., Bert Cunningham, Duke University.

CHEMICAL SECTION

Chairman, L. G. Willis, State College.

Secretary, L. B. Rhodes, State Department of Agriculture.

Councillor, A. S. Wheeler, University of North Carolina.

MATHEMATICS SECTION

Chairman, J. W. Lasley, Jr., University of North Carolina.

Secretary, W. W. Elliott, Duke University.

PHYSICS SECTION

Chairman, W. T. Wright, North Carolina Woman's College.

Secretary, C. C. Hatley, Duke University.

The twenty-eighth annual meeting of the Academy will be held at the North Carolina Woman's College, Greensboro, N. C., in the spring of 1929.

H. R. TOTTEN,
Secretary

THE KANSAS ACADEMY OF SCIENCE

THE sixtieth annual meeting of the Kansas Academy of Science was held at the Municipal University of Wichita, with one session at the Wichita High School, April 13 and 14, 1928. Two sessions on the first day and the forenoon of the second day were devoted to the presentation of papers and to business.

Dr. H. W. Foght, president of the university, gave a short address of welcome. The Wichita Chamber of Commerce sponsored a trip to the airplane factory. Following a banquet at the University cafeteria in the evening of April 13, the annual presidential address of the academy was given by Dr. Mary T. Harman, of the Kansas State Agricultural College. The subject of her address was "The Physical Unit of Life."

Officers were elected as follows:

L. D. Wooster, *president,* Hays State Teachers College.

W. B. Wilson, *first vice-president,* Ottawa University.

Hazel E. Branch, *second vice-president,* Municipal University of Wichita.

L. D. Havenhill, *treasurer,* University of Kansas.

G. E. Johnson, *secretary,* Kansas State Agricultural College.

Additional members of the executive council: E. O. Deere, E. A. White, F. C. Gates, Mary T. Harman.

Thirty-two papers were presented.

The Kansas Entomological Society met on April 14 in conjunction with and became affiliated with the academy.

The academy will meet at the Kansas State Agricultural College at Manhattan in 1929.

GEORGE E. JOHNSON,
Secretary.

THE INDIANA ACADEMY OF SCIENCE

THE spring meeting of the Indiana Academy of Science was held at Logansport, Indiana, on May 17, 18 and 19, with over one hundred members in attendance.

The area along the Wabash and Eel Rivers in this region is a particularly good one for the study of the Silurian stratigraphy and associated coral reefs.

Auto tours in all directions from Logansport gave botanists, zoologists as well as the geologists, ample opportunity for studying the subjects in which they were interested.

Dr. E. R. Cummings and Mr. Robert Schrock, of Indiana University, who have made a special study of the area, acted as guides and explained the geological features.

Dr. Ernest Carman and Dr. Paris Stockdale, of the department of geology of Ohio State University, attended the meeting.

The program committee consisted of Dr. Paul Weatherwax, of Indiana University, *chairman,* assisted by Drs. C. L. Malott, of Indiana University; E. B. Mains, of Purdue University; and W. M. Blanchard, of De Pauw University.

HARRY F. DIETZ,
Press Secretary

SCIENCE

Vol. LXVII JUNE 29, 1928 No. 1748

CONTENTS

The Past Twenty Years of Physical Astronomy: Dr. Walter S. Adams ... 637
Charles Henry Gilbert: Dr. David Starr Jordan ... 644
Scientific Events:
The International Dairy Congress; The Upper Klamath Wild-life Refuge; A Foundation for the Study of Children's Diseases; The American Executive Committee of the World Engineering Congress ... 645
Scientific Notes and News ... 647
University and Educational Notes ... 650
Discussion and Correspondence:
An Old Experiment on Collisions of the Second Kind: Dr. J. Rud Nielsen. *Another Wild Life Preserve near Ithaca:* Professor P. W. Claassen. *Ångström in English:* E. F. B. Fries. *Embryoless Seeds in Cereals:* Mildred E. Lyon. *The Host of the Broad Tapeworm:* Dr. Thomas B. Magath ... 651
Scientific Books:
Goldschmidt and Gordon's Crystallographic Tables for the Determination of Minerals: Dr. Alfred C. Hawkins ... 653
Scientific Apparatus and Laboratory Methods:
An Efficient Dehydrating Apparatus for General Use: Wilbur D. Courtney. *Immobilization of Paramecium:* J. C. Boland. *A Burette Cleaner:* F. H. Fish ... 653
Special Articles:
The Photo-mechanical Changes in the Retina of Mammals: Gordon L. Walls. *Egg Laying of Ixodiphagus Caucurtei du Buysson in Larval Ticks:* Professor R. A. Cooley and Glen M. Kohls ... 655
Science News ... x

SCIENCE: A Weekly Journal devoted to the Advancement of Science, edited by J. McKeen Cattell and published every Friday by

THE SCIENCE PRESS

New York City: Grand Central Terminal.

Lancaster, Pa. Garrison, N. Y.

Annual Subscription, $6.00. Single Copies, 15 Cts.

SCIENCE is the official organ of the American Association for the Advancement of Science. Information regarding membership in the Association may be secured from the office of the permanent secretary, in the Smithsonian Institution Building, Washington, D. C.

THE PAST TWENTY YEARS OF PHYSICAL ASTRONOMY[1]

A complete survey of the progress of physical astronomy during recent years would be so formidable an undertaking that to attempt to cover the entire field would require a whole series of lectures rather than a single evening. So I shall limit myself to the attempt to trace for you the development of only one or two of the more recent conceptions and methods of modern astrophysics and to show how greatly they have enlarged the views which we held, even as recently as the first ten years of this century. From the standpoint both of the results accomplished and the outlook toward the larger problems of astronomy there probably has never been a period quite comparable to that of the past twenty years.

The underlying cause of this remarkable progress has been the intimate relationship which has developed between physics and astronomy, so that important discoveries in the one science have reacted immediately upon the other and found far-reaching applications almost at once. A quarter of a century ago an immense amount of observational material had been collected in our physical laboratories and observatories to the interpretation of which the key was almost entirely lacking. We could hardly hope to understand the behavior of matter in the distant stars when the mechanism of the light given out by a candle flame was still quite unknown to us. So in astronomy, as in physics, a great new field was opened up by the fundamental discoveries of Rutherford, Bohr and many others on the structure of matter and the nature of radiation.

It is a commonplace to say that all our primary knowledge of stars is derived from the light which they give out, where the term *light* is used in a general way to include both visible light and invisible radiation, such as heat or X-rays. From a star's light we can measure its position, its slow movement across the sky, its brightness and its distance, but we can do a great deal more. By analyzing its light we can study its individuality, which is defined almost as uniquely by the faint rays of light which reach us as is the personality of a friend by the actions of his daily life. The main problem of physical astronomy,

[1] Address given in San Francisco on April 16, on the occasion of the presentation of the Bruce medal by the Astronomical Society of the Pacific.

accordingly, is to interpret the inscriptions which we find contained in these stellar records, which we call the spectrum.

To an observer who looks at the stars on a clear night the differences of color are very noticeable. Betelgeuse is red, Sirius is blue-white. If these stars are looked at through a piece of red glass, Betelgeuse still looks bright while Sirius becomes comparatively faint; through blue glass, on the other hand, Betelgeuse is very faint and Sirius remains bright. This means simply that most of the light of Betelgeuse is red light and that of Sirius blue light. If, instead of using colored screens, we look at the stars through a glass prism we obtain all the colors at once drawn out into a band which is known as the spectrum. Red lies at one end and violet at the other, with yellow, green and blue lying between. The red portion of the spectrum of Betelgeuse is very bright and the blue faint, while in Sirius the reverse is the case. We are all familiar with the fact that the color of the filament in the bulb of an electric lamp is red when the voltage is low, and quickly turns to white when the voltage becomes normal. If we should look at its spectrum we should see mainly red light when the filament first begins to glow, and much more blue light as the temperature rises. Hence we can reason directly that the temperature of Betelgeuse is low and that of Sirius very much higher because its blue light is so intense. Actually, the temperature of Betelgeuse is about 3,000° Centigrade (5,400° Fahrenheit) and that of Sirius is about 10,000° Centigrade.

We see then that the band of colored red light which we call the continuous spectrum gives us valuable information regarding physical conditions in the stars. Of much greater importance, however, is the network of dark lines which crosses the continuous spectrum, and which we see when a narrow slit is used in front of our glass prism. A spectrum of lines is formed whenever we heat a gas to the point at which it sends out light. For example, if we look with our prism at one of the long horizontal mercury lamps, used so extensively in the illumination of manufacturing plants, we see a number of colored bright lines. The most intense of these is a green line which is responsible for the rather ghostly color of the light, but there are other lines colored blue, yellow and red. Together these lines form the characteristic spectrum of mercury vapor. In the same way, if we pass an electric current between the ends of two iron rods and form an electric arc, the hot iron vapor gives us some two thousand bright lines, colored according to their position in the spectrum, which are characteristic of iron, and of iron alone. So each element has its own groups of spectral lines which distinguish it uniquely from every other element.

If we now compare directly the lines of the different elements with the dark lines which cross the continuous spectrum of the sun or of most of the stars, we find immediate evidence for the presence of the great majority of the elements in their atmospheres. The lines are dark as seen against the brilliant background, instead of bright as in our laboratory sources, but in number, position and intensity the correspondence is almost perfect. This gives us a means of analyzing the composition of the sun or of the most distant stars which we can observe with our spectroscope. The latest studies of the sun made in this way give definite evidence of the presence of fifty-seven of the elements known to the chemist on the earth. Six have been added to the number within the past few months, and there can be little doubt that all the others are present as well, our failure to observe them being due to physical conditions present in the sun which prevent their spectral lines from appearing with sufficient intensity.

This method of analyzing spectra in a qualitative way has been known for many years. So, too, has the extremely important fact that the spectral lines are displaced by small amounts when the source of light and the observer are approaching or receding from one another. If a star, or the edge of the sun due to its rotation, is approaching us more waves of light reach us in a second than if there were no relative motion. Hence the length of the waves is shortened slightly, and the spectral lines are shifted a trifle from their normal positions toward the violet end of the spectrum. Similarly, if a star is receding from us the displacement is toward the red end of the spectrum. The quantities to be measured are small, but they can be determined with remarkably high precision, and from them we can obtain the motions of the stars toward or away from the earth. This forms one of the most fruitful fields of investigation in all astronomy, for the results derived from it enable us to find at what rate our sun is moving in space, how the motions of the stars in our system are related, and how even the enormously distant universes of stars, the spiral nebulae, are moving with respect to us and to one another. The Lick Observatory was one of the pioneers in this type of research and has maintained its leading position in the accuracy with which it has carried on these difficult and exacting observations. The most recent publication of the Lick Observatory by Dr. Campbell with the collaboration of Dr. Moore forms a landmark in this field, and bears remarkable testimony to the skill and resourcefulness of these two eminent members of our society.

The situation at the beginning of the century as regards the interpretation of spectral lines, how they originate and what information they can give us concerning physical conditions in the sun and stars was much less satisfactory. We knew almost nothing about how an atom gives out light, and the different lines of the spectrum were necessarily classed together in most of our investigations. One important difference, however, had been recognized by Sir Norman Lockyer between some of the lines produced in the electric arc and the electric spark. In the spark spectrum of different elements certain lines were found to be much more intense than in the spectrum given by the arc, and these lines, to which Lockyer gave the name "enhanced," he considered as due to a modified form of the element arising from some sort of decomposition of the atom produced by the high temperature of the spark. In this hypothesis modern research has shown that he was substantially correct.

About 1905 a few studies were commenced which began to throw light upon the differences in behavior among different spectral lines. One of these was made at the Mount Wilson Observatory, and I should like to describe it in some detail, partly because it is of interest historically, but more because it illustrates the extent of the applications which a comparatively simple research may come to acquire. It is one more illustration, so frequent in scientific work, of the old Biblical story of how Saul went out to seek his father's asses and found a kingdom.

One of the earliest photographs of the spectrum of a sun-spot was obtained at Mount Wilson in 1905, nearly all observations before that time having been visual. Now the principal difference between the spectrum of a sun-spot and that of the general surface of the sun consists in the marked change in the relative intensities of great numbers of lines, some being weakened in the spot spectrum and others greatly strengthened. In many cases lines barely visible in the solar spectrum become very prominent in the spot. Many of the weakened lines we soon recognized as being enhanced lines, that is, lines stronger in the spectrum of the spark than of the arc, but we had no adequate explanation to account for the behavior of the strengthened lines. The attempt to find such an explanation was the object of an investigation begun at Mount Wilson a little more than twenty years ago.

As a working hypothesis we made the assumption that the temperature of sun-spots is below that of the general surface of the sun. Our problem, then, was to see whether we could duplicate under conditions of varying temperature in the physical laboratory the observed behavior of the spectral lines in sun-spots. For this purpose we used the iron arc, the supply of electric power on Mount Wilson being at that time quite inadequate for an electric furnace. The method used was to pass a powerful current through the arc and photograph the spectrum: then to reduce the current to as low an amount as possible and on the same plate to photograph the spectrum again. Since the amounts of energy passing through the arc were very different in the two cases it could fairly be assumed that the temperatures were also different. Later we simplified the method by magnifying greater the image of the arc and comparing the spectrum of the outer cooler flame with that of the hotter core near the iron poles.

The study of the photographs at once led to definite results. It was found that many iron lines were relatively much more intense in the flame than in the core of the arc, and that these were without exception just the lines which were strengthened in the spectrum of sun-spots. On the other hand, lines unaffected in different portions of the arc remained essentially unchanged in sun-spots. So we were able to classify the iron spectrum into groups of high and low-temperature lines, and to make an accurate comparison with the corresponding lines in the sun-spot spectrum, which showed remarkably good agreement. Soon afterward some experiments made in Pasadena with an electric furnace of temporary construction showed that the results obtained with the arc were definitely to be ascribed to the effects of temperature, and not to any electrical phenomena present in the arc. Finally, conclusive evidence for the low temperature of sun-spots was afforded by the discovery of the presence of bands in the spectrum, due to the existence of compounds which can exist only at reduced temperatures.

A few years later, when the Pasadena laboratory was completed, a thorough investigation of the spectra of many elements was carried out by Dr. King, and the lines were arranged in classes according to their behavior under known conditions of temperature. These results have confirmed and extended the earlier work at Mount Wilson, and have proved of immense value to all modern investigators who have analyzed spectra and studied the internal structure of the atom.

You will readily see that the discovery of the temperature classification of spectral lines meant much more than a means of interpreting the behavior of lines in the sun-spot spectrum. It formed essentially a new method of attack upon the physical problems of the sun and stars, especially as it was soon supplemented by other results showing the behavior of spectral lines under varying conditions of density and pressure. A partial breach had been in the hitherto almost impenetrable wall surrounding the interpretation of the spectrum.

The fundamental discoveries necessary to the adequate explanation of these results of observation came in the years following 1911 from the physical laboratories of Europe. Sir Ernest Rutherford first suggested that an atom of matter is an electrical structure built up out of natural units of positive and negative electricity. The positive charge is concentrated into an exceedingly minute nucleus; the negative charge extends over a relatively much larger region which, however, is only about one one hundred millionth of an inch in diameter. For a dozen years following the work of Bohr, every one thought of the electrons, the units of negative electricity, as describing tiny orbits around the nucleus, like planets around the sun. Now, since Schrödinger has developed his complicated but very successful "wave-theory," we are much less dogmatic about the exact position and motion of the negative electricity. We know, however, that under increasingly violent disturbance the negative charge can be split off from the atom, one natural unit at a time, to escape as free electrons; and we have good reason to believe that some of these unit charges are held very close to the nucleus and firmly bound, while others are near the outside of the atom and much more loosely held. The number of electrons outside the nucleus ranges from one for the simplest atom, hydrogen, and two for the next, helium, to twenty-six for iron, eighty-two for lead, and ninety-two for the heaviest known atom, uranium. A great many of the properties of atoms can be explained by means of a structure of successive shells of electrons. The laws of atomic structure fix the maximum number of electrons which can go into any one shell, so that a heavy atom like one of iron or lead contains several complete shells of electrons and an incompletely filled one on the outside.

Our immediate interest in the atom is concerned with the way in which it gives out or absorbs light. In an atom in its ordinary or normal state all the electrons are as close to the nucleus, which attracts them strongly, as the laws of atomic structure permit them to be. It is possible, however, by various means to raise one or two electrons into new positions which without serious error we may think of as farther from the nucleus. In this condition, known as an "excited" state, the atom is loaded with energy. If left to itself it will usually change back into a less excited state after something like a hundred millionth part of a second, and to do so it has to unload some of its energy, which is given out in the form of light. By a law of nature which appears to be one of the most fundamental that human science has yet discovered, but which remains utterly unexplained, the number of vibrations a second in the emitted light is exactly proportional to the amount of energy which the atom unloads. If this light is observed with a spectroscope we see a sharp line in a position in the spectrum defined accurately by the energy unloaded by the atoms which produced it. Since even the simpler atoms have dozens of excited states and the more complex several hundred—Dr. Russell has found 364 excited states in the case of the neutral titanium atom—the intricate character of the spectrum of many of the elements is easily understood.

In all these excited states the atom retains all its electrons, but it is possible through more violent disturbance, electrical or otherwise, to remove an electron completely. The atom is then called ionized and can exist in many different excited states. Changes between these states produce a whole new spectrum of lines, not one of which except by chance coincides with a line of the neutral atom. There is abundant evidence to show that the enhanced lines of the various elements come from ionized atoms with one electron missing, and the ordinary arc lines from neutral atoms with all their electrons present. Lockyer's bold hypothesis that the atoms giving the enhanced lines are partly decomposed is, therefore, substantially true, only it is a different kind of decomposition from that known to the chemist. It has been found possible to remove not only one, but two, three, or even more electrons from the atom. In these states, however, the energy emitted is usually so great that the resulting spectral lines lie far in the ultra-violet, where we could not observe them in the stars, or even in the sun.

With one more word we shall be ready to apply our knowledge. The spectra of the sun and stars show dark lines. This means that light has been absorbed by the reversal of the process already described. An atom can pick up energy from light passing by it and become excited, rising from a state of lower to one of higher energy: but it can do this only if the number of waves per second in the light is exactly sufficient to furnish the necessary energy for the change. Hence atoms of a given kind absorb a definite set of sharp spectral lines, identical in position with those which they emit. Any particular atom, however, can not absorb all the lines of the spectrum, but only such as correspond to a transition from its particular state to some other, and can absorb only one of these at once. So when we find thousands of absorption lines in the spectrum of iron, we realize that among the trillions of atoms present in the iron vapor thousands of different processes are occurring. The work of the last five or six years has gone so far in the interpretation of complex spectra that we can take almost any line in a stellar spectrum and say not only what sort of atom produced it, but also, so far as energy transitions go, just what the atom was doing at that time.

Suppose now that we have a long tubular electric furnace in our laboratory and pass white light through it. Inside our furnace is a bit of metallic sodium. At a low temperature, far below a red heat, the sodium begins to vaporize, and in the spectrum of the light which has come through the vapor we find the familiar pair of dark lines in the yellow, as well as others in the ultra-violet. But if we heat our furnace to 2,000° Centigrade we shall find new absorption lines appearing in the orange, the green and the blue, no trace of which could be obtained with the cooler vapor.

The reason is not far to seek. In the cooler vapor practically all the atoms are in the normal state of lowest energy. Such atoms can absorb some of the spectral lines, but not all; and though by this absorption they are raised to excited states each one falls back again so soon that the number of atoms per million which are excited at any given instant is very small. But as we heat our gas hotter and hotter the collisions of its atoms become violent, and as a result a small but steadily increasing fraction of the atoms will be raised to the excited states and absorb other lines.

We see now why the lines belong to different temperature classes and just what these classes mean. The low-temperature lines are absorbed by atoms in unexcited or mildly excited states; the high-temperature lines by highly excited atoms. We see, too, what the relatively great strength of the low-temperature lines in the spectra of sun-spots means. There are more unexcited atoms in the sun's atmosphere above a spot than elsewhere, and this means that the atmosphere there is cooler.

This is not all, however. At a sufficiently high temperature the collisions between the atoms of a gas become so violent as to knock electrons completely off from some atoms and the gas becomes partially ionized. The process is self-limited, since the wandering free electrons will sooner or later meet with other ionized atoms and recombine with them. But the hotter the gas the more numerous will be the ionized atoms and the fewer the neutral atoms. At the temperature of the sun elements which require less energy for the removal of an electron, like calcium or scandium, are very considerably ionized; those which require more, like iron and silicon, are much less ionized. So the enhanced lines of calcium are strong and those of iron relatively weak. Above sun-spots, where the gas is cooler and the proportion of the neutral atoms is greater, the arc lines therefore become stronger, especially for the more easily ionized elements, and the enhanced lines weaker, especially for the elements which are hard to ionize. The combination of these principles affords a detailed and complete explanation of the peculiarities of the sun-spot spectrum which have so long been extremely puzzling.

There is another factor in the process of ionization which is of equal importance in the study of the sun and stars. Let us suppose that we have a mass of gas at a given high temperature. If it is dense the atoms and electrons will be close together, and the chances of their meeting and recombining will be good. But if the gas is allowed to expand and become rarefied the chances of recombination become steadily less. The percentage of atoms which are ionized increases therefore as the pressure diminishes.

This solves a solar puzzle of long standing. At the time of a total eclipse of the sun we can observe its upper atmosphere, the chromosphere, and measure the heights to which the different spectral lines extend. We then find that the enhanced lines of the different elements rise to a much greater height than the low-temperature lines. For example, the H and K enhanced lines of calcium reach a height of seven thousand miles and the blue low-temperature line λ 4227 a height of only three thousand miles. Since the top of the chromosphere should be cooler, if anything, than the bottom, we should expect the low-temperature line to be stronger at the top. The difficulty was solved by Saha, the Indian physicist, in 1920. Though the temperature is probably about the same throughout the depth of the chromosphere, the pressure and density must be far lower at the top than at the bottom. In the lower regions some neutral calcium atoms are present and give the low-temperature line; in the upper regions all atoms are ionized and the line due to the neutral atoms disappears.

One immediate application of this modern theory is to the spectra of the stars. We have every reason to believe that there are no great differences in the composition of the heavenly bodies, and that all the elements recognized upon the earth are present in them. Why, then, do we not see in their spectra the lines of all these elements? The answer is a very simple one. The sun and the stars are too hot or too cold, too rare or too dense to show all the lines at the same time. As we have seen, it takes much more energy to rob some elements of their electrons than it does others. A sun-spot and the red stars are comparatively cool, and the temperature is high enough to bring out strongly only those lines of the elements which require little energy for their excitation. So the low-temperature lines are strong and the lines of ionized elements are weak. At the higher temperature of the general surface of the sun the ionized lines become stronger. When we come to the hottest stars the elements become completely ionized, the lines due to the normal atom disappear and we have a spectrum consisting solely of lines due to very highly excited atoms. The spectra of the hottest stars, accordingly, are very simple, consisting of lines of ionized helium, doubly and triply ionized oxygen, nitrogen and one or two other elements. It would be quite possible to conceive of a star so hot that it had no lines at all, at least in the part of the spectrum we can observe. The temperatures of the hottest stars we know are certainly upward of 30,000° Centigrade (54,000° Fahrenheit), and may in some cases run as high as 100,000° Centigrade. At somewhat lower temperatures the normal helium lines begin to appear, then the lines of the ionized metals, such as iron, calcium and many others, and finally those due to the neutral atom of these elements. The spectra of the cooler stars, therefore, such as our sun, Arcturus, or Betelgeuse, with temperatures ranging from 6,000° to 3,000°, are very complex and rich in lines, the normal atom of iron alone contributing about two thousand lines to the observable part of the spectrum. Hydrogen is the only element to show lines in the spectra of practically all the stars, affording strong evidence of its extreme abundance throughout all space.

If we know the temperature and pressure of a gas the degree to which an element is ionized can be pretty accurately calculated. As we have already seen, the temperatures of the sun and the stars can be determined from such considerations as the color of their light, and by utilizing our knowledge of the intensities of the enhanced lines we can derive the pressures in the stellar atmospheres. In this way we find that the pressure in the sun's atmosphere is not more than one ten-thousandth part of the earth's atmosphere, and that, though it is many hundreds of miles deep, the whole quantity of gas in it is not more than would be contained in a layer of common air a foot or two thick. This is a very remarkable conclusion, but it is confirmed fully by the fact that a layer of gas in the laboratory an inch thick, and by no means all composed of metallic vapor, will give absorption lines stronger than those in the solar spectrum.

The question may fairly be asked why, if the sun's atmosphere is so very tenuous, we see a sharp edge and do not see down deeper into its interior. Ionization and the free electrons produced by it again give the answer. An ordinary gas, like atmospheric air, scatters a little of the light which passes through it, so that distant mountains, even in the clearest weather, are seen through a bluish haze. Various investigations have shown that an ionized gas acts in the same way, but many thousands of times more strongly, and that the haziness increases very rapidly with the density. Consequently, the sun's atmosphere, even at its very low density, becomes filled with an "electron haze," which prevents us from seeing deeply. Such a great flood of energy is flowing through it from the far interior of the sun that this haze appears intensely luminous and gives us the brilliant visible surface.

Recently we have commenced at Mount Wilson an attempt to determine the relative amounts of the various elements in the atmospheres of the sun and stars. For this purpose groups of related lines called "multiplets" are used, in the production of which it is possible to calculate from theory the relative numbers of atoms involved. On comparing the intensities of these lines in the solar spectrum we find that fully a million times as many atoms are active in producing the strongest lines as in giving one which is barely visible.

Using the same principles in the case of several of the brighter stars whose spectra can be photographed on a very large scale, we find that the amount of vapor of iron, titanium and similar metals in the atmospheres of the great red stars Betelgeuse and Antares is something like one hundred times greater per square mile of surface than for the sun. Most of the stars which have been studied so far are, in reality, far brighter than the sun, and have very extensive atmospheres. Procyon, the only star roughly comparable in brightness to the sun, has about the same amount of atmosphere. In the redder stars the low-temperature arc lines are much stronger, in comparison with the high-temperature lines, than in the sun. When the corresponding numbers of atoms are found, a fairly simple calculation gives the temperatures of the star's atmosphere. The resulting values range from 3,000° for Betelgeuse to 9,900° for Sirius and are in excellent agreement with those found from the color of the light.

The enhanced lines of iron and titanium, due to the ionized atoms, are also stronger in Betelgeuse and Antares than in the sun. In view of the much lower temperature we might expect them to be weaker; and it appears that they must be produced in a region of very low pressure; in other words, in the very extensive chromospheres. The hydrogen lines, which are absorbed only by hydrogen in a highly excited state, might be expected to be weaker in these cool red stars. They are actually stronger than in the sun and appear also to arise in the chromosphere. This apparently chaotic set of facts is brought into intelligible order by the modern theory of stellar atmospheres.

Two things determine the equilibrium of a star's atmosphere, the force of gravity and the amount of heat which flows outward per square mile of its surface. The former controls the rate at which pressure increases in the deeper layers, while the latter fixes the temperature of the visible surface and also provides an upward radiation pressure which holds up the atmosphere against gravity and makes it far more extensive even in the sun than it would otherwise be. When gravity at the surface is small the pressure and density in the atmosphere are low and the electron haze is thin. We, therefore, see down through more material, and the total quantity of atmosphere above a given area of the surface is large. At the same time, owing to the lower pressure, the gas is more highly ionized than in the sun, and the enhanced lines are relatively stronger. Radiation pressure, moreover, is stronger in comparison with gravity and can support a more extensive atmosphere in which ionization is high. This still further strengthens the enhanced lines, and also those of hydrogen, which, having the lightest atoms, is easily supported.

The special characteristics which are thus broadly outlined are exactly those of the giant stars, while the much fainter dwarfs show the opposite peculiarities. But why should low surface gravity be associated with great brightness in a star? The answer comes from the famous work of Professor Eddington, which shows that the brightness of a star depends mainly on its mass and increases very rapidly as this increases. For stars of the same mass but different sizes both gravity and radiation pressure diminish as the diameter increases, but in the same proportion, and it can be shown from this that the extent of atmosphere will be a good deal the same for all. But for stars of different mass, whatever their size, the radiation pressure increases much faster than does gravity, and the massive stars should have much more extensive atmospheres and chromospheres than the less massive stars.

This brings us at once to the last application which I shall attempt to make of our theory, that to the determination of the intrinsic brightness and distances of stars. Stars may appear bright to us because they are intrinsically very luminous or because they are very near. For example, the two stars Procyon and Betelgeuse appear in the sky of nearly the same brightness. We know, however, that Betelgeuse is very much farther away, and that if they were at the same distance Betelgeuse would appear at least one thousand times as bright as Procyon. We might then say that if the intrinsic brightness or candle-power of Procyon is 1, that of Betelgeuse is 1,000.

It was nearly fifteen years ago that we made our first attempts at Mount Wilson to learn whether the intrinsic brightness of a star had any influence on its spectrum, the work being a direct outgrowth of our study of the sun-spot spectrum and the temperature classification of spectral lines. Knowing from direct measurement the distances and hence the intrinsic brightness of many stars, we could compare directly the spectrum of a very luminous or giant star with that of an intrinsically faint or dwarf star of nearly the same temperature. This showed at once that many of the enhanced lines and those due to hydrogen were very strong in the giants and weak in the dwarfs, while the behavior of other lines, mainly low-temperature lines, was just the reverse. With the aid of stars of known brightness it then proved comparatively simple to establish a relationship which would give us the intrinsic brightness of a star as soon as the relative intensities of these lines were known. The distance is obtained at once from an easy calculation based on the intrinsic brightness, as compared with the apparent brightness in the sky.

The method has two very considerable advantages. It is rapid, since a single photograph of spectrum will yield a value of the intrinsic brightness and distance of a star; and it is applicable to stars whose distances are so great that the usual direct method of measurement can not be used. The nearest star to us is at a distance of twenty-five million million miles, and most of even the brighter stars are from ten to one hundred times farther away. As seen at these greater distances the earth's orbit becomes almost vanishingly small. In the spectroscopic method, however, the intrinsic brightness of a star can be determined equally well whatever its distance. Hence the method has been used extensively at several observatories during recent years, and has nearly tripled the number of stars for which we know the distance.

A very interesting result of this increase in our knowledge of the real brightness of the stars is the extraordinary range which we find. There is a faint star recently observed by van Maanen which gives out only one fifty thousandth part the light of our sun; on the other hand, the bright southern star Canopus is at least ten thousand times as luminous as our sun, and there are doubtless other stars still brighter or fainter than those which have been observed. So we have a range of at least five hundred million, and probably one thousand million, in the quantity of light which the stars are pouring out.

The spectral differences between giant and dwarf stars and the spectroscopic method of deriving the real brightness of the stars find a satisfactory explanation in the theory we have been discussing. Eddington has shown that the intrinsic brightness of a star is directly related to its mass and increases with it. As we have already seen, the more massive a star is, the more extensive is the atmosphere which it can support by the outward pressure of its radiation. Such an extensive atmosphere of low density favors the ionization of the atoms and we should expect to find the enhanced lines strong. On the other hand dwarf stars of small mass would have shallow atmospheres, and we should expect the enhanced lines to be weak and those due to the normal atom strong. This is in agreement with observation. Our spectroscopic method of finding the real brightness of stars appears, therefore, in the main to be a method of finding their masses. The immense size of such stars as Antares, with a diameter of about two hundred million miles, affords excellent direct evidence for the existence of the extensive atmospheres predicted by our theory.

I realize fully that in this very condensed statement it has not been possible to touch on some of the most interesting developments of modern physical astronomy, such, for example, as the processes which maintain a star's energy, and the source of supply of its enormous radiation. Yet the conception of how modern physics interprets the spectrum and modern astronomy applies it, and how largely both sciences are based upon the ultimate structure of matter and the nature of radiation, is a most illuminating and inspiring one, however inadequately I have been able to bring it before your minds this evening.

WALTER S. ADAMS

MOUNT WILSON OBSERVATORY

CHARLES HENRY GILBERT

DR. CHARLES H. GILBERT was born on December 5, 1859, at Rockford, Illinois, his parents removing later to Indianapolis. He died suddenly at Palo Alto, on April 20, 1928, from a paralytic stroke. His father, Edward Gilbert, came early from Bohemia, becoming an insurance and realty agent and a pillar of the Congregational Church of Oscar McCulloch, widely known as a philanthropist and as a liberal Christian. His mother, Sarah Bean, still vigorous and competent at the age of ninety-three, is a typical representative of the Massachusetts Puritans at their best, and America has no better stock.

Charles was a graduate of the Indianapolis high school, where he found his first scholarly inspiration under Herbert Edson Copeland, a brilliant young naturalist, one of the ablest Cornell has ever sent out, but who died untimely from a fall into White River in January, 1877. From Indianapolis, Copeland transferred him to his intimate friend, the writer, who had become professor of zoology in Butler University at Irvington, then a suburb of Indianapolis. Gilbert took from the University of Indiana in 1883 the degree of Ph.D., the river fishes being his specialty. He had followed Dr. Jordan to the University of Indiana, where he became instructor and later professor in zoology. With the exception of four years as professor at the University of Cincinnati, he was continuously associated with Dr. Jordan, from 1877 to 1928, in Butler University, Indiana University and Stanford University, where he became emeritus professor in 1925.

In 1877, Dr. Gilbert had joined Dr. Jordan in a fish survey of the state of Georgia, a line of research not attempted before. In 1879 he was appointed by Professor Baird as secretary to Dr. Jordan's exploration of the fish fauna of the Pacific Coast, a research occupying most of 1880, and which Gilbert extended to Mazatlán and Panama. For many years the papers of "Jordan and Gilbert" were the most prolific in American ichthyology, their most extended paper being a descriptive "Synopsis of the Fishes of North America" in 1882.

From 1880 to 1928 Dr. Gilbert retained connection with the Fish Commission (later the Bureau of Fisheries). Since the first serious study of the Pacific salmon, by Jordan and Gilbert in 1880, he devoted his scientific work to the five American species of these fishes, until he came to know more of their character and habits than all other men taken together. The demonstration that their individual ages are recorded in their scales is largely his work, though others have made fruitful efforts at the same problem. The clue to his conclusions rests in the fact that in migratory fishes, the rings of growth recorded in the scales are larger and more wide-set during their well-fed life in the sea.

In nearly all the expeditions of Dr. Jordan to various parts of the world, Dr. Gilbert took an active part, as well as conducting others to Alaska, Hawaii, Japan and Panama. The ascent of the Matterhorn in 1881, with Dr. Jordan, Dr. M. B. Anderson and three students, was made at Dr. Gilbert's suggestion. In this adventure he was struck in the face by the fall of a great rock. This kept him, with Jordan, W. W. Spangler and two guides, one the famous Jean Baptiste ("John the Baptist") Aymonod, near the summit all night. His steel-rimmed Derby hat and careful ministrations by his comrades saved his life.

In 1909 Dr. Gilbert assisted the International Fisheries Commission in its salmon investigations, and for the last five summers he devoted himself almost wholly to salmon problems in Alaska.

In 1882 Gilbert was married to a fellow student, Julia Hughes, also interested in zoology and a member of the Matterhorn party. She died in November, 1915. During her life in Palo Alto she was a notable leader in favor of civic betterment. He left three children—Carl Gilbert, an attorney in Santa Fe; Ruth (Mrs. Percy B. Baker), of Atlanta, and Winifred (Mrs. Carl F. Braun), of Pasadena. All these are graduates of Stanford University.

Dr. Gilbert, one of the pioneers of the Stanford faculty, was a man of versatile genius. He had talent as musician and linguist, though his writings and lectures he confined rigidly to aspects of his chosen specialty. He was one of the most careful and accurate of scientific observers, the keenest and ablest critic in natural history I have ever known, and therefore a most helpful teacher. His attitude was wholly modern, though he had little interest in those writers who, as specialists building on fact, add wide deductions as to what may be, and assuming that all these are sound, frame far-reaching theories of consequences of evolution. Results attained too easily, by analogy and imagination, may be more discouraging to actual workers than ever the most rampant of systematized ignorance.

Dr. Gilbert was a man of rather less than average stature, but agile and wiry. In the words of "John the Baptist," "C'est un homme fort et brave" (a man strong and brave).

DAVID STARR JORDAN

SCIENTIFIC EVENTS

THE INTERNATIONAL DAIRY CONGRESS

THE eighth International Dairy Congress, to be held in Great Britain from June 26 to July 12, will be attended by 30 official delegates from the United States. In addition, a large number of unofficial delegates is expected to attend. The delegation sailed on June 16 on the *Leviathan*.

The seventh congress was held in the United States in October, 1923.

The congress will meet with London as headquarters, but excursions, tours and inspection trips will carry the delegates to practically all points in England. Receptions and numerous conferences for the reading of special papers and studies have a prominent place in the program.

The delegates named by President Coolidge to represent the United States are:

R. W. Dunlap, assistant secretary of agriculture, Washington, D. C.

Dr. L. A. Rogers, acting chief, Bureau of Dairy Industry, Department of Agriculture.

Roy C. Potts, chief, dairy marketing division, Department of Agriculture.

Dr. G. E. Sherwood, dairy farmer, Kimball, Minn.

A. J. Glover, editor, *Hoard's Dairyman*, Fort Atkinson, Wis.

J. D. Mickle, state food and dairy commissioner, Portland, Ore.

Professor J. B. Fitch, Kansas State Agricultural College, Manhattan, Kans.

A. M. Loomis, American Dairy Federation, Washington, D. C.

P. H. Kasper, cheese manufacturer, Bear Creek, Wis.

Professor A. A. Borland, Pennsylvania State College, State College, Pa.

Professor O. E. Reed, Michigan Agricultural College, East Lansing, Mich.

Dr. C. W. Larson, director, National Dairy Council, Chicago, Ill.

Dr. H. E. Van Norman, American Dry Milk Institute, Chicago, Ill.

D. M. Dorman, president, the California Dairies, Los Angeles, Calif.

A. L. Haecker, president, Allied State Creamery Association, Lincoln, Nebr.

Harry Bull, secretary, Dairymen's League, Orange County, New York.

Judge J. D. Miller, president, National Cooperative Milk Producers' Federation, New York City.

E. T. Rector, president, Fairmount Creamery Company, Omaha, Nebr.

W. J. Schilling, president, Twin City Milk Producers' Association, St. Paul, Minn.

Fred Rasmussen, secretary, International Association of Ice Cream Mfrs., Harrisburg, Pa.

E. M. Bailey, president, American Dairy Federation, Pittsburgh, Pa.

Dr. Robert S. Breed, bacteriologist, Agricultural Experiment Station, Geneva, N. Y.

T. H. McInnerney, president, National Dairy Products Corporation, New York, N. Y.

Dr. E. B. Meigs, Bureau of Dairy Industry, Department of Agriculture, Washington, D. C.

Frank S. Harmon, director of the Ohio Guernsey Breeders' Association, Cleveland, Ohio.

H. W. Jeffers, Walker-Gordon Laboratory Company, Plainsboro, N. J.

O. S. Jordan, president, Dairy and Ice Cream Machinery and Supplies Assn., New York City.

John Rundall, De Laval Separator Co., Chicago.

Professor George B. Caine, Utah Agricultural College, Logan, Utah.

Professor O. F. Hunziker, Blue Valley Creamery Company, Chicago.

THE UPPER KLAMATH WILD-LIFE REFUGE

BY executive order President Coolidge recently set aside for use as a refuge and breeding ground for birds and wild animals an area in southern Oregon embracing certain unappropriated public lands near the upper end of Upper Klamath Lake. The new reservation will be known as the Upper Klamath Wild Life Refuge and will be administered by the U. S. Bureau of Biological Survey. All the lands involved have been withdrawn for reclamation purposes in connection with the Klamath irrigation project in Oregon and California and, as with other reclamation projects set aside as wild-life refuges, are primarily under the jurisdiction of the Bureau of Reclamation of the Department of the Interior. The reservation of these lands as a bird refuge, therefore, is subject to use by the Bureau of Reclamation for irrigation and other purposes. A federal announcement says:

About 5,200 acres are included in the refuge, which extends as a rather long narrow strip between the Crater National Forest, embracing the high mountain range bordering this part of the Klamath River Valley on the west and Upper Klamath Lake. The refuge area consists mainly of marshland containing a dense growth of tules, sedges and other aquatic vegetation and affording abundant cover for the nesting wild fowl of the region. The marshes and the more open water areas also included will provide important feeding and resting grounds for migratory waterfowl, especially wild ducks and geese.

The establishment of the refuge will be of great importance to the waterfowl of the region, in view of the fact that there has been such extensive drainage of marsh areas in that general section in connection with the reclamation of lands for agricultural purposes. The reservation will be of great interest to conservationists generally as well as to sportsmen who are familiar with the drainage operations that have led to the practical elimination of Lower Klamath Lake, embracing about 80,000 acres and formerly one of the most important breeding grounds for resident waterfowl and feeding and resting grounds for migratory waterfowl in Western North America.

The creation of the refuge at Upper Klamath Lake will in a way serve to offset the disappointment that many felt because of the impracticability of reflooding Lower Klamath to save it as a wild-fowl haven. The development of wild-life refuges in this general section will provide for the needs of the birds on an important migration route near the Pacific Coast.

The new refuge will also extend needed protection to fur-bearing animals. It is unlawful, within the reservation, wilfully to set on fire any timber, underbrush, or grass, or after building a fire to leave it without totally extinguishing it; or to hunt, trap, capture or wilfully disturb any wild animal or bird or the eggs of any wild bird, except under such rules and regulations as may be prescribed by the secretary of agriculture.

A FOUNDATION FOR THE STUDY OF CHILDREN'S DISEASES AT YALE UNIVERSITY

PRESIDENT JAMES ROWLAND ANGELL, of Yale University, has announced that a gift of $1,000,000 has been made by A. E. Fitkin, of New York City. The foundation established by this gift is to be known as the Raleigh-Fitkin Memorial fund, in memory of Mr. Fitkin's son. Under the terms of the gift, a building is to be erected which will be known as the Raleigh-Fitkin memorial pavilion; which will cost $500,000, and which will be dedicated to the care of children. The remainder of the fund will be used as a permanent endowment fund, and will be administered by Yale University to further the objective of Mr. Fitkin's gift.

In announcing the gift, President Angell said:

It is with great gratification that I announce a most welcome gift to Yale of one million dollars, for the establishment of a foundation for the care of children, both from the standpoint of curative and preventive medicine, the study of children's diseases, and the training of men for the achievement of these purposes. It would be difficult to exaggerate the value of this first step in the completion of the plans made by the General Hospital Society of Connecticut and Yale University for the further consistent development here of a medical center of the highest character and of constantly increasing public service. Not only to the children of this community, but to children everywhere, both in the prevention and in the cure of disease, the work of the memorial will be of inestimable value. Reinforced by all the resources of the hospital and the medical school for the alleviation of every form of human suffering, the memorial will be able to multiply by many times its usefulness to the children for whom it is established.

THE AMERICAN EXECUTIVE COMMITTEE OF THE WORLD ENGINEERING CONGRESS

ADEQUATE presentation of America's engineering and industrial story at the sessions of the World Engineering Congress to be held in Tokio next year was discussed at a meeting of the executive committee of the American general committee for the congress held in the Engineers Club, New York, on May 18. Another outstanding feature was presentation of the report of Maurice Holland, executive secretary of the American committee.

Hospitality to be extended in the United States to European delegates in their movement from the Atlantic to the Pacific on the way to the Tokio congress was another subject which came up at the meeting. The entertainment committee reported that local engineering societies already have volunteered their services as hosts to the delegates from Europe.

Importance of careful selection of papers to be read as reflecting the status and tendencies of each of the major branches of engineering in this country was stressed in the report of the technical program committee, headed by Professor Dugald C. Jackson. The program group will call on the societies specializing in the different branches of industry for help in selecting authors for the American engineering papers. Since their acceptance would interfere with adequate presentation of the larger developments of engineering in the United States, miscellaneous papers will not be accepted for reading at the congress.

Professor Jackson announced the following as members, with himself, of the technical program committee: Allen Hazen, *vice-chairman;* H. Foster Bain, Alex Dow, W. F. Durand, J. R. Freeman, Bancroft Gherardi, George W. Fuller, F. L. Hutchinson, Major-General Edgar Jadwin, Dean Dexter S. Kimball, of the school of engineering of Cornell University; A. D.

Little, Fred R. Low, O. C. Merrill, Professor Michael I. Pupin, Calvin W. Rice, George T. Seabury, George Otis Smith and W. E. Wickenden.

Secretary Holland's report covered important phases of the work of the American committee, which is coordinating participation of engineering and industry in the United States in the Tokio sessions. The report went into the matters of coordination of activities, committee progress, financing, promotion and attendance and entertainment. Likewise, the need for further information from Japan on its own engineering and industrial conditions and progress was stressed.

SCIENTIFIC NOTES AND NEWS

DR. JAMES KENDALL, chairman of the department of chemistry, Washington Square College, New York University, has been elected an honorary member of the American Institute of Chemistry. On May 17 the department of chemistry of Washington Square College tendered him a farewell dinner, at which fifty-nine members were present. Dr. Kendall will soon leave to take up his duties as professor of chemistry at the University of Edinburgh.

THE highest award of the American Medical Association for achievement in scientific research, a gold medal, has been awarded to Surgeon Edward Francis, of the United States Public Health Service, for his "thorough and important scientific contributions to the knowledge of tularaemia."

THE Albert medal of the Royal Society of Arts has been awarded to Sir Ernest Rutherford, for his pioneer researches into the structure of matter.

IN connection with the International Geographical Congress in July, honorary degrees of Sc.D. are to be awarded by the University of Cambridge, to General Vacchelli, surveyor-general of Italy, the president of the congress, to Professor E. de Martonne, of the Sorbonne, and to Sir Charles Close, president of the Royal Geographical Society.

DR. GILBERT NEWTON LEWIS, professor of chemistry at the University of California, was the recipient of the honorary degree of doctor of science from the University of Wisconsin at the commencement exercises on June 18.

PRINCETON UNIVERSITY has conferred the honorary degree of doctor of science on Dr. Robert A. Millikan, director of the Norman Bridge laboratory of physics at the Pasadena Institute of Technology, and on Dr. Rudolph Matas, emeritus professor of surgery at Tulane University.

DR. G. CANBY ROBINSON, director of the medical center to be erected by Cornell University and New York Hospital, received the honorary degree of LL.D. from Washington University, on June 5, in recognition of his services to the university and of his contributions to medicine.

DR. HERBERT E. IVES, physicist at the Bell Telephone Laboratories, New York, received from Dartmouth College the honorary degree of doctor of science on June 19.

RUTGERS UNIVERSITY has conferred the honorary degree of doctor of laws on Dr. H. N. Davis, president-elect of Stevens Institute, and the degree of doctor of science on Dr. Frank B. Jewett, president of the Bell Telephone Laboratories, and on Edgar D. Tillyer, optical designer for the American Optical Co.

AT its commencement on June 4, Franklin and Marshall College conferred the honorary degree of doctor of science on Professor David Riesman, of the University of Pennsylvania.

WILLIAM BEEBE, of the New York Zoological Society, received the honorary degree of doctor of science from Colgate University on June 11 and that of doctor of letters from Tufts College on June 18.

THE Republic of France has named Professor G. S. Whitby, of the department of chemistry at McGill University, "officier d'académie," this honor being the first grade of the decoration "officier de l'instruction publique."

DR. E. P. WIGHTMAN, of the research laboratory of the Eastman Kodak Company, Rochester, N. Y., has been elected a fellow of the Royal Photographic Society of Great Britain.

DR. A. M. HANSON, of Faribault, Minnesota, was awarded the prize of $250 by the Minnesota Society of Internal Medicine at its last meeting held in Duluth on May 5. This is an annual prize awarded by the society to the general practitioner in the state who has made the most important contribution to medicine during the year. The prize was awarded to Dr. Hanson in recognition of his work in the isolation of the hormone of the parathyroid gland.

THE first award of the University of Buffalo medal in ophthalmology was made at the recent commencement to Dr. Edmund B. Spaeth, of Philadelphia, for his contributions to the field of ophthalmic plastic surgery. Annual award of the medal is made possible by the gift of a sum of money by Dr. Lucien Howe, professor emeritus of ophthalmology at the university.

DR. RALPH A. FENTON and Dr. Olof Larsell, of the University of Oregon Medical School, were awarded the Casselberry prize of $500 by the American Laryngological Association for work on the pathway of pain referred to the ear in nose and throat diseases.

The second annual award of the orthopedic scholarship of the Hospital for Joint Diseases, New York, of $2,400 yearly, bequeathed by Henry W. Frauenthal, founder of the hospital, was given to a member of the intern graduating staff, Dr. David Sashin.

The first award of the Alexander Brown Coxe memorial fellowship, at Yale University, with a stipend of $2,500, for research in the biological sciences, has been awarded to Dr. Ezra A. Sharp. Dr. Sharp will do research work in immunology and pathology.

After a continuous service of forty years, Dr. George H. Monks has retired from the active teaching staff of the Harvard Dental School. In view of his long-continued, devoted and valuable work for the school and the dental profession, the alumni council has voted that an oil portrait of Dr. Monks be hung in the halls of the school.

Dr. Edward B. Gleason, professor of otology in the University of Pennsylvania Graduate School of Medicine, was guest of honor at the fourth annual dinner of the Physicians' Square Club, on May 25, in recognition of his having completed fifty years in the practice of medicine.

Professor A. W. Porter, F.R.S., is retiring from the chair of physics at University College, London. He was entertained at dinner in the college on June 25 by present and past members of the College Mathematical and Physical Society.

Dr. Frederick E. Breithut, of the College of the City of New York, has been elected president of the American Institute of Chemists.

At the twelfth annual meeting of the National Board of Medical Examiners, Washington, D. C., on May 3, Dr. Evarts A. Graham, professor of surgery, Washington University Medical School, St. Louis, was elected to membership to succeed Dr. John M. T. Finney, Baltimore, whose term expired.

Professor G. S. Whitby, of McGill University, was elected president of the Canadian Chemical Association at the eleventh annual Dominion Chemical Convention held at London, Ontario, from June 6 to 8. This newly-formed association will embrace all local chemical organizations in Canada.

Preston S. Arkwright, of Georgia, was elected president of the National Electric Light Association at the convention held in Atlantic City.

Dr. Hermann J. Muller, professor of zoology in the University of Texas, has been awarded the university research professorship, under the provisions of which he will have most of his time free for research.

Dr. George T. Pack has resigned from his post of professor of pathology and assistant dean of the school of medicine at the University of Alabama, to accept a three-year fellowship appointment at the Memorial Hospital for malignant diseases, in New York City.

Arthur Lowell Bennett, who has been at the Lowell Observatory the past two years, has been appointed to the Thaw fellowship in astronomy at Princeton University.

Dr. Walter N. Ezekiel, formerly National Research Fellow in botany at the University of Minnesota Agricultural Experiment Station, has been appointed to succeed Dr. L. J. Pessin as plant pathologist in the cotton root rot project of the Texas Agricultural Experiment Station.

Dr. Carl O. Lampland, of the Lowell Observatory, Flagstaff, Arizona, has been appointed an exchange professor at Princeton University in exchange for Professor Raymond S. Dugan.

Dr. Clarence F. Jones, of the department of geography at Clark University, and Dr. C. F. Marbut, chief of the U. S. Bureau of Soils, will make a tour of northern South America this summer to make a study of the agriculture of that region.

Alexander Silverman, head of the department of chemistry at the University of Pittsburgh, sailed on May 18 for a three months' tour of Europe. Professor Silverman will accompany the tour of the American Ceramic Society and will later visit educational institutions, museums and glass factories in France, Switzerland, Italy, Austria, Germany, Czechoslovakia, Belgium, the Netherlands, England and Scotland.

F. W. Pettey, senior entomologist of the Union of South Africa, is visiting the United States on behalf of the South African government to study the work of agricultural experiment stations. He will represent South Africa at the International Congress of Entomology in Ithaca, N. Y., in August.

L. E. S. Eastham, lecturer in advanced and economic entomology at the University of Cambridge, has been appointed to represent the university at the International Congress of Entomology.

Dr. T. Shiraki, of the Government Experiment Station at Formosa, who has been spending some time in European museums, recently spent a week at the U. S. National Museum for the purpose of studying type specimens of Japanese and other Oriental insects.

At the thirty-seventh annual general meeting of the Institution of Mining and Metallurgy, held in London on May 17, the Honorable Peter Larkin, high commissioner for Canada, presented to the institution on behalf of Canadian friends and admirers of the late Dr. Willet G. Miller, provincial geologist for Ontario, a replica of the portrait of Dr. Miller which is now hanging in the Ontario Parliament Buildings.

Nature states that one of the houses occupied by Newton when living in London stood on the corner site between St. Martin's Street and Orange Street, where the Westminster City Council is now erecting a new public library, and that the council has decided to commemorate Newton's connection with the site by cutting an inscription on the stone face of the building to read as follows: "Sir Isaac Newton lived in a house on this site, 1710–1727."

DR. ROBERT EDGAR ALLARDICE, emeritus professor of mathematics at Stanford University, died on May 6, aged sixty-six years.

E. T. MEREDITH, editor and publisher of farm journals and formerly secretary of agriculture in President Wilson's cabinet, died on June 17, aged fifty-one years.

THE personnel of the division of chemistry and chemical technology of the National Research Council for 1928–29 will be as follows: George A. Hulett, Princeton, *chairman;* W. C. Geer, New Rochelle, N. Y., *vice-chairman;* Roger Adams, University of Illinois; Marston T. Bogert, Columbia University; R. M. Burns, Bell Telephone Laboratories; W. M. Clark, the Johns Hopkins Medical School; James B. Conant, Harvard; William J. Hale, Dow Chemical Company; Harry N. Holmes, Oberlin College; Charles A. Kraus, Brown University; S. C. Lind, University of Minnesota; Edward Mack, Jr., Ohio State University; H. S. Miner, Welsbach Company; James F. Norris, Massachusetts Institute of Technology; Charles L. Parsons, Washington, D. C.; C. L. Reese, E. I. du Pont de Nemours and Company; C. M. A. Stine, E. I. du Pont de Nemours and Company; W. T. Taggart, University of Pennsylvania; E. W. Washburn, Bureau of Standards; Frank C. Whitmore, Northwestern University.

IN response to an invitation issued by G. Albini, Senator, rector of the University of Bologna, and the president of the organization committee of the International Congress of Mathematicians, the American Mathematical Society has named six persons as follows: Professor R. C. Archibald, Brown University; Professor G. D. Birkhoff, Harvard University; Professor H. F. Blichfeldt, Stanford University; Professor Edward Kasner, Columbia University; Professor Oswald Veblen, Princeton University; Professor Virgil Snyder, Cornell University. Should a chairman be necessary President Snyder has appointed Professor G. D. Birkhoff to act.

FROM May 22 to 24 the Royal Society of Canada met west of Ottawa for the first time. The sessions were held in Winnipeg in the University of Manitoba and the legislative building. Dr. A. H. R. Buller, professor of botany in the University of Manitoba, delivered the presidential address on "The Plants of Canada, Past and Present," and Dr. J. J. R. Macleod, recently appointed Regius professor of physiology in the University of Aberdeen, gave the annual popular address, selecting as his subject "The Air we Breathe." Thirty-eight papers on history and literature, and 179 papers in the various sciences, were communicated to the five sections of the society. M. Camille Roy, of Laval University, Quebec, was elected president, and Professor A. S. Eve, F.R.S., vice-president, for 1928–29.

A CONFERENCE was called by the Federal Horticultural Board at the U. S. Department of Agriculture, Washington, D. C., for June 27, for the purpose of considering the advisability of modifying the requirements governing the interstate movement of five-leafed pines and of currant and gooseberry plants on account of the white pine blister rust. Fifteen states have been designated by the Secretary of Agriculture as infected with this disease, namely: Connecticut, Idaho, Maine, Massachusetts, Michigan, Minnesota, New Hampshire, New Jersey, New York, Oregon, Pennsylvania, Rhode Island, Vermont, Washington and Wisconsin. Five-leafed pines originating in these states are not at present allowed to be moved into non-infected states nor from heavily to more lightly infected ones.

AT the annual meeting of the British Association to be held in Glasgow from September 5 to 12, Sir William Bragg, who succeeds Sir Arthur Keith as president, will deliver an address on the subject of "Craftsmanship and Science" at the inaugural general meeting in St. Andrew's Hall. Dame Helen Gwynne-Vaughan, professor of botany at Birkbeck College, London, has accepted the office of president of Section K (botany) of the association, and will address the section on the subject of "Sex and Nutrition in the Fungi." Professor R. H. Yapp was originally elected president of the section, but resigned when he found he was unable to attend the meeting. Further details of the meeting were printed in SCIENCE for June 15, page 599.

AN international conference on the physical, biological and therapeutical aspects of light will be held at Lausanne from September 10 to 12, and the following day will be spent at Leysin. According to the

British Medical Journal, the subjects to be dealt with include a lecture on the therapeutic, prophylactic and social aspects of heliotherapy, by Dr. Rollier; heliotherapy in Belgium; radiation of food; a lecture on the sun and artificial light, by Professor Leonard Hill, and pigmentation caused by light. Inquiries should be addressed to the Secrétariat Général de la Première Conférence Internationale de la Lumière, Lausanne, Switzerland.

Charles F. Brush, inventor of the arc light, has set aside $500,000 to establish a foundation to be known as the Brush Foundation, in the memory of the inventor's son, Charles F. Brush, Jr., who died a year ago. The income is to be used by a board of managers to finance efforts contributing toward the betterment of the human stock and toward regulation of increase in population, to the end that children shall be begotten only under such conditions as make possible a heritage of mental and physical health and favorable environment. Those named to administer the fund are: Dr. T. Wingate Todd, Western Reserve University; the Reverend Joel B. Hayden, Mrs. Charles F. Brush, Mrs. Roger P. Perkins, Mrs. William H. Weir and Jerome C. Fisher, attorney.

Recently a group of public-spirited laymen, acting through Dr. Edward L. Keyes, president of the American Social Hygiene Association, invited a group of syphilologists and investigators interested in syphilis to meet at the Hotel Plaza, New York City, for the purpose of organizing the Committee on Research in Syphilis. While the importance of syphilis is well known to the medical profession, large funds for the systematic study of the disease have, with the exception of the government appropriations during the war, been exceedingly difficult to obtain. The Committee on Research in Syphilis will distribute annually through its subcommittees the funds made available by the group of donors, to subsidize and develop research in both the clinical and laboratory aspects of the disease. It is the purpose of the committee to expend the sums placed at its disposal in the development of a constructive program of research with planned activities and selected cooperators, and, upon the stimulation through grants, of researches already in progress or about to be undertaken. There will be for the present, at least, no investment in plant.

A gift of $250,000 to the University of Pennsylvania for the establishment of a foundation to study the prevention of diseases of the heart and circulatory system has been made by Edward B. Bobinette, of Philadelphia. It is announced that Mr. Bobinette plans to give additional funds to the foundation.

A research fund of $7,500 per year has been placed in the school of engineering of the Johns Hopkins University by the Utilities Research Commission of Illinois for an investigation of the properties of impregnated paper as used in the insulation of high voltage cables. The work will be under the direction of Dr. J. B. Whitehead, professor of electrical engineering. Dr. Whitehead is chairman of the committee on electrical insulation of the National Research Council, and the work referred to is part of the coordinated plan which is being proposed by that committee. Other similar investigations under Dr. Whitehead's direction are the influence of air and moisture in impregnated paper, supported by the National Electric Light Association, and dielectric absorption, supported by the engineering foundation, with the cooperation of various electrical industries.

The family of the late Fred C. Bowditch has presented his collection of Coleoptera to the Harvard Museum of Comparative Zoology. There are two principal portions: a general collection of Coleoptera of the world based on the G. D. Smith collection, and a special collection of the Chrysomelidae, containing the Jacoby collections (except part of the second), the Tring Museum collection, and an enormous amount of other material. This is said to be the largest private collection of beetles ever made.

UNIVERSITY AND EDUCATIONAL NOTES

President Lowell, of Harvard University, has announced gifts of $6,146,000 made to the university during the past year. This includes $350,000 which has been offered for a new gymnasium, and $350,000 to come from two anonymous donors, gifts not previously made public. President Lowell announces also that the $1,000,000 Arnold Arboretum fund has been fully subscribed.

The $1,000,000 mark in the alumni fund of Princeton University for increasing faculty salaries has been passed. The goal is $2,000,000.

Gifts for Washington University totaling $1,186,444 were made public at the commencement exercises.

Subscriptions totaling $1,000,000 have been received by the University of Southern California for its semi-centennial fund.

The following changes were made relative to the personnel of the faculty of the school of medicine at a recent meeting of the board of trustees of Vanderbilt University: The resignation of Dr. G. Canby Robinson was accepted and Dr. W. S. Leathers, professor of preventive medicine, was elected as dean of the school; Dr. C. Sidney Burwell was made professor of medicine and physician-in-chief of the hospital

Dr. Hugh Morgan was promoted from an associate professorship to a professorship of clinical medicine, and Dr. Horton Casparis was made professor of pediatrics and head of the department.

AT Yale University, Elliott Dunlap Smith, of the Dennison Manufacturing Company, has been appointed professor of industrial engineering in the Sheffield Scientific School; Dr. John Rodman Paul has been appointed assistant professor of medicine, and Dr. Roland Charles Travis has been appointed esearch associate in psychology, with the rank of ssistant professor, in the institute of psychology.

PROMOTIONS which have been recently announced n the department of chemistry, University of Wisonsin, are: from associate professor to professor, Iomer Adkins and Farrington Daniels; from asistant professor to associate professor, George J. Kemmerer, S. M. McElvain and H. A. Schuette.

DR. FLORENCE PEEBLES, lecturer for the extension epartment of the University of California at Los ngeles, has been appointed professor of biology in e California Christian College in Los Angeles.

A. BRAZIER HOWELL, of the U. S. National Museum, as been appointed lecturer in comparative anatomy the department of anatomy at the Johns Hopkins Iedical School.

DR. ERICH VON GEBAUER-FÜLNEGG, assistant proessor at the University of Vienna, has received a milar appointment on the chemistry staff of Northestern University.

R. A. WARDLE, lecturer in economic zoology in the niversity of Manchester, has been appointed to the air of zoology in the University of Manitoba, anada.

ISCUSSION AND CORRESPONDENCE

N OLD EXPERIMENT ON COLLISIONS OF THE SECOND KIND

THIRTY-SEVEN years ago, in the course of an investition on the spectroscopic determination of potasım, F. A. Gooch and T. S. Hart[1] made the interestg observation that the presence of sodium in a flame nds to increase the intensity of the red potassium ublet. A small helix of platinum wire was dipped a solution of potassium and sodium chloride, dried d introduced in the outer cone of the flame of a rge Bunsen burner. The potassium line was obrved in a small spectroscope with the telescope set that the yellow sodium doublet fell outside the field view. The effect of varying the amount of sodium was roughly studied. The phenomenon began to be noticeable when the ratio of sodium to potassium was about ten. With twenty times as much sodium as potassium the potassium line was "much stronger" than in the absence of sodium. The greatest enhancement was observed when the ratio of sodium to potassium was one hundred. A further increase in the amount of sodium decreased the effect, but this decrease may be psychological, due to the strong sodium light scattered into the field of view.

The explanation of this phenomenon, which Gooch and Hart attribute to some, not specified, chemical reaction, is undoubtedly to be found in the so-called atomic collisions of the second kind.[2] Since the resonance potential of sodium is greater than that of potassium, it is possible for an excited sodium atom, colliding with a normal potassium atom, to transfer enough energy to excite the latter. The presence of a large number of excited sodium atoms will, therefore, increase the number of excited potassium atoms and thus enhance the intensity of the potassium doublet.

J. RUD NIELSEN

UNIVERSITY OF OKLAHOMA

ANOTHER WILD LIFE PRESERVE NEAR ITHACA

IN 1919 through the generosity of the late Mr. C. G. Lloyd, of Cincinnati, Ohio, Cornell University obtained what is now known as the Lloyd-Cornell Wild Life Reservation near McLean, N. Y. This preserve comprises an area of slightly over 80 acres and includes several very interesting cold upland sphagnum-heath bogs, grass bogs and an open mud pond, which is now in the process of being slowly filled in. Each year various classes in the biological sciences of Cornell University make excursions to this preserve and in 1926 a report was published on a preliminary survey of the fauna and flora of this preserve.[1]

In 1924 Mr. Lloyd purchased another tract of more than 400 acres of wooded land near Slaterville, N. Y., some 12 miles to the southeast of Ithaca and this has been designated as the Lloyd-Cornell Wild Flower Preserve. This preserve consists of a wooded hilly upland area which is traversed by several streams as well as by a cold spring brook and affords another bit of area in which Nature will be allowed to function without interference from man.

Just before his death Mr. Lloyd made arrangements for the purchase of still another tract of land near

[1] F. A. Gooch and T. S. Hart, *Am. J. Sci.*, 42, 448 391).

[2] O. Klein and S. Rosseland, *Zeitschr. f. Phys.*, 4, 46 (1921); J. Franck, *Zeitschr. f. Phys.*, 9, 259 (1922).

[1] A Preliminary Biological Survey of the Lloyd-Cornell Reservation, by members of the Scientific Staff of Cornell University. Bull. Lloyd Library, No. 27, Ent. Ser. No. 5, 1926.

Ringwood which the limnology classes in Cornell University have frequently for many years. Negotiations for the acquisition of this property have now been completed and this preserve will be known as the Lloyd-Cornell Ringwood Wild Life Preserve.

The Ringwood Preserve lies about 7 miles to the east of Ithaca. It comprises an area of slightly over 110 acres. Situated in the midst of rolling wooded hills, it lies at an elevation of about 1,600 feet. Being of morainic origin the glaciers upon receding have left a series of pot holes which are furnishing some very interesting situations for biological studies. One of these pot holes, known as Winterberry pond, seems to be spring fed and retains approximately the same amount of water the year round. The other pot holes have water in them intermittently. In the spring when the snow begins to melt, the water collects in them to a depth of from 5 to 12 feet, while during the late summer the water becomes lower and lower until in the fall the water disappears entirely. Just to the east of the preserve is found a sphagnum bog which offers a variety of biological forms for study.

The life which is found in these temporary pot-hole pools forms an interesting succession study. Every spring during the latter part of April and the early part of May these temporary pools are fairly alive with the beautiful fairy shrimps, *Enbranchipus gelidus*. Coming back to these pools a week or two later not a single specimen of the fairy shrimp will be noticed. However, another crustacean, *Limnetes gouldii*, is found to be just as abundant as was the fairy shrimp a few weeks previously.

Mr. W. C. Senning, instructor in the department of zoology, has made a study of the plant and animal life of these pools during the last three years so that we have a good beginning of a systematic study of the life in this preserve.

With these three Wild Life Preserves made possible through the generosity of Mr. C. G. Lloyd, Cornell University will always have an opportunity of studying plant and animal life in situations where artificial interference by man has been reduced to a minimum.

P. W. Claassen

Cornell University

ÅNGSTRÖM IN ENGLISH

Is it not unreasonable to muster the letter E, as appears imminent, into duty for almost any vowel? Something may be said for the simplification achieved in using E for the sounds represented in the original German, Swedish, etc., by Ä (or in Latin by AE). But it seems to be overdoing the point to render the ō sound of the Swedish letter Å with an E, as is done (through a misprint?) in "engstrom units" appearing above the name of Alfred F. Hess on page 334 of Science (March 30, 1928). Preservation of the original spelling of Ångström's name is perhaps too much to expect, especially of American typewriters. Nevertheless, to convert it to *engstrom* is unduly to succumb to a somewhat prevalent ignorance of the fact that *ongstrum* is in English the nearest phonetical rendering of the physicist's name (cf. Webster's New International Dictionary). Perpetuating the error fails to simplify international scientific intercourse.

E. F. B. Fries

EMBRYOLESS SEEDS IN CEREALS

Of interest in connection with the theory of doubl fertilization in angiosperms is the discovery of em bryoless seeds in wheat, rye and bald barley. Suc seeds develop endosperm which is perfectly normal but they show no trace of embryo tissue. The abnor mality is not apparent on casual observation, bu upon closer examination the lack of embryo is evi denced by a depression at the proximal end of th seed. Microscopic examination of sections also show embryo tissue and the epithelial layer to be absent.

Pope and Harlan reported the occurrence of fiv barley seeds in which the embryo was entirely lackin among many thousands examined. The writer find that embryoless seeds occur in wheat in the propor tion of approximately 0.1 per cent. Sufficient add tional work has been done to indicate that this sam proportion holds true for both bald barley and rye.

Mildred E. Lyon

Botanical Section,
Colorado Experiment Station

THE HOST OF THE BROAD TAPEWORM

The recent article by Vergeer[1] prompts me to ca attention to my experiments on *Diphyllobothriu latum* (the broad tapeworm) which was published *Minnesota Medicine*, October 1927, page 614. Sin my report was the first demonstration of the fact th North American fishes act as hosts for this worm, Ve geer's report may be looked upon as confirmation my findings. In my report it was indicated that I h evidence of the fact that there was an endemic ar in and about Winnipeg, Manitoba. Since then I ha obtained wall-eyed pike from Lake Winnipeg and ha found larvae in a great percentage of them, whi when fed to dogs produced typical tapeworms of t species *D. latum*. The importance of this is appare when one learns that a great proportion of the wa eyed pike sold in the middle western markets com from Canadian Lakes and that a large proportion

[1] The *Journal of the American Medical Associati* 90: 673–678.

the fresh fish sold on the Winnipeg market comes from this lake.

A full report of my investigations will be published shortly.

THOMAS B. MAGATH

MAYO CLINIC,
ROCHESTER, MINN.

SCIENTIFIC BOOKS

Crystallographic Tables for the Determination of Minerals. By VICTOR GOLDSCHMIDT (Heidelberg) and SAMUEL G. GORDON (Philadelphia). Philadelphia, Pa., Special Publication No. 2, The Academy of Natural Sciences of Philadelphia, 77 pp., 4 figs., 16 tables, 1928.

THIS is a complete presentation of the most modern methods of dealing with crystal identification by means of two-circle goniometric measurements. In earlier days Professor Federov, of Petrograd, Russia, wrote a "Dictionary of the Mineral Kingdom," which has been published by the Petrograd Academy of Science. This work is a sort of crystallo-chemical analysis of over ten thousand compounds, both organic and inorganic, which had been previously investigated as to crystallographic details; but unfortunately it is much involved with Ferderdov's theories of crystal structure.

The present work is intended for treatment of the unknown crystal which has been measured on the two-circle goniometer. It is very concise. First, it is necessary to identify the crystal system to which the unknown crystal belongs; then its complete identification is accomplished by means of the angles and polar elements as given in the tables. These tables are especially useful because any normal orientation of the crystal will give sufficient data for identification.

Since isometric crystals can not be distinguished from one another by crystal measurement, they are arranged according to luster, then by chemical composition, and lastly according to increasing specific gravity. The tetragonal minerals are arranged according to tangent relations, orientation with reference to either first or second order prism position being allowed for. For the orthorhombic crystals we may use either the linear or polar elements, the tangent or the cotangent. In this connection a supplementary table (Table 7) is used to make the work more complete for every possible orientation. Monoclinic minerals are classified according to prism angles and tangents of these, since the prism zone usually can readily be identified. Triclinic crystals are listed according to projection elements, polar elements and linear elements, and a special table is also provided to aid in correct orientation.

In every table there are cross references to other tables. The index at the end of the book refers directly to the minerals, of which a total of 1,710 species are listed. The book should be very useful to crystallographers in general.

ALFRED C. HAWKINS

RUTGERS UNIVERSITY

SCIENTIFIC APPARATUS AND LABORATORY METHODS

AN EFFICIENT DEHYDRATING APPARATUS FOR GENERAL USE[1]

SOME animal tissues are very difficult to dehydrate without disastrous shrinkage, which is due to sudden changes in alcoholic concentration. Many devices have been prepared to overcome this problem, with various degrees of success. While searching for a method which was easy to procure, simple to operate and sure of positive results, the apparatus here figured has proved very efficient. While designed especially for the dehydration of plant nematodes, excellent results were also obtained with other animal and plant tissues preparatory to embedding and sectioning. As its application seems quite general, it is hoped that its use may prove as beneficial to workers in other fields as it has here the past months.

The apparatus is made by using a separatory funnel (1) to which is welded a lead tube which in turn is bent up and welded into the end of a small test-tube (5), thus formed into the magazine tube. Near the top of the test-tube is inserted the overflow tube (2), which is bent down and drawn out at its end. It will be noted that the insertion of this tube is on a level, or a bit above, with the stop-cock of the separatory funnel, so the apparatus can not run dry. The unattached end of the magazine tube is left open for ease of loading and unloading of material to be dehydrated. Evaporation is minimized by placing a cork in this open end. At the bottom of the bend in the lead tube, a drain tube (9) is welded in, which is fitted at its open end with a glass stop-cock. This allows for quick and complete drainage when an entire change of fluids is desired. All rubber connections are avoided, so there would be no difficulty when such fluids as xylol are to be used. The glass used is Pyrex, due to the fact that soft glass is hard to manipulate, especially in burning the necessary holes through the magazine.[1]

As used by the author, the entire apparatus is mounted on a ring stand by using suitable clamps

[1] The author is indebted to Mr. George Pettengill, of the Oregon State Agricultural College, department of chemistry, who made many valuable suggestions and did the glass work for the apparatus.

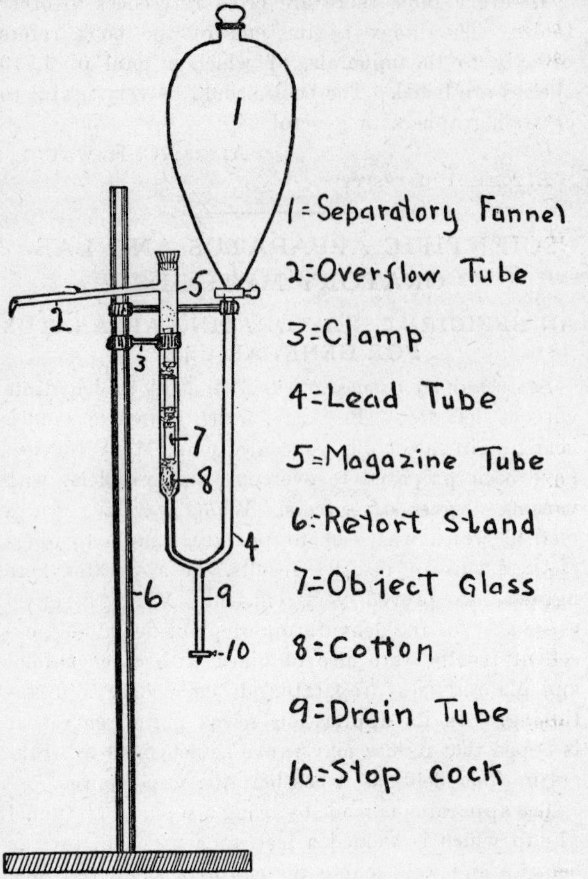

and filled with the appropriate fluid. A small piece of absorbent cotton was placed at the bottom of the magazine tube for the lower object-glass to rest on, and also to aid in gradual change in the strength of fluids. The object-glasses are made in the usual way, by selecting a piece of glass tubing a bit smaller in diameter than that of the magazine tube, and cutting into suitable lengths. The ends of the object-glasses were prepared in either of two ways. When the object-glasses were of small diameter, *i.e.,* to be used for very small objects, they were fitted with glass tube-stoppers which had a bit of bolting-cloth stretched across the inner open end. If the object-glasses were of larger diameter, *i.e.,* to be used for larger objects, the ends were heated and slightly flanged so that cheese-cloth, or cloth of suitable mesh, could be tied over the ends. Inside each object-glass a small bit of paper was placed with the record written in waterproof India ink.

The prepared object-glasses were then placed in the magazine tube, one on top of the other. With larger tissues the magazine tube was often filled with small cheesecloth bags, each bag containing the desired tissues and label. The stop-cock of the separatory funnel was then turned so that the fluid passed through the tissues, out the overflow tube and into a dish. The passage of fluid can be controlled so that any amount passes through—from a few cc per day to liters. The dilutions varied 10 per cent., from water to absolute alcohol, and the time of immersion in each dilution was the same. These two factors being constant, the dehydration rate was very gradual, with a minimum of shrinkage of the tissues.

The change of xylol for objects to be mounted in gums, dissolved in that medium or to be imbedded in paraffin, was made a gradual one by using similar methods. The strengths of xylol in absolute alcohol were 10, 25, 50, 75 and 100 per cent.

Wilbur D. Courtney
Department of Zoology,
Oregon State Agricultural College

IMMOBILIZATION OF PARAMECIUM

Various methods have been suggested from time to time for the immobilization of active ciliates for the purposes of study.

In some recent preliminary experiments on Paramecium with ultra-violet radiation it was observed that cultures of this infusorian, exposed in small embryological dishes filled to a depth of 0.5 cms, were in some cases immobilized to such an extent as to permit of detailed study of ciliary activity, vacuole contraction and formation and the general activities of the organism.

The apparatus employed was an ordinary quartz mercury vapor-lamp, DC voltage 90, current 3–4 amperes. The cultures were placed at a distance of 10 cms from the source of light and exposed for a period of eight minutes.

After one such exposure, the result seemed to offer possibilities for rapidly securing immobilization of Paramecium for class study, and so four other cultures were similarly treated with identical results. This simple procedure may prove a satisfactory means of immobilizing this much-used infusorian for class study.

J. C. Boland
Department of Biology,
Rensselaer Polytechnic Institute,
Troy, N. Y.

A BURETTE CLEANER

I have used a burette cleaner for ten years, but have never seen the method explained in print. In school-work, where there are anywhere from one hundred to one thousand burettes in use during the year, often we find several which will not clean up with chromic acid. After trying chromic acid, which is oxidizing in nature, the burette will become clean very easily if the following method is used:

Wash once with a little 95 per cent. ethyl alcohol and drain. Add about 2 cc of ethyl alcohol 95 per cent., and stand upright under a hood. Now add about 5 cc of concentrated nitric acid, and place a large test-tube over the open end of the burette to prevent any liquid from spatting out. In a very few minutes the reaction begins and throws the contents repeatedly up the full length of the burette. After the reaction has gone to completion, the burette will be clean and the contents are easily washed out.

F. H. FISH
VIRGINIA POLYTECHNIC INSTITUTE,
BLACKSBURG, VA.

SPECIAL ARTICLES

THE PHOTO-MECHANICAL CHANGES IN THE RETINA OF MAMMALS

AT various times attempts have been made to demonstrate the occurrence of pigment migration and positional changes of the visual cells in the retinae of mammals. Conflicting results have been obtained on certain forms, and in only one or two cases, notably that of the ape (Cercopithecus)[1] and that of the dog,[2] have measurable differences in pigment or cone position been observed after light and dark exposures.

The band of retinal pigment is very narrow in most mammals, and in all that I have studied the pigment needles are relatively pale, never having the almost black color observed in fishes and amphibians. In the ape mentioned above, Garten reported a pigment band two or three granules wide in the dark- and three or four granules wide in the light-adapted animal. This slight difference has been accepted by subsequent workers in this field as definitely proving the existence of pigment migration in at least this one member of the mammalian group. The suggestion made by Garten and reaffirmed by Arey[3] that the photomechanical changes occur so quickly in mammalian eyes as to fail to be "caught" by the fixative seems to be invalidated by the work of Detwiler[4] on nocturnal animals, for he was always careful to excise and fix the eyes of dark-adapted animals under faint red light and got negative results.

It has seemed to me that the slight differences found in the pigmentation of the retinae of oppositely-adapted mammals might well have existed before the experiments, and it occurred to me that it would be better to experiment on a single individual, first light-adapting one eye and removing it, then dark-adapting the other eye. Casting about for a form in which it would be easy to remove one eye without much shock or blood loss to the animal, the deer-mouse (Peromyscus maniculatus) was chosen. The eye in this form is very large and protrudes well from the surface of the skull.

My thanks are due to Dr. H. W. Feldman, of this laboratory, who supplied the animals used from his breeding stock and assisted in the operations.

Two animals were used. One was placed in darkness overnight to obtain a standard and for practice in a technical way.

The other, or experimental animal, was placed in diffuse daylight supplemented by the light from a 60-watt lamp and reflector, for five hours. Under ether, one eye was pulled out slightly in its orbit, the optic stalk was ligated with silk thread and the eye snipped off distal to the ligature. The blood loss was negligible, and the animal was allowed to recover in total darkness in which it was kept for twenty hours. At the end of that time the animal was again etherized and the second eye removed under faint red light.

The eyes from both animals were fixed in Perenyi's fluid, embedded in Parlodion and cut 7.5 μ. Sections from both eyes of the experimental animal were mounted on the same slide for convenience, but were not stained. The pigment bands in the two eyes were identical in all respects. They were five or six granules in width, quite uniform in all parts of the eyeball and showed no measurable differences attributable to migration. No attempt was made to measure cone positions, since cones, if present, are indistinguishable from rods in mouse retinae.[4]

I believe this method to be superior to that employing separate animals for the two exposures, and that skilled operators might apply it to other forms in the attempt to settle once and for all this long-standing question as to whether the retinal pigment migrates in mammals and "consequently" in man.

I should like to suggest a more or less philosophical reason why pigment migration should after all not be expected in mammals. If the photo-mechanical changes in the retina be considered from a comparative standpoint, their story is one of degeneration. In the fishes the phenomena are rapid and pronounced; in the amphibians they are less rapid and in general less marked, though still obviously of functional value; in the reptiles only long exposures have resulted in measurable differences in pigment and cone positions in light and darkness. In the mam-

[1] Garten, S., 1907, "*Graefe-Saemisch Handbuch der ges. Augenheilkunde*," Leipzig, Aufl. 2, Bd. 3, Kap. 12, Anhang; 130 pp., 5 Taf., 49 Textfig.

[2] Chiarini, P., 1906, *Arch. Ital. de Biol.*, Tom. 45, Fasc. 3, pp. 337–352, 8 fig.

[3] Arey, L. B., 1915, SCIENCE, n. s., Vol. 42, pp. 915–916.

[4] Detwiler, S. R., 1924, *J. Comp. Neur.*, Vol. 37.

mals, the phenomena seem to have practically disappeared.

Correlated with this backward orthogenesis is the forward progress in the development of the iris reaction—the familiar dilation in dim light and contraction in strong light of the pupil of the eye. In the fishes the pupil is practically stationary; in the amphibians it expands and contracts within narrow limits; in reptiles the response is about the same as in amphibians, while in the mammals and man the response is very rapid and very extensive. Ophthalmologists are agreed that the chief function of the pupil reaction is to protect the sensitive retina from too strong light and to make available to the retina all the illumination possible in dim light.

Arey[5] has summed up the surmises of previous workers, added his own and evolved an inclusive theory of the adaptive significance of the photomechanical changes based on this very idea—the protection of the sensitive and delicate rods by the pigment and the exposure of the color-perceptive cones in strong light.

It seems to me that we have here one of the not infrequent instances of the replacement of one mechanism by another of similar function through the course of evolution. Certainly the rapid pupil reaction, measured in seconds, is a decided improvement over the sluggish pigment and cell movements whose minimum reaction time at best, in certain fishes, is many minutes.

It must be admitted that the situation in nocturnal animals where both kinds of phenomena are lacking, and in the birds, where both kinds of phenomena are present to a marked degree, is disturbing to this suggestion, but the nocturnal animals have little or no need for either mechanism, and the eyes of birds are so aberrant in many respects that perhaps we are safe in dismissing them in this instance.

GORDON L. WALLS

UNIVERSITY OF MICHIGAN

EGG LAYING OF IXODIPHAGUS CAUCURTEI DU BUYSSON IN LARVAL TICKS

IN connection with experiments in rearing and liberating the French tick parasite (*Ixodiphagus caucurtei* du Buysson) at the Hamilton Laboratory of the Montana state board of entomology, the junior author, who is locally in charge of the work, in conducting an incidental and minor experiment uncovered surprising facts.

Both *I. caucurtei* and *Hunterellus hookeri* Howard, so far as is known, develop only in the nymphal stage of their host ticks, and effective egg-laying in certain experiments conducted by Dr. E. Brumpt, of Paris, and H. P. Wood, of Dallas, Texas, was found to occur only in the nymphs of ticks. Following such egg laying, development has always been found to be immediate and continuous.

Having at hand an abundance of fed larvae of *Dermacentor andersoni* Stiles and a plentiful supply of fresh adults of *I. caucurtei,* the junior author placed about 350 of the former with about ninety of the latter (mixed males and females) in a small glass jar at "room temperature" and in the direct sunlight on August 20, 1927. They were left thus for a period of three hours, when the fed larval ticks were placed in a thermal cabinet at 19° C. for incubation, which is our usual method in rearing ticks. By September 22 all the fed larvae had "molted" to the nymphal stage and the resulting "flat" nymphs were placed in a longevity tube out-of-doors in the "tick yard" under conditions simulating nature. On November 11 these nymphs were placed on a rabbit in the laboratory for feeding and seventy-eight fed nymphs were later recovered. These fed nymphs were placed in a thermal cabinet at 19° C., after which they were examined from day to day. On December 5 it was observed that a few showed the usual mottled appearance characteristic of parasitism, and thirty-two nymphs or 41.02 per cent. of the whole number were eventually isolated as parasitized. From these, nine yielded adult parasites in due time. Nine out of thirty-two is an unusually small proportion to come through to the adult condition and there may or may not be special biological meaning in the small number, since a loss of adult parasites is rather common, especially if the conditions of moisture and temperature are not correct, particularly the humidity.

From the foregoing it is shown that (a) under the conditions stated *I. caucurtei* will deposit eggs in fed larvae; (b) that, while in the case of eggs deposited in nymphal ticks, development of the parasites begins promptly and in suitable temperatures will proceed to the maturing of the parasites, in the case of eggs deposited in fed larval ticks development is delayed; (c) that the living parasite is carried through the quiescent period of the fed larva and is alive in the next stage; (d) that the parasite may remain alive through a resting period of the unfed nymphs prolonged for fifty days (September 22 to November 11); and finally (e) that on the nymphs being fed the parasites will develop to maturity.

These findings suggest the possibility of a more or less established adaptation which had not been suspected.

R. A. COOLEY
GLEN M. KOHLS

BOZEMAN, MONTANA

[5] Arey, L. B., 1919, *J. Comp. Neur.*, Vol. 30.

SCIENCE NEWS

Science Service, Washington, D. C.

SOME PAPERS PRESENTED AT THE NASHVILLE MEETING

DR. R. G. AITKEN, who is in charge of the Lick Observatory of the University of California, delivered the address as retiring vice-president of the astronomical section of the American Association for the Advancement of Science. Taking Dr. Barnard, who was a native of Nashville, and whose astronomical career largely began at the previous meeting of the association there in 1877, as the subject of his address, Dr. Aitken related many personal reminiscences. "On September 17, 1881, he found a comet and he sent word of the discovery to Lewis Swift, and through him to astronomers generally. This comet was therefore carefully observed and is known, in the annals, as Comet 1881 VI. This discovery had important consequences quite other than its bearing upon his reputation as an observer. Mr. H. H. Warner, of Rochester, New York, had offered a prize of $200 for each unexpected comet discovered by an American observer. This prize came to Barnard for the discovery of Comet 1881 VI; Mrs. Barnard felt that the money must be used for some definite purpose, and with her encouragement, and faith that later payments would be met "somehow," and that they would "manage," it was accordingly used as the first payment for a house. Faith backed by hard work had its due reward, for Mr. Warner's offer was continued for several years, and Barnard actually won enough prizes for cometary discoveries to pay for the 'Comet House,' as it is still known here in Nashville and to all astronomers." Upon the founding of the Lick Observatory in 1887 Barnard, then at the age of thirty, joined its staff. Later he went to the Yerkes Observatory, in Wisconsin. Among the many important discoveries which he made were those of the fastest-moving known star, and also the second closest, the first moon of Jupiter to be found since 1610, the "Gegenschein" or faint glow of light that appears in the sky opposite the sun, as well as numerous comets and double stars. As a great astronomer, concluded Dr. Aitken, Barnard was "honored by astronomers throughout the world. Barnard, the modest, simple-minded, unselfish, kindly man was loved by every one who knew him."

THE millions of dollars invested in the movies and the pleasure of the millions of people who daily attend them is based on chemical impurity in gelatine. This announcement, in effect, was made in a lecture given in conjunction with the meeting, by Dr. C. E. K. Mees, director of the Research Laboratory of the Eastman Kodak Company. "It has recently been found," said Dr. Mees, "that the sensitiveness of films is not due to the grains of silver bromide only, but is in some way connected with the presence on those grains of specks of some other substance, and the Kodak Research Laboratories after a long and careful study have found that these specks are produced by an accidental impurity present in the gelatine. This impurity is derived from the plants eaten by the animals from whose skins the gelatine is made. There is only a very small amount of it, but it is a compound which contains sulphur, and when the gelatine is used for making the film, the sulphur reacts with the silver bromide and produces specks of silver sulphide on the crystals. In some way or other these specks increase the effectiveness of the light to which the film is exposed in the camera and enable the light to change the silver bromide so as to form a trace of metallic silver. Then this silver acts during development as a nucleus on which more silver can deposit by the chemical process until the whole of the silver bromide crystal is turned into silver. Each of the original crystals of the film therefore, after exposure to light, becomes a grain of silver in the developed film, and it is of these grains of silver that the image projected on the screen is composed."

AN immediate investigation of the earthquake situation in the Mississippi Valley was urged by Commander N. H. Heck, in charge of the seismologic work of the U. S. Coast and Geodetic Survey, who spoke before the American Association for the Advancement of Science. Calling attention to the fact that one of the great earthquakes of all history occurred in the New Madrid region of the Mississippi Valley in 1811–12, Commander Heck intimated that there was a possibility that history would repeat itself, although it can not be foretold what the future will bring. Occasional minor earthquake shocks have been felt in the Mississippi Valley and along the Ohio River in past years and one of the sharpest of these shocks was on April 9, 1917. Another occurred at the time of the great Mississippi flood. Probably the fact that flood and earthquake came at the same time was merely a coincidence that serves to call attention to the damage that would be done by a major earthquake in that region to-day. "Thorough examination of the situation in the entire Middle Western region subject to earthquakes is desirable," Commander Heck said. "There is little doubt that the first investigation should be confined to the area surrounding the New Madrid region. Dr. James B. Macelwane, S. J., director of the Jesuit Seismological Association, has proposed such a plan, and it is endorsed by Dr. Arthur L. Day, chairman of the advisory committee of seismology of the Carnegie Institution of Washington, who is in charge of the earthquake investigation in California which is being made with the cooperation of the national government, various state institutions, including the universities, various other groups and the citizens of California. This organization has all that it can take care of in the California problem and the government activity as carried on by the United States Coast and Geodetic Survey is fully occupied with taking care of earthquake information for the United States and the regions under its jurisdiction, and operating its own observatories so that it is left for the Middle West to work out its problem. Its rapidly-growing cities make it important that this problem be attacked.

X-RAYS played a highly important part in the discussions of the biologists at the meeting of the association and its affiliated societies. Within recent months many workers in various parts of the field have discovered this type of radiation to have almost miraculous powers to change the course of events in the development of living organisms, and to leave so deep an impress on their substance that their descendants for many generations will show the effect of their ancestors' experience. Professor Winterton C. Curtis and Raymond A. Ritter, of the department of zoology at the University of Missouri, told of their researches on the effects of X-rays on the development of growing tissue. They experimented on a small marine animal related to the jelly-fish, which reproduces itself by constantly budding off new individuals very much as a tree produces branches. After exposure to the X-rays for ninety minutes the animals lost the power of producing new individuals, although the original parent portion remained alive. Professor H. J. Muller, of the University of Texas, who recently startled the scientific world by speeding up evolutionary processes over a hundred-fold with heavy X-ray doses applied to a small insect, the fruit-fly, reported further on his work and displayed specimens showing the results of his technique. Professor Frank B. Hanson, of Washington University, St. Louis, who has been collaborating with Professor Muller, reported the effects of the rays on the rapidity with which the insects reproduce. Professor Robert T. Hance, of the University of Pittsburgh, told of some of the first results of X-ray experiments on warm-blooded animals. The hair color of mice exposed to very light doses of the rays in his laboratory was radically changed. Normally "mouse-colored" mice of mixed ancestry went completely white after being rayed, while pure-bred mice of the same color changed in the opposite direction and became darker. Dr. H. J. Bagg, of Memorial Hospital, New York City, and Dr. Clarence R. Halter, of Cornell University Medical College, working in collaboration, were also among the first to obtain positive results with warm-blooded animals. Their mice developed certain marked bodily defects, such as possessing only one kidney instead of two, abnormal eyes, and legs in bad condition at birth. Such defects occur among mice bred under ordinary conditions, but not so often as among X-rayed animals.

PLANTS as well as animals respond to X-ray treatment. Professor T. H. Goodspeed, of the University of California, has obtained results in the breeding of X-rayed tobacco plants which are comparable with those of Professor Muller on fruit-flies. The new varieties produced in this way have a stronger growth and produce more flowers than their cousins descended from un-rayed parents. Professor L. J. Stadler, of the University of Missouri, has conducted similar experiments with corn and barley. In these, as in all the other animals and plants on which the treatment has been tried, the hereditary units or genes have been knocked out of place and more or less violently rearranged, resulting in forms of life wholly new to the universe.

ULTRA-VIOLET radiation, now widely used for the promotion of human health, has been shown to be able to promote plant growth as well, and to increase the production of valuable plant ingredients. Experiments in this field were reported before the Botanical Society of America by Adelia McCrea, of Parke, Davis and Company, Detroit. Miss McCrea planted two crops of foxglove plants, from which the widely-used drug digitalis is made. Part of each crop was started under ordinary glass, which shuts out ordinary light, and the rest under special glass which transmits ultra-violet. The young plants under the ultra-violet responded at once, forming new leaves faster than the others did. After they were transferred out of doors and grown to maturity under similar conditions, both crops were put through the process for extracting the drug. The irradiated plants yielded an extract of notably higher potency than the untreated controls; in the second crop the increase amounted to as much as 35 per cent.

ULTRA-VIOLET rays can sometimes be too much of a good thing, especially to the lowlier forms of animal life. Some of the effects they have were discussed by Professor E. E. Just, of Howard University. Eggs of Nereis, a sea worm, were exposed to ultra-violet rays by Professor Just. Normally the eggs of this animal possess 28 chromosomes, or bearers of hereditary qualities. After irradiation they were found to have 70. Since multiplication of these important bodies in any living organism is apt to be followed by the development of freak forms in the adult stage this discovery may come to have considerable importance in genetics. The rays have other effects on the eggs also. They lose a jelly-like substance on raying. When they begin to undergo cell division, the first partition always starts from the spot where the rays hit their covering membranes, and the young worms usually show certain localized defects traceable to their experience while in the one-cell stage. Professor Just and his students also presented papers on the fertilization of eggs of Arbacia, another lowly sea animal, in water containing potassium cyanide, and demonstrated the presence in ordinary mayonnaise dressing of structures usually claimed to be present only in living protoplasm, and thought to be of importance in life processes.

ULTRA-VIOLET light has the power to kill as well as cure. Experiments were reported by Professor A. Brooker Klugh, of Queen's University, Kingston, Canada, showing that the short length ultra-violet radiations of the sun are deadly to the minute crustacea that furnish food for the fish of commerce. For many years biologists have puzzled over the question why these tiny relatives of crabs and lobsters remained at a depth of 90 feet or more under the sea during the day and came to the surface only by night. A long series of experiments conducted at the Atlantic Biological Station, St. Andrews, New Brunswick, during the past summer has demonstrated that this particular form of food for the fishes is really fatally affected by ultra-violet light. Consequently they keep down at a considerable depth below the surface of the sea while the light from the sun is intense.

WHILE the biologists attending the meeting were listening to accounts of newly-discovered ways in which X-rays affect living tissue, the physicists heard about another new property of these rays. Dr. Fred Allison, of the Ala-

bama Polytechnic Institute at Auburn, told the American Physical Society how he had found that they change the effect of certain liquids and other substances on light. Many liquids, such as a sugar solution, have the property of turning the plane of polarized light. Ordinary light consists of vibration in an indefinite number of directions, but when polarized, the vibration is confined to one particular plane. If a beam of such light is passed through a sugar solution, it is still vibrating in one direction when it emerges, but in a different direction from that when it went in. Dr. Allison has found that even liquids which do not ordinarily have this power gain it when exposed to X-rays. When liquids, or glass, are placed in the field of a powerful magnet, they gain this property, as discovered many years ago by Faraday. When X-rays are used in addition, says Dr. Allison, the rotatory powers of the liquids are increased, while in glass, it is made to rotate in the opposite direction.

ANOTHER newly-discovered effect of X-rays, by which they impart on certain chemical substances the power of glowing when slightly heated, was described to the meeting of the American Physical Society by Dr. Frances G. Wick, of Vassar College. Dr. Wick told of work that she had done in collaboration with Miss Mabel K. Slattery, research assistant at Cornell University. Some substances, such as fluorite and calcite, have long been known to possess the property of shining in the dark after being moderately warmed, she stated. However, the investigators have found that chemicals which do not have this power acquire it when exposed to X-rays. One of these is calcium sulphate, of which gypsum is a form, mixed with a little manganese. The phenomenon is called thermoluminescence, and is of two kinds. One dies out quickly, but with the other, the power to glow when heated may continue for months.

HOW a thin layer of atoms of caesium on the filament helps the vacuum tube of a radio set to work better was described by Dr. J. A. Becker, of the Bell Telephone Laboratories in New York. Dr. Becker told of work that he had done in collaboration with D. W. Mueller, of the same laboratories. The operation of a radio tube, he explained, depends on the copious emission of electrons from the hot filament. When coated with caesium, in the form of caesium oxide, the atoms of the metal arrange themselves over the filament in a single layer. But the atoms are ionized, which means that each of them has lost one of its quota of electrons, and so is positively charged. This atomic layer is then able to act in the same way as the grid of the tube, but being so close to the filament is particularly efficacious in pulling the electrons out of the tungsten of which it is made.

THE path traced by a moving spot of light in a special vacuum tube reveals the quality of a quartz crystal to be used in keeping broadcasting stations on a constant wave-length At the meeting of the American Physical Society Dr. Karl S. Van Dyke, of Wesleyan University, told of his researches which may play a useful part in the production of these important crystals. These piezo-electric crystals, as they are called, usually consist of plates of quartz, cut from larger quartz crystals. At present, it is usually necessary to try several of them in order to find a satisfactory one, as a large number may not work at all. Some may be considerably improved with a little grinding. With the use of the cathode ray oscillograph, as the special vacuum tube is called, a stream of electrons, or cathode rays, falls on a screen, where it makes a spot of light. The motion of the stream of electrons causes the spot to trace a curve, and quick inspection of this curve reveals the quality of the crystal.

VITAMIN A, the substance needed for normal growth and health, is present in green vegetables, but the much-sought-after blanched garden products do not have it. This has been proved to be true in the case of asparagus, at least, by Dr. John W. Crist and Dr. Marie Dye, of Michigan State College, who reported their experiments before a session of the American Association. Young white rats were fed on a diet lacking in the growth-promoting vitamin. Some of them were given, as a supplementary ration, a small amount of green asparagus tips every day, while a second lot of rats, as "controls," were fed on blanched tips. The asparagus was fed both fresh and cooked. In all cases the animals receiving the green asparagus grew and throve normally, while the ones on the blanched tip diet dwindled and died. Even doubling the amount of blanched asparagus fed to one of the rat groups failed to save them.

FISH blood has its sugar radically reduced by the diabetes-curing drug, and if only the normal concentration of sugar is present the fish goes into convulsions, just as a man or a warm-blooded animal would, and may die as a result, unless a counteracting dose of glucose is injected after the insulin. These results of researches on the blood-sugar physiology of fishes were reported by Dr. Irving E. Gray, of Tulane University. Only one species of fish, the puffer, resisted the action of the insulin and did not go into convulsions. This fish normally has a very low concentration of sugar in its blood.

THERE has been a marked decrease in the incidence of hookworm in the states of North and South Carolina in recent years according to Dr. W. G. Gamble, of Charleston. After reading some of the early surveys of hookworm infestation in the southern states, especially in the Sand-Hill regions and Coastal Plains in the Carolinas, Dr. Gamble said, one wonders what the inhabitants did except to raise razorback hogs, hookworms and drink moonshine. Some of the figures for the period from 1910 to 1915 gave as high as 50 per cent. infection. In the period from 1920 to 1923 the rate was much less. Recent surveys made by Dr. Gamble and the Hygienic Laboratory at Columbus, S. C., show 17.8 and 21.8 per cent., respectively, for infestation with all intestinal parasites, a marked decrease from years ago. Hookworms still lead the list, with round worms, a poor second. Children, women, men, white and colored in the order named, showed the greatest percentage of infection.

NEW SCIENTIFIC BOOKS

The Oxford University Press, American Branch, New York

THE ELECTRONIC THEORY OF VALENCY. Nevil V. Sidgwick. pp. xii + 310. $5.00.

This book aims at giving a general account of the principles of valency and molecular constitution, founded on the Rutherford-Bohr atom.

QUALITATIVE ANALYSIS. W. F. F. Shearcroft. 71 pp. $0.35.

Particular attention has been paid to the theory underlying qualitative analysis, and the student is given a reason for every operation outlined.

Harper & Brothers, New York

THE SCIENCE OF HEALTH AND DISEASE. Howard W. Haggard. pp. xii + 538. $4.00.

A physiological text-book, but it also extends over the whole field of modern medicine. The nature of health and the chief causes and processes of disease are described. For the student and the general reader.

The Draughtsman Publishing Company, London

AN OUTLINE OF STELLAR ASTRONOMY. Peter Doig. 183 pp. $2.00, post free.

The main features are outlined of the present state of knowledge of the constitution, dimensions, motions and distribution in space of the stars and nebulae. Since books on astronomy quickly become out of date, the author has appended bibliographical notes indicating where will be reported the results of future investigations.

SCIENCE NEWS

Science Service, Washington, D. C.

ADVANCES IN MEDICINE IN 1927

THE 1927 Nobel prize for medicine was awarded Prof. Julius Wagner-Jauregg, of Vienna, for his treatment of paresis by inoculation with malaria.

Cancer in the chicken can be rendered inactive by small quantities of aluminum and calcium salts, according to Mrs. Margaret R. Lewis and Dr. Howard B. Andervont.

A "heart hormone," or internal secretion that stimulates the heart to keep it beating, was discovered by Dr. Ludwig Haberlandt, of the University of Innsbruck.

Thyroxin, the hormone of the thyroid gland, was made synthetically in the laboratories of University College, London, by Dr. C. R. Harington and Professor George Barger.

Dr. J. J. Abel, of the Johns Hopkins University, has prepared a crystalline insulin which appears to be a pure hormone necessary for the maintenance of normal sugar metabolism.

"Synthalin," a German preparation designed to supplement or replace insulin in the treatment of diabetes, was at first widely hailed, but proved a disappointment.

Discovery of a new drug, "myrtillin," as a valuable treatment for diabetes was announced to the American Medical Association, by Dr. Frederick M. Allen, of Morristown, N. J.

Liver extract can be used to cure pernicious anemia, Drs. George R. Minot, William P. Murphy and E. J. Cohn, of Harvard University, announced; also the latter extracted from liver an extract which produces red corpuscles which is probably the active ingredient.

A diet that simulates a condition in the body brought about by starvation, has been found by Drs. F. B. Talbot, K. M. Metcalf and Margaret E. Moriarty at the Massachusetts General Hospital in Boston, to give very successful results in treating epileptic children.

Vitamin C, the substance that wards off scurvy, is present in milk as well as in the fresh vegetables usually relied on to supply it, was the report by Professor L. F. Meyer, following extensive experiments at the University of Berlin.

Ergosterol was declared to be the really active and essential substance in the antirachitic vitamin, by a number of investigators working independently of each other.

Dr. Alfred F. Hess, of New York, reported that dried milk that has been treated with ultra-violet light is the most practical of the irradiated foods that have been used to prevent rickets in babies.

Preventive vaccination for smallpox and typhoid, large quantities of quinine and elaborate mosquito control measures contributed to checking outbreaks of disease epidemics in the South after the Mississippi flood.

Drs. E. G. Wakefield and W. W. Hall, of the U. S. Navy Medical Corps, completed a systematic survey of heat injuries and one of the first investigations into the physiological reactions underlying sunstroke.

Scientists at Berlin have shown that it is possible to change simple embryonic tissues into malignant tissue by exposing the former in tissue cultures to the action of arsenic.

Discovery of the germ causing trachoma, a serious disease of the eye that has been especially troublesome among the Indians, was announced by Dr. Hideyo Noguchi, of the Rockefeller Institute, N. Y.

A curative antitoxin for erysipelas, first developed by Dr. K. E. Birkhaug, of Rochester, N. Y., has been tried out with highly successful results at the Bellevue Hospital in New York, which has one of the largest erysipelas clinics in the world.

Streptococcus germs isolated from skin lesions of erysipelas are capable of causing sore throat without any skin affection, it was found by Drs. George F. and Gladys H. Dick, at the John McCormick Institute for Infectious Diseases.

Progress in the work of developing a serum to fight the African sleeping sickness was announced by Dr. William H. Taliaferro, of the University of Chicago.

A color test for tetanus and diphtheria toxins has been worked out by Drs. Lucy Mishulow and Charles Krumwiede, of the New York City Health Department, that will greatly speed up the commercial production of these products. Hitherto toxins have had to be tested out on live guinea pigs, a time-consuming and not altogether accurate procedure.

Dr. Florence B. Seibert, of the University of Chicago, has produced an active protein in crystalline form which represents a step nearer the solution of the actual chemical nature of tuberculin.

Statistical evidence that the first-born child in a family is more likely to have certain malformations of mind and body than later children, and that such malformations are not likely to recur in later births in the same family, was presented by Dr. G. F. Still, professor of children's diseases at King's College, London.

The utility of X-ray photographs of the head as a positive means of identification was demonstrated by Drs. William L. Culbert and Frederick M. Law, of New York, when they identified an unknown body with their aid.

Heart disease occurs less frequently in children who have had their tonsils removed than in those who have not, said Dr. A. D. Kaiser, of Rochester, N. Y., before the American Medical Association.

An extract from the liver of dogs that will keep blood from clotting was discovered by Dr. W. H. Howell, of Johns Hopkins University.

A new anesthetic known as avertin that lacks many of the undesirable features of the anesthetics now in use, is being tried out in German hospitals.

A new and accurate chemical test for drunkenness, by which the subject's breath is passed through a chemical solution, was demonstrated to the American Medical Association by Dr. Emile Bogen, of the University of Cincinnati.

The Metropolitan Life Insurance Co. announced that their statistics showed that America has had more deaths from alcoholism since prohibition than before.

RELATIVITY

ONCE again photographic plates, exposed at the time of a total eclipse of the sun, help to substantiate the theory of relativity, as proposed by Einstein. This time it is the moon's diameter which is being measured. On plates made at the January, 1926, eclipse, which they went to Sumatra to observe, Dr. John A. Miller, director, and Dr. Ross W. Marriott, of the Sproul Observatory of Swarthmore College, find that the moon is just as large as at other times.

One of the possible experimental tests of Einstein's theory, announced in 1915, was on account of the fact that he considered light to have mass. This would result in its being pulled out of a straight line as it passed a heavy body such as the sun. Stars can only be observed near the sun at the time of a total eclipse. At such a time the stars around the sun should appear closer together than if the sun were not there. In 1919 English astronomers actually observed this effect at an eclipse visible in Brazil, and it was again verified at the Australian eclipse in 1922 by Dr. W. W. Campbell, of the Lick Observatory.

Another possible cause of this shift of star images on eclipse plates other than the one given by Einstein was proposed by Professor Charles Lane Poor, of Columbia University. He pointed out that the shadow of the moon in the earth's atmosphere during an eclipse forms a cone of cooler air. The observers are inside and as the light from the stars has to enter this cone, it might be deflected in the same way. As the edge of the moon is clearly seen during an eclipse, the light that grazes it should be similarly affected. This would mean that the moon's diameter, as measured on eclipse plates, should be less than the diameter of the moon at other times.

After unsuccessful attempts to make satisfactory plates at the eclipses in Mexico in 1923 and in New England in 1925, Dr. Miller and Dr. Marriott succeeded in 1926. A large camera, 65 feet long, with which the moon's diameter on the plate was about 7½ inches, was used. The night before the eclipse one of the plates was exposed on some stars, then, the next day, on the eclipse. The stars, their positions being accurately known, gave points from which to measure the moon's diameter.

After months of careful measurement, Dr. Miller and Dr. Marriott have found that the plates show the moon's angular diameter, as it would appear from the center of the earth, to be 2001.30 seconds, with an uncertainty of .18 second. The most accurate figure for this diameter, from measurements made at other times, is 2001.35 seconds, with an uncertainty of .1 second. As the difference, which is much less than expected by Professor Poor, is less than the uncertainty of each, Dr. Marriott has announced that there "is no measurable effect."

DR. BESREDKA'S EXPERIMENTS IN IMMUNIZATION

PILLS of dead bacilli are taken before breakfast for three days in the simple method of immunization against typhoid, dysentery and cholera now being used by people in large sections of Europe and Asia. The pills are preceded by doses of ox bile in the typhoid and cholera vaccination. This means of immunization which grew out of animal experiments made at the Pasteur Institute by Professor A. Besredka is becoming increasingly popular, according to Dr. Harry Plotz, his American assistant. It is being used extensively in France, Russia, Italy, Spain and India.

American workers in this field regard Dr. Besredka's figures as interesting and encouraging, but are of the opinion that they can not be accepted at their face value alone. Interpretation of such fundamental experiments, they maintain, is not entirely acceptable without further confirmation.

According to Dr. Plotz, "vaccination by the mouth is much simpler and easier for the patient. There are no disagreeable after-effects such as often follow vaccination under the skin and which, in the case of dysentery, proved so disastrous that the subcutaneous method was abandoned. It is also more rapid in its immunizing power. We have proved experimentally that immunization takes place a day or two after the last dose of vaccine is given."

Moreover, he stated, the new method is quite as effective as the old. Statistics show that in various typhoid and cholera epidemics where both methods were used, vaccination by the mouth was equally effective, and, in some cases, more so. Just recently Lieutenant-Colonel A. J. H. Russell, in a report to the medical section of the League of Nations, showed that he had found vaccination by the mouth and vaccination under the skin to be of equal effectiveness for cholera. He drew these conclusions after extensive vaccinations in towns in India, using both methods. Colonel Russell is director of Public Health, Madras, India. Vaccine by the mouth was given 4,982 persons. Of these 18 contracted the disease, with 4 deaths resulting. In other words, the percentage attacked was 0.36 with the deaths 22.2 per cent. of those. Among 11,004 unvaccinated controls, 222 contracted cholera and 93 died, making the percentage 2.02 attacked of which 41.9 per cent. died. Vaccine under the skin was given 8,485 persons of whom 31 contracted the disease, 2 dying. The percentage attacked was then 0.37 and the mortality 6.5. Of 29,254 unvaccinated controls in this experiment 489 contracted the disease, 184 dying. The percentage attacked was 1.67 and the percentage of mortality 37.6.

Professor Besredka's theory, which led him to experiment with oral vaccination, is simply that it is logical to vaccinate the organ that is infected during the course of the disease. In the case of dysentery, typhoid and cholera, the germ enters by way of the mouth and pro-

duces the disease in the small intestine. Then why not vaccinate by the mouth and emulate mother nature as much as possible? This is a far more direct way for the vaccine to reach the intestine than through the skin.

But to immunize against typhoid and cholera Professor Besredka found that it is necessary to administer ox bile first. Bile prepares the mucous membrane of the intestinal wall to receive the dead bacteria which are given by the mouth. It removes the mucous and prepares for the absorption of the vaccine which might otherwise slip through the intestinal tract. In the case of dysentery, however, the bacteria in the vaccine are capable of performing this function.

THE YIELD OF TOBACCO IN THE RIO GRANDE VALLEY

HEALTH-RESORT sun and river irrigation water combine to produce in the middle Rio Grande Valley a yield of tobacco much greater per acre than that grown anywhere else in the United States. The nicotine content of the plants is twice that of crops produced elsewhere, according to R. G. Mewborne, chemist, who is president of a local tobacco company.

The extraordinary yield in this region of the Southwest it attributed to the fact that New Mexico receives more actual hours of sunshine in a year than other sections of the country. Sufficient food from the soil in the form of potash, for which tobacco has a greater appetite than most other plants, is supplied by the waters of the Rio Grande River which irrigate the valley farms.

The Rio Grande Valley qualified as a tobacco country in a series of experimental plot tests. The heavy trial yield justified the establishment of a tobacco-growing industry in this region.

While the various smoking types of tobacco show large increases in weight per acre, a species known as rustica, whose high nicotine content was developed by the U. S. Bureau of Plant Industry, is the chief commercial crop. This tobacco, as grown in the Rio Grande Valley, has such marked insecticidal properties that it is unnecessary to extract the nicotine as is ordinarily done. The whole plant is dried, pulverized and separated into different classes of insecticidal products, some for animal parasites, particularly for dipping sheep and cattle, and others for spraying and dusting insects in orchards, gardens and farms. The supply of insecticidal nicotine in the United States was formerly limited to waste material swept up in tobacco factories.

ITEMS

HEALTH and nutrition may play a part in determining keenness of hearing, according to an investigation made by Dr. Dana W. Drury, of Boston. Using an audiometer, Dr. Drury measured the acuity of hearing of four groups of children. The best hearing was found among a group of boys in a school where care is taken to maintain high physical and nutritional standards. The next best hearing average was made by children at an institute for the blind. One hundred children from the Boston public schools average just a little lower than the blind children, and a group of children in a Massachusetts institution for state wards who are crippled and deformed had the least keen hearing of all. Of the numerous groups of different ages studied by Dr. Drury, the Harvard football squad at the close of the playing season exhibited the highest level of auditory keenness.

WHY some motormen and bus drivers have the hard luck of getting their car into accidents, while others sail along without much trouble has been investigated by two psychologists of the Personnel Research Federation. A connection between health and accidents was discovered among older drivers, the psychologists, Dr. Walter V. Bingham and C. S. Slocombe, report. Men over 50 years of age with abnormal blood-pressure had on the average more than twice as many accidents as men of the same ages and experience whose blood-pressure was normal. "It has not been generally recognized," they state, "that excessive blood-pressure, even when it is not so high as to indicate danger of a sudden collapse, may, nevertheless, be a symptom of incipient nephritis or of some systematic condition which affects general health and temperament to an extent which may seriously interfere with safe driving."

AN archeological find, throwing light on the little-known period following the withdrawal of the Roman legions from the German frontier early in the fifth century A. D., has been made by Dr. Fritz Fremersdorf, of the Wallraff-Richartz Museum at Cologne. It consists of an ancient Frankish graveyard, which was discovered during excavations in an athletic park in one of the suburbs of the city. Thus far 35 burials have been uncovered, consisting of skeletons of both men and women. The latter have articles of household gear about them, and the men are equipped with their warriors' weapons. These consist for the most part of the typical Frankish battleax, the long sword and the lance. One skeleton has the head of a long lance beside its right foot, and on the left side extending from shoulder to knee, was the blade of a magnificent sword.

DRIED whites of eggs, when included in the diet of rats, produces a curious new type of disease, Dr. Margaret A. Boas, of the Lister Institute, has found. "After two or three weeks, red scaly patches appear at the corners of the animal's mouth, the coat becomes rough and sticky, and the long hairs fall out. The red patches then spread, and the baldness increases. There are also nervous symptoms. In all cases the rats lose weight progressively and soon die, although rats on the same diet, but with fresh instead of dried egg-white, live quite contentedly in perfect health." Dr. Boas does not consider that the disease is caused by a toxic substance, but believes that it is due to the deficiency of some essential food factor which is probably destroyed when the egg-white is dried. The dried egg-white can be rendered quite harmless, she has found, by adding some other substances to the diet, such as potatoes or arrowroot.

SCIENCE NEWS

Science Service, Washington, D. C.

MAN-LIKE FOSSIL REMAINS

EXTREMELY ancient fossil bones, which may be those of the Heidelberg race of man or of even earlier man-like creatures, have been found in the same region that yielded the famous Mauer jaw, the sole relic of this extinct human species so far accepted as authentic. The discoverer of the new fossils, Dr. Wilhelm Freudenberg, of Frankfort-am-Main, states in a communication to the British anthropologist, Sir Arthur Smith Woodward, that he has eighteen bone fragments of men or man-like apes, all collected in sand pits in the river deposits near Heidelberg.

One of the fossils, a shin-bone, is short, very heavy, and decidedly curved, resembling the corresponding bone in a gorilla. There is also the fragment of a thigh-bone with gorilline characteristics. A foot-bone shows some resemblance to that of a chimpanzee. Associated with other bones of undoubted apes and monkeys were several which Dr. Freudenberg states are more strongly human in their shape, and which he considers to be the remains of a forerunner of Neanderthal man.

Scientists in London are inclined to be somewhat conservative until all the evidence is in. *Nature* comments editorially: "Paleontologists and anthropologists will await with great interest Dr. Freudenberg's detailed description of his finds. Remains of monkeys of Pleistocene age are known from Norfolk, the Thames Valley, France and Germany, but no trace of the man-like apes has hitherto been discovered in Europe of later date than the lower Pliocene. If Dr. Freudenberg's results are confirmed, the search for the earliest ancestors of man in Europe is not so hopeless as it is commonly supposed to be."

A single tooth, declared by its finder to be human or at least human-like in character, has been dug up in China, in a geological formation of about the same age as the one in which the German fossils were discovered, Dr. Davidson Black, of Peking Union Medical College, reports. It was found by Dr. Birger Bohlin, a paleontologist attached to the Geological Survey of China, at the same site that last year yielded other fossils claimed to be human. Dr. Black states that the new find is a molar tooth from an individual in the same stage of development represented by that of an eight-year-old modern European child.

A DISAPPEARING ISLAND

FALCON ISLAND, in the Goro Sea, southwest of Apia, Western Samoa, and between the Fiji and Tongan Islands, is again above water after years of submergence. This is indicated by word received by Dr. Andrew Thomson, director of the Apia Observatory. Heralded by a slight earthquake on September 30, great columns of smoke were observed from Nukualofa in the Tongan Islands issuing from the sea on October 4. Three days later the site was visited by the British warship *Laburnum*, and a new island was found about 300 feet high at its central point and three miles in circumference.

Puffs of smoke shot up about every 20 minutes to a height of from 4,000 to 5,000 feet, the tops of the smoke columns being lost in the clouds. With each outburst ashes and cinders were thrown into the air, to fall back and build up the central cone. Late in the fall the island was reported to be erupting steam at intervals of about once a minute along its entire length.

"The island was discovered in 1865 by the British cruiser *H. M. S. Falcon*, when it was a low-lying reef," says Dr. Thomson. "In 1885 an eruption took place, which built up a cone, which in 1889, after four years' weathering, was found to be over 150 feet high. A slight volcanic outburst occurred in 1895. Since then the island, which was composed entirely of cinders and ashes, gradually slipped down into the sea.

"The area around the little South Sea Kingdom of Tonga is of great seismic activity. The earthquakes equal in intensity and frequency those of Japan. Some of the earthquakes are directly due to submarine volcanoes; others are caused by a readjustment of the earth's crust along a line of great ocean depths, which stretch from the Samoan Islands to New Zealand."

THE VIVARIUM IN PARIS

WHAT might be called an insect zoo has just opened in Paris where the public is turning its attention from the lions and tigers in the menageries to see the new vivarium in the Jardin des Plantes. Here it has the extraordinary experience of watching insects in their natural environments, each group shown in an indoor glass cage fitted up to seem like home to the inhabitants.

This somewhat unique accomplishment has not been so easy as it might seem. The insects come from various climates and their requirements are naturally vastly different. Thus a complicated heating system is necessary to simulate the African desert in one cage and a coolish temperature in the next. Heat, humidity and light have all formed tremendous problems solved by the ingenuity of Dr. Jeannel, director of the vivarium.

In some cases it has been necessary to fool the insects for the benefit of the public. In their desire to establish the closest possible contact with objects about them, the scorpions, if left to their own devices, would completely disappear from sight by burying themselves and leave the public to look at a seemingly empty cage. However, they seem very well satisfied to hide beneath plates of transparent glass through which they can easily be seen.

A pair of giant phasmas have shown that hens are not the only ones whose reproduction is affected by electric light. For two months they failed to reproduce, but the day an electric light was put in their cage they responded accordingly.

Several cages are devoted to exhibits of insect mimicry. There are the giant phasmas just mentioned which look like the green leaves they feed upon, and others which exactly resemble the straw-colored branches to which they are clinging. The observer must watch closely for some movement to tell which is which.

The vivarium is for the purpose of exhibiting all cold-blooded animals in their natural environments, but the insect exhibits are the most unusual part of the program.

MOUNTAIN SHEEP IN YELLOWSTONE PARK

M. P. Doyling, a government engineer, describes an interesting battle of bighorn mountain sheep he saw a short time ago in Yellowstone National Park.

"Although they were not more than fifty feet from the edge of the road, they didn't pay the slightest attention to the car I was in, and I sat for about fifteen minutes, and witnessed a most unusual and interesting sight," he reports.

"There were two young rams fighting an old and somewhat heavier one. What surprised me most was their method of attack in which they were 'true gentlemen.' They would stand about twenty feet apart and both start at precisely the same time, coming together, always, directly head on. Only after one has seen the size of the horns on the little animals and knows the speed at which they travel can one imagine the terrible shock it must be to them, at each such encounter.

"I expected to see them butt each other in the sides and rear, but in every instance they waited for the other to get set and then always came head on. After each such encounter they would stroll around for a minute or two, sometimes even taking a few mouthfuls of grass, before going through exactly the same performance again. If one tried to lie down, as did happen several times, the other would be over immediately and bother him until he got up.

"In one encounter one of the rams was on higher ground than the other but, apparently, to counteract this condition the one on the low side reared up on his hind legs and came down just in time to hit the other square in the center between the horns. After a bit one of the young rams strayed away a couple hundred feet and, after pawing away the dirt on the side hill, became, for the time being, an interested spectator. The other young one kept at the old ram, however, and every minute or two they would have another encounter.

"I doubt very much if the old ram could stand this relay of encounters for a great period as he was panting heavily and blood was coming from his nose when I left the scene of action."

VITAMIN D

Vitamin D, the radiation-generated something that prevents the development of the bone-disease, rickets, in children and young animals, has been traced to a new source by Dr. Walter A. MacNair, of the U. S. Bureau of Standards, and Dr. C. E. Bills, of Evansville, Ind.

Recent research has shown that vitamin D is produced when a substance known as ergosterol is subjected to the invisible ultra-violet rays. Not the whole range of the ultra-violet is thus able to generate the vitamin, but only certain zones or bands of wave-lengths. These wave-length bands are also able to prevent rickets in young animals when turned directly on them, instead of on the food which is later fed to them.

Ergosterol is a comparatively new substance, which is extracted from cholesterol, a material that has been known for a long time. It occurs associated with the fats in animal bodies. It was formerly thought that cholesterol was the seat of vitamin D activity, but after the art of extracting the ergosterol from it was perfected, the cholesterol seemed to be inert and unable to form the vitamin even when subjected to ultra-violet raying. The conclusion, therefore, was that ergosterol could form vitamin D, and that the cholesterol from which it had been extracted could not.

But now Dr. Bills has been able to obtain some degree of vitamin D activity from cholesterol, freed from ergosterol, and on examining the effects of the rays with a spectrograph Dr. MacNair has found that certain wave-lengths of ultra-violet light are absorbed by it. This may indicate that cholesterol after all has some capacity for forming vitamin D, although Dr. MacNair inclines to the opinion that it is more likely that it still contains as an impurity another substance as yet unextracted and unidentified, possibly of the same order as ergosterol.

LOSS OF APPETITE AND VITAMIN B

Professor J. C. Drummond, vitamin specialist, and Dr. S. K. Kon, of University College, London, have found that there is a close relationship between the amount of vitamin B in the diet and the total amount of food taken. Pigeons fed a diet adequate in all respects except that it lacked vitamin B gradually lost all appetite for the meals presented to them. Another group of pigeons kept under observation as controls, fed as much food as they wanted along with an ample ration of vitamin B, grew healthily and retained normal appetite. A third group, fed only the amount of food that the first group actually ate plus a plentiful supply of the vitamin in question, showed loss of weight due to slight starvation.

From their results, Professor Drummond and Dr. Kon concluded that the loss of weight that is always associated with lack of vitamin B is simply caused by partial starvation; the pigeons lose their appetites and refuse to eat the deficient food, and hence lose weight.

Since vitamin B occurs in only minute quantities in different foods its presence becomes of increasing importance. Consequently an elaborate study of this question has been taken in hand at the chemical department of St. Thomas's Hospital Medical School, London, by Dr. R. H. A. Plimmer and his colleagues. They tested a number of cereals by feeding them to pigeons for a long period. They found that none of the cereals examined contained such a rich amount of vitamin B as dried yeast. Wheat, barley and rye contained more vitamin B than maize or oats. These investigators, like

Professor Drunmmond and Dr. Kon, found that young animals need more vitamin B than adults and that the first important symptom is loss of appetite, which leads to loss of weight.

COFFEE AS A BEVERAGE

COFFEE drinkers will welcome the tidings, announced by Professor Ralph H. Cheney, of the biology department of New York University, that coffee is not only harmless but beneficial.

"Evidence derived from my study of the effect of coffee on animals and man," Professor Cheney declared recently, "indicates that the properly prepared beverage is highly advantageous with respect to over 90 per cent. of normal individuals. Judging from the effect of aqueous solutions of caffeine or of the coffee beverage taken through the stomach in the 1.5 grain quantities such as exist in the average coffee cup, the reasonable use of coffee is a great blessing to man. To be sure, caffeine is a drug and its use can be abused, but acute injury, as far as the caffeine content is concerned, would necessitate the consumption of over 150 cups which is, of course, ridiculous.

"Psychological responses of amiability and a sense of well-being and good cheer are undeniable accompaniments of the coffee beverage and the physiological effects are also non-injurious and gratifying. Temporary relief from hunger and fatigue is a general result, and light headaches, due to other than gastric disturbances, are commonly alleviated. Coffee serves as a mild stimulant of the heart, brain and muscles, thereby accomplishing greater power and coordination in mental and physical endeavors.

"The outstanding fact to be heralded in favor of coffee is the absence of any after effect or subnormal, recuperation period. It does not seem to be habit-forming since satisfactory stimulation does not require continually enlarged quantities. No other beverage produces equal stimulation without deleterious after-effects. On this basis, it is safe to say that coffee, prepared by subjecting the ground bean to water just below the boiling-point for 5 minutes or even somewhat longer in most household percolators, is not injurious to adults in normal health who show no acute idiosyncrasy regarding caffeine or other substances in the beverage."

Coffee is an impressive example of a plant, Professor Cheney pointed out, whose economic importance has been raised to great heights by its successful planting in a locality entirely foreign to its natural distribution since it is indigenous to Africa and Asia and is raised principally in Brazil and Colombia. The United States is the largest consumer, coffee imports being exceeded only by sugar and raw silk.

ITEMS

THE cotton crop losses from the boll-weevil in 1927 were about 1,487,000 bales, according to estimates reported to the American Association by Dr. R. W. Leiby, of the North Carolina Department of Agriculture. Losses sustained by the states of Texas, Arkansas, Florida, Georgia, South Carolina, Mississippi, Louisiana and North Carolina amounted to $148,700,400, Dr. Leiby declared. "The unusual injuries caused by the weevil during 1927," the entomologist explained, "are attributed to a rapid multiplication of the weevils under favorable weather conditions, the climate during the summer in most sections of the cotton states having been only moderately warm and rather rainy."

THE corn borer has spread its domain in Canada over 95,650 square miles, according to L. S. McLaine and H. G. Crawford, entomologists of the Canadian Government. An outbreak was discovered at New Liskeard, Ontario, practically the northern limit of corn growing and 385 miles north of the original outbreak in southern Ontario. Infestation in Quebec is still less than one per cent., but has increased in Ontario. The pest has not yet been found in Nova Scotia or New Brunswick, it was stated. Control operations in Ontario were, on the whole, a success, but were seriously handicapped by a wet spring and fall.

FOWLS that have been rendered completely sexless are substantially identical, regardless of their original sex, Dr. Lincoln V. Domm, of the University of Chicago, reported at the meeting of the American Association. Hens, deprived of their characteristically feminine organs, develop rooster-like plumage, spurs and small combs, but never attempted to crow, the scientist stated. In general they resembled capons both in behavior and appearance except for their consistently smaller size.

HUGE mounds of snail shells are evidence that prehistoric men in North Africa depended chiefly on snails for food, according to Dr. George L. Collie, director of the Logan Museum of Beloit College, speaking to anthropologists at the meeting of the American Association. A shell mound 300 feet long and eight feet high has been excavated by an expedition from the Logan Museum. Among the snail shells and kitchen ashes of the dump piles are found some bones of animals and once in a while a human skeleton. Excavators also unearthed flint arrow points and scrapers and hammer stones lost or thrown away by Stone Age men and women thousands of years ago. Small bone tools with fine, delicate points are the most common of the bone implements in the shell mounds, and some archeologists believe that they were used as picks or forks to remove snails from their shells.

MANHATTAN'S smoke screen cuts out 42 per cent. of the morning sunlight. At noon the loss is 18 per cent. The figures for this indictment of the smoke nuisance in large cities have been compiled by experts of the U. S. Public Health Service. Loss of efficiency from decreased lighting is not the only result of excessive smoke in manufacturing centers. It also cuts out to a large extent the ultra-violet rays necessary for good health. The importance of getting rid of smoke is emphasized for the preservation of eyesight and health generally, as well as for the prevention of accidents. On foggy days the loss of light runs even higher than the figures quoted.

SCIENCE NEWS

Science Service, Washington, D. C.

NATURAL, CULTURE AND ARTIFICIAL PEARLS

TRUE pearls derive their origin from the accidental introduction of an irritating foreign substance into certain cell tissues of the pearl oyster or other pearl-bearing mollusc. This foreign substance—parasitic worm, water-mite, grain of sand—which finds its way by accident into the tissues of the oyster becomes the nucleus of a natural pearl, the most prized and most valuable of the three classes. The cells of the oyster proceed at once to imprison the foreign substance, surrounding it with layer upon layer of nacreous material, of the same iridescent character as the inside shell of the oyster.

Since the discovery of the origin and growth of natural pearls, man has been striving to produce these results by artificial means, that is, to grow culture pearls. Simple as the process may seem, it was not until 1894 that Kokichi Mikimoto in Japan developed a satisfactory method for inducing the development of culture pearls. The success of this venture is attested to by the fact that he was able to produce an annual output valued at $600,000 in 1921.

Imitation pearls are a synthetic product manufactured in large quantities from pearl essence—a product derived from fish scales. Formerly the source of supply was a small Europeon minnow, the iridescent effect being discovered by accident by Jaquin, a French rosary maker, about 1656. Jaquin noted that the water in which the fish had been washed contained a highly lustrous substance which, when concentrated and applied to small globes of alabaster, produced remarkably good imitations of pearls. During the War, the European source of supply of fish scale essence or pearl essence was cut off. Experiments with the scales of native American fishes resulted in the development of an entirely new industry in this country. Some two million pounds of the scales of such fishes as our north Atlantic sea herring and river herring are used annually, the uses for fish scale essence are steadily increasing and the cost of producing excellent imitation pearls is decreasing. Large sheets of celluloid are also given a coating of imitation mother-of-pearl and used as backs for brushes and many other toilet articles.

But to return to the question of the means for distinguishing between the three classes of pearls under discussion, as pearl essence is usually applied as a thin coating, little difficulty will be experienced in ascertaining whether your possession is an imitation pearl. The celluloid coating can be cut or peeled off or dissolved off with amyl acetate or acetone.

As between culture pearls and natural pearls the problem of differentiation is a most difficult one. Yet, because of the difference in sales value, one buying a natural pearl wishes to assure himself that he is getting what he is paying for. In perfection of form and lustrous beauty there are no distinguishable differences. There is no chemical difference, the same cells of the oyster function after the same manner in producing a pearl. When the culture pearls began appearing there was considerable litigation in France and the courts concluded that culture pearls possessed all the specific characteristics of real pearls and their quality could not be questioned.

Since 1923, a small group of Japanese investigators acting on the suggestion of Professor Nakamura have been studying the problem, and have recently published the results of these investigations in the Proceedings of the Imperial Academy of Tokyo, Japan.

By the use of the X-rays they were able to distinguish between culture pearls and natural pearls. In the former, a perfectly spherical nucleus of shell is introduced into the oyster and around this the oyster builds the pearl. An examination of natural pearls, of culture pearls, and of the nuclei used in culture pearls by the expert in X-ray analysis and a comparison of the patterns produced for different orientations of the primary X-rays revealed valid differences between the two classes of pearls. It will undoubtedly be comforting to many to know that a method of differentiation has been evolved.—*Louis Radcliffe.*

THE DESIGN OF AIRPLANES

THERE is no "best" type of airplane, it all depends on what it is expected to do; and the plane should be as simple as possible, for then there are less chances for things to go wrong. This is the belief of the Honorable Edward P. Warner, assistant secretary of the Navy for aeronautics, and former professor of aeronautics at the Massachusetts Institute of Technology, expressed in an address in Philadelphia before the Franklin Institute.

"The quest for a universally applicable formula, for a hard and concrete statement of what is 'best' in design, has been persistent and unavailing. One of the many committees which has investigated the aeronautical activities of the government of the United States made a special effort to secure some sort of a 'yardstick' whereby statesmen comparatively uninstructed in the purely technical aspects of aviation could rate the merits of aircraft, but the effort was, and would be likely always to be, in vain.

"What is 'best' depends upon the end to be accomplished. Neither monoplane nor biplane has proved itself definitely and generally superior to the other. Machines with external bracing have neither driven from the field nor been overcome by those with the structure contained within the wings. Airplanes with one engine and those with two engines and those with more exist side by side."

In Mr. Warner's opinion, the design of airplanes is pretty well stabilized, and will probably not suffer any fundamental change for many years to come.

"It would not do to ignore or deny the possibility of invention producing a fundamental modification in the whole mode of operation of heavier-than-air craft," he

said, "but whatever happens the laws of aerodynamics will remain unchanged and will continue to govern the behavior of every machine that flies, however the details of its means of propulsion and of support might be changed.

"Anything may happen, but for myself I am not among those sanguine spirits who expect to see the airplane as we now know it displaced by some radically different machine capable of vertical ascent or descent, or other valuable novelties of performance. Such devices deserve the most serious consideration and examination and they may well prove of great usefulness in certain employments, but they are subject to fundamental difficulty in that they all involve some continuously moving parts within the structure. A rigid structure can be designed so that its chance of collapse is infinitesimal, but as soon as bearings and moving parts are introduced, even with the most careful design and the most watchful maintenance, there exists the chance for something to go wrong.

"If the upkeep is as slack as it is likely to become in the hands of the average private owner the chance is multiplied.

"To complicate the structure is to make the minimum conditions of safety less simple and sure, and it is because most of the proposals for radical modification in the fundamental method of operation of heavier-than-air craft are suggestions for increasing complication and for introducing new working parts that I view them as a whole with a considerable skepticism."

THE CHRONOTEINE CAMERA

Feeding movie film through a camera at the rate of three miles a minute to slow down rapidly moving machinery to about one two-hundredth of its normal speed is the feat accomplished by C. Francis Jenkins, of Washington. At the meeting of the Society of Automotive Engineers in Detroit Mr. Jenkins told of the "chronoteine camera," one of his latest inventions, and how it may be applied to the study of automobile engines.

Instead of the sixteen pictures a second, taken by the ordinary movie camera, or the 128 taken by the "ultra-rapid" camera now frequently used in filming athletic events, the chronoteine takes 3,200 pictures a second at its normal rate. If desired, it can be speeded up even further, and take as many as 10,000 a second. When these are projected in the ordinary machine at the speed of 16 a second, the apparent speed of the motion is correspondingly reduced. When taken at 3,200 per second, the reduction of speed is 200 times, and at the higher speeds it is of course greater.

In the usual type of motion picture camera, the film is stopped for each exposure, so that it stops and starts sixteen times a second. At such high speeds as those employed in the chronoteine camera this is impossible, for the film would be torn to pieces. Therefore it is moved through in a steady stream.

A further difficulty is introduced, because with a single lens extremely short exposures would have to be made. Otherwise the picture would be blurred, just as if the object itself were close to the camera and moving at such a high speed. Mr. Jenkins has avoided this difficulty by providing 48 lenses, set in the periphery of a 13-inch disc, which turns at a speed of 4,000 revolutions per minute. The film moves back of one side of this disc, so that the images formed by the lenses move right along with the film. In fact, the exposures overlap, as the exposure is begun through one lens before that through the preceding lens is completed. At 3,200 exposures a second, each one is about one twenty-five-hundredth of a second in length. With the rapid lenses used, and sensitive film, this is easily sufficient for a fully timed negative in bright sunlight. In the ordinary movie camera, at 16 a second, each exposure is about one thirty-second of a second in duration.

Mr. Jenkins calls attention to the good photographic quality in the pictures, which is unusual in such high-speed studies. "The pictures are true photographic pictures having half-tone values like other motion pictures, not mere shadowy outlines of grayish silhouettes," he says. "They are made out of doors as well as in the laboratory, of large subjects or small subjects, and from a moving vehicle as readily as from a fixed platform.

"The chronoteine camera is an instrument for the study of many problems in science and engineering, some of which are not possible of accurate determination in any other way. Some additional applications of this instrument which immediately suggest themselves are a study of gun recoil, shell trajectories and plate impacts, airplane propellers and landing-gear action, bursting of balloons and air hose, tire action over obstructions, water streams, propagation of flame, engine-valve rebound at high speed, cam-roller jumping, crank-shaft whip; transformer explosions and circuit-breaker arcs; shuttle thread-knots and bobbin action, brake-shoe and draft-gear application, in fact, anything that moves too fast for the eye to follow can be shown slowed down and can be examined in detail at leisure and repeatedly."

THE MOSQUITO FISH

Gambusia, the little fish that is such an enemy of "wigglers" that it has earned for itself the honorable title of Mosquito Fish, reverses the usual order of nature, in that the "gentler sex" is the male. The world's rude buffets kill off male mosquito fish as they grow up, until when a given brood arrives at maturity there are from two and one-half to eleven times as many females as there are males, although they started out in life in equal numbers. So states Dr. Samuel F. Hildebrand, director of the U. S. Fisheries Biological Station, who has been studying the survival rates of these little but economically and hygienically important fish. The sex ratios vary according to the season, being about 2.5 females to 1 male in June, and 11.3 females to 1 male in August.

The reasons for the higher death-rate among the young males have not been fully worked out, but it is suggested that inasmuch as they are considerably smaller than the females they fall easier prey to carnivorous fish. Moreover, the females themselves frequently attack and

SUPPLY DEPARTMENT
Open the Entire Year

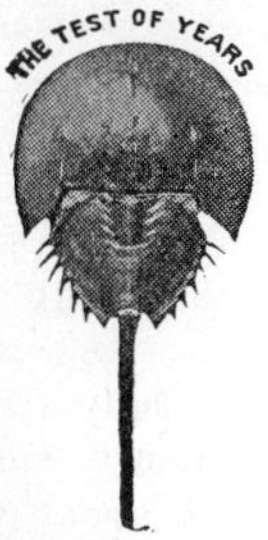

BIOLOGICAL SUPPLIES

For the classroom, museum or collector.

First class preparations.

Send for new (1926) Catalogue No. 1. Zoological and Embryological material, Life Histories and Habitat Groups.

Catalogue No. 2, Botanical Material
Catalogue No. 3, Microscopic Slides

Address all correspondence regarding material and catalogues to:

GEO. M. GRAY, Curator

THE MARINE BIOLOGICAL LABORATORY
Woods Hole, Mass.

THE MICROSCOPE

By SIMON H. GAGE, of Cornell University

Revised, Dark-field Edition (1927) now Available.
The Old and the New in Microscopy, with a special chapter on Dark-Field Methods and their Application.

Postpaid, $3.50

COMSTOCK PUBLISHING CO., ITHACA, N. Y.

SCIENTIFIC PERIODICALS

Chemical, Medical and allied subjects. Complete files, volumes and copies, bought and sold. Kindly send us a list of your wants and items of which you may wish to dispose.

B. LOGIN & SON
29 East 21st Street New York, N. Y.

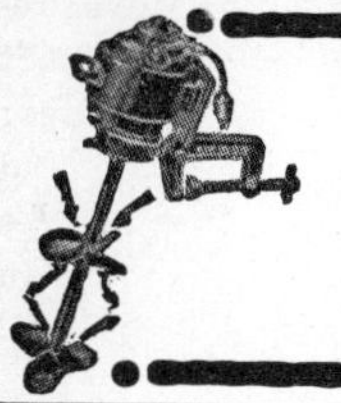

Hy-Speed Mixers

Clamp to any tank, operate from light circuit, mix all kinds of liquids. Also used for even temperature baths. Thousands in use.
Write for circular.
ALSOP ENGINEERING CO.
47 W. 63rd St., New York

PROFESSOR

Your manuscript or notes can be published by the photographic-zinc-plate process. We print on both sides of a page, reduce to desired size and bind in book form. Write for our booklet and prices.

SHELWOOD-HILL, Inc.,
50 Church St., N. Y. C.

A Personal Service for INVENTORS

I maintain an unexcelled organization and thoroughly equipped laboratories, to render the following services:

I PREPARE APPLICATIONS for patents for filing in the United States and foreign countries.

I PLACE INVENTIONS with responsible manufacturers, with whom I am acquainted, under arrangements that are made profitable to the inventor.

I SPECIALIZE in Electrical, Mechanical, Chemical and Radio Devices.

I INVITE CORRESPONDENCE with reputable Inventors, Scientists, Chemists and Physicists, regarding their inventions and uncompleted experiments.

H. R. VANDEVENTER
Registered Patent Attorney
Licensed Professional Engineer
342 Madison Avenue, New York City

PHOTO-ELECTRIC CELLS
THE BURT CELL

Without Fatigue—Highly Sensitive
Absolutely Reproducible—Instantaneous in Response

The **BURT-CELL** is made by a new method and should not be confused with any other photo-electric cell. By a special process of electrolysis, the photo-electric metal is introduced into a highly evacuated bulb directly through the glass wall of the bulb, giving photo-electric material of absolute purity. The superiority of the **BURT-CELL** is due to these features, making possible results never before obtainable.

Described in Bulletin No. 271

QUARTZ CELLS—We are pleased to announce that we are manufacturing reproducible quartz photo-cells for measurement of ultra-violet.

We also manufacture the **STABILIZED OSCILLOSCOPE**—the only **VISUAL OSCILLOGRAPH** having a linear time axis and no inertia—giving an accurate picture of high frequency wave forms. This is a most powerful tool for the study of periodic phenomena.

Write for Bulletin 273

DR. ROBERT C. BURT
Manufacturing and Consulting Physicist
327 S. Michigan Ave., Pasadena, Calif.

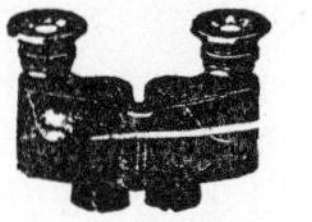

MIRAKEL BINOCULARS

The new 7-Power, weighs only 6 oz. Can be carried in vest pocket or ladies' bag. A wonderful high-grade Jena Prism Binocular for every use $35

Hensoldt New "Dialyt"—6 x 30—13 oz.	$58
Zeiss Wide-Angle "Deltrintem"—8 x 30	$66
Prismiris Pocket Binocular. 6 Power	$16
Compass—U. S. Engineers, Floating Dial	$3.50
Sleeping Bags: Fiala Pat., Light Weight, Sanitary, Scientifically Correct	$25
Mannlicher-Schoenauer Rifle, with Zeiss Telescope, Noske Mount, Very Fine	$142
Barometer: Mahogany, for Wall, Accurate	$5
Hygrometer: Every House Needs one	$3.50

Scientific Instruments, Tents, and Complete Outfits
Write for FREE Catalog "A"

ANTHONY FIALA, 25 Warren St., N. Y. City

LIVING BULLFROGS

Safe delivery guaranteed

Teach Biology with live specimens where practicable

We have the only complete live materials establishment in America. Live plants and animals representing all types are kept on hand under semi-natural conditions at all seasons.

Also headquarters for preserved specimens of all types, microscopic slides, life histories, demonstrations, osteological preparations, insect collections. We specialize in many important southern species not obtainable elsewhere.

All material guaranteed without reservations.

SOUTHERN BIOLOGICAL SUPPLY CO., INC.,
Natural History Building, New Orleans, La.

kill the males, which seem to be too chivalrous or else too timid to bite back. Finally, experiments indicate that unfavorable environmental factors, such as lack of oxygen in the water, affect the males more severely than the females.

In spite of the predominance of females it is not belived that the breeding rate is held in check, for the fish are highly polygamous.

MUMMIES IN NEW MEXICO

THE discovery of some interesting mummies has been announced by Frank Pinkley, superintendent of southwestern monuments for the National Park Service. At the Aztec Ruin, in New Mexico, excavation work has been in progress for the purpose of getting daylight down into a row of prehistoric rooms being used for museum purposes. In the course of this work two child burials were taken from the floor, one with a very interesting black obsidian pendant, two decorated dippers, a mug and two dishes containing food. This mummy was first wrapped in feather cloth and then in matting, and in addition had beneath it a large reed screen and over it a large mat.

The body itself was wrapped as a large package and tied with yucca cord. The pendant had slipped from the package, and it is believed by George L. Boundey, custodian of the monument, who made the excavation, that there are other ornaments within the wrappings. He did not open them, however, as the whole is in such a good state of preservation and is an excellent museum exhibit.

The other child burial found at Aztec had with it an ax, a basket, a flat board, and about a pint of corn ears. One ear, of red corn and just as fresh looking as though from last year's crop, has about half the kernels still in place. Mr. Boundey states this is unlike any corn he ever saw before. In the hard dirt floor of the lower story of rooms in the ruin five soft breaks were noticed. One of these was partially dug out and disclosed some peculiarly carved sticks and three pots.

Montezuma Castle National Monument, in Arizona, also yielded a prehistoric infant burial, which has been added to the museum at that place. The child had been buried with eleven shell bracelets over one arm and a string of shell beads around the neck. This mummy was discovered by Mrs. Martin L. Jackson, wife of the custodian of Montezuma Castle. She also unearthed two fine fragments of lace or embroidered cloth.

ITEMS

THE general death rate of the industrial population of the United States and Canada for 1927 will probably be the lowest ever reported, according to figures already available from the records of the Metropolitan Life Insurance Company. The chief factor in bringing about this decrease is the drop in the influenza death rate to about half that of 1926, with an accompanying decline in pneumonia mortality. Deaths from tuberculosis probably will reach a new low level in 1927, it is stated, attaining a point that would have been regarded as nothing less than visionary as short a time as ten years ago. Whereas the rate was 224.6 deaths for every 100,000 of the company's policyholders in 1911, the indications are that for 1927 it will not exceed 90 per 100,000. The year just past, however, will show no decrease in the number of accidental deaths over the last three or four years. The rising toll of the automobile, the statisticians report, along with considerably more suicides and a small increase in homicides all combine to make the 1927 record of violent deaths decidedly depressing.

THE ability of a living diphtheria bacterium to pour poisons into the blood stream of humans bears a relation to the size of the charge of electricity which each bacterial cell carries, according to Drs. I. S. Falk, L. B. Jensen and J. H. Mills, of the University of Chicago. Their electrical measurements can be made in a few minutes and with simple apparatus on cultures thought to be capable of producing toxin. The results are obtained much more rapidly than by time-consuming methods of animal experimentation. The electrical method is based on the fact that the power of the bacterium to excrete poisons depends on the porosity of its outer wall. This, in turn, affects the electrical charge on the cell as a whole. The observation is made by placing the suspected organisms in a small chamber between metallic plates charged to a definite electrical potential. The rate at which the bacteria cross the electrical field is then watched through a microscope. The virulence of the germs can be calculated by reference to the rate of "migration" of a stream of diphtheria of known toxin-producing power. This new method is expected to speed up detection of cases of diphtheria, and to facilitate release from quarantine.

NEW light has been shed on the problem of getting the marten, an animal of the mink family whose skin is highly prized for fur, to produce offspring during captivity. Research conducted by Frank G. Ashbrook and Karl B. Hanson, of the U. S. Biological Survey, at a federal fur farm in the foothills of the Adirondacks indicates that contrary to general belief martens of opposite sex will live together in peace and harmony during most months of the year. The males, however, fight ferociously whenever they come in contact. The normal breeding season, Mr. Ashbrook declares in a report in a forthcoming issue of the *Journal of Heredity*, is late summer rather than during the winter as was previously supposed. The normal gestation period, moreover, may require as long as eight months instead of the two or three that naturalists have assumed in the past.

THE puncture vine, whose sharp-pointed burrs cause endless trouble to motorists in California, has made its appearance in Australia, it has just been learned. The Australian authorities are endeavoring to stamp it out by piling refuse on it and burning both vine and seeds. Botanists have given the vine the appropriate name *Tribulus terrestris,* which means "trouble of the earth." It is stated that its original home was in the Mediterranean region, but like many ill weeds it has become a great traveler.

SCIENCE NEWS

Science Service, Washington, D. C.

BROADCASTING PHOTOGRAPHS

In broadcasting photographs from Station WEAF, in New York, and receiving them in a private home 25 miles away from the transmitting station, radio engineers have gone a step farther towards the day when broadcasting of pictures of events, as well as the events themselves, will be as common as broadcasting of music.

The sending apparatus developed by Dr. E. F. W. Alexanderson, of the General Electric Company, and used in the recent demonstration from WEAF, is essentially similar to that used by the Bell Telephone Company in sending photographs across the country by telephone wires, as that used by the Radio Corporation of America in transmitting photographs across the ocean by radio, and as that invented by C. Francis Jenkins, of Washington, and used by the Navy Department to send weather maps to ships at sea. Another form of the same apparatus has been developed by *Radio Broadcast Magazine*, which recently conducted the first sending of photographs by radio for reception on a set that could be built at home.

In all these methods, the heart is in the so-called photoelectric cell. This device takes a beam of light that falls on it, and converts it to electricity. It depends on the fact that when a film of metal, such as potassium or sodium, is illuminated, it gives off electrons. These are the tiny atoms of electricity, of which the atoms of matter are supposed to consist. Their motion inside the cell results in a minute electric current. Vacuum tubes like those in ordinary radio receivers can amplify this minute current millions of times, if necessary.

In the Alexanderson transmitter, the photograph to be sent is wrapped around a cylinder which revolves in the same way as the old-time cylindrical phonograph records. But instead of the needle and sound box of the phonograph, a lens focusses a spot of light from a tiny lamp on to the cylindrical picture. A toothed revolving disc breaks the reflected light up into a series of impulses bright or faint, depending on the brightness of the part of the picture illuminated at the time. These impulses of light fall on the photoelectric cell, which produces a varying electric current corresponding to the picture. This apparatus is connected to the radio transmitter replacing the microphone, and so the radio impulses go out from the aerial, carrying the picture with them.

In the device for receiving the picture any standard radio set can be used for converting the radio waves back to electrical impulses. But instead of feeding these impulses into a loud speaker to emerge as sound waves, they go to a box where they are amplified further. Then they go to a Moore neon lamp, a form of electric bulb in which the light is furnished by glowing neon gas, instead of a tungsten filament. Unlike the tungsten light, which takes a brief time to start glowing after the current is turned on, and which remains glowing for an instant after the current is off, the neon lamp goes on and off instantaneously. On account of this advantage it has been extensively used in phototelegraphy and television. Forms of it were employed in the Bell laboratories system of television, demonstrated last April, and in Dr. Alexanderson's own television system, which had its public début a few weeks ago.

In this way a beam of light is obtained from the neon lamp that varies as did the beam reflected from the cylindrical picture in the transmitter. This beam is focussed on a sheet of sensitive photographic paper, which is wrapped around a cylinder revolving like the cylinder at the transmitter. Both cylinders slowly move in the direction of their length as they turn, covering the whole picture. About 90 seconds of broadcasting time is required for a 4½- by 8-inch picture. The photographic paper is taken from the receiving cylinder and developed in the same manner as any ordinary print, made from a snapshot negative. It is a facsimile of the original picture.

Other forms of apparatus for transmitting pictures by wire or radio have been demonstrated from time to time. Their chief differences are in the method of varying the light in the receiver. In the Bell apparatus, by which any one with the price can wire a photograph in a few hours from New York to San Francisco, a "light valve" takes the place of the neon lamp. An electric bulb of the ordinary type provides the light, and its intensity is varied by the valve, which in turn varies according to the current reaching it from the distant transmitter. The Cooley "rayfoto" device, that was demonstrated at the recent New York radio show by *Radio Broadcast Magazine*, uses an electrical discharge playing directly on the sensitive paper to form the image. In the Radio Corporation's radiophoto system, the amount of ink sprayed pneumatically on ordinary paper is regulated by the incoming current.

GAME ANIMALS IN THE SOUTHWEST

Manage your game animals and your livestock the same. This is the advice given to New Mexico sportsmen and ranchers by J. Stokley Ligon, of the U. S. Biological Survey. The once abundant wild life of the Southwest can be restored on the same basis as the deflated cattle industry by scientific range management and control of predatory animals, Mr. Ligon contends in his report on the wild life of New Mexico recently published by the state game commission.

"As an asset to the Southwest, wild life in the future can be made equal to a stabilized livestock industry," said Mr. Ligon. "It is one of the most valuable crops that can be produced; yet it has and continues to be the most recklessly abused. For the same reason that the Southwest is the leading year-around open range cattle and sheep country in the land, it is one of the best year-around game sections. The varying topography of the

state ranging from plains at less than 3,000 feet to mountain peaks at 13,600 feet results in the widespread distribution of more than fifteen distinctive game animals, ten species of resident land game birds, the many species of fish and a great variety of non-game birds.''

It is man's domestic animals rather than his shot-gun which have nearly exterminated the native wild life in the Southwest, says Mr. Ligon. In the early days of free range the country was so heavily overstocked with cattle that the forage was badly depleted. This resulted in starvation for the game animals and birds and loss of the protective shelter of browse. While the stock suffered as much in a few years by these methods as the wild animals, the latter were able to find natural refuges in the rugged mountainous areas into which the stock could not penetrate. For this reason big game is still found all over the state except in the Navajo country which was completely hunted out before state game laws became effective. Deer, turkey and quail are now the principal residence game. Mr. Ligon recommends the restocking of depleted areas with native game, reintroducing such exterminated species as buffalo, elk and sage grouse, the establishment of refuges and the enforcement of strict game laws.

THE ART OF INSANE PATIENTS

Art critics of Paris are interested in an exhibit of painting and sculpture by patients afflicted with mental disease, according to reports received by the American Medical Association from its French correspondent.

It is a difficult matter, apparently, to choose between the psychopathic art and the products of the ultramodern school, futurists, cubists and the like. Only the work of patients who were not artists before their admission into institutions, it is stated, are included in the exhibition.

This does not necessarily mean that the ultramoderns, who paint voluntarily the impressions of the subconscious mind, are insane, in the opinion of Dr. August Marie, a well-known French expert on mental disease. Such artists contend that they give free rein to their emotions and depict their inmost dreams without the control of reason very much after the manner of spontaneous art of savage tribes and prehistoric races.

The insane merely describe the vagaries of their subconscious minds and hallucinations for the satisfaction they get out of it. Most of them have no notion of technique, yet one painted in quite unearthly colors, roaring flames and waves of fire worthy of Turner. This picture was bought by a wallpaper manufacturer to serve as the basis of a new wallpaper design. A psychopathic priest depicted a pope blowing soap bubbles before an assemblage of swooning frogs.

The French expert believes that some of the paintings, if removed from their environment and placed in the collections of a reputable dealer, would command high prices.

ITEMS

One of the largest group of spots observed in recent months is now crossing the face of the sun, according to Professor George H. Peters, of the U. S. Naval Observatory. Professor Peters takes photographs of the sun every clear day, and he first noticed the spot, as it came around the eastern edge of the sun, on January 17. On Friday, January 20, he photographed it again, and estimated its size as approximately 125,000 miles, or about half of the distance from the earth to the moon. Sunspots shoot out rapidly moving electrons, or ''cathode rays,'' and when directly pointed towards the earth, the earth receives them. Under the influence of the earth's magnetic field, they cause the rarefied gases in the earth's upper atmosphere to glow, thus producing the aurora borealis, or ''northern lights.'' Professor Peters pointed out that several years ago he predicted that the maximum of the approximately eleven-year period, during which the numbers of sun-spots wax and wane, would be reached late this year and that it now looks as if this prediction would be fulfilled.

Dr. S. Bayne-Jones, of the University of Rochester Medical School, has taken motion picture reels of thousands of generations of bacteria that enable a spectator to follow them through many days of growth and activity in a few minutes. Micromovies will aid biologists in working out obscure growth processes of many rudimentary forms of life, it is said, and in addition, classroom reels may be made for the instruction of students of medicine and industrial bacteriology. One of the chief difficulties which had to be overcome was to maintain the microscope in accurate focus, which required elimination of vibration from the camera part of the apparatus. Most of the negatives which have been made to date call for one exposure a minute, and when the positives have been prepared they are run through the projector at the rate of 16 pictures a second, which gives the effect of compressing the life histories of the microscopic plants and animals.

American automobile owners can save gasoline by using engines that operate at a constant instead of a variable pressure, Professor H. M. Jacklin, of Purdue University, has reported to the Society of Automotive Engineers. Present auto engines operate so that the volume of the gaseous fuel exploded is constant. Professor Jacklin's experiments were made upon an experimental engine constructed with a movable cylinder-head that was used to reduce the volume of the cylinder as the speed of the engine decreases. This maintained the same pressure within the cylinder at all speeds. No adjustment of spark was necessary. Gains of up to 50 per cent. in miles per gallon might be expected if the new type engine were substituted for the ordinary engine now in use. Fuel bills would be cut a third, according to Professor Jacklin's computations. Assuming a complete substitution of the constant compression engine in the 20,000,000 cars now running 6,000 miles a year on 20 cents per gallon gasoline, Professor Jacklin sees the possibility of conserving our natural resources and the national pocketbook to the extent of some four hundred millions annually.

saw mills and pulp mills have had to move to more and more remote locations from their markets.

"Lest the corn production should decrease, the fertility of the soil must be maintained. It has been learned that this can readily be done by growing soya beans as the 'rotation' crop. The soya bean is a strong nitrifier of the soil. After extracting the oil from the bean, the refuse, including the stalks and meal, can be plowed back into the soil. The income from the oil, which has many uses, will partially offset the lack of income from corn in the years of change of crop. Thus the cycle would become complete by the chemistry of nature, and the energy of the sun would be converted perennially to many uses of man.

"Depletion of forests and of mineral resources and advances in chemistry and engineering will have much to do with the measures of success which may be achieved in turning these agricultural wastes into wealth. At best, it will take much time, research and development.

"More than research, engineering, industrial development and financing will be required. Useful and valuable new commodities may be produced, but successful production at a fair price may not bring economic success. As has well been said: The fight for recognition for a new product is almost as hard to wage as is the fight for a new idea."

THE CORN BORER MENACE

THE corn borer, which has swept over the northeastern states and during the past season made its first serious inroads into the great mid-western corn belt, may lose its terror as it spreads westward into the less humid prairie regions. Researches by Professor E. N. Transeau and Professor H. C. Sampson, of the Ohio State University, indicate that the pest tends to accumulate in really destructive numbers mainly in areas of naturally high soil and atmospheric moisture, and that its presence in drier places is less likely to be a serious matter.

Professor Transeau's studies began in Ohio and Ontario, but were carried forward last summer by visits to the principal corn-raising regions of Europe, where the borer has been known for more than a century. In the analysis of the Ohio and Ontario data, it was discovered that the most serious borer infestation occurred in parts that were once covered by swamps and swamp forests. Fields that had been won from the former beech forests were also infested, but less seriously, and the areas that got off most easily were those that had once been covered by oak-hickory timber. The significant thing about this difference, Professor Transeau points out, is that the beech forest was a formation of relatively moist lands, whereas the oak-hickory was a dry type of forest.

In Europe, the Ohio botanist found that conditions bore out his preliminary observations in this country. The heaviest infestations were found in what were once swamp forest regions, while corn growing in drier and better drained hilly areas was much less troubled. In particular, he found that the great corn-growing areas of Rumania and southern Russia, which are naturally open grasslands instead of forests, are not greatly troubled by the borers, in spite of the fact that the farmers of these two countries probably take fewer clean-up precautions than do the corn growers of any other part of Europe.

Since the richest part of the American corn belt, reaching from central Illinois across Iowa into Nebraska, was originally a grassland, it is hoped that conditions here will be as unfavorable to the borer and as favorable to the corn as those of the European grasslands seem to be. It is true that the situation is not exactly parallel, for the long-grass prairies of Illinois and Iowa have no counterpart in southeastern Europe, whose grassy steppes are more like the mixed prairie and short-grass plains of Nebraska and Kansas. The long-grass prairies in part originated from sloughs and swamps, and in part developed on well drained uplands. The swamp prairie lands appear to be favorable to the corn borer. The upland long-grass prairies on the other hand fit into the series between the oak-hickory forest and the short-grass steppes or plains; and the relatively slight borer infestation of both regions gives rise to the hope that when the pest finally reaches the heart of the corn belt it will not everywhere have the disastrous effects on the principal American grain crop that were at first feared from its behavior in the vicinity of Lake Erie.

ULTRA-VIOLET RAYS AND MINERAL SALTS IN PLANTS

ULTRA-VIOLET rays, used to prevent the bone disease, rickets, in young children and animals by raising the calcium and phosphorus content of the blood, have a parallel effect on plants. This is indicated by the results of experiments by Herbert C. Beeskow, a graduate student at the University of Chicago.

Mr. Beeskow grew groups of soy bean plants in solutions of known mineral composition. He subjected different groups to ultra-violet radiation for varying periods of time, keeping other groups away from the rays as "controls." Then he dried the plants and analyzed them for calcium and phosphorus. In each case it was found that the irradiated plants had noticeably higher contents of these important minerals than the corresponding unrayed controls.

The effects of irradiation with ultra-violet light were not all beneficial to the plants. Soy beans grown in the greenhouse and subjected to direct ultra-violet raying for as short a period as one minute every other day showed a distinct reddening in the parts of the stem and leaves struck by the rays. This coloration increased with increases in dosage. In cases where the under side of the leaves was exposed to the rays the reddening action was much more in evidence.

Plants grown in darkness and subjected to the rays showed this red color much more distinctly than plants grown in daylight and permitted to become normally green. Heavy overdoses of the rays simply killed the plants.

THE VOLTAGE OF VACUUM TUBES

USING a radio vacuum tube backwards in order to reduce the voltage and increase the power at the same time is the trick described at the Institute of Radio Engineers.

In a paper by Frederick E. Terman, of Stanford University, California, it was stated that the plate and the grid of a tube could be made to interchange their functions.

In the ordinary vacuum tube, as used in the usual receiving set as an amplifier, the feeble electrical impulses that form the signals are fed into the grid. The electrons that travel across from the filament to the plate produce an electrical current, much larger than the current entering the tube, but varying in conformity with it. However, the outgoing current is also higher in voltage, as well as more powerful, than the incoming.

Mr. Terman has found, however, that the voltage can be reduced by interchanging the plate and grid. He feeds in the current to be amplified to the plate instead of the grid, and takes it out from the grid.

"It is relatively simple," he states, "to construct an inverted vacuum tube with wide clearances between the plate and the rest of the tube, so that potentials of hundreds of thousands of volts can be applied at the plate, while the effect of this high voltage stepped down in almost any desired ratio is obtained in a low potential circuit."

The chief use of the inverted tube, Mr. Terman stated, is in studying the waves formed by high voltage alternating currents, using an oscillograph. In this way, the current variations can be studied without consuming any appreciable amount of the current. No immediate use of the device in ordinary radio sets is foreseen.

RADIO RECEIVERS

SHEETS of metal such as iron, gold or platinum, so thin that ordinary type can be read with ease through them, may find use in radio and phonograph reproducers. Ordinary diaphragms for this purpose are so heavy that they dampen some of the overtones and so coarsen the sounds. These thin metal sheets are the result of research by Dr. Carl Mueller, of the Charlottenburg Laboratory, near Berlin. His method of preparing them is to electroplate the metal on the surface of some soluble substance, such as rocksalt, and then dissolve away the support. A ring of thicker metal can be used to support the films, of which two and a half million would have to be piled to make a stack an inch high.

Such films have been made of iron, nickel, gold, silver and platinum, and it is found that although the nickel is much less transparent to visible light than gold, it readily transmits the shorter ultra-violet rays. The films are very elastic, and will bulge out for as much as a tenth of their diameter without breaking. Another curious thing about them is their high electrical conductivity. Electric current is carried only along the surface of a wire, and as these are practically all surface, a strip of film containing no more metal than in a round wire one hundredth of a millimeter in diameter—scarcely visible to the naked eye—will carry enough current to light several lamps. If the same current were passed through the wire, it would be instantly melted.

ITEMS

SEEDLING trees of a species that represents the vegetation of Florida a hundred thousand years ago, during the glacial epoch, have been added to the collection in the New York Botanical Garden as the result of a scientific tour of the state by Dr. John K. Small. The trees, which are known as Torreya, or locally as Savern, belong to the botanical genus *Tumion*, and occur naturally in a small strip of territory along the east bank of the Appalachicola River, in the Florida Panhandle. They occur nowhere else in the world, though related species are found in California, Japan and China. They resemble yew trees in some ways, and can be cultivated under the same sort of climatic conditions that favor the yew. In addition to the Torreya seedlings, Dr. Small also obtained a collection of native Florida iris species, which are being carried through the winter in the garden of Mrs. A. C. James at Coconut Grove, Florida. A part of this collection will be brought north to the New York Botanical Garden in the spring.

THE largest telescope in Italy, with a mirror 40 inches in diameter, is now in use at the Merate Observatory, in the foothills of the Alps. Ordered in 1923, when the dust and smoke of Milan made it necessary for the observatory to move to a better location, the new instrument embodies all the latest improvements. It is a reflecting telescope, in which the 40-inch concave mirror takes the place of the convex lens in the more familiar type of telescope. The moving parts of the telescope weigh over 18 tons, yet so perfectly are they balanced that a one half horsepower motor is adequate for turning the instrument to follow the stars across the sky. The instrument was built by the Carl Zeiss Optical Works, in Jena, Germany.

"A LOVE of luxury is everywhere in the world tending to produce fewer marriages and fewer births," according to Dr. Charles V. Chapin, who for almost 40 years has supervised the collection of the vital statistics of Providence, R. I. The city's birth rate last year was the lowest since records were first kept. "In most of the advanced countries of Europe for several years the tendency of both marriages and births has been downward. I believe this is generally due to the fact that people don't feel they can afford to either marry or have children. They would rather have fur coats and automobiles." Of the children born here last year, 3,089 were boys and 2,049 girls.

A SELF-WINDING clock, run by what is virtually a glycerin thermometer, has been invented by a Swiss engineer, Karl Heinrich Meier. It utilizes the energy captured by the daily fluctuations in temperature to raise the weights that drive its mechanism, and it is stated that one of the clocks has been kept going for a year on a daily range of not more than eight degrees Fahrenheit. The essential mechanism consists of a long coiled tube filled with glycerin, connected with a cylinder into which a piston is fitted. When the glycerin is warmed and expands, it forces out the piston, which in turn lifts the clock weight. It is expected that this device will be especially useful in operating outdoor clocks in public places. The types now in common use are usually electrically driven and are therefore expensive to install, besides requiring frequent attention.

laboratory were improved by being subjected to doses of oscillating electricity produced by vacuum tubes similar to those used in radio sets.

The frequencies used by Dr. Schereschewsky in his experiments ranged from 8,300 to 135,000 kilocycles per second, a range that expressed in the more familiar language of radio corresponds to wave-lengths below about 40 meters. The most effective frequencies were found to be at about the middle of the extremes used, and more deaths of the mice occurred at the high and low ends of the frequency range. Some of the mice treated suffered a shriveling of the ears and tail due to the current to which they were subjected, but many were perfectly normal after the treatment that had a beneficial effect on the cancers.

The dosage of electricity used by Dr. Schereschewsky were much more than any one could possibly receive from radio broadcasting, and public health officials discounted in advance any ideas or suggestions that the speed of radio would by this means aid in the treatment of cancer. They also emphasized the fact that the method was still in its early experimental stage upon animals only, and that treatment of human beings is still far in the future.

The investigations are being supported by the U. S. Public Health Service, with laboratory space furnished by the Harvard Medical School. They are now being pushed on account of the promising results and the unique methods that have been developed.

MEASUREMENTS OF THE SUN'S DISTANCE

A DEFINITE check on the distance of the earth from the sun is being made by University of California astronomers through observations of stars that will form a background for the planetoid Eros when it makes its remarkably close approach of 16,200,000 miles to the earth in 1931.

Many of the observations already have been completed by Dr. R. H. Tucker from the Lick Observatory on Mount Hamilton.

The positions of 821 stars were accurately determined in the series of observations thus far completed, according to Dr. Tucker. In the second series of observations, of 402 stars, about 2,100 checks were made during the course of 77 nights of work during the best observing season at Lick Observatory in 30 years.

The positions of the fixed stars, it is explained, appearing in the same portion of the sky as will the planetoid Eros during the coming approach, although at an infinitely greater distance away, will aid in the determination of the distance of Eros from the earth, both in terms of miles and in terms of a common astronomical unit, the mean diameter of the ellipse which the earth describes about the sun once each year.

By determining the exact distance of Eros in terms of both miles and of the unit of distance set by the earth's orbit about the sun, it will be possible also to compute the latter unit of distance in miles more accurately than ever before.

Eros' approach in 1931, astronomers state, will be its first close approach since its discovery in 1898. It is a small body, some fifteen or twenty miles in diameter, one of the host of such bodies known as the asteroids, but departing from the path followed by most of the group sufficiently to bring it in close proximity to the earth once in about 36 years.

SNAILS AND FRESH WATER FISH

THE humble pond snail has been indicted as one of the criminals whose activities have interfered with the peace and welfare and the family life of our fresh-water fishes. Ichthyologists generally have been unable to explain why so few of the hundreds of thousands of eggs laid by each female among the fresh-water fish ever reach maturity.

In a life-history study of the long-eared sunfish, carried on at the Indiana University Biological Station at Winona Lake, Indiana, observations were made each day of the troubles of a vigilant male sunfish trying to guard his nest with its precious eggs.

This sunfish had very little trouble with the larger fish. They had seemed to learn their lesson of the purpose and use of the fin spines and remained at a respectful distance. Minnows lingered in a persistent swarm and darted into the nest every time the warrior's attention was diverted, but their activities were more of a nuisance than a vital menace.

The greatest difficulty the harassed father sunfish had was the insidious advance of the tank corps of snails. The sunfish could not kill the snails because of their protective shells, but had to pick them up and carry them away from the nest one at a time. By the time he was transporting one half a dozen others would crawl in among the eggs and eat their fill.

Several thousand eggs and a few snails were put in a bucket over night. In the morning all the eggs had disappeared, and an examination of the snails' stomachs did not leave even a scientific doubt as to where they had gone.

THE DEATH RATE OF 1927

THE healthiest year in history was 1927. Only 8.4 deaths for every 1,000 persons is the record for a group of insured wage-workers that numbers one seventh of the total population of the United States and Canada.

If the death rate of 1926 had prevailed, 8,808 persons among the insured group now living would have died, and if the rest of the population improved its health as much, some 50,000 lives were saved. If the death rate of sixteen years ago, 1911, had not been reduced 33 per cent. to the present figure, last year's death list would have numbered 72,570 more among the insured group.

These facts are shown by the statistics of the Metropolitan Life Insurance Company reporting the mortality of its industrial policyholders which had been found to reflect the trends of the whole population.

The outstanding health fact of 1927 was the big drop in the tuberculosis mortality, the rate of 93.5 per 100,000 representing a decrease of 4.8 per cent. from the previous minimum of deaths from the great white plague. Recent surveys have shown that this reduction applies to all parts of the country, rural and urban, colored and

white, and extends to all occupations and branches of industry.

Three of the diseases of childhood, measles, scarlet fever and whooping cough, had encouragingly low death rates, while influenza and pneumonia reached unexpected low records. Never, except in the years immediately following the big influenza epidemics of 1918 and 1919, has there been as big a drop in the number of deaths from these much-dreaded plagues.

To counterbalance these gratifying returns, the toll of cancer was higher than ever before and that of diabetes remained the same as last year in spite of the increasing use of insulin. This, however, is no ground for drawing the conclusion that insulin is ineffective. Statisticians declare that the average age of diabetics at death has increased, and that without insulin the diabetes death rate would undoubtedly run even higher than it now is.

The automobile continued its guilty rôle in 1927 as principal cause of fatal accidents. Almost as many wage-earners' children lost their lives in 1927, it was pointed out, from automobile accidents as from measles, scarlet fever and whooping cough combined, while the number of motor car fatalities as a whole was double that of ten years ago.

RELIGION AND ZOOLOGY

FUNDAMENTAL religion is supported by the scientific truths of zoology, although that science often finds itself unable to substantiate the claims made by the various sects and churches, especially when these are made by men who may be authorities in theology, but have no scientific background.

This was the position taken by Dr. Charles Wardell Stiles, secretary of the International Commission on Zoological Nomenclature, in an address before one of the leading church audiences of Washington.

Fundamental religion might be summed up in one word, "obligation," as exemplified in the golden rule and the famous definition of St. James: "To visit the fatherless and widows in their affliction, and to keep himself unspotted from the world." Special assertions about the existence and nature of God at once carry one beyond the constitution of religion and into a discussion of its by-laws, he said, and since these differ with different religions and sects, science is unable to agree with all of them, and may not be able to agree on certain points with any.

Obligation, the foundation of religion, might further be expressed in the phrase of the school-yard, "Play the game," and it is in inculcating the necessity of playing the game with one's fellowman, fairly and squarely, that zoological facts most strongly support religious teaching. Our hospitals and prisons are crowded with men who have failed to "play the game" according to the rules of nature no less than according to the rules of religion; they preach a more powerful sermon than can be heard from any pulpit on the effects of the sins of the fathers on the third and fourth generations.

It is only when the theologian fails to stick to his last, and wanders over into a field where the zoologist knows more than he, that apparent conflict arises between science and one of the religions, Dr. Stiles declared. The current controversy over evolution offers a good example of this difficulty. And really, the speaker continued, the anti-evolutionists among the churches are more radical evolutionists than the zoologists themselves, for they acknowledge the development of all the religions of the world to-day from the one religion that must have prevailed in the Garden of Eden. And on the physical side, if all the races of the world have arisen among the descendants of Noah since the flood, this is carrying on human evolution at a far faster rate than any zoologist would dare to claim before a scientific audience.

ITEMS

THE "ether drift" which, if it exists, would force the abandonment or radical modification of the Einstein theory, is declared to be non-existent by two Swiss scientists, Dr. A. Piccard and Dr. E. Stahel, of the University of Freiburg, as the result of experiments performed at the summit of the Rigi, a lofty peak in the Alps. The first effort to show a drifting motion, relative to the earth, of the hypothetical ether in which light waves travel was made about a half-century ago, by two American physicists, Dr. A. A. Michelson and Dr. S. G. Morley. Their results showed a small positive effect, but were not regarded as conclusive. During the past few years Dr. Dayton C. Miller, of the Case School of Applied Science, Cleveland, has been repeating the experiment with improved apparatus at the summit of Mt. Wilson, Calif., which has about the same altitude as the Rigi. His results have been definite and positive, but have nevertheless been the subject of much controversy.

BLACKBOARDS of translucent ground glass lighted from behind are proposed as a substitute for the opaque black surface familiar to every school child. Professor W. Weniger, of Oregon Agricultural College, has demonstrated this new blackboard and is using it in teaching his physics classes. The old type of blackboard is difficult to illuminate so that all the room can see, Professor Weniger found, while the ground glass lighted from the rear electrically allows everything chalked upon it to be seen from all parts of the room even when a combination of daylight and artificial illumination is being used. Erasing on the new "blackboard" is easy. It can also be used as a stereopticon screen and chalk talks can be interspersed with lantern slides without changing the lighting of the room.

THAT watercress, the familiar garnish for meat and salad, is a remarkably rich source of the vitamin necessary for growth and of the scurvy-preventing vitamin C, has been found by Dr. Katherine H. Coward and P. Eggleton, of the University of London. It boasts of small quantities of vitamin D as well in its small green leaves. The green shows considerable seasonal variation, however, in its growth-promoting properties, being more effective with laboratory animals in this respect in spring and summer than in winter.

SCIENCE NEWS

Science Service, Washington, D. C.

A SEISMOGRAPH TO RECORD MINOR EARTHQUAKES

A NEW seismograph that records the less violent tremblings of the earth's crust, undetectable by the human senses, is now installed and in operation at Stanford University. As a part of the fundamental plan for an intensive study of the California earthquake situation, this station has been established by the business men of San Francisco and Oakland as one of four, which are so located as to record the local shocks in the vicinity of that metropolitan center. The central station is at the University of California and the auxiliaries at Lick Observatory, Stanford University and the California Academy of Science in Golden Gate Park. The instruments and arrangement are patterned on the plan of observation inaugurated by the Carnegie Institution of Washington for southern California to keep track of the minute earthquakes that are constantly occurring and which indicate the development of strain that leads to the greater ones. Four little shocks were recorded recently at Stanford on the new instruments. There is no occasion for alarm, however, since this is merely the normal activity of the earth's crust, not only in California, but also in any region where earthquakes have occurred. Vibrations of the solid earth are as unknown as were those of the atmosphere before radio showed them up. Protection against earthquakes will not be achieved unless we secure a better understanding of their development during the long periods that elapse between severe shocks.

The seismograph installed at Stanford was placed on a ledge of rock that was selected because of its apparent solidity, but the first records showed an extraordinary number of microscopic vibrations, not exactly like those of earthquakes. They were most continuous on windy days and are attributed to a large oak tree which stands about fifty feet away from the instrument piers. The roots evidently extend into the crevices of the rocks, where they find water during the long dry season, and the swaying of the tree shakes the massive ledge of sandstone. The oak will probably have to be cut, to the regret of those who, because of its beauty, sought to include it in the Seismograph Park which has been set aside in perpetuity.

CORN WASTES

A BILLION dollars of new wealth for the corn belt, through the annual utilization of its two hundred million tons of corn stalks and twenty million tons of cobs, now wasted, is the promise of engineers and chemists to the American farmer.

How the greatest agricultural waste, corn stalks and cobs, can be made into some three hundred useful products is told in a report to the Engineering Foundation by Professor O. R. Sweeney, of Iowa State College. In a decade or two they will be utilized on a large scale, he predicted.

''Before the many products of promising usefulness could be made even on a small scale in the laboratory,'' Professor Sweeney said, ''years had to be spent in patient, ingenious, fundamental researches to determine the exact chemical and physical natures of these raw materials and their constituents. Not only agricultural, but also industrial and economic problems had to be solved with the aid of engineering research, supplementing the work of the scientist. Much remains to be done.

''Iowa State College, in the midst of the corn belt, has been a leader in the attack. Knowledge being gotten in the cornfield will be useful also to growers of other grains, peanuts, flax and cotton, who have similar waste materials. Civilized men will be able to continue to feed and clothe the increasing populace and to supply many of their other wants by successful solution of just these problems.

''What does the laboratory offer to industry from these raw materials now wasted? Paper of several grades, papier maché, wallboard and other substitutes for building lumber, substitutes for hard woods used in furniture and finish, rayon, acetic acid, acetone, a sugar that can be used by diabetics, maple-sugar flavoring to be combined with cane- or beet-sugar to make 'maple-syrup,' oxalic acid, plastic materials, electrical and heat insulation and furfural.

''Furfural was a laboratory chemical not many years ago, scarce at $50 a pound. Now it is produced in large quantities at 14 cents. With increasing production, improved methods and development of co-products, even the latter price may be more than cut in half. Furfural is a fluid heavier than water, having many and various uses in plastics, dyes, paint removers, antiseptics, anesthetics, germicides, embalming fluids and motor fuels. It burns in lamps with a more brilliant flame than kerosene and has not the unpleasant odor of the latter.

''If the chemist and engineer and farmer can solve the economic problems, new industries may dot the prairies. Among these problems one of the foremost has been the cheap collection of the stalks and cobs to a few places where they will be subjected to the first steps toward becoming saleable commodities. Special machines have been devised for gathering up the cornstalks in the field, or for cutting the standing corn, husking the ears and shredding the stalks. Another problem is the safe and inexpensive storage of the raw materials throughout the year, in order that the industrial operations may be continuous.

''As contrasted with forests, which, once cut, are not quickly replaced, and commonly in America are not replaced at all, the corn wastes would be produced year after year in great quantities within the same areas. As nearby forests have been consumed, for example, the

SCIENCE NEWS

Science Service, Washington, D. C.

ENGINEERING AND THE EVOLUTION OF SOCIETY

IN man himself, and in his behavior as a unit in the great superorganism into which society is developing, lies the chief obstacle to future social evolution. This was the keynote of an address given in New York on February 15 by General John J. Carty, vice-president of the American Telephone and Telegraph Company, in accepting the John Fritz Medal of the American Institute of Electrical Engineers. Only by adequate support of scientific research, he declared, can the human obstacle be surmounted.

"If seeking the truth and applying the truth to the affairs of men, is a spiritual thing, then the engineer must be absolved from the charge of materialism," said General Carty. "He is an advocate for truth. His works must be tried in the inexorable court of nature, where no errors are committed and no exceptions granted. The work of the engineer is dedicated to the use of mankind, and the pecuniary compensation which he himself obtains is slight compared with the great benefits received by society."

Future evolution of present-day man into a superman, even if it should occur, will be too slow to be of any immediate benefit. There is another kind of evolution that is preeminently under the control of the engineer. Quoting Professor E. G. Conklin, Princeton University biologist, General Carty pointed out that "the evolution of man, the individual, is no longer limited to his body or mind; but by adding to his own powers the forces of nature, man has entered upon a new path of progress. The differentiations of various members of a colony of ants or bees are limited to their bodies and are fixed and irreversible. But in human society, differentiations are no longer confined to the bodies of individuals. Although he is not as strong as the elephant, nor as deft as the spider, nor as swift as the antelope, nor as powerful in the water as the whale, nor in the air as the eagle, yet by his control of the forces of nature outside his body, man can excel all animals in strength and delicacy of movement, in speed and power, on land, in water and in air.

"The true object of engineering is not to create machines to which man would be bound by the chains of necessity, or mechanisms to which they would become slaves. The mission of the engineer is to obtain such a mastery in the application of the laws of nature that the forces of the universe will be employed in the service of man.

"The use of the spoken word to convey ideas distinguishes man from all other created things. It is the function of the engineer to provide for the extension of the spoken word by means of electrical systems of intercommunication which will serve to connect the nervous system of each unit of society with all the others, thus providing an indispensable element in the structure of that inconceivably great and powerful organism which I believe is to be the ultimate outcome of the marvelous evolution which society is to undergo.

"There is one element, and only one, which stands in the way of the realization of this inspiring vision. That is man himself, for he is the unit or cell out of which the new organism is to be evolved.

"Already, the applications of science to human affairs have far outrun the ability of man to use them wisely. The engineer has provided agencies of incalculable value in time of peace, but they are also endowed with prodigious powers of destruction which can be loosed in time of war. Unless we solve the problem encountered in man himself, the outlook is dark indeed, and it may even be questioned whether our civilization will endure. Human behavior presents the most formidable and the most important problem of all the ages. Its solution can be achieved only by concentrating upon it all of the knowledge and wisdom and resources at the disposal of man."

GEOPHYSICAL EXPLORATION FOR ORES

PROBING into the depths of the earth, inaccessible to the miner's eye or drill, the geologist is now determining the location of valuable oil and minerals through the use of instruments and methods that up to a few years ago were not known outside of scientific laboratories.

Engineers, gathered in New York City for the sessions of the American Institute of Mining and Metallurgical Engineers, discussed the application of these modern "divining rods" to the discovery of new mineral riches.

Gullible miners and landowners have been fooled and humbugged in past years by unscientific diviners who claimed to be able to locate hidden oil, coal and minerals by rods or devices that they held in their hands. Farmers have hired these rural mystics to determine where to dig wells. Such methods of prospecting have been discredited. Through the use of the principles of physics, however, the geophysicist has realized the wishful claims of the impostors and now by an array of complicated instruments can advise the mining engineer where to drill or dig in order to try for oil or metal.

Prospecting by geophysical methods is possible because the rocks and other deposits in the earth have different physical properties which can be detected by suitable apparatus at the surface, according to Dr. Hans Haalck, scientific expert for German and American exploration companies, speaking before the meeting. Geophysical prospecting is now possible practically by gravimetric, magnetic, seismic and electric methods.

Masses of light or heavy materials within the earth affect the gravitation of the earth nearby and can be detected with a pendulum, or gravity balance, like the Eotvos torsion balance. Such information about internal

NEW SCIENTIFIC BOOKS

George Routledge and Sons, Limited, London

An Introduction to the Theory and Use of the Microscope. C. R. Marshall and H. D. Griffith. 32 illustrations. pp. viii + 90.

It is expected that this book will prove of value to all students who require a microscope as well as to those amateur microscopists who desire to understand the fundamental principles on which microscopy is based. There is a chapter on the elementary mathematical treatment of certain problems.

E. P. Dutton and Company, New York

Thermionic Phenomena. Eugène Bloch. viii + 145. $2.50.

A summary of our knowledge concerning the emissions from heated bodies. The value of the book is increased by a chapter giving an account of some of the applications of thermionic phenomena.

Ginn and Company, Boston

Education through Manual Activities. Anna M. Wiecking. pp. vi + 351. $1.80.

This book is designed for teachers of kindergarten and primary grades and should also have an interest for parents from the point of view of its bearing on home play and the employment of leisure.

The Peking Union Medical College, Peking, China

Bibliography of the Publications of the Peking Union Medical College and Hospital.

This includes all the scientific papers published by members of the staff of the institution during the year from July, 1925, to June, 1926.

Contributions from the Department of Anatomy. Volume IV. Collected Papers Numbers 58–83.

A collection of reprints of papers written by members of the department staff, many of which would otherwise be difficult of access.

University of Colorado, Boulder

Colorado Plant Life. Francis Ramaley. Volume II. pp. viii + 299. $2.00.

A presentation in simple form of some of the larger facts of plant life in Colorado, for the man or woman who is not trained in botany, but who wishes to gain an appreciation of nature. The book is well illustrated.

Geology and Natural Resources of Colorado. Russell D. George. pp. xv + 228. $2.00.

Some of the subjects discussed are: Rocks and Minerals, Typography and Drainage; Metals and Mining; Structural and Industrial Materials; Water Resources, Soils; Mineral Waters, National Parks, Fish and Game; Climate and Scenery; Geologic Eras.

Zoology of Colorado. Theodore D. A. Cockerell. pp. vii + 262. $2.00.

A semi-technical discussion of living and fossil animals and fishes and of birds, insects and reptiles native to Colorado.

structure aids the geologist to determine where to drill for oil, for instance. Various kinds of rocks have different degrees of magnetization and consequently vary the magnitude and direction of the earth's magnetic field. Refined forms of the compass and similar instruments allow the geologist to measure any magnetic irregularities and speculate upon the cause.

Artificial earthquakes can be caused by small explosions and recorded on seismographs in order to determine the difference in elasticity of the underlying rocks. This information gives clues to mineral deposits and formations in some instances. Electric currents passed through the earth sometimes give valuable information since different kinds of rocks have different conductivities. Other methods not yet in wide practical application include: Radioactivity measurements, transmission of radio waves, temperature records, measurement of natural earth currents, etc.

President Max Mason, of the University of Chicago, was among those who spoke on geophysical exploration for ores, and other reports revealed that the new methods are being used for oil prospecting in the mid-continent fields, in the lead and zinc district of Missouri, Arkansas and Oklahoma, in England, in the Lake Superior copper country and elsewhere.

SCIENTIFIC METHODS IN THE STEEL INDUSTRY

THE city of Youngstown, Ohio, to-day lies in the midst of one of the greatest industrial battles in years—the battle iron and steel manufacturers are waging to retain a reasonable margin of profit. In this struggle, scientists are bringing forth many new ideas as weapons against loss. Some of their ideas, if successfully applied, may revolutionize the whole industry. Others seek to cut off a cent from the cost here and another cent there and little by little to keep the production cost down.

Much money is spent by the industry for improvement. Unfortunately, in some instances cost of production is advanced so rapidly by adverse economic conditions that the profit gained through improvements can hardly keep abreast.

It was said that one of the most substantial improvements made recently lies in the use of electricity as a source of motive power. The Youngstown Sheet and Tube Company is installing high pressure boilers to run electric generators at a plant in Ohio. The boilers will be fired by the waste gas from coke ovens. Electric motors used for driving rolling mills, conveyors and other machinery are more economical because they permit the operation of one unit at a time. They increase the flexibility of the mill operation and thereby save time and labor, it is said.

Plants located near sources of water-power are calling upon it to furnish electricity for more economical operation.

In the struggle against advancing costs, iron and steel manufacturers are adopting a more diversified output. They are taking advantage of the fact that if the market for rods and strips slumps they can keep their mills going by turning out tinplate.

Chemists and metallurgists are eyeing the blast furnace critically. "This business of shipping iron ore down here from way out in Minnesota seems to be a waste of money," say some, "Why can't we ship iron down here instead of ore with all its impurities?"

With the use of the blast furnace, iron and steel plants must have a means of manufacturing coke. This entails the operation of a gas plant in most cases. The University of Minnesota has been experimenting with the combination of gas plant and blast furnace. They mix the ore with coal and put the mixture into a coke oven similar to those used in the manufacture of coal gas. They heat the mixture. The iron comes out in a crumbly form and is pressed into cylindrical blocks for shipment to steel plants. It is declared that iron produced in this manner near where it is mined costs a few cents less after shipment to Pittsburgh than iron manufactured in blast furnaces at Pittsburgh.

A process similar to this for the elimination of the blast furnace is being tried by the United States Steel Corporation in its plant at Lorain, Ohio. Metallurgists are reluctant to predict how successful this experiment will be.

More economical methods in the use of fuel are being sought. It has been found that the admonition "cleanliness is next to godliness" holds true in the manufacture of iron and steel as well as in human life. More care is being taken with the cleaning of coke before it goes into the blast furnace. Cleaning of coke eliminates ash. As little as one per cent. of ash taken from the coke takes twenty cents off the cost of production of pig iron.

Attention is being given to purifying the gas from the blast furnace of all particles of dust. Some plants have installed electric precipitators across the path of the gas. The dust particles become charged electrically and can no longer be carried along by it.

Manufacturers are seeking greater fuel economy in the open-hearth furnace where the greatest steel tonnage is manufactured. Before gas and air in this furnace reach the charge that is to be melted down, they pass through heated chambers stacked with fire-brick. These chambers comprise the regenerator. In an effort to make the operation of the regenerators more efficient, the bricks are being stacked in new arrangements to get as much heating surface as possible in a small space. Bricks made of carborundum, which will withstand a higher temperature, also are being tried.

Engineers who have many problems to solve in the rolling mill have not been idle. The United Engineering and Foundry Company, at Pittsburgh, has perfected mills for the continuous rolling of sheet metal. Heretofore, rolling has been a comparatively slow process. The metal has had to be sent through the mill to be rolled for one thickness, backed up and rolled again if a greater degree of thinness is desired. One of the new continuous rolling mills will take a 63,000-pound ingot 8¾ inches thick and roll it down to a sheet of No. 20 gauge metal 41 inches wide at the rate of a ton a minute.

MULTIPLE WALLS FOR THE ABSORPTION OF SOUND

MULTIPLE-LAYERED walls are the most efficient absorbers for deep musical sounds, Dr. E. C. Wente and E. H. Bedell have discovered as a result of experiments at the Bell Telephone Laboratories.

Radio studios, auditoriums and other places, where echoes are troublesome and must be carefully controlled, can be made to have better acoustic properties through the use of a thin, perforated partition, set a short distance out from the main wall.

Formerly such sound studies had to be made in a large room, with good-sized pieces of the material to be tested. Dr. Wente and his associate have invented a way of testing in a small tube, and they claim that it gives results as satisfactory as with the older method. At one end is a telephone receiver to furnish the sound of any desired pitch. Sliding in the other end is a piston, with which the material undergoing test is covered. The echoes formed are studied with a still smaller tube that goes into the main tube at the end near the telephone receiver. On the outside, at the end of this small tube, is a telephone transmitter with which the sounds can be picked up and analyzed.

Sounds of high pitch are largely absorbed by layers of felt, porous "acoustic tile" or wood fiber mixed with felt. Deep or low frequency sounds pass through rather easily. But if the wall is covered with felt, and then, an inch away, a piece of perforated building board is placed, the low frequency sounds are much more completely absorbed. Still better is the effect of two layers of building board, with two air spaces.

Somewhat similar to this is the method recently adopted by engineers of the National Broadcasting Company in designing the new studios of station WRC in Washington. In order to make a sound-proof window between the studio and the control room, three layers of glass of different thicknesses are used. Each piece has its natural frequency, and sounds of a similar pitch would be transmitted. But sounds that get through the first layer are stopped by the second, while any that might still leak through are stopped by the third.

THE TRANSPLANTATION OF SMELT

THE transplanting of fresh-water smelt from eastern Maine to the waters of Idaho is planned in an experiment now being tried out by the United States Bureau of Fisheries, the Forest Service and the Idaho State Game Commission.

Smelt is the natural food of the land-locked salmon, and the object of introducing the Maine smelt in Idaho is to produce an abundant and suitable forage fish to serve as food for salmon and trout. The smelt live principally on minute forms of life which ordinarily occur in abundance in deep-water lakes and turn this into a readily available trout food. Salmon has been introduced in the Redfish Lake section of Idaho, and it is believed that the planting of the smelt will make favorable results much more certain.

The smelt, ordinarily growing to about six inches in length, is remarkably prolific and runs in large schools in the deep waters of the lake. In the early spring these little fish ascend inlets to spawn, the spawn being very minute and adhering to rocks and sticks. The eggs develop readily and hatch in from two weeks to a month, the tiny young migrating immediately to deep water.

The main difficulty encountered in transplanting this fish from the East to the Far West is due to the rapid development of the eggs. The eggs to be shipped to Idaho will be surrounded by a layer of ice and packed in an insulated box, for sending by express. If this method of transportation is not successful, it is planned to attempt a small shipment by air mail.

ITEMS

A NEW type of loud-speaker, that can give out sounds 300 times as loud as any of the older types, has been invented by engineers at the Bell Laboratories. However, there is no danger that this will form a new source of annoyance to apartment-house dwellers, for the horn is so large that it is not adapted for use with ordinary radio sets. It is intended particularly for out of door public address systems, and for talking motion pictures in large theaters. The new device is the invention of Dr. E. C. Wente and A. L. Thuras. It employs a moving coil, in which the entire electromagnet that all such sound reproducers contain, moves back and forth according to the current flowing through it. In small speakers, the magnet is fixed, and moves a small armature attached to the vibrating diaphragm from which the sound waves start. This is not new, but Dr. Wente and his associate have worked out improvements in the design, and in the way the diaphragm is connected to the horn. As a result, 30 watts of electrical power can be used in the horn, instead of about 5 watts, the previous maximum. Its efficiency, in converting this electrical power to sound, is about 50 times greater than older speakers, so that good reproduction can be obtained about 300 times as loud as formerly.

THE only case of rickets that experts from the U. S. Children's Bureau found in a recent survey of 600 Porto Rico babies was in an infant that had spent five of its six months in a cellar lighted only by electricity. The survey was undertaken under the direction of Miss Grace Abbott, chief of the bureau, to determine the effect of the tropical sun on rickets, the disorder of the mineral chemistry in the bodies of young children that is prevented by the action of ultra-violet rays. It is especially desirable, Miss Abbot pointed out, to have a series of X-ray pictures of the bones of babies who live in the tropics, because they normally spend most of their waking hours with their little bodies completely exposed to the beneficial action of the sun. The photographs will be used to compare with those of children in temperate climates so that some sort of a standard can be obtained of what the healthy bones of a growing child should look like.

SCIENCE NEWS

Science Service, Washington, D. C.

SOME PAPERS PRESENTED BEFORE THE NEW YORK MEETING OF THE AMERICAN PHYSICAL SOCIETY

AT the meeting of the American Physical Society, in New York, which opened on February 24, Dr. Ernest O. Lawrence and Dr. J. W. Beams, of Yale University, told of their studies of the length of time required for this "photoelectric effect." Less than a three billionth of a second is all the time that it takes an electron to be knocked out of a film of potassium metal when light strikes it in a photoelectric cell—the device that has made television and radio photographs possible. In the photoelectric cell there is a film of potassium, and another electrode. When light strikes the film the electrons travelling from the film to the other electrode cause a minute electric current, which can be amplified by means of vacuum tubes. In this way a current of any desired magnitude, but one which varies with the illumination of the cell, can be obtained. Because the response of the cell is practically instantaneous, it can be used in television and wire and radio photographic service.

MEMBERS were able to see by wire through walls and around corners when they were given a special demonstration of the process of television developed by the Bell Telephone Laboratories. This was the process that was used last April in the first successful long-distance television tests, when Secretary Hoover spoke in Washington and was seen in New York. At a session of the society at the Bell Laboratories, Dr. Herbert E. Ives, under whose direction the method was developed, explained its operation, and the recent improvements that have been made on it.

STUDY of such devices as radio loud-speakers on the basis of the sound waves that come to the listener's ear is now possible with an instrument invented by Dr. Dayton C. Miller, of Case School of Applied Science, Cleveland. Dr. Miller described this new use of his apparatus, which he calls the "phonodeik." He made the experiments in conjunction with John R. Martin. The phonodeik makes a photographic record of the sound wave as it is received by the ear. Dr. Miller's method is to connect the loud-speaker undergoing test to a microphone, then to record the output on the phonodeik. A similar record can be made of the original sound, and by comparing the two, the characteristics of the speaker determined. When a vacuum tube voltmeter is substituted for the speaker, the experimenter can determine how much distortion is introduced by the electrical system, and make allowances for it.

NECKTIE and clothing manufacturers probably still have plenty of colors left with which to add to the brilliance of life. Altogether there are slightly over two million separately distinguishable colors possible. This is the conclusion by George B. Welch, of Cornell University, who spoke before the society.

BOWLING enthusiasts will now have available a scientific study of their favorite pastime. Dr. L. W. Taylor, of Oberlin College, told of apparatus that he has developed to study the motion of the ball in a bowling alley. A recording device registers to the hundredth of a second the passage of the ball at half-meter (about 20-inch) intervals. Instead of rolling the ball by hand, a catapult is used, so that the force used can accurately be controlled. Studies already made with the device indicate that the accepted theories of the ball's motion are not quite correct, but that the friction seems to vary with the ball's speed.

STELLAR EVOLUTION

A STAR that exploded, and is now changing to a nebula, in reverse of the usual process of stellar evolution, is the rare spectacle being observed at the branch station of the Harvard College Observatory at Bloemfontein, South Africa. This unconventional behavior of Nova Pictoris, as the star is called, was discovered by Dr. J. S. Paraskevopoulos, who is in charge of the branch station, Dr. Harlow Shapley, director of the observatory, announced through Science Service. Confirmation of the discovery has just been received from the Observatory of LaPlata, in Argentina.

Until the spring of 1925 this star was too faint to be seen with the unaided eye. Then it suddenly flared up as a nova, or "new star," and was discovered by R. Watson, a South African amateur astronomer. The star is in the constellation Pictor, the painter, a group not visible from northern latitudes.

"The evolution of stars," Dr. Shapley explained, "is generally thought to be in the direction from nebula to star, but in this instance, and in two or three others, the transformation is in the opposite direction, and astronomically speaking, is very rapid. All of these reversed cases are associated with the so-called novae, or new stars.

"Examination of earlier plates in the great collection at the Harvard Observatory, in Cambridge, where the southern photographs are stored, showed that before its outburst, it had been of the twelfth magnitude, and astronomers believe that it will gradually return to that same degree of faintness.

"Dr. Paraskevopoulos' discovery was based on photographs of the star, made under various conditions, with the rapid photographic telescopes which he has recently transferred from the former Harvard station in Peru to the new site in South Africa. A ring or shell of nebulous matter appeared around the outer edge of the image of the star, and has gradually grown larger and more dis-

tinct. The phenomenon clearly indicates that the outburst of the nova, and its rapid increase three years ago to ten thousand times its former brightness, was actually an explosion of the star, which blew its outer parts away from the nucleus.

"The ring of nebulosity now observed is the former outer portion receding with a velocity of several hundred miles a second. Future observations will show whether the explosive transformation will result in one of the permanent typical 'planetary' nebulae of which a hundred or so are known among the stars, or whether the receding atmospheres will gradually dissipate into space, leaving the nucleus as a typical star.

"The normal course of stellar evolution," Dr. Shapley stated, "is believed to be in the direction of contraction, and for perceptible progress requires billions of years; but these suddenly expansive transformations are in the reverse sense, require but a few years, and may be exceedingly important in knowledge of the development of celestial bodies."

The observation from the University of LaPlata, which confirmed the Harvard astronomer's detection of the expanding gaseous shell around Nova Pictoris, was made by Professor Hartmann, director of the National Observatory of Argentina. His observations were made visually with a large refracting telescope. He cabled that the angular diameter of the ring is now one second of arc. Dr. Paraskevopoulos' description of his observations is being published by the Harvard College Observatory.

MOUNT LASSEN

Mt. Lassen, America's principal active volcano, is still asleep, but the spectacular effect produced by blowing clouds of snow, mixing with the steam that the crater is continually emitting, may give the illusion of a return to activity. The effect is especially striking when it occurs near sunrise or sunset, according to R. H. Finch, associate volcanologist of the U. S. Geological Survey, whose work it is to keep his finger on the pulse of the slumbering volcano. That it is merely slumbering, and not dead, is indicated not only by the steam, but by frequent earthquakes. Sometimes several shocks occur on the same day.

Evidence of subterranean activity also comes from Glass Mountain, about seventy-five miles north of Lassen Peak, and in the Modoc lava beds. Fairly recent lava flows are to be found nearly all the way between Glass Mountain and Lassen Peak, and Forest Service officials in the vicinity report about half an acre of land covered with pumice which is very hot. By digging but a little way into the pumice much higher temperatures are reached, and near the pumice bed is a deep fissure emitting steam.

With George L. Collins, of the National Park Service, Mr. Finch attempted to make temperature measurements and to take photographs on the mountain, about 7,850 feet high, during January, but were driven back by a heavy snow storm. They are now planning to conduct further explorations in the spring.

According to the Indians the heat of Glass Mountain has been known for many years, and earthquakes originating in the mountain and accompanied by rattling noises have been noted by Forest Service officials for at least fifteen years.

MAN-MADE EARTHQUAKES

Man-made earthquakes, recorded some distance away upon a simple form of seismograph weighing only a few pounds, are helping Russian engineers to survey the site of the proposed Turkestan-Siberian railroad.

The method is to detonate charges of explosives underground and to record the travel of vibrations through the ground in different directions. By a minute study of the records so obtained it is possible to secure data on the geological formation of the locality.

The new seismograph invented by Professor Paul M. Nikiforov, director of the Physico-Mathematical Institute of the Russian Academy of Science at Leningrad, is similar to one recently invented in the United States by Dr. John A. Anderson, of the Mt. Wilson Observatory in California. Its main part, the pendulum, is a small vertical cylinder of pure gold suspended a little off center on a pair of fine wires. Whenever there is any vibration the cylinder turns slightly in proportion to strength of the shock. A tiny mirror attached to the pendulum reflects a beam of light on a constantly advancing sheet of photographic paper. Every turn of the cylinder, no matter how small, shifts the light spot considerably and it traces a wavy black line. Several of the new instruments are now installed on earthquake stations in Turkestan and Crimea and give complete satisfaction.

THE DETECTION OF FLAWS IN CASTINGS

Using radium rays so penetrating that they can go through pieces of metal—15-inch pieces of metal—to test for hidden flaws in large castings is one of the latest accomplishments of the Russian State Radium Institute.

These "gamma rays," as they are called, are similar to X-rays, but are of much shorter wave-length. They are more penetrating and can pass through pieces of metal too thick to be examined with the X-rays. Examination by radium is said also to be cheaper than with X-rays, because the same radium can be used over and over for an indefinite time. Large and expensive photographic plates are not required, since the rays, after passing through the object, act upon a special, sensitive electroscope. The test record is preserved for future reference in the form of a simple diagram automatically traced. Another advantage is that the gamma rays speed up the inspection—it may be cut down to a couple of minutes for a large casting—while X-rays require a very long exposure, often of several hours, when metal is more than two or three inches thick.

The apparatus, as developed by the Russian scientists, is very simply constructed. A tiny glass capsule with a radium preparation is inserted into a deep hole bored in a large lead ingot. This stops all rays, except a narrow strong beam that goes along the bore. This beam pierces the casting and encounters two filaments charged with electricity and enclosed within a copper cage. There is an air space between the filaments and the cage which act normally a perfect insulator, allowing no electric cur-

rent to pass through it. But as soon as gamma rays have a chance to get in the cage they ionize the air and turn it into a conductor.

Electricity from a battery flows from the filaments to the copper cage and from it passes through a galvanometer and back to the battery.

As intensity of the rays changes with thickness of metal pierced by them, the rate of ionization varies accordingly. Therefore the flow of electric current exactly mirrors the shape of the object under test. Any deviation at once shows that some imperfection is present.

A NEW TYPE OF HEAVY LOCOMOTIVE

A NEW type of locomotive, the heaviest yet used in Europe, is being built in Germany. It is especially designed to haul heavy freight trains over tracks cursed with many curves, and through regions where water is scanty.

The Garrat locomotive, as the new engine is called, shows a radical departure from the usual types of locomotive design. The driving wheels, of which there are two sets of six each, are not placed under the main body of the locomotive at all, but under the tenders. Of these there are two, one of them pushed ahead of the engine and the other pulled behind in the usual position. The cylinders are as far apart as possible, the forward pair being under the forward end of the front tender, while the rear pair is under the opposite end of the rear tender. This necessitates long steam lines, but the builders claim that they are able to deliver steam at 189 pounds pressure with entire success.

This type of construction makes the locomotive a three-section affair, articulated by two pivots. Although total length is 75½ feet, it can turn in a circle of 300-foot radius.

The forward tender carries nothing but water, the rear one both water and fuel—either oil or coal. In addition, there is a third supply of water carried in a tank slung under the boiler, in the space usually occupied by the driving mechanism. In all about 27 tons of water can be carried, and about 15 tons of fuel. The unusual capacity for water is designed to permit the locomotive to operate in arid regions.

The total weight when ready for service is 206 tons.

ITEMS

A NEWLY-INVENTED German machine, designed to do for Occidental grain fields what Chinese coolie labor has done for centuries in the rice fields of the East, is attracting considerable attention on the part of British agriculturists. Instead of sowing seed like an ordinary grain drill, it sets out sprouted and rooted seedlings at the rate of 12,000 plants per hour, one to every square foot. It is claimed that this method of raising grain requires only one thirtieth as much seed as now used, and that it will yield from three to five times as many bushels to the acre. This is said to be the result of the greater freedom each plant has to develop a more vigorous root growth beneath the soil, and especially to tiller, or "stool out," above its base. From 30 to 40 stalks per plant are usually developed.

MEDIEVAL cathedral builders, if they could come back to life, would probably regard with superstitious awe the modern power-driven saws, drills and planes that speed up the shaping of the thousands of tons of stone used in the construction of Washington cathedral, now going up on Mount Saint Alban. Each of the 260,900 stones that the builders' estimates call for must be separately designed and shaped for its particular place. As soon as the architect determines the specific shape and dimension, each of the stones that weigh from 300 to 500 pounds apiece, is numbered. These numbers appear on all drawings, on the individual time cards, which record the progress of each stone through the cutting plant, on the completed stone and on the plan followed by the mason. The cost of the stones varies from $10 for the plain ones, used for the basic construction, of which 146,000 will be needed, according to the estimate, to $300 each for the 5,000 elaborately sculptured ones. In addition to this, thousands of molded and carved stones at $50 and $100 apiece will go into the complete structure.

NEW finds of fossil footprints in the rocks of the Grand Canyon of Arizona, but this time on the north rim, fourteen miles from the site of previous discoveries on the south rim, are reported by Dr. Charles W. Gilmore, of the U. S. National Museum, and Glenn E. Sturdevant, government naturalist of Grand Canyon National Park. Slabs bearing the foot imprints of small reptiles or salamander-like amphibians were found at two levels, one in the Coconino and one in the Supai formation. These correspond with two of the three formations on the other side of the canyon in which tracks have been found during the past few years, but further exploration and examination of specimens will have to be carried on before it can be determined whether the levels match up exactly and whether the tracks represent the same kinds of feet. The fossil footprints from the south side of the canyon thus far discovered represent 36 species, distributed among 28 genera.

EVIDENCE that stone age man lived in Ireland, hitherto lacking, is now supplied by J. P. T. Burchell, of London. Mr. Burchell has discovered a rock shelter typical of the Mousterian period, when Neanderthal man roamed Europe, on the Sligo coast, and beneath it and along the beach he has found large quantities of the roughly flaked flint implements which these ancient savages made. No bones have been turned up as yet, but the quantity of tools and weapons leaves no doubt that some one was in Ireland to make them. Like other sites of the same culture, this shelter was inhabited during an interlude between two advancements of the ice of the most recent glacial epoch. Evidence on this point is cited by Mr. Burchell in two forms: the layer in which the implements are found is buried under 35 feet of boulder-filled clay, such as glacial deposit; and one of the largest of the stone implements is scarred with glacial striae or scratches, indicating that it was caught under a glacier and scraped over other rocks. The finds have been examined by J. Reid Moir, one of the foremost of British authorities on the stone ages, who pronounces them authentic. A complete technical report will probably be published in the near future.

SCIENCE NEWS

Science Service, Washington, D. C.

CHANGES IN THE EARTH'S ROTATION

EVERY day the earth changes a little in its rate of rotation.

This is the opinion of Dr. Benjamin Boss, director of the Dudley Observatory at Albany, and director of the department of meridian astrometry of the Carnegie Institution of Washington. Furthermore, this variation appears to be related to the frequency of earthquakes, and so further investigation of it might aid in the study of quakes.

Dr. Boss has found evidence for this apparent variation in a long study of star positions. At the Dudley Observatory an exhaustive catalog of star places is in preparation, and in the work on this it has been found that a considerable correction, which varies annually, is needed for the right ascension of the stars. The right ascension is the celestial equivalent of longitude. As a telescope permanently placed on the earth would point to different right ascensions in the sky as the earth turns, any change in the rate of the earth's rotation would affect the right ascensions of the stars.

For sometime, says Dr. Boss, it has been known that the sun, the moon and the planets Venus and Mercury undergo changes indicating the variable rotation of the earth over long periods of years.

The annual change in the star positions can be explained by daily variation in the rate of rotation of the earth. Possible evidence in favor of such a variation is suggested when checking clock time with the stars, for it has been found that there is a daily variation in the clock rate, which indicates that the earth may change daily in the rate of its rotation.

That the changes in the moon and stars are both due to the same cause is indicated by the fact that when the minor fluctuations in the moon's path, and the variation in star positions, are plotted over a long period of years, the curves are closely similar. About 1860 both curves reached a minimum, while about 1900 they were both at a high mark. Since that they have been going down, until 1920, when the moon fluctuation reached a minimum. For the last ten years the figures for the star variations have not been completed, but they also seem to have reached a minimum about the same time. Dr. Boss believes that this indicates very strongly that the two variations are due to the same cause.

What this cause may be is not certain, but Dr. Boss thinks that it is very likely to be the result of tides in the earth. This view is supported by the fact that Dr. A. A. Michelson, of the University of Chicago, has actually obtained experimental evidence of earth tides. Ocean tides are not sufficient to account for the observed phenomena, but if the outer crust of the earth is in a condition such as recent investigation supposes it to be, tidal friction might appreciably affect the rate at which the earth turns.

According to Dr. Boss, the tide might produce the long period changes by the fact that the crust of the earth, lifted at high tide, fails to settle back to its original position. Thus the earth's diameter is gradually increased, slowing its rotation. When a critical point is reached, it gradually starts to settle, speeding up rotation.

AUTOMATIC CONTROLS

A FEW turns of copper wire around an iron core is able, in many places, to do the work of a man! With the recent demonstration of a "mechanical man" to unveil a portrait of George Washington by a telephoned signal attention has been called to other ways of performing routine tasks either by remote control of an operator, or even without any operator at all.

The televox, by which the portrait was unveiled, depends upon a device that responds to a sound of certain frequency, but not to another. Stand in front of a piano, put your foot on the loud pedal, and whistle a note. Then stop whistling, and you will hear the piano continue to emit the same note. This is because the sound waves of your whistle set in vibration the piano string tuned to that particular note. Other strings, tuned to other notes, or to air waves vibrating at a different rate, fail to respond, just as a radio set will not bring in a broadcasting station unless it is tuned to waves of the proper frequency. With the televox, the receiving apparatus is tuned to a particular frequency of sound. A musical note, either from a tuning fork or a whistle, is telephoned to it. A relay, which is simply an electromagnet with a movable armature arranged to come against it when the current flows through the coils of the magnet, operates when the proper note is sounded. This in turn may start a motor, turn on or off a light, or do any one of a number of mechanical operations. By having several units of the apparatus, each with its relay, a complicated performance may be gone through by sending a series of different notes. These may, if wished, be so adjusted that the notes form a tune.

So far this particular device has only been used with land telephone lines, but it could be easily adapted to radio. Experiments have been made for many years with radio-controlled automobiles and other machinery, but in many cases these devices used several radio wavelengths, instead of different sounds, each performing a certain task.

Entirely automatic operation has in many instances made it possible to dispense with the human element completely. For instance, lights on buoys and light-houses have been operated with a selenium cell, with which light regulates the flow of an electric current. As soon as darkness comes, the light is turned on, when daylight breaks, the light goes off.

Another form of automatic control has been used in electrical substations, where formerly it was necessary

NEW SCIENTIFIC BOOKS

The Macmillan Company, New York

A Short History of Western Civilization. Alan F. Hattersley. pp. ix + 246. $2.75.

Tracing the origin and growth, in its essential features, of our present civilization. The book treats of past conditions rather than events. The standard of civilization, the economic growth of communities, the development of governmental institutions and the religious beliefs of the masses have been selected as the truly significant factors in human history.

University Bookstore, Bloomington, Indiana

Experimental Radio. R. R. Ramsey. pp. xii. + 229. $2.75.

This new, third edition has been enlarged and revised in order to keep up with the rapid changes in radio. Simple tests are given which will bring out fundamental principles. 150 figures and diagrams.

The Century Company, New York

Research in the Humanistic and Social Sciences. Frederic Austin Ogg. 454 pp. $2.50.

Being a report of a survey conducted for the American Council of Learned Societies. It covers the research work done by learned societies, colleges, universities, bureaus, foundations, business houses and individuals.

Harper & Brothers, New York

Plane Trigonometry. With Tables. N. J. Lennes and A. S. Merrill. Edited by H. E. Slaught. $2.20 with tables. $1.60 without tables. Tables alone $1.20.

Particular attention has been paid to cumulative reviews as an aid to students whose habits of thought are not well organized, and to the provisions made for the stronger students by which they may be encouraged to do more than the rank and file of the class.

to keep an operator in constant attendance. Electric current comes over the lines from the power plant to the substation, from which it is redistributed, perhaps at a lower voltage, to the users. When the load is heavy, certain transformers may have to be turned on, while different ones would be required when so much current is not needed. In such cases relays can be used so adjusted that when the load reaches a certain point, the necessary switches are closed, while they are turned off when the load is lightened.

THE SHORT-WAVE, HIGH-POWER VACUUM TUBE

A VACUUM tube with a power of 15,000 watts, sending out radio waves of only six meters length, that can light electric lamps without wires or socket, produce a warmth in nearby spectators reminiscent of prohibited stimulants, and cook sausage in a glass tube without fire, is one of the latest radio wonders. It has just been demonstrated at the General Electric Company's research laboratory.

The new tube, known as the ZT-6, looks harmless enough. It is about five inches in diameter, and two feet long, set in a wooden cage and surrounded by a network of wires, condensers and meters. With its great power of 15 kilowatts, it is at least fifty times as powerful as any short-wave tube previously constructed. Through a coupling system it is connected to a copper bar about three meters, or ten feet, long, which acts as the tuned aerial circuit, radiating the full 15 kilowatts into space.

When an ordinary electric lamp is touched to the copper bar, it lights up brilliantly. A loose copper rod, lying on the floor, is picked up, and, though cold, it blisters the hand. When a person approaches the apparatus, he first feels a warm glow, then pain in the limbs and joints. Artificial fever, as much as 100 degrees Fahrenheit, is induced after standing close to it for 15 minutes.

This may indicate one of the future applications of the tube, says Dr. W. R. Whitney, director of the laboratory. "If we had a perfectly harmless method for warming the blood it might have value," he stated, "because fevers are sometimes artificially produced in order to start convalescence, and it may well be, as asserted, that raised blood temperature, or fever, is one of nature's factors in the recovery from infectious diseases."

Another feat of the apparatus, which also involved the heating of animal tissue without fire, was the cooking of a sausage in a glass tube, suspended from a wire some distance from the transmitting aerial. An apple was placed on the end of this receiving aerial and in a few minutes it was thoroughly baked to the core.

One of the most spectacular "stunts" performed was the imitation of the famous but seldom observed "ball of fire" reputed to accompany tropical thunderstorms. When the end of the radiating aerial was touched with a metal-tipped pole, a greenish-white arc arose to a height of a foot or more. This arc remained, even after the pole was removed, like a plume of fire, sputtering and sending out molten copper in all directions until it was blown out. As many as three of these standing arcs, each without any visible return circuit, were established along the bar at once.

ADVANCES IN TELEVISION

A SMALL crystal of quartz, less than an inch thick, has now simplified television by taking the place of a complete telephone line or radio transmitting and receiving equipment. This is the latest achievement of the Bell Laboratories, which perfected a process of television first demonstrated nearly a year ago.

With practically all methods of television so far invented it is necessary to have a disc at the receiving end rotate in exact synchronism with a similar disc in the transmitter. When first demonstrated, the Bell system did this with a separate synchronizinz circuit. Over land telephone lines, this consisted of a special pair of wires connecting Washington and New York, separate from the two lines used for carrying the actual image and the spoken words. With the radio television, a special signal was sent out over its own wave-length for the purpose.

Only two telephone lines, instead of three, or only two wave-lengths, are now required, as the result of the work of W. A. Marrison and J. W. Horton, in making quartz crystal oscillators capable of holding the rate of vibration constant to within one part in ten million.

The control of the picture on the television screen is now as simple as that of a motion-picture image on the movie screen. Sometimes the motion-picture image becomes "out of frame" when the pictures on the film are out of step with the mechanism. The effect is that the top of the picture is seen at the bottom of the screen, and the bottom at the top. At the touch of a lever by the operator this can instantly be corrected.

With the television apparatus, the failure of the two discs to keep in step produces a similar effect, except that the picture is displaced laterally, instead of vertically. The remedy is also very simple. Connected with the receiver are two buttons. When one is pushed, the whole picture slowly moves to the right, while the other moves it to the left. The operator merely touches one of the buttons until the picture is in the proper position, then the quartz oscillator holds it in place for a long time. In an hour, it is stated, the image will not wander more than one third of its width.

Despite this great simplification, which represents a step well in advance of anything yet accomplished in television, the engineers point out that it is still full of such complexities that its field of application is still quite restricted.

THE CONTROL OF ERYSIPELAS

ERYSIPELAS may now be added to the list of diseases controlled by man, Dr. Konrad E. Birkhaug, of the University of Rochester School of Medicine, told the American College of Physicians meeting at New Orleans.

As a result of four years of work, Dr. Birkhaug has developed an antitoxin treatment for use in the early stages of erysipelas that gives results commensurate with those obtained through the use of diphtheria antitoxin in the early hours of that disease.

The erysipelas treatment reduces to half the time that the patient must spend in the hospital. The mortality in adults has been reduced from twelve to only four per cent., while recurrent attacks of erysipelas have been

SCIENCE NEWS

Science Service, Washington, D. C.

PHOTOGRAPHS OF THE SUN'S CORONA

LONG and expensive expeditions of astronomers to distant parts of the earth to photograph the fleeting phenomena of a total eclipse of the sun may be avoided in the future. The sun's corona, the outer layer of which until now has only been observable when the moon obscures the bright solar disc, has been photographed in full daylight by Dr. G. Blunck, the German astronomer.

In the past many experiments have been made by astronomers to achieve the photography of the corona without waiting for an eclipse, but they have all failed. For ordinary colors, the brightness of the corona is just about the same as that of the sky itself around the sun, so that photographs can not show where one stops and the other begins. The sky itself gives off light largely of blue and the shorter, invisible, ultra-violet, while a large part of the corona's light is in the red, and the longer wave, invisible, infra-red. Accordingly, efforts have been made to take the corona's picture with red, or infra-red, light. So far, these have also been unsuccessful.

Dr. Blunck explains that the reason for these failures is that the previous experiments have been made with rays that were not long enough. For a wave-length of 7,000, which is in the visible red part of the spectrum, the corona is only eight tenths of a per cent. brighter than the sky. This is scarcely enough difference to permit a good picture. However, for infra-red light of 8,500, the corona is 1.7 per cent. brighter than the sky, while at 9,500, it is 2.5 per cent. brighter, which should be enough difference to permit a photograph to be made.

The difficulty comes in securing photographic plates sensitive to these longer waves. Ordinary plates are most sensitive to the blue, hence they are developd in red light. Special plates sensitized before use by immersion in a dye called neocyanin are most sensitive to light of wavelength of 8,000. Dr. Blunck tells of a new dye, called procyanol, that he has used, with which the plates can be sensitized to light at 8,500, and it is with these plates that his efforts have been successful.

Photographs made last year by Dr. Blunck show details that make them appear to be of the actual corona. As a test of his method, however, it has been suggested that the method might be tried at a partial eclipse of the sun, while the moon obscures part of the sun, and part of the corona. If Dr. Blunck's method is really successful, then he should obtain on his plates the outline of the moon, even where it is not in front of the actual solar disc.

THE EFFECTS OF SUNSPOTS ON RADIO

FUTURE radio engineers may be able to look at the sun through a telescope and then tell how the presence or absence of spots will affect the transmission of radio waves as a result of an investigation now under way, at Cambridge, Mass., with the cooperation of physicists and astronomers.

There has just been installed in the Harvard Astronomical Laboratory, under the direction of Dr. Harlan T. Stetson, professor of astronomy, apparatus to study the relation of spots and radio. Greenleaf W. Pickard, Boston radio engineer, designed the apparatus, and installed it for use in cooperation with studies that he has been carrying on for several years. Each day the sun is photographed to give the size and number of spots.

It is not yet possible to say whether or not combination of radio data, with observation of the sun, can ever be used to predict earthly weather conditions. However, according to Dr. Stetson, observations are beginning to make us feel confident that there is a direct connection between conditions in the solar atmosphere and certain atmospheric disturbances on the earth. It seems not unlikely that with the further study of the bearing of sun-spots upon radio reception it will be possible to make allowances for the solar disturbances and by so doing discover more closely than ever before the correlation of radio reception with temperature, pressure and other meteorological phenomena.

Just what happens on the earth when a sun-spot appears on the side of the sun towards us is not fully known. It is believed that electrified particles discharged from the disturbed region on the sun, hurling through space, bombard the upper atmosphere of the earth and are responsible for an increased ionization of the latter which is responsible for the modification of the intensity of the radio waves.

The station from which the signals will be sent, which are measured at the Harvard Laboratory, is WBBM, Chicago. The apparatus, which automatically records signal strength, as received in Cambridge, is carefully calibrated each day and makes it possible to record the measurement in absolute units of electrical intensity.

Dr. Stetson explained the apparatus was so designed that it would measure the intensity of the carrier wave and would scarcely be affected at all by superimposed modulations caused by the broadcasting of music.

3,600,000 VOLTS OF ELECTRICITY

THREE million, six hundred thousand volts of electricity can now be stored in artificial "clouds" and discharged in a ten millionth of a second, thus imitating in the laboratory the effects of lightning more accurately than ever before. This feat has been accomplished at the laboratory of the General Electric Company, at Pittsfield, Mass., by F. W. Peek, Jr., who spoke before the recent regional convention of the American Institute of Electrical Engineers at St. Louis. Such a voltage is seventeen times as great as that carried over even the highest voltage power lines.

As these sparks last but a ten millionth of a second, and as light travels about 100 feet in that time, the blinding flash is all over when seen by a person only a hundred feet away. Yet the flash appears to be there when he sees it!

Although these voltages frequently have a duration of less than a millionth of a second their rate of rise and fall or wave shape has been accurately measured by an instrument using a beam of electrons as a pointer and known as a cathode ray oscillograph.

The object of the study is to secure scientific information on the nature of electricity and to obtain further engineering information on the protection of life and property against lightning, to build transmission lines, transformers and other electrical apparatus to resist lightning voltages. Lightning is one of the greatest foes to electrical apparatus and much has already been done in this laboratory to produce lightning-proof apparatus. The present generator produces higher voltages than ever produced by natural lightning on transmission lines.

THE OX5 AIRPLANE ENGINE

To those in aviation OX5 means the Curtiss water-cooled 90-horsepower engine that has powered so many airplanes in the decade since the war. Last year during the boom in aircraft production that accompanied the extraordinary development of airways, flying fields and aviation exploits, 65 per cent. of the estimated 1,653 airplanes produced for commercial use were powered by OX5 engines.

For the OX5 was the airplane engine produced in quantity for war use. Probably no other airplane engine has had such quantity production. Some 17,000 were in storage at the end of the war. They were sold cheap, cheaper than they can now be produced to-day. And that is the secret of airplanes being quoted on the market at the cost of a medium-priced automobile. You can buy an airplane, f.o.b. the flying field, for as little as $2,500.

The supply is about exhausted. Airplane manufacturers estimate that the last of the easily available, cheap OX5's will be installed in airplanes to be built by the end of this month (March). The threatened engine shortage may have a tendency to slow down the booming airplane production that has been stimulated by the quickening aviation interest in this country. One manufacturer last year produced more than one airplane per working day of one OX5-engined type alone, and the production possibilities of this plant are now said to be as high as eight airplanes a day. Several other manufacturers are contemplating large-scale production.

Realizing the need of a cheap and reliable engine to take the place of the OX5, several engine manufacturers are producing experimentally on a small scale low-powered motors, most of them air-cooled. Nine established engine manufacturers are producing in this country, but many of them are occupied with the production of the larger engines for transport, mail and military airplanes and have not yet entered the low-price field. Some see in the Ford aircraft activities a promising future source of inexpensive engines for the aircraft that Americans are beginning to demand in much the same spirit that they bought automobiles in the early years of the century.

THE ANTARCTIC ICE

ANTARCTICA, whose desolate ice fields will soon reecho the roar of Commander Byrd's motors, has enough ice to cover the whole earth to a depth of 120 or 130 feet, and has been gathering this vast store of solidified cold for a quarter of a million years or more.

This is the opinion of Professor W. Meinardus, of the University of Göttingen, who has been engaged lately in an endeavor to estimate the bulk of the ice that covers the south polar continent. He is of the opinion that only a small part of the elevations of from 6,000 to 10,000 feet reported for the surface of the Antarctic plateau can be made up of solid land. Most of the mass, he thinks, consists of accumulated ice, piled on a foundation of rock not more than about 2,000 feet in mean elevation. Professor Meinardus derives this estimated land height of Antarctica from an average of the mean elevation of the nearest continents, South America, Africa and Australia. Everything above that is ice.

Multiplying the estimated average thickness of this massive sheet by the area of Antarctica, Professor Meinardus obtains a total of twenty-six quadrillion (26,000,000,000,000,000) cubic yards of ice, weighing about twenty quadrillion tons. There is enough ice there, he says, to cover all Europe to a depth of over 6,500 feet, or to blanket the whole earth under a layer between 120 and 130 feet thick. Melted down, it would raise the world's general ocean level approximately 100 feet.

From the slowness of glacial movements in the Antarctic region, Professor Meinardus has come to the conclusion that at least part of the southern ice mass has been there since Pleistocene geological times. This is variously estimated at from 250,000 to 400,000 years ago, so that the ice of Antarctica has been in cold storage at least a quarter of a million years.

THE CORN BORER IN RUSSIA

THE European corn borer, on which the United States is now waging costly war, is an old and troublesome story in Russia. It is a pest throughout the southern half of European Russia, and occurs in less destructive numbers in an additional stretch of territory to the north. Its northernmost extension carries it to the latitude of the Gulf of Finland, which is as far north as Hudson Bay in the western hemisphere. At this latitude in Russia it is not counted especially bad, but serious outbreaks occur in the new Baltic nations, formerly a part of the old empire.

The borer plague is felt especially in the south, where the cornfields of Russia merge with those of Roumania, and swing eastward across the shores of the Black Sea and up the great river valleys. In the eastern part of the south Russian grain belt corn gives way to millet, which is better adapted to the drier steppes; but the borer afflicts the millet as well as the corn, and efforts are now being made to find varieties less susceptible to its attack.

Russia has no measures against the pest that have not already been recommended in the United States. The best means are the most laborious: a thorough clean-up and burning of all stalks that are not fed to cattle. The burning must be thorough, too, for according to A. Dobrodeyer, a well-known agricultural scientist, borers have often been seen emerging from stalks that were charred black on the outside, apparently none the worse for the experience. He has also seen borers coming out

of stalks that had been left lying about in farm yards after the feeding of cattle, although these had been tramped about for weeks in snow and frozen mud.

The great increase in corn borer infestation in Russia seems to have taken place shortly before the World War. In 1908 a 20 per cent. infestation was observed in the fields of the Government (State) of Ekaterienoslav. This initial infestation took approximately an additional 20 per cent. of the stalks in each of the following years, until by 1912 practically every stalk in the afflicted fields had its borers.

INOCULATION FOR CHICKEN POX AND MEASLES

CHICKEN-POX may be added to the list of diseases that can be prevented by vaccination. Dr. Jean V. Cooke, of the Washington University School of Medicine at St. Louis, Mo., has reported to the American College of Physicians, meeting in New Orleans, that inoculation of exposed children with serum from convalescent patients has successfully prevented cases of both chicken-pox and measles.

Though the former is sufficiently mild, a disease not to require general protective measures, its appearance in epidemics in institutions causes considerable difficulty, especially in the very young children affected. Of a total of 369 cases of exposed children, vaccinated for chicken-pox described in medical literature, Dr. Cooke declared, only 74, or 20 per cent., developed chicken-pox. Of 206 unvaccinated exposed children observed as controls, 158, or 77 per cent., contracted the disease. Such immunity is temporary but serves to protect orphanages and schools from an epidemic.

The preventive treatment for measles should be concentrated on account of the danger of complications on infants and young children under five years of age. Results with this method show, he stated, that almost 90 per cent. of children given convalescents' serum during the first week after exposure fail to develop the disease.

ITEMS

THE probabilities that the influenza epidemic now ravaging Japan will afflict this country are not great, in the estimation of public health officials. Until this disease appeared in Japan the world in recent months had been comparatively free from it. The epidemic is expected to die out with the coming of spring and the warmer weather that checks the respiratory diseases. Fall and winter are the influenza seasons and, unless this tricky disease takes a new turn, health specialists consider a spring and summer epidemic unlikely. As the spring is now further advanced in Japan than in this country, reports of the subsidence of the epidemic are expected shortly.

TURQUOISES and other rare and beautiful objects which were buried beneath an altar in Chichen Itza some 700 years ago have been discovered by Earl Morris, archeologist of the Carnegie Institution of Washington. A telegraphic report from Mr. Morris states that the space beneath the altar has not been fully explored, but articles which have been removed from their hiding place prove it to be the most important cache of Maya objects known in Yucatan. A magnificent mosaic disk, containing one thousand beautifully cut and polished turquoises, is pronounced the most elaborate and beautiful product of the Maya civilization that has ever been discovered. The altar find was made in the Temple of the Warriors, which is one of the masterpieces of Maya architecture. Each column in the temple is graven with the figure of a warrior in full regalia, and it is believed that the eighty or more warriors are all portraits of real Maya heroes. The temple, however, was built in honor of the Plumed Serpent, an important Maya deity.

SPRAYING on paint with a gun, a process that has practically revolutionized finishing in the automobile industry in recent years, is under indictment as a source of considerable health hazard. A representative committee, appointed by the National Safety Council, has just reported upon an investigation of twenty-nine plants and groups of workmen, including automobile and vitreous enamel concerns as well as contracting painters. Several workmen gave evidence of benzene poisoning acquired from spraying benzene lacquers, while the indications of lead poisoning were called "distinctly significant." The danger of silicosis from silica dust particles in the air was apparently not so great though three positive cases were found. As a remedial measure the committee suggested the use of what is known as the positive pressure respirator for the general protection of paint sprayers. Persons spraying compounds of lead or benzene should receive periodic medical examination, the committee declared. It also recommended that manufacturers of paints, lacquers, shellacs and vitreous and varnished enamels to be used in spray coating should eliminate as far as possible benzene, lead and free silica from their products.

CASABA and honeydew melons have been added to the list of fruits which can be given the color and texture of ripeness by treatment with ethylene gas, as a result of researches carried on by Dr. J. T. Rosa at the University Farm at Davis, Calif. Partly ripe melons, with rinds still green and flesh still hard, were subjected to the gas at a concentration of one part in 4,000. They assumed the orthodox "ripe" color, and their flesh became soft. The sugar content, however, was not raised by the treatment. For this reason the hastening gas treatment is not recommended for fruits picked before a fairly advanced stage of maturity.

LOCUSTS, one of the causes of the famines that periodically threaten the great grain-raising plains of Russia, are being fought with the latest means of chemical warfare from the air. During 1927, Soviet agricultural officials report, nearly 77,000 acres of agricultural lands were sprayed with chemicals from airplanes, as compared with only 2,700 acres in 1925.

SCIENCE NEWS

Science Service, Washington, D. C.

DARWINISM

THE frequent statement of critics of the evolutionary hypothesis, that Darwinism is dead and that scientists are rejecting evolution wholesale, is sharply challenged by Professor T. H. Morgan, of Columbia University, one of the foremost of living biologists.

Writing in the April issue of the *Yale Review*, Professor Morgan states that this misconception apparently has arisen out of a confusion over the several distinct meanings that Darwinism has come to have. In its broad sense, as meaning evolution in general, the doctrine is becoming more firmly entrenched every year.

In its more strict sense, as meaning evolution caused by natural selection at work on small, fluctuating variations in a given plant or animal stock, Darwinism has come in for more or less criticism from scientists, though even this does not mean that it has been totally rejected. It merely means that scientists have recognized certain difficulties that were not clearly seen in Darwin's own day. Professor Morgan calls attention to one of these, which makes it difficult to derive one species from another. He says:

"If any particular character, such as size or color, is measured in a large number of individuals of a race or species, it is found to vary. Some of the individuals will be smaller or fainter in color; others, larger or darker; but the great majority will be average or middle class. If the smaller individuals are destroyed and the larger ones become the parents of the next generation, the resulting population will again show a wide range of variability, but the middle class will be a little taller than was that class in the parental population. Suppose again in the next generation, the smaller individuals are destroyed and only the larger ones left to breed. The same result follows, and the average may again be somewhat larger. Experience has shown, in fact, that the average population may in most cases be changed by eliminating consistently certain kinds of individuals through a few generations. But then the process slows down rather quickly and soon comes to an end. Further selection fails to produce further change. The upshot has been not to produce a new race in which all the individuals are taller than the tallest of the original race, but only a race in which the average individual has become taller. The tallest may be no taller than before. This fact was not known to Darwin, or at least, if vaguely known, it was not given due weight."

Professor Morgan is inclined to believe that the force which gets new species past the limits of the old is to be sought in the phenomenon of mutation, in which sudden and relatively large changes occur. When such changes are hereditary, as they frequently are, they provide material on which the process of natural selection can work in the manner postulated by Darwin. Students of evolution have concentrated too much attention on the "survival value" of visible body structures, such as claws and teeth, at the expense of less tangible but perhaps more important things, such as inherited ability to withstand cold or drought, or to run or fly fast, which are of obvious importance in the struggle for survival.

VITAMIN F

THE day when we will live on synthetic concentrated pills of food is yet far distant. Yet the latest attempts to raise laboratory animals on an artificially devised diet of pure foods have led to the discovery of the new vitamin F, recently announced by Dr. Herbert M. Evans, of the University of California.

When a diet of purified food elements consisting of casein and recrystallized cane sugar, certain necessary salts and the five recognized vitamins, A, B, C, D and E, were fed to rats in the laboratories of the department of anatomy, the animals failed to reach more than half size. Theoretically this diet contained all the elements necessary for the health and happiness of rats, but actually something else was necessary. Growth stopped altogether and the animals remained sexually immature. Natural food had to be resorted to, to supplement what might be called a chemically pure menu in order to reawaken their growth and convert them into healthy adult animals.

"Among the natural foods, lettuce and liver were the most potent," declared Dr. Evans, "and they, therefore, almost certainly contain a new sixth member of the vitamins, to which designation F will be given."

Lettuce when heated and dried failed to give the good results of the fresh product, the investigation showed.

Dr. Evans has to his credit also the discovery of vitamin E, at one time known as vitamin X, a lack of which brings about sterility. Oil from the germ of the wheat grain is thus far the most potent source of this necessary food factor.

DISEASES OF THE CALIFORNIA FIG CROP

WARFARE against a plant disease that threatens California's huge fig industry is being waged at Fresno by a unique scheme of campaign. It all centers around keeping a certain small insect, a little wasp no bigger than a gnat, aseptically clean. If the fig-wasp can be kept clean the figs will be saved.

This tiny wasp, called Blastophaga by scientists, looms so large in the fig business because she is the only creature than can pollinate the Smyrna fig, which is the most valuable variety raised in California.. The Smyrna fig, being exclusively female, produces no pollen itself, and the wasp is depended on to transfer pollen to it from an exclusively male fig variety, known as the "caprifig," which produces inedible fruits, but plenty of good pollen.

The Blastophaga wasps breed only in the fruits of the caprifig, and emerge from them as adult insects covered with pollen. Fig growers fasten caprifig branches in their

NEW SCIENTIFIC BOOKS

The McGraw-Hill Book Company, New York

A GUIDE TO THE CONSTELLATIONS. Samuel G. and William H. Barton. pp. x + 74. Illustrated. $2.50.

Devoted exclusively to naked-eye, observational astronomy and written for beginners and as a supplement to the regular text-books. Because of the many large charts included, the book will also be helpful as a source of reference.

The Macmillan Company, New York

COLLEGE TEXT-BOOK OF HYGIENE. Dean F. Smiley and Adrian G. Gould. pp. xiv + 333. $2.00.

Based throughout on those facts of hygiene which have been demonstrated as valuable by modern scientific research. The plan of the book has been developed gradually during the past seven years in the courses in personal and community hygiene for Cornell University students.

University Press Association, Honolulu

THE MATRIX OF THE MIND. Frederic W. Jones and Stanley D. Porteus. 457 pp.

In writing this book the authors have had a very definite aim—the blending of the subject-matter and viewpoints of two sciences which have the same physical structures as a basis, namely, psychology and neurology.

Oxford University Press, London

ELEMENTARY BUILDING SCIENCE. Alfred Everett. 159 pp.

No new science is implied in this title, but rather the application of physics and chemistry to building and building materials and related problems. Some of the chapters are: Measuring and Weighing; Transference of Heat; Hard and Soft Water; the Barometer, Pumps and Siphons; Building Materials.

Microtome Knife Sharpener

Designed by J. A. Long, Ph.D., *University of Calif.*

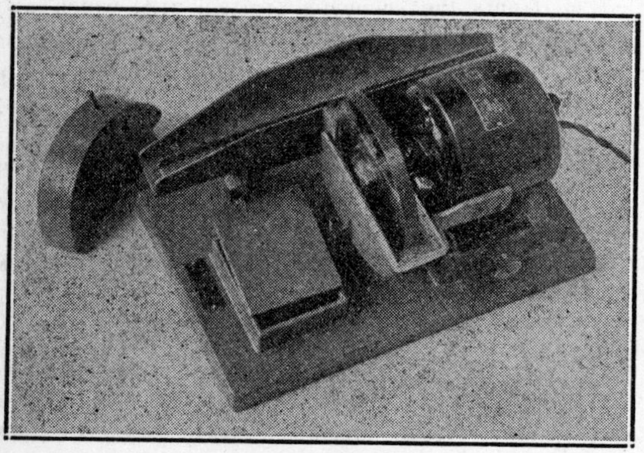

A machine of precision, simple and substantial in construction

It consists essentially of a motor-driven, accurately ground wheel of glass running in water which carries an abrasive in suspension. The knife is held by hand in a guide made adjustable for any desired angle, and is moved to and fro against the wheel.

Eliminates the use of hones and strops.
Soon saves its cost in greatly reduced time and labor.
Results unexcelled by any other method.
The result of over ten years' trial and use.
In use in over 25 university and research laboratories.
Descriptive circular and prices on application.

RELIABLE MANUFACTURING CO.
734 Dwight Way Berkeley, Calif.

WANTED--ANATOMIST

An M.D. or Ph.D. with thorough training in microscopic and gross anatomy. Beginning salary $2,500. Address, D. J. L. Worcester, University of Washington, Seattle, Washington.

THE MICROSCOPE

By SIMON H. GAGE, of Cornell University

Revised, Dark-field Edition (1927) now Available.
The Old and the New in Microscopy, with a special chapter on Dark-Field Methods and their Application.
Postpaid, $3.50

COMSTOCK PUBLISHING CO., ITHACA, N. Y.

SCIENTIFIC PERIODICALS

Chemical, Medical and allied subjects. Complete files, volumes and copies, bought and sold. Kindly send us a list of your wants and items of which you may wish to dispose.

B. LOGIN & SON
29 East 21st Street New York, N. Y.

A Personal Service for INVENTORS

I maintain an unexcelled organization and thoroughly equipped laboratories, to render the following services:

I PREPARE APPLICATIONS for patents for filing in the United States and foreign countries.

I PLACE INVENTIONS with responsible manufacturers, with whom I am acquainted, under arrangements that are made profitable to the inventor.

I SPECIALIZE in Electrical, Mechanical, Chemical and Radio Devices.

I INVITE CORRESPONDENCE with reputable Inventors, Scientists, Chemists and Physicists, regarding their inventions and uncompleted experiments.

H. R. VANDEVENTER
Registered Patent Attorney
Licensed Professional Engineer
342 Madison Avenue, New York City

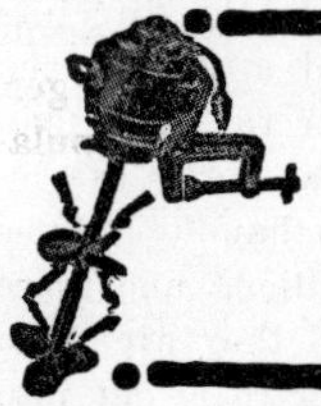

Hy-Speed Mixers

Clamp to any tank, operate from light circuit, mix all kinds of liquids. Also used for even temperature baths. Thousands in use.
Write for circular.
ALSOP ENGINEERING CO.
47 W. 63rd St., New York

LIVING BULLFROGS

Safe delivery guaranteed

Teach Biology with live specimens where practicable

We have the only complete live materials establishment in America. Live plants and animals representing all types are kept on hand under semi-natural conditions at all seasons.

Also headquarters for preserved specimens of all types, microscopic slides, life histories, demonstrations, osteological preparations, insect collections. We specialize in many important southern species not obtainable elsewhere.

All material guaranteed without reservations.

SOUTHERN BIOLOGICAL SUPPLY CO., INC.,
Natural History Building, New Orleans, La.

Smyrna trees, and the wasps, attempting to enter the immature Smyrna figs, accomplish their fertilization. The resulting seeds in the Smyrna figs give them their special value and the medical properties which are claimed for them.

Thus for many years the little fig-wasp has been a vital factor in the prosperity of California fig growers. Now she threatens to be the agent of their ruin, because a serious outbreak of a brown-rot disease has occurred among the figs, and the fig-wasp has been shown to be the unwitting carrier of its germs. Every fig it pollinates it also infects with the virus of destruction, for the pollen-providing caprifigs are infected, and the wasp carries off the infection when it carries off the pollen.

To break this vicious circle a drastic and elaborate clean-up campaign has been necessary. Instead of letting the fig-wasp breed and over-winter in its natural way, the stock of insects that are to fertilize this year's crop has been concentrated in a newly built "insectary" near Fresno, and fig-growers have been required to ship every single caprifig fruit there. Millions of insects and tons of caprifigs, have been assembled.

The wasps are brought out of their over-wintering condition in special incubators, and are allowed access to the caprifig pollen only after the fruits containing it have been carefully sterilized to kill the brown-rot germs. Then the wasps are induced to enter special mailing tubes which are sent to the fig growers. Released in the orchards, the little pollen-carrying insects proceed to the Smyrna fig flowers and complete their fertilization.

State officers inspect all orchards to see that no caprifig fruits, containing possible infection, are left on the trees. If the clean-up campaign can be made 100 per cent. complete for a few years, it is believed that the disease will be completely stamped out.

LIVER FOR FISH FARMS

THE high cost of liver, due to recent medical discoveries of its high value in the human diet, puts the directors of fish hatcheries up against a new and stiff problem. Young fish like liver; it is probably better for them than any other kind of meat they can get. Hatcheries are increasing their facilities so that they can handle billions of fry and fingerlings instead of mere millions, and there is a tendency to hold the little fish until they are from four to ten inches long instead of turning them out into a rough and predatory world while they are still of mere minnow size, as formerly.

All this means a vastly increased demand for fish fodder, and fish men are looking the market over with considerable care and anxiety.

To ascertain the quantity, kinds and costs of fish foods used in the United States, the U. S. Bureau of Fisheries recently made a canvass covering about 200 private and state hatcheries in addition to the 44 federal hatcheries. The results of this survey indicate a consumption of about 3,500 tons of fish food, valued at $275,000 per annum.

The principal fish foods now used are sheep plucks, horse meat and other fresh meat, beef liver, beef lungs, pig liver, cereal products and fish, arranged in order of their importance.

Beef liver is generally recognized as one of the best fish foods, its use being limited by its high cost. Feeding tests conducted by the Bureau of Fisheries at their Holden, Vermont, station during 1927, reveal that much better results can be obtained from feeding brook trout beef heart for the first four or five weeks and then changing to a mixture of equal parts beef heart and beef liver than by using either alone. An unusually low mortality resulted from the use of this combination. Feeding tests in which clam meal was used gave very promising results.

THE STUDY OF BIRD MIGRATION

BIRD enthusiasts who want to help solve the problems of bird migration will have plenty of employment trying to get returns on the 270,000 birds that have been banded under the auspices of the U. S. Biological Survey. Returns on banded birds, according to Frederick C. Lincoln, in charge of this activity of the survey, now amount to 10,338 cases. Knowledge of the movements of the bird after its initial banding, gained from these return reports, enables ornithologists to get precise information concerning bird migration.

Ducks furnish the most returns, undoubtedly due to the fact that many banded waterfowl are taken by the millions of hunters in the field during the hunting season.

Prominent among the bird problems of economic interest which banding may be expected to solve, Mr. Lincoln pointed out, is the control of red-winged blackbirds that do much damage to the rice crop of the South and of California in late summer and early fall. Poison bait has proved ineffective in the rice fields, so that control measures must be undertaken at other times and other places.

"The question, therefore," Mr. Lincoln explained, "that confronts the economic ornithologist, which may be at least partially answered by banding red-winged blackbirds, is whether the individuals in the flocks that are so destructive in fall are the same as those that may be readily destroyed elsewhere at other seasons."

Observations made at one banding station have shown, he added, that the "budding" of fruit trees by purple finches has had no bad effects on their bearing, but might have been responsible for an actual increase in the yield of fruit.

THE ST. FRANCIS DAM

A SHORTAGE of water and electricity in the regions around Los Angeles, California, will be the chief effects of the breaking of the St. Francis dam. Since the dam drained into the ocean through a valley entirely separate from that in which Los Angeles was located, the city itself was in no danger from flood.

The dam was part of the Los Angeles municipal system and, while it was not used for hydroelectric power, one of the two largest of the city-owned power plants was in the San Francisquito canyon below it and was put out of business by the flood. As only a part of the city's power is obtained from these plants, a large amount being purchased from private companies, the loss in power could be taken care of.

About 1,655,000,000 cubic feet of water was impounded in the reservoir behind the St. Francis dam, before the

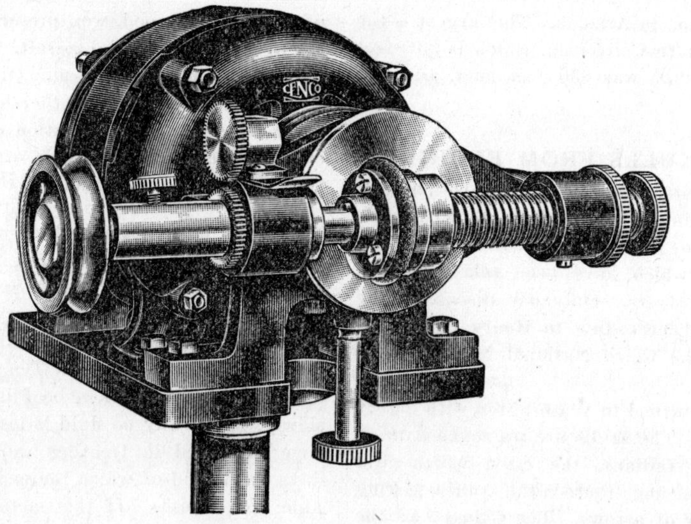
CENCO

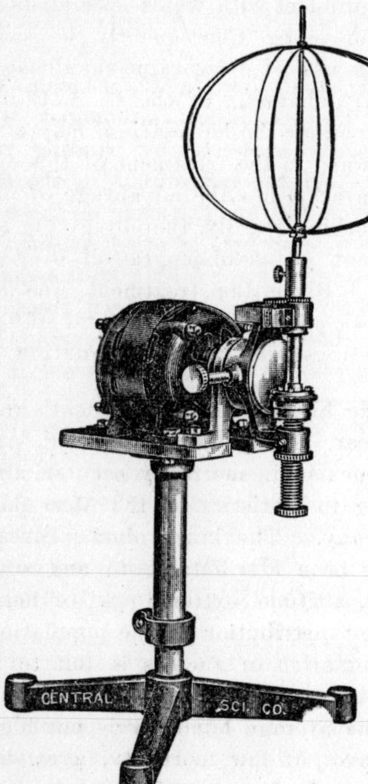
CENTRAL
SCI. CO.

heavy rains burst it and emptied the water down the valley, to the Santa Clara River, and thence to the Pacific near the city of Ventura. Though not the country's largest dam, it was in the front rank as far as size was concerned. It was 205 feet high, as compared with 280 feet for the Roosevelt dam, in Arizona. The largest is the Exchequer dam, in northern California, which is 330 feet high. The St. Francis dam was 650 feet long, and 169 feet thick at the base.

PREHISTORIC SKULLS FROM FLORIDA

PREHISTORIC inhabitants of southern Florida may not have known the fountain of youth that the Spaniards sought in Florida, but they were an extraordinarily healthy lot, judging by bones which have been taken from a burial mound near Ft. Myers. Only one diseased bone was found in the mound, according to Henry B. Collins, Jr., anthropologist of the U. S. National Museum, who excavated at the site.

Mr. Collins has just returned to Washington with eighty skulls from this mound. The skulls are pronounced those of the famous Calusa Indians, the tribe which first greeted Ponce de Leon and routed the youth-seeking Spaniards with a shower of arrows. The Calusa had the reputation of being cannibals and fierce warriors, but they were among the first Indians to be wiped out by the white man, and by the time of the American Revolution they were practically extinct.

"Remains of these extinct Indians have been extremely rare, and very little has been known about them," said Mr. Collins, in describing his expedition. "The skulls show that the Calusa were not particularly large or powerfully built people, as were tribes of northern Florida."

A strange discovery from the mound was that only half a dozen of the eighty burials were children. Whether this means that these Indians were more successful than most tribes in raising their children, or whether babies who did not survive were disposed of in some other way, can not be determined.

No Indian possessions were found in the burial mound, with the exception of some fragments of pottery. These broken pieces of pots and jars had been stuck in the ground all around the heads of most of the Indians, probably with some magic rite.

The burial mound was outlined by a border of conch shells over two feet wide, the white shells making a sharp contrast against the black muck of the mangrove swamp. Further excavations were made in a number of large shell heaps, some of them 30 feet high, but these kitchen dumps of the Calusa revealed no traces of cannibalism or other unusual practices.

ITEMS

IN an endeavor to check the mosaic disease of sugarcane, which is one of the most destructive of tropical plant diseases, the State of Rio de Janeiro, Brazil, has offered a prize of approximately $1,200 to any scientist who, before the end of the current year, will ascertain its cause and determine an effective method for combatting it.

SALT mines that were operated on an extensive scale, with very "modern" shafts, tunnels and drifts, more than 500 years before Christ, have lately been explored near Hallstadt, Austria, by Dr. Adolph Mahr, of the Vienna State Museum. In addition to knowledge of the mining methods of these prehistoric men of the early Iron Age, the exploration yielded also numerous articles of leather and wood, well preserved against decay during the ages by their burial in salt. These finds included pick handles, torches, wedges, mine timbers, felt caps, shoes of wood, leather and felt, leather hand-protectors, and many other articles. The exploration was backed by two Americans, Professor F. W. Bade, of the University of California, and Major Gotshall.

BRITISH scientists have been at work to make palatable the famous roast beef of England that has to come in these days from Australia or South America. The freezing process necessary to carry the meat on its long journey dries up all the natural juices. It has been found, however, at the Low Temperature Research Station at Cambridge that when beef is frozen and thawed very slowly, practically no fluid is lost. In one experiment the time consumed in freezing and thawing took nearly 80 days at the end of which the meat was hardly distinguishable from fresh. If this method can be applied in industry, it may be of considerable commercial importance.

A NEW combination of chaulmoogra oil with benzocaine has enabled several lepers at the National Leprosarium, at Carville, Louisiana, to receive the benefits of the curative drug with a minimum of pain. The discomfort which accompanies the administration of chaulmoogra oil is a problem with which specialists in leprosy have struggled for years. Consequently the success which has attended the use of benzocaine-chaulmoogra oil by Dr. Frederick A. Johansen,, of the U. S. Public Health Service, on 24 lepers at the leprosarium may mark an important step forward in the treatment of this ancient disease. This preparation has the advantage of not causing pain, and of absorbing readily, thereby giving the patient a uniform amount of chaulmoogra oil over a definite period of time. Since the treatment was started 36 patients have been added, making a total of 60 who are taking the injections semi-weekly as routine treatment.

MARCH has the highest pneumonia death rate of any month in the year. Frequently more than one seventh of the annual pneumonia mortality occurs in this single month, according to statistics of the Metropolitan Life Insurance Company. The large number of pneumonia deaths have not been attributable to any single cause, such as latitude, altitude, extreme cold or heat, high or low humidity, age distribution of the population or occupation. A combination of factors is felt to be responsible for the high mortality of this disease. A cold climate where the average humidity is not high appears to operate in favor of low mortality, a condition illustrated by the very low pneumonia rate for the western provinces of Canada. Oregon and Washington, also, have fewer pneumonia deaths than the average while Pennsylvania, New York and New Jersey in approximately the same latitude consistently register some of the highest rates.

SCIENCE NEWS

Science Service, Washington, D. C.

ELECTRICITY FROM THE AIR

ELECTRICITY of nearly two million volts, capable of jumping gaps of nearly 15 feet, has been obtained from the air by Drs. A. Brasch, F. Lange and C. Urban, three members of the staff of the Physical Institute of the University of Berlin.

Mount Generoso, in Switzerland, near Lugano, was the scene of these experiments and the experiments will soon be resumed. This mountain is noted for the frequency of electrical storms upon it, and also it has the advantage of being easily accessible.

It was found impossible to make use of kites for the purpose of collecting the atmospheric electricity, because use was made of a wide-meshed wire net having an area of several hundred square yards. It was out of the question, they found, to suspend this from kites or balloons, because such means would be particularly undependable during a storm, when the experiments were made.

In order to get the net as far as possible above the earth, they hung it on a cable between two mountain peaks. The span was about 1,800 feet, and the height of the net above the ground about 250 feet. At each end were chains of insulators capable of withstanding as much as 3,000,000 volts.

Another problem was to prevent what are called brush discharges, in the conductors which carried the current from the net to the measuring instruments. The intensity of these discharges is less, the greater the radius of curvature of the conductor, so that the discharges would be less from a large hollow cylinder than from a smaller solid wire, with the same amount of metal. As long cylindrical conductors would have been difficult to transport to the mountain, Dr. Brasch and his associates made use of a string of short, round-ended cylinders.

From a lightning-proof metal house the observations and measurements were made. The spark gap, under the last of the short cylinders, could be regulated from this post, and, from the length of the gap across which the spark would jump, the voltage was determined.

As the chief electrical storms of the neighborhood are in the summer, and as the apparatus was not completed until last August, the best storms had to go unused. One storm occurred after it was completed, and indicated the success of the method. The spark gap could not be made larger than about 15 feet, but the sparks easily jumped across it at the rate of about one per second and continued for thirty minutes at a time. Also, it was found with an auxiliary collecting antenna, and with distant storms that affected the main station, that a discharge of once a second was possible at all times.

During the winter months, the experiments were discontinued, but the apparatus was left in place. The scientists are now preparing to return, to take full advantage of the storms this season. With the antenna about three hundred feet above the earth, a height that could easily be obtained, voltages as high as thirty million would result.

Dr. Brasch and his colleagues credit Benjamin Franklin with being the pioneer experimenter in the field in which they are working. One possible use of these huge voltages, they say, is to generate extremely rapid cathode rays, similar to those formed in the tube recently developed by Dr. W. D. Coolidge, of the General Electric Company. These are similar to one of the principal radiations from radium, but with 30 million volts, the artificial rays would travel even faster than those emanating from radium itself.

AN ECLIPSING VARIABLE STAR

THE star epsilon Aurigae in the constellation of the Charioteer, near the bright Capella, which is now directly west in the evening, is now getting fainter, several months ahead of the schedule, according to a report made by Dr. Joel Stebbins, director of the Washburn Observatory of the University of Wisconsin.

Epsilon Aurigae is one of a class of stars known as eclipsing variables, that periodically change in their brilliance. They consist of two separate globes, one brighter than the other, which revolve around their common center of gravity. When the dark one comes between the brighter orb and the earth, the light is diminished.

When at its brightest, epsilon Aurigae is of the 3.4 magnitude, but when eclipsed diminishes to magnitude 4.1. With the naked eye, on a dark night, stars down to about the sixth magnitude can be seen. The average period between the times of minimum brightness of the star in Auriga is about 9,900 days, one of the longest known periods for a star that so changes in brightness.

With his colleague, Dr. C. M. Huffer, Dr. Stebbins has been studying the changes in brightness of various stars with the photoelectric cell. This device converts the faint light from the star into a minute electric current, which can then be measured with a delicate galvanometer.

Not until later in the year was epsilon Aurigae expected to begin to diminish in brightness. Observations made on four nights since January 22 by Dr. Stebbins and Dr. Huffer show that in that time the star's light has decreased more than a tenth of a magnitude, so that it is now changing at the rate of about eight hundredths of a magnitude per month.

Just what might cause this unexpected change in brightness is uncertain, but Dr. Stebbins expects to continue observing the star in the hope of learning more about its queer behavior.

PROTECTION FROM LIGHTNING BY TALL BUILDINGS

TALL buildings and lightning rods mounted on high towers protect neighboring structures from lightning, pro-

vided they are not so high as to extend out of the cone of protection. This protected area extends around the base of the high building for a distance of between two and four times its height. Imaginary lines drawn from the top of the building to the edge of the protected area define the protected cone, says F. W. Peek, Jr., in charge of the General Electric Company's high voltage investigations at its laboratory at Pittsfield, Mass.

Mr. Peek's investigations have been made with artificial lightning at pressures of as high as three and a half million volts. These man-made flashes have been used on small models of buildings. However, confirmation of his discoveries was obtained by studying a natural electrical storm that occurred in New York last summer, and during which the New York World building was struck. Though this building is close to the Woolworth Tower, and is in the 1,100 foot circle around its base that is protected, the dome of the World building extends for about a hundred feet outside the cone, and that is the reason that it was struck, explains Mr. Peek. If it had been 200 feet closer to the Woolworth building, it would have been protected.

Practical application of these experiments, says Mr. Peek, has already been made in California, in safeguarding oil storage tanks from lightning. Several tall rods, placed outside the big reservoirs, provide overlapping cones of protection and reduce the danger to a minimum.

HOW TO LIGHT PAINTINGS

PHYSICS has come to the aid of the artist in showing how paintings can be hung to best advantage in picture galleries.

If pictures are to be seen as the artist meant them to be seen, according to Dr. J. W. T. Walsh, of the National Physical Laboratory, the lighting should be as much like unaltered daylight as possible. In cases where natural lighting is used, the windows through which the light passes, and the glass in front of the pictures should be practically colorless. Also the decorations of the roof and walls should be neutral in tone, especially where they are liable to receive direct sunlight.

One of the practical difficulties in the arrangement of old paintings is that the old paints may tend to fade. Ultra-violet light is now thought to be to some extent responsible for this condition, and to prevent it one should allow no direct sunlight to shine on the pictures.

Another great difficulty often encountered in picture galleries is the reflection of spectators in the picture glass, or a reflection of the pictures on the opposite wall. The former type of reflection can be avoided by having a roof design in which the windows are so arranged that no direct light falls on visitors, although the pictures receive full illumination. Reflections of pictures opposite are of course best prevented by not having any pictures on the opposite wall, and some modern galleries are designed with pictures on one wall only. If this is impossible, reflections can be avoided by erecting a screen the whole length of the room.

THE OXYGEN-CARRIER OF THE BLOOD

AN important step toward the understanding of how the process of breathing sustains life has been made by Professor Otto Warburg who, in an address before the Kaiser Wilhelm Association for the Advancement of Science at Berlin, demonstrated the constitution and action of the ferment in the blood which controls the conveyance of the oxygen of the air from the lungs to the muscles. So minute an amount of this ferment or catalyst is present in the blood that it can not be isolated, yet it is an essential factor in the supply of vital energy to all animals. Its chief constituent is haemin, a chemical compound which has been known for the last seventy-five years, but which was first made artificially in the laboratory a few months ago by Professor Hans Fischer. It contains iron and is a component of the familiar red coloring matter of the blood, haemoglobin.

But the ferment is ten thousand times more sensitive to light than haemoglobin. The color of the light makes more difference than its intensity. Rays of a certain frequency will be absorbed while light of another wavelength will not affect it. These iron-containing compounds of the blood are tuned to react to select radiations like a fine radio apparatus. One of the derivative compounds can act as a sensitizer to sunshine so that a person taking a dose of it would be light-struck, perhaps fatally, by ordinary daylight, while he would be all right so long as he remained in a dark room. Pigs are sometimes so sensitized by eating buckwheat as to be sickened by sunlight.

The "breath-ferment" described by Warburg is beneficially affected by light, for when it is poisoned by combination with carbon monoxide such as may come from automobile gases, the combination is readily broken up by faint light, and the ferment can then resume its function of carrying oxygen.

GLUCOSE FOR ENCEPHALITIS

THE treatment of encephalitis by the injection of glucose has awakened considerable interest among specialists at St. Elizabeth's Hospital for the Insane. Dr. Walter Freeman, who has made many researches on encephalitis, states "that even though the way in which it works is uncertain, this mode of treatment undoubtedly offers something of importance in the treatment of nervous diseases."

The improvement of acute cases of encephalitis by glucose injections was recently announced by Dr. Leland B. Alford, of St. Louis, Mo. The action of the glucose is not well understood, but it is believed that the compound exerts a protective action on the nervous system.

The first clue to the beneficial action of glucose, according to Dr. Alford, came from its administration as nourishment to an encephalitis patient who was delirious and refused food. This took place in November, 1926. To the surprise of every one the patient began to improve. On Christmas day she recovered her senses and by New Year's day returned home and has remained well ever since. Glucose seemed the most probable factor in

this unprecedented recovery and so was given a trial in another acute case which likewise registered rapid improvement.

The method was followed up with good results in as many as forty acute cases. The injections have no harmful effects, it was stated. It has, however, brought about only slight improvement in chronic cases. The chronic form of encephalitis is particularly stubborn and to date few ways have been found of combatting it.

It will be many years, Dr. Freeman pointed out, before the glucose treatment can be properly evaluated but, he added, any method that gives hope of relief in dealing with this unfortunate disease, is worthy of trial and further research.

FAST TRAVEL IN THE ORIENT AND THE CONTROL OF DISEASE

AIR lines and bus routes in the Orient make hard work for the European health officials whose job it is to hold in check the time-honored diseases of the East.

In Iraq two new lines of communication, according to Dr. C. P. Thomson, president of the Egyptian Conseil Sanitaire, now have to be taken into consideration when cholera breaks out.

The first is the weekly airplane trip from this city to Basra by way of Palestine and Bagdad. Only 12 hours are required to reach Bagdad from Cairo, and 27 to reach Basra, since the planes do not fly by night. When this route has been extended to Karachi in western India, Dr. Thomson pointed out, a potential cholera victim from an infected center in that country could easily be on board ship at Port Said in three and a half days, before the incubation period of the disease would be completed.

The second avenue of contact is by the motor route from Bagdad to Beirut *via* Damascus, which takes only 29 hours. The traffic on this line is increasing constantly while pilgrims, always a fertile source of epidemic spreading, have already made use of it to the number of 2,000.

Medical authorities of Syria control the motor traffic while that of the airway is under strict medical surveillance by Palestine and Egypt. Travelers coming from the infected territory may be released from quarantine at the aerodrome if they can show they have received two injections of cholera vaccine, the last administered at least six days before.

During the cholera epidemic in Iraq in the summer of 1927, a supply of cholera vaccine sufficient for 700,000 doses was provided, from which about 40 per cent. of the inhabitants of infected towns were vaccinated.

ITEMS

CORONIUM, the mysterious substance in the sun's corona that only manifests itself in spectrum photographs made at the time of a total solar eclipse, is probably due to argon, third most abundant gas in the air. This is indicated in researches carried on at the Ryerson Physical Laboratory of the University of Chicago by Dr. Ira M. Freeman. "Coronium" was first found in 1869 when, in the eclipse of that year, astronomers noticed a strange line of a green color in the spectrum of the corona. This is the extremely rarefied outer layer of the sun that is visible only when the central disc of the sun is obscured by the moon. Ever since that time physicists have been trying to find the cause of it and a group of unknown lines that were later discovered. Dr. Freeman has found that 18 of these lines can be identified as those of the element argon, which occupies nearly one per cent. of the atmosphere. Other observations of the sun with the aid of the spectroscope have never shown the presence of argon, but, Dr. Freeman points out, it may well be that it is present but that it is quite possible the conditions on the sun are not just right for it to be in evidence ordinarily.

THE aid of ultra-modern chemistry has been invoked to salvage another relic of the remote past. An ancient leather roll of Egyptian writing had lain unopened for 50 years in the British Museum because it was so brittle that no one dared unroll it. Experiments with a broken fragment of the leather in the museum's laboratory, however, finally gave scientists a clue as to how to handle the mysterious manuscript. Several thin coatings of celluloid were soaked into the pores of the leather, after which it was cemented with strong celluloid on to a piece of celluloid-treated cheesecloth. In this way it was unrolled without a break and pressed flat between two glass plates to dry. It remained perfectly flat after drying and can now be read with ease.

ROMAN artisans in England only two to three centuries after the time of Christ knew how to weld iron and how to join or "solder" two pieces of iron together with copper, the Institute of Metals was told at its meeting by Professors J. Newton Friend and W. E. Thorneycroft, of the Technical College, Birmingham. The specimen examined by them was a deep iron ferrule, like a modern napkin ring, that was unearthed during excavations of the Roman city of Uriconium located on the river Severn and destroyed about A. D. 380. Lead pipe manufactured and laid in Rome's water system 1,800 years ago was pronounced to be in perfect condition by William A. Cowan, chemist of the National Lead Company, Brooklyn, N. Y., in a communication to the institute. Analysis showed that the same lead was used by the Romans in England and Italy.

THE Ruhr industrial region, recently restored to normal operation following the withdrawal of the French, has given a striking illustration of the damage wrought by factory smoke not only to trees and gardens in the cities, but to the farm crops throughout the countryside. When the French occupied the region in 1923 the Germans adopted a policy of "passive resistance," closing down all the factories. With the air cleared of its load of smoke and acid fumes, the farms of the Ruhr Valley yielded full crops for the first time in many years. Then the French withdrew and the chimneys started smoking again, and now the crops have dropped back to their previous low level.

SCIENCE NEWS

Science Service, Washington, D. C.

OXYGEN ON MARS AS AN INDICATION OF LIFE

THE presence of oxygen gas in the atmosphere of Mars is the best evidence to date of life on that planet, according to the opinion of Dr. Henry Norris Russell, of Princeton University, who spoke recently at the University of California at Los Angeles.

The concentration of oxygen about Mars is only about fifteen per cent. of that over the earth. This was recently shown by measuring the wave-length of certain radiation passing through the moving atmosphere of the planet. So dilute an atmosphere would not support life in animals of the earthly type. There is no very good reason, however, why an entirely different animal evolution should not produce creatures whose venous blood or other bodily fluid could absorb oxygen at low air pressure. Nevertheless, as a matter of simple logic oxygen still does not prove the presence of animal life.

In the vegetable realm oxygen tells a more convincing story. Dr. Russell points out from the chemical viewpoint that free oxygen gas is utterly out of place in the advanced stages of a dead world. In particular, the ferrous iron minerals, present in vast quantities in the various planets, by the laws of the chemist should long ago have absorbed all oxygen gas in sight. In such chemical action the minerals are normally converted into the ferric iron of common red soils. It is only the reverse chemistry of a growing plant which could possibly restore a supply of the active gas.

Extensive gray-green bands on the planet Mars—sometimes called "canals"—are thought by Dr. Russell to consist of vegetation. The extreme distance of the planet, however, renders evidence of animal life so far impossible of detection.

The very existence of a planet such as the earth with so favorable a combination of physical and chemical conditions is regarded by the astronomer as an extremely rare accident. Accordingly there are likely very few inhabited worlds in proportion to the total number of heavenly bodies in existence. Nearly all are either too hot, too cold, too small to hold an atmosphere by force of gravitation, too dry, or have the wrong kind of atmosphere. Moreover, it is equally unlikely that any great number of inhabited worlds would happen to develop during the period of time in which we live.

BELGIAN ELEPHANT FARMS

PLOWING by elephant in the Belgian Congo has proved fourteen times less costly than plowing by tractor. Since maintenance of the great beasts, including food, two attendants each, medication and depreciation, works out to about twenty-five cents a day and a trained elephant brings about $2,400, at the present value of the franc, the government elephant farms at Bas-Uele and Haut-Uele in the Kongo district are expected to be soon on a self-supporting basis.

On account of the havoc brought upon horses and cattle by the tsetse fly, the government began experimenting with the training of wild elephants as far back as 1902. Indian mahouts and domesticated Burmese elephants were imported but both soon succumbed to the climate. The ferocious African elephant is not easily transformed into a gentle domestic servant, though there is some evidence that the famous elephants in Hannibal's legions were from his native continent.

Before the Burmese mahouts departed, however, they taught the African natives some of the age-old Burmese elephant songs and a few apt pupils picked up the art of elephant management. Certain fierce tribes found elephant hunting a pleasant substitute for killing their neighbors so that the experiment went on after the war with redoubled interest. The black mahouts were soon singing the Burmese elephant songs to Niam-Niam tunes, but the big pachyderms seemed to understand.

Only baby elephants, from approximately two to ten years old, are singled out from the wild herds for capture. They are trained under the tutelage of skilled elephant men and older elephants known as "moniteurs," wise in the ways of breaking in the younger ones of their kind. Some idea of the rate of elephant growth can be gathered from the case of one elephant that has grown from four feet two inches when he was captured in 1902 to eight feet three inches at the present time.

It is estimated that one elephant will plow two and a half acres in two days and is an otherwise valuable asset in pulling stumps, piling timber and such arduous tasks, necessary in bringing a new country under cultivation.

DISEASE OF THE GROUSE

THE grouse disease that has made the partridge literally a rare bird in sections of the northeast, where his drumming was once as familiar as the robin's call, is proving a difficult problem for science to unravel.

Under the direction of Dr. A. A. Allen, of Cornell University, research has been carried on for three years with the object of locating the cause and possible cure of the scourge. Progress has been hampered by the fact that ruffed grouse are delicate and high-strung birds to handle in the laboratory. Some of the difficulties can be appreciated from the fairly typical results obtained by one game preserve officer, who succeeded in raising only 50 birds from 394 eggs laid in captivity.

Attempts made to identify the germ of the malady responsible for the large losses throughout the northern states and Canada have not yet succeeded, though a vast amount of useful information has been collected concerning the parasites that infect the birds and certain fungus diseases that affect the lungs. It has been found that one parasite produces changes in the blood that bring about the deposit of waste products in the feathers, causing patches of them to turn black.

The tick that transmits tularemia, the rapidly spreading disease of wild rabbits and man, is also suspected of infecting grouse. Dr. R. R. Parker, of the Spotted Fever Laboratory at Hamilton, Montana, has found the tick on grouse but has been handicapped in further research on the problem from lack of funds with which to secure live birds for experiment. One species of grouse has definitely been infected artificially in the laboratory, but whether this dreaded disease is actually prevalent among birds in the field is not yet known.

RICKETS IN BIRDS

FEATHERS may be still another source of the much-discussed antirachitic vitamin D. Hawks and owls raised by Dr. William Rowan, of the University of Alberta, Canada, in captivity and fed only on "livers and lights" from the butcher shop developed rickets and in many cases died before reaching maturity. His experiments are reported in *Nature*. Two young owls, however, that had been fed mice and sparrows almost exclusively, were not affected. This suggested the addition of chicken heads with feathers and an occasional sparrow to the menu of the rest of the survivors. Thereafter rickets ceased to give trouble.

The preen gland of the domestic fowl, Dr. Rowan points out, is known to be a rich source of cholesterol, one of the parent substances of vitamin D, a condition that may apply to feather oil. As further evidence for his suggestion, he cited the case of a merlin under his observation several years ago that fed her offspring on birds that were plucked before they were brought to the eyrie. Only occasionally did she bring home a victim with the feathers still on, from which she fed the young birds mouthfuls of feathers only. Her offspring apparently objected to the "dose" because it had to be thrust well down their throats before it would go down.

"Possibly," said Dr. Rowan, "it is true that there is nothing new under the sun, and we may here be witnessing a crude method of administering the antirachitic vitamin D that has, no doubt, been in practice for countless centuries."

THE DOG'S WORLD

THE average dog owner could write an enthusiastic book about his pet's intelligence and keenness. But scientists have only begun to penetrate into the dog's world, to find out carefully and exactly how much a dog sees and understands.

Experiments so far made indicate that the average dog has far more faulty vision that most dog-lovers suppose, according to a survey of what is known about dog psychology made in *The Quarterly Journal of Biology* by Dr. C. J. Warden and L. H. Warner, psychologists of Columbia University.

Laboratory experiments in Russia and other countries have led most psychologists to believe that the dog has little or no ability to see colors. A puppy that seems to know red from green may be responding to a difference in the brightness of the two colored objects, or some other clue that his human friends overlook. A dog's vision for still objects appears to be decidedly inferior to that of a man, but he is keenly sensitive to moving objects.

A dog's sense of smell appears to be far superior to that of a man. A German shepherd dog, for example, was able in every instance to pick out a small piece of pine wood that had been handled by her keeper, even when the piece of wood was placed with as many as twenty other pieces that he had never touched. Two seconds' contact between the keeper's hand and the object was sufficient to insure the dog's identifying the keeper with the object.

On the other hand, police dogs were tested in Germany by giving them the glove of a person and telling them to pick out the owner from a row of men. The dogs all failed on this test and on a number of other tests intended to prove their usefulness in police work. As a result of the tests the use of dogs in criminal detection was forbidden by the Prussian Government. It is not clear whether the dogs really "understood" what was wanted of them in these tests.

Whether dogs recognize words as a human being does, or whether they respond to sounds, or merely to tones and inflexions of the voice, is not agreed upon by experimenters. In tests with the thoroughbred German shepherd dog, "Fellow," recently made by Dr. Warden and Mr. Warner, the dog responded to 400 words used in various commands given by his master Jacob Herbert, of Detroit. In some cases, Mr. Herbert gave the commands from an adjoining room with the door closed, thus showing that the dog did not depend on watching his master's face or gestures for clues. Taking commands through a closed door was new to "Fellow," and the voice was muffled, but he made a good record though not a perfect one.

One of the chief reasons why scientific men disagree on the dog's capacities is that all sizes and sorts of dogs have been used in experiments, from highly bred bull terriers to an assortment of mongrels. The authors suggest that a representative breed of dog should be settled upon for systematic study.

THE KENTUCKY MOUNTAINEERS

A LITTLE over a century ago, the mountaineers of eastern Kentucky were probably slightly superior to the average American in intelligence. To-day, these disappearing American highlanders rank considerably lower than average.

To find the cause for this striking decline in mentality, Dr. Nathaniel D. M. Hirsch, of Duke University, has visited three counties of the mountain country and has tested almost 2,000 young highlanders.

According to Dr. Hirsch, environment is responsible for only about 25 per cent. of the sub-average mentality; heredity is the cause of 75 per cent. For a hundred years migrations have played a large part in lowering the intelligence level. Long ago, when game and fish became rare in eastern Kentucky, the people who had settled in the mountains were faced by the problem of trying to farm the steep hillsides, or of moving. A migration of the restless and foresighted took place about 1820 to 1840.

Two more waves of migration struck the mountain region, one about the time of the Civil War and again in 1880. Now, since 1903, there has been a fourth migration, which has probably not yet reached its height, carrying away chiefly the more energetic, ambitious and intelligent groups.

Dr. Hirsch concludes that very close intermarriage of the depleted stock that has remained in the mountains is another cause for the falling level of intelligence. The outlook, however, is good. The gifted sons and daughters of the mountains, who have moved to more desirable surroundings are contributing their pure blood and sturdy character to American life in a wider field. "The nation is bettered by their spread," says Dr. Hirsch. "The communities to which they move are biologically and morally enriched."

The mountains that they left are being rapidly developed industrially for the hidden resources of oil, gas, soft coal, mica, kaolin. More changes have taken place there in a few years than in a whole century preceding. The unique civilization of isolated pure-blooded highlanders will soon be lost by the intermingling of mountain families with the Italian and Hungarian laborers that are coming in to dig in the mines, run the railroads and work in lumber camps.

ITEMS

BUTTERFLY breeders, who have built up a respectable little business in Germany as well as in the United States, have their work simplified for them by a simple trick described by Julius Stephan, a German naturalist. Many butterflies have the habit of emerging from their cocoons at night, so that breeders have had to sit up with their charges until all hours in order to prevent them from fluttering about their cages and damaging their delicate wings. Herr Stephan avoids this nocturnal labor by artificially hastening nightfall. At two or three in the afternoon he transfers the cocoons to a dark, cool place, and the insects soon begin to display their normal night-reäction. By seven o'clock all that are due to emerge that day will have put in their appearance.

THE latest available figures of the U. S. Public Health Service show that there are 250 more cases of smallpox in the last reported week in March than there were in the corresponding week of last year. In spite of the fact, however, that smallpox is more prevalent this year in the country at large, it has just been reported to the American Medical Association that not a single case of the disease has been contracted in the public schools of St. Louis, Mo., for thirty-three years. Systematic vaccination with subsequent inspection and reinspection of vaccinations on the part of the city division of health and the hygiene department of the public schools are considered the agents that have made possible this remarkable record.

ULTRA-VIOLET light can be used to take photographs to reveal alterations in documents, according to a report of Professor Carlo Bonàcini to the *Rivista Fotografica Italiana*. He has found that writing on a paper which had been erased by chemical means, and was entirely invisible to the eye, had altered the fibers of the paper, a fact which was shown by the ultra-violet photographs. Professor Bonacini has also confirmed previous reports that if writing is done in ink of the ordinary kind, and the paper is placed in contact with an ordinary photographic plate or film for a time, the plate loses its sensitivity where it touches the writing. Then, if it is briefly exposed to the light, and developed, the writing appears transparent on a gray background. He has found that this works even if the writing has been bleached by chemicals, so that the method offers another way of detecting altered checks or other documents.

A DIET high in protein or meat increases the activity of laboratory rats but makes them easily frightened. These are some of the results of an attempt to find the effect of food on the temper made by Professor Emil Abderhalden, of the University of Halle, who has been making determinations of the psychological behavior of rats fed on different diets. One series of rats was fed on a diet that was rich in protein and poor in carbohydrates, while a control series of similar rats was fed on a more usual diet, with abundance of carbohydrates. The experiment was continued for a considerable time, and observations were made of rats' dispositions while fed on the prescribed food. It was found that the variation of the diet had a striking effect on the behavior. The rats which received little carbohydrate and a great deal of protein showed distinctly abnormal characteristics. They were much more active and were more resistant to the ill effects of alcohol. Together with these more or less desirable changes was a decidedly undesirable one, namely increased susceptibility to fright.

THE use of charcoal for producer-gas as a propellant for motor vehicles is being seriously considered in Great Britain. The Forests Products Research Laboratory has already conducted preliminary experiments on various methods of preparing charcoal for this purpose. So far it has investigated two French types of portable kilns, and also the more ordinary type of bee-hive kiln. Arrangements have been made with the Fuel Research Station to carry out tests on the charcoal prepared from various species of timber, and to determine its value for producer-gas.

SOLID bubbles of selenium, the element that transmits electricity when light shines on it, though at other times it offers great resistance to an electric current, can be blown with the aid of a glass tube, according to a report in *Nature*, by Charles E. S. Phillips. The selenium is melted and then when the tube is dipped into it, withdrawn and blown through, a rather sausage-shaped bubble can be blown. A curious effect reported is that when two bubbles, even twenty-four hours old, are brought into contact, they come violently together and can not again be separated. The method is said to be a convenient one of getting flakes of selenium for experimental purposes.

SCIENCE NEWS

Science Service, Washington, D. C.

COPPER AS AN ANEMIA PREVENTIVE

COPPER, the red metal, is an essential factor in the diet to keep the blood red and the body vigorous, a group of University of Wisconsin chemists headed by Dr. E. B. Hart, announced recently at the meeting of the American Society of Biological Chemists.

Copper may become acknowledged as one of the more essential requisites in human nutrition and livestock feeding. The Wisconsin experiments indicate that it exerts a tremendous influence on anemia in rats, a disease similar to anemia in children who have been fed exclusively on milk. The malady in both rat and child is caused by a deficiency of hemoglobin in the blood stream.

A shortage of iron has been credited with being responsible for the disorder, and, although iron compounds are still limiting factors, their effectiveness, according to Wisconsin investigators, depends on the presence or absence of copper. The investigations covered four years, and Dr. Hart was assisted by his colleagues, Drs. H. Steenbock, C. A. Elvehjem and J. Waddell.

Because milk is notoriously low in iron and hemoglobin is rich in the mineral, it has always been assumed that the way to correct anemia was to add iron to the milk diet.

In the case of animals this plan proved ineffective. The daily feeding of iron, administered as chloride, sulfate, acetate, citrate or phosphate, all prepared from pure iron wire, did not check the decline in the hemoglobin content of the blood. Rats suffering with anemia were not improved.

However, when a supply of iron was obtained by feeding dried liver, or the ash of dried liver, corn or lettuce, the hemoglobin was raised to normal and the stricken rats immediately restored to health. In ashing the foodstuffs, the investigators noted a pale, bluish color, the typical hue produced when copper compounds are burned. Observation of this peculiar color, in addition to the fact that copper is known to be present in the respiratory pigment, hemocyanin, of certain crustacea, led the chemists to use copper sulfate as a supplement to pure ferric chloride in the whole milk diet.

Striking cures resulted. Rats, so anemic that their days appeared to be numbered, recovered immediately and the hemoglobin in their blood was brought to normal.

"What about pernicious anemia in man?" the chemists asked. Patients suffering with anemia have been told to eat liver, advice which has evidently made a wide impression, judging from the rise in price of what was once poor man's meat. However, some sufferers find liver unpalatable, especially when eaten in large quantities. Harvard University scientists have prepared a liver extract which has proved exceedingly efficacious in abating the disease. In the Wisconsin experiments, this product was ashed and fed the anemic rats. When fortified with ferric chloride, it also proved effective in correcting the ailment. Thus this product which has been most successful in treating man corrected the deficiency in rats.

Copper's rôle in plant and animal tissue is not clearly understood. It is found in milk, in small quantities. Its function in producing hemoglobin is, as Hart states, unknown. Hemoglobin may not contain copper, at least no evidence to the contrary has yet been produced. In this connection, copper may act as a catalyzer, an agent which starts an action without being changed itself. It may promote the building of hemoglobin. Iron functions in a similar manner in the production of chlorophyll, the green pigment of vegetation, although it is not a constituent of the chlorophyll molecule.

Experiments with the use of copper in the diets of anemia patients will be undertaken in the near future at certain leading hospitals. If this inorganic substance plays the part in the human system that it does in the life of white rats, nutrition specialists will probably give as much consideration to the copper content of foodstuffs as is now paid to some other elements, such as phosphorus, calcium and iodine. Future experiments at Wisconsin will also approach the problem from this standpoint, as the copper content of animal feeds is known to vary widely.

THE BORAX INDUSTRY

EXPLOITATION of the kernite (also called rasorite) deposits in the Mohave Desert, Kern County, California, probably will result in killing off the mining of other borate minerals elsewhere in this country and in other countries so that the United States will have a complete monopoly, according to Dr. Waldemar T. Schaller, of the U. S. Geological Survey.

So far as is known, kernite, an entirely new mineral, exists nowhere else in the world. The deposit lies but three to four hundred feet beneath the surface, is more than 100 feet thick and extends at least 500 feet in every direction. It was discovered in 1926 and mining operations were begun approximately a year ago.

Kernite is virtually pure sodium borate. The material mined is over 75 per cent. pure mineral, the remainder being clay. To prepare it for the market it is only necessary to dissolve it in water, filter off the clay, and permit recrystallization to take place. Marketable borax is sodium borate plus ten molecules of water. Kernite is the same sodium borate plus four molecules of water. During the refining process six molecules of water are added so that one ton of kernite makes 1.4 ton or nearly a ton and a half of borax. There is probably no other commercial mineral that increases its marketable bulk in such a fashion through the process of refining.

Previous to the discovery of kernite the world's borax supply was derived principally from the minerals borax, colemanite and ulexite. Italy procured it from volcanic steam containing boric acid. In each case the process involved was complex and expensive. In this country borax was formerly secured from mineral deposits in and near Death Valley, under dangerous circumstances, and

had to be hauled from the mines by the familiar "twenty-mule team," to a distant railroad.

The kernite mines are within four miles of the Santa Fé main line and a spur track, built at small expense across the intervening alluvial flat, has made transportation simple. It is estimated that enough of the mineral already has been blocked out to supply the market for some time and millions of tons for future needs require only to be shoveled out of the ground, dissolved in water, and recrystallized.

CAMOUFLAGED TRAPS

CAMOUFLAGE patterns are now used for mouse traps. At the office of the United States Biological Survey in Washington, clever devices, designed to catch the most wary of mice, are on exhibit.

For the field mouse who robs the corn crib there is a trap made by hollowing out the center of a corn cob and wiring it. The mouse who boldly chews the papers on your desk makes his last predatory excursion the night he examines what appears to be an ordinary steel wire paper-clasp.

One clever trap will reset itself and capture as many as six or eight mice in an evening. When the mouse enters, the small metal door falls shut. Seeking a way out, he ascends a miniature passageway which leads to a plunge in a half-gallon can of water. The trap is so constructed that it automatically resets itself when the victim plunges into the water.

Still another trap, one that any boy could make, is fashioned out of an ordinary tin can. The top has been carefully cut all the way around, rewired in place and equipped with a simple spring. When set, it appears to be nothing more harmful than the usual tin can whose top has been incompletely mashed in. But when the mouse investigates he finds that the top springs into place with surprising quickness, leaving him locked inside.

These traps, and many others designed for larger and more dangerous prey, such as mountain lions and wolves, have been collected by the survey during its long campaign to eradicate predatory animals. Economic experts of the bureau estimate that rodents alone, such as mice, rats, prairie-dogs, ground-squirrels and jack-rabbits, are responsible for a crop-production loss of approximately $500,000,000 each year. In addition some of them, such as rabbits and rats, have been found to be carriers of disease and therefore dangerous from the standpoint of public health.

LOSS IN INDUSTRY FROM COLDS

COLDS and their relatives, such as pneumonia, influenza and bronchitis, are responsible for more lost time in industry than any other group of diseases.

Statisticians of the U. S. Public Health Service have found that over half, 54 per cent. to be exact, of the illnesses of the men employed by a large industrial firm throughout a period of ten years were caused by colds and other respiratory infections. Furthermore, the reports of a group of sick-benefit associations show that 47 per cent. of the illnesses lasting eight days or longer among male members were due to the same causes.

"From the effect upon the absence rate in industry, no other disease group," declared Dean K. Brundage, assistant statistician in the Public Health Service, "approached in importance the respiratory diseases. Among employees of the industrial firm described above, diseases of the respiratory system caused more absences from work than all other diseases put together. The sickness records of the company revealed an annual loss of 3.23 calendar days of disability from respiratory diseases per male employee, compared with 6.92 calendar days of disability from all causes of sickness per man on the pay roll.

"In view of the frequency of disability and the amount of time lost from work on account of the respiratory diseases even a small degree of success in their prevention would contribute enormously to the sum total of physical and mental energy, to the number of days that the industrial population is physically able to work, and, accordingly, to an enhanced national prosperity."

Careful scientific analysis of records, it is believed, will cast some light on the causes of these two prevalent infections. One of them, lobar pneumonia, is being subjected at the present time to special investigation by the Public Health Service in an attempt to evaluate the more important factors influencing its incidence and high death rate.

THE TARANTULA

THE common tarantula of the southwest achieves a ripe old age and can easily go without food for periods as long as a month or six weeks.

Professor W. J. Baerg, of the University of Arkansas, well-known authority on spiders, has kept tarantulas in his laboratory under observation for nine years, until the life cycle of this member of the spider family, not previously known to science, is now fairly clear.

The male tarantula is approximately eleven years old before he attains maturity, declared Professor Baerg in a report to appear in a forthcoming issue of the *Quarterly Review of Biology*. Since a tarantula only locates his food by touch and sits serenely at the door of his burrow in the earth, waiting for his dinner to walk by in front of him, he is equipped to withstand long periods of starvation. Consequently the period at which the spider attains all the attributes of adulthood is probably determined in a measure by the amount of fasting his lethargic habits have caused him to endure. The same statement probably holds good for the female as well.

"They locate their prey entirely by sense of touch," Professor Baerg explained. "Thus a cricket may come within a centimeter of where the tarantula is waiting, and be perfectly safe; however, as soon as one touches the other, the cricket is very speedily brought in reach of the fangs and consumed." Grasshoppers, cockroaches and caterpillars vary the spider menu in the laboratory, but if they are kept in a cold room they will not require any food from early in October until late in March.

For many years scientists were puzzled because, in spite of diligent search, no males were seen out-of-doors in the field except at the mating season in September and October. Professor Baerg's hand-raised tarantulas, however, have furnished the answer. During the eleven years it takes the male to grow up, he changes his skin 22 times, and only after the last is distinguishable from the female. Soon after the mating season the males decline and die, rarely surviving to see another season.

The females, on the other hand, present a very different picture. After attaining sexual maturity at 12 or 13 years of age they continue to live on till they are at least 20 and probably much older.

Professor Baerg's observations, he pointed out, have not been made on one individual tarantula from hatching time until death, but on several of various ages that have been under observation at different stages of development.

PLANT ROOTS

WHEN you pull up a radish from your spring garden you are gathering in materials that were once scattered around through the soil to distances of more than a foot on either side of the little pungent globe in your hand, or buried two feet or so underneath it. Later on, when you gather your first ears of sweet corn, you will be getting the benefit of work done by roots through a circle five feet in diameter and three or four feet deep. Roots are the world's greatest miners.

The wide-spread activities of the roots of garden vegetables, hitherto suspected but never intensively examined, have been the subject of research by Professor John E. Weaver and Dr. William E. Bruner, of the University of Nebraska. Their work has involved much hard digging in the literal as well as the figurative sense, for a five-foot trench had to be excavated alongside of each plant studied, and the details of the roots' travels followed with hand tools.

Annual vegetable crops like radishes, beans, melons and turnips will occupy in their few weeks of growth a great deal more space in the soil than their tops occupy in the air, and their roots will drill a great deal deeper than their stalks go high. Longer-lived plants, such as rhubarb and asparagus, do not send their roots a great deal deeper, but tend to solidify their holdings, by penetrating the soil much more thoroughly with their bushier branching systems. A four-year-old rhubarb plant, for example, was found to occupy a cylinder of soil eight feet in diameter and eight feet deep, with some of the longer roots straggling downward an additional two or three feet. A ten-year-old plant of horseradish reached out only eighteen inches or so on either side of its crown, but its roots drilled downward to a depth of more than fourteen feet.

CALIFORNIA TREES

YELLOW pine trees from all over the United States are being tested and cross-pollinated at the Eddy Tree Breeding Station, at Placerville, Calif., in an effort to obtain choice varieties of forest trees that will grow faster than the present wild stocks and hence produce a crop of timber in fewer years. Nursery plantings made last season include seedlings of 49 species and 9 varieties, from seed obtained in 17 different countries; and extensive additions are now in hand as part of this season's program.

The program of the station includes gathering tree stocks from as many different localities as possible, comparing geographic races of the same species, selection of the best individuals in native stands as breeding stocks, and artificial pollination both within given species and between species in an effort to produce hybrid varieties. Cross-pollination thus far has yielded hybrids of Western yellow pine with Swiss mountain pine and with the digger pine of California.

The second tree genus on which the experimenters intend to work is the black walnut. They now have a stock of the black walnut species of northern California established, but have not yet reached out for the Eastern and Old World walnuts, due to their preoccupation with the pine work. Eventually they wish to add other timber trees to the two now on their experimental schedule.

The work of the station is under the direction of Lloyd Austin, a graduate of the University of California.

ITEMS

COLLECTORS of old china will be interested to know that the authenticity of certain types of old porcelain can now be determined by chemical tests. Under the direction of Dr. Alexander Scott tests have been worked out in the laboratory of the British Museum that have helped classify several doubtful pieces in the museum collections without disfiguring the specimens. Old patent acts were consulted to determine the chemical composition of Old Bow and Chelsea china, while tests were then resorted to to detect the presence of various phosphate components known to have been used in its composition.

THE people of the United States are to be the beneficiaries of a patent obtained by E. N. Bates, of the U. S. Department of Agriculture, on a seed-cleaning machine operating on an entirely new principle, which the inventor calls an "aspirator." The device consists essentially of a funnel-shaped hopper into which the grain, seeds or other material is poured. From this it is allowed to fall in a thin circular stream into a chamber beneath, flowing over a wide, cone-shaped valve. As the grain trickles down, a current of air is sucked upward through it by a motor-driven fan. In this air current all dust, light seeds, bits of straw and chaff and, in general, all particles lighter than the seeds being cleaned are carried off into a side chamber, where they are deflected into a receiving cup. The cleaned grain meanwhile falls into a receiving pan on its own side. Mr. Bates has constructed two different types of his aspirator, one for large-scale use on a threshing separator and the other for laboratory use in seed-testing and similar work. The machine is covered by Public Patent No. 1524012. Under the terms of American patent law, any article so patented may be manufactured and used in the United States by any citizen without the payment of royalty.

SCIENCE NEWS

Science Service, Washington, D. C.

THE MEANING OF EVOLUTION

"The meaning of evolution is probably more misunderstood than any doctrine of science. The misunderstanding has arisen from ignorance of the subject, from misinterpretation of the statements of scientific men, and from what may be called a medieval attitude of mind. It has been a shock to educators to realize that there still remains such a mass of untrained minds that can be imposed upon by eloquent ignorance."

With these sentences Professor John M. Coulter, of the Boyce Thompson Institute, Yonkers, N. Y., and formerly head of the botany department at the University of Chicago, opened his lecture March 31, at the New York Botanical Garden.

Opponents of evolution who state that the doctrine has been cast aside by scientists are either self-deceived or deliberately deceiving others according to Professor Coulter. What is being cast aside is not the idea of evolution itself, but many of the formerly accepted explanations of how it came about. Evolution becomes more firmly entrenched every day in the minds of scientists as new facts continue to accumulate, but while these new facts make the probability of the evolutionary process ever stronger, they are themselves so many and present such complicated problems that the question of how evolution happens becomes ever more difficult to answer.

The teaching that acquired characters can sometimes be inherited, long denied, is now beginning to find friends again, Professor Coulter stated. This doctrine of evolution was advanced by Lamarck, long before Darwin's time, but seemed to have been shoved aside by Darwin's alternative doctrine of constant, small, spontaneous variations acted upon by the process of natural selection. The force of natural selection is still admitted, at least in part, but the usefulness of small variations has been called in question by many biologists.

The mutation theory of DeVries, which substitutes sudden origins of new forms at a single leap for the slow variations conceived by Darwin, is still widely accepted, but doubts have been thrown on its validity in many instances, and even its own author has accepted some cases of apparent mutations as being due to the sorting out of hybrid characters.

Yet in spite of all doubts and questions as to method, the fact of evolution remains unshaken, the speaker declared. With evolution, the living world is a single unified picture; without it, creation is chaos, and no single fact has any necessary relation to any other fact.

In conclusion, Professor Coulter cited the great practical value which the study of evolution has had in its applications to the bread-and-butter problem of agriculture.

The statement was made that during the ten years preceding the great war our population had increased twenty per cent. and our food production about one per cent. It was certainly an alarming outlook. Under these circumstances plant crops began to be studied from the standpoint of genetics, and plant breeding became a science.

The lack of crop production arose chiefly from three causes, namely, lack of adaptation of crops to environment, destruction by drought, and destruction by disease. The same races of plants were being cultivated everywhere, and only in certain places was the maximum result obtained. A study of races of crop plants throughout the world, and of the environment necessary for maximum yield, resulted in such an adjustment of crops to conditions that total food production was enormously increased.

The problem of drought is being rapidly solved by the discovery or development of drought resistant races, not only insuring against loss from this cause, but also enormously increasing the possible area of cultivation.

The problem of disease has been attacked in the same way, and disease resistant races of most of the important crops have been developed, much reducing loss from this source.

As a result, food production is now beginning to overtake population, and we may thank the persistent study of evolution for the result.

ANCIENT MAN IN AMERICA

Dr. Aleš Hrdlička, of the U. S. National Museum, expresses serious doubt as to the high antiquity of the hu-
presses serious doubt as to the high antiquity of the human inhabitation of America, in spite of such evidence as the recent finding of arrow-heads and human bones in Florida, apparently associated with the remains of animals that lived during the Ice Age.

Dr. Hrdlička is not as inclined to place great emphasis on finding human and animal remains in the same strata as are the paleontologists, or scientists who study ancient animal life. Except for accidental introductions, man alone, among all the forms of animate existence, has the custom of burying his dead; and this must often have introduced his bones, and the tools placed with them as funeral gifts, into strata containing the remains of animals that died many thousands of years earlier. And it is not always possible, he says, to tell whether or not the overlying earth has been dug out and then shoveled back in.

Another point is that, because an animal is extinct, it is not necessarily ancient; it may have lived up to a few thousands of years ago and been a contemporary of the earlier American man, without thereby making the latter very ancient.

A further difficulty, from the anthropologists' point of view, is that so very few of these supposedly ancient human remains and implements have been found in America, as contrasted with the literally millions of flints, bones and similar objects showing human handiwork, together with scores of human skulls and skeletons that have been found in the old Stone Age caves and

sites of Europe. Although experienced anthropologists have been working for many years among the cliff and cave dwellings in the Southwest and elsewhere, they have not found underlying these comparatively recent structures a single implement or a bone of either human being or animal that would indicate the presence of a paleolithic race on this continent.

Another weighty point advanced by Dr. Hrdlička is that the European deposits show a more or less orderly evolution of human skill, from the earliest rough-chipped flints to the perfected stone implements that just preceded the use of metals, whereas the American finds, even those associated with the bones of extinct animals, are all of culturally far advanced types. But the same is true of all the American skeletal remains of man claimed to be ancient—they are all of modern types. This would mean that while man was developing both culturally and in bodily characteristics from the earliest to modern forms in Europe, here in America he started at the top and made no progress at all. And Dr. Hrdlička considers this highly improbable.

AVIATION HAZARDS

Flying is becoming safer. Aviation accidents, in proportion to the mileage flown throughout the whole United States, are diminishing, according to statistics compiled by Dr. Frederick L. Hoffman, consulting statistician of the Prudential Life Insurance Company.

During the year 1926, there were 160 fatal accidents in air operations, including pilots, mechanics, passengers and others. Five of these were women, one a negress, a professional aviatrix. The number was probably somewhat less during 1927, while the air mileage during the year increased considerably.

It is estimated that in 1927 there were about 1,500 licensed pilots, among whom there occurred 11 fatalities, a rate of about 7 per 1,000. Even if the rate were 10 per 1,000 it could not be considered excessive considering the novelty of flying over new air routes and the rapid growth of the industry.

Dr. Hoffman is making a comprehensive survey of aviation hazards in this country and abroad to determine among other things what percentage of aviators die, and what constitute the primary factors in aviation accidents. In the course of his investigations, statistics of military, mail and commercial aviation have been consulted, while personal flights have been made to the extent of over 10,000 air miles in this country, Canada and Europe.

The Imperial Airways of London during the three years ending with 1927 carried about 52,000 passengers without a fatality. The air mileage flown was not quite 2,500,000 and, as stated, without a single death to mar the record. By the way of contrast Dr. Hoffman pointed out that in 1842, according to the London *Times,* the number of passengers carried on the eight railway lines of the United Kingdom numbered 10,000, while the distance traveled was 3,500,000 miles. The number of passengers killed that year was 22. Yet air transportation has vastly greater difficulties to contend with.

This summer Dr. Hoffman expects to fly from Boston to the Pacific Coast and return by the southwestern route, giving special attention to airports, radio reporting, plane and engine performance, comfort, safety and medical examination of pilots. The trip will extend over about 6,000 miles of established airways.

A STATISTICAL SURVEY OF THE INCIDENCE OF CANCER

"If, in some manner or other, malignant tumors of the alimentary tract and of the reproductive organs could be prevented, cancer would retire at once to a relatively unimportant place among the causes of death."

This statement was made by Dr. Raymond Pearl, director of the Institute of Biological Research of the Johns Hopkins University, after the completion of a statistical survey, made by himself and Miss Agnes Latimer Bacon, on necropsies performed on fatal cancer cases in the Johns Hopkins Hospital.

In summarizing the results of the survey, a report of which will appear in a forthcoming issue of the *Archives of Pathology,* he stated that in men malignant tumors occurred more frequently than anywhere else in the organs of digestion, such as the stomach, intestines, gall bladder and liver. In the women the cancers were found in the reproductive organs. These conditions are in general agreement with the cancer figures of the U. S. Census Bureau.

"The greatest discrepancy between the general population and the necropsy statistics is in respect cancer of the skin," added Dr. Pearl. "Patients with cancer of the skin die at home rather than in a hospital relatively more frequently than do patients with cancer of any other organ system. This fact means that such cases tend to the under-represented in necropsy statistics. The patient who enters a hospital with cancer of the skin in an early stage is discharged cured. But for the patient who lets his cancer of the skin go without treatment, or with the supposedly palliative treatment of quackery, until it is destined shortly to be fatal, a hospital has little to offer."

From these studies it appears that more of the different organ systems of the body are susceptible to cancer in white people than in colored. On the other hand, a relatively larger proportion of the cancers of colored people occur in the digestive system and in the reproductive system than is the case in whites. The average age at death of people with tumors that had produced secondary growths or metastases, as they are known to medicine, was found to be from one to three years earlier than in cancer cases without such secondary growths.

HAY FEVER

The spring hay-fever season is officially started. Maple and elm trees, oaks, hickories, and walnuts have announced the open season for sneezing by broadcasting their pollen on the April air. And in return the first faint hay-fever sneezes have promptly been set off.

Spring hay fever, caused by the pollen from trees, is less likely to be recognized than the summer hay-fever due to weeds and grasses, according to Dr. Harry S. Bernton, associate professor of preventive medicine of the Georgetown University Medical School. Many people who start sneezing about this time of year attribute their symptoms to colds due to the fickle changes of spring weather.

Hope for some of the baffling cases of hay fever due to grass pollen is held out this year by Dr. Bernton, through new analyses of the pollen grains. It has been customary to find out the kind of pollen that irritates the nasal tissues of each hay-fever victim, and then to treat the patient with injections of that particular pollen extract until he becomes immune. Recently by analyzing the pollen, it has been found that a person may be sensitive to one substance in a grain of pollen and not to the rest of the material packed in the tiny grain. Some cases that have stubbornly resisted treatment are due entirely to a sensitiveness to the albumen fraction in the pollen. Albumen makes up only about one ninth of the extractable protein in the pollen grain. So when these patients were treated with pollen extract they did not get big enough doses of albumen to help them. This year, Dr. Bernton is reinforcing the extract of albumen to see if these puzzling patients can be rendered sneeze-proof.

Foresighted sufferers from summer hay-fever are now having the usual pollen injections to render their noses invulnerable by the time the summer pollens get on the air. The newer method of having injections twice a month throughout the year, instead of taking a steady series of freatments before each hay-fever season, is slowly gaining favor. This method seems to produce a more permanent immunity to the disease, but the average hay-fever sufferer likes to forget his sensitive nose entirely in the months when he can breathe freely.

THE USE OF GOAT SERUM TO PREVENT MEASLES

When measles broke out in the children's ward of the Cook County Hospital, Dr. Louis J. Halpern, resident physician, undertook to stem the disease with goat serum first developed by Dr. Ruth Tunnicliff, of the John McCormick Institute for Infectious Diseases of Chicago.

This serum is produced by immunizing goats by means of cultures of a coccus which Dr. Tunnicliff believes to be the causative germ of measles. It has been used on a previous occasion to prevent measles but only with a small number of cases.

Fifty children, ranging in age from a few weeks to twelve years old, who had never had measles before were treated with the serum, said Dr. Halpern in a report to the American Medical Association. Five of the young patients were ruled out of the series by death from the diseases from which they were suffering when admitted to the hospital. None of these, however, developed measles or showed any signs of serum sickness.

Of the remaining 45, 28, or 63 per cent. were successfully protected, while 17 developed the disease, but the majority of these experienced it only in an attenuated form. None of the children suffered from the after complications that make measles a severe menace to very young children.

As a result of this experience, it seems evident that goat serum gives efficient protection in a large number of cases and offers the advantage of being more readily available than human convalescent serum, which has seen considerable application for the same purpose, since it can be produced in quantities to meet all necessary demands.

ITEMS

"Astronautics" is the latest name to be introduced for a branch of science. It has recently been adopted by the French Astronomical Society to indicate the problems of voyaging through space to other heavenly bodies. To encourage development of this new "science" the society has been given funds for an annual prize of 5,000 francs (about $200) to be awarded in 1928, 1929 and 1930 to the "author of the best original work capable of bringing a realization of one of the numerous scientific desiderata tending to the final goal of astronautics," namely, of actually traveling from the earth to another celestial body. The funds for the prize have been donated by Robert Esnault-Pelterie and André Hirsch, and is known as the Rep-Hirsch prize. It is under the control of a committee of leading French astronomers and physicists, including General Ferrie, former president of the society and head of the telegraphic system of the French army; Professor Jean Perrin, Nobel prize winner in physics; Professor Charles Fabry, director of the Optical Institute; Professor Henri Deslandres, director of the Paris Observatory, and others.

An example of evolutionary effects in a breed of domestic poultry originally noticed by Darwin, the white-faced Spanish fowl, has gone on evolving rapidly under the guidance of artificial selection, according to a British student of poultry, F. Finn, who writes in *Nature*. When Darwin knew the breed, Mr. Finn states, its face and the sides of its head were covered with white skin, and its earlobes were prominent and pendulous. This white skin has developed even more extensively during the half-century since Darwin called attention to the birds, and the earlobes have vanished as such, having been merged in a sort of horizontal delap that hangs across the cock's throat.

A plant that generates gas which can be lighted with a match is described in the British scientific journal, *Nature*, by Dr. W. A. Hamor, assistant director of the Mellon Institute of Industrial Research, of Pittsburgh. The plant is known botanically as *Dictamnus albus*, and in common speech as dittany; it grows in southern Europe and central Asia. It is covered with glands that secrete a volatile oil, which in hot weather apparently evaporates, making the air about the plant inflammable.

SCIENCE NEWS

Science Service, Washington, D. C.

THE EFFECT OF SUPER-SONIC WAVES ON BLOOD CORPUSCLES

SUPER-SONIC waves which are sound-waves vibrating too rapidly to be heard, have now been brought under such control that observers can watch their effects through a high-power microscope. Using a small electrically driven crystal to produce these waves at a rate of 406,000 a second, Professor E. Newton Harvey, of Princeton University, and Alfred L. Loomis, of Tuxedo Park, N. Y., have watched blood corpuscles warp, twist and disintegrate, and have seen the living protoplasm in plant cells whirl in a dance of death, faster and faster until it has separated into spinning bits, broken and disorganized.

The apparatus used in these experiments is a refinement, on almost a jeweler's scale, of an earlier form devised by Mr. Loomis and Professor R. W. Wood, of the Johns Hopkins University. It takes advantage of the fact that when a rapidly alternating electric current is fed into a quartz crystal cut in a certain fashion, the crystal vibrates at the speed of the electrical oscillations, producing sound-waves. By cutting the crystal small, and using an electrical oscillator of the type employed in radio stations, it is possible to produce sound waves twenty times as fast as the 20,000-per-second waves which represent the upper limit of human hearing ability. And these extremely rapid waves, at high enough intensities, have a tearing, killing effect on living substance. They have been nicknamed "the death whisper."

"Observing under a high-power microscope," Professor Harvey and Mr. Loomis state, "it has been possible to follow the progressive destruction of frog blood corpuscles. The oval cells at first become warped and twisted. Strained areas appear and the color fades, leaving a pale distorted shadow. Human blood corpuscles are likewise twisted and sometimes broken up into many small globules like an emulsion of oil."

Vibrations on the leaves of a water-plant, in which the living protoplasm usually keeps up a constant circulation around the wall of each cell were also investigated. "High frequency waves of low intensity passed through these cells caused the protoplasm to rotate very much as in the normal rotation. Increasing the supersonic intensity increases the movement until the whole cell is a rapidly whirling mass of protoplasm, fragments of which are torn loose and rotate as small balls in the vacuole. The effect is very striking.

"The microscopic method offers a promising means of attack upon the problem of influencing the development of eggs of various species, as forces can thus be applied inside an egg at different stages of its development without the necessity of puncturing the cell wall or enveloping membrane. The results immediately suggest the interesting possibility of converting an egg with determinate cleavage into an indeterminate one by thoroughly mixing and redistributing the organ-forming substances of its interior. We are now engaged upon this and allied problems, the results of which we expect to publish in due course."

TESTS OF HEARING

HOLDING a watch near the ear to test hearing may soon be a thing of the past. Ear tests developed by scientists of the Bell Telephone Laboratories, New York, make use of accurate instruments which, with psychological aids, determine a person's exact degree of hearing. False claims of either deafness or exceptional hearing are of no avail, for the truth can now be easily discovered.

A push-button on the instrument which measures the tone emitted for the test permits the interruption of the sound at any moment. If a patient says he hears a tone, and then claims that he still hears it when it has been cut off, it is evident that he has been deceiving himself.

Another device makes it possible to switch the sound to either ear or both. A loud tone in either ear causes the eye nearer it to blink slightly, though the patient may claim that he hears nothing.

The patient is made to read aloud in his normal voice in another test, while a tone is switched from ear to ear. The intensity of the voice is regulated by the sound of the voice and this can be drowned out. One who has normal hearing in both ears will, however, be able to hear his voice with one ear while the tone is switched to the other, and he will not change the level of his voice as the tone is switched back and forth. If he is deaf in one ear, he will raise his voice every time the tone sounds in his normal ear.

When the tone is switched on and off both ears, a person with normal hearing will raise his voice each time the tone is turned on, while one who is deaf will continue to read without changing his voice.

To detect a false claim of deafness in one ear, the tone is switched repeatedly back and forth between the ears at varying intensity, and the patient is asked to signal each time he hears a sound. A truthful signal can be made almost instantaneously, but if the patient must stop to decide each time in which ear he hears the sound, much more time is required and he quickly becomes confused, thus betraying himself. These tests are expected to prove valuable in compensation cases where loss of hearing is involved.

PROBABLE FLOODING OF THE WHITE AND BLACK RIVERS

THE low-lying areas along the White and Black Rivers in Arkansas and Missouri are in danger of another flood. Heavy rains which fell in that region on April 20 will so swell the waters of these rivers that rises of one to six feet above flood stages were expected, beginning on April 21 in the upper portion and extending to the lower parts of the White River the first few days of May. These predictions are made by Dr. H. C. Frankenfield, in charge

of the rivers and flood division of the U. S. Weather Bureau.

These areas suffered severely in the great Mississippi Valley flood of last year and the farmers have not yet fully recovered. Moreover, high water caused them damage and concern about two weeks ago. News of hardship and privation are therefore to be expected from this region in the next few weeks.

The Mississippi River will feel the influence of these floods in its tributaries, but on the whole this great river is behaving itself this year.

There are no large cities along the White and Black Rivers, but towns which were expected to feel the flood include: Batesville, New Port, Georgetown, DeValls Bluff, Clarendon, all in Arkansas and on the White River, and Poplar Bluff, Missouri, on the Black River.

Heavy rains in the lower basin of the Ohio River, some of them having sent to earth as much as three inches of rain in the last twenty-four hours, will cause a considerable rise in that river. It is, however, expected that the excess water will flow down to the Mississippi without great trouble.

A REMEDY FOR SEASICKNESS

Seasickness may cease to be the voyager's bugbear if experiments of Drs. J. Frank Pearcy and Daniel Hayden, of Chicago, are substantiated by further tests.

The possibilities of the new remedy came to light when the doctors were making experiments to determine the depressant effects of the common drug, sodium nitrite, on the mechanism of the middle ear that controls the balancing of the human body. The experiments were reported to the American Medical Association.

"Believing that seasickness is due mostly, if not completely," the authors explained, "to overstimulation of the vestibule (of the middle ear), we felt that the nitrites offered a direct attack at the long-sought but never attained cure for the terrible malady of the ocean voyage."

So when Dr. Hayden was about to take a trip abroad he sought to put his theory to the test, but none of the passengers on the trip going over the Atlantic accommodated him by becoming ill. On the return voyage, however, he had better luck. Sixteen succumbed and were divided into two groups of eight each, one of which received the nitrite treatment while the others were kept under observation as controls. Every attempt was made to have patients with equally acute symptoms in each group.

The controls were prostrated for about two days, but the others who received from three to five grains of sodium nitrite every two hours until they were relieved were comfortable on deck and able to eat meals in four hours. There was no recurrence of symptoms.

Although the work has a sound experimental basis, the actual tests having been adequately controlled and 100 per cent. cures obtained, the authors expect to use nitrites in a much greater series before drawing final conclusions. They are certain, however, that they will cure many cases of seasickness, but it is also possible that there are cases that will not be cured.

ITEMS

The U. S. Bureau of the Census is waging a campaign to bring every state in the Union into the birth and death registration area before 1930. The registration area is slowly growing, with some expansion in 1927, but federal health officials feel that it is extremely important for the country's warfare against disease that accurate information concerning the birth and death records of the entire nation be available to epidemiologists and health workers. The birth registration area at present covers 40 states and the District of Columbia, which takes in 87.3 per cent. of the total population of the country. In the death registration area are 40 states, the District of Columbia and 21 cities in non-registration states of the death registration area. This gives information on the cause of death of 91.3 per cent. of the population of the United States.

North sky light, long accepted as the perfect standard of white light for examining colors, has been found to vary in intensity and color, not only from day to day but also from hour to hour. The American Institute of Electrical Engineers reports that north sky light is not white, but blue and the examination of colors under such light exaggerates blues and minimizes reds and yellows. It is claimed that noon sunlight and not north sky light should be accepted as the standard, and that artificial white light for color discrimination purposes should approximate noon sunlight.

Victims of Addison's disease and other conditions associated with adrenal insufficiency may be greatly benefited by a method of treatment now under development by Drs. J. M. Rogoff and G. N. Stewart, of Western Reserve University, according to an announcement made at the meeting of the Federation of American Societies for Experimental Biology at Ann Arbor. By means of injections of extracts made from adrenal glands obtained from the slaughter house, Dr. Rogoff has enabled dogs completely lacking the adrenal glands to survive for periods from 18 to 78 days. This extract when sufficiently purified can be used to treat Addison's disease, a condition in which the function of the adrenals is greatly impaired. Progressive anemia develops in this disease, which usually results in death. The functions of the adrenal gland are obscure at the present time and the work by Drs. Rogoff and Stewart will probably lead to new developments in the treatment of other serious ailments associated with adrenal insufficiency.

Far under the feet of pedestrians who are serenely unaware of what is happening, two parallel subway tunnels are being blasted and bored through the bed rock of Manhattan. At the rate of twelve feet per day, the tunnels are pushing their way, ninety feet below Fifty-third street. At the East River they will meet tunnels dug under the East River from Long Island. The rock taken out of the tunnels in Manhattan is being used to fill in deep spots in the river where the tunnels pass. The same rock will thus be dug out for a second time before being finally disposed of. The use of electrical machinery in this remarkable operation is eliminating almost all manual labor in tunneling.

SCIENCE NEWS

Science Service, Washington, D. C.

THE "NEW" SOUTHERN STAR

NOVA PICTORIS, the star that flashed out from previous obscurity in May, 1925, and has since proved more and more puzzling to astronomers, may be an example of an event which occurs, on the average, once in ten billion years—the actual encounter of two stars. So thinks Dr. Harlow Shapley, director of the Harvard College Observatory.

New stars, with which this outburst was first classed, are rather common. Every year half a dozen or more are observed, though one reaching the first magnitude does not occur nearly so often, perhaps there are not more than five or six in a century. But even this frequency has been thought to effectually dispose of one theory of their origin, namely, that when two faint stars happen in the course of their wanderings to collide, the explosion results in a temporary object far brighter than either. So thinly are the stars scattered through space that it has been figured that such a collision of stars could not happen oftener than about once in ten billion years on the average. Therefore this theory can not account for the ordinary nova, or new star.

In the case of nova Pictoris, which is so called from its position in the constellation of Pictor, the painter, a group not visible from northern latitudes, a number of things have occurred to show that it is no ordinary nova. The first noticed peculiarity was that it was changing much more slowly than the ordinary new star. They usually rise from very faint to very bright within a few hours. Nova Pictoris was discovered on May 25, 1925, and was then of the second magnitude. A photographic plate was then found, taken 42 days before its discovery, that showed it to be of the third magnitude on April 13. For years before it had been of the thirteenth magnitude. Though it could not be determined just when the increase in brightness began, it was, for a nova, very slow.

After discovery it continued to brighten and, by June 7, was of the first magnitude. Then it should have quickly diminished in brightness, but by the beginning of September it was still of the third magnitude. Even now, three years after discovery, it is of the seventh magnitude, and appears as if it might never return to the original brightness.

Another unusual feature of nova Pictoris was the appearance, a few months ago, of a companion body beside it, which was discovered by South African astronomers. In the opinion of Dr. Spencer Jones, a British government astronomer at the Cape of Good Hope, this indicated that there had been an actual encounter of two stars. The latest peculiar feature has been the discovery around it of a series of rings. The outer one, discovered by Dr. J. S. Paraskevopoulos, Harvard astronomer in South Africa, was about a tenth of the diameter of the full moon, while inside it are now seen two smaller rings. The inner rings were discovered by Dr. Harry E. Wood, of the Union Observatory at Johannesburg. As the star became bright after discovery, diminished, and then increased, then diminishing and increasing to maximum a third time, these rings may consist of material thrown out at each outburst, and just now getting sufficiently clear of the star to be visible from the earth.

The star has been found to be at a distance of 540 light years, a light year being the distance (some six trillion miles) that a beam of light will travel in a year. Hence the nova is being viewed by light that has been on its way for more than five centuries. The explosion, or collision, occurred about the year 1390, but earthly astronomers are just learning about it. This distance, not extraordinarily great for a star, shows that the rings are not due to light traveling outward from the star and illuminating successive rings of previously dark stuff around it, for in that case the rings would have appeared much more shortly after discovery. A ring that was observed around a nova seen in 1901 was ascribed to such a cause.

According to Dr. Shapley, the outer ring is now about six billion miles in diameter, and the stuff is traveling outward from the star at a speed of about 60 miles a second. All these peculiarities of nova Pictoris indicate, in his opinion, that the nova is most unusual, and that it might be the once-in-ten-billion-years encounter of two stars that we are witnessing.

IRRADIATED ERGOSTEROL

IRRADIATED ergosterol, the potent new rickets remedy, one ounce of which will do the work of six tons of cod-liver oil, is one of the most powerful specific substances which has thus far been isolated.

Dr. Alfred Hess, of Bellevue Hospital, New York City, told the American Pediatric Society meeting in Washington on May 1, that one twenty-five thousandth of a milligram of this parent substance of vitamin D, an amount almost inconceivably small, is sufficient to protect a rat from rickets when added to his daily ration.

The curative effects of irradiated ergosterol were discovered about a year ago by the combined efforts of Dr. Hess and Professor A. Windaus, of the University of Göttingen in Germany. English investigators working independently also achieved the same results at about the same time.

Dr. Hess has been using the new remedy in his clinical work and reported to-day that babies that receive from two to four milligrams a day are almost regularly cured of rickets.

"The question arises," declared Dr. Hess, "as to whether this substance may not to a large extent replace cod-liver oil in view of the fact that it can be given in any desired potency and that it has the advantage of being tasteless and odorless. Subsequent clinical tests carried out during the past year have served only to emphasize the practical usefulness of this new remedy. It is an absolute specific for rickets as well as for tetany, disorders which are so often associated, and it brings about healing of the bones more quickly than any sub-

stance which has heretofore been used. The appetite and general condition of the child also show a marked improvement.

"A word of warning should be uttered in this connection. Irradiated ergosterol is so powerful that there is a temptation to use it in exceedingly large doses. It is being frequently prescribed in doses which are 100, or even 500, times greater than cod-liver oil. Such amounts are quite unnecessary and may even be harmful. A remedy which is so potent for good may, when given in excess, bring about changes which are as yet unknown and unsuspected."

A VITAMIN VIRUS

THE formation of the antineuritic vitamin B somewhere in the digestive system of laboratory rats that have previously been deprived of this necessary factor is an unexpected development in vitamin research recently reported in London.

Dr. L. S. Fridericia and a group of workers at the university department of hygiene at Copenhagen found in the course of working with rats deprived of vitamin B that one rat did not die as usually happens with animals on this deficient diet. While making observations on this unique specimen it was discovered that other rats weakened by lack of vitamin B recovered if they fed on secretions from the immune rat that had gotten well spontaneously.

After large numbers of experiments, Dr. Fridericia came to the conclusion that the apparently spontaneous cure is infectious, just as diseases are infectious. He believes that the rats are cured by being infected with a virus which forms vitamin B in the rat's alimentary canal. In this way, the rat is really obtaining a supply of vitamin B, although it is completely absent from its diet. From the evidence that large numbers of undigested starch grains are found in the secretions of the cured animals it is thought that the action of the virus is also linked up in some way with the digestion of starches.

Independent work by Miss Margaret Roscoe, at the Lister Institute, London, and by Dr. R. Adam Dutcher, at State College, Pennsylvania, has confirmed some of the remarkable results of the Danish investigators. While the significance and application of these various experiments is not yet clear, they are so contradictory to all that has yet been learned about vitamins that it is felt that they will have an important bearing on future developments in vitamin research.

ITEMS

THE Food Investigation Board, a government bureau under the direction of the British Department of Scientific and Industrial Research, reports that the refuse from fish may amount to as much as 30 per cent. of the total quantity of material brought on board. At present it is thrown back into the sea and wasted, but it is hoped that future arrangements will be made for utilizing it on land as a feed for animals. One of the objections to the present method of dumping the refuse in the sea is that this drives the fish away from the area, rendering it useless from the fisherman's point of view. Work on fish meal and fish oils is at present in progress under the Food Investigation Board at the Imperial College of Science and Technology, London, and at Liverpool University.

AIRPLANE photographs taken by two officers of the Royal Air Force flying over Oxfordshire have disclosed a number of evidences of buried archeological remains whose existence has never been suspected, though the fields where they are situated have been in cultivation for many years. The bird's-eye view effect of a photograph taken from the air enabling the observer to perceive as a whole what can be seen from the grounds only as obscured details, is credited for the discovery. Two great circles, one within the other, lying under a field planted partly in barley and partly in beans, were among the finds. The bean-field portions of the circles were discovered first, for the rest was concealed by the growing grain. Near the circles was a rectangular enclosure which had no relation to existing field divisions. A semicircular enclosure, possibly prehistoric, and a track some forty feet wide of Roman-British origin, were also shown up on the plates.

IF the open season for taking fur-bearing animals were limited to the comparatively brief period when fur is at its best, more money would actually be realized and the killing of many valuable animals would be appreciably decreased. This concrete argument for the preservation of wild life was advanced at the meeting of the American Society of Mammalogists by Dr. Ernest P. Walker, of the U. S. Biological Survey. It would be possible to adjust the hunting and trapping seasons so that a greater profit could be derived from a small number of animals taken at the proper time than would be made by killing a larger number of animals when their pelts are not at their best. Thus it is possible for 950 mink taken in Southeastern Alaska in a two-months open season to be worth $8,693.75, whereas 1,000 taken in the same region over a three-months' season would be worth only $7,868.75, or $825 less.

THE danger of introducing hoof-and-mouth disease infection by means of bone marrow imported in the bones of chilled meat and bacon, was discussed by Sir George Courthope, at a recent meeting of the Council of Agriculture for England. It has been found that the virus of hoof-and-mouth disease remains active for exceedingly long periods even when the meat has been chilled, frozen or salted. Since chilled meat has been coming into England evidence is continually being piled up which shows that the bone marrow is frequently infected with the disease. Since the chilled meat trade of England amounts to some $250,000,000 annually, an embargo is not practicable. Sir George urged that the bones should be removed from all chilled meat in the country of origin, thereby confining this source of infection to areas already infected. One large packing firm in Argentina, he said, is already following this practice.

SCIENCE NEWS

Science Service, Washington, D. C.

ELECTRONS AND WAVE MATTER

SO-CALLED "solid" matter—the bricks of our homes, the sidewalks we walk on, in fact, even the tissues of our own bodies, may consist ultimately of waves, or vibrations. Such is one of the startling conclusions that might be drawn from experiments at the Bell Laboratories by Dr. C. J. Davisson, in collaboration with his colleague Dr. L. H. Germer. An extended account of the researches will be given by Dr. Davisson in an article to appear shortly in the *Journal* of the Franklin Institute.

The experiments indicate that electrons—one of the important parts of the atoms of matter—may really be waves, and not the infinitesimally tiny particles that previous scientists have supposed them. What Dr. Davisson and his associate have done is to study the way that a beam of electrons, given off from a glowing electric light filament, is reflected from a crystal of nickel. They found that the electrons were reflected in the same way that light waves would be reflected. That is, if the beam hit the face of the crystal at an angle of 45 degrees, for example, it left at the same angle. "The angle of reflection being equal to the angle of incidence."

At first glance, says Dr. Davisson in his forthcoming article, this might not seem inconsistent with the theory that the electrons are actual particles. But the electrons are supposed to be so small that some 25 million million would make a row an inch long. The size of the atoms is about a hundred thousand times as great, for only about 250 million of them are required to fill an inch. Furthermore, the distance between the adjacent atoms, in the nickel crystal, is something like 250,000 times the diameter of an electron.

"The difficulty of picturing the regular reflection of particles as small as electrons from a surface made up of bodies as large as atoms is at once evident," says Dr. Davisson. "If we were to fire a load of birdshot against a pyramid of cannon balls, we should not expect to find a little cloud of shot moving off in the direction of the regular reflection from the face of the pyramid. A surface made up of cannon balls is much too coarse-grained to serve as a regular reflector for particles as small as birdshot.

"The analogy is not such a good one, really, for we do not think of electrons rebounding from the surface of an atom in the way that shot rebound from a cannon ball. We have been accustomed to think of the atom as rather like the solar system—a massive nuclear sun surrounded by planetary electrons moving in closed orbits. On this view the electron which strikes into a metal surface is like a comet plunging into a region rather densely packed with solar systems."

Dr. Davisson points out that if the electrons were waves, their behavior would be perfectly understandable, for X-rays, which are supposed to be waves, are likewise reflected from a crystal in the same way. Another experiment brings out the similarity to X-rays in an even more striking way.

"We direct a stream of electrons against a target of ordinary nickel—a target made up of many small crystals instead of one large one—and we never under any circumstances find any indication of regular reflection. Electrons are not regularly reflected from a target of ordinary polycrystalline nickel.

"It seems curious that electrons should be reflected only from a crystal-face—and then we remember that this is true also of X-rays. X-rays may be regularly reflected from the face of a crystal, but not from a polycrystalline mirror. The difference between light and X-rays in this respect is due, as we know, to a difference in order of wave-lengths. The lengths of light waves are great compared to the distance between atoms in solids while the X-ray wave-lengths are comparable with these distances."

Since scientists also have good reason for supposing that the electrons are particles, there is a conflict of ideas that he can not explain. The so-called Schroedinger wave mechanics, named after its German inventor, has suggested that electrons are either made up of, or accompanied by, a system of waves and this, he thinks, may help explain the difficulty.

"Are electrons waves?" he asks. "The easiest way of answering this question is to ask another. Are X-rays waves? If X-rays are waves, then so also are electrons. But we are no longer so certain as we used to be that X-rays are waves. The Compton effect and the photoelectric effect are most simply described by supposing that there is some sense in which X-rays are particles. It is all rather paradoxical and confusing. We must believe not only that there is a certain sense in which rabbits are cats, but there is also a certain sense in which cats are rabbits."

PHOTOGRAPHS OF STELLAR SPECTRA

GIGANTIC stars that could engulf the whole solar system are transported from their far distances of hundreds of trillions of miles and set beside our own sun as a result of the latest researches of astronomy.

Spectral messages are received by a combination of the world's largest stellar spectrograph and the world's largest telescope, the 100-inch on Mt. Wilson, Calif. They are interpreted by Professor Henry Norris Russell, of Princeton University, who worked with Dr. Walter S. Adams, director of the Mt. Wilson Observatory.

The powerful spectrograph, just put in commission, gave stellar spectra photographs almost as detailed as the standard spectra of the sun, the earth's nearest star. Hundreds of lines in these fingerprints of the stars were revealed for the first time. These spectrum lines allow the astronomer to analyze the stuff of stars, take their temperature and probe their atmosphere.

"For the giant red stars, such as Antares and Betelgeuse, the total quantity of material above a square mile of the visible surface is apparently about a hundred times as great as in the sun," Professor Russell said.

"Procyon, a dwarf star only a little brighter and probably no larger than the sun, has an atmosphere comparable with the sun's in extent."

The lines of the new photographs tell the proportion of excited atoms loaded with energy and thus determine the temperatures, which range from 3,000 to 10,000 degrees Centigrade for the stars studied.

THE GREEN SUNSET RAY

INTENDING voyagers to Europe during the next few months should carefully watch the setting sun, and they may be able to see the "green ray." This is the brilliant green coloration that the sun assumes just before its last narrow sliver disappears behind the horizon. A really satisfactory sight of it is rather rare, said Professor R. W. Wood, professor of experimental physics at the Johns Hopkins University. On thirty crossings of the Atlantic he has looked for it every time there was a clear sky and no haze or clouds near the horizon at sunset, but has only seen it three or four times. Only once, he said, was it really striking. At that time it appeared a brilliant emerald green, about the color of a railroad signal.

The cause of the green ray is generally supposed to be that the rays of light are bent as if by a prism when they pass through the atmosphere of the earth. This enables us to see the sun for a short time after it is below the line of the horizon. As the red and orange rays are bent least, they disappear first behind the horizon. This leaves the green, blue and violet rays still visible. Blue and violet affect the eye much less strongly than green, and so the green color predominates.

Dr. Wood accepts this theory of the origin of the ray, but proposes a new theory to explain why it is not always seen at sunset. At the time that he saw the ray so well, the air and ocean were at approximately the same temperature. Through the rest of the voyage, when it was not seen, the ocean was much warmer than the air. He thinks that when the water is warm and the air cool, the layer of warm air right in contact with the sea would cause the light rays of all colors to be bent less, and so the sun would set abnormally early. When the air is warmer than the water, the curvature of all the rays would be increased, and so the atmospheric dispersion that causes the ray would have a longer time to act.

THE MEASUREMENT OF ULTRA-VIOLET RAYS

RADIO amplification now is to be of service in the field of medicine. Professor Ernst A. Pohle, roentgenologist of the University of Michigan, in collaboration with Walter S. Huxford, of the physics department, has designed a measuring device for ultra-violet rays, independent of other radiation which comes from quartz lamp or other light source.

In recent years ultra-violet light has come to be recognized as a cure for rickets and possibly for other diseases, but there has been no accurate means of measuring the quantity with which the patient is treated.

Up to the present time the photo-electric cell, one means of measurement, has required precision apparatus too complicated for the average physician to handle. Professor Pohle and his associate have designed one that is simple and dependable. In it a radio amplifier is used to magnify an extremely small electric current so that it can be read on an ordinary switchboard galvanometer. The current comes from a photo-electric cell, which turns light into electricity.

Only ultra-violet rays between certain definite wavelengths are believed to have any beneficial effect upon the patient, so it was necessary to develop apparatus which would measure only light of that wave-length, disregarding both longer and shorter waves. For this purpose the metal cadmium has been utilized by Dr. Pohle and Mr. Huxford because it is most sensitive to the waves long enough to affect the skin. The glass which they use in their cell cuts off longer light waves.

Dr. Pohle and Professor Ralph A. Sawyer have also succeeded in calibrating the photo-electric cell in absolute units. This makes any recorded dose reproducible.

A RADISH-CABBAGE HYBRID

A CROSS between a radish and a cabbage, considered to be about the most difficult feat in plant breeding so far on record, has been made by Dr. George D. Karpechenko at the botanical institute at Detskoje Selo, in Russia. The Russian botanist's work is reported by Professor William Seifriz, of the University of Pennsylvania, who recently visited a number of scientific laboratories and experiment stations in the Soviet union.

Although the new plant has no economic significance at present, its development is of much interest to plant breeders because of the remoteness of the relationship between the two parents. The great bulk of our hybrids, both plant and animal, are between varieties of the same species, or even between strains or races of the same variety. Hybrids between two species within the same genus are usually hailed as out of the ordinary; the crossing of the lime and the kumquat to produce the limquat was such a hybrid. There are, however, certain crosses between species that are very common, such as the mule.

But the hybridization of radish and cabbage means that two quite distinct genera have been combined to produce something entirely new under the sun. The more remotely related the parents, the more difficult the cross is to make; and in this instance the parents are believed to be more distantly related than any plants from which successful hybrid offspring has yet been secured.

A MAGNETIC SENSE

AT the sessions of the Congress of American Physicians and Surgeons, in Washington, Dr. Frederick Tilney, professor of neurology at Columbia University, mentioned experiments now in progress on a hitherto undiscovered animal sense, the power that allows the homing pigeon to find its loft, the migrating bird its far distant summer home, the animal its burrow. This sense may prove to be magnetic. The retina of the eye was suggested by Dr. Tilney as the organ of the body in which the sense resides.

Mere men have long marveled at the abilities of animals to find their way home through strange surroundings. Aviators need compasses and intricate instruments to navigate as efficiently as the birds of the air. Such phenomena as these gave impetus to Dr. Tilney's researches.

One clue in the search that is now under way is the fact that animals are greatly disturbed by any change of direction of their surroundings. Mice that are taught to run intricate mazes, a feat that is not dependent upon ordinary senses of sight and smell for instance, are completely baffled when the mazes are moved and oriented geographically in a different direction. They have to learn the mazes all over again.

Dr. Tilney was careful to point out that as yet his researches are in a preliminary stage. Both his own laboratories and those of the department of psychology at Columbia University are at work. If this magnetic sense is confirmed by his experiments, it will be the ninth sense. Five senses, sight, hearing, touch, taste and smell, which are the result of contact of the nervous system to environment, are familiar to every one. Then there are what Dr. Tilney called the skeletal sense and the visceral sense, both of which reside in the body itself. As the eighth, Dr. Tilney lists what he calls the hurt or pain sense, which is protective instead of guiding like the others.

THE ETHNOLOGY OF ST. LAWRENCE ISLAND

THE belief that ancient men bridging the gap between Asia and America may have left clues to their identity and their manners near Bering Strait is taking Henry B. Collins, Jr., ethnologist of the U. S. National Museum, to St. Lawrence Island, which lies just south of Bering Strait. Mr. Collins left for Seattle on May 4. He will be the first scientist to excavate in the island, though Eskimos living there have dug up a number of very old ivory harpoons and ornaments used by their forerunners. Mr. Collins will spend most of the summer locating ancient Eskimo villages and digging where excavation seems most likely to reveal traces of early inhabitants.

St. Lawrence Island would be rather south of the direct line of travel across Bering Strait. But some of the prehistoric men who found their way across the short cut between Asia and America, thousands of years ago, may have wandered to the island or stopped off there. At any rate, it is known that men have inhabited the island for many centuries.

St. Lawrence Island is about 100 miles long, but it is now inhabited by only a small group of Eskimos. Prior to 1880, the population was much larger, but in that disastrous year the Eskimos drank a good deal of bad whiskey and neglected to hunt and store up a food supply. When winter came, hundreds died from famine, and the island never regained its former importance.

Mr. Collins plans to spend some time in conducting excavations along the mainland of Alaska just south of the Arctic Circle and in making studies of the physical type of the natives.

ITEMS

M. SCHELENZ, of the Carlsruhe Museum, writing in *Naturforscher*, states that museum specimens of fish can be prepared in such a way as to be as bright and interesting and attractive as the mounted animals or birds. One side of a freshly killed fish is cleaned of its coat of mucus. The specimen is embedded in modelling clay, leaving the cleaned side projecting, melted paraffin is poured over it, forming a solid block and impregnating the fish with the wax. The paraffined fish is next removed, leaving an exact mould of itself in the clay. Into this mould fine plaster-of-paris is poured and allowed to harden. The clay is then dissolved and the plaster cast of the fish remains, with every detail of skin and scale and fin. White plaster models, "aged" for some weeks, are then coated successively with shellac and with silver or gold leaf. Finally, life colors and markings of the fish are painted by hand, and the model is given a protecting coat of varnish.

AS a result of his investigations of the common magpie, E. R. Kalmbach, biologist of the division of food habits research, states that the magpie eats more insects than any other member of the crow family and must also be credited with the destruction of a number of small rodents. These virtues, however, are counterbalanced by destruction of poultry and beneficial wild birds and their eggs. The magpie likewise preys on sick and injured cattle and has proved a nuisance and a hindrance in anti-coyote campaigns by stealing bait and tripping the traps. Poisoning is the cheapest and most effective method of destroying the magpie.

THE country around the town of Geestemuende, in Hanover, has recently suffered from an outbreak of vipers. These snakes are troublesomely poisonous, though their bites are not often fatal. The farmers' best snake-alarms were their hens, which invariably set up a clatter when a viper appeared. A number of cases were reported of battles between a snake on one side and a flock of hens on the other, in which the reptiles were invariably pecked to death.

To be eligible for the presidency of the French republic a man must be the father of at least seven children, is one of the provisions of a bill proposed by M. Jean Rameau, with the idea of increasing the dwindling population of France. A Frenchman who aspires to be a cabinet minister would have to have at least six children, according to the proposed law. If he had only five in his family, he could rise no higher than the senate. With four he might aspire to the Chamber of Deputies. To be mayor of a French town a man would have to have two children, and even a town councilor would be required to have one child, as one of his qualifications for office. The author of the plan, relying upon the aspirations of his countrymen for political careers, estimates that such a law would increase the French population by 10,000,000 in ten years.

would attain great speeds because of the lack of air resistance.

The Opel rocket auto looks like a multiple-barreled piece of light artillery in speedy retreat. From the rear of the car project twelve large tubes arranged in a rectangle. From these tubes the exploding gases emerge with terrific kick which sends the car racing along the track. Any highly explosive mixtures can be used such as light gasoline, alcohol, or even pure hydrogen and oxygen mixtures which give the greatest expansion for the least weight.

LIVER DIET FOR ANEMIA

THE liver treatment for pernicious anemia recently developed in America has given great success in the hands of British physicians.

Drs. Stanley Davidson, J. G. McCrie and G. Lovell Gulland, of Edinburgh, have announced through *The Lancet* that in their experience the feeding of liver and liver extract has helped anemia patients more promptly and regularly than any former method.

"The most important point," they declare in their report, "is that recovery is more complete. Formerly one had too often to be content with a count of about 3,500,000 red blood corpuscles (per cubic millimeter); now an extra million or more may be confidently expected; the whole blood picture returns to normal with much greater frequency and certainty, and apparently remains so indefinitely, so long as the treatment is persevered with."

The benefits of a liver diet for pernicious anemia were put before the medical world about two years ago by Drs. G. R. Minot and W. P. Murphy, of Boston, Mass. The method has sprung into wide-spread use with the result that calves' liver now retails in the United States for ninety cents a pound.

Half a pound of liver daily, however, is for many patients a gustatory impossibility. Many acquire a distaste for it that can not be overcome even to recover from a hitherto incurable disease. To surmount this difficulty, Dr. E. J. Cohn and a group of collaborators at Harvard University have endeavored to isolate the active principle in liver in a liver extract. Five to fifteen grams of this concentrated form is equal to 200 grams, or approximately 6 ounces, of whole liver and produces corresponding effects. Liver extracts from the United States, Germany and Great Britain are now on the market and give about equally good results. Since the extracts are soluble in water a single dose, equivalent to nearly 30 ounces of whole liver, can be given to a patient too weak to take solid food.

SERUM FOR ALL TYPES OF PNEUMONIA

A NEW serum for treating pneumonia, developed by Dr. L. D. Felton, of Harvard University, has given very promising results in combatting this highly fatal disease. The serum marks an advance in that it can be used for all four of the recognized types of pneumonia, according to Dr. Russel L. Cecil, of the Bellevue Hospital, New York City, who has obtained very efficacious results from its use in the pneumonia clinic of that hospital. It works best with types one and two, the two groups that comprise the majority of pneumonia cases. The recoveries after its use with type one have been very encouraging, indeed, Dr. Cecil declared, though the deadly type three, which always has had a very high death rate, has proved the least amenable of any group.

Pneumonia serums used in the past have been specific for each type. Since certain laboratory procedures have to be followed out before the type from which the patient is suffering can be determined, precious time often has to be lost before the doctors know which serum to give. The Felton serum of mixed cultures can be administered on admission to the hospital and frequently a gain of many hours can be made in checking the course of the disease.

CATNIP OIL AS A BAIT

BOBCATS, mountain lions and lynxes, which assist in destroying from $20,000,000 to $30,000,000 worth of game and livestock each year, are being baited on a large scale with catnip oil, according to the United States Biological Survey.

Prior to the discovery that catnip makes an effective bait the taking of mountain lions particularly presented a serious problem to hunters and trappers. They frequent rough, inaccessible country and had to be trailed with dogs and shot after being driven into caves or up trees. Last year literally hundreds were lured to traps and poisoned bait with catnip oil.

Dr. A. K. Fisher, in charge of economic investigations, is credited with the discovery. Walking through the National Zoo, with a sprig of catnip in his pocket, he noticed that a mountain lion woke up when he passed by and that a tiger next door, reputed to be dangerous, seemed to be courting his friendship. It minced up to the bars and tried to follow him.

Dr. Fisher tossed the catnip over the fence. The tiger purred and sniffed and rolled over on it, licked the fur where it had touched, located the sprig on the floor, pounced upon it and finally ate it up. He reported this singular conduct to the survey and an investigation was begun to determine whether the plant could be used effectively as bait. The fact that oil of catnip was not produced anywhere on a commercial scale at first delayed the experiments. The Bureau of Chemistry reported that only minute quantities had ever been extracted, but a small amount was finally procured from which it was determined that the oil carried the characteristic odor and that this odor would persist for several months in the open air.

A catnip garden was then planted on the Experiment Farm at Arlington, from which enough oil was secured for field experiments. These proved so successful that additional crops were planted by the government at Saratoga Springs, New York.

Some hunters have reported taking every "cat" that came within the vicinity of traps baited with the catnip and the result is that the oil is now being distributed and used on a large scale.

NEW SCIENTIFIC BOOKS

McGraw-Hill Book Company, New York

Comparative Morphology of Fungi. Ernest A. Gaumann. Translated and revised by Carroll W. Dodge. pp. xiv + 701. Illustrated. $7.50.

The introductory chapters contain a discussion of the most important points of view and the basic forms, assuming previous knowledge of a text-book. The last part of the book describes modifications of the basic forms.

Macmillan Company, New York

Human Values and Verities. Henry Osborn Taylor. pp. xiv +282. $2.75.

Some chapters are: The functioning of faculty; Human values; Human validity; Values and validity in history; Cleavage between science and philosophy; Philosophy's validity and value; The imaginative arts; Art's value and verity; The active life.

Geological Survey of China, Peking

Palaeontologia Sinica

Fusulinidae of North China. Series B, Volume 4, Fascicle 1. Jonquei S. Lee. pp. vii + 172. 24 plates, 21 figures.

Discusses the distribution of fusulinidae in North China, gives the terminology of the common structural elements in boultonia, fusulinella and fusulina and describes the various species contained within these groups.

Revised Determinations of some Tertiary Mammals from Mongolia. Series C, Volume 5, Fascicle 2. Gerrit S. Miller, Jr. pp. vi + 20.

Some of the mammals described are: scaptochirus primaevus; crocidura kormosi; hyaena; martes anderssoni; aplodontia asiatica; allactaga wimani.

The Biological Laboratory

Cold Spring Harbor, Long Island, N. Y.

Now open the entire year for
Research
in any branch of Biology

***Fundulus* and other marine material abundant for embryological and physiological investigation.**
Special Equipment for mammalian work.
Fee for private laboratory $75, table $50.

Instruction

Six weeks, June 27th to August 8th. Courses in Field Zoology, Physiology, Surgical Methods in Experimental Biology, Endocrinology, Field Botany and Plant Ecology. Tuition, $75.

A marine littoral location, in rolling, forested country, with close proximity to brackish and fresh water collecting grounds, yet only an hour from the center of New York City, with access to its splendid museums, institutions and libraries.

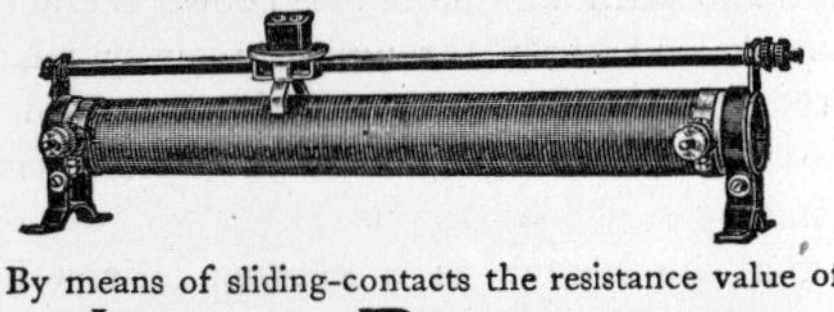

By means of sliding-contacts the resistance value of

JAGABI RHEOSTATS

can be varied from zero to full rating in exceedingly small steps.

They are eminently suited for, and are largely used in Educational, Research and Industrial Laboratories.

Write for illustrated Bulletin 1140-S

JAMES G. BIDDLE, PHILADELPHIA
1211-13 ARCH STREET

THE MICROSCOPE

By SIMON H. GAGE, of Cornell University

Revised, Dark-field Edition (1927) now Available.

The Old and the New in Microscopy, with a special chapter on Dark-Field Methods and their Application.

Postpaid, $3.50

COMSTOCK PUBLISHING CO., ITHACA, N. Y.

THEORY OF CONTINENTAL DRIFT

An international symposium on the origin, structure and movements of the earth's crust. Foreword by E. DeGolyer. Authors—van der Gracht, Willis, Chamberlin, Joly, Molengraaff, Gregory, Wegener, Schuchert, Longwell, Taylor, Bowie, White, Singewald and Berry. 240 pp., 29 figs. 6 x 9 inches. Cloth. Price, $3.50, postpaid.

American Association of Petroleum Geologists
Box 1852, Tulsa, Oklahoma, U. S. A.

PROFESSOR

Your manuscript or notes can be published by the photographic-zinc-plate process. We print on both sides of a page, reduce to desired size and bind in book form. Write for our booklet and prices.

SHELWOOD-HILL, Inc.,
50 Church St., N. Y. C.

SCIENTIFIC PERIODICALS

Chemical, Medical and allied subjects. Complete files, volumes and copies, bought and sold. Kindly send us a list of your wants and items of which you may wish to dispose.

B. LOGIN & SON

29 East 21st Street New York, N. Y.

FOR SALE

Complete set of **SCIENCE**, 1906 to 1927, unbound; a few numbers missing; also complete volumes for 1888 and 1889. Complete sets from beginning to date: Chemical Abstracts (without decennial index); Jour. Ind. and Eng. Chem.; all unbound. Journal of Amer. Chem. Soc. from 1893 to 1927, 1893 to 1906, bound in half leather; 1907 to 1927, unbound.

Complete set "Orig. Communications International Cong. of Applied Chem.," 29 vols., unbound; Amer. Chem. Research, 1899 to 1906, bound in 3 vols. Address,

C. H. EHRENFELD
57 S. Beaver St., York, Pa.

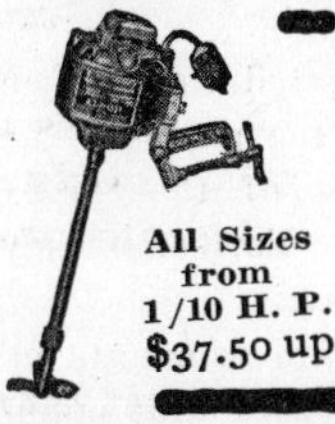

All Sizes from 1/10 H. P. $37.50 up

Hy-Speed Mixers

Clamp to any tank, operate from light circuit, mix all kinds of liquids. Also used for even temperature baths. Thousands in use.

Write for circular.

ALSOP ENGINEERING CO.
47 W. 63rd St., New York

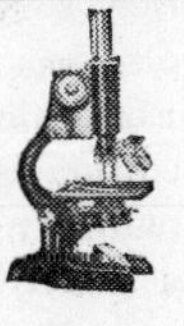

LIKE NEW AGAIN
Microscopes

Rebuilt Reconditioned Repaired

Moderate Fees

Physicians' Supply & Drug Co.
427 S. Honore St. Chicago

Last year 246 lions, 3,677 bobcats and 41 Canada lynxes were taken by hunters employed by the Biological Survey and, while some of these were probably caught by the old method, hundreds were victims of their taste for catnip.

CHILDREN'S READING HABITS

THE extent to which a child buries his nose in his book when he reads or studies is determined to a considerable extent by his imitation of other readers that he sees. This is the belief advanced by E. B. Notson, of the University of Arkansas, in a report to *School and Society*.

From measurements made during two years, Mr. Notson concludes that the average first grader holds his primer about eight inches from his eyes. This distance increases rather steadily a little less than an inch a year until at high-school age he is holding his Latin book and his algebra thirteen inches away. After that, there is only a small and slow increase to manhood.

The change in distance can not be attributed to the chief ocular features involved, which are accommodation and convergence. "The most influential factor seems to be imitation. Children imitate the reading posture of older children and adults and consequently, as they grow, their books naturally grow farther from their eyes until adolescence, when both physical growth and reading distance slow up and eventually become stationary. Such an explanation may at first seem absurd, but when all the data are in this conclusion will be inevitable."

Measurements made by Mr. Notson are cited as showing that the usual recommendation for children to hold their books 14 inches away is actually very little followed. Whether the normal tendency of children to hold their books closer to the eyes is best for the children's sight is yet to be determined.

EXPEDITION TO RUSSIAN TURKESTAN

FRAGMENTS of a lost race of white men, marooned on lofty mountain ranges in interior Asia among a sea of Mongol folk, are among the objectives of an expedition participated in by German, Austrian and Russian scientists. The group goes into territory hitherto never explored by Europeans, under the leadership of W. Rickmers, of Bremen, who conducted a German expedition into Turkestan some years ago.

The mountain regions to be investigated are known as the Transalai and the Seltau. They are parts of the Himalaya uplift, lying to the northwest of the "roof of the world," in Russian Turkestan. Formerly they were lumped together under the name Pamir.

It is believed that their inhabitants are remnants of Indo-Germanic races, descendants of the stock that populated India and Europe. The theory is that they sought refuge in these mountains when the Mongols overran Asia during the Middle Ages, and have remained there ever since. One of the members of the expedition is a specialist in the structure of languages; he will try to gain some clue to the ancestry of the mountain folk from their speech.

Other members of the party will represent the sciences of geology, geography, meteorology and natural history. Four expert mountain climbers will accompany the party for the purpose of scaling the more difficult peaks and making a study of the high glaciers.

ITEMS

SOME of the dreaded after-effects of scarlet fever may be lessened by new tests developed by Dr. A. A. Osman, of Guy's Hospital, London. The cases of scarlet fever that are likely to develop kidney complications, one of the most serious of the consequences that scarlet fever leaves in its wake, can be detected by these tests in the early stages of the disease and preventive treatment administered in the shape of doses of simple alkaline compounds. The number of cases of kidney complications has been reduced by Dr. Osman by means of these methods from 5.5 per cent. in an untreated control group of 316 to .6 per cent. in a treated group of 620.

CHILDREN may have to welcome an undesired addition to the whooping cough and measles afflictions they have to undergo in the process of becoming grown up. Several cases of a new eruptive disease which does not fit into the category of either measles or German measles, though it resembles both, have broken out in Paris, according to reports received from the French correspondent of the American Medical Association. "The fifth disease," as French physicians have christened the new malady of children, does not provoke symptoms of a serious character though certain changes in the number of cells in the blood have been noted. Many of the children who have "taken" the disease have histories of both types of measles and of scarlet fever.

BIG predatory locusts, that prey on their own fellow-insects instead of on growing grain crops, are being tried out in Greece as one means of combatting the pest of ordinary locusts now threatening the fields, according to word received from Athens. These modern descendants of one of the plagues of Egypt have been causing serious losses to Greek agriculture during the past few years, and the Ministry of Agriculture is preparing to spend 16,000,000 drachmas (approximately $3,200,000) in a campaign against them.

A MACKEREL with an unbroken rubber band running over its back and right through the lower part of its body is the zoological puzzle recently examined and reported by Dr. E. W. Gudger, of the American Museum of Natural History. The fish was purchased on a market stall, so that its history is unknown. Dissection indicates that the band must have been snapped around the fish's body, and that its pressure and friction forced it upward through the tissues of the abdomen. These later healed shut beneath it, leaving it apparently "wove through" the living fish. Other mackerel have been reported with rubber bands placed around their tails by unknown persons, but this is the first case recorded where the band went through the body.

SCIENCE NEWS

Science Service, Washington, D. C.

RADIO MOVIES

Rods of quartz, through which light is transmitted like water through a hose, make possible the latest method of television—the radio movies demonstrated by C. Francis Jenkins, Washington inventor. As a result he is able to substitute a seven-inch drum for the two- or three-foot disc that previous methods of television have employed.

If light is allowed to shine into one end of a rod of fused quartz, it is reflected back and forth as it goes through it. Practically none is lost by leaking out the side, but all emerges through the end.

In the Jenkins home radio movie receiver, which may soon become a common attachment to radio sets, the current from the set, instead of operating the magnets of a loud speaker, causes a glow of a small metal plate sealed in a bulb containing the rare gas, neon. Such a neon lamp glows immediately, as soon as the current is turned on, and is extinguished as soon as the current is turned off. The ordinary filament of the incandescent lamp continues to glow for an instant after the current stops, and so can not respond to the rapid changes required by the television receiver.

In previous methods of seeing by radio, either of movies, or actual objects, the person viewing the received image gazed directly at the surface of a neon lamp. A revolving disc with a spiral row of holes obscured all but the proper spot of the neon glower. These spots of light, seen in rapid succession, were built up into the complete picture seen by the observer, just as the successive pictures of a movie film shown in a theater merge together into a continuous view on the screen.

Mr. Jenkins employs a cylindrical glass tube, in which there is a row of small neon glowers. This is at the center of a revolving drum, seven inches in diameter. Around the surface of the drum is a helical row of small holes. Extending from these holes, inside the drum, to an inner cylinder, almost in contact with the neon lamp, there are a number of the quartz rods, about two inches long, somewhat resembling the wire spokes of a bicycle wheel.

An ordinary electric motor, which is arranged to run in synchronism with the motor at the transmitter, spins the drum around at a speed of 3,600 revolutions a minute. A revolving contact, or commutator, attached to it serves to connect the separate glowers in the neon tube, and so enables the current from the radio receiver to light them at the proper time. The light from the glowing neon tube is carried by the quartz rods out to the round surface of the revolving drum, where the picture is actually seen. Thus a small neon lamp is made to serve the purpose of a much larger one, one as large as the drum itself. The drum turns on a horizontal axis, so a slant mirror and a large magnifying lens enable the persons viewing it to see the picture vertically, as on a movie screen.

In his demonstration Mr. Jenkins used a motion picture film as the original object, and this was reproduced both by wire, in another part of his laboratory, and by radio, in his home some miles distant. However, he claims, the apparatus is just as applicable to the broadcasting of views of actual persons or objects. The received picture is a silhouette, and does not show gradations of light and shade. This, he thinks, is not a serious objection, but it is one which he expects to overcome. "At present," he says, "the apparatus is in the 'crystal set stage.'" Future developments, he promises, will bring it to the perfection of present-day radio or movies.

A NEW METHOD OF TRANSPORTATION

A new method of transportation with the motive power furnished by spurts of expanding gases, like the trail of a Fourth-of-July rocket, is about to make a bid for practical success.

After secret experimental development, a rocket automobile has been given speed tests at the racing track of the Fritz Opel motor car factory at Russelsheim near Frankfort, where it was built. Speeds of slightly over 60 miles an hour were attained eight seconds after the start.

A demonstration before experts at the Avus racing track in Berlin is scheduled for the near future. As the speeds on this track are limited to a hundred miles an hour, plans are under way to utilize later a stretch of railroad track which has been offered for this purpose by the German States Railways.

The theoretical investigations which inspired this rocket-propelled automobile were begun by Professor R. H. Goddard, American scientist, who designed a rocket that would travel to the moon. Later mathematical studies were made on the same problem by Professor Max Vallier, of Munich, and Albert Mueller, whose results were available to the Opel Company's designing engineer, Sander.

Tests of the rocket automobile are believed to be merely preliminary to the construction and launching of a rocket airplane capable of arising to heights that ordinary propeller-driven airplanes can not possibly attain. Journeys to other planets across the great distances of airless space are theoretically possible through the use of the rocket exhaust kick as the motive power. For experiments show that the kick of the exploding rocket charge is just as effective in a vacuum where there is no air as it is under ordinary conditions where there is plenty of atmosphere. Propellers of ordinary airplanes need the air to work against. The rocket is effective in vacuum for the same reason that a rifle fired in an airless chamber would have the same sort of kick that it would in air.

The rocket airplane, once it reached the airless outer space or the upper rarefied portion of the atmosphere,

SCIENCE NEWS

Science Service, Washington, D. C.

RED ARC LIGHT FOR FOG

A BRILLIANT red arc light that makes use of the rare atmospheric gas neon, and which can shine through thick fog, has been developed at the research laboratory of the General Electric Company. The new lamp is the result of the work of Dr. Clifton G. Found, in collaboration with J. D. Forney, of the Cooper-Hewitt Electric Company, and was recently demonstrated by them to engineers.

Airplane landing fields will probably be among the first to make use of the lamp, for by outlining the fields with them aviators flying above through fog will be enabled to make a safe landing. Such an occurrence as that of Commander Byrd on his flight to Paris, when he actually flew over Le Bourget, but could not see to land, would probably be prevented.

Docks in harbors may also be marked with the lamp. According to Dr. Found, the light has been tested for this use when one was recently placed on a pier in the Hudson River. "Observations from boats during fog," he says, "have shown that it was possible to pick up the red neon light before any of the other lights in the same vicinity were observed."

Earlier forms of neon tubes, which give the characteristic red neon light that is now so common in advertising signs, suffer from what is called the "cathode drop." This is the great difference in voltage between the electrode through which the electric current enters the tube, and the near-by gas. On account of it, also, tubes must be operated with a high voltage, and must be made quite long in order to be efficient. Another disagreeable effect is that the gas is made to gradually disappear.

The new tube of Dr. Found and Forney heats the cathode, or the electrode through which the current enters the tube, by means of an additional electric circuit. This causes it to give off the electrons which cause the neon gas to glow, but without the high voltages that are needed in the older tubes. By such means an extremely efficient source of brilliant red light can be obtained. Light of this color is best for penetrating fog.

Another possible use of the lamp is in photography, especially in colors. The mercury vapor-lamp, which gives a characteristically violet-colored light, has often been used for ordinary photography, but the unnatural pallor which it causes is a disadvantage, especially where colors are concerned. By combining the neon light with the mercury vapor-lamp, the former supplies the red rays which are lacking in the latter, and the result is a good approximation to white light.

SYNTHETIC SUGAR

THE synthesis of sugar by two Swiss chemists, Professor Ame Pictet and Hans Vogel, has aroused great interest among the chemists in this country. For this is a problem on which investigators have worked in vain for over fifty years because of its scientific interest and possible commercial importance. Sugar of the common sort, extracted from cane or beet, is easily split up, or, as it is called, "inverted," by weak acids, forming two other sugars. One of these is glucose, which is now manufactured in the United States from corn. The other half is fructose, which can be manufactured from Jerusalem artichoke, as has recently been demonstrated by the U. S. Bureau of Standards.

But to bring these two sugars together so as to form sugar of the common or table variety has hitherto been impossible. Professor Pictet has discovered that the difficulty has come from the fact that fructose exists in two forms identical in composition, but differing in the arrangement of their atoms. By transforming the normal fructose over into what is called the "gamma" form he was able to combine this with an equal amount of glucose and get sucrose or common sugar. This he accomplished by first joining to each molecule of glucose and fructose four molecules of acetic acid, the acid of vinegar. After the two sugars have been combined the acid is easily eliminated by alkali.

Since this is a difficult and expensive process it could not be employed on a commercial scale, but it is important as proving that it is possible to make sugar artificially and it suggests the possibility of inventing new kinds of sugar which are not to be found in nature. Some of them might prove to be sweeter than common sugar or safer for the use of diabetics.

Professor Pictet, of the University of Geneva, is now seventy-one years old and has long been one of the world's leading authorities on the constitution of sugar and cellulose. Within the last two years he has succeeded in synthesizing two other of the double sugars, lactose, which occurs in milk, and maltose, which occurs in malt.

PHOTOGRAPHS ON STEEL

SHOOTING a photograph into the hardest of chrome steel with the aid of high explosive nitrogelatin, and so making a photographic record as permanent as the steel itself, is the feat that has been accomplished as a result of the "Munroe effect." This effect was the discovery of Dr. Charles E. Munroe, of the U. S. Bureau of Mines. An incidental result of the work is the proof that the blacks in a photographic print are due to varying thicknesses of finely divided silver, the thicker the deposit, the darker being the shadow in the photograph.

The steel photograph was made recently by G. St. J. Perrott, superintendent of the Bureau of Mines Experiment Station at Pittsburgh, and sent by him to Dr. Munroe. To make it, a photograph of Dr. Munroe was laid on a piece of steel about two inches in diameter and an inch thick. On top of this was placed a disc-shaped piece of the nitrogelatin explosive, which was then fired. Though the paper photograph was completely destroyed, when the steel cooled sufficiently to be handled, the profile of Dr. Munroe was found impressed on the surface. Where the photograph had been black, that is, in the

shadows, the surface of the steel was raised, and where there had been high lights, the steel was incised.

Another example of the effect that is in Dr. Munroe's possession now was made by W. O. Snelling, director of research of the Trojan Powder Company. In this case the words "Munroe effect" were impressed into the surface of a block of the explosive, so that the letters were in intaglio. When this was exploded on a disc of the steel the letters appeared on it. However, they were also in intaglio on the steel. This is the opposite from what would be obtained with a die, for then the intaglio letters on the die would come out in relief on the finished product.

Dr. Munroe explains the effect by saying that when the detonation of the explosive occurs, the entire amount of the solid is converted to gas. This volume of gas, however, momentarily has the same size and shape as the original block of the explosive, and is therefore extremely compressed. Where there was a cavity in the original explosive is the line of least resistance for the escape of the rapidly moving gas molecules. In seeking to escape, they collide with each other, producing a vast number of tiny molecular drills, which bore into the hardest steel.

Using the same principle, Dr. Munroe once blew a hole in a safe with a hollow cylinder of dynamite. He took a bundle of sticks of dynamite, then, by pushing a tin can through the center, he pushed out the center sticks, and bound together the other ones so as to form a ring. This he exploded in a vertical position upon a safe. The result was a hole in the top of the safe corresponding to the hollow center in the ring of dynamite sticks. This hollow cylinder had acted as a gun to fire the gas molecules through the steel.

Any thin objects, such as a leaf, or photograph, can be reproduced on steel in this way, and so a permanent record can be obtained. The explosion has the effect of greatly magnifying slight differences in thickness, such as between the layers of silver in the shadows and highlights of the photograph.

ZINC AND BORON FOR PLANTS

THE common metal zinc, together with boron, the chemical basis of borax, are needed by plants if they are to live and grow in full health, according to Miss A. L. Sommer and Professor C. B. Lipman, of the University of California, as described in an article in *The Scientific Monthly*. The amounts needed are exceedingly minute; one part of each in two million parts of the solution surrounding the roots will suffice, but without these microscopic quantities plants drag out a dwindling, sickly existence or even perish altogether. These minerals, together with several others needed in equally minute amounts, are likened by the experimenters to the almost undetectably small amounts of the vitamins needed by man and the lower animals.

To test the response of plants to such low concentrations of the two elements, most elaborate precautions had to be taken, the two researchers report. Even the dust of the air might carry enough zinc or boron to feed a plant otherwise kept completely deprived of it by specially refined chemicals dissolved in double-distilled water; so a smaller greenhouse was built inside a large one, and all the air used in ventilating it carefully filtered. Since ordinary glass contains a little zinc, the jars used in part of the experiments were made of pyrex glass.

A number of different kinds of plants were grown in the culture jars. One set was given a properly balanced ration of mineral nutrients, but no zinc. Another set was similarly deprived of boron. Other plants were supplied with a full ration plus both boron and zinc, in the very low concentration of one part of each to two million parts of water. The plants supplied with both boron and zinc made a healthy and flourishing growth, while those that lacked either of the two elements showed only a fraction of normal growth or even failed to advance beyond the seedling stage.

THE RECENT PACIFIC EARTHQUAKE

BY means of records obtained on seismograph instruments at observatories as distant as Massachusetts, Alaska, Hawaii and the Philippine Islands, and gathered by Science Service, the earthquake experts of the U. S. Coast and Geodetic Survey have located the center of the quake on May 14. It was at latitude 8.0 degrees south and longitude 80.5 degrees west, and occurred at 5 hours 14 minutes 20 seconds P. M., Eastern Standard Time. This location is in the Pacific Ocean about 70 miles off the Peruvian coast. Fortunately for residents of this region, the slip of the ocean bed which produced it was mostly in a horizontal direction. Had the shaking been up and down, a severe tidal wave would doubtless have been the result.

At Guayaquil, Ecuador, nearly four hundred miles to the north of the center of the shake, severe shaking was reported. This, and the fact that seismograph observatories at such distant points recorded it, shows that it was a quake of great severity.

The seismograph stations that reported their records of the quake to Science Service were those of the U. S. Coast and Geodetic Survey at Tucson, Arizona, Sitka, Alaska, Honolulu, T. H., and Chicago, Ill.; of the Jesuit Seismological Association at Georgetown University, Washington, Fordham University, New York; Regis College, Denver; Loyola University, New Orleans, and St. Louis University, St. Louis; and the stations of Harvard University, Cambridge; the Dominion Observatory, Ottawa, Canada, and the Manila Observatory in the Philippine Islands.

THREE ECLIPSES IN ONE MONTH

THREE eclipses in a single month, one of the moon and two of the sun, the first of the trio happening on Saturday, May 19, form the coming celestial program. This is the first time that three eclipses have followed at such short intervals since 1924, and the last time that it will happen until 1931, say astronomers at the Nautical Almanac Office of the U. S. Navy Department.

Since an eclipse happens when the shadow of the moon, cast by the sun, falls on the earth, or when the moon itself gets into the earth's own shadow which stretches

out into space, an eclipse can not happen any oftener. It takes two weeks for the moon to travel from a position between the earth and sun, to one where the earth is between the moon and the sun. An eclipse occurring at the former position is of the sun, and one at the latter is of the moon.

On May 19, the moon's shadow swept across a small area about a thousand miles south of South Africa, just on the edge of the Antarctic region that Commander Byrd will explore next year. As the eclipse was extremely brief, and the region where it was visible most inaccessible, no astronomers traveled to see it.

Two weeks later, by June 3, the moon will be half way around its orbit encircling the earth, and then will enter the earth's shadow. As the moon is lighted by the sun, it will then be temporarily darkened. Unfortunately for most American observers, this eclipse happens after the moon has set for all but the extreme western states, and so will not be visible over the greater part of the country. From Hawaii and the Philippines, as well as eastern Asia, it will be possible to view it.

When another two weeks have passed, on June 17, the moon will again be between the sun and earth, and then part of its shadow will cross the Antarctic region. During this eclipse, at no part of the earth's surface will the sun be completely covered by the dark lunar disc. Therefore, like the first of the trio of eclipses, this one will be completely without scientific importance.

Unfortunately for astronomers, eclipses that are really satisfactory for observing can not occur as often as this. When the moon's shadow lands squarely on the earth, by the time the moon travels around its orbit again, the shadow will miss the earth completely. The next eclipse that Americans can observe without leaving the country will be on August 31, 1932, and will be seen in parts of Maine, Vermont, New Hampshire and Massachusetts.

ITEMS

A CURIOUS crop is described in a bulletin of the Missouri Botanical Garden. It consists of a tomato vine grafted on a potato stock, which yields tomato fruits above and potato tubers below. The graft is fairly easy to make, it is stated, requiring no more skill than is needed for a similar operation on an apple twig. Apparently the first one on record was made over a century ago by an amateur scientist named De Tchudi, who reported his experiments to the Horticultural Institute at Fromont in France. Neither partner in this double plant body seems to have any influence on the other. The tomatoes are like those of sister plants grown on their own roots, and the potatoes differ in no way from those grown in the ordinary way from other eyes cut from the same parent tuber.

ANCIENT mythologies tell of gods slain by their worshippers; and something of the kind is happening in the Big Tree grove of Mariposa County, where thousands of tourists are unconsciously destroying that which they come hundreds of miles to admire. At the request of the National Park Service, Dr. E. P. Meinecke, U. S. Forest Service plant pathologist, has investigated the present status of the cherished sequoias and has reached the conclusion that long-continued and heavy tramping of human feet has destroyed the root endings and finer roots of many of the trees. Without these of course the trees are unable to absorb water and mineral nutrients from the soil. The rescue of Grizzly Giant, one of the finest Big Trees in existence, from a similar fate about 25 years ago, is recalled. Trampling had destroyed its endings, and friends of the trees were at a loss to know what to do. Finally it was suggested by George T. Harlow, at that time guardian of the grove, that the soil surrounding the tree be loosened somewhat and that additional soil be placed around the tree and over the roots to a height of three or four feet. The experiment, though ridiculed at the time, proved entirely successful, and the old tree was restored to health.

A COUNTRY ZOO, where tired animals of the London Zoo can go for a holiday and where sick animals can go to recuperate, is proposed in a bill considered by the British Parliament. The estate which would be set aside for the animals covers 480 acres and provides enough room for the animals to exercise in surroundings somewhat like their natural home country. The holiday home for the wild animals would be about 40 miles from London.

YELLOWSTONE PARK headquarters at Mammoth Hot Springs will have a house built of elk antlers to display to visitors during the coming season, as part of the exhibits of the park museum. It will be only a little house, containing a single room six by eight feet and seven feet high, but even so its construction will require some thousands of pairs of antlers. Each year every adult male in the 20,000 elk in the park herds sheds a pair of antlers, so that large quantities of these have been easy to obtain. Enough have been brought to Mammoth Hot Springs to provide walls and roof for the "house of horn," which Chief Ranger Sam Woodring has undertaken to construct.

THE insect-catching leaves of a southern species of pitcher plant are sometimes borrowed by tree frogs for their own insect-catching purposes, according to Professor E. A. Andrews, of the Johns Hopkins University. On several occasions, during a sojourn in North Carolina, he found these little yellow-green frogs ensconced inside the narrow, trumpet-shaped hollow leaves of the pitcher-plant, whose color almost exactly matched the color of the froglets. Inasmuch as the leaves of the pitcher-plant normally serve as traps for insects, whose remains apparently nourish this predatory vegetable, it seems that the frogs were in a way playing the part of parasites, by robbing the plants of their rightful prey as it tumbled in at the mouths of the pitchers. In a few instances the frogs were in their turn cheated, for he observed frog-inhabited leaves across whose openings spiders had spun their webs, so that any insect undertaking to enter the inviting mouth of the trap would reach neither the frog's stomach nor the plant's digestive pit at the base of the leaf.

SCIENCE NEWS

Science Service, Washington, D. C.

TWO FORMS OF YELLOW FEVER

NOT for months and perhaps years will the medical world be able to estimate the importance and value of the varied researches undertaken by Dr. Hideyo Noguchi, internationally known bacteriologist and latest addition to yellow fever's long list of scientific martyrs.

From the germ cultures he has left, perhaps from samples of his own blood that he insisted be taken from his body for inoculation of monkeys, it may be found whether or not there are two forms of the disease, one American and one African. It may be that when his assistants who are at work on his material have their results ready to give the world, the ancient controversy will be settled and it will be established whether the dread "yellow jack" was one of the New World's questionable gifts to humanity or whether it was brought over from Africa with the importation of slaves.

During work on yellow fever in South America, in 1918, Dr. Noguchi isolated a germ believed to be the cause of yellow fever. From it he developed a preventive vaccine and a causative serum that proved fairly efficacious if used within two or three days after the onset of the disease. Campaigns against the deadly stegomyia mosquito, carrier of the disease, practically stamped out the infection in the Western Hemisphere. Nevertheless, it continued to be a serious menace in West Africa.

Epidemiologists stress the importance of suppressing yellow fever in the west of Africa before a transcontinental railway is opened up to carry the disease to the East. The stegomyia flourishes in the warmer countries of the Orient, and once these mosquitoes became infected the havoc that a disease like yellow fever would wreak amid the unsanitary conditions of India and southern China would be appalling and should be prevented at any cost.

Anxious to smother the disease before it could spread afresh from its last stronghold, the international health division of the Rockefeller Foundation established a laboratory at Lagos, Nigeria, where a trained staff has been at work on the problem for many years. In South America, Dr. Noguchi was able to transfer the disease to monkeys and even guinea-pigs, but workers in Africa found it impossible to inoculate any animals for a long time, a condition that argues in favor of two distinct entities for the disease in the two countries. In all outward aspects, however, they are much alike. Finally Dr. Adrian Stokes, a British investigator at the laboratory at Lagos, succeeded, along with a group of colleagues, in infecting monkeys of the variety known as *Macacus rhesus* with typical African yellow fever. Dr. Stokes also succumbed to the disease. But his work constituted an important step, since it did away with the necessity in studying the African form for volunteer human victims, such as were called for by the U. S. Army Commission in Havana years ago. At the same time the workers were unable to find the causative Leptospira in the patient's blood. It almost seemed as if the two diseases had different origins.

Since Dr. Noguchi was generally conceded to know more about this particular group of germs than any other living person, he undertook the African trip last fall to see if he could personally sort out the two diseases. Perhaps his skilful crippled hands, famous throughout the realm of bacteriology for their technique with test-tube and microscope, could demonstrate *Leptospira icteroides* where others had failed, or even show an entirely different cause. While at work he contracted the disease and died. Whether or not he found what he sought, authorities at the Rockefeller Foundation refuse to affirm or deny. Only after his coworkers and assistants have some concrete results to show from his research will the world know. In the meantime the work at Lagos goes on.

HIGH-FREQUENCY X-RAYS

EXTREME high-frequency X-rays, generated in a million-volt tube, are the next item of promise on the program at the California Institute of Technology. Allied to the investigation of the cosmic rays, which has recently yielded such interesting results, is the attempt, long under way at the institute, at the artificial production of very short waves, and therefore very penetrating radiation. In the hands of C. C. Lauritsen and R. D. Bennett this work has already yielded some promising results.

As yet no apparatus can be devised for handling the terrific electric potential required for the artificial production of cosmic rays. For intermediate rays of about one-twenty-billionth of an inch wave-length, however, there seem to be experimental possibilities. Such rays are much shorter than the surgeon's X-rays and much more difficult to produce.

The X-ray "tube" used in the new work is several yards long, made in sections similar to the glass cylinders used in gasoline dispensing apparatus. Before operation all but one billionth part of its air content is pumped out. A water-cooled anode raised to a potential of a million volts pulls electrons bodily and violently out of the nearby cathode by the application of the principle of "field currents" studied intensively for some years past at the Norman Bridge laboratory by Millikan, Eyring and Lauritsen. Under this terrific force the electrons attain a speed very near to 186,000 miles per second, the velocity of light. Striking the anode at this enormous speed the electrons generate X-rays like the gamma rays naturally emitted by radium.

In preliminary trials now being run in the high tension laboratory of the institute, where a million-volts to ground at a thousand kilowatts is available to the experimenters, Lauritsen and Bennett have succeeded in obtaining continuous operation of their new tube at voltages that have approached the million mark. The high-frequency rays produced were observable through the steel doors of the laboratory more than 100 feet away.

The physicists of the institute make no pretense of any immediate project beyond an extension of spectrographic studies, long a part of Millikan's program. It is suspected, however, that these new and very difficult experiments are a preliminary skirmish in a further campaign on the nucleus of the atom. It is well-known that the gamma rays of radium are intimately connected with nuclear disintegration and transmutation of elements. The structure of the nucleus is a profound mystery, but there is plausible evidence of enormous forces connected therewith. Electrically the problem is one where voltage is counted in seven and eight figures. Economically the problem suggests fabulous power values as yet wholly within the domain of fancy.

THE EMERGENCY ASSOCIATION OF GERMAN SCIENCE

A German scientific association, originally organized in the post-war and post-revolutionary emergency to help out hard-pressed scientists and impoverished laboratories, has developed into one of the most active agencies for the promotion of science to be found in Europe.

It still keeps the now somewhat inappropriate name, "Notgemeinschaft der deutschen Wissenschaft," that is, "Emergency Association of German Science." But its present functions, now that times have become a little less stringent, have expanded far beyond its original work of rescue in distress. It is backing half-a-dozen promising ventures in science, in widely varying fields.

Of greatest interest to Americans, perhaps, is the plan now under discussion for the creation of a school for research into the physiological improvement of human beings by means of sports and games. Germans have always been much interested in physical culture, and since the war have taken increasingly to track and field athletics on the American plan. It is the ambition of German athletes to offer a really serious challenge to America for first place in this year's Olympics.

In the realm of industrial science the Notgemeinschaft is supporting research in metals and their properties, under Professor Schenk, of Muenster, Westphalia. He is engaged in examining the plasticity and other properties of metals which offer possibilities of development for science and for the metallurgical industries.

Another field is the investigation of the nutritive physiology of plants, especially questions of manures and fertilizers, and the growth and cultivation of grains and other economic plants.

Exploratory expeditions of purely scientific character are also under way. One goes to Transbaikalia in cooperation with Russian scientific institutions, under Professor Wilmans, of Heidelberg. Another expedition, in association with the Russian Academy of Sciences, is to be sent to the Altai regions on the borders of Siberia and Tibet.

The Notgemeinschaft has interested itself in archeological finds at the ancient town of Trier or Treves, which was once a Roman garrison city. During the construction of a new high school there the foundations of a large Roman building were unearthed, which were shown to constitute a temple area and a praetorium. It is hoped to gather new light here concerning Roman culture in Western Germany.

Similar problems engage attention in the East, where prehistoric earthworks and fortifications have been excavated. Professor Unverzagt, of the Ethnological Museum, Berlin, well known for his excavations at Lossow, near Frankfurt on the Oder, has been working in this field.

STUDY OF THE HARESKIN INDIANS

The prospect of studying a primitive culture, which has been maintained for thousands of years untouched by outside contacts, is taking Cornelius Osgood, graduate student of ethnology at the University of Chicago, on a 15 months' expedition to the Canadian Barren Grounds, the region around Great Bear Lake. He is *en route* to Waterways, where he leaves the railroad. The 1,000-mile trip from Waterways will be made by canoe and dog team. He expects to reach Ft. Norman, the last outpost of civilization in that region, sometime in August.

Almost nothing is known of the Hareskin Indians, which he will study, except that they are sullen and inhospitable. Two white missionaries who tried to convert them were murdered. Mr. Osgood hopes, if it is possible, to live with them during the long winter season, getting first-hand observations of their manners and customs. The difficult language of the Hareskin tribe presents a problem, but Mr. Osgood expects, if he receives a friendly reception, to make himself understood by using Athabascan word stems. The Hareskin tribe is a member of that linguistic group.

Professor Edward Sapir, University of Chicago anthropologist, believes that this expedition presents "an almost unparalleled opportunity of studying a primitive people who have been uninfluenced by outside cultures." It is hoped that a complete knowledge of this tribe will shed light on the development of other Athabascan tribes, particularly the Navajos, in Arizona and Mexico.

The Barren Grounds lie almost wholly within the Arctic Circle, more than 300 miles from Ft. Norman. The hardships of a winter in this region induced Mr. Osgood to make a 1,300-mile preliminary trip on the rivers north of Edmonton last summer, in order to learn what he may expect. The expedition is being financed by the National Museum of Canada.

THE ROCKET AUTOMOBILE

With fire-spurting rockets instead of engine-furnishing power, the Opel rocket car made trial runs on the Avus race course in Berlin, on May 23, reaching speeds of 90 to 120 miles an hour. The small, slightly-built automobile was piloted by Fritz V. Opel. To stabilize it during its speedy travel it has a plane or fin on each side.

A battery of slow-burning rockets, filled with powder, by discharging into the air at the rear of the car, furnished the impulse that drove the car forward. The driver controlled the burning of the rockets and therefore the speed of the car by an ignition foot lever.

Each rocket was about a yard long and three inches in diameter and metal cases were used as containers. The curves of the two-mile track were taken without difficulty or danger. Tests of this new sort of automobile are understood to be preliminary to the trials of a rocket airplane designed to reach high altitudes where an ordinary air propeller airplane could not obtain traction. The rocket, operating upon the same principle as the kick of a rifle, does not need the air in order to produce its effect. The rocket principle is, therefore, the method of power that could be used in airless outer space that must be traversed on a journey, a la Jules Verne, to the moon or the planets.

Although interested in the Opel rocket auto tested in Berlin, scientists in Washington point out that for land or air transportation the rocket car will not prove economical when compared with the usual internal combustion engine autos and airplanes. The rocket applies effectively only a small percentage of the fuel's energy, about five per cent., as compared with four to six times that percentage for ordinary automobiles operated on gasoline. For use where there is no air the rocket provides propulsion where other methods can not apply. The idea of applying rocket power to automobiles is not new, for in the past extensive tests have not been made.

THE SEVENTEEN-YEAR "LOCUSTS"

THE seventeen-year cicada, often called the seventeen-year locust, is booked to appear during late May and early June through a wide stretch of territory east of the Alleghenies, from North Carolina up to the Hudson Valley and the Long Island Sound region. In a few spots in the middle west, in southern Indiana and southern Michigan, it is also expected to emerge.

These remarkable insects, which are the longest-lived of all the six-legged hordes that crawl the earth, spend over sixteen years under ground, clinging to plant roots from which they suck their nourishment. Then, in the spring of the seventeenth year, they emerge from their burrows, shed their pupa cases, and spend a few weeks as fully developed adults, mating and depositing eggs to provide for the next generation.

During the four or five weeks of their above-ground existence the seventeen-year cicadas make their presence known by the incessant shrill song of the males. The chorus of millions of tiny saw-like voices is very disagreeable to many persons. The Pilgrim Fathers didn't like it. Governor Bradford spoke of it as "a constante yelling noyes, as made all ye woods ring of them and ready to deafe ye hearers."

The immense number of these rather large insects sometimes causes alarm, but they are really comparatively harmless. They feed very seldom or not at all, depending on the reserves accumulated during their long underground life. The principal mischief is caused when the females lay their eggs, which they deposit in furrows cut into the green bark of young twigs. This causes a temporary defoliation of many trees, but no permanent harm in the forests. It may be very damaging at times, however, in orchards and nurseries.

There are 17 "broods" of the seventeen-year cicada, distributed in various parts of the country. One brood comes out each year. The one emerging this year is designated as Brood II. Brood III, which is due in 1929, has its headquarters in the prairie states, especially Iowa, In addition to the seventeen-year species there is an allied thirteen-year form which ranges principally in the lower Mississippi region. This is divided into 13 broods, so that an outbreak of this insect also is to be expected somewhere in the South every year.

ITEMS

ACCORDING to Dr. M. Blaschke, a German ceramic chemist, glass windows were in use in ancient Rome. Most of the panes did not exceed 12 by 16 inches in size, though a few larger ones have been found. Glass-making, known for many centuries in Egypt, came to Rome relatively late. During the time of Cicero, who died in 43 B. C., glass objects of any kind were rarities, and glass windows were unknown. A hundred years later most households owned some, and by the time the Empire was well established glass was fairly common. The famous mosaics of the later Empire, notably at Ravenna and Constantinople, were made largely out of bits of glass.

A 120,000-pound master truck scale of the plate-fulcrum type, used for weighing railroad trucks, was this month installed and housed on the Chicago Belt line in Chicago by the United States Bureau of Standards. Since the scale has a sensitivity to one tenth of a pound and so is accurate to the millionth point under full load, the bureau believes that it will do much for standardization in heavy weighing. The scale is so sensitive that the atmospheric barometric pressure causes different registrations of weight for one object. It is the purpose of the bureau to have different railroads bring their different type cars to this scale, have them weighed, and then send these cars back to the scales of the railroad for a checkup of differences. In this way, a standard weight can be established and maintained from coast to coast for the first time.

APPARENT "earthquakes" accompanying a great meteor, such as that which flashed over Georgia and South Carolina recently, are really due to air waves from the speeding celestial projectile. This is the opinion of Professor Charles P. Oliver, of the University of Virginia and recognized authority on meteoric astronomy. It is not possible for such a meteor to cause an actual tremor of the earth, he stated. However, as it passes through the earth's atmosphere, it causes air waves, similar to those caused by a projectile from a large gun. The meteor may travel as fast as 25 miles a second, or around fifty times the speed of the shell from the gun, and so the air waves are much stronger. As they strike houses and buildings, they cause them to vibrate, even breaking window panes and cracking plaster walls. To a person within such a building, the effects are practically indistinguishable from those of an earthquake.

SCIENCE NEWS

Science Service, Washington, D. C.

COMETS AND METEORS AROUND STARS

EVIDENCE that many, if not all, stars are surrounded by meteors and comets like those that we see in the solar system, and that they may serve as fuel to keep the stars going, is the announcement just made by Dr. Harlow Shapley, director of the Harvard College Observatory. If this is correct, it would explain how the stars may survive for a far longer time than the one hundred trillion years that astronomers have recently supposed to be their maximum life.

By means of the spectroscope, which breaks their light up into a rainbow-like spectrum, crossed by numerous dark lines and bands that indicate the constituent elements, Dr. Shapley has studied a large number of stars. Though they are of varying temperatures, and supposed to be of different ages, they all show a band which indicates the presence of cyanogen. This is a gas composed of carbon and nitrogen and which is used terrestrially for killing insects.

Probably, he believes, this cyanogen is not actually in the stars themselves, but rather is it provided by meteors and comets that surround them. Comets and meteors that have come within range of observation have been found to contain carbon and nitrogen as separate elements. When these fall into a star, the high temperature would cause the elements to combine to form cyanogen.

One important aspect of this hypothesis concerns the life of the stars. The generally accepted theory now among astronomers is that the energy of the stars comes from the actual disintegration of their matter into energy. Matter and energy, according to the ideas of modern physics, are both the same, and so one can be changed to the other. In this way, the matter in the average star will keep it running for about 100,000,000,000,000 years. However, if more and more fuel is constantly being shoveled on the stars, in the form of meteoric material, the star might survive almost indefinitely.

A NEW EXPLOSIVE

RADIUM atomite, the explosive said to be more powerful than T.N.T. or dynamite, is now engaging the attention of army engineers in Washington. The report of Lieutenant-Colonel L. M. Adams, who tested the new explosive at the California Institute of Technology at Pasadena, has just been received, and has been referred to the Board of Engineer Equipment of Troops, at Fort Humphreys.

No details of the composition or samples of the explosive have been received in Washington. Lieutenant-Colonel Adams reported that it is a light greenish powder, dry and very finely divided. The inventor, Captain H. R. Zimmer, of Los Angeles, former army officer, claims that it can be produced for one half the cost of T.N.T. It is declared more stable than T.N.T., and unaffected by dampness, a serious fault of the latter.

In the tests by Lieutenant-Colonel Adams, the power of radium atomite was compared with T.N.T. and 80 per cent. dynamite. A lead cylinder, 12⅛ inches in diameter, 14½ inches high, with a hole 1⅛ inches in diameter and 9¼ inches deep, was used with each. The entire cylinders each weighed about seven hundred pounds. An ounce of the explosive was placed in the bottom of the hole and covered with three ounces of sand, then the explosive was detonated electrically.

Before explosion, the holes each had capacities of 125 cubic centimeters. T.N.T. enlarged the hole 1,002 cubic centimeters, dynamite 1,255, and radium atomite 1,370.

Tests were also made of the speed of explosion, or how fast the explosive reaction travels through it. This is about 10,721 feet per second for radium atomite, 16,082 for T.N.T. and 8,300 for 60 per cent. dynamite. For general use, it was stated by army engineers, this range makes no practical difference.

Officials of the engineer corps were unable to state whether or not the explosive will be adopted. After the board that is now considering the report is through, they may either request Captain Zimmer to furnish them with samples for additional tests or else invite him to Washington for the purpose.

STANDARDIZATION OF METERS

STANDARDIZATION of meters for gas, electricity and water was urged by W. T. Henrichson, meter inspector of the state of Texas, in a report to the Conference on Weights and Measures held in Washington. In Texas, meters are supervised both before and after installation. Testing equipment cost only $1,481.36, but led to savings of thousands of dollars each year for the people in some communities.

Inaccuracy in meters, said Mr. Henrichson, is usually due to incompetent men and neglect on the part of the utility company rather than any deliberate intent to defraud.

Before the passage of the law, a gas company in a Texas city sought to raise rates, Mr. Henrichson related, but the city council decided that the existing rates were adequate to net a fair profit. During one of the meetings, a council member suggested that there should be other ways for the gas company to increase its earnings besides increasing the rates, no doubt having in mind increased efficiency and economy. The gas company acted on his suggestion and increased its earnings. It speeded up every meter in the entire city and increased gross receipts about 25 per cent.

On the other hand, a small gas company was on the verge of bankruptcy. After spending a week testing meters, the speaker found that 25 per cent. of those in service were not registering the gas flowing through them. A much higher percentage of the meters were "slow" and registered only a portion of the gas used. This investigation showed the directors why they were not making money.

In one community where gas bills had suddenly jumped, investigation showed that the meters were correct, but whereas the company had been delivering gas of 1,000 British thermal units per cubic foot, they were found to be delivering gas of 575 British thermal units per cubic foot. This was equivalent to speeding up all the meters about 74 per cent.

ANCIENT SKELETONS FROM ALGERIA

WHILE Cro-Magnon man ruled Europe, twenty-five thousand years ago, he had as neighbors in Africa a race who used tools and weapons like his own, but who in their bodily makeup so closely resembled men of to-day that they may fairly be called "modern." This great backward extension of the history of the "modern" type of human beings is the most significant point about the recent discovery by American and French anthropologists of a number of ancient skeletons in a shell mound at Mechta, Algeria. This opinion was expressed by Professor Fay-Cooper Cole, of the University of Chicago, in response to an inquiry by Science Service.

For the past three years Beloit College has been conducting excavations in France and North Africa, under a fund given by Dr. Frank Logan, Chicago philanthropist. Dr. George Collie, directeor of the museum at Beloit, has spent much time in the field, while active excavation has been carried on by graduate students in anthropology from the University of Chicago.

Last year Alonzo Pond, one of the American workers, found the skeleton of a child in a shell-heap of Cro-Magnon age at Mechta. This year another worker, Paul Nesbitt, took out three more skeletons, while previously a Frenchman named Debrugge had secured a skeleton there.

A careful study of the shell mound and its contents indicate that it seems to be like the Old Stone Age finds of Europe of twenty-five thousand years ago. No New Stone Age objects occur in the site, and no bones of any domestic animals were found—domestication of animals is a "modern" accomplishment. "We seem to be justified in saying that the site is pre-Neolithic, and is probably as old as the Aurignacian," Professor Cole concludes.

The skeletons are neither Neanderthal nor Cro-Magnon. One skull, a woman's, shows negroid characteristics, but the others appear to be rather close to the Mediterranean type, though somewhat more primitive. Fuller details will be announced when the material shall have arrived in America.

THE PROLONGATION OF LIFE

INSTEAD of using alchemy, or the numerous supposed "elixirs of life" in order to retain youth, the late Dr. A. C. Eycleshymer, of the University of Illinois Medical School, points out in a manuscript left in incomplete form by his death that the quest for youth is not less popular to-day than it has been for countless ages, but the search to-day is becoming more and more scientific, and so is coming nearer to success than any of the older processes. This article was prepared for publication in the *Scientific Monthly* by Dr. Eycleshymer's friend, Dr. E. P. Lyon.

The idea of an elixir of life dates back to Biblical times, when the "tree of life" is introduced in the Garden of Eden. Adam was sent from the Garden, "lest he put forth his hand and take also of the tree of life, and eat, and live forever." This idea that there must be somewhere a tree which was intended to preserve man from disease and death prevailed for ages.

Stars were the next attraction and it was believed that the planets possessed either good or evil qualities which were given to those born under them. Since metals were thought to be intimately associated with the planetary bodies, amulets or figures which had been cast, stamped and submitted to the influence of stars, therefore becoming charmed, became popular. Alchemy succeeded astrology. Liquid gold, when made, would be life. But it was never made. Then came blood transfusion. When in 1667, Denys, of Paris, transferred about a pound of calf's blood into the veins of a maniac, and repeated the process twice, resulting in the death of the patient, transfusion was prevented by law.

To-day, through the avenues of empirical medicine and sanitary science, the expectancy of life has been greatly increased. The average span of life was increased about four years during the seventeenth and eighteenth centuries, about eight years in the first three quarters of the nineteenth century, and about sixteen years since 1875.

"While we have thus made much progress," Dr. Eycleshymer states, "we still lack information in easily accessible fields. While there is always interest shown in plants and animals, the study of man, with a view of preserving and accentuating, in the offspring, the sterling qualities found among the ancestors, has not received serious consideration. Yet we know that heredity is one of the chief factors in longevity."

POLAR RESCUE EPICS

IF the passing hours prove that the *Italia*, with Nobile and his party aboard, is lost in the Arctic somewhere between the North Pole and Spitsbergen, there may be enacted one of the heartrending tragedies of attempted Arctic rescue such as history records. To-day, although the ice is as merciless as ever, circumstances are different from the days when Franklin was lost, when Greely and his brave band starved, or even when the more recent Wrangel Island tragedy was revealed.

In the days when Arctic explorers were limited to difficult sledging over ice, when only a few miles a day could be traveled, the rescue party knew in what general locality to search. If the *Italia's* radio remains silent and gives no clue of the location of that ill-fated ship, Amundsen and his aides in the relief expedition have a difficult task before them. A dozen dirigibles in the best of weather might scour the icy wastes without sighting the landing place of the *Italia*. If the radio brings news of Nobile and his party and gives their location, even then rescue over ice will be difficult enough.

Up until the *Italia's* latest voyage, recent aerial exploration of the Arctic has been singularly without serious mishap. But the first airplane venture pole-

ward by Amundsen and Ellsworth gave the world some anxious moments while their airplane was down in the Arctic and out of communication. When the *Norge* landed at Teller, Alaska, after its successful trip across the North Pole and the great Arctic blind spot, the news of success was slow in reaching civilization and some at that time thought that dirigible lost.

But the first attempt at Arctic exploration by air, made in 1897, ended disastrously. The Swedish balloonist, S. A. Andree, and two companions, set out for the North Pole in a large free balloon. The start was made from Danes Island, in the north of Spitsbergen, on July 11, 1897. Five tons of supplies were carried. In an hour the balloon was out of sight. That night, seven and a half hours later, a message buoy, found later, was dropped. This was the last trace of the expedition, although years afterwards various unconfirmed rumors of finding the balloon have come out of the Arctic regions of Siberia and Canada.

The Franklin expedition of 1845–48, from which not one of the 129 officers and men returned alive, is probably the most famous of Arctic tragedies. Not until a decade later did searching parties discover the fate of Sir John Franklin and his men and of their accomplishment of the Northwest Passage and other geographic discoveries.

Living in retirement in Washington to-day, there is a survivor of another rescue epic of the north. General A. W. Greely is now eighty-four. In 1881, when a lieutenant, he commanded an expedition the remnants of which three years later were rescued at the point of starvation. Notable scientific explorations were accomplished. Only six returned out of the twenty-five who started, but records, instruments and collections told the story of the efforts of those who perished.

TREATMENT OF MONGOLOID IDIOTS

MONGOLOID idiots—those baffling cases of defective reclaimed from their smiling, contented state of idiocy and in some cases they may even reach practically normal intelligence. This was the encouraging report made on June 1 by Dr. Walter Timme, of New York, before the American Association for the Study of the Feebleminded, meeting in Atlantic City.

The cause of Mongolism and how to treat it are still children that look like flat-faced oriental dolls—may be uncertain, though it is generally recognized as a gland disorder. Dr. Timme described his theory, which traces many of the symptoms of Mongolism to faulty development or lack of development of the fore section of the pituitary gland. This gland is located at the base of the brain and its secretions enter both the blood and the cerebro-spinal fluid.

Working on this theory, Dr. Timme stated that he has been feeding Mongoloid patients pituitary substance, both of the whole gland and particularly of the fore lobe of the gland. Hypodermic injections of the gland solution have also been given and in addition the patients have been given the usual thyroid treatment.

"As a result of ten years of this work, I have brought many of my Mongoloid patients to much higher levels than we have heretofore been able to do," he said.

Some of these children, who had started in life with the prospect of remaining idiots, unable to dress themselves, talk properly or even eat like normal children, learned to do arithmetic up to multiplication by three or more figures and long division. They also learned to write letters and do oral arithmetic, which is remarkable achievement for these cases.

One of the patients, described by Dr. Timme, has attained an intelligence quotient of 90, which brings this child up to average intelligence. Not all the children treated have attained this degree of improvement, but Dr. Timme declared that "we have with these means accomplished more than by any previously known treatment, so far as I am aware."

ITEMS

No diphtheria deaths in 1927 puts Cambridge, Mass., at the head of the list in diphtheria prevention, of all the cities with populations over 100,000 in the United States. Only once in the last five years, according to the American Medical Association, has any city gone a year without a single death from diphtheria. The previous diphtheria record breaker was Duluth, Minn., in 1925. Seven cities with more than 100,000 inhabitants had no typhoid deaths last year, the medical association's statistics show. New Haven, Conn., Springfield, Mass., Yonkers, N. Y., Paterson, N. J., Richmond, Va., Canton, Ohio, Kansas City, Kan., make up the typhoid honor roll, which is the largest known since studies of typhoid death rates were started in 1913.

THE pronghorn antelope of Nevada and Oregon have been given a new lease on life with the recent acquisition made by the National Association of Audubon Societies of a 380-acre ranch in northern Nevada. These beautiful and hard-pressed animals of the semidesert regions of the West were gradually being killed off, due mainly to lax game law enforcement. At a recent national conference, the association was appointed to take the lead in securing congressional action, but political interference at the behest of nomadic sheep-herding interests caused this project to fail.

A SURVEY of two centuries of rain in England shows that the rainfall of 1927 was 124 per cent. of the normal and was exceeded by only eight other years. The records, dating back to 1727, show that the three years 1768, 1852 and 1872 were markedly wetter than 1927, with 136, 137 and 144 per cent., respectively. There was no year so dry as 1921 with only 69 per cent. of the normal since 1788. The reports show that there were nine consecutive wet years from 1875 to 1883, while the longest run of dry years was only six, from 1800 to 1805. A remarkable feature of the rainfall of recent years is that in all but two of the last fourteen years the fall has been below average.

SCIENCE NEWS

Science Service, Washington, D. C.

THE COLD LIGHT OF SEA ANIMALS

MAN will face new and important ways of controlling nature when he succeeds in demonstrating the mechanism by which tiny organisms of the sea produce light without appreciable heat, Dr. Charles A. Kofoid, of the University of California, said in his presidential address before the Pacific division of the American Association for the Advancement of Science at Claremont, Calif., on June 13.

Dr. Kofoid described the occasional outbreaks of luminescence in the ocean by night, when each breaking wave is accompanied by an outburst of flaming light, and the path of a vessel becomes an illuminated trail across the water. By day, the water of the luminous sea is rusty red, and mottled with patches of color. The luminous outbreak brings death and destruction to tons of sea creatures, and has baffled attempts of scientists to plumb the mystery to its exact source.

The epidemics of light have been definitely traced to tiny sea animals with the long name of dinoflagellata, which sometimes develop and multiply with what seems like an astonishing ambition to cover the ocean. But what causes such enormous flares of growth is still to be explained.

The fact that the outbreaks occur so frequently off the Pacific coast of this country rather than off the Atlantic is a clue that local conditions of weather and sea geography may play their part in the mob drama of the dinoflagellata. Chemical analysis of sea-water patiently made over long periods of time is also expected to reveal some evidence of the exact kind of water in which the creatures flourish. It is also possible that the organisms themselves produce some substance which favors their own growth, and that they flourish and multiply until the food supply becomes inadequate and then the surplus hordes starve.

The task of handling and experimenting with these delicate organisms is extraordinarily difficult, Dr. Kofoid said, because they are attuned to an environment of great constancy, and the changes in their environment which cause them to respond are slight compared with other creatures of the animal world.

"The secret of the production of light without appreciable heat is locked up in the metabolism of these simple organisms of the sea," Dr. Kofoid said in conclusion, pointing out that some of the most inviting problems of biology are involved in understanding the relations of these organisms to the solar radiations on which they depend and in demonstrating the mechanism by which they release their stored-up reserves of energy.

CHEMICAL BONDS AND LIGHT WAVES

THE chemical bonds between particular kinds of atoms are tuned precisely with certain wave-lengths of light, according to recent discoveries of Dr. Joseph W. Ellis, physicist in the University of California. Instead of cooperating with the light radiation, however, these chemical attachments nullify or absorb the special light waves to which they are attuned. Dr. Ellis thus identifies the bonds by noting the kind of light which does not get through the substance he is investigating.

For decades chemists have been able to tell what elements are present in a substance, and in most cases how many atoms of each. The pattern by which the atoms are tied together in compounds, however, is known or guessed only on circumstantial evidence. Nevertheless the pattern is all-important. Dr. Ellis' experiments show which atoms are directly bonded together.

Chemists would gladly accomplish all this by magnification and direct photography of the molecular structure. Unfortunately this is impossible with atoms only one two hundred millionth of an inch in diameter, and light waves five thousand times as wide.

By the new methods infra-red, or low frequency, rays are passed through simple chemical compounds like aniline, alcohol, etc., whose structure is already known and undisputed. Accurate measurement is made at the odd places in the spectrum where a stoppage of light is caused by particular chemical bonds. Dr. Ellis is able to specify with high numerical accuracy just what wave-length, or color of light will be absorbed if a substance under examination contains, for example, a nitrogen atom attached to a hydrogen atom. Nitrogen and hydrogen atoms scattered about in other relations and tied to other atoms give no such response. Similar data have been obtained for the carbon-hydrogen and sulfur-hydrogen bonds. Many additions to the list are expected with further research.

By combining a spectrograph and camera with electrical accessories, the physicist simply tests his substance down the gamut of the spectrum from blue to infra-red. Each chemical bond automatically records its presence by a dent in the photographic line record. Just as a piano wire may respond to sounds in more than one octave, so the chemical bonds give over-tone records which confirm the proof desired.

Even greater value may lie in the possibility of calculating the strength of a chemical bond. Dr. Ellis is enabled through mathematical physics to show how firmly a substance is bonded on a basis of the wave-length chosen. From such a computation it may be possible to predict in some degree the possibility of some desirable chemical reaction taking place.

EMISSION OF RAYS BY PLANT CELLS

THE latest sensation in scientific circles in Berlin is the discovery that the apex of certain rapidly growing vegetable and animal tissues emit some sort of invisible radiation which has the power to stimulate the growth of living matter with which it is not in contact. When this was first announced in 1924 by Professor Alexander Gurwitch, of Moscow, it was received with considerable

NEW SCIENTIFIC BOOKS

P. Blakiston's Son and Company, Philadelphia

A TEXT-BOOK OF ORGANIC CHEMISTRY. Joseph S. Chamberlain. pp. xxx + 901. $4.00. Second edition.

An expression of the author's teaching experience, the book is written primarily as a text-book for the undergraduate student and instructor, but it is hoped that those who have already studied the subject may find it of value for its general presentation.

The Williams and Wilkins Company, Baltimore

SIR ISAAC NEWTON. Edited by F. E. Brasch. pp. ix + 351. $5.00.

A series of essays giving a modern interpretation of the great English physicist through American eyes. Discusses Newton as a physicist, mathematician, chemist, astronomer, philosopher, etc.

The McGraw-Hill Book Company, New York

ELEMENTARY ORGANIC CHEMISTRY. Homer Adkins and S. M. McElvain. pp. xi + 183. $2.25.

A summary of facts such as students might be expected to note down, leaving to the individual instructor the vitalization of the subject. Intended for a one-semester course in colleges, normal schools and summer schools.

The Cambridge University Press,

The Macmillan Company, New York

WILLIAM BATESON, NATURALIST. pp. ix + 473. $8.40.

A collection of his essays and addresses together with a short account of his life by Beatrice Bateson.

The Macmillan Company, New York

AN OUTLINE OF PHYSICS. Albert E. Caswell. pp. xiv + 773. $4.25.

The effort of the author has been to make the subject-matter more vital and more stimulating. He first brings together essential facts from the whole field of physics, then coordinates these facts by well-established theories and finally brings to light new facts presented by the theories.

The University of Chicago Press, Chicago

TRIGONOMETRY. Ernst R. Breslich and Charles A. Stone. pp. ix + 122. $1.85.

The arrangement of the course is such that every new concept is immediately employed in practical situations as soon as its meaning is understood. Tables of common logarithms, of natural functions and logarithmic trigonometric functions are given, together with full instructions for their use.

ABSTRACTS OF THESES. Science Series. Volume IV. pp. x + 440. $3.00.

The University of Chicago requires publication of all theses accepted for the degree of Doctor of Philosophy, and the present book contains abstracts of theses submitted in the various branches of science during the period from September, 1925, to June, 1926.

BY-PRODUCTS IN THE PACKING INDUSTRY. Rudolf A. Clemen. pp. xi + 410. Illustrated. $4.00.

The technical and economic phases of the by-products of meat packing are described and evaluated. Hides and skins, wool and hair, soap, pharmaceuticals, fats and oils, glue, gelatin and all other by-products are traced through various stages of manufacture.

Oxford University Press, American Branch, New York

METEOROLOGY. David Brunt. 110 pp. 19 illustrations. $1.00.

A brief sketch of the physical principles underlying the phenomena which constitute the "weather" in so far as this is possible without mathematical analysis.

THE MIND OF THE GROWING CHILD. Edited by Viscountess Erleigh. pp. xii + 229. $1.75.

Consists of lectures by experts in child welfare and gives the mother definite, concrete aid in handling the problem of correct bringing up of children. Such important subjects as heredity and environment, fear and the backward child are discussed.

skepticism here, but now it has been confirmed by German investigators who are eagerly prospecting the new field of research in various directions.

Gurwitch found that if the tip of one of the rootlets of an onion or turnip was fixed so as to point at right angles to the side of another root, though as much as a quarter of an inch away, the cells in the side nearest the tip would multiply more rapidly than elsewhere and so bend the root away. That this influence was not due to the emission of some gaseous emanation from the root tip was proved by the interposition of a thin sheet between the two roots. Glass and gelatin sheets stopped the transmission of the growth stimulation power but quartz did not. This is characteristic of ultra-violet rays and Gurwitch concludes that the radiation from the root tips has a wave-length of 180–200 millimicrons, which would place it among the ultra-violet rays of high frequency.

The German botanist, N. Wagner, has repeated these experiments with bean and onion roots and measured the effect by counting under a microscope the number of new cells produced in the roots acted upon. The increase is as high as 70 per cent. in some cases. Old cells that have ceased growing show the greatest relative increase.

The German bacteriologist, M. A. Baron, has found that the radiation from onion roots will likewise accelerate the growth of anthrax bacillus and other bacteria. The growing tip of toadstools gives off these same growth-generating (mitogenetic) rays.

The Siemens Electrical Company has taken up the question and Doctors Hauser and Vahle working in these laboratories report that certain growing animal tissue, such as cancer, emit such rays.

These results, if confirmed, will radically revolutionize present theories of life and growth. It has hitherto been assumed that the impulse to cell subdivision was somehow due to the direct contact of certain chemical substances transmitted through the tissues, but it now seems that an energy agency is active in vital processes, an immaterial radiation of the nature of light but of too high a frequency to be detected by our eyes.

PUBLIC HEALTH AND THE PHYSICIAN

Care of the public health is the particular province and special responsibility of the physician, said Dr. William Sidney Thayer, of Baltimore, new president of the American Medical Association, in his inaugural address on June 13 at the annual meeting of the association in Minneapolis.

"In the first place we should use every means in our power to maintain the character of our public health officials," said Dr. Thayer. "Conditions have changed for the better but we are still treated too often to the humiliating spectacle of a mayor who appoints his family physician or some friend who has tired of practice to the position of commissioner of health."

Speaking to the 6,000 physicians who have assembled here, representing the organized medical profession of the country, Dr. Thayer reminded them of the object of their association as stated in its constitution: ". . . to promote the science and art of medicine and the betterment of public health." It is this altruistic attitude that marks the difference between medicine or any other profession and trade which has financial gain as its primary object. The true physician will not forget this difference and while he must earn a living, "if his main interest be not in his profession or if financial gain be his sole object, he will accomplish little and his name will be soon forgotten."

Of a physician's functions, the first, and most obvious, according to Dr. Thayer, is the individual care of his patients, after which comes prevention of epidemics, which requires attention to every detail involved in the spread of disease including cooperation with local boards of health by reporting communicable diseases, enforcing quarantine regulations, etc.

"Too early specialization is one of the great faults of modern American education," declared Dr. Thayer, speaking of the future of medical education. "The medical school is not the place for the training of specialists . . . the specialist who has not had a good basic medical training is a danger to society." Dr. Thayer also voiced the feeling current in many medical schools to-day that too much is being crowded into the four years' course. In this connection Dr. Thayer expressed the hope that "such elementary methods as a prescribed four years' course" will disappear from our medical education, schools of medicine in the future will be organized so that the student will be treated as a man and not as a schoolboy.

SENSITIVITY TO SUNBURN

Whether or not you sunburn easily may now be tested in a doctor's office, without going to the seashore. At the meeting of the American Physical Society in Claremont, Calif., on June 15, Dr. Robert C. Burt, of Pasadena, told of a new instrument that he has invented and calls the "erythemameter." It measures sensitivity of a person to erythema, as the physician terms painful sunburn.

Erythema, or sunburn, is caused by the ultra-violet rays in the sun's light. It can also be caused by ultra-violet light from a quartz tube mercury vapor lamp, or one of the other forms of lamp now being used in the treatment of rickets and other diseases. In Dr. Burt's instrument such a quartz lamp is contained in a light-tight box from which the ultra-violet rays can escape through a hole about two inches square. This opening is placed directly against the bare skin of the person being tested.

A set of filters in back of this hole cuts off more and more of the rays so that the skin at one edge gets the full benefit of the rays from the lamp, while that at the opposite edge receives none. After being exposed to this apparatus for ten minutes, the untanned skin of any one becomes burned at the side receiving the most rays. The distance that the burned area spreads measures the person's sensitivity.

As it is also desirable to measure the effect of varying exposures on sunburning, a shutter is provided behind

the opening also. This moves across the hole in a direction at right angles to that at which the intensity varies. When the exposure is complete it has moved completely across. The result is an actual curve drawn on the subject's skin which shows how long an exposure he can stand to ultra-violet rays of any intensity.

The instrument is expected to be useful to physicians who are now using ultra-violet rays in the treatment of disease. Over-exposure of a sensitive person to them may be very harmful, and by making a test with such an instrument, serious effects can be prevented.

Dr. Burt also described another instrument of his invention that measures intensity of ultra-violet light, either from the sun or an artificial source. It makes use of a photoelectric cell, in which light is converted to electricity, but a cell made of quartz, instead of glass, which is opaque to the rays.

"The instrument is so portable and easy to use," says Dr. Burt, "that the day may come when up-to-date bathing beaches will have an observatory giving out the intensity of the sunburn light in the sun, so that each person may stay out just long enough to become a delicate brown, without becoming severely burned."

TREE GROWTH AND THE WEATHER

A NEW theory regarding the period of greatest growth of California's big trees, or *Sequoia gigantea*, has recently been advanced by Walter Fry, commissioner for Sequoia National Park and for 40 years a student of natural conditions in the big tree park area.

Most scientific men have for years held the theory that the greatest growth of the trees was made in wet years or the years of the most snow. Judge Fry disagrees with this, contending that the Sequoia makes its greatest growth during dry seasons, and its least growth when the ground is covered with snow until late in June. Superintendent White, of Sequoia National Park, agrees with this latter theory.

The growing season of the Sequoia, occurring at elevations varying from 5,000 to 8,000 feet, is necessarily short. The judge points out that the big trees do not begin to bud until the snow has disappeared and the sun begins to warm the ground. In years when the snow remains late on the ground the growth of the trees is retarded, while in winters of light snowfall the ground is free of snow early and the trees have a longer growing season and the rings therefore have a greater growth in the dry years.

Judge Fry, to prove this contention, has counted the annual rings on a large number of down trees. The largest of all that he has counted, a fallen monarch of the Converse Basin near the park, has 3,226 annual rings. According to the judge a study of this tree shows that it had its fastest growth in the years between 400 and 250 B. C., and its smallest growth in the years between 650 and 800 A. D.

His years of investigation and study among the big trees lead the judge to believe that the climate of that portion of California in which they thrive has remained practically the same throughout the life of the Sequoias, although 1923–24 appear to have been the dryest years known to man.

ITEMS

FOUR Antarctic sea elephants, among the rarest of all large animals, have been brought to Hamburg by the great animal-importing firm of Carl Hagenbeck Company. At the present time no European zoo can boast the possession of a specimen. Other importations from the Antarctic include 25 king penguins and 35 gold-crested penguins. South America has contributed two very rare animals, the maned dog and Magellan's wolf, in addition to better-known creatures such as tapirs, ant-bears and jaguars. From Africa a new subspecies of chacma, a kind of baboon, has been brought for the first time.

A PROCESS for getting oil out of steam condensation water has been developed by Fritz Hoyer, a German scientist. It is expected to replace the mechanical methods for removing the troublesome residue of oil now in use. Most of the oil which is used for lubricating steam pistons and gearing is atomized and carried away in the waste steam. As a result of this a very stable milky emulsion is formed on the condensed water, and the problem of separation of oil and water is an extremely difficult one. In the Hoyer process a direct current is passed through the water, which collects the oil in small foam flakes, thus destroying the emulsion and making filtration possible. The consumption of electricity is about one kilowatt hour for five cubic meters of water.

THE relationship between lack of sufficient food and tuberculosis has been definitely proved by Dr. Harry Schutze and Dr. S. S. Zilva, of the Lister Institute. In their experiments with tuberculosis in guinea-pigs during the last six years they have found that diet is a very important factor. They divided their animals into two sets; one set was given a complete normal diet, with abundance of food, and the other set had a similar diet but restricted in amount. The guinea-pigs on the restricted diet did not put on weight, whereas the others did. After two and one half months of dieting, all the animals were inoculated with a living culture of tubercle bacilli, in order to test their resistance. In each case the animals on the abundant diet lived twice as long as those on the restricted diet.

WHILE to-day walruses are practically confined to the little-visited Arctic seas, within historic times they have been common as far south as the Gulf of St. Lawrence and the recent finding of a skull on Georges Bank, off the coast of Massachusetts, seems to indicate that these mammals did come down as far south as northern United States waters perhaps no longer than two or three hundred years ago. This interesting specimen, consisting of the fore part of a walrus skull with the tusks still in place, was recently dredged up by the steam trawler *Mariner* at a depth of eighty fathoms. Colonel J. M. Andrews has turned the skull over to the Boston Society of Natural History.

SCIENCE NEWS

Science Service, Washington, D. C.

THE PLANETARIUM

WITH the vanguard of the thousands of American tourists who will visit Germany during the coming months now reaching Berlin, the planetarium is attracting large crowds. Many of the Americans wish to see in operation this device that reproduces the night sky on a white dome, and which will soon make its debut in the United States when one is installed in Chicago.

Since the first planetarium was erected in 1924 in Jena, on the roof of one of the buildings of the Carl Zeiss optical works, its manufacturers, fourteen other German cities have installed them, including Munich, Berlin, Hamburg, Hanover, Dusseldorf, Barmen, Leipzig, Stuttgart, Nuernberg and Mannheim. One has been installed in Vienna; Mussolini has ordered one for Rome, which will be opened this fall; while the Soviet Government has also ordered one for Moscow.

The planetarium is a huge instrument, consisting of a long cylinder, with two spherical ends. Imbedded in the spheres, and also along the cylindrical parts, are a number of lenses, 119 in all. These act as magic lanterns to project the images of the naked eye stars, the Milky Way, the sun, moon and planets on the white cloth-lined dome. So realistic is the effect that when the room is darkened and the visitor has become used to the dim light, the stars appear as in the actual night sky. The visitor does not seem to be in a 90-foot dome, but under the stars themselves on a cloudless night.

The mechanism of the machine, all controlled by the lecturer from a single switchboard, will enable it to reveal the stars as seen from the North Pole, the South Pole, or any place between. The "great year," of 26,000 ordinary years, can be duplicated in a few minutes, and the heavens shown as they appeared thousands of years ago. Five thousand years ago our present pole-star was not in that prominent position, but it was occupied by the star we call alpha Draconis. At that time also, the Southern Cross was visible from the present latitude of New York. This can be shown with the planetarium. When desired, the names of the constellations can be flashed on the sky in the proper places, as if on huge electric signs!

The phases of the moon as it spins around the sun, along with the earth, are displayed. So are the motions of the planets. These can be speeded up so that the events of a year take place in a few seconds. The sun speeds across the dome with Mercury and Venus looping around it. The alternate forward and backward motion of Jupiter and Saturn, hardly visible in reality because of their slowness, become immediately apparent. Yet so accurate is the mechanism that, if the planets are shown as they would appear 5,000 years hence, Mercury, the fastest moving of them, is out of its proper place less than the diameter of the full moon.

Most of the German planetariums are operated by the school boards of the respective cities, but for general visitors an admission charge of one mark is usually made. Despite this, the popularity of them has been so great that in the four years since the first one more than a million paid admissions have been recorded in Germany. This has gone far towards paying the cost. The instrument itself sells for about $40,000, and the cost of the building is from about $150,000 upwards.

By this time next year, Chicagoans will be able to see, without leaving the city, the first planetarium in the western hemisphere. Max Adler, former Sears-Roebuck official, has just given $500,000 to the city for one of these instruments and the building to house it. An island in Lake Michigan, near the Field Museum, has been selected as the site. Mr. Adler will shortly leave for Germany to study the instrument at Jena, home of the Carl Zeiss optical works where it is built, as well as other German cities, and will personally supervise its erection in Chicago.

RECENT INDIAN MOUND-BUILDERS

THE last traces of the old idea that the mound-builders were a mysterious ancient race who vanished before the coming of the Indians have been very effectually destroyed by the discovery in Joliet, Ill., of a mound filled from bottom to top with the skeletons of buried Indians, each skeleton provided with funeral gifts of European manufacture as well as the more usual stone, bone and shell objects of native workmanship. Professor Fay-Cooper Cole, of the University of Chicago, states that so far as he is aware this is the first wholly post-European mound discovered in this country.

The mound is one of the so-called Fisher group, which have been subjected to excavation during the past few years by George Langford, a factory executive of Joliet. The other mounds have yielded Indian relics of pre-European date, one of the cultures represented being very primitive and possibly very ancient. A few articles of white man's manufacture were found near the top of one of these larger mounds, linking the history of the Indians of this region with that of French Colonial trading in the Mississippi Valley.

The mound which Mr. Langford has just finished exploring had been given a somewhat superficial going over by an earlier group of amateur diggers, who found a considerable number of silver objects, including a crucifix, several spoons, bangles and other ornaments. It was thought that everything had been removed, but when Mr. Langford dug into the mound again he discovered that the previous excavation had done little more than remove the surface. He found burials with European and Colonial funeral gifts throughout the mound and down into the ground to a depth of five feet beneath its base.

The finds include a couple of brass pots in excellent condition, one of them with a close-fitting lid, a pair of scissors, a large number of knives bearing a French trademark, several silver spoons and quantities of beads, but-

NEW SCIENTIFIC BOOKS

The Institute for Government Research, Washington, D. C.

The Problem of Indian Administration. Lewis Meriam and associates. pp. xxii + 872.

Report of a survey of the economic and social conditions of the American Indians, containing the following sections: A General Policy for Indian Affairs; Health; Education; General Economic Conditions; Family and Community Life and the Activities of Women; Migrated Indians; Legal Aspects of the Indian Problem, and Missionary Activities.

Longmans Green and Company, New York

Intermediate Electricity and Magnetism. R. A. Houston. pp. x + 170. 155 diagrams. $1.75.

Treats of the fundamental facts of magnetism, magnetic measurements, terrestrial magnetism, electrostatics, Ohm's law, electrolysis, induced currents, cathode rays, X-rays and radioactivity. An additional chapter on electrical oscillations and waves is included.

The D. Van Nostrand Company, New York

Storage Batteries. Morton Arendt. pp. v + 285. Illustrated. $4.50.

Such material as can be readily applied to every-day problems relating to the manufacture and assembling of storage batteries, to questions having to do with their upkeep and care, and to their application and usage comprise the scope of this book.

Prentice-Hall, New York

General Chemistry. Azariah T. Lincoln and George B. Banks. 133 figures. pp. xxii + 681. $3.50.

Suited for a first-year course in college. The material is so arranged that several sizes and types of courses can be offered, depending on the group of students concerned and the amount of time available.

Allyn and Bacon, Boston

Second Course in the New Mathematics. Edward I. Edgerton and Perry A. Carpenter. pp xi + 369. $1.20.

This is the second-year volume of a mathematics series for junior high schools. The first part of the book is devoted to saving time in the use of fundamental processes. The second part makes specific application of the New Mathematics to business.

Boni and Liveright, New York

Growing into Life. David Seabury. pp. xviii + 715. $5.00.

The author finds alarming the large number of young people and children who have become mental cases, through ignorant training given by parents and faulty ethics. He shows the causes of mental difficulties, the cure and prevention of them. For parents and teachers and every one interested in the welfare of children.

tons, pins and other trinkets. Brass seems to have been a favorite metal; every skeleton had some brass object with it. These modern mound-builders unquestionably did a lot of business with the French traders.

One of the most remarkably well-preserved specimens is a combination pocket compass and sun-dial in a brass case. The "floating" compass card swings freely on its pivot, the glass cover is unbroken, and the gnomon of the sun-dial can still be turned on its hinge.

A change in the type of burial may possibly be due to European influence. All the adult skeletons in this post-European mound lay flat on their backs, heads west, feet east. This resembles the white man's method of burial. All the other deep burials at the Fisher site, whose funeral gifts do not include European objects, were turned over on one side and drawn up into a crouching position, as primitive peoples are wont to sleep in cold weather.

ARCTIC EXPLORATION AND THE "ITALIA"

General Nobile's *Italia,* now down in the Arctic, was too small and slow for serious Arctic exploration, and German authorities warned him against using it. This is the opinion of Dr. Walter Bruns, general secretary of the International Society for the Exploration of the Polar Regions by means of the Airship, generally known as "Aeroarctic." The society is particularly interested, as several of its members are with the Nobile expedition. Also, Aeroarctic is itself planning extensive polar explorations next year in the *LZ–127,* the gigantic Zeppelin now nearing completion at Friedrichshafen. This ship is six times as large as the *Italia,* and even larger than the American *Los Angeles.*

"In spite of its great sympathy towards the undertaking," said Dr. Bruns, "the Aeroarctic has had, from the very beginning, serious concern regarding the expedition. It was pointed out to Nobile that, after the wonderful flight of the sister ship *Norge,* too distant a goal for a new expedition this year should, before all things, be avoided for this very small type of airship. We know from our Berlin conferences with General Nobile that, because of the small size of the airship, the mass of the necessary reserves of ballast (in case the ship were covered with ice), and the polar equipment requisite for a possible forced landing, had to be reduced greatly on account of the great distance.

"The small speed (about 53 miles per hour) of the airship required that General Nobile spend the month of April and the first half of May, the most precious time for polar work, awaiting favorable meteorological conditions. Already the flight to Nicholas II Land (Leninland) had demonstrated that it was really too late for further undertakings because of the prevalence of summer fogs. In addition to the unpromising meteorological conditions, General Nobile had to fix the base of his operations at Kings Bay in the Arctic itself, owing to the small radius of action of his airship. This again made him not only dependent upon the general weather conditions but also upon the local storm phenomena (winds, snowstorms, etc.) which are often very troublesome. The snow even penetrated the hangar and made it very inconvenient for the airship in its shelter.

"The very favorable flight to the Pole justified the hope that the return trip would likewise be propitious. Under good weather conditions, the journey from Kings Bay to the Pole and back is no great undertaking for an airship. This, however, is not the case, in view of the small speed of the *Italia,* as soon as a moderately strong contrary wind arises, as apparently took place on the return trip. That General Nobile on approaching Spitzbergen met with strong adverse winds is, from a meteorological standpoint, not strange, since the region of Spitzbergen is in the area of storm paths which take their course from the North Atlantic along the Norwegian Coast and only gradually die out in the inner Arctic, *i.e.,* become less dangerous for flights.

"Our society has, therefore, as is generally known, held firmly to the opinion that the solution of Arctic problems should not be attempted with too small an airship. In order to be independent of the especially unfavorable storm conditions of Spitzbergen, one should, before all else, establish his base for Arctic exploration as far distant as possible from the Arctic. For this reason we plan for next year's expeditions, anchorages in Leningrad, and perhaps at Murmansk in Kola, and at Nome in Alaska. We wish also, in spite of the very great cruising radius of the new Zeppelin-airship which may be three times that of the *Italia,* to establish anchorages on both sides of the Arctic in order to be approximately independent of meteorological factors during our journeys covering several days."

TUBERCULOSIS

The need for careful supervision of tuberculosis patients discharged from sanatoriums as cured was described as an economic as well as a sociologic need by Dr. H. Longstreet Taylor, of St. Paul, in the presidential address before the annual meeting of the National Tuberculosis Association which opened in Portland, Oregon, on June 17.

Every relapse doubles the original cost of the care of the patient, a burden that generally falls on the community at large, said Dr. Taylor. A third period of treatment, the "cure to end the cure," was recommended as having but trifling cost compared to that of caring for relapses. Figures from the Metropolitan Life Insurance Co. showed that of 896 patients who had this after-care, 80 per cent. were at work seven years after discharge from the sanatorium. On the other hand, a survey of unsupervised patients in New York City revealed that 52 per cent. had suffered relapses within one year after leaving the sanatorium.

Of 148 cases of pulmonary tuberculosis during the last seven years in which surgery was used, 41 per cent. were cured and 33 per cent. improved, Dr. William H. Thearle, of Denver, reported to the meeting of the association. By this method of treatment, known as thoracoplasty, part of the ribs are cut away. The lung collapses, so that it is completely at rest and thus has a chance to heal. The results with this method of treat-

ment were characterized as "brilliant" by Dr. Thearle. However, proper selection of cases for this procedure is of great importance and further progress along this line will depend on the degree of cooperation between internist and surgeon.

The task of the industrial physician in determining whether or not a worker contracted tuberculosis as a result of his occupation, and was thus entitled to compensation, was described and difficulties pointed out to members of the association by Dr. John B. Hawes, 2nd, and Frank Kiernan, of Boston. In eleven of 76 cases considered by the Industrial Accident Board of Massachusetts during the last two years, there had been direct exposure to tuberculosis for many years through another member of the family.

Present training for public health work is of three types. The first is the standard nurses' training, the second supplements the nurses' training with a period of training in social work, the third adds to the training of nurse and social worker such academic and cultural training as may be obtained by a regular college or university course and finishes with specialized training for research in social health work. This last type is still in the experimental stage and all the types are constantly undergoing change and improvement, members of the association were told by Dr. Philip A. Parsons, of Eugene, Ore.

Light is a valuable factor in the cure of tuberculosis, but it must not be considered as the sole agent. There are other and more important ones, such as diet, rest and fresh air, Dr. Clarence L. Hyde told members of the National Tuberculosis Association at their meeting. "Heliotherapy is much more than a bath in sunlight," said Dr. Hyde. Treatment with artificial lights, while it may reproduce the rays, can not equal actual sunlight treatment which is accompanied by changing air currents, differences in atmospheric temperature and humidity, and constant variations in the sunlight itself. These features all have importance in the value of sunlight treatment. A method of using an open flame carbon arc, which Dr. Hyde considered the most satisfactory substitute for sunlight, was described.

ITEMS

A HOUSE without a single sliver of wood in its construction is being built in Gary, Ind., for the president of a local steel company. The framework is made of angle-irons with a complete system of diagonal bracing. Both bolting and electric welding is used to fasten the steel together. Concrete is used in the foundation and for the floors, while stairs, sills and interior trim are all steel.

THE quantity of water underground, beneath the crust of the earth's surface, is nearly one third the total volume of the oceanic waters, according to estimates of Dr. Chester A. Reeds, of the American Museum of Natural History, who has just completed investigations of buried rivers and caves. The earth's ground water extends to great depths, perhaps six miles, and has been accumulating for countless ages. This great mass of water percolates slowly through the porous and jointed rocks to form great systems of underground drainage, creating such beauty spots as the Mammoth Cave, in Kentucky, and the Endless Caverns, in Virginia. In the limestone regions, where so many of these unfamiliar streams are found, the formations of huge stalactites, stalagmites, columns and stony curtains in the cavernous depths remind one of the artistic handiwork of ancient artisans on the Renaissance palaces.

WHETHER or not flowers will reproduce may be traced to the size and general appearance of the pollen grains, according to a report to the western division of the American Association for the Advancement of Science. Miss Laura E. Shaw, of the University of Southern California, separated pollen grains into four groups according to size and found that the third group, containing grains of from three to four thousandths of an inch and comprising half of the grain studied, gave the highest percentage of germination, the rate being 75 to 80 per cent.

FOOD is digested, absorbed and made available for doing the body's work just as effectively when liquid petroleum is added to the diet as when inert laxative oil is not taken with the food, according to a report to the American Medical Association by Dr. Alfred B. Olsen, of Battle Creek Sanitarium, who reported experiments on dogs and human beings.

THE hard-worked liver diet is to have an assistant in curing patients of pernicious anemia. Ultra-violet rays which have been used both with and without the liver have caused a marked improvement in the condition of these patients, according to Dr. David I. Macht, of Baltimore. An increase in hemoglobin and number of red blood cells resulted from the use of these rays. The toxic effect of the blood serum, which is believed to be a causative factor in this disease, decreased.

WHEN the rogues' gallery of plants causing hay fever has been checked over, the paper mulberry tree which flourishes in back yards and vacant lots has always been pronounced innocent. But now, Dr. Harry S. Bernton, specialist in this disease, has reported the first cases in which hay fever was traced to the baleful pollen of the paper mulberry. Three cases have been found by Dr. Bernton in the past two years.

MEASLES, whooping cough, digestive ailments and other diseases attack more boys than girls under 10 years, according to a survey made by the U. S. Public Health Service. However, after the boy is 10 years old, unless he breaks a collar bone or suffers other injury in the course of his more venturesome activities, he will spend less time in bed sick than his sisters of the same age. This bears out the previous morbidity and mortality experience of health officers which gives male infants a handicap over girl babies, but reverses the condition during adolescence and maturity.

SCIENCE NEWS

Science Service, Washington, D. C.

COAST GUARD EXPEDITION TO THE ARCTIC

DOES a branch of the Gulf Stream dive to the bottom of the Atlantic Ocean and emerge again far north in Baffin Bay? Is the Labrador current a continuous overflow from the Arctic Ocean? Does the east Greenland current stretch all the way across to Labrador? Why is the west coast of Greenland so much warmer climatically than Baffin Land in the same latitude?

These are some of the outstanding questions of Arctic oceanography that may be solved during the coming summer. About July 10 the U. S. Coast Guard vessel, *Marion*, will sail from Boston for Sydney, Nova Scotia, on the first leg of an expedition to the region between the coast of Labrador and Greenland, an area where the icebergs are supposed to originate. Oceanographically, very little is known about this region at present.

The *Marion* will be under the command of Lieutenant-Commander Edward H. Smith. He has had ten years' service in the ice patrol work, and is also a trained oceanographer, for he spent two years in Europe and several more at Harvard University in oceanographic research. Lieutenant N. G. Ricketts is his first officer, and he also has had extensive experience in the ice patrol.

After April 15, 1912, when the White Star liner *Titanic* struck an iceberg off the Grand Banks of Newfoundland, and went to the bottom with the loss of 1,500 lives, an international convention "for the safety of life at sea" was held at London. From this there resulted the Ice Patrol of the U. S. Coast Guard. Every March two staunch Coast Guard vessels sail from Boston to the ice fields, and remain there until the dangerous season is over, usually about the middle of July. Twice a day these boats broadcast by radio to near-by liners the location of all the ice in the vicinity, so that they can head southward to safety. Since the Coast Guard began this work fourteen years ago only three lives have been lost by collision of a ship with ice.

The science of oceanography has helped to a great degree in solving the problem of making ships more safe in the ice field, Commander Smith told Science Service. "Little was known," he said, "before 1912–14 regarding the drift of the bergs, their rate of melting, and the degree of danger which they formed to passing traffic; except for the fact that they mostly came from Greenland, and that they finally melted in the offshore waters of the Atlantic, which appeared considerable of a mystery.

"Over 3,000 observations," he continued, "have been compiled during the last ten years by the ice patrol vessels. The program has consisted in securing observations of temperature and saltiness at various depths in various positions, carefully selected in the danger area. The ocean currents have been computed from these data in accordance with a mathematical formula. It is based upon the principle that ocean currents are due to differences in the specific gravity of the water. Water will flow from the place where it is relatively light to another region where it is proportionately heavy. This, combined with the fact of earth rotation, permits us to issue regular weekly current maps, similar to the better known weather maps issued daily by the U. S. Weather Bureau.

"In the course of this work we have secured quite a correct picture of current and ice conditions in the immediate area south of Newfoundland, and near the steamship tracks, but little is known of the wild and unexplored stormy region northward between Labrador and Greenland. Our expedition will enter these foggy waters and, it is hoped, will snatch from them a long-contained mystery."

At present the ship is at New London, Conn., where she is being fitted for the expedition. She will be equipped with apparatus for measuring the temperature and saltiness of the ocean water, for observing the ocean currents, and other apparatus unusual in such a boat.

One of the most important instruments with which she will be provided is the sonic depth-finder. With this an accurate measurement can be made of the depth of the water, with far more precision and speed than with the old type sounding-line. This consists of an oscillator, operated electrically and located on the ship's hull, which sends out sound-waves. These travel to the bottom, and are reflected as an echo. Microphones located elsewhere on the ship's hull pick up this echo. The speed of sound-waves through water is well known, and so, from the time it takes the waves to return, the depth can be measured.

Every half hour, day and night, on her cruise, a measurement will be made of the depth. The expedition will sail over an area of 50,000 square miles where no sounding has ever been made and the results will be of great scientific importance.

The Coast Guard expedition will not be alone in this area during the coming months, for the Danish Government is sponsoring a similar exploration with which the Coast Guard will cooperate. The Danish party, on the steamer *Godthaab*, has already sailed from Copenhagen. It is in charge of Commander Riis-Cartensen, of the Royal Danish Navy. Both biological and oceanographical in its scope, it will cover the entire range of west Greenland waters.

TESTING FIREPROOF SAFES

Two buildings, one five stories high, in the heart of Washington, and within less than a mile of the White House, were burned to the ground on June 17 while firemen stood by and watched. No effort was made to save the buildings, though they contained large amounts of lumber and other material, as well as 35 safes, filled with records. The fire was started by S. H. Ingberg, Bureau of Standards scientist.

This unusual fire was made as a scientific experiment, part of a series made by the fire protection section of the Bureau of Standards, of which Mr. Ingberg is in

charge. Previous tests have been made in a large concrete chamber of the bureau, but never before has it been possible to make a careful study of conditions at a full-sized fire, for which preparation had been made months in advance.

With the demolition of many old buildings in Washington, in the triangle south of Pennsylvania Avenue, in order to make way for the government's extensive building program, the idea was conceived of burning one or more as an experiment. Thus the expense and trouble of wrecking them by the ordinary means was saved, and at the same time data of great value to manufacturers of safes, engineers and architects have been obtained.

The two buildings were at 1007 and 1009 Little B Street, opposite the north side of the National Museum, and between the Capitol and the White House. One was two stories high, 22 feet wide and 75 feet deep, while the other was five stories high and 30 by 75 feet. Both had brick walls, and open joisted wood floors, about an inch thick, and very few partitions. The elevator shafts were open and the stairways inadequately protected. According to the bureau officials they were typical of the non-fire resistive type of structure built some years ago, and still very common in American cities. Until last fall they had been used as warehouses.

All the surrounding buildings had been completely demolished several months ago. The two under test were loaded with waste lumber and such material, the weights varying from 7½ to 30 pounds per square foot of floor area. Thirty-five safes, submitted by various manufacturers, were placed at different locations in the buildings. These were numbered inside the doors to permit of identification. They were filled with useless records, so as to determine the degree of protection that they afforded. Each safe also contained a thermometer to record the highest temperature within during the fire, and a clock arranged to stop with a heavy jar. These give records of the time at which each safe fell through the burned-out floor to the ground below.

Mr. Ingberg and his associates observed the fire from a "dugout" in an old boiler room near-by. By means of thermocouples placed in open spaces at 50 advantageous points within the burning buildings, and at 45 points in the débris, connected by wires with instruments in the dugout, the temperatures were measured electrically.

For days after the experimental fire temperature observations were being continued. Several days after the fire the thirty-five safes were still among the débris and too hot to permit them to be removed and opened.

Within an hour after starting the fire the buildings were completely gutted and temperatures estimated to be as high as 3,500 degrees F., above the melting-point of iron, had been reached. Within 15 minutes after the start of the fire some of the thermocouples in the building, by which the temperatures were measured electrically, had reached 2,800 degrees, at which point they melted, and stopped working.

THE MEXICAN EARTHQUAKE

PROBABLE damage and loss of life at Oaxaca and other towns in southern Mexico as the result of an earthquake at 10:14 P. M. Saturday, June 16, was announced by Science Service on Sunday, within 20 hours of the time of the quake, and before reports from the most greatly damaged area had reached the United States. This announcement was made possible by earthquake wave messages received at six American and Canadian seismological observatories, relayed to Science Service by telegraph and interpreted by the U. S. Coast and Geodetic Survey.

This Science Service earthquake-reporting network allowed the locating of the center of the quake at latitude 14 degrees north and longitude 95.5 degrees west. This point is in the Pacific Ocean about 125 miles off the coast of the state of Oaxaca, and close to the Isthmus of Tehuantepec, in which great damage was reported. Vera Cruz, which first reported shakes, was some distance from this center. The Dominion Observatory at Ottawa, Canada, reported that the tremors continued for six hours, while the Meteorological Observatory at Victoria, B. C., characterized it as "very severe." Other stations reporting their records were those of Georgetown University, Washington; St. Louis University, St. Louis; the University of California, Berkeley, and the U. S. Coast and Geodetic Survey at Tucson, Ariz.

A severe earthquake occurred at very nearly the same center on March 22, and other shocks, also reported by Science Service, were felt in the same region on April 13 and 17. One of these quakes broke open a tomb in the mysterious city of Monte Alban, near Oaxaca, revealing valuable jewel treasures that Mexican archeologists believe will help solve the enigma of the strange prehistoric race that lived there.

EUROPEAN ROADS

EUROPEAN roads, which fifteen years ago were superior to the American automobile trails of those days, are now far inferior to the hard-surfaces available for touring here in America, Tore Franzen, of Detroit, told the Society of Automotive Engineers recently.

The main roads of the Old World, once the trade routes of the civilized world, have deteriorated as a result of war and lack of proper maintenance. The old stone roads that in many cases date back to the Romans are durable, but very rough, narrow, highly crowned and surfaced with cobblestones and slabs. Other roads are of dirt, rutted and rough, with only the most necessary repairs made by the peasants who live alongside them.

There are two kinds of European motorists, Mr. Franzen discovered in surveying the situation. The dashing sportsman drives his own car and insists upon speeding over poor roads. Most European car owners, however, employ chauffeurs and desire to travel in safety and comfort.

American automobiles are sometimes criticized because they shimmy and shake on European roads. Rough roads and the low tire pressure used cause the springs to deflect deeply and give the riders severe jolts. Thin oil plentifully applied is considered in Europe to be a universal cure for any slight spring or shock-absorber squeaks. But the oil simply puts most shock-absorbers out of commission and makes the springs weak. Mr.

SCIENCE NEWS

Science Service, Washington, D. C.

A NEW FORM OF COPPER

FOLLOWING on his announcement that he has produced big crystals of copper differing from ordinary samples of the metal, is the discovery by Dr. W. P. Davey, research physicist of the General Electric Company, that the metal prepared in this way possesses increased electrical conductivity to the extent of 13 per cent. Dr. Davey reported his investigations at the meeting of the American Physical Society held in affiliation with the American Association for the Advancement of Science at Washington on December 31.

While the use of single crystal copper is at present not a commercial possibility, the time is in sight when electrical machinery and conducting wires will be made of the new copper, thereby cheapening the cost of new power lines, and releasing a proportion of the metal which would otherwise be tied up in cables. Another way of regarding the superconducting copper is to consider that with conductors maintained at their present weight, energy losses on transmission lines would be reduced by 13 per cent., or, if the losses are permitted to remain the same, then smaller conduits could be used for underground work, and lighter towers could be erected for the support of overhead wires.

When Professor P. W. Bridgman, Harvard University, discovered that copper could be produced in relatively large crystals by the process of heating gradually in an electric furnace, and cooling down again equally slowly, Dr. Davey set himself to make copper crystals of appreciable size, and he succeeded in producing pieces nearly an inch in diameter and six incres long.

It was at once observed that these specimens could be bent without effort, but that they could not be straightened again. This is due to the fact that the distortion upset the balance of the atoms of copper, and they readjusted themselves into small crystals, so that the bar was to all intents and purposes, a piece of ordinary copper, and quite as inflexible.

Dr. Davey proved by X-ray examination that the treated copper really was just one big crystal, with the atoms arranged in regular rows from end to end, and he found that one of the axes of the cubic form in which copper crystallizes, ran through the single-crystal rod. Knowing that different axes of a crystal possess different electrical conductivities, he decided that his new copper should also conduct differently in different directions, and when the measurement was made it turned out that the resistance of the metal in the direction of its long axis was 13 per cent. less than before it had been treated. In order to make sure that there was no flaw in the argument, the crystal was hammered and them annealed, so that its uniform structure was spoiled, and then its conductivity was found to be the same as an untreated piece of copper.

Commercial copper was used in the test, and it was found that it would submit to the warming and cooling process. The important result was obtained, however, that single-crystal, commercial copper conducted better than the purest obtainable samples of the metal which had not been processed, and it exceeded even silver in the facility with which it permitted the passage of the electric current. Silver is the best conducting metal known.

THE CLIMATE OF MARS

THE climate on Mars is such that it may support life, mosses and lichens or trogdolytic animals able to withstand a freezing night and a thawing midday on that ruddy planet. These are the conclusions presented to the American Physical Society by Dr. W. W. Coblentz, of the U. S. Bureau of Standards, who, with Dr. C. O. Lampland, of the Lowell Observatory, Flagstaff, Ariz., has measured radiation from this planet and determined its temperatures accurately.

The north pole during the Martian winter has a temperature of 94 degrees below zero, Fahrenheit, and in summer the south pole is 76 degrees below zero. An estimated value for the night side of the planet is 112 degrees below zero, Fahrenheit. In the equatorial regions of the planet, higher temperatures corresponding to those on earth are attained during the day, reaching 41 degrees Fahrenheit. In the equatorial regions of the planet, higher temperatures, corresponding to those on earth, are attained during the day, reaching 41 degrees Fahrenheit in the bright regions and 59 degrees Fahrenheit in the dark regions. The integrated temperature of the whole disk is 22 degrees below zero.

"What about life on Mars?" Dr. Coblentz said: "That depends upon our point of view; whether we think of palm trees growing in our tropics, or mosses and lichens which grow on the apparently bare piles of volcanic cinders of Arizona and under our Arctic snows.

"The foregoing measurements show that for a few hours at noonday on the equator of Mars the surface temperature is not unlike that of Washington on some bright day in March. But consider the exceedingly cold nights and the great daily variation in temperature, amounting to perhaps 180 degrees Fahrenheit. Water is not present on Mars in sufficient quantity to form permanent lakes.

"Hence, with noonday temperatures of only 40 to 60 degrees Fahrenheit, even on the hottest spots on the equator, and with temperatures so low that probably all the water vapor freezes out of the atmosphere at night, it is evident that while vegetable and perhaps animal life appears to be possible on Mars it must be adapted to withstand prolonged drought and intense cold. Moreover, with such rapid temperature changes the reactions must be rapid. With most of the surface at Arctic temperatures it is reasonable to assume that if vegetable life similar to ours can exist on Mars, it must be like the mosses and lichens which thrive under our Arctic snows. Similarly, animal life must be trogdolytic, able to bur-

row deep and hibernate; or able to withstand the intense cold in a benumbed state, as do, for example, the torpid grasshoppers, wasps and ants one finds on warm days in winter.''

ATMOSPHERIC NITROGEN

DIFFICULTIES in the path of those who would capture the nitrogen gas of the atmosphere, famous for its aversion for other chemicals, were brought to the attention of the American Chemical Society at its meeting in Washington by Dr. J. A. Almquist, of the Fixed Nitrogen Research Laboratory. Among the most promising of the methods so far introduced for accomplishing this result, which would cheapen fertilizer, is the making of synthetic ammonia. This pungent gas, formed by the union of three atoms of hydrogen with one of nitrogen, would then serve as the starting point for the manufacture of other nitrogen-containing substances.

Nitrogen and hydrogen can be caused to unite by the agency of catalysts, which are substances capable of producing reactions between chemicals unwilling to unite, although the catalysts themselves do not actually form a part of the new substance. This is the method to which Dr. Almquist has devoted his attention.

''We have made an extensive investigation of catalysts for this reaction,'' he said. ''Observations with materials of the iron type have shed light on the nature of the process involved.'' Just why the presence of one substance will set off a reaction between others when none of it is used up in the operation, is a point which still puzzles chemists, and one which is the subject of much investigation.

Dr. Almquist and his associates have found, in the case of the iron catalyst in ammonia synthesis, that the pressure under which the nitrogen and hydrogen gases are kept influences the efficiency of the catalyst; they find that the absorption of the product, ammonia, slows up the operation. It was previously thought that the iron had to take up some of the ammonia before it would work, but the experiments now show that this view is wrong.

Another difficulty in the way of large scale application of the technic is the fact that nitride of iron may be formed on catalysts which cuts down the surface at which the union between the two gases takes place.

ARTIFICIAL FAT AS A FOOD

TESTS under way at Teachers College and Columbia University for the purpose of deciding whether intarvin, an artificial fat for cases of chronic diabetes, exerts a harmful effect on the body, have shown to date that no evil results follow the inclusion of the material in the diet of rats, according to the report of Hattie L. Heft, Max Kahn and William J. Gies to the American Society of Biological Chemists meeting this week in Washington.

This material was invented recently for the purpose of providing a utilizable fat for persons suffering from acute diabetes who could not eat fat from natural sources. Sugars and fats are built upon a framework of strings of carbon atoms, to which atoms of oxygen and hydrogen are attached, and the surprising feature about the compounds containing a large number of carbon atoms, arm in arm, is the fact that nature invariably makes the chains out of an even number of links. It is on this point that the success of the artificial fat swings.

When a natural fat is utilized or ''burned'' in the body of a person afflicted with diabetes, substances such as acetone are formed which have for a backbone a chain of three carbon atoms, and then the breakdown process stops, instead of being carried on to the ordinary harmless end-products, water and carbon dioxide. But the diabetic products are poisonous and consequently the sufferer has to cut down on fat as well as on sugar. The inventors of intarvin decided to prevent the formation of these unfavorable materials by providing in place of natural fats an artificial one, containing an uneven number of carbon atoms. The idea stood the test of experiment. Artificial ''odd carbon'' fat was found edible and nourishing, and its manufacture is now carried on by the ton, the principle of the method being to knock one of the carbon atoms from the end of the chain which occurs in stearin, a common natural fat with an 18-carbon chain.

Consequently, intarvin is an alternative to insulin for coping with diabetes, the difference being that a special food is substituted for periodic injections of the hormone, insulin. In order to find out whether any deleterious effects may result in the long run from feeding on the synthetic fat white rats were provided with a natural, balanced diet, to which was added up to twelve per cent. of intarvin for half of the subjects of the experiment, while the remainder received instead an equivalent quantity of rendered lamb fat.

Mating was permitted between the corresponding animals in the two groups, in such a way as to prevent inbreeding, and, after seven generations, the rats eating synthetic food have shown themselves to be in every way the equals of those provided with natural fat. ''There have been no discernible effects on the animals treated with intarvin,'' these workers said. ''Their fecundity has not been impaired.

''Our study of the beneficial effects of intarvin in the treatment of diabetes has confirmed the earlier indications of its utility, and also of its lack of toxicity.''

THE ANTIRACHITIC VITAMIN

FURTHER clews in the tracking down of the mysterious accessory food factor or vitamin which prevents rickets were pointed out to the American Society of Biological Chemists by Drs. Alfred F. Hess and Mildred Weinstock, of New York, who are on the trail of the component of cod liver oil now well known as an effective substitute for the ultra-violet rays of sunshine in the banishing of bow legs, bad teeth and bending bones.

Cod liver oil supplies a curative and preventive principle, which is absent in vegetable oils, such as olive or cottonseed oils. But these oils, as well as green vegetables, such as lettuce or wheat, can be likewise endowed with the power of preventing rickets by exposing them

to the rays of ultra-violet light from a mercury vapor or carbon arc light. The power so acquired is not immediately lost, but is retained by the lettuce for several days.

Further, according to the statement of the authors, the property imparted to otherwise inactive oils by the exposure to ultra-violet rays is of a permanent nature, and is retained for many months. "While it is impossible to state definitely that the substance which is formed is the same as that which is responsible for the remarkable curative value of cod liver oil, it has been found by means of chemical examinations that cod liver oil can be separated into two definite portions—one which is of value and one of no value in curing rickets," they stated. "The vegetable oils which have been exposed to the ultra-violet rays can likewise, and by the same chemical means, be separated into a portion which is of no value, and another which acts as a specific in warding off or curing rickets. It would, therefore, seem that a substance has been formed in the vegetable oils by the action of the ultra-violet rays, similar to that which is naturally present in the oil of the liver of the cod."

NUTRITIVE CONDITION AND HABIT FORMATION IN RATS

FEED a rat an imperfect or insufficient diet, and you sharpen her wits. Drs. Arthur H. Smith and John E. Anderson, who reported their experiments to the Washington meeting of the American Psychological Association, speak of their animals as "she's", not by analogy to the catty tribe, but because they chose female rodents in their studies of the relation between nutritive conditions and habit-formation. They thereby side-stepped the issue as to the relative brain power of the females and males.

They put a number of female rats into a maze, and noted the time they required to effect an exit. Next they divided their performers, by this time familiar with some of the wrong turnings in the maze, into three groups so that each one contained approximately an equal number of smart ones and slow ones, and each group was given a different diet for another month.

One third were given as much as they desired of food known to be adequate for health and growth; an equal number had a full supply of fat, sugars and vitamins, but were restricted in their nitrogenous food to a single source; and the rest were given just enough of a menu which included all the essentials that would maintain their weight. At the end of the training period, Group 1 had thrived, Group 3 were stunted and Group 2 showed that something was wrong with their food. When the animals were put into the maze again, it was found that those which had been partially starved were quickest to find their way to freedom and food, and similarly, the poorly fed rats won the race to find the way out of a new and different maze.

The new maze brought out the difference that the stunted rats made more mistakes on the new maze, even though they found the door first, and thus, although their starvation treatment had sharpened their intellects to the extent of refreshing their memories about the maze which they previously knew, it made it harder for the poorly developed ones to learn the route out of the new blind alley, even though the desire for food made them hustle along the wrong paths to such an extent that they got out first in the end. When all the rats were given normal rations again, they were equally adept in solving the puzzle.

The experiments indicate that habit formation is akin to physiological processes in the body, according to Drs. Smith and Anderson, and the results of these will be presented to the American Physiological Society shortly.

"The normal functions of the organs concerned with the process of habit formation are interfered with by the same alterations in nutritive conditions as have been found to bring about the well-known disturbances in metabolism, growth and reproduction."

ITEMS

ARE "peculiar properties" of a chemical substance simply an exaggeration of a quality possessed by many of its chemical cousins, due to special physical conditions, such as a favorable temperature, under which it finds itself? This was the question raised by the report of Dr. Russell S. Bartlett, of Yale University, to the American Physical Society meeting in Washington. The electrical resistance of the metal, selenium, is known to vary with the amount of illumination which its surface receives, and this peculiarity is finding increasing practical applications in the construction of cells which vary an electrical current to a measurable degree when different amounts of light are allowed to fall on them. Among uses to which they have already been put is the turning off of beacon lights in the day time and the electrical transmission of photographs. Dr. Bartlett now finds that this is a property which many other metals possess, if they are kept at the temperature of liquid air. Bismuth was found to decrease in resistance to an electric current, when light shone on sheets kept in this extreme cold. Copper and platinum behaved similarly. "These results were first predicted from theoretical considerations," the physicist stated. Perhaps selenium's mysterious power is no more mysterious than the fact that mercury is unique among metals in existing in the liquid state at ordinary temperatures. Other metals are fluid when heated, while a mixture of the two metals, sodium and potassium, remains liquid.

METHODS for getting purer extracts of chlorophyll, or the green coloring-matter of leaves, for use in medicine, industry and science, were described before the American Association for the Advancement of Science by Dr. Frank M. Schertz, biochemist of the U. S. Department of Agriculture. Chlorophyll is important in medicine as the basis for a remedy used in anemia. It is used in industry as a coloring for foods, toilet articles, soaps and leather. A pure extract is important in biochemical study because plants depend on chlorophyll and sunlight in the making of foods. Dr. Schertz's method involves the use of successive extractions and separations by means of acetone, petroleum ether, alcohol and distilled water.